Surgery of
Spine Trauma

Surgery of Spine Trauma

Edited by

Paul R. Meyer, Jr., M.D.

Professor, Department of Orthopaedic Surgery
Northwestern University Medical School
Director, Spine Injury Center
McGaw Medical Center of Northwestern University
Chicago, Illinois

Illustrated by Kathryn A. Sisson, A.M.I.

Churchill Livingstone
New York, Edinburgh, London, Melbourne   1989

Library of Congress Cataloging-in-Publication Data

Surgery of spine trauma/edited by Paul R. Meyer, Jr.
   p.   cm.
  Bibliography: p.
  Includes index.
  ISBN 0-443-08122-0
  1. Spine — Wounds and injuries. 2. Spine — Surgery.   I. Meyer,
Paul R. (Paul Reims), date.
  [DNLM: 1. Spinal Cord Injuries — diagnosis. 2. Spinal Injuries-
diagnosis. 3. Spine — surgery.   WE 725 S9615]
RD768.S79 1989
617′.482044 — dc19
DNLM/DLC   88-23790
for Library of Congress   CIP

© **Churchill Livingstone Inc. 1989**

Distributed in the United Kingdom by Churchill Livingstone, Robert Stevenson House, 1–3 Baxter's Place, Leith Walk, Edinburgh EH1 3AF, and by associated companies, branches, and representatives throughout the world.

Accurate indications, adverse reactions, and dosage schedules for drugs are provided in this book, but it is possible that they may change. The reader is urged to review the package information data of the manufacturers of the medications mentioned.

The Publishers have made every effort to trace the copyright holders for borrowed material. If they have inadvertently overlooked any, they will be pleased to make the necessary arrangements at the first opportunity.

Assistant Editor: *Nancy Terry*
Copy Editor: *Margot Otway*
Production Designer: *Angela Cirnigliaro*
Production Supervisor: *Jocelyn Eckstein*

Printed in the United States of America

First published in 1989

To my wife, Eileen, whose initial and sustained encouragement led to the acceptance of the challenge and to the ultimate accomplishment — its completion; to my physician father, Paul R. Meyer Sr., who placed the dream of medicine in front of me and, with self-determination, allowed it to happen; to my children, Kristin, Holly, Paul, and Stewart who, through this book, though the language be strange, come to know and understand their father; to my teachers, professors, partners, and colleagues, whose knowledge, patience, guidance, tolerance, encouragement and support made this effort a wonderful opportunity for learning. Finally, I dedicate my thoughts, thanks, and continued concerns to the many patients who unselfishly, through the management of their injuries, have contributed to my knowledge. It was their experiences, successes, and failures that made the writing of this textbook, a reality.

Contributors

Julian E. Bailes, M.D.
Clinical Instructor, Department of Surgery, Division of Neurosurgery, Northwestern University Medical School, Chicago, Illinois

Roy D. Cane, M.B.B.Ch. (Rand), F.F.A. (S.A.)
Professor of Clinical Anesthesia, and Associate Director, Division of Respiratory/Critical Care, Department of Anesthesia, Northwestern University Medical School, Chicago, Illinois

Leonard J. Cerullo, M.D.
Associate Professor, Department of Surgery, Division of Neurosurgery, Northwestern University Medical School; Director, Chicago NeuroSurgical Center; Chief, Section of Neurosurgery, Columbus-Cuneo-Cabrini Medical Center, Chicago, Illinois

Herbert H. Engelhard, M.D.
Assistant Professor, Department of Surgery, Division of Neurosurgery, University of Louisville School of Medicine, Louisville, Kentucky

Mark L. Harlow, M.D.
Instructor, Department of Anatomy and Cellular Biology, and Resident, Department of Orthopaedic Surgery, Medical College of Wisconsin, Milwaukee, Wisconsin

Steven Heim, M.D.
Attending Orthopaedic Surgeon, Central DuPage Hospital, Winfield, Illinois

Antoun Koht, M.D.
Assistant Professor of Clinical Anesthesia, Department of Anesthesia, Northwestern University Medical School, Chicago, Illinois

Paul R. Meyer, Jr., M.D.
Professor, Department of Orthopaedic Surgery, Northwestern University Medical School; Director, Spine Injury Center, McGaw Medical Center of Northwestern University, Chicago, Illinois

John B. Nanninga, M.D.
Associate Professor, Department of Urology, Northwestern University Medical School; Attending Urologist, Northwestern Memorial Hospital; Urology Consultant, Midwest Regional Spinal Cord Injury Care System, Chicago, Illinois

Terrie L. Nolinske, O.T.R./L., C.O., M.A.
Assistant Professor, Department of Occupational Therapy, Rush University, Chicago, Illinois; Clinical Editor, *O.T. WEEK*, Alexandria, Virginia

Lee F. Rogers, M.D.
The Drs. Frederick J. Bradd and William Kennedy Professor, Department of Radiology, Northwestern University Medical School; Chairman, Department of Radiology, Northwestern Memorial Hospital, Chicago, Illinois

James C. Russ, C.O.
Associate Professor, Department of Orthopaedic Surgery, Northwestern University Medical School, Chicago, Illinois

Barry A. Shapiro, M.D.
Professor of Clinical Anesthesia, and Director, Division of Respiratory/Critical Care, Department of Anesthesia, Northwestern University Medical School, Chicago, Illinois

Tod B. Sloan, M.D., Ph.D.
Assistant Professor, Department of Anesthesia, Northwestern University Medical School; Director of Neurophysiologic Monitoring, Northwestern Memorial Hospital, Chicago, Illinois

J. Richard Toleikis, Ph.D.
Assistant Professor, Department of Anesthesia, Northwestern University Medical School; Director, Evoked Potential Laboratory, Northwestern Memorial Hospital, Chicago, Illinois

Preface

This text distills the experience of myself and others in the management of vertebral column fractures, especially the experience of the Northwestern University Spine Injury Center and the Midwest Regional Spinal Injury Care System (MRSICS). It has been an often frustrating challenge to record this experience; whenever the task seemed clear-cut, a patient would be admitted with a new fracture or an unanticipated neurologic pattern, or a new internal fixation technique would be introduced.

Innovations in emergency care (discussed in Chapters 1 and 2) have been central to the dramatic improvement in patient care achieved by the MRSICS. The new breed of highly trained prehospital and hospital medical professionals, including paramedics, trauma coordinators, helicopter pilots, and emergency room trauma teams, have greatly reduced patient transport and admission times. The admission time for the MRSICS, which serves a catchment area more than 200 miles in radius, has dropped from months or weeks to a median post-trauma time of 6.4 hours. Largely as a result of rapid admission to a specialized Category I center, the first-year mortality at the Northwestern University Spine Injury Center has dropped from 11 percent in 1972 to 2.2 percent in 1986.

These factors have also resulted in a phenomenal decrease in the number of complete neurologic injuries admitted to the Northwestern University Spine Injury Center — from 75.8 percent in 1972 to 22.1 percent in 1986 — and a complementary increase in the number of patients who have an incomplete neurologic injury or are neurologically intact. We have found that a higher percentage of neurologic improvement (9.7 percent) occurs in patients admitted within 72 hours of injury than in patients arriving later (5.8 percent).

These improved results were detectable within five years of the founding of the Northwestern University Spine Injury Center. Patients began to arrive at the Center so soon after their injury that the usual alterations in neurologic function (normally considered to be the result of spinal cord edema) had not appeared. As a result, we have been able to observe in detail the progression of neurologic deficiency after trauma, both with and without surgery. For example, we found that the neurologic deficit may spread by one or more vertebral levels within hours of injury, and that this neurologic function will often return spontaneously over a few weeks as spinal cord medullary blood flow recovers. In the past, such recovery was often attributed to surgery.

The past two decades have seen a revolution in surgical stabilization of the spine. Fundamental to this revolution is the realization that surgical stabilization of the injured spine is not only legitimate, but may enhance patient recovery by speeding rehabilitation. The revolution has been accompanied, of course, by dramatic innovations in spine surgery instrumentation, starting with the introduction of the posterior Harrington rod in 1958, and continuing through the appearance of transpedicular screw fixation in 1986.

This text is organized into several sections, covering various aspects of the management of spinal cord injuries. Chapters 1 and 2, as mentioned above, deal with emergency care. Chapters 3 through 5 discuss the relevant developmental, vascular, and neurologic anatomy of the spinal cord and vertebral column. Chapters 6 through 13 cover the role of various specialties—neurology, anesthesia and life support, radiology, urology, and orthotics—in the management of spinal cord injured patients. Finally, Chapters 14 through 19 discuss in detail the general and surgical management of traumatic spine fractures. The text concludes with a general bibliography organized by subject.

I wish to extend my warmest thanks to the following people. First, I thank Ms. Marianne Kaplan, academic office and Spinal Cord Project Administrator-Manager, who, in addition to all her other duties, served as manuscript coordinator, typist, and editorial manager for this book. Without question, this text could not have been completed without her untiring dedication and years of effort. Second, I must express gratitude to Dr. Giri Gireesan, my partner, who shouldered the burden of patient care during my frequent absences to write and edit, and maintained a standard of excellent patient care. To the many orthopaedic residents and Spine Fellows who contributed time and effort to the pre- and postoperative care of the patients, and who assisted greatly by providing radiologic and follow-up patient data, I extend great thanks. To Mr. Vernon Keenan, who conceived and established the Spinal Cord Center data base in preparation for this book, and to Mr. Joe Schreiner, who made it happen, I extend deep appreciation. Special thanks and appreciation are extended to the book's artist, Kathy Sisson, and to her able assistant, Lori Vaskalis. Their contribution is unmatched, and they showed great patience and competence in the face of my numerous revisions. To Jessica Lowy, Jill Klein, and Jennifer Cromar, my office staff, who found themselves too often serving as liaison between myself and unseen patients, running bibliography errands to the library, and tempering the seemingly constant state of confusion, I express my deep appreciation. Finally, to the fantastic Acute Spinal Cord Injury nursing and unit staffs, my neurosurgical colleagues, and to the physician staffs of the other medical and surgical specialties, who provide what I believe to be the most outstanding patient care given anywhere, I "tip my hat," and give my unfeigned thanks.

Paul R. Meyer, Jr., M.D.

Contents

RETRIEVAL AND ASSESSMENT

1. Acute Injury Retrieval and Splinting Techniques: On-Site
    Care   1
    Paul R. Meyer, Jr.

2. Emergency Room Assessment: Management of Spinal Cord
    and Associated Injuries   23
    Paul R. Meyer, Jr.

ANATOMY

3. Embryology and Developmental Anatomy of the Nervous
    System and Vertebral Column   61
    Paul R. Meyer, Jr.

4. Vascular Anatomy of the Spinal Cord   85
    Paul R. Meyer, Jr.

5. Neuroanatomy   107
    Paul R. Meyer, Jr.

SPECIALTY MANAGEMENT AREAS

6. Evaluation of Spinal Cord Function by Means of Evoked
    Potentials   121
    Tod B. Sloan, J. Richard Toleikis, and Antoun Koht

7. Neurologic Assessment and Management of Head Injuries   137
    Julian E. Bailes, Leonard J. Cerullo, and Herbert H. Engelhard

8. Anesthesia for Spinal Cord Injury   157
    Antoun Koht and Paul R. Meyer, Jr.

9.   Pulmonary Effects of Acute Spinal Cord Injury: Assessment
     and Management   173
     Roy D. Cane and Barry A. Shapiro

10. Radiologic Assessment of Acute Neurologic and Vertebral
     Injuries   185
     Lee F. Rogers

11. Anticipated Urologic – Sexual Dysfunction   265
     John B. Nanninga

12. Orthotic Management of the Spine   279
     *Mark L. Harlow, Terrie L. Nolinske, James C. Russ, and
     Paul R. Meyer, Jr.*

13. Orthotic Management of the Neurologically Involved
     Upper and Lower Limb   305
     Terrie L. Nolinske, Mark L. Harlow, and James C. Russ

GENERAL AND SURGICAL MANAGEMENT OF FRACTURES

14. Cervical Spine: Overview and Conservative Management   341
     Paul R. Meyer, Jr.

15. Surgical Stabilization of the Cervical Spine   397
     Paul R. Meyer, Jr. and Steven Heim

16. Fractures of the Thoracic Spine: T1 to T10   525
     Paul R. Meyer, Jr.

17. Surgery of the Thoracic Spine   573
     Paul R. Meyer, Jr.

18. Indications: Anteroposterior Surgical Approach to the
     Thoracolumbar Spine   625
     Paul R. Meyer, Jr.

19. Fractures of the Lumbar and Sacral Spine: Conservative
     and Surgical Management   717
     Paul R. Meyer, Jr.

BIBLIOGRAPHY   823

INDEX   853

Acute Injury Retrieval and Splinting Techniques: On-Site Care

Paul R. Meyer, Jr.

This chapter discusses the care of accident victims with acute spinal cord injuries, at the accident scene and before admission to a hospital or trauma center. In Illinois, the general methods used for treating and transporting persons with acute spinal cord injuries were developed by me as founder and director of the Midwest Regional Spinal Cord Injury Care System (MRSCICS). Recommended management protocols for the care of patients with acutely injured spines have been developed by the spine center and widely disseminated.

MRSCICS comprises two Northwestern University-affiliated hospital institutions, Northwestern Memorial Hospital and the Rehabilitation Institute of Chicago. Since 1972, when MRSCICS was established as Illinois' primary trauma center for the treatment of persons with acute spinal cord injuries, it has admitted more than 2,700 patients. Patients are transported to the center from distances as great as 300 miles from a six-state region (Illinois, Missouri, Wisconsin, Iowa, Michigan, and Indiana). Generally, patients are transported to the center by helicopter or ambulance and travel an average distance of 25 to 50 miles (Fig. 1-1). The median admission time for the total population is 6.2 hours.

Absolutely essential to the delivery of appropriate, highly specialized spinal cord injury care is the interest of medical and paramedical personnel, who are responsible for managing the patient from the scene of the accident to admission to the trauma center institution. These include the highway patrol, police and firemen, paramedics and emergency medical technicians, flight personnel, and, medically, the emergency room physician, the anesthesiologist, the respiratory critical care physician, the general surgeon, the orthopaedic surgeon, the neurosurgeon, and the physical medicine physicians as well as the allied health personnel, which include the nurse, the occupational and physical therapist, and the social service worker.

MULTIPLE TRAUMA – SPINAL CORD INJURY MORTALITY STATISTICS

Forty-three percent of persons with traumatic spinal cord injuries sustain multiple trauma to areas of the body other than the spine. Consequently, the death rate in this patient population is high.[1] In a study by Kraus in 1972 to 1973, it was estimated that 50 persons per million sustain a spinal cord injury each year.[1] Of those, one third, or 15 per million, die within 1 year of the accident, and of those 15 per million, 90 percent, or 13.5 per million, die enroute to the first emergency room. The remaining 10 percent expire within the next 360

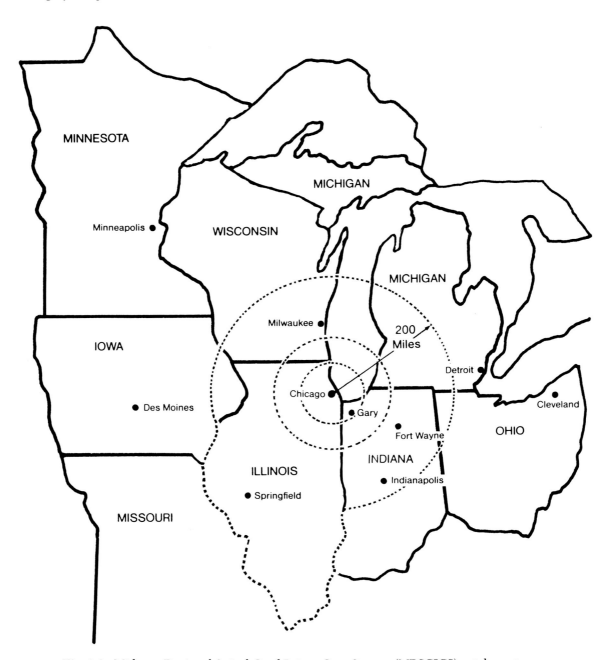

Fig. 1-1. Midwest Regional Spinal Cord Injury Care System (MRSCICS) catchment area.

days. This leaves a working figure of 32 spinal cord injuries per 1 million population per year that survive 1 year after injury. The average mortality rate from June 1972 through December 1986 for the first year after injury (from **MRSCICS** statistics) was 4.2 percent. The rate varied between 1.6 and 13.6 percent. The average mortality rate from 1979 to 1986 was 3.7 percent.

These statistics reflect several changes: (1) an increased awareness of, and participation in, emergency medical (trauma) services by the medical and paramedical professions; (2) an increase in the number or availability of community hospital trauma centers; (3) a greater involvement of state and local authorities in providing emergency medical services and educating emergency medical paraprofessionals and professionals. This involvement has increased the chances for survival of those who sustain serious spinal cord and multiple trauma injuries.

Incidence statistics allow for the computation of projected annual spinal cord injury admissions per unit size (national, state, county, or city). As an example, Chicago has a population of 3.0 million. At an annual rate of 32 spinal cord injuries per million, 96 new spinal cord injuries may be anticipated in Chicago each year. The actual average annual admission rate over the past 5 years was 255 patients (145 with spinal cord injuries). Since MRSCICS serves a 15-million-person catchment area (480 new cord injuries per year), MRSCICS serves approximately 30 percent of all new cord injuries in the central midwest region of the United States. During 1986, the acute center admitted more patients (299) than during any preceding year. The reason for this increase is interpreted to be more appropriate utilization of specialized medical facilities (acute spine center) by area and regional hospitals (Fig. 1-1).

INCIDENCE OF MULTIPLE TRAUMA

The benefit of the immediate availability of care by a sophisticated tertiary trauma center (whether provided by comprehensive or regional facilities) is obvious. Analysis of patients with acute spinal cord injuries admitted to the Northwestern University spinal cord injury center from 1972 to 1986 revealed the incidence of multiple trauma to be 42.9 percent (Fig. 1-2). The incidence of multiple trauma is: head and facial injuries, 26.2 percent; chest (hemo/pneumothorax, fractured ribs), 16.1 percent; extremity and pelvic fractures, 8.5 percent; abdominal (viscera-bladder), 10.0 percent. Medical experience gained during the Korean and Vietnam wars revealed that the mortality rates in each, respectively, were 2.5 percent and 2.6 percent. In World War I, the mortality rate was 18 percent, and during World War II, it was 4.5 percent.[2-5] Experience has shown that critically injured patients who receive immediate first aid by trained paramedical personnel and who are then rapidly transported to a facility capable of providing aggressive, comprehensive, experienced lifesaving management have a much higher chance of survival. Trunkey and Lim[6] and West et al.[7] each have demonstrated high trauma survivability in areas where trauma systems and trauma centers are in place and patients with critical injuries are rapidly retrieved. In the study conducted by West and colleagues in 1974 to 1975 in Orange County, California, where at that time trauma care was poorly organized, 60 percent of non-central nervous system related deaths were classified as potentially preventable and 33 percent of CNS-related deaths were classified as potentially preventable.[7]

In 1971 to 1972, Illinois developed a statewide trauma program under the Illinois Categorization Law of 1972.[8] The law established a three-tier trauma system across the state, with sufficient numbers of trauma facilities so that no one suffering a life-threatening illness would be more than 20 to 25 miles from a trauma center. Trauma center hospitals were classified in the following manner.

Local trauma center (located in small communities). A local trauma center has both a physician and a trauma nurse on duty in the emergency room 24 hours a day. The type of spinal trauma victim admitted to a local trauma center would be one whose injury does not reveal evidence of spinal column instability or the presence of neurologic injury.

Area trauma center (located in larger rural communities and serving as a referral hospital for the smaller local trauma centers). An area trauma center has other critical medical and surgical support staff, available to the hospital within 30 minutes of the initial call. In addition to an emergency room physician and trauma nurse on duty 24 hours a day, other necessary support facilities such as the medical laboratory, radiology, and surgery are available upon request, 24 hours a day. The type of spinal trauma victim admitted to an area trauma center would be one whose spinal injury does not include neurologic injury.

Regional or comprehensive trauma center (normally a university-affiliated institution located in a large suburban or urban area). This is the highest category of trauma facility, with a house staff in all medical and surgical specialities available 24 hours a day, along with all ancillary support facilities on

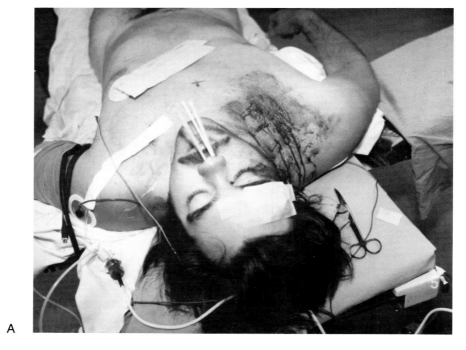

A

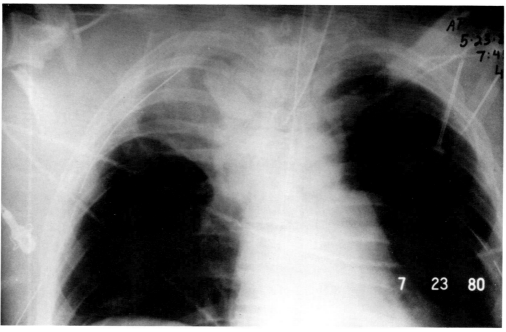

B

Fig. 1-2. Multiple trauma patient. (A) Operating room photograph of acute spinal cord injury patient who sustained fracture dislocation of the thoracic spine (T4 to T5) from a motorcycle accident. Note head injury, injury to right shoulder and right chest, and neurologic level marked on anterior chest. (B) Anteroposterior (AP) chest radiograph showing chest tube in left chest for hemopneumothorax, fractured right clavicle and right scapula, and hemothorax in superior lobe of right chest. *(Figure continues.)*

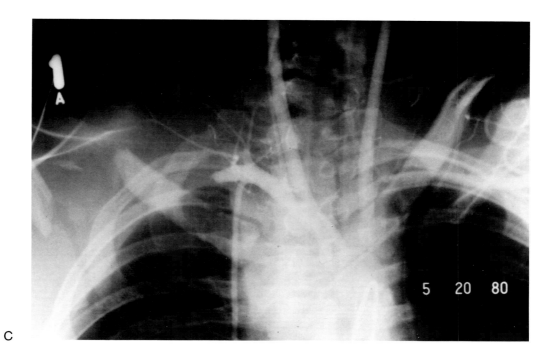

C

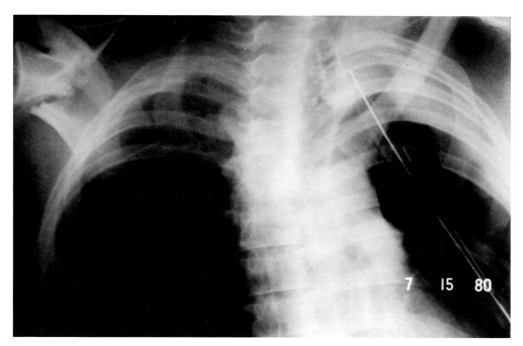

D

Fig. 1-2 *(Continued).* **(C)** Arteriogram demonstrating occlusion of right subclavian artery just lateral to internal mammary artery. Note fractured right clavicle and scapula. **(D)** AP chest radiograph demonstrating compression of T4 and T5. Thoracostomy tube is seen in left chest. Neck of right scapula is fractured. *(Figure continues.)*

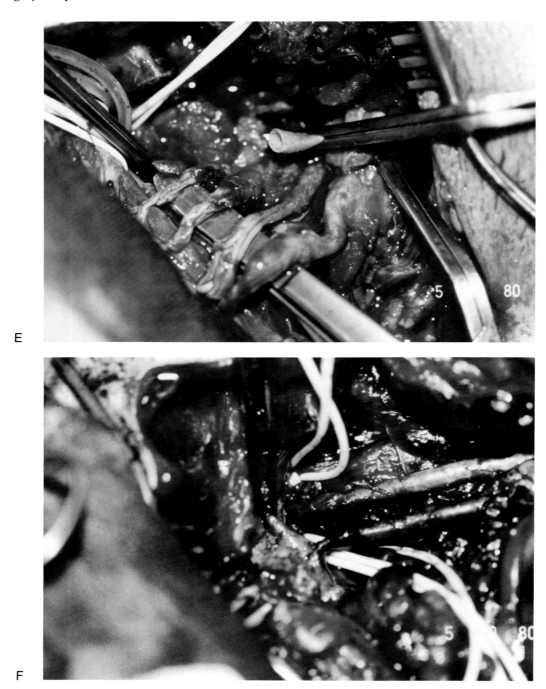

Fig. 1-2 *(Continued).* **(E)** Operative photograph demonstrating complete avulsion of brachial artery and vein and avulsion of right brachial plexus. **(F)** Operative photograph showing repair of brachial artery and vein and excision of avulsed portions of brachial plexus. Patient was T5 paraplegic complete with complete right brachial plexus injury.

an immediately available basis. A regional or comprehensive trauma center should have designated trauma teams for the management of specific types of trauma and should have facilities to communicate with paramedics in the field, to provide medical assistance and medical control. This type of institution should have established protocols for the management of all types of trauma. The regional trauma hospital should have an annual admission rate of 300 to 400 trauma patients (critically injured) each year to maintain a high degree of trauma team proficiency, judgment, and coordination.

Patients with all categories of spine trauma are eligible for admission to a spine trauma center: those with fracture, without instability; those with unstable fractures without neurologic injury; and those with both neurologic injuries and vertebral column instability.

INITIAL PATIENT ASSESSMENT

Evaluation of the patient at the scene of the accident begins with a primary survey, paying particular attention to the ABCs.[9] During this phase of the initial evaluation, life-threatening conditions are identified, and when necessary, simultaneous management is initiated:

A. Airway maintenance with care and control of the cervical spine
B. Breathing
C. Circulation with hemorrhage control
D. Disability: observing for neurologic disability or an altered state of consciousness
E. Exposure: as soon as possible the patient should be carefully but totally undressed, and skin surfaces observed for injuries not otherwise identifiable.

Airway, Cervical Spine, and Breathing

If the initial evaluation of an accident victim reveals a ventilation problem, it must be addressed expeditiously and carefully. In managing the upper airway, one must be certain to look for maxillofacial trauma. If such trauma is evident, one should be highly suspect of an associated cervical spine injury and take great care of the neck while providing airway management. Absence of neurologic deficit does not rule out injury to the cervical spine. Although an accident victim may not reveal signs of head or facial injury, the identification of ventilation difficulties should alert the examiner to the likely presence of neurologic injury arising from injury to the cervical spinal cord (C1 to C4), and, in turn, the muscles of respiration in the chest and diaphragm. Manual ventilation at the accident scene may be required. One person should assume and maintain control of the head and neck position, maintaining straightaway cervical spine traction and alignment. If possible, the head and neck should not be hyperflexed or hyperextended while the airway is being established, but establishing the airway takes precedence. Ventilation may be provided by one of several methods. If the patient is unconscious and the upper airway is otherwise clear, insert a plastic airway-tongue depressor, a nasal tube, or an esophageal oral airway (EOA) and connect it to a bag-valve device connected to a mask. If the above method does not provide adequate ventilatory support, the patient may require nasotracheal (the best method for a cervical spine injury) or endotracheal intubation. Oxygen must be administered by whichever airway system is developed.

Three other diagnoses that should be considered when respiratory difficulties are identified at the accident scene are tension pneumothorax, closed pneumothorax, and flail chest (with multiple rib fractures) and associated pulmonary contusion. Tension pneumothorax requires that the chest cavity be evacuated of free air as soon as possible with a needle or chest tube. If an open chest wound exists, it must be tightly covered, and the flail chest must be supported.

Circulation

Maintenance of peripheral perfusion and oxygenation is vitally important from the standpoint of the heart, the brain, and the spinal cord. Tissue aerobic metabolism is ensured by perfusion of all tissues with well-oxygenated red blood cells. Thus, maintenance of blood pressure and volume ensures perfusion and prevents metabolic acidosis.

Generally, as a guide:

If the radial pulse is palpable, systolic pressure is approximately 80 mmHg.
If the femoral pulse is palpable, the systolic pressure is approximately 70 mmHg.
If the carotid pulse is palpable, the systolic pressure is approximately 60 mmHg.

Bleeding

Hemorrhage may be overt or covert. If obvious, the most effective means of control is direct pressure to the wound. Tourniquets should not be used, except in life-threatening situations or when bleeding must be controlled before going on to perform another life-saving task.

When bleeding is occult, there may be hemorrhaging into the chest or abdominal cavities or into the areas of closed fracture and muscle injury. As a rule, one unit of blood is lost for each major long bone fracture or for each major site of a pelvic fracture. Two units of blood are lost at a femoral fracture site. Pneumatic splints may be useful in controlling bleeding at a fracture site, whereas hemorrhage into the abdominal cavity may be partially controlled or tamponade may be significantly reduced by using the PASG (pneumatic antishock garment).

Disability (Neurologic) Evaluation

A rapid neurologic assessment should be performed to ascertain the patient's level of consciousness. Pupillary size and reaction should be simultaneously noted. Is the patient alert, responding to verbal commands, responding to painful stimuli only, or unresponsive?

When time permits, a more careful assessment of a patient's conscious state may be made by using the Glasgow coma scale (Table 1-1). One should be aware of the possible presence of an epidural or subdural hematoma, a depressed skull fracture, or some other intracranial complication that may produce a progressive deterioration in the patient's neurologic function.

Table 1-1.   Glasgow Coma Scale

Eyes open	Spontaneous	4
	To sound	3
	To pain	2
	Never	1
Best verbal response	Oriented	5
	Confused conversation	4
	Inappropriate words	3
	Incomprehensible words	2
	None	1
Best motor response	Obeys commands	6
	Localizes pain	5
	Flexion withdrawal	4
	Abnormal	3
	Extension	2
	None	1

(Teasdale G, Jennett B: Assessment and prognosis of coma after head injury. Acta Neurochirurg 34:45, 1976, with permission.)

A more thorough neurologic evaluation of the remainder of the patient's other functions may have to be delayed until the patient's arrival at the initial receiving hospital facility. If the patient is alert, a cursory assessment may be made by asking

Table 1-2.   Neurological Function: Level of Intactness

Motor–Sensory Response	Intact Level
Motor	
Diaphragm	C3,4,5
Shrug shoulders	C4
Deltoids (and flex elbows)	C5
Extend wrist	C6
Extend elbow/flex wrist	C7
Abduct fingers	C8
Active chest expansion	T1–T12
Hip flexion	L2
Knee extension	L3–L4
Ankle dorsiflexion	L5–S1
Ankle plantarflexion	S1–S2
Sensory	
Anterior thigh	L2
Anterior knee	L3
Anteriorlateral ankle	L4
Dorsum great-second toe	L5
Lateral side of foot	S1
Posterior calf	S2
Perianal sensation (perineum)	S2–S5

the patient questions relevant to sensation and asking the patient to make minor movements at the terminal ends of the upper and lower extremities. Although the information obtained may be sketchy and incomplete, it may be very valuable in establishing whether further neurologic injury or deterioration has occurred between the first evaluation at the accident scene and the patient's arrival at the receiving hospital. These initial findings may serve as the basis for all subsequent treatment. Table 1-2 describes the correlation between the level of neurologic function (motor and sensory) and the neurologic complications (see also Emergency Room Neurologic Assessment, below).

EMERGENCY ROOM NEUROLOGIC ASSESSMENT

A careful neurologic evaluation in the emergency room is the responsibility of the admitting service. Additional, confirmatory examinations will be performed by the consulting services (neurosurgery, orthopaedics, the respiratory service, the nursing service, and the general surgery service). Any loss of neurologic function observed by the nursing service or other examining physicians should be immediately reported to the managing services.

Perianal Neurologic Examination

Because the perianal area of the body is the lowermost dermatomal representation of the nervous system, the perianal neurologic examination is valuable (Fig. 1-3). The initial emergency room assessment of the patient must include an examination of the perineum (Table 1-3). This examination is important because the findings relate to, and substantiate, residual neurologic function, that is, whether a patient's neurologic injury is complete or incomplete. It is not possible to validate statistically any combined significance in the prognostication of neurologic recovery or lack thereof by the presence or absence of perianal sensation, bulbocavernosus reflex, or priapism.

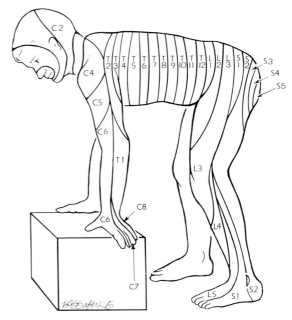

Fig. 1-3. A human in the "quadruped" stance. Note the sensory distribution of C5–T1 nerve roots into the upper extremities and of L2–S2 into the lower extremities, and the concentration of S2–S5 into the "saddle" or perianal region. When a human is in the upright, bipedal position, the perianal region represents the lowermost portion of the nervous system.

The best prognostic indicators are the presence of perianal sensation about the rectum and the presence of voluntary function within the perianal musculature. The perianal region serves as an indicator of present neurologic function. The fact that a patient has residual sensory or motor function below the level of neurologic or bony injury is a hopeful sign, and as such indicates an incomplete injury to the intervening neurologic tissue. When this is present, potential neurologic recovery (varying from minimal to great) is possible, but it cannot be accurately prognosticated and its extent cannot be estimated. What may be stated more emphatically is that in the absence of perianal sensation, perianal voluntary motor function, and peripheral reflexes (i.e., patellar or achilles), with or without priapism or a bulbocavernosus reflex, in all likelihood, the neurologic injury is complete and recovery is not likely.

Table 1-3.   Perianal Neurologic Assessment

Neurologic Injury	Perianal Sensation	Voluntary Perianal Motor	Bulbocavernosus Reflex[a]	Perianal Wink[a]	Priapism
Complete	−	−	+ − peripheral nerve lesion (flaccid paralysis)	+ − peripheral nerve lesion (flaccid paralysis)	+[b] − peripheral nerve lesion
Incomplete	+ sensory intact (anterior cord syndrome) − motor intact (posterior cord syndrome)	+ motor intact (posterior cord syndrome) − sensory intact (anterior cord syndrome)	+ with intact reflex arc	+ with sensation − without sensation	−
Intact	+	+	+	+	−

[a] Same reflex arc.
[b] Cervical spine injuries.

When performing the perianal neurologic examination, one should test for perianal pain and sensation, voluntary anal sphincter motor function, and intra-anal proprioception. Intra-anal proprioception is another valuable indicator of incomplete neurologic injury. Intra-anal proprioception should be determined in addition to the presence or absence of pinprick pain or perception around the anus. Intra-anal proprioception indicates that the patient has an incomplete neurologic injury with reference to abolition of the posterior columns. Similarly, the presence of active and voluntary perianal motor function (even in the absence of sensory function) points to an incomplete neurologic injury. Without evidence of neurologic improvement within the first 24 hours after injury, there is not likely to be any significant neurologic recovery.[10] In the MRSCICS total patient population of 2,710 patients, only 4.3 percent diagnosed on admission as having a complete neurologic injury demonstrated any neurologic improvement during their admission.

The presence of an anal wink has no prognostic significance. A perianal wink is a reflex motor contraction of the perianal muscles (the levator ani and external sphincter ani muscles) produced when the skin surrounding the anus is stimulated (a pain stimulus). The production of "pain" (not perceived by the cerebral sensory cortex owing to an injury of interruption between the sacral segments of the nervous system and the cerebral cortex) in the presence of a reflex arc both into and out of the spinal cord (assuming that the sensory and motor portion of the spinal cord below the spinal injury has not been injured) will produce a perianal wink (see Table 1-3).

Another neurologic finding in the area of the perineum is the bulbocavernosus reflex. This is a reflex similar to the anal wink reflex, and travels through the same neurologic pathway. To produce this reflex, a gloved finger of one hand is placed in the rectum, while with the other hand, the glans penis (in the male) is squeezed, or the indwelling catheter in either the male or female bladder is gently tugged. Either action stimulates the pelvic floor and bladder, producing an anal muscle contraction that will be felt by the examining finger in the rectum. The contraction, a positive bulbocavernosus reflex, indicates that this portion of the reflex neurologic system is out of spinal shock.[10] It is frequently associated with the presence of priapism. Priapism has long been associated with complete neurologic injury; according to the studies of Edwin Smith, the association was recorded some 2,500 to 3,000 years BC. According to these records priapism in the presence of a spinal injury was tantamount to a complete neurologic injury,[11] "and the patient not to be reckoned with."

EXTRICATION TECHNIQUES

At the scene of an accident, confusion prevails, particularly when a victim demonstrates acute cardiorespiratory distress. This confusion often contributes to further patient injury, particularly with a drowning. First, there is the realization that a drowning has occurred. Immediately, and simulta-

neously, everyone tries to help. Persons at the scene fail to appreciate that the victim may have sustained a cervical spine (diving) injury, resulting in neurologic injury. Were this identified, however, the patient's course might be altered.

For the inexperienced, uninitiated, or untrained, fright overrules good judgment. Someone dives into the water, extricating the victim by dragging

Fig. 1-4. (A) Simulation of typical position of a victim of a motor vehicle accident involving sudden deceleration. The hazard here is inappropriate extrication of the victim before suspecting a spinal injury. The victim should be managed as though a spine injury is present. (B) Correct extrication by paramedics after the victim has been appropriately splinted and secured to a fracture spine board.

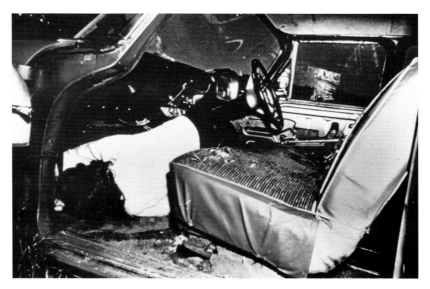

A

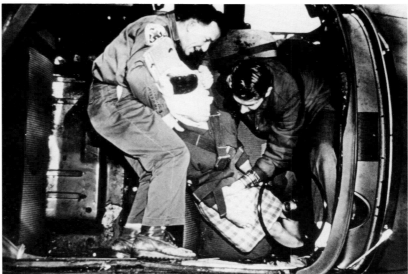

B

him or her to dry land or out of the water, without any attention to the cervical spine. Similar attempts at assistance often occur in motor vehicle accidents. The victim is assisted or extricated (implying inability to do so by oneself) out of a severely damaged vehicle, with little or no thought given to the sudden, positive deceleration that the victim just experienced (particularly in the absence of seatbelt restraints) (Fig. 1-4). The accident results in the victim's head and face striking the windshield or dashboard, forcibly driving the head and neck into either flexion or extension (Fig. 1-5). The unsplinted victim becomes highly susceptible to further injury or to a worsening of the already present injury when assisted by untrained individuals without concern for and splinting of the spine. Thus, extrication, whether from a vehicle or a swimming pool, requires awareness of the possible presence of a serious spinal injury.

The use of appropriate extrication techniques is as important as any other aspect of acute spinal cord injury care. This may be attested to by the increasing number of high-level quadriplegics arriving (indicating survival) in the spinal injury center and the decreased incidence of complete neurologic injury (62 percent incidence of complete injury in 1972, 21 percent incidence of complete injury in 1986).

Cervical Spine

For suspected cervical spine injuries, it is paramount throughout the extrication period that the cervical spine, the neck, and the thorax always be maintained in "straightaway" alignment. In the review of the etiologies, falls and motor vehicle accidents are the two primary causes of spinal injury and gunshot wounds are third. Other primary causes of injury are diving, motorcycle, and pedestrian accidents.

The accident site somewhat dictates the extrication method. If the injury occurs in a swimming pool and injury to the cervical spine is likely, care should be taken to bring the victim to the surface by the hair, with a straight pull upward in line with the torso, or to take the victim's head and hold it between the retriever's hands. Once on the surface of the water, if help is available, one person assumes control of the head and neck, while the others control the remainder of the body. If shallow water is available, one person, other than the individual holding the head and shoulders, should initiate mouth-to-mouth resuscitation, if required.

The patient should be left in the water until a long bath towel, a long backboard, or at least five people are available to lift the victim to the side of the pool (Fig. 1-6). During this period, the head

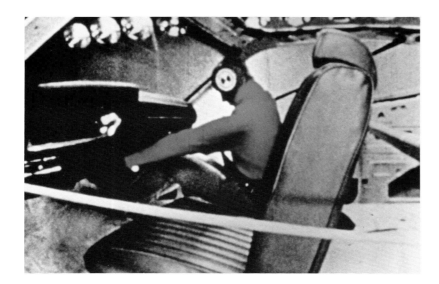

Fig. 1-5. Instrumented laboratory dummy showing beneficial effect of seat belt restraint at the moment of vehicle impact.

and neck must be maintained in mild traction and in straightaway alignment with the torso. Once the victim is on the pool deck and a long backboard is available, the patient should be secured in place on the board with the head tied in place to prevent any side-to-side motion. Rolled towels may be placed adjacent to the head, on either side, and fixed in place. A common question is whether a rolled towel should be placed beneath the nape of the neck, to maintain the "normal" cervical lordosis.

Fig. 1-6. Retrieval from the water of a victim with suspected cervical spine injury. **(A)** Victim found motionless at bottom of pool. **(B)** Rescuer approaches victim from the rear, places his arms and hands under the patient's axillae, and supports the head and neck from either side. *(Figure continues.)*

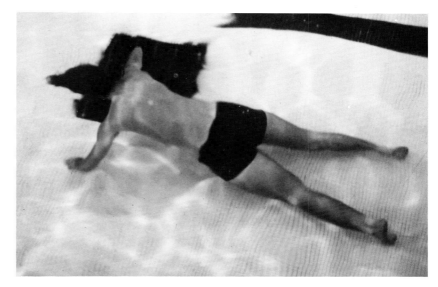

A

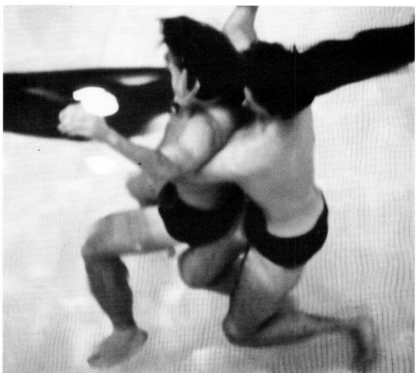

B

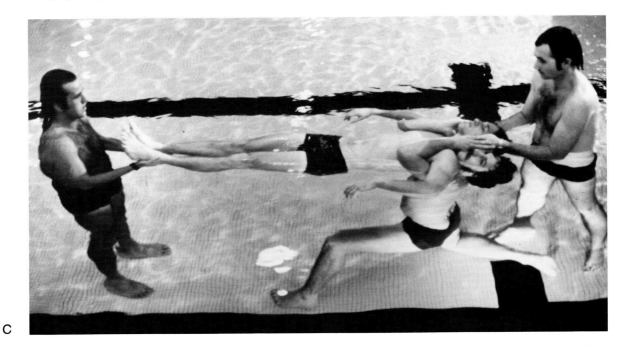

C

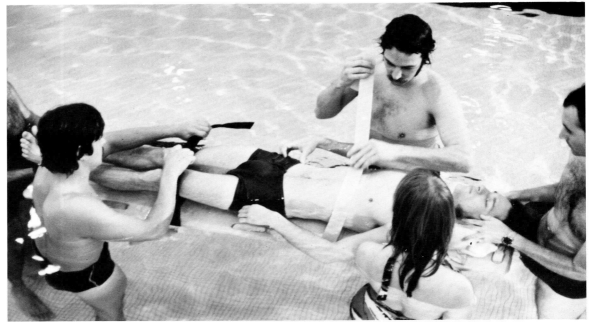

D

Fig. 1-6 *(Continued)*. **(C)** Patient and rescuer at the surface. Assistants take each end of the victim, one supporting the head, neck, and back, the other the lower extremities. If the victim requires resuscitation, the rescuer is free to perform mouth-to-mouth. **(D)** If a spine board is available, it can be slipped under the patient and the patient appropriately stabilized. If a board is not available, a large beach towel can be placed under the patient to extract him from the pool. One person supports the head and neck.

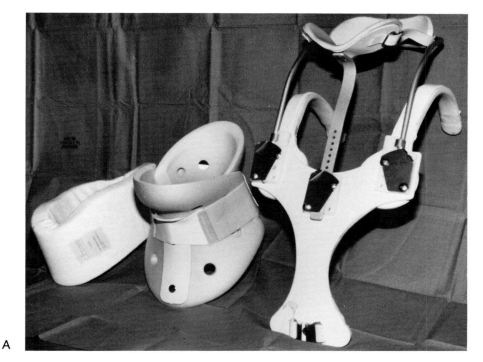

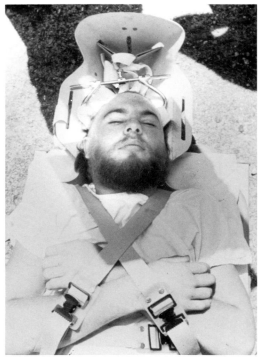

Fig. 1-7. Cervical support devices used for patient transport. (**A**) Three cervical orthotic devices commonly used for supporting the cervical spine. The soft collar (left) is the least acceptable. A similar plastic collar (not shown) would also be less than desirable. The Philadelphia collar (center) or the SOMI (sternal-occipital-mandibular immobilizing) orthosis (right) are better for patient transport. (**B**) The Meyer cervical orthosis (Zimmer U.S.A., Inc.) in place on an acute quadriplegic patient with C5 complete injury with skeletal tong traction. Note that the paralyzed arms have been placed under straps (see Fig. 1-8).

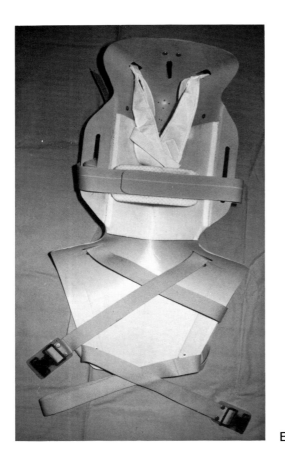

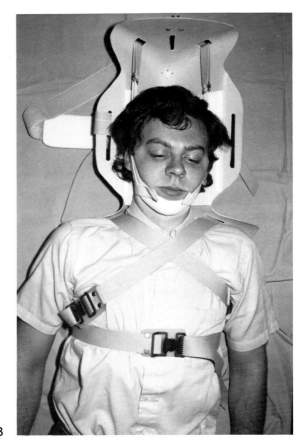

A

B

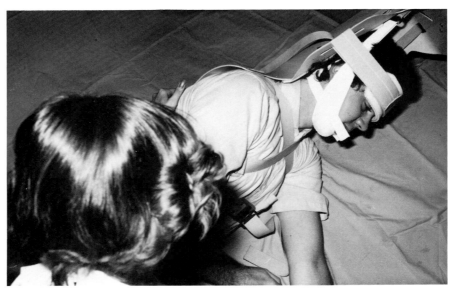

C

Fig. 1-8. Meyer cervical orthosis (Zimmer U.S.A., Inc.). **(A)** The orthosis is constructed of light plastic, allowing it to be slipped easily beneath or behind a sitting or lying patient. **(B)** The orthosis applied to a patient, with the head halter traction strap in place. Traction is applied through elastic straps attached to the halter. **(C)** The device allows the patient to be turned on his or her side for emesis while maintaining the relationship of head, neck, and chest and the airway. *(Figure continues.)*

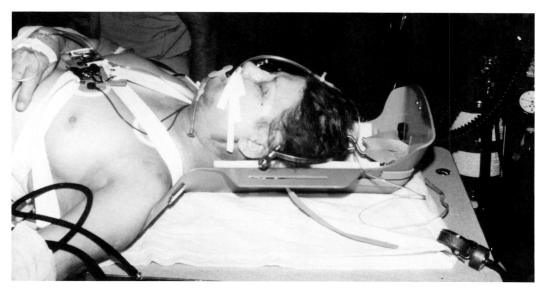

D

Fig. 1-8 *(Continued).* (**D**) The orthosis can be used to move a patient in traction from the fracture frame to the operating table while maintaining the traction. Note that this patient has Gardner-Wells tongs in place and is intubated.

This is not necessary, and in fact, because most injuries to the cervical spine are flexion injuries (42 percent flexion, 20 percent axial, 15 percent rotation, 6 percent extension, remainder unclassified), and with 20 percent of all spine injuries occurring at the C5 level, the use of a roll may be detrimental to the flexion-dislocated spine. However, the skin in the area of the occiput becomes very painful when the victim's head is tied down to a spine board for a prolonged period. Care must be taken if *anything* is placed beneath the occiput to relieve pressure. A *thin*, soft sponge or pad between the occiput and board (without elevating the head or neck) may be comforting if the patient will be required to remain on the board for any great period.

Another question that is somewhat more controversial is whether the application of light cervical traction, either by means of a cervicohead halter or through traction on skull tongs, may be harmful before an accurate (radiologic) diagnosis of the cervical spine injury is made. Because the majority of injuries to the cervical spine occur in flexion (42 percent), applying light traction is more likely to bring about some improvement in the overall alignment of the cervical spine. This motion may be sufficient to reduce the deleterious effects of a sub-luxation-dislocation and may be sufficient to decompress the anterior aspect of the spinal cord. The principal anatomic structure to be salvaged in this area is the anterior spinal artery (see Ch. 4). This converse is also true — beware of flexing the cervical spine. This motion may produce significant injury.

Other methods of splinting the cervical spine are the short spine board (similar to the long board, but one-third the length); a soft collar (Fig. 1-7); a firm plastic collar; or an orthosis such as the one developed at Northwestern University (Meyer cervical orthosis, Zimmer U.S.A., Inc.) in 1974. This latter device is most frequently utilized by ambulance and trauma services throughout Illinois for the transfer of patients with suspected cervical spine injury. This orthosis maintains alignment of the cervical spine with the neck and the thorax (Fig. 1-8).

Never transport a patient suspected of having sustained a cervical spine injury in either the *sitting* or *prone position*. Airway management and suctioning for emesis cannot be accomplished with the patient in the prone position (Fig. 1-9).

It should be axiomatic that unconscious patients should be intubated (orally or nasally) as soon as

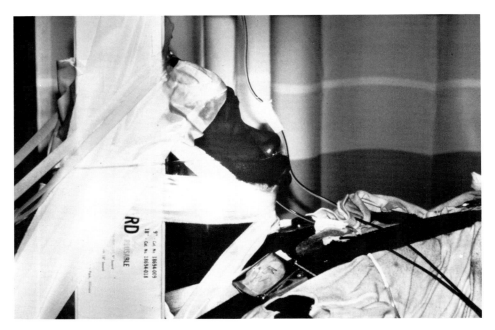

Fig. 1-9. Inappropriate splinting of the cervical spine after trauma. The patient's head and neck have been placed in an inappropriate "splint them where they lie" position. Note the acute hyperflexion of the head and neck. The patient's injury was C5–C6 subluxation with significant C5–C6 incomplete neurologic lesion. Neurologic recovery began as soon as the patient was removed from the splint and the head and neck placed in a "straightaway" position. Neurologic function returned to normal over the next 3 weeks.

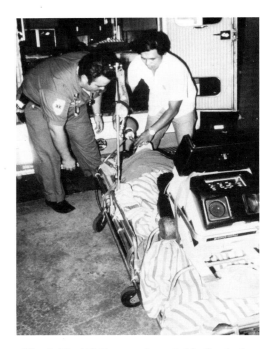

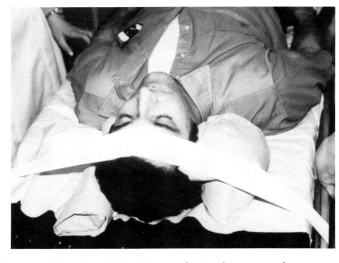

A   B

Fig. 1-10. **(A)** Unconscious child after being struck by a car. Note the rigid collar, intubation by paramedics, and one paramedic maintaining head and neck control. **(B)** Suspected spine injury patient in emergency room. Head and neck are taped in position until the radiographic examination and diagnosis are made.

possible after injury to support the airway, and always before being transferred between hospital facilities (Fig. 1-10).

Thoracolumbar Spine

Most injuries to the thoracolumbar spine are the result of axial and flexion load forces. A third mechanical factor producing injury is rotation. The principal etiologic factors producing injury are falls and falling objects (41 percent), followed by motor vehicle injuries (32 percent) and gunshot wounds (12 percent).

The patient should be extricated in a horizontal plane. If in a vehicle and originally found in a sitting position, the patient may be first splinted with a short backboard or Meyer orthosis, followed by placement into a supine position on the seat. (No patient should ever be transported in the sitting position or in a prone or face-down position. Should emesis occur, the airway could not be adequately supported.) Changing the patient from the prone to the supine position requires the help of several individuals. One person should assume control of the head and neck, while the others simultaneously "log roll" the victim. The patient should then be firmly secured to the spine board for transport (and turning, should it be required for emesis or clearing of the airway).

MODE OF TRANSPORT

Patients requiring immediate life-saving medical or surgical techniques require transportation from the scene of the accident to an initial care facility by the most appropriate and expeditious method. The two most important factors are the patient's medical condition and the distance (or time en route) from the accident site to the closest or most appropriate receiving hospital. Whether the initial institution is the most appropriate for the identified problem is not an immediate concern.

There are several guidelines for determining the most appropriate means of patient transportation, assuming that any mode requested would be available.

Land transport may be utilized when the time between dispatch and patient arrival at the receiving hospital is 45 minutes or less. This rule may not be applicable in the following circumstances: high-density urban or suburban traffic; the patient is a multiple trauma victim; extended time was taken at the accident scene because of prolonged patient extrication; or the severity of the injury requires rapid air transport, plus the presence of an aeromedical support team.[12]

Helicopter transport should be used for patients whose injuries are relatively stable and who require transport over extended distances (15 miles to 100 miles) or through high-density traffic.[12] If the patient's condition is unstable, an aeromedical team and working space must be available.

Fixed-wing transport should be used for patients in need of tertiary medical care who are more than 100 miles from the required tertiary facility. They should be transported first to the nearest receiving hospital, stabilized, and then transferred to the tertiary care institution. (Having an aeromedical team on board extends the distance over which this mode of transportation may be used.)

The transport scheme used by the acute spinal trauma center of Northwestern University differs from that described above for the following reason: no patient with spinal cord injuries should be transported to the tertiary facility (spinal injury center) initially, unless by chance this becomes the first available facility. The spinal cord management protocol suggests that because of the high incidence of multitrauma (42.9 percent), patients with spine injuries should be evaluated first in a receiving hospital and then, if physiologically stable, transported to the appropriate tertiary facility[13] (Fig. 1-11).

Between 0 and 45 miles, the patient may best be transported by land ambulance. Although this mode of transport may not be appropriate during peak traffic periods, with qualified paramedics and numerous receiving hospitals in the urban setting, it is the most reliable.

Between 45 and 75 miles, the most expeditious mode of transportation is the helicopter. Generally, the patient will be retrieved at an airport or hospital heliport, rather than at the accident scene. Problems encountered in the urban setting include lack of landing sites, high buildings, and inclement weather.

MODE OF TRANSPORTATION PLAN

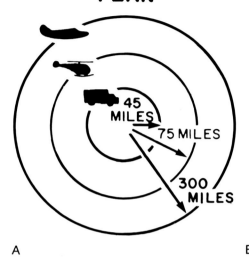

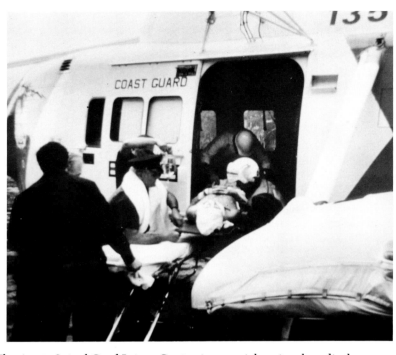

A   B

Fig. 1-11. (A) Patient transfer protocol. The Acute Spinal Cord Injury Center is a special regional medical facility receiving patients from a catchment area 200 miles in radius centered on Chicago (see Fig. 1-1). The region has a population of 15 million. To retrieve patients appropriately and as quickly as possible, the severity of the injury, the distance from the Center, and the traffic density must all be considered. (B) Air transport of spine-injured patients to the Center is a cooperative, integrated system that involves the Chicago metropolitan police, the State of Illinois, private air transport systems, and the Federal Government.

Patients requiring transport over long distances (75 to 300 miles) frequently require more time and greater planning. Also, the patient's condition may require space and specialized equipment and personnel.

It is appropriate to review the success of the Northwestern University transportation scheme. Over the past 14 years, this system of transportation selection has been used to transport patients over distances ranging from 1 to 300 miles. Although all patients are retrieved from an accident scene and taken to a receiving hospital for initial evaluation (and remain there for various periods), followed by transport to the tertiary (spinal cord injury) care institution, the average admission time to the acute spinal cord injury center, for all patients over this 15-year period, is 6.2 hours after injury.

If there is any disadvantage to the above plan, it is that generally one and often two short distances (one on either end) will require ambulance transportation between the accident scene and the initial hospital and between the airport facility and the trauma center. Designated trauma facilities should have, as a prerequisite, heliport (or helistop) facilities either on or in close proximity to the trauma center.

REFERENCES

1. Kraus JF, Franti CE, Riggins RS et al.: Incidence of traumatic spinal cord lesions. J Chronic Dis 28:471, 1975
2. Swan K, Swan RC: Gunshot wounds: pathophysiol-

ogy and management. P.S.G. Publishing, Littleton, MA, 1980

3. Neel S: Helicopter evacuation in Korea. US Armed Forces Med J 6:691, 1955

4. Neel S: Army aeromedical evacuation procedures in Vietnam: implications for rural America. *JAMA* 204:309, 1968

5. Neel S: Medical support of the US Army in Vietnam 1965–1970. U.S. Government Printing Office, Washington, D.C., 1973

6. Trunkey DD, Lim RC: Analysis of 425 consecutive trauma fatalities: an autopsy study. J Am Coll Emerg Phys 3:368, 1974

7. West JG, Trunkey DD, Lim RC: Systems of care. Arch Surg 114:455, 1979

8. Illinois Categorization Law, Senate Bill 568, Public Act 76-1858, October 1972

9. Advanced Trauma Life Support Course, Instructors Manual. Committee on Trauma, American College of Surgeons, 1984

10. Holdsworth FW: Review article: fracture, fracture-dislocations of the spine. J Bone Joint Surg 52-A:1534, 1970

11. Elsberg CA: The Edwin Smith surgical papyrus, and the diagnosis and the treatment of injuries to the skull and spine 5,000 years ago. Am Med Hist 3:271, 1931

12. Baxt WG: Aeromedical emergency care. p. 131. System Approach to Emergency Medical Care. Appleton & Lange, Norwalk, CT, 1983

13. Meyer PR: System approach to the care of the spinal cord injured. p. 404. System Approach to Emergency Medical Care. Appleton & Lange, Norwalk, CT, 1983

Emergency Room Assessment: Management of Spinal Cord and Associated Injuries

Paul R. Meyer, Jr.

Instead of presenting a broadly based overview of existing knowledge on emergency room assessment, this chapter emphasizes lessons learned and knowledge gained through the development and operation of the largest acute spinal cord injury trauma center in the United States, over the 14 years from 1972 to 1985.

The acute spinal cord injury center at Northwestern University was first initiated in 1968 at Northwestern Memorial Hospital. The acute spinal program, the Midwest Regional Spinal Cord Injury Care System (MRSCICS) at Northwestern University, received federal sponsorship from the Division of Rehabilitation Services Administration, Department of Health, Education and Welfare, in June 1972 and, at that time, became the first acute care spinal cord injury center in the United States and the first such center directly attached to a major acute comprehensive rehabilitation hospital, the Rehabilitation Institute of Chicago. This system provides each patient admitted to the spinal cord injury center with appropriate spinal care from the time of the accident to the patient's eventual re-entry into society (Fig. 2-1).[1]

The development of the spinal cord injury program at Northwestern University was stimulated by the simultaneous development of the Illinois State Emergency Medical Service (Trauma) Program in 1971 to 1972.[2-6] From this program, national awareness grew concerning the benefits of available, strategically located urban and suburban regional (comprehensive) trauma centers and community-identified area and local trauma center hospitals, each capable of responding appropriately to the needs of the gravely injured patient. Nonetheless, today the concept of trauma centers is still controversial. However, the controversy ought not to be whether the trauma center concept is viable — it has been proved to be so — but rather, which hospitals are best suited to become trauma centers; what makes an institution eligible; and, what does comprehensive trauma care imply? I define a trauma center as an institution having the physical presence of all medical and surgical specialties on a 24-hour basis with the simultaneous availability of all required support services (operating rooms, computed axial tomography [CAT] scan, magnetic resonance imaging [MRI], tomography, somatosensory evoked potential monitoring, angiography, etc.) (Fig. 2-2).

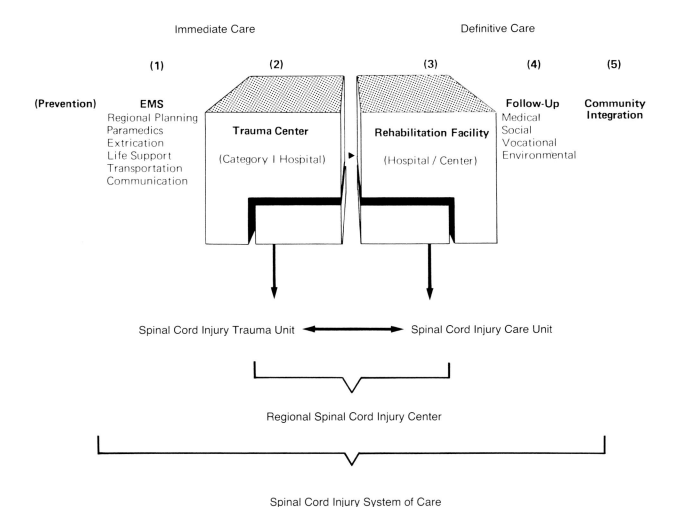

Fig. 2-1. Components of a spinal cord injury care system. (From American Spinal Injury Association/Foundation,[1] with permission.)

SPINAL CORD INJURY

Normally, the definition of "spinal cord injury" is an injury to the spinal cord that results in some form of neurologic deficit. While this definition is correct, it is also restrictive, and the hazard then becomes upholding the definition. Patients who have suffered injury to the spine may, on initial evaluation, have either unidentified associated injuries or a spine injury whose severity is underestimated. In either case, the resulting misdiagnosis may lead to the onset of neurologic injury. In a series of 2,710 patients admitted to the Spine Injury Center between 1972 and 1986, 187 (9.3 percent) had neurologic injury without spinal fracture (Table 2-1).

Many trauma patients simply receive care in the emergency room, a situation that limits the opportunity for immediate identification of all potential problems. The admission of a spinal injury patient to a designated spinal cord trauma center, however, is likely to reduce the occurrences of unattended or undiagnosed complications for three reasons: a trauma center has a greater awareness that the patient is likely to have a particular asso-

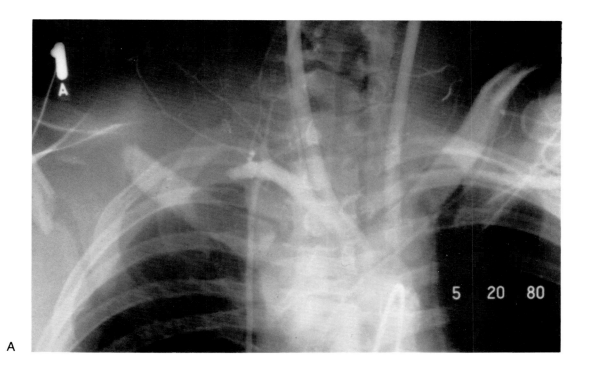

A

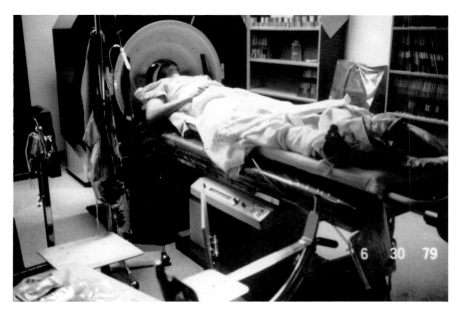

B

Fig. 2-2. Evaluation of the multiple trauma patient. **(A)** The incidence of pulmonary trauma in association with spine trauma is 15 percent, vascular injury, 2 percent, orthopaedic trauma, 9 percent. Radiograph demonstrates fractured clavicle and scapula, occlusion of subclavian artery, and compression fracture at T6. At surgery, patient had complete avulsion of brachial plexus. **(B)** Incidence of head trauma with spine trauma is 26 percent. Scene demonstrates need for radiologic capabilities allowing for immediate assessment of head trauma victim with spine trauma. Note patient in EMI scanner on Stryker wedge frame back support. *(Figure continues.)*

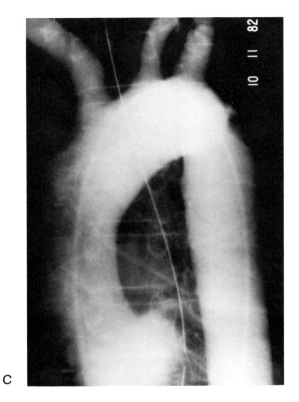

C

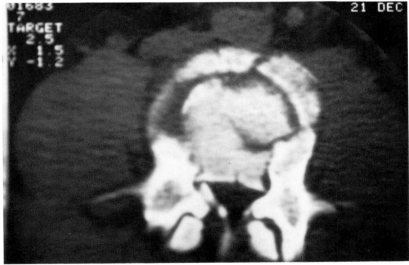

D

Fig. 2-2 *(Continued)*. (**C**) Anteroposterior (AP) subtraction angiogram of the aorta in a 77-year-old man involved in a motor vehicle accident. Patient sustained an extension injury to the cervical spine with fracture at C6–C7. Note a tear in the adventitia just to the right of the arch of the aorta superiorly. The aorta required immediate repair. The neck was in Gardner-Wells traction. (**D**) CAT scan of 35-year-old man who fell 30 feet and sustained a burst fracture of L2 with neurologic compromise. He required immediate anterior decompression and posterior stabilization.

Table 2-1. Extent of Neurologic Injury by Location of Spine Fracture at Northwestern University Acute Spine Injury Center, 1972 to 1986

Level of Spine Fracture	No. of Cases	Intact		Incomplete		Complete		Missing	
		No.	Percent	No.	Percent	No.	Percent	No.	Percent
No Fracture	515	152	29.5	160	31.1	81	15.7	122	23.7
Cervical	1372	352	25.7	567	41.3	437	31.9	16	1.2
Thoracic	323	37	11.5	83	25.7	201	62.2	2	0.6
Thoracolumbar	430	126	29.3	179	41.6	124	28.8	1	0.2
Lumbar	63	26	41.3	36	57.1	1	1.6	0	0.0
Sacral	7	0	0.0	7	100.0	0	0.0	0	0.0
Total	2710	693	25.6	1032	38.1	844	31.1	141	5.2

ciated injury (through experience derived from managing a large number of similarly injured patients); a trauma center's medical and nursing team is skilled and proficient in treating patients with spinal cord injuries; and most importantly, a trauma center undergoes constant program analysis, re-evaluation, and peer review, constantly seeking to improve its performance.

The association of multiple trauma with spinal column and spinal cord injury is very high. Between 1972 and 1986, 2,710 patients with acutely injured spinal cords and spinal columns were admitted through the emergency room to the acute spinal cord unit. Their median admission time posttrauma was 6.2 hours, and they were retrieved from a surrounding catchment area of 300 miles. Sixty-nine (42.9 percent) were victims of multiple trauma.

After the presence of a spinal injury, the next most frequent sites of associated trauma were as follows: the head and face, 26.2 percent; fractures of long bones and pelvis, 8.5 percent; the chest (hemothorax, pneumothorax, multiple fractured ribs, fractured clavicle or scapula, and occasionally, major vessel injury), 16.1 percent; and intraabdominal injuries to the spleen, liver, or viscus, 10.0 percent (Table 2-2). The incidence of neurologic injury in this multiple trauma population was 75.2 percent of the 1,163 multiply traumatized patients (Fig. 2-3).

Table 2-2. Vital Sign Changes in Trauma Patients

Vital Sign	Spinal Cord	Head Injury	Hemorrhage Injury
Bradycardia	+	+	−
Hypotension	+	−	+
Hypothermia	+	+	−
Depressed respiration	+		−
Diaphoresis	−	−	+
Tachycardia	−	−	+
Hypertension	−	+	−
Depressed consciousness	+	+	−
Mental confusion	−	+	+
Agitation	−	+	+

EMERGENCY ROOM PATIENT ASSESSMENT AND MANAGEMENT

An important component in the overall success of a trauma center is a system of communication that informs the appropriate medical personnel when an accident victim is being transferred to the trauma center. The MRSCICS established the position of trauma coordinator to help the facility identify patients requiring the care available in a particular trauma center and to expedite the retrieval and transport of that patient to the appropriate care facility in the shortest time. This position was initially established in each of the state's designated trauma programs, but when the program passed

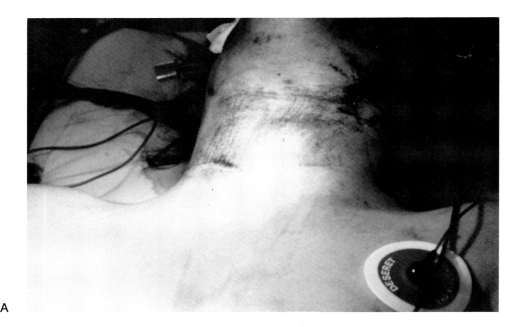

A

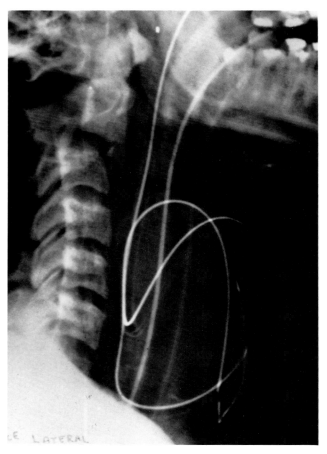

B

Fig. 2-3. Anterior injury to neck. The patient was riding a motorcycle when he struck a wire object across the anterior neck. **(A)** Clinical appearance. **(B)** Lateral radiograph revealing coiled nasogastric tube in anterior neck and fracture through posterior element of C2 (hangman's fracture). Patient was neurologically intact. *(Figure continues.)*

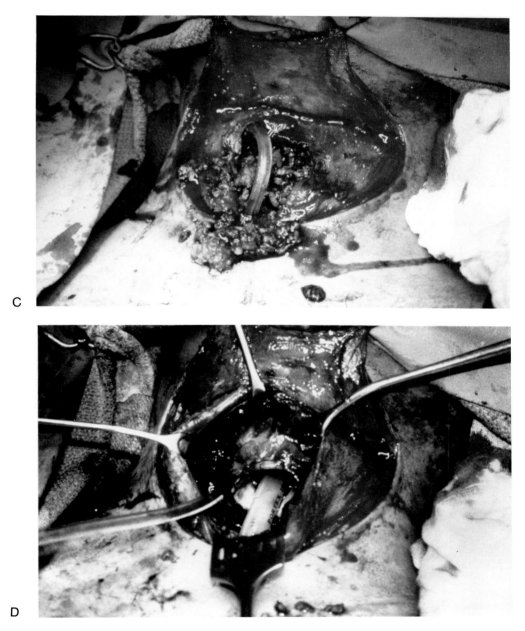

Fig. 2-3 *(Continued)*. **(C)** Operative exploration of anterior neck reveals rupture of esophagus, with extravasation of nasogastric tube and food particles. **(D)** The trachea is also transected. Endotracheal tube can be seen traversing gap. *(Figure continues.)*

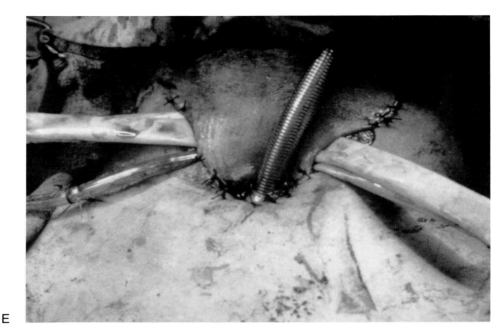

E

Fig. 2-3 *(Continued)*. (E) Postoperative repair of trachea, esophagus, and skin flap. Cervical spine was managed by cervical tong traction until neck tissues healed, and then by a halo vest for 3 months. Patient had normal neurologic function.

from a state government-supported activity to one supported by individual hospitals, many hospitals discontinued the position. However, MRSCICS maintained the trauma coordinator.

The trauma coordinator's responsibilities include the following:

1. To serve as the first communication link between the referring institution and the receiving trauma center.
2. To gather all pertinent information concerning the patient's medical condition.
3. To convey this information to the attending physician whose service will be the primary service responsible for the management of the patient (i.e., spinal cord trauma to the spinal cord service; head trauma to the neurosurgery service; mass trauma to the general surgery service, etc.).
4. To transmit to the referring institution specific pretransfer medical or surgical recommendations, made by the respective attending physi-

cian and directed through the coordinator (physician-to-physician communication may be appropriate in instances in which specialized management regimens are required or requested, e.g., peritoneal lavage, insertion of a chest tube, fracture debridement before transfer, etc.).

5. To make or confirm all transportation arrangements, as overseen by particular members of the medical or nursing staff.
6. To monitor the progress of the transfer and inform the emergency room and the appropriate medical-surgical teams of the patient's estimated time of arrival.

A prerequisite in the administration of a trauma center program is the immediate availability of the medical-surgical attending teams for patient care. This aspect of the emergency room administration is managed on one-call roster, rather than on individual physician's or service's monthly medical specialty call rosters.

SPINAL CORD AND GENERAL TRAUMA TEAMS

At the spine trauma center at Northwestern University, the spine service is the emergency surgical service most frequently called upon. Upon the arrival of trauma patients, the orthopaedic, neurosurgery, anesthesia-respiratory therapy, and general surgery services are present. To facilitate patient management, the services are divided into separate teams:

Routine Spinal Cord Trauma Team. For all acute spinal cord admissions to the emergency room, three services routinely examine the patient and write history and physical exam notes: orthopaedic surgery, neurosurgery, and respiratory-critical care (Fig. 2-4).

General Surgery Trauma Team. This fourth service team attends all acute spinal cord patients with known multiple trauma and those patients as requested by the spinal cord team. The team comprises a general surgeon (captain), orthopaedic surgeon, neurosurgeon, and anesthesiologist.

The center admits patients to either a neurosurgeon or an orthopaedic surgeon on an alternate-day basis (but always to the spinal cord service). This scheme equalizes participation of all services and reinforces the use of a common management protocol. The primary admitting service becomes the managing service, the other the consulting service. On the next day, the roles of the two services are reversed.

EMERGENCY ROOM PROTOCOL

When the spinal cord patient is admitted to the emergency room and while still on the initial transfer backboard or ambulance cart, an immediate, cursory physical and neurologic examination is performed.[7] Once the trauma team is satisfied that the airway is clear and the cardiovascular system is stable, the patient can be transferred (with the help of the emergency room staff) to an awaiting Stryker wedge frame or an appropriate bed surface. The patient with spinal cord injuries should be removed from a backboard as soon as possible after arrival in the emergency room. Frequently, the patient will have been on the frame for several hours during the transfer. With the loss of sensory and motor function, the areas of the buttocks, heels, scapulae, and occiput are immobile and consequently, within 3 to 5 hours, they may develop skin pressure irritation and potentially break down.

Under the care of a trauma system, a patient will usually have in place before transfer and arrival at the trauma center one and preferably two large-bore intravenous (IV) lines (with lactated Ringer's solution running). If not, they are immediately inserted, along with an arterial line to obtain baseline blood gas values and an SMA-16 (including electrolytes). Baseline arterial blood gas values should be immediately obtained and compared with previous readings, if available, because the most com-

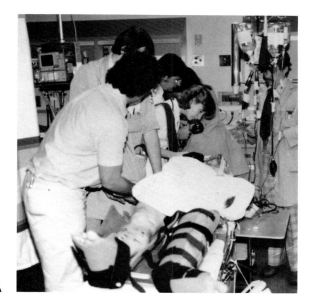

A

Fig. 2-4. Spinal cord-injured patients with multiple trauma. (A) Emergency room view of aircraft accident victim with cervical spinal cord injury. This patient required immediate surgical care by neurosurgeon, general surgeon, orthopaedic surgeon, and anesthesiologist. Each of these services sees every spinal cord patient who has evidence of multiple trauma in the emergency room. Each service is present in the emergency room when the patient arrives. *(Figure continues.)*

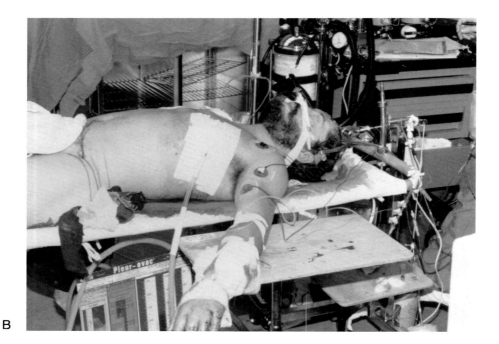

B

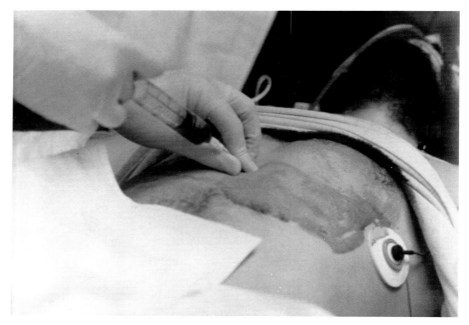

C

Fig. 2-4 *(Continued)*. **(B)** Victim of motor vehicle accident who required immediate bilateral thoracostomy tubes, pericardiocentesis, and debridement of fractures of all four extremities. Note the abdominal tap as well. **(C)** Patient who required pericardiocentesis in the emergency room. The patient had pericardial tamponade with narrow pulse pressure, associated with bilateral chest trauma.

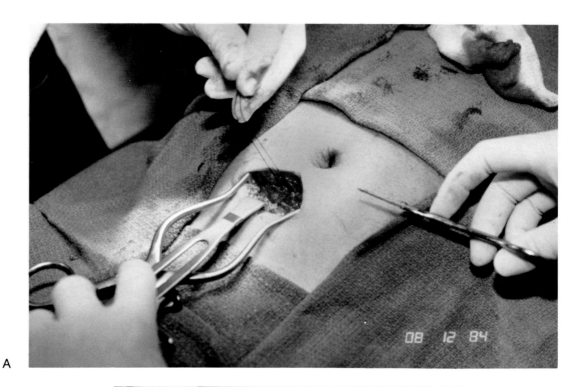

A

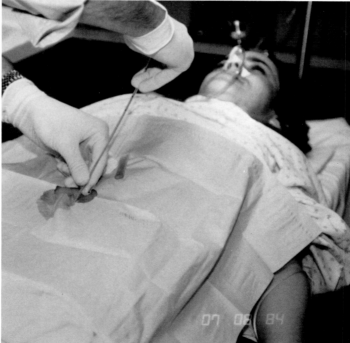

B

Fig. 2-5. Patient with acute abdominal trauma and possible intra-abdominal injury. (**A**) Under local anesthesia, a midline incision was made allowing exposure of the peritoneal sheath. (**B**) An Intracath catheter being inserted into the peritoneal cavity for peritoneal lavage.

mon problem identified in the quadriplegic patient (secondary to neurologic injury) is neurologically related difficulty with pulmonary ventilation. Often, this problem is insidious in its onset and difficult to detect. Consequently, the respiratory-critical care service always evaluates every patient. Blood gas values are serially obtained and monitored throughout the next 24 to 36 hours (in the spinal cord intensive care unit, to which the patient will be transferred from the emergency room). With any uncertainty of pulmonary compliance, the patient should be intubated and supported on demand ventilation or on an intermittent mechanical assist (**IMA**) of 6 to 8 × 1,000 ml/min, regulated up or down depending on the maintenance of near normal arterial gas values (see Ch. 9).

It is important to constantly remember that the patient with acute spinal cord injuries (having an absence of motor sensory function) may not be able to identify all sites of associated multiple trauma. Therefore, areas where skin and visceral sensation may be absent below the level of the injury require particular attention. In the neurologically traumatized patient, it is not unusual to find a surprisingly negative abdomen to external evaluation. It is for this reason that a minilaparotomy is suggested in the emergency room for the patient with signs of lower chest trauma (fractured ribs) or upper abdomen trauma (Figs. 2-5 and 2-6). Similarly, should the patient not have external evidence of bleeding, yet reveal a falling hematocrit, a minilaparotomy and peritoneal dialysis are indicated. If these are negative, concern for a major intra-abdominal injury can usually be lessened, and the search for other sources of blood loss may be extended to areas such as the long bones or the chest (Fig. 2-7).

Another major system requiring careful monitoring is the pulmonary system. Not only is this area susceptible to neurologic dysfunction secondary to injury to the cervical spinal cord (the C4 nerve root being the primary innervator of the diaphragm) (Fig. 2-8), but also the chest is a frequent site of hidden trauma (multiple fractured ribs) that may result in a hemopneumothorax (Figure 2-9). It is not at all unusual for this type of injury to go undiagnosed or unreported before transfer of the patient to the spine trauma center. For this reason, serial blood gas values must be obtained along with serial chest radiographs before the transfer and upon arrival, particularly in the patient with injury to the upper thoracic spine and spinal cord. Frequently, radiographs of the chest will reveal a fracture of the first or second vertebra, a fracture of the clavicle, multiple rib fractures, a fractured scapula, or an associated fracture-dislocation of a thoracic vertebra. This information should accompany the transfer. The receiving institution should seek specific evidence of changes in pretransfer blood gas values and chest radiographs. If there is evidence before transfer of blood gas deterioration, the transfer should not proceed without the patient being cleared by either a general or a thoracic surgeon.

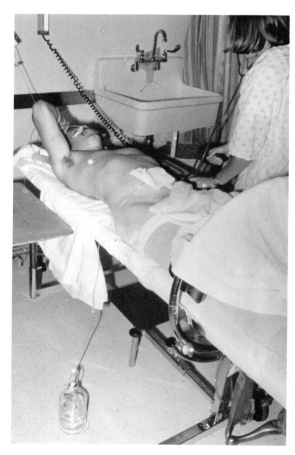

A

Fig. 2-6. Peritoneal lavage. **(A)** Patient with acute cervical spine injury with passive (gravity) drainage of intraperitoneal 500-ml 0.5 N saline lavage. The lavage was negative. *(Figure continues.)*

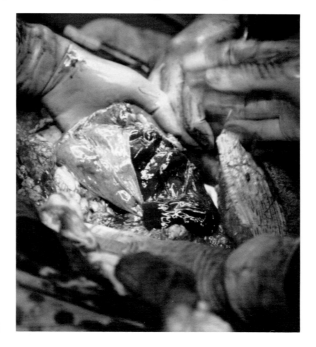

B

C

Fig. 2-6 *(Continued)*. (**B**) Patient with compression fracture of L1. Admission hematocrit was 32. Follow-up hematocrit was 28. Abdominocentesis was positive for nonclotting blood. Patient underwent splenectomy. (**C**) Patient with compression fracture of L2 and positive abdominal peritoneal cavity lavage underwent exploratory laparotomy. Note blood in abdominal cavity (just under upper retractors) secondary to viscus injury and retroperitoneal hemorrhage.

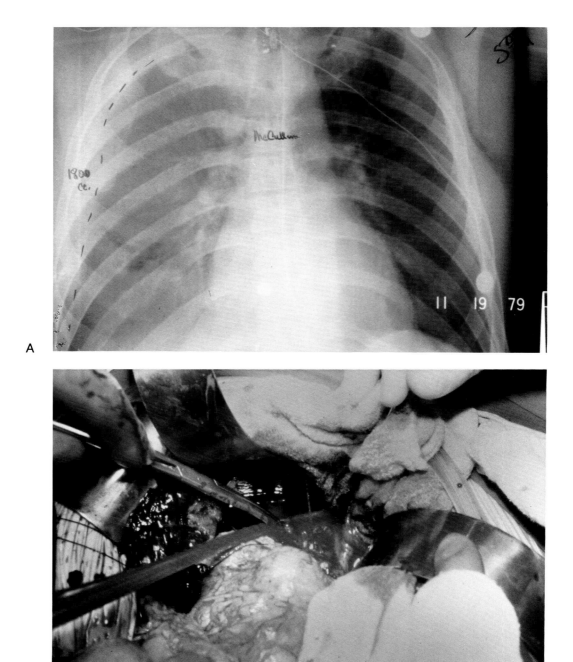

Fig. 2-7. (A) Supine AP chest radiograph in a multiple trauma patient with a cervical spine injury. Subcutaneous emphysema in the left axilla and hemothorax involving the right chest are clearly seen. This patient had a progressively falling hematocrit due to bleeding into the right chest. (B) Operative view of a patient admitted with a hangman's fracture of the cervical spine. Shortly after admission, the patient showed a falling hematocrit associated with an acute abdomen. Subphrenic air was identified on lateral abdominal radiograph. In the middle of this photograph an active posterior duodenal arterial bleeder can be seen. This duodenal ulcer was most likely stress induced.

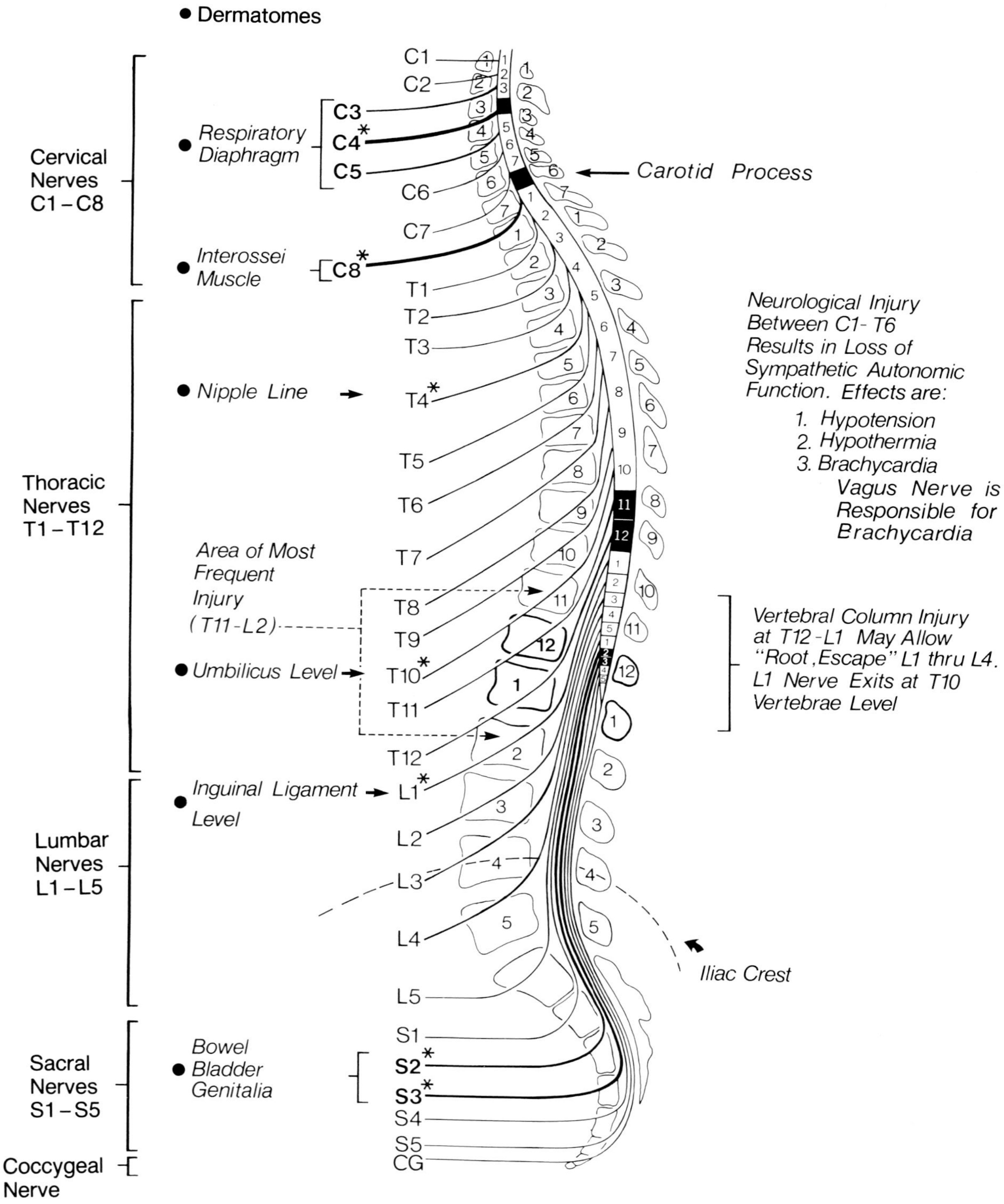

Fig. 2-8. Spinal nerves. Asterisks indicate the primary innervating nerves or specific levels of neurologic importance.

Hematology evaluations of each patient upon admission include a substance abuse screen and a urine drug screen. These two studies are helpful in gaining a full and thorough interpretation of the patient's state of consciousness on admission. Routinely administered, these tests allow for the differentiation between symptoms of head trauma, intoxication, and sociopathic behavior.

If not already in place, an indwelling urinary catheter should be inserted. Although the inherent potential for urinary tract infection exists, the catheter is nonetheless a valuable monitor of renal func-

tion and urinary output. To combat the infection problem, the indwelling system should be converted to an intermittent catheterization as soon as possible.

INTERPRETATION OF VITAL SIGNS

The trauma physician is accustomed to changing vital signs in the trauma patient and having to adjust or respond in an appropriate manner. In spinal

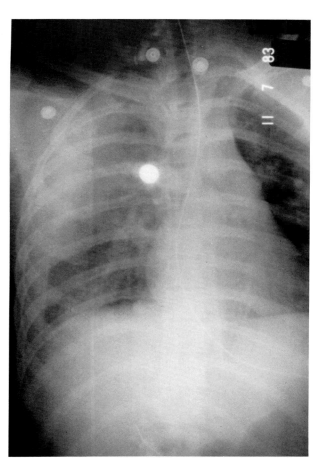
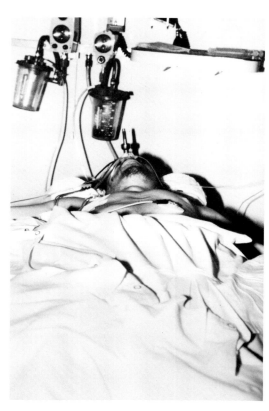

A   **B**

Fig. 2-9. Patient with multiple trauma, including chest trauma and a C5–C6 cervical spine injury causing incomplete quadriplegia. The patient is on a Stryker wedge frame and in Gardner-Wells tong traction. **(A)** Supine AP chest radiograph shows significant hemothorax involving the right chest. **(B)** Photograph of the patient from the foot of the Stryker wedge frame shows depression of right chest and compensatory hyperexpansion of left chest. *(Figure continues.)*

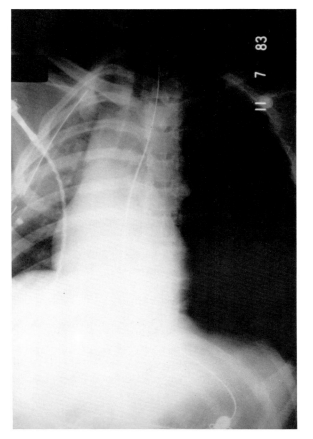
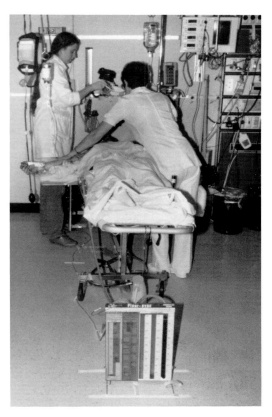

C   D

Fig. 2-9 *(Continued).* **(C)** Supine AP radiograph after insertion of right thoracostomy tube. If the patient had remained unstable after insertion of the right chest tube, right pulmonary atelectasis or foreign body in the right mainstem bronchus, or a tension pneumothorax in the left chest, would have been suspected. Neither was present in this case, and within 2 hours the right chest re-expanded. **(D)** The patient on a Stryker wedge frame in the Spinal Cord Intensive Care Unit. Note the Pleur-evac at the foot of the frame, to which the right chest tube is attached. (20 cmH$_2$O suction).

cord injury, however, owing to altered cardiovascular reflexes resulting from neurologic injury, flexibility in management frequently does not always result in improvement, particularly if the patient sustains a spinal cord injury above the level of T6. Such an injury interrupts the nervous system's ability to respond to the outflow of the thoracic sympathetic nervous system. Thus, the latter system loses its control over the peripheral vascular system, which prevents the cardiovascular system from responding to trauma (as a result of the traumatic sympathectomy). Thus, the peripheral vascular system demonstrates peripheral vasodila-

tation and is responsible for the presence of hypotension.

Simultaneously, with a similar loss of sympathetic influence over the heart via the superior cardiac nerves, the remaining (parasympathetic and vagal) neurogenic influence on the heart produces a slowing of the heart rate, or bradycardia. A third response to the loss of the sympathetic control over the peripheral vascular system is the pooling of blood in the dilated peripheral vessels close to the surface of the skin. This results in a loss of body heat through the skin and hypothermia. Thus, even in the absence of hemorrhage, the three changes in vital signs that are automatically associated with a fracture of the cervical spine and neurologic injury anywhere above the level of T6 are hypotension, hypothermia, and bradycardia (see Table 2-2).

Thus, when these vital sign changes are present along with blood loss (hypovolemia), the pulse will be slow rather than rapid and thready, because of the effects of the vagus nerve in the absence of the sympathetics. Because the heart is unable to respond to the decreased blood volume, bradycradia persists, along with hypotension. With a head injury, other vital sign influences may be present. For example, head injury is more likely to produce a slow rise in the peripheral blood pressure (a reflex mechanism providing increased perfusion to the cerebral vessels) rather than hypotension (see Table 2-2). When shock is present, in addition to a head injury, one must look elsewhere for the cause (e.g., abdomen, extremities, etc.).[8] Similarly, the pulse will be normal or somewhat slowed. Of course, these "normal" abnormal vital signs will occur only with an intact peripheral nervous system. In the presence of neurologic injury, the total picture will be confusing. Other vital sign changes associated with a head injury (with increased intracranial pressure) are a depressed level of consciousness, unequal pupils, and a slowly falling respiratory rate.

Because the interpretation of vital signs in the multitrauma patient is very often confusing, adherence to a management protocol is the ideal means of ensuring that the multiply traumatized patient with spinal cord injuries is appropriately managed. Personnel working in the emergency room and those working with the neurologically injuried patient should understand that the vital signs of multiple-trauma patients with spinal cord injury often do not match the extent of their trauma. The irregular signs will often be the result of neurologic injury and will be accompanied by the absence of the normal conpensatory neurologic reflexes (i.e., vasoconstriction or tachycardia). To counter this problem, all spinal cord-injured patients having a multisystem injury should be managed with the assistance of treatment algorithms. The following spinal cord-multiple trauma management algorithm is suggested:

1. Splint, protect, or place in traction the cervical spine (Fig. 2-10).
2. Start two no. 16 gauge (Intracath) IVs.
3. Insert a central venous catheter (or Swan-Ganz catheter when adequate cardiac compliance is questioned).
4. Type and match the blood to give the patient four to six units of packed cells. While waiting, the following fluids may be administered as required:
    a. 0.5 percent normal saline or lactated Ringer's solution.
    b. Albumin for greater vascular tree expansion.
    c. In an emergency situation, give type-specific (first) or O-negative blood for immediate needs.
    d. Do not administer Plasmanate.
    e. Be careful not to overload the vascular system with fluids not able to carry oxygen.
    f. Observe the presence of cardiac fluid overload and congestive heart failure.
5. Insert a nasogastric tube (if not in place) and connect to low suction.
6. Insert urinary catheter to observe and monitor urinary output.
7. A minilaparotomy should be performed in the emergency room when the question of intra-abdominal injury exists or an unexplained fall in hematocrit is identified. (Fig. 2-5).
8. In the presence of hemothorax or pneumothorax or both, insert a 28/32 chest tube and connect to a 20-cm water suction (Pleur-evac) or water bottle system (Fig. 2-9A, D).
9. Splint all extremity fractures temporarily. Open fractures require surgical debridement but take second priority to the presence of chest, abdominal, vascular, or central nervous system-neurologic injury. Remember, one unit of blood is lost at the fracture site of each major pelvic fracture and each long bone fracture, except the femur, where two units of blood may be lost. Do not fail to include retroperitoneal hemorrhage.
10. Administer broad-spectrum antibiotics in the presence of open fractures.
11. Administer 250 mg of human hyperimmune

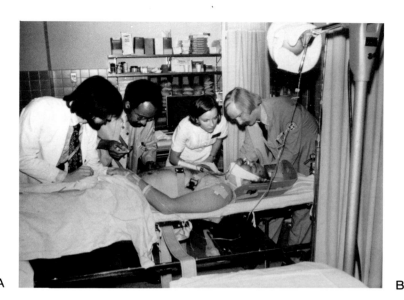

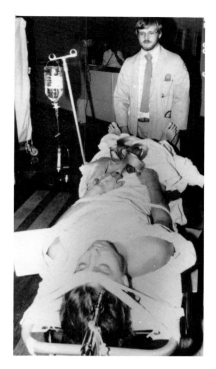

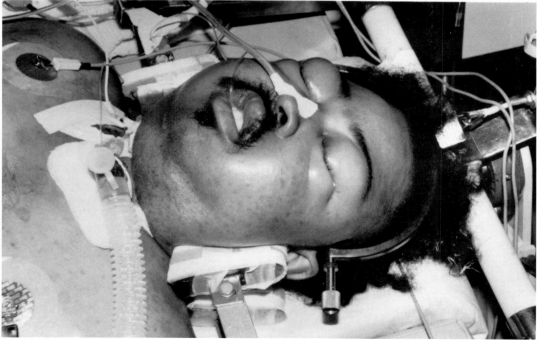

Fig. 2-10. Supporting the cervical spine during initial patient assessment. (A) Emergency room evaluation of patient with C5 fracture dislocation. The patient's cervical spine is stabilized in a Meyer cervical orthosis (Zimmer U.S.A., Inc.). This orthosis is used in the transport of patients with cervical spine fractures. (B) Patient being transported from the emergency room to the radiology department by a physician. Note that both the head and the intravenous line are taped in place. (C) Patient in Gardner-Wells tong traction, on Roto-rest frame. Note subcutaneous emphysema secondary to pulmonary and mediastinal injury.

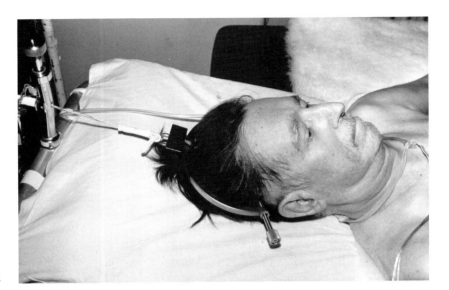

A

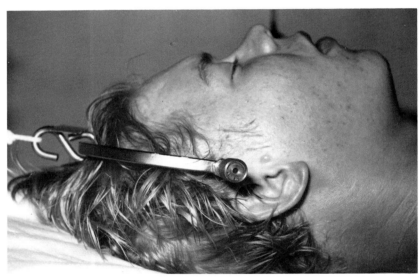

B

Fig. 2-11. Placement of Gardner-Wells cervical tongs. (A) Gardner-Wells tongs in place with rope traction. Patient is supine on a Stryker wedge frame. Tongs are positioned in line with the center of the pinna to give straight traction. (B) Gardner-Wells tongs positioned slightly anterior to and above the center of the pinna. This position produces extension of the cervical spine.

tetanus antiserum in the presence of an open fracture.

12. If surgery is required, the patient should be maintained on a Stryker wedge frame.

13. As a guide for the application of weights to the cervical spine-skeletal traction apparatus: 5 lb of weight per level of injury (as an example, for a C6 injury, $6 \times 5 = 30$ lb) (Figs. 2-11 and 2-12).

14. Make every effort to obtain a reduction of the spine dislocation while the patient is in the emergency area (particularly for the cervical spine) by direct traction through the skeletal tongs. Reduction of thoracolumbar dislocations may be attained by postural positioning on the frame or by closed manipulation under rare circumstances and with specific criteria (see Ch. 16) (Figs. 2-13, 2-14, and 2-15).

15. Obtain frequent repeat lateral radiographs after the application of the initial weights or additional weight to prevent cervical spine fracture overdistraction (Fig. 2-16).

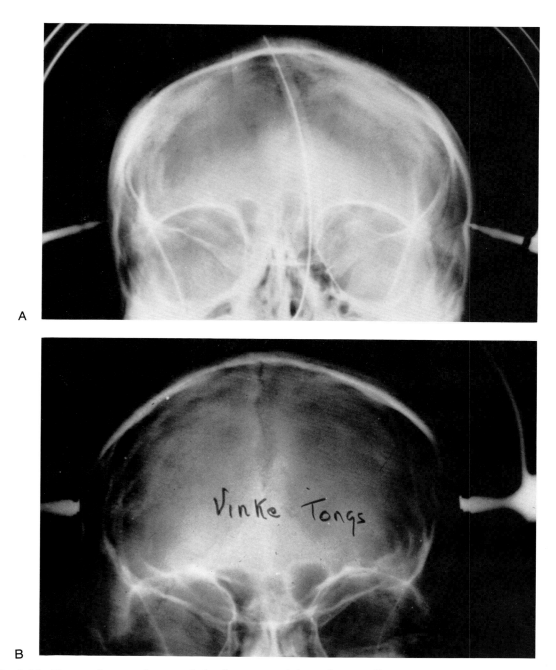

Fig. 2-12. Types of cervical spine skeletal traction. **(A)** Gardner-Wells tongs. These tongs are applied directly through the skin, and require only skin preparation and local anesthetic. They are stable. **(B)** Vinke tongs. Insertion of these tongs requires skin preparation, local anesthetic, skin incision, and drilling a hole in the outer table of the skull. The pin of the tong locks between the inner and outer tables of the calvaria. The tongs are stable. *(Figure continues.)*

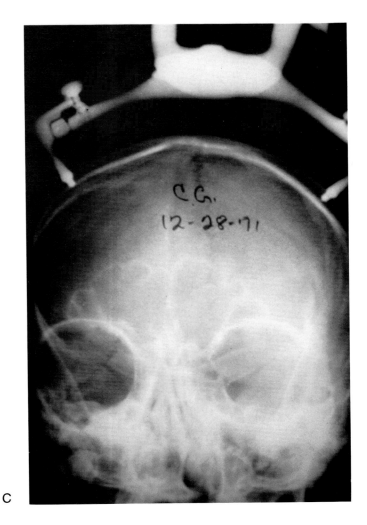

C

Fig. 2-12 *(Continued)*. (C) Crutchfield tongs. Insertion of these tongs requires skin preparation, local anesthetic, incision, drilling of holes, and careful placement of tongs. The tongs are unstable.

SPINE REDUCTION IN THE EMERGENCY ROOM

As with dislocations involving major joints of the body (e.g., the hip[9,10] and shoulder[11,12] joints), reduction as soon as possible after injury gives the most favorable outcome. Failure to attain early hip joint reduction results in the onset of avascular necrosis of the femoral head. In the shoulder, failure to obtain an early reduction of an anterior dislocation is likely to result in either a permanent axillary nerve palsy with paralysis of the deltoid muscle or vascular compromise.

Cervical Spine

Injuries involving the cervical spine are, of course, very serious. Only 26 percent of all fractures occur without neurologic injury, with 32 percent resulting in complete neurologic injuries and 41 percent resulting in incomplete neurologic injuries (from a series of 2,710 patients with spine injury at Northwestern University from 1972 to 1986). According to Bedbrook, in the cervical spine the spinal canal can be compromised as much as 50 percent before any compression of the cervical spinal cord occurs.[13] It is not the compression that commonly produces irreversible neurologic

Fig. 2-13. Bilateral facet dislocation. Lateral radiograph of cervical spine showing bilateral facet dislocation at C3–C4. In bilateral facet dislocations, the superior vertebra overrides the inferior vertebra by more than half the width of the vertebral body.

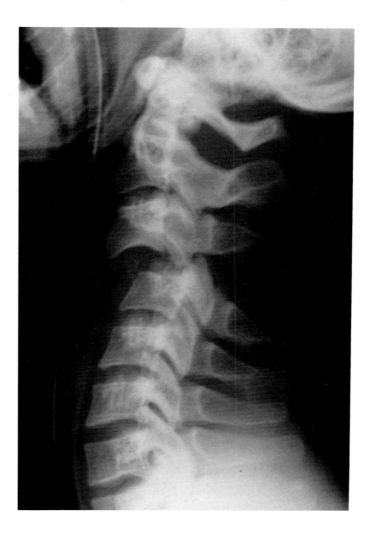

injury, but the crushing, stretching, and rotational shear forces exerted on the cord during the moments of trauma. Thus, a dislocated facet, a fracture-dislocation, or a similar mechanism of spinal injury may not be the single most important etiologic factor contributing to neurologic injury, but may in fact be just one of a series of events producing the resulting pathology. The resulting neuropathology is believed to be a time-oriented event and the extent of injury to be commensurate with the severity of the initial trauma. Radiographs of the cervical spine may not reveal neural canal compromise, but as noted in Chapter 4, the presence of unseen edema and spinal cord swelling may compromise the spinal cord's neurovascular blood sup-

ply and contribute to further loss of spinal cord function, particularly in the presence of mechanical compromise (Fig. 2-17, spinal cord swelling). Therefore, it is imperative that realignment of the spinal column be attained in the shortest period of time. Although this concern applies to all areas of the vertebral column, it is particularly relevant in the cervical spine owing to the anatomic narrowness of the cervical neural canal.

The type of skeletal tongs routinely utilized is the Gardner-Wells tongs (Fig. 2-11). They are uncomplicated tongs requiring no predrilling and can be rapidly inserted into the area 1 cm superior to the middle of the pinna of the ear, after an appropriate skin preparation and infiltration with a local

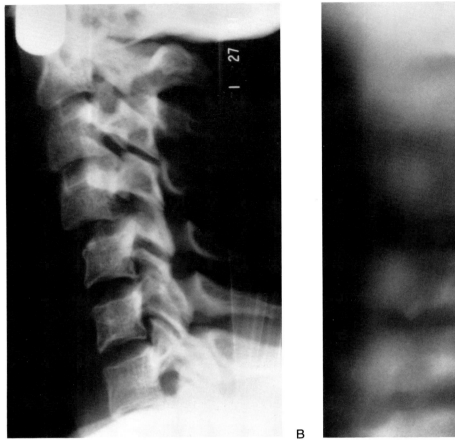

A   B

Fig. 2-14. Unilateral facet dislocation. **(A)** Lateral radiograph of cervical spine showing unilateral facet dislocation at C4–C5. Note that the C4 vertebral body overrides C5 by *only 25 percent* (indicative of unilateral rather than bilateral facet dislocation). **(B)** AP tomogram of same case. Note the rotation (malalignment) of the spinous process at the level of the facet dislocation (left in this view).

anesthetic agent (3.5 ml of 0.5 percent Marcaine). This entire process requires no more than 5 minutes. The cervical spine may now be looked on as reasonably stable, and other important management activities may be done. As soon as the patient's overall condition is stable and other priorities are met, any spinal malalignment that persists should be addressed. Every effort should be made to achieve reduction either in the emergency room or within the spinal cord intensive care unit. If the patient's neurologic injury is incomplete and reduction is unattainable, surgical reduction must be considered. All patients with acute spine injuries should be observed in

an intensive care area for the first 24 hours after admission.

Following a brief observation period in the emergency room, after having obtained a set of post-tong-traction cervical radiographs to evaluate position, alignment, or reduction, if no change in cervical spine alignment has occurred, more weights are applied at 5-lb increments. As they are added, new radiographs must be obtained. It may be necessary to augment the reduction by gentle manipulation of the cervical spine (always with the patient awake), by carefully turning the head and neck to the side *away* from the direction the chin is pointing, in the case of a unilateral facet dislocation

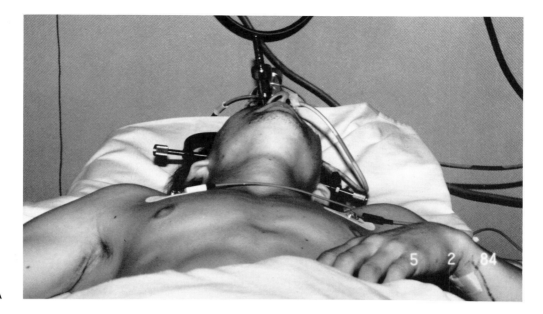

A

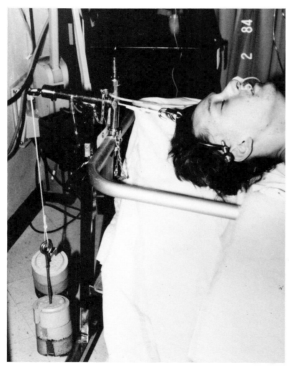

B

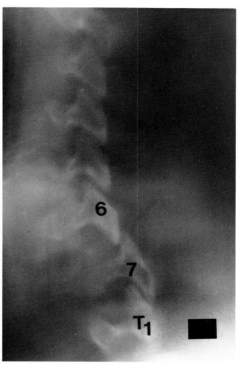

C

Fig. 2-15. Patient with a C6–C7 unilateral facet dislocation. (**A**) Note the position of the head and chin. In the presence of a unilateral facet dislocation, the face and chin will point to the side opposite the dislocation. Note also the position of the Gardner-Wells tongs, in line with the center of the pinna for straightaway traction. (**B**) View of the patient under Gardner-Wells traction. Note the amount of the initial weight (5 lb per level of injury: six 5-lb weights = 30 lb). If more weight is required, the weights should be supported by two ropes to prevent sudden loss of weight. Care must be taken to keep the weights off the floor, and the Gardner-Wells tongs must be well tightened. (**C**) Lateral radiograph showing facet dislocation at C6–C7. *(Figure continues.)*

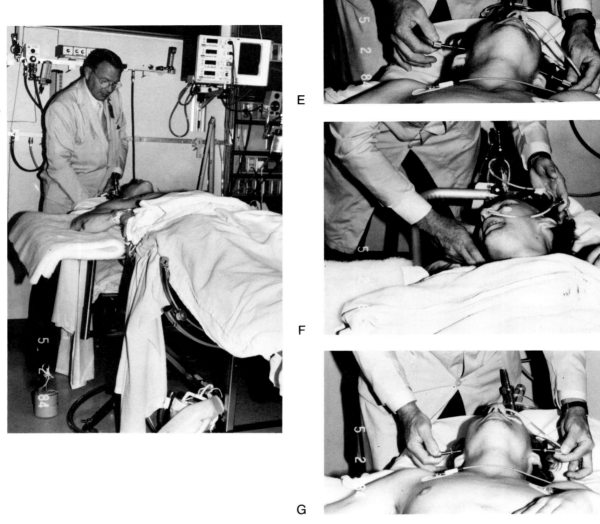

Fig. 2-15 *(Continued).* (**D–G**) Closed reduction of unilateral facet dislocation of cervical spine. (**D**) Patient in Gardner-Wells tong traction (30 lb). To maximize the effect of the weights, the head of the Stryker wedge frame is elevated, allowing the patient's body weight to counter the cervical traction weights. Additional weights should be available. In the absence of a history of loss of consciousness, intravenous diazepam (Valium) and morphine sulfate may be used as muscle relaxant and analgesic. (**E**) Before the cervical spine is manipulated the Gardner-Wells tongs should be tightened. (**F**) With premanipulation medications given and tongs tightened, the cervical spine is turned in the direction opposite the "facing" of the chin (which is opposite the side of the dislocation, as seen in **A**). When reduction occurs, patient will report a palpable "snap" and sudden relief of pain. The physician may palpate the "snap." (**G**) If the dislocation has been reduced, removing all force from tongs should allow the head and neck (chin) to return to center alignment. Check radiographs should be obtained. If reduction cannot be obtained with the addition of weights up to 80 lb, no further weights should be added. Additional time or medication may be helpful. Failure to obtain reduction of unilateral facet dislocation with a reasonable amount of weight indicates the likely presence of a fractured facet that cannot be reduced by traction and requires open reduction. In this case, the patient is maintained in 15 lb of traction until surgery.

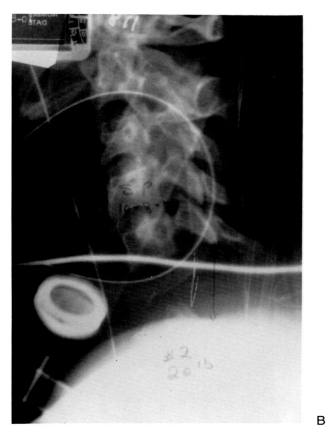
A

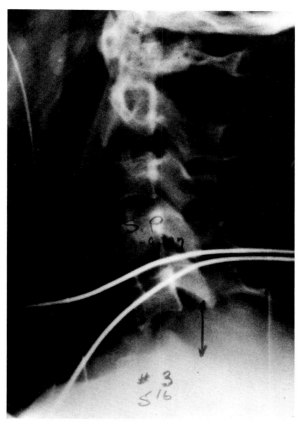
B

Fig. 2-16. Cervical spine injury with evidence of gross instability. **(A)** Significant soft tissue separation between bony elements of C5 and C6 in cervical traction. Rule of thumb of 5 lb per level of injury revealed instability. Note separation with only 20 lb. **(B)** Note separation at C5 – C6 with only 3 lb of cervical traction. Surgical stabilization is indicated.

(in which the head and neck are rotated away from the affected side). If there has been no history of head injury associated with loss of consciousness and no significant alteration in ventilation, the reduction may be facilitated and relaxation augmented with morphine sulfate (8 mg), and diazepam (10 mg) (Figs. 2-14 and 2-15A,F). When reduction occurs, either the patient and the physician will palpate a "snap" or the patient will report hearing a "snap," which frequently brings an immediate reduction in the degree of pain. New radiographs must be obtained, and the reduction must be confirmed. If reduction has occurred, the amount of cervical traction weight is reduced to a maintenance level of 10 to 15 lb. New radiographs are obtained to ensure that the reduction is maintained.

A constant consideration is whether the patient's neurologic condition is stable (i.e., complete and no change, or incomplete and no evidence of further deterioration). If change has occurred, the patient care process must be accelerated, and all studies (tomogram, CAT scan, myelogram) completed as soon as possible, so that the etiology of the change may be determined. If it is vascular in origin alone, conservative care is advised. If it is a vascular compromise secondary to encroachment by bone or malalignment, surgery is indicated (see Emergency Surgical Indications and Protocol, below).

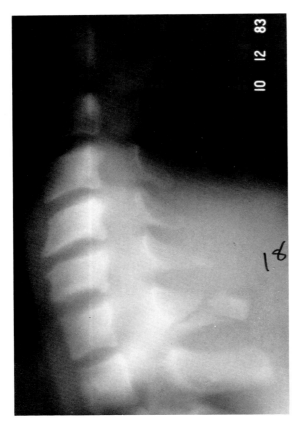
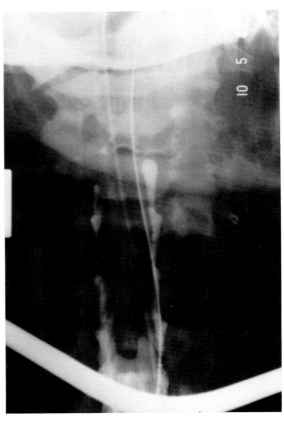

A   B

Fig. 2-17. (A) Lateral tomogram of the cervical spine in a patient who sustained a motor vehicle extension injury to the cervical spine with resulting fracture of the posterior element of C7. Neurologically, the patient had a central cord lesion with loss of function in the C6–C7 dermatomes and maintenance of function in both lower extremities. (B) AP radiograph shows cervical spinal cord swelling on myelogram. No obstruction of the flow of contrast medium was noted. The patient was managed conservatively.

Thoracic Spine

Because the neural canal is narrow in the thoracic spine, very few injuries to this area of the spinal column occur without neurologic injury (62 percent complete, 26 percent incomplete, 12 percent intact; Table 2-3). At the level of T6, the neural canal is as large (round) in size as the size of the distal end of an adult index finger (Fig. 2-18). The thoracic spinal cord varies in thickness, but measures 6.1 mm at the T6 level and is surrounded by the dura and an anatomic space of approximately 1 to 2 mm. With fracture of a thoracic vertebra in which there is associated injury to the vertebral body, the spinal canal is frequently compromised. The usual mechanisms of injury are flexion, axial load, and rotation, which produce an oblique fracture through two vertebrae seen in the coronal plane (Fig. 2-19). Here, there is likely to be an associated lateral translation of the upper vertebral segment on the lower segment, and in the lateral plane, where the primary mechanism producing injury is axial load, there is likely to be anterior or posterior shearing of one vertebral body or another, further compromising the neural canal. Most of the time, the result is complete neurologic injury.

Occasionally, injury to the thoracic spine is so severe that the vertebral segments are displaced with each breath (seen during surgery) (Fig. 2-20).

Table 2-3.   Neurologic Injury Secondary to Spine Trauma

Spine Trauma	Percent Complete	Percent Incomplete	Percent Intact	Percent Missing	No.
Cervical	32	41	26	1	1372
Thoracic	62	26	12	1	323
Thoracolumbar	29	42	29	0	430
Lumbar	2	57	41	0	63
Sacral	0	100	0	0	7
No fracture	16	31	30	24	515
Total					2710

The importance of this observation is in the recognition that the thoracic vertebral column is greatly enhanced in strength by the rib cage.[14] Although this is the case, it should not be assumed that the thoracic spine is inherently stable, as multiple rib fractures most certainly reduce the stability of the thoracic vertebral column.

In the presence of an incomplete or normal neurologic examination, when significant malalignment of the thoracic vertebral column has occurred, great care must be taken in bringing about a reduction and stabilization. Generally, when this is the case, it has occurred because the posterior ele-

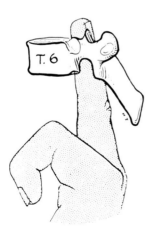

Fig. 2-18. Index finger shows how small is the neural canal of the T6 vertebra. The small size of this canal and the limited space available for the spinal cord can be clinically important. (From Anderson JE: Grant's Atlas of Anatomy. 7th Ed. Williams & Wilkins, 1978. With permission.)

ments have fractured outward (due to an axial load), producing a traumatic laminectomy. As a result, the margin of error in attempting a reduction is too great. As stated above, immediate surgery is indicated by a changing or deteriorating neurologic condition in a grossly unstable spine and by a dislocation that cannot be reduced (if the patient has an incomplete injury). In the absence of neurologic function, surgical stabilization greatly reduces recovery time by allowing the patient to be mobilized and by reducing the chances of secondary complication that accompany inactivity.

The safest immediate method of managing fractures of the thoracic spine is on a fracture bed of the Stryker wedge frame variety. By positioning the patient on pillows on the frame, spinal realignment can be greatly improved. In the emergency room, with the patient in a supine position, a pillow is placed between the patient (thoracic, thoracolumbar, and lumbar spine injured) and the frame, opposite the level of the gibbus or prominent spinous process (indicating the level of the fracture). Similarly, when the patient is prone on the frame, pillows are placed in two areas: opposite the sternum and opposite the lower abdomen-pubis. This technique positions the spine into extension when the patient is prone or supine on the Stryker wedge frame and allows the patient to be turned prone and supine with less of a concern for fracture instability between vertebral segments. This is not the case when managing the patient on the Stryker circle electric bed. Because this latter bed requires the patient to pass through a vertical position on the way from a prone to a supine position, many spines have demonstrated significant vertebral element

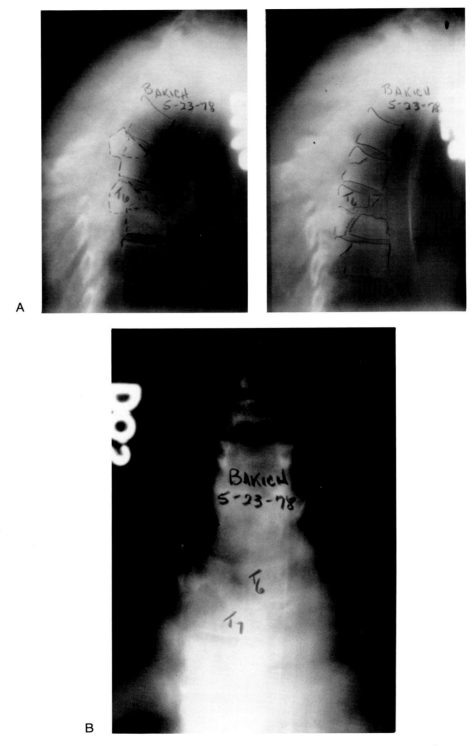

Fig. 2-19. (**A**) Lateral radiograph of the thoracic spine showing an axial load compression fracture involving the vertebral bodies of T5, T6, and T7 and posterior elements. Note intrusion and posterior luxation of T6 on T7, typical of axial loading injuries. (**B**) AP view demonstrating impaction of T6 on T7 with characteristic lateral translation of the upper segment. This injury is produced by three mechanical forces: axial load, flexion, and rotation.

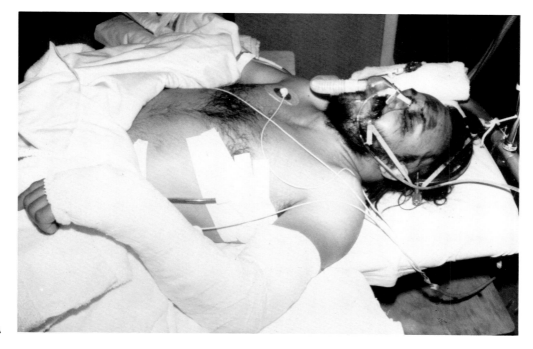

A

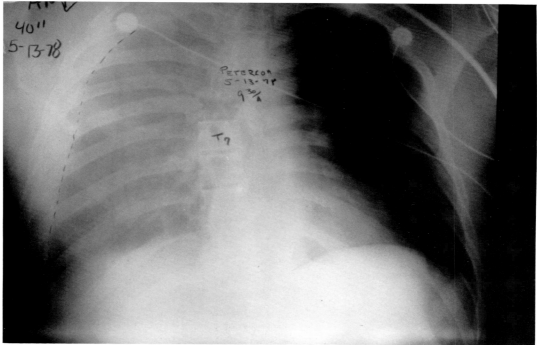

B

Fig. 2-20. Patient who sustained multiple trauma in a motorcycle accident including closed fracture dislocation of T6–T7. **(A)** Emergency room photograph. Note associated head, face, and upper extremity injuries and thoracostomy tube in the left chest. **(B)** AP chest radiograph showing cloudiness in the left chest and evidence of hemothorax. The injury to the spine is obscured by the clouding. A thoracostomy tube was inserted and the hemothorax evacuated; the chest cleared immediately. *(Figure continues.)*

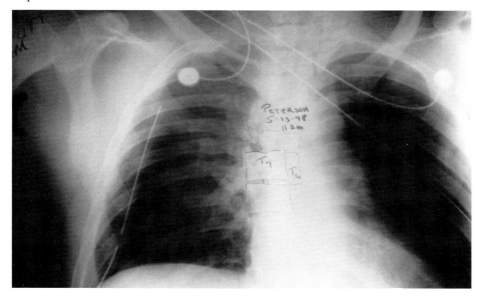

C

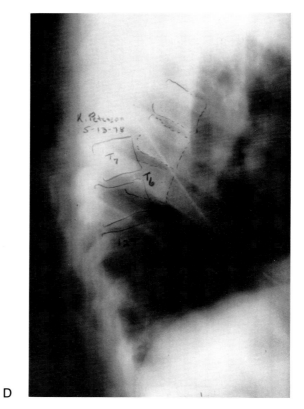

D

Fig. 2-20 *(Continued).* **(C)** AP radiograph of cleared chest showing fracture dislocation of T6 on T7. The patient had a T6 complete neurologic injury. **(D)** Lateral radiograph clearly demonstrating significant fracture dislocation of T6 on T7. *(Figure continues.)*

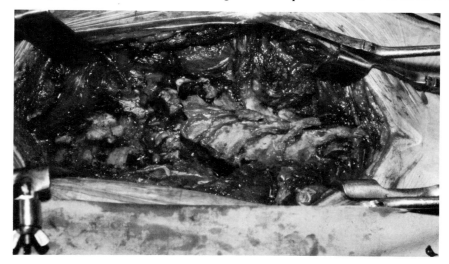

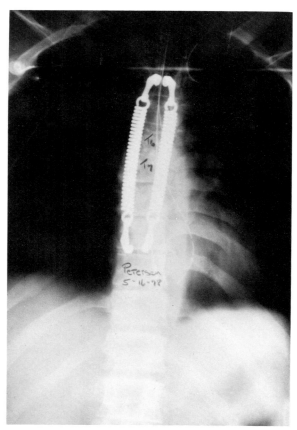

Fig. 2-20 *(Continued).* **(E)** Operative photograph showing complete disruption of the posterior elements of the thoracic spine, T5 through T8. The spinal cord can be seen lying in the wound just above the fractured posterior elements. The spine moved freely with each breath. **(F)** AP radiograph showing spinal realignment under compression after insertion of compression (Weiss) springs from T4 to T9. *(Figure continues.)*

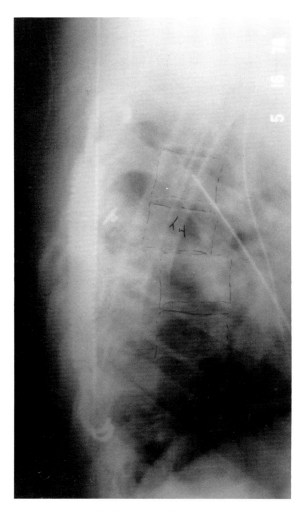

G

Fig. 2-20*(Continued).* (**G**) Lateral radiograph of spine showing reduction of fracture dislocation.

shift secondary to instability in the vertical position. Also, neurologic changes during this transition have been reported.

It is important to remember that injury to the lower thoracic spine (T10 to T12) may result in vascular injury to the lower thoracic spinal cord, via interruption of the vessel of Adamkiewicz.[15] This phenomenon has been recognized by the occurrence of an ascending neurologic deficit without loss of spine position (usually within the first 12 hours after injury). Surgical intervention may be considered; however, it will not influence the neurologic outcome because the loss is vascular in

origin. When this is the case, because of the watershed nature of the spinal cord vascular pattern, the neurologic level may ascend as high as T4 (see Ch. 4).

Lumbar Spine

Because one of the two normal anatomic enlargements of the spinal cord occurs at the junction of the thoracic and lumbar segments of the nervous system, the neural canal at the level of T12–L1 is enlarged. This area accommodates the conus medullaris and the cauda equina (Fig. 2-21). The conus medullaris of the spinal cord is very important in the male: it is the area of neurologic control of bowel, bladder, and sexual function. Therefore, the most appropriate method of attempting to improve the alignment of the unstable lumbar spine is to position the patient on the Stryker wedge frame in the following manner: with the patient in the supine position, place a pillow between the patient and the frame, adjacent to the level of the gibbus or prominent spinous process (the level of fracture displacement) when in the supine position; with the patient in the prone position, place one pillow horizontally across the chest at the level of the patient's sternum and another transversely at the level of the lower abdomen-pubis. These pillows assist in producing hyperextension and correctly maintaining spinal alignment while the patient is being managed on the Stryker frame. They also allow the patient to be turned supine and prone with less concern for anterior-posterior shift of the vertebral segments while turning.

Very seldom is immediate surgery required for injuries to the lumbar spine. Normally, one can wait for several days to complete the evaluation and allow the effects of trauma to disappear (9 to 14 days). However, injury to (dislocation of) the lumbosacral joint often produces an incomplete neurologic injury, with the principal neurologic injury being to the sacral segment (Fig. 2-21). Because of the neurologic implications to the bowel, the bladder, and sexual function (S2–S3), and because large segments of L5–S1 disc can be extruded (Fig. 2-22), early myelography and surgery are often indicated. In two patients with dislocations at the junction of L5–S1, findings at surgery indicated that early surgical intervention is recommended.

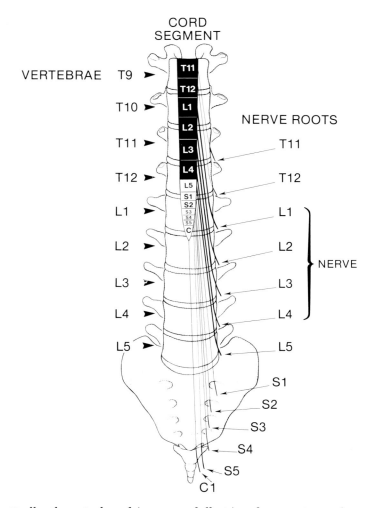

Fig. 2-21. Diagrammatically, the spinal cord (conus medullaris) ends posterior to the vertebral bodies of T12–L1. Because the conus medullaris portion of the spinal cord contains the anterior horn (motor) cells of L5 to S5, it is possible for injury to the spine at L1 to destroy bowel and bladder function (S2 neurologic injury), while preserving L1 to L4 lower extremity function ("root escape"). Note that the L1 nerve root exits the spinal cord at the vertebral level of T10.

EMERGENCY SURGICAL INDICATIONS AND PROTOCOL

The criteria for emergency surgery are restrictive. There are very few indications for surgery within the first hours after injury. In the recent past, many surgeons performed a laminectomy or a spine-stabilizing procedure on the day of patient admission. A careful analysis of surgically managed war injuries to the spine during the Korean conflict failed to demonstrate recovery attributable to surgery.[16] In my experience, several patients deteriorated after surgery performed within the first days after spine trauma. Analysis of the circumstances in which neurologic deterioration did occur revealed several contributing factors: (1) it should have been suspected that the patient had residual spinal cord edema in the area of injury; (2) the administration of an anesthetic cannot be regarded as physiologic;

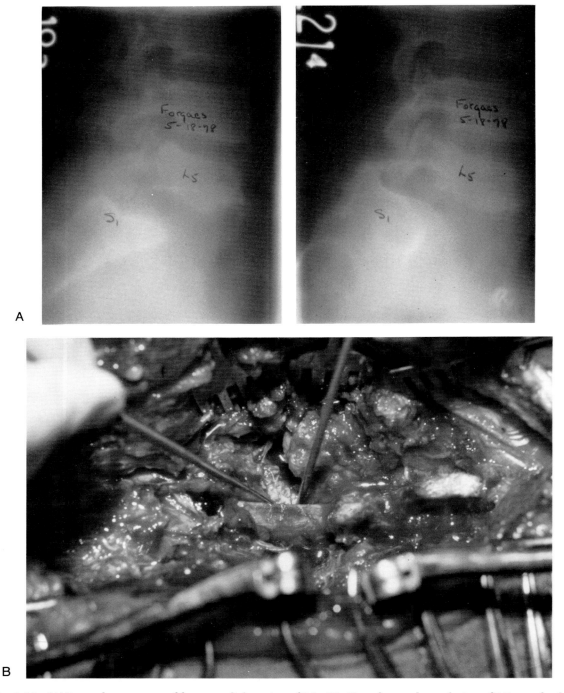

Fig. 2-22. (**A**) Lateral tomogram of fracture-dislocation of L5–S1. Note forward translation of L5 vertebral body on S1. (**B**) Operative view of open reduction of fracture-dislocation seen in **A**. Note dural sac visible in center of picture. The sacrum is to the left. Immediately above the dura, between two Penfield elevators, is a large segment of extruded L5 intevertebral disc.

(3) the patient's blood pressure during surgery is always affected to some degree (occasionally with only minor alterations, a major vascular change in neural tissue circulation has occurred); (4) turning a patient from the supine to the prone position onto an operating table (even with great care) may result in neurologic change (possibly related to spine instability); and (5) the surgical procedure, no matter how carefully performed, may cause alterations in the patient's homeostasis. Because of these known or suspected causes for potential neurologic changes accompanying surgery, the spine service adheres to the practice of not performing surgery on a patient before 9 to 14 days after trauma, except in cases of either overt evidence of neurologic deterioration between the admission and the subsequent evaluation or evidence of an incomplete neurologic injury in the presence of an unreducible spine dislocation.

In these instances, immediate or early surgery may be indicated, and the following procedural protocol should be followed preoperatively:

1. Obtain a myelogram (metrizamide or Pantopaque).
2. Obtain tomograms of the affected areas of the spine.
3. Perform CAT at the level of obstruction to myelographic flow.
4. Perform, if available (in place of tomograms and CAT scan), magnetic resonance imaging (MRI), if not injurious to the patient (because of transfer to the examination table).
5. Obtain, or utilize when available in the operating room, somatosensory cortical evoked response monitoring.

For the patient requiring surgery, the team members vary. For management of the cervical spine, the team should include an orthopaedic surgeon and a neurosurgeon. For surgery of the thoracic or lumbar spine, in which the posterior approach is the only approach to be utilized, an orthopaedic surgeon is needed. For a transpleural thoracotomy (for an anterior decompression of the thoracic vertebral column and dura) or transperitoneal (abdominal) approach to the lumbar spine, the surgical team includes the chest service, for the initiation of the approach; the orthopaedic service, for exposure of the vertebral column, decompression, and fusion; or the assistance of the neurosurgery service for the anterior decompression. For the flank approach to the lumbar spine; the team should have a general surgeon or urology services. For the anterior approach to the lumbosacral spine, a general surgeon or the vascular service should be present.

REFERENCES

1. Guidelines for Facility Categorization and Standards of Care: Spinal Cord Injury. American Spinal Injury Association/Foundation, Chicago, IL, 1981
2. Boyd DR, Dunea MM, Flashner BA: The Illinois plan for a statewide system of trauma centers. J Trauma 13:24, 1973
3. Emergency Medical Services System Act of 1973, P.L. 93–154, Amended 1976, P.L. 94–573
4. Accidental Death and Disability: The Neglected Disease of Modern Man. National Academy of Science–National Research Council, Washington, D.C., 1966
5. Categorization of Hospital Emergency Capabilities. American Medical Association, 1971
6. Illinois Categorization Law, Senate Bill 568, Public Act 76–1858, Oct. 1972
7. Meyer PR: The spinal cord injured patient. p. 311. In: Critical Care for Surgical Patients. MacMillan, New York, 1982
8. Chusid JG: Trauma to the CNS. p. 339. In: Correlative Neuroanatomy and Functional Neurology. 17th Ed. 1979
9. Epstein HC: Traumatic dislocations of the hip. Clin Orthop 92:116, 1973
10. Gregory CF: Early complications of dislocation and fracture dislocation of the hip joint. In American Academy of Orthopaedic Surgeons: Instructional Course Lectures. Vol 22. CV Mosby, St. Louis, 1973
11. Bankart ASB: The pathology and treatment of recurrent dislocations of the shouldser-joint. Br J Surg 26:23, 1938
12. Rowe CR: Prognosis in dislocations of the shoulder. J Bone Joint Surg 38–A:957, 1956

13. Bedbrook GM: Some pertinent observations on the pathology of traumatic spinal paralysis. Paralegia 1:215, 1963

14. White AA, Panjabi MM: Functional spinal unit and mathematical models. In: Clinical Biomechanics of the Spine. JB Lippincott, Philadelphia, 1978

15. Lazorthes G, et al: Arterial vascularization of the spinal cord. J Neurosurg 35:253, 1971

16. Comarr AE, Kaufman AA: A survey of the neurological results in 858 cord injuries. A comparison of patients treated with or without laminectony. J Neurosurg 13:95, 1956

Embryology and Developmental Anatomy of the Nervous System and Vertebral Column

Paul R. Meyer, Jr.

As a basis for understanding the development, performance, behavior, and defects that can affect the development of the spinal cord and spinal column, this chapter reviews the basics of human embryologic development. This discussion of embryologic development, beginning with conception and carried through fetal growth to term, brings together the work of several authors. I have attempted to outline the development of the pre-embryo, the embryo, and the fetus all the way up to epiphyseal maturation in a natural progression. This procedure enables the reader to follow each new embryonic process (Table 3-1) from fertilization to the complete development of the nervous (spinal cord) and skeletal systems to end with a miraculously constructed normal newborn infant. Although developmental errors, single and multiple, do arise and terminate in birth deformities, this chapter describes only those that result in a spinal or neurologic deformity and thus influence function or contribute in some manner to the effects of trauma.

PRENATAL DEVELOPMENT

All osseous structures begin as a mesenchymal condensation early in the developmental, or embryonic, period and are derived from the primary germ layers. There is an apparent influence that pervades the tissue, directing its maturation by either mechanical or chemotactic means. This influence results in the appearance of cellular condensations that then develop directly into osseous structures through intramembranous ossification (facial bones, clavicle, cranial vault), or, as in most of the skeleton, that undergo transformation of the mesenchymal models into a cartilaginous analogue that subsequently ossifies through the process known as endochondral ossification.

Bones and joints are relatively self-differentiating. They attain their initial anlage form, the contour of which is often very similar to the final mature shape, through factors intrinsic to the developing cell mass. Skeletal development may be

Table 3-1. Sequence of Embryonic and Fetal Developmental Events

Event	Time
Conception	Zero time
Embryo (two-layer disc; ectoderm-entoderm)	2nd week of gestation
Formation of notochord	Late 2nd to 3rd week
Formation of neural plate	3rd week of gestation
Mesoderm forms 3rd layer of disc	End of 3rd week
Closure of rostral neural tube	Early 4th week
Somite development (29) Skeletal-muscle-integument systems Neural tube, ganglia, ectoderm, dermatome, myotome, sclerotome	Early 4th week
Complete somite formation (44)	5th week (10 days)
Neural crest, spinal ganglia	5th week
Chondrification of vertebral centrum (2)	6th week
Ossification of vertebral arches	8th to 10th week
Primary center ossification (ribs)	9th week
Ossification of centers of each vertebra 3 primary, 3 secondary	15th to 24th week
Fusion of vertebral arch with centrum	Newborn to 50 week
Closure of posterior fontanel	25 to 52 weeks postnatal
Fusion of two odontoid centers	50th to 52nd week
Closure of the anterior fontanel	2 years
Ossification of vertebral body apophysis	2nd decade
Fusion of 2nd and 3rd centers of vertebral arch	2nd decade
Secondary center ossification (ribs)	2nd decade
Fusion of odontoid with centrum	2nd decade
Fusion of sacral neural arch and alae	2nd to 3rd decade

divided into two stages: morphogenetic and cytodifferentiation. In the former, cellular movement and cellular interactions determine the resulting skeletal shape. The latter phase is concerned with the differentiation of the extracellular matrix, primarily composed of hyaluronic acid, chondroitin sulfate–protein complexes, and collagen. The development of mesenchyme into cartilage and then into bone is a complex one. A careful balance exists between chondroitin sulfate and the enzyme hyaluronidase. As chondroitin sulfate increases during the cartilage stage, hyaluronic acid is removed by an increase in the production of hyaluronidase. Hyaluronic acid seems to be necessary for cellular aggregation and may be essential for the accumulation of a sufficient number of precartilage cells to precipitate a transition from the morphogenetic phase to the differentiation phase (see Rationale for Occurrence of Congenital Deformities of the Spine, below). The intercellular molecular component chondroitin sulfate is required to interact with collagen and is important in structural integrity, particularly in the area of cell columns within the growth plate. Thus, early genetic, teratogenic, or hormonal variations may disrupt one or more of the normal, basic biochemical processes and result in aberrant skeletal development.

The classification of bone development as membranous or endochondral refers only to the initial mechanism of ossification. In many instances, both forms of ossification occur in the development of a single bone (e.g., the diaphysis of long bones, the distal clavicle, and the posterior elements of the spine, etc.).

MEMBRANE BONE FORMATION

Membrane bone formation occurs in the cranial vault, the facial bones, and in portions of the clavicle and mandible. The axial skeleton and appendicular bones involve only in endochondral bone formation. Membrane-derived bones form directly from the proliferation of mesenchymal tissue condensations. A biochemical characteristic of these cells is first an increased alkaline phosphatase production, followed by calcification and then by ossification of the fibrous matrix.

Development of the Cranial Vault

Beginning in the ninth or the tenth fetal week, bones within the cranial vault begin to ossify. The first is the frontal bone, followed by the parietal bones. The overall result is a dense mass of bone that comprises the primary ossification center. This center expands by two mechanisms: extension along the outer periphery and coalescence of small islands of bone arising in the more peripheral region of the fibrocartilage anlage. As outward expansion of the cranial vault slows, a new osteogenic induction tissue, periosteum, arises on its external surface. The outer surface is a thick, fibrous layer. The inner area is composed of a fibrovascular layer with many mitotic cells and an innermost layer composed of mature osteoblasts. This layer results in periosteal osteogenesis as the principal mechanism of growth and the principal mechanism of cranial vault accommodation for the growth of the brain (Fig. 3-1). As the inner surface of the cranium undergoes resorption, the outer surface of the cranium undergoes bone deposition. The intracranial portion of the periosteum becomes the dura mater and retains its osteogenic potential. This is identified by the occasional deposition of abnormal bone on the inner surface, as in the presence of tumor (e.g., meningioma).

The clavicle is the first of the membrane bones to ossify, and this generally occurs by the eighth week of development. It is followed closely by the mandible. There are two fibrous open spaces overlying the superior aspect of the calvarium. They provide for cranial growth and development. The fibrous tissue that forms the fontanels undergoes modulation to ossification and closure of the posterior fontanel between months 6 and 12 after birth. The anterior fontanel does not close until sometime during the second year of life. Because the fibrous tissue overlying the presumptive cranial sutures also has the potential for bone production, it is possible for this area to produce intercalated (wormian) bones, which are characteristic of long bone formation, in which the periosteum contributes to the diametric growth of the diaphysis. This osteogenic potential of the periosteum is retained throughout life, and is stimulated to form new bone by fracture, occasional soft tissue disease, or bone-producing tumors.

ENDOCHONDRAL OSSIFICATION

Endochondral ossification is the primary process by which axial and appendicular skeletal segments are developed. This same mechanism continues throughout life in the normal process of bone remodeling and fracture callus formation and healing. Through this process the cartilage anlage is replaced by osseous tissue. The sequence of events begins with the appearance of a condensation of mesenchyme, followed by hyaline cartilage enlargement of the central cartilage cells and the development of an osseous collar by the conversion of the perichondrium into the periosteum.[1] The early osseous collar is penetrated by fibrous and vascular tissue and results in a bony replacement of the calcified central chondrocytes. As this inner and outer shell process proceeds toward the ends of the anlage, primary centers of ossification develop, forming the diaphysis and the metaphysis. Although the secondary chondroepiphyses ossify in the distal femur just before birth, elsewhere they do not do so until the postnatal period.

Ossification of the vertebral column is very similar to that of tubular bones. The neural arch, however, develops principally by periosteal appositional growth.[1]

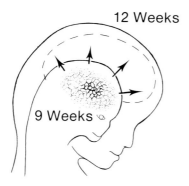

Fig. 3-1. Developmental changes in the cranial vault from 9 to 12 weeks.

SEQUENTIAL GESTATIONAL DEVELOPMENT

Conception

The development of the fetus begins with fertilization (or conception) on approximately day 14 of the menstrual cycle. From that point until delivery, development proceeds with growth, and mass increases with time. The stages of fetal development have been variously described. Ogden,[1] in his chapter on the development and growth of the musculoskeletal system, arbitrarily divided his remarks concerning development into the prenatal (embryonic and fetal) and postnatal periods.

Streeter and colleagues[2] divided the human embryonic period into 23 stages, calling each a "horizon." Both Ogden[1] and Streeter et al.[2] defined the embryonic period of development to include the first 8 weeks of gestation. During this period, the embryo grows from 1 mm in length at 3 weeks to 27 mm to 31 mm by postovulatory day 56 (approximately 2 months). The importance of this period is that by week 8, virtually all major differentiation processes are complete. The remainder of the gestation period, the fetal period, is characterized by continued growth of the now well-differentiated organ systems, and the fetus reaches a crown-rump measurement of 360 mm to 370 mm at full term.

Lonstein[3] subdivides the fetal period into three stages. The first 3 weeks after fertilization Lonstein calls the pre-embryonic period. During this period implantation occurs, followed immediately by development of the three primary germ layers, the ectoderm, mesoderm, and entoderm (Fig. 3-2). The second period, the embryonic period, lasts from week 3 through week 8. During this most active period of embryonic and fetal development, all organ differentiation occurs. At the end of this period (6 weeks), the embryo appears human, weighs 1 g, and measures between 27 and 31 mm (Fig. 3-3). Lonstein's third stage (synonymous with Ogden's second stage) is known as the fetal stage. It extends from week 8 until term. During this period, all structures and organs enlarge (Table 3-2).

Second Week of Gestation

Development of the Notochord
As the embryo enters the second week of gestation, it reaches the two-layer stage of development. One layer is the ectoderm (dorsally located and on the side of the amniotic cavity); the other is the entoderm (on the ventral side, which is the side of the yolk sac) (Fig. 3-2A). An area of proliferating and laterally migrating cells, the primitive streak, appears caudally at the midline of the ectoderm.

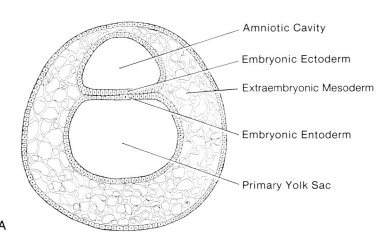

A

Fig. 3-2. Development of germ layers: primitive streak, primitive knot, notochord, and appearance of neural groove. *(Figure continues.)*

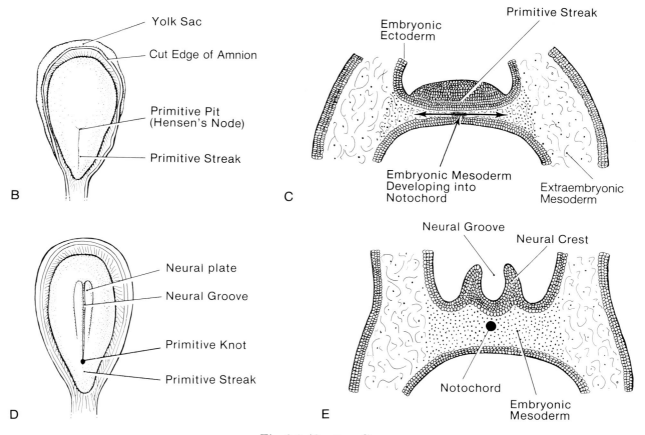

- Yolk Sac
- Cut Edge of Amnion
- Primitive Pit (Hensen's Node)
- Primitive Streak

B

- Embryonic Ectoderm
- Primitive Streak
- Embryonic Mesoderm Developing into Notochord
- Extraembryonic Mesoderm

C

- Neural plate
- Neural Groove
- Primitive Knot
- Primitive Streak

D

- Neural Groove
- Neural Crest
- Notochord
- Embryonic Mesoderm

E

Fig. 3-2 *(Continued).*

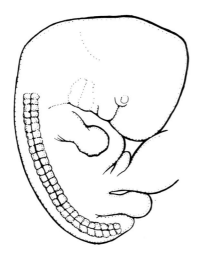

Fig. 3-3. Human embryo at 6 weeks (12 mm).

Table 3-2. Major Stages of Embryonic and Fetal Development

Pre-embryonic stage (weeks 1 to 3)	Conception, implantation, development of 3 germ layers
Embryonic stage (weeks 4 to 8)	Rapid growth and differentation; formation all major organic tissues
Fetal stage (weeks 9 to 52)	Further growth and development of the organs and systems formed in the prior stages

Here, between the ectoderm and the entoderm, lies the mesoderm (Fig. 3-2). At the cranial end of this trilaminar embryonic disc, proximal to the primitive streak where the ectoderm and the entoderm are in contact, there appears an invagination in the ectoderm known as the primitive pit. The invagination continues to extend proximally between the ectoderm and the entoderm to become the all-important notochord (Fig. 3-4). On either side of the invagination is an area of proliferating ectoderm, Hensen's node (Figs. 3-2D, 3-4A). The dorsal portion of the notochord remains in close contact with the ectoderm. On the ventral side, however, the portion of the notochord formerly in contact with the entoderm disappears. The notochord is now open to the dorsal surface and the amniotic cavity through the primitive pit or knot

(Fig. 3-4B). On the ventral side, the notochord lies on top of the yolk sac, producing a ridge in the roof of the sac known as the notochordal plate. As the embryo begins to fold laterally, the lateral portion of the entoderm begins to form a solid plate across the embryo's ventral surface and, consequently, the tubular gut as well. The now solid notochord, by virtue of its position, lies dorsally and in close proximity to the newly forming neural plate (see Fig. 3-7A).

Third Week of Gestation

As noted above, the third, or middle, layer of the embryonic disc—the mesoderm—is forming during week 3. It lies between the dorsally located

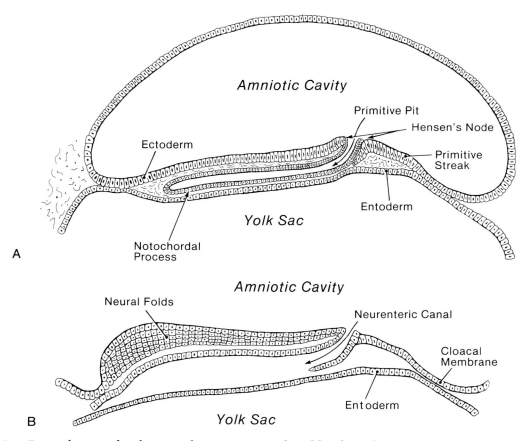

Fig. 3-4. Pre-embryonic developmental stage: 16 to 20-day-old embryo demonstrating progressive development in longitudinal and transverse section. Early organization of major germ layers: ectoderm, mesoderm, notochord, and neural tube. *(Figure continues.)*

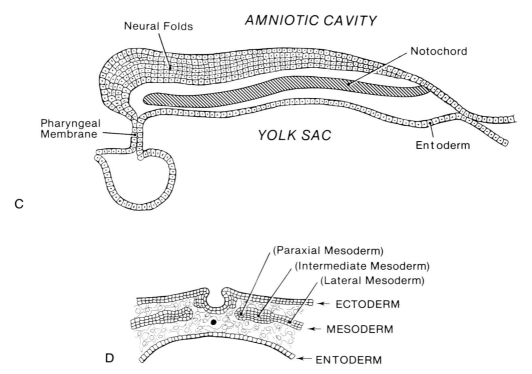

Fig. 3-4 *(Continued)*.

ectoderm and the ventrally located entoderm. The mesoderm does not exist, however, in the area of the pharyngeal and cloacal membranes and in the area of the notochord in the midline (Fig. 3-4).

The mesoderm differentiates into two distinct layers and directions: mediolaterally and craniocaudally. With marked cellular activity along the paraxial lateral sides of the notochord, these two parallel, proliferating, and undifferentiated sheets of cells form tubular structures, one on either side of the notochord (Fig. 3-5A). Continued lateral proliferation of the mesoderm results in the further development of an intermediate column and a more lateral mesodermal plate, which terminates into two separate areas: the dorsal (somatic) mesoderm and the ventral (splanchnic) mesoderm (Fig. 3-5B). From the somatic layer will arise the muscles of the ventrolateral body wall. From the splanchnic layer arises the muscular layer of the gut, and the intermediate mesoderm forms the urogenital system.

Third and Fourth Weeks of Gestation

With the lateral bending of the embryo and the closing of the ventral entodermal plate, the notochord migrates toward the dorsal surface, and finally toward the developing neural crest. The neural tube develops next, beginning as an enlargement of the ectodermal midline. The neural tube's development begins dorsally, in the middle of the embryo, and then continues both proximally and distally. The newly developed neural tube is open at both ends (Fig. 3-6A). At approximately the fourth week of gestation, the cranial (or rostral) end begins to close. As stated earlier, there are 42 to 44 somites from which the embryo develops. Only 33 to 34 pairs, however, will eventually form the adult spine. At the fourth week of embryonic life, the embryo passes through the 18- to 20-somite stage. By the time the caudal neuropore closes (Fig. 3-6B,C), the embryo will have reached the 25-somite stage of development. Failure of the

(7 SOMITES)   (22 SOMITES)

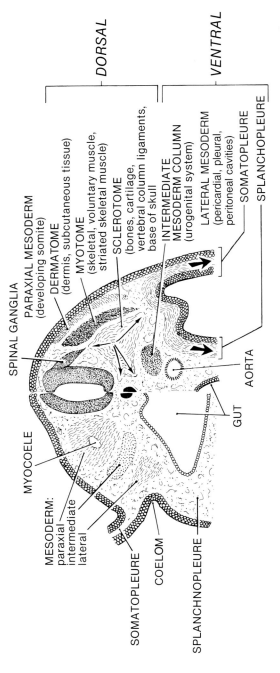

MESODERM:
paraxial
intermediate
lateral

SOMATOPLEURE

COELOM

SPLANCHNOPLEURE

MYOCOELE

SPINAL GANGLIA

PARAXIAL MESODERM
(developing somite)

DERMATOME
(dermis, subcutaneous tissue)

MYOTOME
(skeletal, voluntary muscle,
striated skeletal muscle)

SCLEROTOME
(bones, cartilage,
vertebral column ligaments,
base of skull)

INTERMEDIATE
MESODERM COLUMN
(urogenital system)

LATERAL MESODERM
(pericardial, pleural,
peritoneal cavities)

SOMATOPLEURE

SPLANCHOPLEURE

GUT

AORTA

DORSAL

VENTRAL

Fig. 3-5. Cross section of embryo at 7 somite stage (3 weeks) (left) and 22 somite stage (right). At the 7 somite stage, the mesoderm is proliferating mediolaterally and craniocaudally to form two parallel, paraxial, undifferentiated sheets of cells along the notochord. By the 22 somite stage, the mesoderm has differentiated further into intermediate and lateral mesodermal plates, from which will arise the muscles of the ventrolateral body wall and the muscles of the bowel and urogenital system.

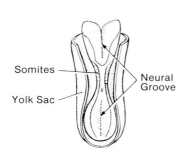

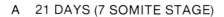

Somites

Yolk Sac

Neural Groove

A   21 DAYS (7 SOMITE STAGE)

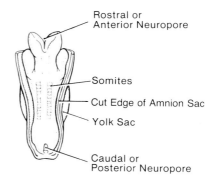

Rostral or Anterior Neuropore

Somites

Cut Edge of Amnion Sac

Yolk Sac

Caudal or Posterior Neuropore

B   22 DAYS (10 SOMITE STAGE)

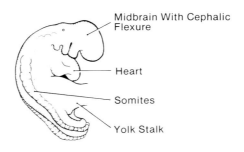

Midbrain With Cephalic Flexure

Heart

Somites

Yolk Stalk

26 DAYS
(25 SOMITE STAGE)
C

Fig. 3-6. Human embryo. **(A)** 21 days (7 somite stage). The neural groove is open at both ends. **(B)** 22 days (10 somite stage; 1.0 to 2.0 mm in length). The neural groove is closed at the caudal end. **(C)** 26 days (25 somite stage). The increase of dorsal growth over ventral growth results in the characteristic fetal curve or position. The characteristic structure of the embryo is identifiable at this stage.

ends to close results in the two major neurologic congenital anomalies: failure to close proximally results in anencephaly (failure of the brain to develop and of the cranial vault to close); failure to close distally results in myelomeningocele (failure of the posterior neural arch to form, resulting in a less than normally developed spinal cord and nerve roots at the level of the uncovered defect).

Formation of the Nervous System

Nerve Roots; Spinal Cord; Autonomic Nervous System.[1,4]   As the neural tube closes dorsally, another group of cells is differentiating from the neuroectoderm to form the neural crest. The neural tube will differentiate primarily into the central nervous system, and the neural crest will become the dorsal root ganglia and the peripheral nervous system including the autonomic nervous system (Fig. 3-7).

The walls of the neural tube become thin at the roof and the floor plates, while the lateral walls thicken and narrow the central canal. The lateral thickening forms two distinct masses, the alar (dorsal) plate and the basal (ventral) plate (Fig. 3-7D). These will become, respectively, the afferent and the efferent areas of the spinal cord. These two plates are separated by a shallow, longitudinal groove, the sulcus limitans. The alar plate cells will form a portion of the dorsal roots, which will become the dorsal root ganglia. The basal plate en-

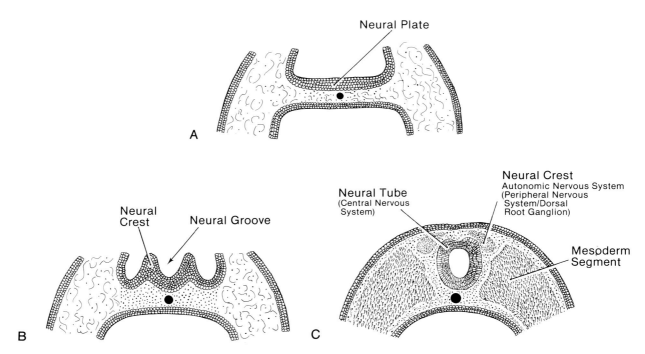

Fig. 3-7. Formation of the nervous system. **(A)** The cells surrounding the neural groove proliferate and form the neural plate. **(B)** The neural plate differentiates to form the neural crest and neural groove. **(C)** The neural tube closes, and separates from the neural crest. *(Figure continues.)*

larges to form the anterior roots and will contribute to the spinal nerves (Fig. 3-7E).

At the cellular level, the walls of the neural tube contain neuroepithelium that will differentiate into neurons and macroglial cells (or astrocytes and oligodendrocytes). Three zones develop: the inner ependymal layer around the central canal; the outer marginal layer, which will become the white matter of the spinal cord as axons grow in from other areas of the spinal cord, the dorsal root ganglia, and the brain; and the central zone, which is the most cellular. The central zone becomes the central gray matter of the spinal cord, made up of neuroblasts. These cells become multipolar and develop dendrites and one long neurite (or axon). The end of this axon makes synaptic contact with adjacent cells. The axons from the alar neuroblasts remain inside the spinal cord or central nervous system but synapse with other neuroblasts in both the alar and basal laminae. Axons from the basal neuroblasts are induced to grow beyond the finite limits of the neural tube and become the ventral roots of

the nervous system, synapsing with either muscles or autonomic neurons (Fig. 3-7E).

The neural crest develops two dorsolateral columns paralleling the neural tube. These columns are continuous at first, but they become segmented and form the anlage of the spinal ganglia (Fig. 3-7D). Some cells detach and migrate to become the sympathetic and parasympathetic ganglia and neurons (Fig. 3-8). The remainder of the spinal root ganglia (the neural crest derivatives [primitive neurocytes] form bipolar neuroblasts with peripheral and central processes) completes the dorsal roots of the spinal nerves (Fig. 3-8B). These nerves synapse with various receptor mechanisms in the musculoskeletal system, establishing the reflex arc (Fig. 3-8C). The central processes enter the developing neural tube, initially traveling in the white matter, synapsing with neurons in the alar (dorsal) and basal (ventral) laminae. In the spinal ganglia, each peripheral and central process fuses to form a single process entering the cell body, thus creating a unipolar neuron.

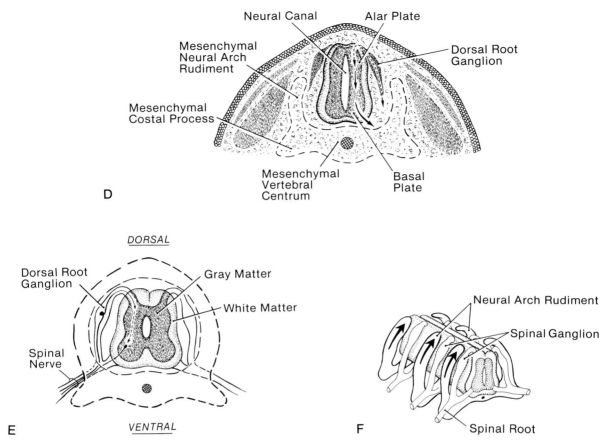

Fig. 3-7 *(Continued).* **(D)** The neurectoderm differentiates further into dorsal and vertebral (basal) plates. These become respectively the afferent and efferent areas of the spinal cord. **(E)** Progressive maturation of the neural crest and the dorsal and ventral plates leads to formation of the dorsal root ganglia and the anterior roots and spinal nerves. Meanwhile **(D,E,F)**, cells from the sclerotome migrate to the area around the notochord, where they differentiate to form the vertebral bodies, neural arches, and intervertebral discs.

Fourth and Fifth Weeks of Gestation

Development of Somites, Neural Tube, and Sclerotome[4]
Somites, which consist of highly specialized tissue masses condensed into pairs, arise from the craniocaudal differentiation of the paraxial mesoderm (Fig. 3-5A). Their ultimate function is the development of the major structures composing the skeletal, muscular, and integument systems. The first somites appear during the fourth embryonic week near the cranial end of the embryo, which will

eventually be the occipital region of the skull. The development of the somites progresses in a rostral (cranial)-to-caudal direction, and by the end of the fourth week, 29 paired somites will have developed (all within 10 days). By the end of the fifth week, all 42 to 44 somites will have developed. These differentiate on each side of the neural tube into the following: 4 occipital, 8 cervical, 12 thoracic, 5 lumbar, 5 sacral, and between 8 and 10 coccygeal paired somites. The first paired occipital somites disappear, as do the last five to seven coccygeal somites. The remaining occipital somites co-

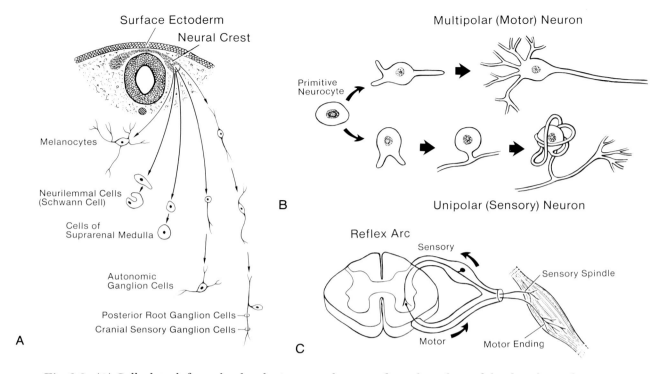

Fig. 3-8. (A) Cells detach from the developing neural crest to form the anlage of the dorsal spinal gangia. From these cells arise the sympathetic and parasympathetic ganglia and neurons. (B) The primitive neurocytes arising from the spinal root ganglia form bipolar neuroblasts having either central or peripheral processes, which form the dorsal roots of the spinal nerves. (C) These cells synapse with motor cells within the spinal cord to give rise to the basic reflex arc.

alesce to form the base of the skull and the craniocervical articulation (Fig. 3-9).

As noted in Figure 3-5A,B, the cells of the somite are centered about the periphery of the myelocele cavity. As the cells within these somites increase in numbers, they also develop three distinct layers. An outer layer of cells adjacent to the ectoderm becomes the dermatome — the cell mass that ultimately contributes to the development of the skin and the subcutaneous tissue. A middle layer becomes the myotome, which later gives rise to the development of somatic striated skeletal muscle along the dorsal, or posterior, lateral body. A third layer becomes the sclerotome. These cells lie along the anterior and medial wall of the somite, migrate in the direction of the notochord and the developing neural tube, and give rise to the future vertebral bodies, neural arches, and intervertebral discs (Figs. 3-7E,F; 3-10B; 3-11).

Development of the Vertebral Column

Sclerotomal cells first aggregate in the dorsolateral area of the early embryo and later migrate in a cranial and caudal direction.[1] Between the two areas of cells, a fissure develops, producing a sclerocele. The cells closest to the fissure migrate toward the notochord and then surround it with a perichordal ring (Fig. 3-11A). The perichordal ring in turn becomes the anulus fibrosus (Fig. 3-11B). The notochord then expands to become the nucleus pulposus. The two cellular areas described above migrate further and assume a cranial and a caudal orientation.[9] Those cells that migrate toward the notochord encompass it, thus appearing to be under the influence of the ventral half of the neural tube and the influence of inducement of the notochord.

In the midst of the cellular migration described above, the caudal cell mass from one sclerotome

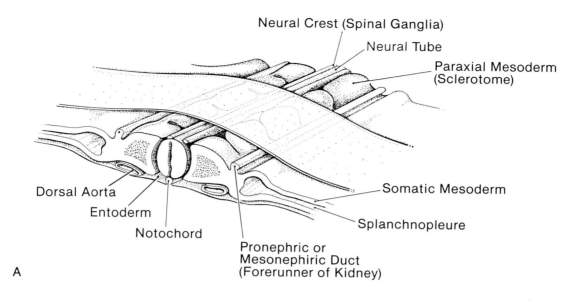

Neural Crest (Spinal Ganglia)

Neural Tube

Paraxial Mesoderm
(Sclerotome)

Somatic Mesoderm

Splanchnopleure

Dorsal Aorta

Entoderm

Notochord

Pronephric or
Mesonephiric Duct
(Forerunner of Kidney)

A

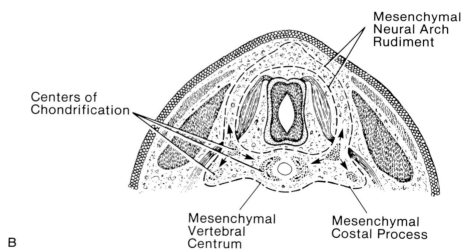

Mesenchymal
Neural Arch
Rudiment

Centers of
Chondrification

Mesenchymal
Vertebral
Centrum

Mesenchymal
Costal Process

B

Fig. 3-9. Further differentiation of the somites (see Fig. 3-5).

begins to fuse with the adjacent cranial sclerotomal cell mass (Fig. 3-11A). This same process occurs throughout the 44 somites and results in the development of the vertebral column, with each vertebra separated by an intervertebral disc. When the two sclerotomal cell masses fail to fuse, congenital abnormalities arise.

Those cells that are more dorsally located and later become the neural arch appear to be under the influence of the neural crest. This indicates that the two segments of the spine (the vertebral body and the neural arch) are under the influence of two different inducers (Fig. 3-10B).[1] More important, though, failure of segmentation in one area is not likely to induce abnormal development in the other area. Thus, the presentation of a congenital fusion between two vertebral bodies need not be associated each time with a fusion between the same posterior elements.

Somite formation occurs simultaneously with the

development of dorsal root ganglia, which arise from the neural crest and are situated opposite the medial surface of each myotome, resulting in a "one nerve–one somite" relationship. Consequently, each muscle arising from a particular somite will have its nerve innervation arising from that same level of spinal ganglia. For example, despite the migration of the diaphragm muscle, it is innervated primarily by nerves originating from the spinal ganglia (C3 to C-5) opposite the developing somite from which they arose. As noted in the discussion on the development of the vertebral bodies from the sclerotome, which in turn rose from the ventral and medial wall of its somite, these cells migrate toward and encircle the notochord (Fig. 3-11A). This circle of cells separates the notochord from its close relationship with the neural tube. At first, these cells are equally distributed longitudinally, with the separation of the somites being marked by the presence of an intersegmental blood vessel. A fissure then develops in the middle of the sclerotome, dividing it into a cranial half and a caudal half. The cells circumscribing the notochord reveal alternating areas of varying density. The denser areas (i.e., near the sclerotomal fissure and when migrating toward the notochord) form the perichordal disc opposite the developing spinal nerve. As the cells continue to migrate, the denser

area fills the cranial two-thirds of the caudal sclerotome half and the caudal one-third of the cranial sclerotome half (Fig. 3-11A). This dense area is ventrally contiguous with the neural arch rudiment and the rib rudiment (Fig. 3-10B). The area around the perichordal disc forms the intervertebral disc, and the less dense area of cells forms most of the vertebral centrum (Figs. 3-11A, 3-10B).

Development of the Atlas-Axis (C1-C2) Anlage
The formation of the atlas and the axis differs from that of the rest of the vertebral column. As noted earlier a number of occipital somites play a major role in the development of the occipital portion of the lower skull and the upper cervical spine (Fig. 3-9). The caudal half of the fourth occipital somite (O4) fuses with the cranial half of the first cervical somite (C1) to form in humans the ligamentous attachments between the base of the occiput and the odontoid process. The major cell mass contributing to the development of the odontoid process is derived from the caudal half of the first cervical somite (C1) and the cranial half of the second cervical somite (C2). These same somites, when fused together, contribute to some of the supporting ligaments between C1 and the odontoid process (Fig. 3-9) and to the anterior bony arch of C1.

The centrum of C2 is derived from the caudal

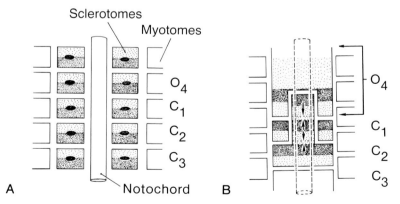

Fig. 3-10. (A) Three cell concentrations arise from the mesoderm: paraxial, intermediate, and lateral (see Fig. 3-5A). From the paraxial cell mass arises the sclerotomes, the forerunners of the vertebral and skeletal systems (see Fig. 3-5B). Condensed paired areas of highly specialized sclerodermal paraxial tissue make up the somites, which will form the vertebral column. By the end of week 5, all 42 to 44 somites have formed: 4 occipital, 8 cervical, 12 thoracic, 5 lumbar, 5 sacral, and 8 to 10 coccygeal. (B) Diagram showing the coalescence of somites O4, C1, and C2 to form the foramen magnum, the ring of C1 (without a vertebral body), the ligamentous attachment between the base of the occiput and the odontoid process, and C2 (with both a vertebral process and the odontoid process).

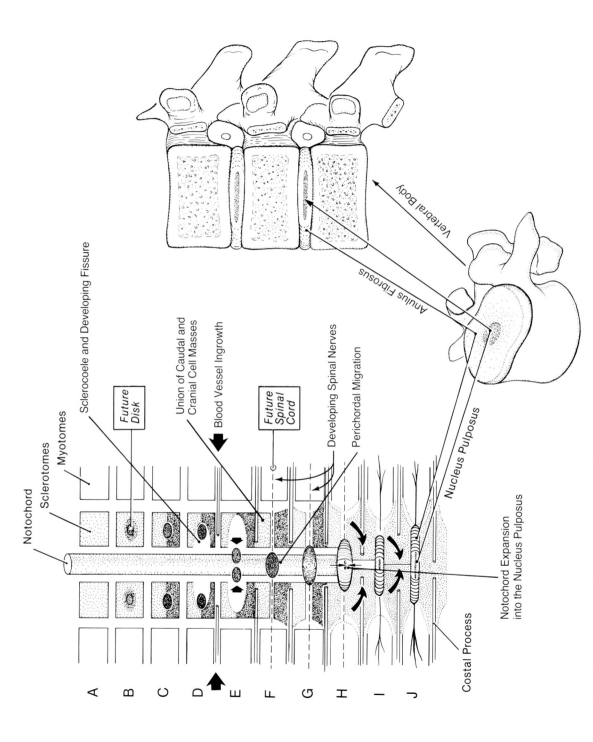

Fig. 3-11. These diagrams depict the coming together of laterally aligned paraxial somites along the notochord. The somites fissure and recombine. Blood vessels develop from each myotome, arising from the paired dorsal aorta. They lie between the somites, and eventually come to pierce the centrum of each vertebral body. As somite "regeneration" occurs, a dense area within the developing sclerotomal fissure migrates to become the intervertebral disc, with a nucleus pulposus and annulus fibrosis. The craniocaudal separation and recombination of adjacent somites leads to the formation of the vertebral processes (neural arch and rib rudiments) and the vertebral body.

half of the second (C2) somite and the cranial half of the third (C3) somite. The normal resegmentation process (sclerotome melding) is incomplete in the second (C2) cervical somite and thus allows the centrum of C1 and the centrum of C2 to fuse without involving the entire sclerotome. This fusion may hinder the normal development of the odontoid process. Were the process of resegmentation to proceed as it does elsewhere in the spine, congenital variants would result (see Rationale for Occurrence of Congenital Deformities of the Spine, below).

While the cells composing the sclerotome that eventually will develop into the vertebral centrum migrate (Fig. 3-10B), another group of cells begin to migrate. These cells are positioned laterally and migrate both dorsally and ventromedially. The dorsal cell mass divides into two areas, one more dense than the other. The cells in the dense area are contiguous with the dense perichordal disc, migrating dorsally between the developing spinal ganglia and the myotome, to give rise to the neural arches (Fig. 3-10B). The arches migrate upward, around the neural tube, but incompletely. The roof of the arches, along with the meninges, arise from local tissue adjacent to the neural tube.

Development of Vertebral Body Vascular Supply

Discussion of the development of the vascular pattern of the vertebral column would not be complete without also discussing the development of the vertebra (Fig. 3-11A). The intersegmental derivation of the vertebra helps explain the development of the vascular pattern. Blood vessels arising from paired segmental branches off the paired dorsal aorta (Fig. 3-10A) course from the myotomes toward and between the somites. As resegmentation occurs, each vessel takes a position within the centrum of the vertebral body (Fig. 3-11A).

The intimate relationship between developing blood vessels and vertebral bodies can be best shown by depicting first the developing vertebral column; second, the pathologic analysis of healing vertebral fractures; and third, the relationship between a particular disease process and its effect on the spine (e.g., tuberculosis, which affects solely the vertebral body (affecting the vertebral end plate and intervertebral disc only secondarily) (see

Chapter 4). With little question, the vertebra's vascular pattern also influences how metastatic disease invades the vertebral column (Batson's plexus). The vascular supply to each vertebral body enters at its midportion (the area surrounding the nutrient vessel). Although in cases of bacterial infection the mechanism of gaining entry to the vertebral body remains the same, the location of the vertebral body pathology is different. Under these circumstances, the affected vertebra reveals destruction of the cartilaginous end plate (probably the result of enzymatic dissolution of the vertebral cartilaginous end plate and the disc [nucleus pulposus and anulus fibrosus] by the action of hyaluronidase liberated by the bacteria (streptococci, staphylococci, and gonococci).

Fifth and Sixth Weeks of Gestation

As the neural tube closes, cells along the interface between the neural plate and the ectoderm begin forming the neural crest (Fig. 3-7C). These cells arise as a parallel column along the dorsolateral surface of the neural tube and become the anlage of the spinal ganglia (Fig. 3-7D) (each lying opposite a developing somite). In time, adjacent to these cells, there will arise the beginning of the ganglia and neurons of the sympathetic and parasympathetic nervous systems. Because the embryo grows and lengthens more dorsally than ventrally, it takes on a C-shaped posture for the remainder of fetal life (Fig. 3-6C).

Sixth Week of Gestation

As noted earlier, the third week of gestation is marked by extensive cellular differentiation and the development of three basic cell layers: the ectoderm, mesoderm, and entoderm. In the ensuing weeks, these layers continue to mature. By the sixth week, the skeleton and a mesenchymal anlage of the vertebrae have resegmented. In addition, two centers of chondrification, one on each side of the notochord, appear in the vertebral centrum. These fuse to form a single centrum. Two more chondrification centers appear on each side of the neural arch and extend laterally into the articular (facet) and transverse process areas. Another two centers of chondrification appear lateral to the junction of the centrum and the neural arches, in the area that will be the rib rudiment.[5] Eventually, all the centers fuse, forming a single, solid, cartilaginous model of the vertebra (Fig. 3-12A). The notochord becomes totally surrounded by the vertebral centrum. In the area within each vertebral centrum it degenerates and disappears. In the area between the centra of successive vertebrae, where the intervertebral discs will form, the notochord undergoes mucoid degeneration, creating the nucleus pulposus[6] (Fig. 3-11B). Finally, the surrounding perichordal cells differentiate to assume the role and form of the anulus fibrosus (Fig. 3-11).

Eighth Through Tenth Week of Gestation

Several events take place during this period. The two ossification centers in the developing vertebral arches appear between the eighth and the tenth week of gestation. There is some controversy as to where they first appear. Some believe they appear first in the cervical region; others believe they appear lower in the thoracic spine, from where ossification progresses both cranially and caudally. According to Bagnali et al.,[7] there does not appear to be any regular order of ossification in the nine most proximal arches. Their research demonstrates that the sequence of neural arch ossification spreads from two basic regions: the cervical and the lower thoracic–upper lumbar regions. It seems that there is no regular sequence of ossification in the nine most proximal or cephalic neural arches and that the earliest stages of ossification are located in the lower thoracic (T11, T12) and upper lumbar (L1) region and spread cephalically and caudally until all the ossification centers of the centrae are established.

Ossification centers lie at the base of each lamina. Ossification begins in the spinous processes, then in the articular processes (Fig. 3-12A,B), and finally in the transverse processes. In the ribs, as previously discussed, beginning in the ninth week of gestation, a primary center of ossification appears near the future angle of the corresponding rib. The cartilaginous rib ossifies in a proximal and distal direction, the distal end of the thoracic ribs

always remaining cartilaginous. With the ossification of the cartilaginous rib (which precedes ossification of the vertebral centrum), a joint is formed between the head of the rib and the vertebral element[2,9] (Fig. 3-12B). Also during the ninth week, the primary centers of ossification within the sacral centra of S1 to S3 form.

15th Through 24th Week of Gestation

The vertebral body begins to ossify about the 15th to 16th week of gestation with the development of primary and secondary centers of ossification. By the 24th week, ossification is complete. Each vertebra contains three primary and three secondary centers. Each vertebral body except the atlas (C1), the axis (C2), and the sacrum ossifies in a similar manner. Before ossification, the cartilage cells hypertrophy and their matrix calcifies. Ossification then occurs as small blood vessels migrate in.

Ossification first occurs in the lower thoracic or upper lumbar vertebral centrum and advances both cranially and caudally. Ossification of the vertebral centrum begins from a single center and spreads throughout the vertebral body, with the exception of the two cartilaginous end plates that lie along the vertebral body's superior and inferior margins. These two plates form the epiphyses from which growth by endochondral ossification continues. The cartilage plates become vascularized, but vessels do not enter the anulus fibrosus, which remains avascular throughout life. As noted in the discussion on the ninth week of gestation, the sacral primary centers appear at different times. During the 24th week, the primary centers of S4 and S5 appear.

Birth Through Week 50

The neurocentral chondrosis is an area of cartilage that lies between the ossified arches posteriorly and the ossified centrum of the vertebral body. It lies anterior to the junction of the vertebral body and the lamina (Fig. 3-12C). The centrum and the adjacent posterior portion of the neural arches fuse to form the definitive vertebral body. Fusion begins in the upper lumbar spine in the late fetal

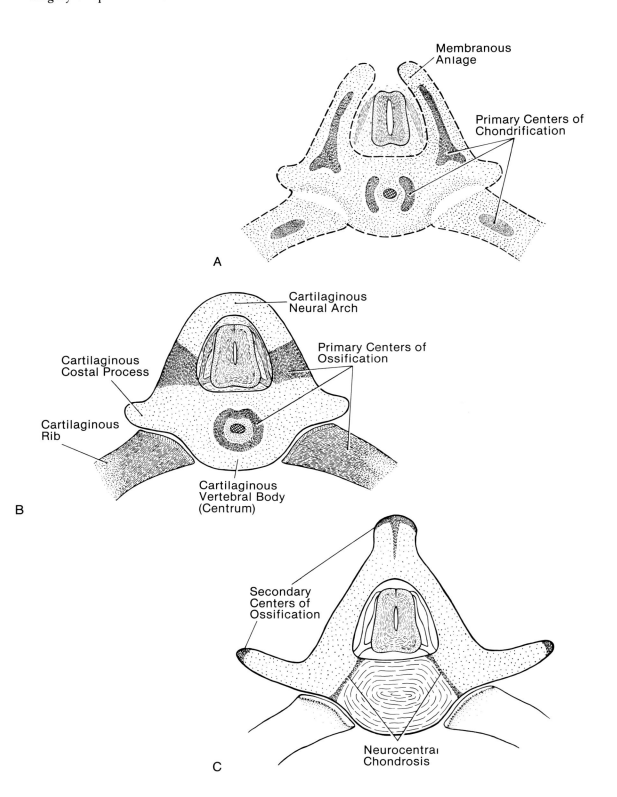

period and continues in the newborn.[2] Fusion of these centers in the lumbar spine becomes complete within the second decade of life. Failure of fusion results in the development of spondylolisthesis.

As explained in the section on the fourth to fifth week of gestation, the atlas, axis, and sacrum form differently from the other vertebrae. The atlas has five primary ossification centers (three anterior and two for each of the neural arches). The axis has five primary centers and two secondary centers of ossification. Because the odontoid process arises from more than one sclerotome, there are two additional laterally placed centers in the odontoid process (Fig. 3-13). These two odontoid centers fuse near term (52 weeks). The remaining odontoid synchondroses between the centrum and the odontoid do not fuse until about the second decade.

Second and Third Decades

As noted above, the odontoid process and the vertebral centrum do not completely fuse until sometime in the second decade, as does the sacrum. Ossification of the sacrum begins in the primary centers of the vertebral centrae that have rudimentary epiphyseal plates, without ring apophyses. The sacral neural arches form from two centers. Three additional laterally placed centers develop to produce the sacral alae. Fusion of the sacral neural arches and the sacral alae begins in early adolescence and is complete by the third decade. The coccygeal vertebrae do not have a neural arch; therefore, they form only a single, primary ossification center.

The vertebral arches have three secondary ossification centers that develop during adolescence: one for the tip of the spinous process and one for each transverse process. Additional secondary centers may appear in the cervical vertebrae and occasionally in the lumbar vertebrae, where the costal process may have been incorporated into the vertebra. The ribs develop as mesenchymal condensations growing out from the primitive vertebrae and later separate from the costal process of each vertebra. Joints then form between the head of the rib and the vertebral body and between the tubercle of the rib and the transverse process. Secondary centers of ossification for the ribs appear in the second decade: two in the tubercles and one in the head of the rib. In the cervical spine, the costal process usually regresses and becomes the anterior half of the vertebral artery foramen. In the lumbar spine, the costal process forms a large portion of the transverse process. Both the cervical and lumbar spine have the potential of producing accessory

Primary Ossification Centers

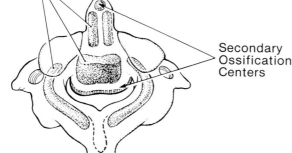

Secondary Ossification Centers

Fig. 3-13. Ossification centers of the axis (C2).

Fig. 3-12. (A) By the 6th week of gestation, the skeleton and mesenchymal anlage of the vertebra have resegmented. A paired center of chondrification arises on either side of the notochord, and grows to form the vertebral centrum. Another pair of centers of chondrification appears in the area of the neural arch, and grows laterally to form the articular facets and transverse processes. A third pair of centers of chondrification forms the rib rudiments. (B) Ossification occurs first in the ribs, forming a joint between the head of the rib and the vertebral element. (C) By the 50th week after the beginning of gestation (13th month), the neurocentral cartilagenous chondrosis between the posteriorly ossified neural arches and the anteriorly ossified vertebral centrum lies anterior to the junction between the vertebral body and the lamina. Fusion of these areas results in the formation of the definitive vertebral body (complete by the 2nd decade). Failure of fusion results in spondylolisthesis.

ribs. In the sacrum, the costal process forms the anterior portion of the sacral ala.

RATIONALE FOR OCCURRENCE OF CONGENITAL DEFORMITIES OF THE SPINE

Congenital defects may result from aberrations occurring during the embryonic (developmental), the fetal (growth), or both stages.[1] For example, hemimelia may result from primary failure of the fibrous or cartilage anlage to form (developmental error) or from primary failure of specific collagens or mucopolysaccharide moieties that will allow further cellular changes to synthesize appropriate

amounts at the appropriate time, or from secondary failure of biochemical syntheses resulting from a delay in differentiation. Because the development of the various skeletal components is interrelated and interdependent, a single developmental failure in one area of the skeleton may result in developmental failures in other skeletal regions.

As noted above, quantitative deficiencies in particular enzymes and chemical substrates may prolong the phase of cellular transition, leading to skeletal reduction deformities. For example, the onset of the development of the cartilage collagen is important to the formation of the skeletal anlage. Also, the timing of the numerous stages of skeletal development is crucial.

Spatial development is equally important. For instance, a change in structure or function must accompany each change in collagen type, such as

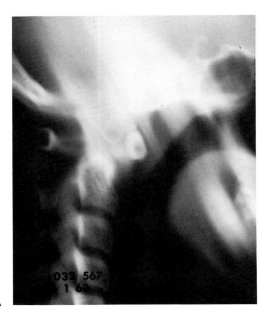
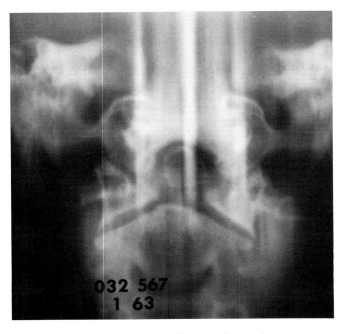

A   B

Fig. 3-14. (A) Lateral radiograph of child's skull and cervical spine demonstrating failure of union between proximal odontoid and base of odontoid (os odontoideum). (B) AP radiograph of occiput (C1–C2) demonstrates absence of odontoid waist. The odontoid arises from two primary ossification centers (extending vertically from the body into the odontoid). The most proximal tip arises from a secondary ossification center. This radiograph reveals failure of segmentation between occipital somite 4 and cervical somites 1–3.

when two different collagen types separate within the mesenchyme to develop into cartilage, bone, fibrous tissue, or muscle.[1]

There is some controversy whether congenital defects occur before or during chondrification or ossification. It is generally accepted, however, that defects occurring early during the embryonic (developmental) period tend to produce multisystem abnormalities, whereas those that develop during the fetal (growth) period tend to result in more localized abnormalities. A good example of the former is that cited by Winter et al.[3] and Rivard et al.[8] Abnormalities occurring during the stage of membrane development of a vertebral element remain through the period of chondrification and ossification. Failure of segmentation bilaterally or the formation of a ''bar'' between two segments is responsible for producing one of the following abnormalities: congenital scoliosis,[1] hemivertebra, a cleft vertebra, or a wedge or congenital fusion between vertebral segments. Therefore, it may be

conjectured that once an aberrant cellular structure reaches the cartilage stage, the deformity remains. This supports the argument that defects occur early with chondrification and that ossification is passive and proceeds only in the direction already established by the cartilage cellular structure.

A common abnormality that may be discovered coincidentally in the evaluation of a patient with an acute spinal cord injury is a benign abnormality (os odontoideum) found in the C1 to C2 area (Fig. 3-14). Distinguishing this benign abnormality from trauma-induced pathology is often difficult. Two congenital developments that fall in this category are the complete, rather than the normal and appropriate incomplete, sclerotome fusion at the C1 to C2 level, resulting in a pseudoarthrosis between C2 and the odontoid process; and the failure of the C1 centrum to separate into the anterior arch and odontoid, in conjunction with complete sclerotome formation in the second cervical somite (C2).

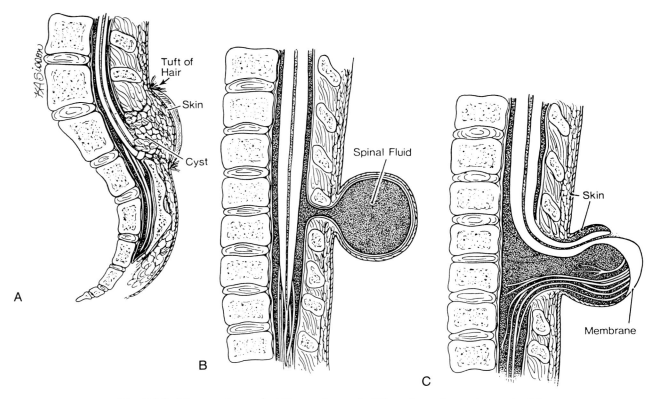

Fig. 3-15. Lipomeningocele (**A**), meningocele (**B**), and myelomeningocele (**C**).

This latter defect causes the absence or hypoplasia of the odontoid process.

Probably the most frequently occurring deformity of the spine, and a clear indicator of failure of fusion between the ossification centers of the neural arch, is spina bifida occulta. Some studies report the incidence of this deformity to be at 20 percent,[1] although most contend that the deformity is less common (6 percent). Most commonly, this defect occurs at the level of either L5 or S1, although it may appear anywhere. Spina bifida occulta is rarely, if ever, associated with neurologic involvement.

Unlike spina bifida occulta, meningomyelocele (Fig. 3-15) — a failure of fusion of the posterior neural arch — is always associated with neurologic involvement (Fig. 3-16). Often extensive, it results in loss of both motor and sensory functions in large areas of the lower extremities. The etiology of this congenital defect has not been absolutely established. Often, the various spinal cord coverings are herniated through the incomplete posterior arch containing cerebrospinal fluid only (meningocele). In other situations, the neural tissue is contained within the meningocele, forming a meningomyelocele, but it is not clear whether the defect results from the failure of the posterior neural arch to close or from the failure of the neural plate to develop. The above-mentioned developmental defect's exclusive association with spina bifida suggests that complete closure of the neural arch depends on the complete closure of the neuropore and neural tube. Similarly, a defective differentiation of the neural crest may play a role in arch failure. By the same reasoning, some vertebral anomalies may be caused by primary neurologic defects, which in turn are responsible for the maldevelopment of the associated vertebral centrum and/or neural arch.[1]

Finally, a tumor that is encountered occasionally is the chordoma. It is easily recognized by its pathologic cells, the very gelatinous physaliphorous cells. This is a residual cell of the degenerated notochord, which persists most often in the basisphenoid (base of the skull) or the sacrococcygeal regions.

CONCLUSION

An effort has been made in this chapter to construct the embryology of the newborn from conception through birth and into the second decade of life when bone maturation occurs. The sequence of events of nervous and skeletal system development have been detailed diagrammatically, with the hope that the required three-dimensional conceptualization of the fetal growth process was facilitated.

The rationale for the inclusion of embryonic and fetal embryology is that as the fetus progresses through the growth period between conception and term, at each stage, developmental errors could arise. It is this chance occurrence that gives rise to such defects as congenital amputation, meningomyeloceles, hemivertebra, and the os odontoideum.

REFERENCES

1. Ogden JA: The development and growth of the musculoskeletal system. p. 41. In Albright JA, Brand RA (eds): The Scientific Basis of Orthopaedics. Appleton & Lange, New York, 1979

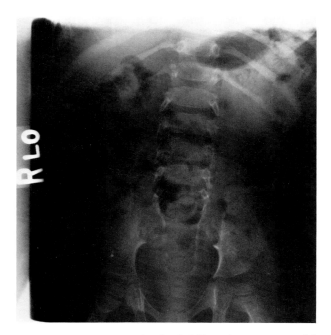

Fig. 3-16. AP radiograph of a child less than 10 years old who has a defect involving L1 through S5. This defect is caused by failure of the neural tube to close.

2. Streeter G, Henser C, Cornor G: Development horizons in human embryos. Contrib Embryol 230:166, 1951

3. Winter RB, Lonstein JE, Leonard AS, Smith AE: Spine embryology. p. 1. Congenital Deformities of the Spine. Thieme, New York, 1983

4. LaRocca H: Embryology of the musculoskeletal system. In: Lovell WW, Winter RB (eds): Pediatric Orthopaedics JB Lippinott, Philadelphia, 1978

5. Wyburn GM: Observations on the development of the human vertebral column. J Anat 78:94, 1944

6. Parke WW: Development of the spine. p. 1. In: Rothman RH, Simeone FA (eds): The Spine. WB Saunders, Philadelphia, 1975

7. Bagnali KM, Harris PF, Jones PRM: A radiologic study of the human fetal spine. The sequence of the development of ossification centres in the certebral column. J Anat 124:791, 1977

8. Rivard CH, Narbaitz R, Uithoff HK: Congenital vertebral malformations. Orthop Rev 8:135, 1979

4

Vascular Anatomy of the Spinal Cord

Paul R. Meyer, Jr.

The arterial vascular supply of the spinal cord is the single most important consideration in the management of all spinal deformities, whether congenital or caused by trauma or tumor. The concern is injury to, or alteration in, the arterial vascular supply to the spinal cord during correction of spinal deformity or fracture reduction and instrumentation. In cases of significant trauma to the spinal column with resulting malalignment, bone fragmentation, and spinal cord compression, the principal pathologic process that results in neurotissue injury or ischemic necrosis is a loss of spinal cord blood supply. This loss occurs either in microscopic form — subtle loss of capillary blood supply associated with post-traumatic edema — or macroscopically after spinal column trauma resulting in subluxation or dislocation. Under traumatic conditions at the time of injury, the actual extent of spinal displacement cannot be known; thus, the actual origin of the loss of the blood supply cannot be known and may follow vascular stretching, tearing, tissue pinching, or entrapment. The effects are swelling and hemorrhage of spinal cord neural tissue.

The most recognizable cause for obstruction of the spinal cord's blood supply, principally the anterior spinal artery, is direct pressure of bone fragments or intervertebral disc material posteriorly against the spinal cord (Fig. 4-1), with greater than 50 percent compromise of the neural canal (Fig. 4-1B). The result is temporary, permanent, or progressive loss of circulation to a highly sensitive tissue that is incapable of surviving extended periods (4 hours[1]) of oxygen deprivation. Because of the close relationship between the metabolic requirements of the spinal cord and its blood supply, the balance is precarious at best and barely adequate for the spinal cord's minimal needs.[2,3]

ETIOLOGY OF SPINAL CORD VASCULAR EMBARRASSMENT

Trauma need not be the sole cause of vascular embarrassment to the spinal cord. Surgical correction of abdominal vascular problems and spinal deformities has been cited as a cause of alteration in the spinal cord blood supply.[4] The resulting effect is a deterioration in neurologic function. Not infrequently, for example, alterations in spinal cord function occur during the surgical instrumentation and correction of a severe scoliotic curve. The cause is assumed to be temporary loss of spinal cord blood flow from cord stretching. Why this occurs in some cases and not others is unknown. Schneider[5] reports a rather extensive amount of "available" cord stretch, as do White and Paniabi.[6] Embarrassment of spinal cord blood flow and loss of neurologic function are related to

the extent or severity of the deformity (greater than 30 degrees) to be corrected[3]

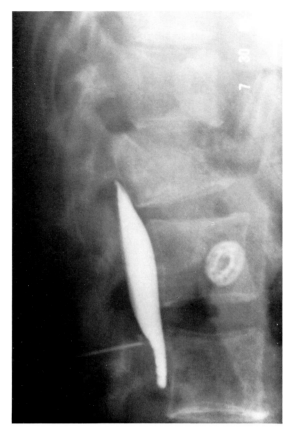

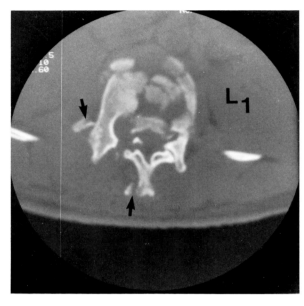

A   B

Fig. 4-1. (A) Lateral radiograph of lumbar spine showing comminuted compression fracture of vertebral body L1 with retropulsion of posterosuperior segment and posterior wall into canal. Myelogram demonstrates obstruction to flow of contrast material at L1. Area under compression is conus medullaris portion of spinal cord. (B) Computed axial tomography (CAT) scan demonstrating comminuted burst fracture of vertebral body L1. This injury is the result of flexion axial load mechanical forces.

the rigidity of the spinal deformity (correctable only with extensive soft tissue resection and high distraction pressure)

the etiology of the deformity (congenital [hemivertebrae] or trauma)

the length of time the deformity or disease process has been present

whether previous anterior surgery (with resection of anterior segmental vessels) or bone resection surgery has been performed

whether the curve is unstable, pliable, and easily overdistracted (as with trauma)

These factors, plus surgery, each influence the hazard of injury to the spinal cord and its vascularity. Interestingly, numerous investigators[4,7–9] with extensive experience in anterior spinal surgery report a low incidence of complications as a result of interruption of the anterior vertebral segmental vessels (Fig. 4-2). Dommisse[7,10] reports personal communication with Professor Hodgson of only one occurrence in more than 100 procedures (1972). He advised careful attention to details at the anterior spine at the level of T10 (Fig. 4-3). It is at this level that the artery of Adamkiewicz[11] enters the neural canal via the neuroforamen and provides the primary blood supply to the thoracic cord via the anterior spinal artery (see Arterial Vascular Supply: Cervical Spinal Cord, below). The prevention of inadvertent injury to these vessels is best accomplished by awareness; maintenance of an

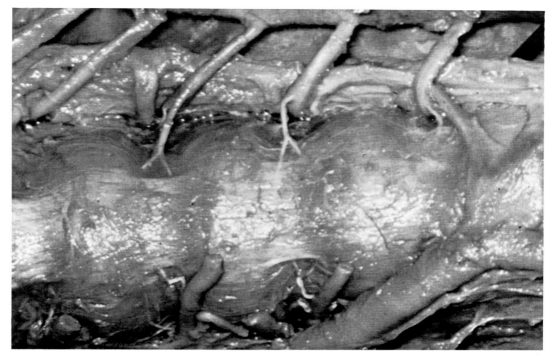

Fig. 4-2. Anterior vertebral segmental vessels. (From Dommisse,[10] with permission.)

elevated or above normal blood pressure during surgery, by administration of a high fluid load during surgery; the use of the wake-up test[12,13] if neurologic injury is suspected and somatosensory evoked potential monitoring is not available; when possible, the use of somatosensory evoked response monitoring preoperatively (for baseline purposes) and during the performance of the surgical procedure (see Ch. 6).

MANAGEMENT OF POTENTIAL VASCULAR INJURY TO SPINAL CORD DURING SURGERY

During surgery, should any reduction in neuro-response occur, the following routine is utilized on the spine service:

1. Steroids (50 mg dexamethasone) should be administered as an intravenous (**IV**) push, followed by further administration of steroid (10 mg) q 6 hours on a graduated, reducing scale over the next several days.
2. Any internal fixation that was just inserted and that might be responsible for vascular stretching is removed.
3. The anesthetic agent being used is evaluated, and the patient "lightened" and placed on 100 percent oxygen.
4. The ambient temperature of the operating room is checked.
5. The patient's core body temperature is checked. If cold, the patient should be warmed with a warming mattress (the placement and use of a temperature mattress should be planned for preoperatively).
6 If the patient's core temperature is low (below 36°C), fluids administered to the patient (including blood) are warmed.

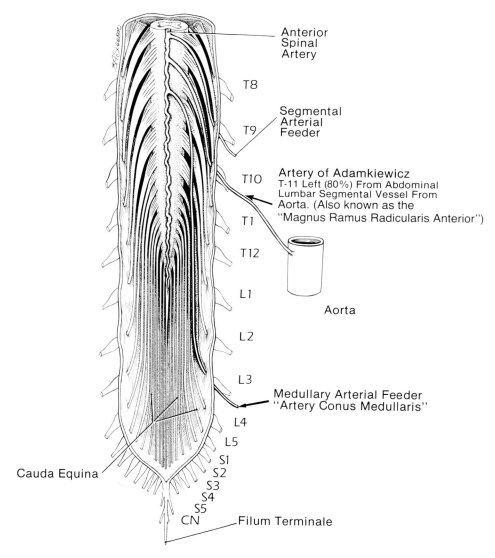

Fig. 4-3. Arterial vascular supply to the thoracolumbar and sacral spinal cord.

SPINAL COLUMN VASCULAR ENCROACHMENT

The etiology of insidious loss of spinal cord function after known trauma to the vertebral column is frequently difficult to immediately identify or diagnose. The gradual changes in neurologic function that most frequently appear include progressive extremity weakness, hyper-reflexia, clonus, loss of coordination, changes in bowel and bladder function, and a decrease in sensory function (less often an early symptom). Disease entities that must be ruled out include the presence of primary intramedullary or extramedullary-intradural spinal tumor with progressive neurologic tissue encroachment, extradural metastatic tumor, bacterial infection or tuberculosis involvement with abscess formation, primary neurologic disease such as multiple sclerosis, neurotoxic drugs, and neural tissue vascular embarrassment secondary to tumor encroachment of vertebral column malalignment secondary to trauma or disease. Depending on residual motor and sensory function, one should be able to identify the location of the lesion and the type of neurologic deficit (motor, sensory, vibratory, proprioception, etc.), the severity of the symptoms, the extent of loss function, and the length of time the symptoms or vascular compromise have been present. Knowing each of the above will be helpful in determining the outcome. Prognostically, the more sudden the onset, accompanied by loss of motor and sensory function for greater than 24 hours,[14] the less likely is neurologic recovery.

COMPLICATIONS FROM VASCULAR SURGERY

The literature reveals the occasional onset of paraplegia after the performance of an abdominal vascular procedure. It has also been reported[15] after a standard flank (sympathectomy) approach.[16] Analysis of the complication revealed that the onset followed the ligation of the 12th intercostal artery during the approach. This vessel was obviously the major contributor to the segmental vessel of Adamkiewicz.[7,10,11] A second oc-

currence I am aware of followed temporary cross-clamping of the lower thoracic aorta for resection of an abdominal aortic aneurysm (personal communication, L. Michaelis, Chicago, IL).

Analysis of the thoracic vascular anatomy reveals that the vessel or artery of Adamkiewicz *magnos ramus radicularis anterior* exits the aorta (80 percent) at the level of T10–T11 on the left and, in 75 percent of specimens, arises from level T9, T10, T11, or T12, accompanying one of the nerves. In 10 percent of persons, the vessel exits between L1 and L2, and in 15 percent of persons the vessel exits between the T5, T6, T7, or T8 dorsal nerves. In the latter situation, a supplementary artery occurs lower down, known as the *arteria conus medullaris*.[17]

A spinal cord (anterior spinal artery) vascular insult may be suspected whenever there is a loss of neurologic function inconsistent with either the history of trauma or the physical or radiologic findings of vertebral column trauma. The occurrence of this phenomenon is not as unusual as one might believe. In my series of 514 admissions (1972 through 1986) without any spinal fractures, 103 (20 percent) exhibited some neurologic deficit at the thoracic, lumbar, or sacral level. Of 525 thoracic injuries, 5 patients (1.0 percent) had neurologic deterioration. Within 36 hours of injury, ascension of the neurologic level occurred. In each, the investigative evaluation produced negative contributory findings. The assumption was neurologic change secondary to an insidious anterior spinal artery thrombosis or the occurrence of spinal cord edema with loss of spinal cord capillary blood flow and a resulting neural tissue ischemic necrosis. Confirmation of the occurrence of neural tissue ischemia as the cause of lost function comes with the appearance of a flaccid peripheral paralysis rather than a spastic peripheral paralysis (indicates an absence of a spinal cord reflex arc secondary to cord ischemia and necrosis).

The history of a patient demonstrating neurologic injury that is probably secondary to vascular changes within the spinal cord is the presence of a known injury (fall or motor vehicle accident), a flexion injury to the lower thoracic spine, or a hyperextension injury to the cervical spine (particularly in the older patient with significant cervical spondylosis). With injury to the lower spine, vertebral fracture may occur. With injury to the neck, a hyperextension injury to the cervical spine with anterior disruption of the anterior longitudinal ligament, a tear through the anulus fibrosus, and a widening of the intervertebral disc space may have occurred (Fig. 4-1B). Under either circumstance, the spinal cord may become momentarily pinched or contused between anterior vertebral fracture fragments, intervertebral disc, or posterior vertebral body osteoarthritic spurs and the posterior interlaminar calcified ligamentum flavum. The spinal cord becomes edematous and undergoes central hemorrhage (hematomyelia) or occlusion of the anterior spinal artery. In the latter case, as noted in the thoracic spine because of the "watershed" vascular supply to the spinal cord from T10 to T4 (the higher level being dependent on the blood supply from below), spinal cord ischemia insidiously occurs as the blood supply from below is lost and that from above is unable to compensate. The result is a creeping ascending paraplegia.

This same pathologic process occurs in the cervical spine. A not infrequent occurrence is the patient with vertebral column injury at the C5 to C6 level (Fig. 4-4) with a complete C6 neurologic injury. Within 24 to 36 hours of injury, evidence of neurologic deterioration appears. Usually the first sign of change in neurologic function in a patient with spontaneous ventilation who was previously noted to have adequate spontaneous ventilatory parameters (tidal volumn, vital capacity, respiratory rate, etc.) will be changes in subsequent arterial blood gas values, including a fall in PO_2, an increase in PCO_2, an increase in blood pH, a decrease in percent of oxygen saturation, etc. Left unattended, the patient will continue into respiratory acidosis, rapidly deteriorate, and terminate in respiratory or cardiac arrest.

The pathologic events after spinal cord tissue injury are edema of the spinal cord itself followed by hemorrhage into the spinal cord, necrosis of both the central gray matter and the peripheral white matter, and loss of motor (anterior horn) cells and sensory (posterior horn) cells as well as peripheral white matter (long tract) function. In those with neurologic injuries above the level of T6, a loss of peripheral autonomic (sympathetic) function also occurs. This condition results in the heart being sympathetically unbalanced and singularly under the influence of the vagus nerve (producing a

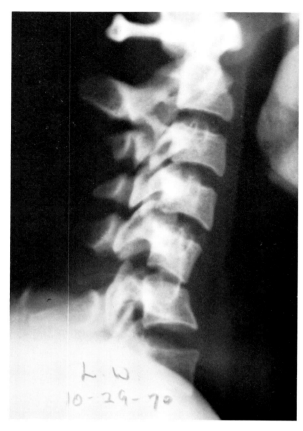

Fig. 4-4. Lateral radiograph of cervical spine demonstrating flexion distraction injury at C5–C6. Note wide diastasis between the posterior elements of C5 and C6, indicating disruption of all posterior stabilizing structures. Patient admission diagnosis was C6 injury complete. Over the ensuing 36 hours, the patient deteriorated to a C4 neurologic level.

bradycardia). Similarly, with the loss of sympathetics the peripheral vascular tree is in a state of vasodilation (producing hypotension) (see Ch. 5). The resulting changes (from spinal cord vascular ischemia) are sufficient to result in four potential ascending neuropathologic processes, either temporary or permanent:

Complete sensory and motor neurologic injury at and below the level of injury
Anterior cord injury (loss of motor function, preservation of posterior column function, i.e., proprioception, vibration, light touch

Central cord injury (loss of motor function at the level of injury with maintenance of long tract function beneath that level)

On rare occasions, posterior cord lesion (loss of posterior dorsal column function) with maintenance of anterior motor function (locally and long tract).

Braakman[18] reports that posterior column lesions more frequently follow acute hyperextension injuries to the cervical spine. To the contrary, I have noted that the type of neurologic injury that follows an extension injury to the cervical spine, particularly in patients more than 50 years old, is a central cord syndrome (14.5 percent), anterior cord syndrome (9.7 percent), or complete cord injury (14.5 percent). Twenty-six percent of these patients were neurologically normal. The neurologic injury is probably due to pinching of the spinal cord between anterior bone osteophytes and posterior calcified ligamentum flavum.

A concern that must be kept in mind during the first hours after trauma is the extent of cervical spine instability. Stability relies on both ligamentous and bony structures. When there is a frank vertebral element subluxation (Fig. 4-4) or dislocation (Fig. 4-5A), instability should be suspected (Fig. 4-5B). When gross but unrecognized instability is present, what normally would be insufficient traction suddenly produces gross overdistraction (Fig. 4-5). The presence of this type of instability

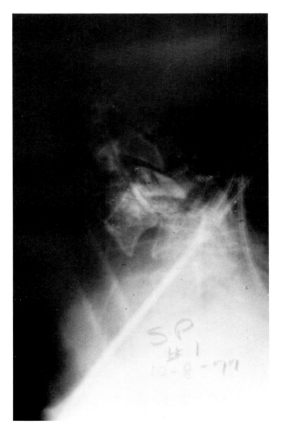
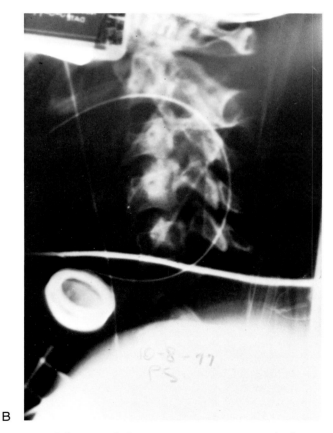

A   B

Fig. 4-5. (A) Lateral radiograph of cervical spine of patient with fracture dislocation at C5–C6. Patient had complete C5 neurologic lesion. After this radiograph was taken, the patient was placed in Gardner-Wells traction and 25 lb (5 lb per level) were applied before the next radiograph was taken. (B) Lateral radiograph after applying 25 lb of traction. Note gross distraction. This radiograph demonstrates the need for careful radiographic evaluation after adding each weight. Unrecognized gross instability like this is sometimes the reason for severe vascular injury.

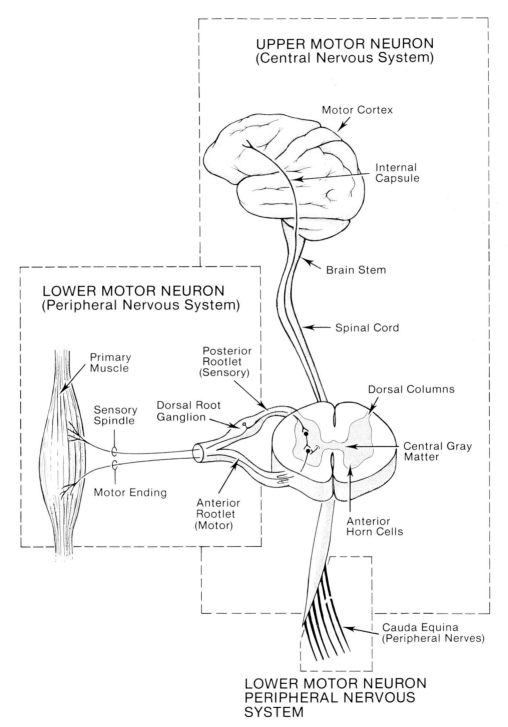

Fig. 4-6. Basic communication between central nervous system and peripheral nervous system.

and distraction is sufficient to further compromise an already embarrassed spinal cord vascular supply. Care must be exercised during the acute application of weights (by frequent repeat radiographs) to rule out vertebral column instability.

A final example of what likely is an expression of post-traumatic altered spinal cord blood supply is the following. A patient has an injury to the lower thoracic spine. Upon admission, the neurologic injury is consistent with the level of spinal column injury (T12). The initial findings reveal absent motor and sensory function below T12 and a positive bulbocavernosus reflex (see Ch. 1). The presence of the bulbocavernosus reflex has two important interpretations: first, that portion of the nervous system is out of spinal shock (the bulbocavernosus reflex frequently returns within 45 minutes of trauma, while the remainder of the nervous system below the level of injury continues areflexic for a period of 3 to 6 weeks); second, the reflex loop is intact (i.e., injury to the motor cells and the dor-

sal sensory ganglion of the conus medullaris has not occurred). With gentle pulling on an indwelling urinary bladder catheter, the bladder wall will be stimulated via sensory afferents to the conus medullaris portion of the spinal cord (Fig. 4-6). With synapses between and by means of internuncial neurons, a motor impulse passes out of the anterior horn cell area of the conus, at the same level, to produce an anal wink or perianal sphincter muscular contraction. This reflex has no significance for prognosis. It does reveal an intact reflex arc and indicates that the conus medullaris portion of the spinal cord contains viable cells that are functioning on both the sensory and motor sides. After 36 hours, the patient's sensory level had ascended from T12 and terminated at the T4 neurodermatomal level. Simultaneously, repeat of the anal portion of the neurologic exam revealed an absence of this previously present bulbocavernosus reflex. The most logical cause in the absence of spinal cord neurologic level trauma was post-traumatic inter-

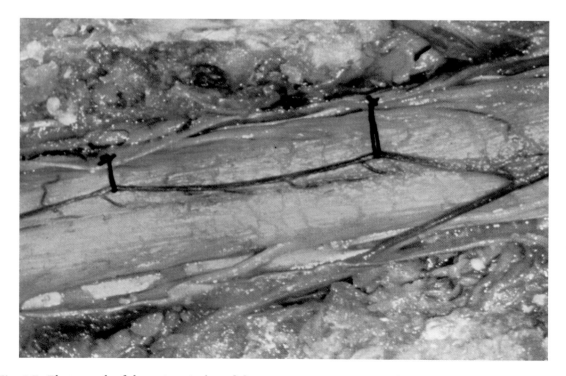

Fig. 4-7. Photograph of thoracic spinal cord demonstrating anterior spinal artery and anterior sulcus perforating arteries. Note scarcity of vessels, which explains the high incidence of complete neurologic injuries in the mid-thoracic spine even with minor injuries. (From Dommisse,[10] with permission.)

ruption of the blood supply to the thoracic spinal cord.

Because of the variations in its anatomic occurrence, the artery of Adamkiewicz cannot always be the accused structure, but it is a very likely candidate. Dichiro et al.[19] noted in rhesus monkeys no decrease in lower spinal cord function with ligation of the vessel of Adamkiewicz, but they did consistently find that ligation of the anterior sulcus artery below the entrance of the vessel of Adamkiewicz caused paraplegia. This evidence does substantiate the concern for the presence of a watershed blood supply within the thoracic spinal cord. It is also recognized by Dommisse[7,10] that the blood supply to the thoracic cord between T4 and T9–10, and occasionally T11, is the poorest, with the fewest in number and the smallest in diametric size of perforating arteries into the central sulcus from the anterior spinal artery (Fig. 4-7). This condition coincides with the least volumetric space in the spinal canal, the area from T4 to T9, T10, T11. This zone has been labeled the critical vascular zone of the spinal cord.

Dommisse's anatomic review of the vascular supply of the total spinal cord, in particular, the thoracic portion, revealed the following salient ele-

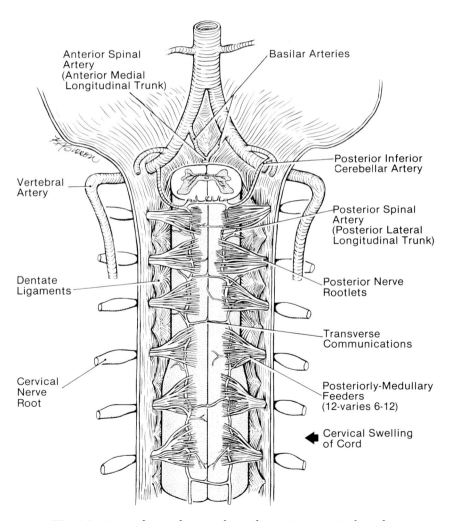

Fig. 4-8. Arterial vascular supply to the posterior spinal cord.

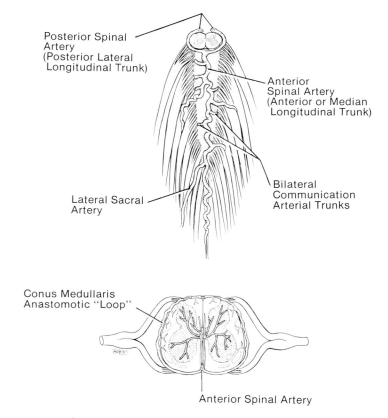

Posterior Spinal
Artery
(Posterior Lateral
Longitudinal Trunk)

Anterior
Spinal Artery
(Anterior or Median
Longitudinal Trunk)

Lateral Sacral
Artery

Bilateral
Communication
Arterial Trunks

Conus Medullaris
Anastomotic "Loop"

Anterior Spinal Artery

Fig. 4-9. Arterial vascular supply to the anterior aspect of the conus medullaris.

ments. There are two rings of circulation (Figs. 4-8, 4-9), the inner arterial circle, composed of the three longitudinal arterial channels (an anterior median longitudinal trunk (anterior spinal artery) and two posterior lateral trunks [posterior spinal arteries], and the outer arterial circle (Fig. 4-10) in the extradural space and in the extravertebral tissue planes. The outer arterial circle has an abundance of anastomoses, which are lacking in the inner circle. These anastomoses vary, however, and are found at irregular levels. Although this abundance is recognizable, the outer arterial circle can only support or supplement the inner circle through the existing outlet points — the perforating sulcal arteries and pial arteries to the cord. It is important to repeat the statement of Woollam and Millen, "man has just as much nervous system as he can supply with oxygen and no more." [3]

SPINAL CORD VASCULAR SUPPLY

There are numerous reviews of the vascular supply of the spinal cord. Most, in one way or another, substantiate the principal vascular patterns. To bring reason out of variations, two sources on the subject of spinal cord blood supply were selected for scrutiny because of their clarity and consistency. What was also consistent on the part of each of the authors was a lack of understanding as to the reliability of the spinal cord's supplemental sources of secondary blood supply. Each author reports three consistent findings:

The major spinal cord vessels remain the same (i.e., anterior spinal artery; vessel of Adamkiewicz).
The cervical and lumbar enlargements of the spinal

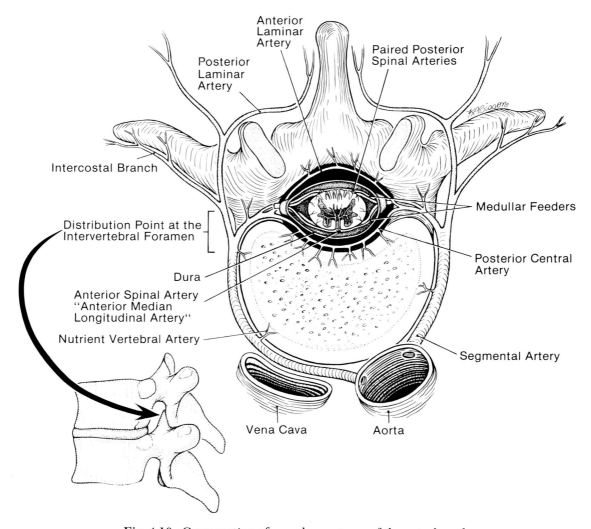

Fig. 4-10. Cross section of vascular anatomy of the spinal cord.

cord have a very rich blood supply. Despite this, the clinical question remains why there is such a high incidence of irreversible clinical neurologic injury.)

The thoracic spinal cord has a poorer blood supply from T4 to T9.

It is interesting to note that the variations in the spinal cord size follow the size of the spinal canal closely and, like the cervical spinal cord, vary from cephalad to caudad. In the upper cervical spine, the canal is quite spacious, particularly at C1 and C2[20] (Fig. 4-10). The anterioposterior cord-to-canal allowance is not great in the mid-cervical spine (0.6 to 0.7 cm), the lateral extension for accommodation of the nerve root is large.[20] The same is true for the lumbar spine. In both areas, the spinal canal demonstrates an enlargement that correlates with the large number of rootlets exiting and entering the spinal cord at these levels. In the thoracic region, there is a marked narrowing of the semielliptical neural canal from T4 to T9. This narrowing coincides with the area of the spinal cord where the blood supply is the poorest and the spinal cord is the smallest. The sacral canal is flat anteriorly to posteriorly, but is very flat and wide to accommodate the roots of the cauda equina.

ARTERIAL VASCULAR SUPPLY: THORACIC AND LUMBAR VERTEBRA

Arbitrarily I select the T12–L1 level of the spinal column as the most representative level for demonstration of the cross-sectional vascular supply to both the vertebral column and the spinal cord because of its size, ease of demonstration, and vascular consistency (Fig. 4-10). The specimen in Figure 4-10 is viewed from above, facing posteriorly from its anterior border.

In front of the thoracolumbar vertebral column lie the two major vessels (on the diagrams to the right, the aorta, *1*, and on the diagrams to the anterior left, the inferior vena cava). Passing posteriorly around the sides of the waist of each vertebral body are segmental arteries, taking their origin from the aorta at each corresponding vertebral level. Although these vessels are known as segmental arteries in the thoracic and lumbar areas, they are also known as the intercostal or lumbar arteries. In reality, the intercostal vessel exits or enters the intervertebral neuroforamen with the corresponding nerve root.

Along the way, the segmental vessels contribute small branches to the vertebral body in the form of nutrient arteries, as well as joining a network of small perivertebral arteries that provide a rich network of anastomosing vessels with the ipsilateral and contralateral sides. As the segmental vessel reaches the point posteriorly in the vicinity of the intervertebral neuroforamen, the vessel trifurcates. This area, as described by Dommisse,[7,10] is the distribution area. The surgeon is reminded that this area is "noxious" because of the potential hazard of injury to that portion of the segmental vessel that will contribute to the vascular support of the spinal cord despite a recognized collateral blood supply to the spinal cord. As the vessel passes into the vertebral foramen, it branches into two circles. The extradural, extravertebral outer circle is composed of the posterior central artery across the posterior surface of the vertebral body, which provides nutrient arteries to the vertebral body and from which metastatic disease to the vertebral processes arise; and the anterior laminar artery along the anterior inside of the lamina, posterior to the spinal cord, which provided nutrient arteries to the

lamina. The inner circle is also divided into two very important vessels. One is the anterior spinal artery, also known as the "anterior median longitudinal artery." A branch from either side joins to form this single vessel. The anterior spinal artery passes into the anterior median sulcus of the spinal cord proper by way of perforating arteries (Fig. 4-10) that not only supply the adjacent pia mater, but also the anterior white matter and all the central gray matter. There is essentially no medullary communication within the substance of the central gray matter between perforating vessels from the anterior and posterior spinal arteries. The other important vessels are the posterior spinal arteries, also known as the "posterolateral longitudinal trunks." The posterior arteries are paired. They supply small perforating arteries to the pia mater and the posterolateral and posterior white matter. Only at the level of the conus medullaris (vertebral bodies T12–L1) is there an obvious connection between the anterior and the two posterior spinal arteries. Here, they form a trident known as the anastomotic loop of the conus medullaris[17] (Fig. 4-9).

Just outside of the intervertebral foramen is the posterior extension of the segmental artery, which passes with the respective nerve root, known as the intercostal or lumbar branch arteries. From this vessel passes a more posterior arterial branch, lying in close proximity to the facet and over the transverse process. This vessel bifurcates into the two terminal arteries, the branch nourishing the muscles (the musculocutaneous artery) and the most posterior branch nourishing the posterior lamina, spinous process, and paraspinous muscles, the posterior laminar artery. As with the other vessels, similar branches arise from each side.

ARTERIAL VASCULAR SUPPLY: CERVICAL SPINAL CORD

The vascular supply to the cervical spinal cord is extremely intricate and represents a vast network of anastomoses from multiple levels and several sources. As one would anticipate, the root lies with the aorta and its major branch on the right, the subclavian artery (Fig. 4-11). Arising from these two vessels are the vertebral arteries, which pass cephalad through the vertebral foramen of the cervical vertebra beginning at C6 and bending around the posterior ring of C1 to enter the cranium via the foramen magnum. Here, over the anterior aspect of the pons, these vessels join to form the basilar artery. From the vertebral vessels distal to the basilar artery two medullar feeders course anteriorly, one from each vertebral artery, and join over the me-

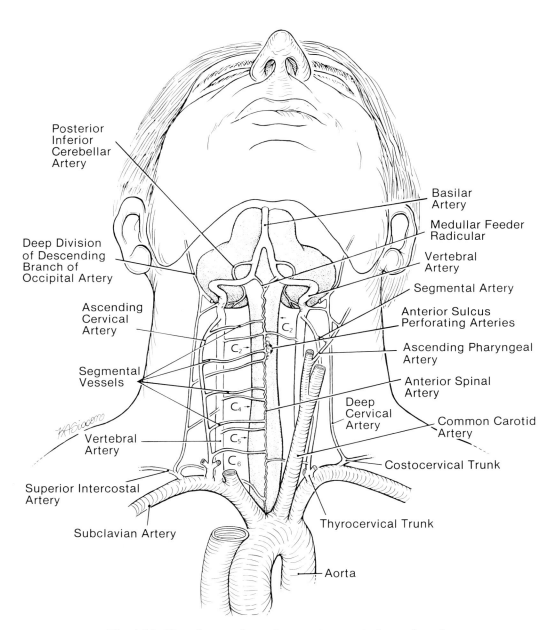

Fig. 4-11. Vascular supply to the anterior cervical spinal cord.

dulla oblongata to form the all-important anterior spinal artery or anterior median longitudinal trunk.

Dommisse prefers to call the two branches from the vertebral arteries the anterior spinal arteries and the vessel formed by their fusion, the *anterior medial longitudinal trunk*.[7,10] For the sake of clarity and uniformity, I will call the primary anterior spinal cord vessel by its popular and most frequently used name, the anterior spinal artery. It is this vessel that henceforth will take the reliably permanent role of providing the major blood supply to the whole of the anterior aspect and central gray matter of the spinal cord throughout its extent, down to the conus medullaris. Although many other vessels send tributaries to the anterior spinal artery at various levels to support its efforts, vascular focus of attention is the anterior spinal artery.

Passing posteriorly around the medulla oblongata on each side are two vessels that also originate from the vertebral arteries, the posterior inferior cerebellar arteries. These vessels will assume the role of primary contributor to the development of two posterior spinal arteries (posterior lateral longitudinal trunk) (Fig. 4-8) to lie one on each side of the posterior spinal cord. Suffice it to say, the posterior spinal cord vascular supply is much less sophisticated and has very few major reliable contributing vessels.

Anteriorly, the other major arterial branches contributing heavily to the cervical spinal cord's vascular supply are the ascending cervical artery arising from the thyrocervical trunk, a branch off the subclavian (primarily on the left), and the deep cervical artery from the costocervical trunk of the subclavian artery.

Providing the interconnection between each of these principal vessels and the anterior spinal artery are medullar feeders or radicular branches. They arise from the vertebral artery on both sides, appearing at various levels, but most constantly at the C2 and C6 levels on the left and the C2, C4, and C5 levels on the right. Although the average number of medullary feeders is around 8, this number varies from 2 to 17. From the ascending cervical artery and the deep cervical artery arise segmental vessels. It is reported in approximately 60 percent of Dommisse's specimens that there existed a contribution of segmental vessels from the ascending

pharyngeal artery, a branch off the external carotid artery.[7,10] In the neck, the vertebral artery provides 80 percent of the medullary or segmental feeders to the anterior spinal artery. The remainder come from the deep cervical and the superior intercostal artery, with occasional support from the ascending cervical artery.

The anterior spinal artery, which lies in the anterior median sulcus of the spinal cord, has many closely located central perforating vessels. On the average, there are 45 of these in the cervical spine (5 to 8 per centimeter); 80 in the thoracic region; 35 in the lumbar region (5 to 12 per centimeter); and 25 in the sacral region. The density is greatest in the cervical and lumbar regions of the spinal cord. In the thoracic spinal cord, these vessels are extremely small. This size accounts for the deficiency in the vascular supply throughout the thoracic spinal cord.

The anterior spinal artery contributes, along the anterior median sulcus, small radicular branches all along the way that nourish the pia mater and the peripheral spinal cord tissue, the white matter. More centrally are the perforating branches, which enter the median sulcus deeply and contribute almost the entire blood supply to the central gray matter. Like the anterior spinal artery, each of the posterior spinal arteries (posterior lateral longitudinal trunk) (Fig. 4-8) contributes to the circulation of the pia mater, but contributes minimally if at all to the circulation of the central gray matter. Again, this configuration explains the almost total dependence of the spinal cord, particularly the thoracic spinal cord, on the anterior spinal artery.

POSTERIOR VASCULAR SUPPLY OF THE SPINAL CORD

For the most part, the posterior spinal cord blood supply is derived from two sources: the right and left branches of the respective vertebral arteries and the posterior inferior cerebellar arteries. Although the branches from the posterior inferior cerebellar arteries bilaterally are consistent in their positions, the *right and left posterior spinal*

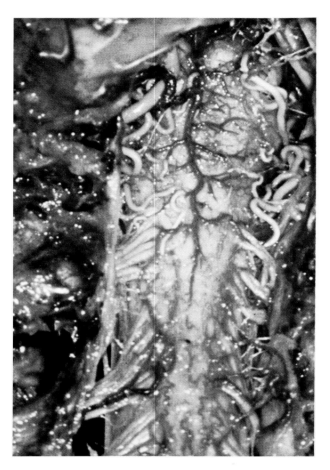

Fig. 4-12. Posterior view of cervical spinal cord showing undisplaced descent of right and left posterior spinal arteries. Note wavy course of vessels in and out of area of posterior cord rootlets. Note also abundant accompanying veins. (From Dommisse,[10] with permission.)

VASCULAR SUPPLY OF THE THORACOLUMBAR AND SACRAL SPINAL CORD

The vascular supply of the spinal cord below the level of the mid- and lower cervical cord is derived from five or six consistent sources: the anterior spinal artery; the two posterior spinal arteries; and a series of vessels described by Dommisse and Lazorthes as intercostal and lumbar segmental vessels (Fig. 4-13).

The *anterior spinal artery* and the *first or superior intercostal artery* arise in the lower cervical spinal cord. The superior intercostal vessel originates from the thoracic aorta and assists in supplying the lowermost cervical region and the upper thoracic spinal cord. Below this level in the thoracic region of the spinal cord, there is a less than uniform entry of from one to five *segmental vessels* (average of two). These vessels arise from corresponding levels of the thoracic aorta. The thoracic cord extends from T2–T3 to T8–T9. Posteriorly, there are even fewer vessels, widely spaced, making this area of the spinal cord very vulnerable to trauma. Further distally and anteriorly arises the artery of Adamkiewicz (correctly described by Lazorthes as the *"magnus ramus radicularis anterior)"* (Fig. 4-3). Though there is great variance in its origin, Dommisse[7,10] and Lazorthes et al.[17] found that this vessel more often arose at the level T9 to T11. Suh and Alexander[21] found the level to be T10 80 percent of the time, whereas Lazorthes et al. noted a 75 percent occurrence varying between T9 and T12, 15 percent between T5 and T8, and 10 percent between L1 and L2. Both author agreed that the blood vessel leaves in company with one of the nerve roots. In those cases in which the vessel arose from a higher level, a supplementary artery arose below (sacral segmental vessels) known as the *arteria conus medullaris*. This latter vessel arises from one of three sources: the lateral sacral vessels, entering with a cauda equina nerve root; L5; or the iliolumbar artery (Fig. 4-3).

At the level of the conus medullaris, or that portion of the spinal cord anatomically located behind the vertebral body of T12–L1, there exists an unusual but constant vascular pattern. Here, with

arteries (posterior lateral longitudinal trunk) are serpentine and weave in and out of the posterior nerve rootlets with little discipline and, therefore, show little regularity as to position (Fig. 4-12). Throughout the spinal cord, but of particular importance in the thoracic region, is the presence of transverse communication vessels. These vessels lend assistance from one side to the other. Also supportive, but in a much more indirect manner, are the extradural space arterials. Some offer alternate pathways to the segmental arteries, from which medullary feeders arise.

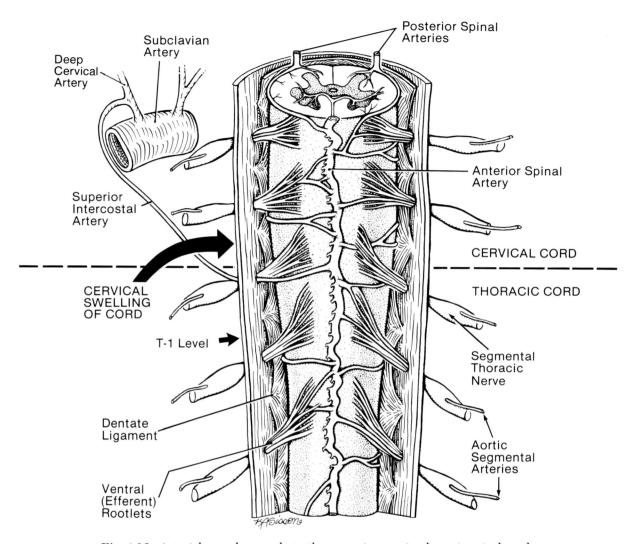

Fig. 4-13. Arterial vascular supply to the posterior cervicothoracic spinal cord.

great uniformity, there occurs a constant trident of anastomotic connections uniting the *anterior spinal artery* with the two *posterior spinal arteries*. The interconnection between the three major vessels is known as the *anastomotic loop of the conus medullaris* (Fig. 4-9). Dommisse noted that the number of *anterior medullary feeder vessels* to the sacral segment of the conus medullaris varied between zero and seven, the average being three, with a preponderance occurring on the left and arising from two sources; *the aortic segmental arteries* at their corresponding level and the *lateral sacral arteries*. Many of the *anterior feeders* come from below the conus, passing upward to join the anterior spinal artery.

Dommisse noted that the *medullary feeders* posterior to the sacral segment of the conus medullaris, number between one and nine.[7,10] The average is four, with a preponderance arising from the right side, similar to the medullary vessels in the thoracic spinal cord.

VENOUS DRAINAGE OF THE SPINAL CORD

Venous drainage of the spine is more difficult to define clearly than the arterial supply because of technical problems related to the dissection and study of the venous system. It is well recognized that the venous system is more haphazard in its pattern and thus highly variable.

Probably the best known work in this area is that performed by O.V. Batson of the University of Pennsylvania.[22,23] Dommisse[10] calls attention to a distinction that must be made between two sets of veins, those of the spinal cord and those that fall under the whole of the plexiform network of Batson. The spinal cord veins are only a small component of the whole and drain into the plexus of Batson.

There are two reasons for reviewing the venous segment of the spinal cord circulation. First, infectious and tumorous metastases to the spine are not uncommon. The more familiar occurrence is the development of a disc space infection in the lumbar region of the vertebral column after manipulation of the genitourinary tract. Although gram-negative bacteria were most commonly suspected as the offending organisms, it has since been noted that gram-positive infections are equally likely. Similarly, metastasis to the spinal column from carcinoma of the prostate occurs often enough that it has been a subject of frequent concern and study. Consequently, the venous drainage of the pelvis has been highly suspected as playing an important role in the spread of disease to the spine. Whether other tumors metastasize to the spinal column in a similar manner is not absolutely known, but because of the extensiveness of the venous network of the vertebral column it is possible. Finally, a review of the venous drainage of the spinal column and spinal cord completes the review of the vascular supply to this area of the neurovertebral complex.

Batson's Plexus

Batson's plexus is a large and complex venous channel. It is the venous system that extends from the basiocciput of the skull to the coccyx at the lower end of the vertebral column. This venous system communicates directly with the superior and inferior vena caval system and the azygos system and forms an integral part of the venous drainage of the brain and the spinal cord (Fig. 4-14).

The longitudinal venous trunks of the spinal cord are the anterior and posterior venous channels, which are counterparts of the arterial trunks (Fig. 4-12). Anteriorly lies a single trunk in the anterior median sulcus, deep to the arterial trunk. Draining into this anterior venous trunk are the central perforating and pial perforating veins along with nu-

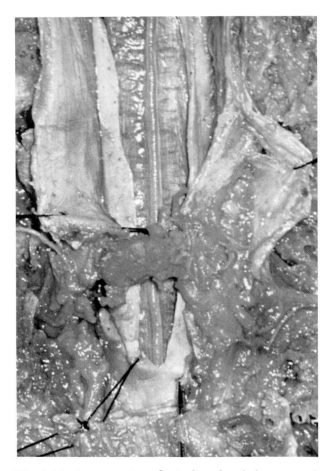

Fig. 4-14. Anterior view of spinal cord with dura incised to reveal the anterior spinal artery. In the middle of the picture over the external surface of the dura there is an extensive venous plexus. (From Dommisse,[10] with permission.)

merous radicular venules at each segment. At the cervical and lumbar enlargements lies a complex system of abundant venous channels resembling arteriovenous malformations. Posteriorly, a single midline trunk may be replaced in whole or in part by duplicated or ramifying vessels. The longitudinal venous trunks of the cord drain into the inner, central portion of Batson's plexus (the extradural vertebral venous plexus that occupies the extradural space of the spinal cord and extends from the basiocciput to the coccyx).

The medullary veins of the spinal cord are the counterpart of the medullary feeder arteries. They accompany the nerve roots in their exit from the dural sac at levels not related to medullary feeder arteries. They are the largest and most consistent at the cervical and lumbar enlargements.

The vertebral venous plexus is the plexus of veins that surrounds the vertebral artery within the transverse foramen of the cervical spine. It communicates with the cervical portion of the extradural plexus at every segmental level. It also communicates with the veins of the neck, both deep and superficial.

VEINS OF THE SPINAL CORD

Abrams[24] described the direction of spinal cord drainage as the "foreign azygos system." It was interpreted that his definition of vertebral veins coincided with those in the spinal theca that drained directly through the vertebral veins into the extradural veins of Batson's plexus. Herlihy,[25] like Suh and Alexander,[21] agreed that the venous system is much greater in volume than the arterial system, that there are often two veins occurring with each artery, and that as a rule, veins are larger than arteries. The implication is the fact that venous outflow is greater than arterial inflow and probably is based on venous reflex. Dommisse[7] disagreed with the view of venous reflux within the spinal medulla for two reasons: medullary veins are not abundant, and the axillary pouches of the dural sac, where veins make their exit with each segmental nerve root, appear to serve the function of a

venous valve. A third factor against venous reflux into the spinal cord is the opinion stated by Stephen and Stillwell[26] that in the brain, and probably the spinal cord, neural tissue metabolic activity is high and oxygen consumption is approximately ten times greater than that of any other area in the basal state. Thus, the circulating blood volume is proportional to demand, allowing no room for storage of venous blood in either the brain or the spinal cord.

VENOUS PLEXUS OF BATSON

Batson[22] demonstrated the spread of metastatic emboli from the pelvis to the brain via the extradural vertebral veins. He noted that these veins had connections with the veins in the spinal canal; around the spinal column, and within the bones of the column. His proof of this intricate interconnection was the injection of a radiopaque material into the dorsal vein of the penis of an adult cadaver. The material bypassed the inferior vena cava and reached the base of the skull and cranial cavity by way of the veins about the dura, as well as those in and around the vertebrae. This study completed a composite picture of the metastatic pattern of carcinomatosis in the prostate. He was also able to demonstrate the passage from breast to brain via the venous channels of the vertebral column, as well as the direction of blood flow and the potential for blood-borne spread of metastatic emboli by way of the venous plexus. He also revealed a reversal in flow from the brain distally. Batson's conclusion was that the vena cava offered normal drainage under conditions of trunk muscle inactivity, whereas the vertebral system was responsible for some of the drainage under conditions of increased intra-abdominal pressure as in coughing or straining. The three components of Batson's plexus are the extradural vertebral venous plexus; the extravertebral venous plexus that includes the segmental veins of the neck, the intercostal veins, the azygos communications in the thorax and pelvis, the lumbar veins, and the communications with the inferior vena cava system; and the veins of the bony structures of the spinal column.

Herlihy,[25] in summary, described the functions of the vertebral venous plexus as follows:

A storehouse of blood via dilations

A pool for receiving backflow from adjacent veins and anastomoses

Redistribution of blood from other parts with the backflow from other regions accommodated in its immensity — "It reminds us of the invaders of China, who were absorbed until they themselves became Chinese!"

Unequal pressure in adjacent veins is quickly equalized

The system has no inherent pressure, hence it is a pressure absorber

The system has no direction of flow, thus making possible quick adjustment and accommodation to a sudden inrush of blood

Both Batson and Herlihy, according to Dommisse,[10] conclude: "We have a vast system of veins which, on the grounds of anatomic injections, animal experiments and simple logic, is constantly and physiologically the site of frequent reversals of flow." During these reversals, a pathway exits up and down the spinal column that does not involve the heart or lungs. Dommisse reminds us that these comments are only applicable to the plexiform network around the vertebral column; the spinal cord veins as such do not have such a capacity.[7,10]

CONCLUSION

The spinal cord, like the brain and the heart, is totally dependent on an ever present intact vascular system. Any interruption in the vascular supply results in neurologic injury to the area of ischemia. The extent of damage depends on the extent and length of time the tissues are compromised. Allen[1] demonstrated that direct injury to the spinal cord resulting in hemorrhage and edema in the area of the central gray matter caused within 4 hours an expansion of the hemorrhagic process outward to the peripheral white matter to the pia mater. After this elapsed time period, irreversible neurologic tissue changes occurred. From this early neuropathology research came the first indications of the pathologic process that follows direct trauma to the spinal cord as well as the optimum period of time for possible intervention.

The two principal vascular structures providing the primary blood supply for the whole of the spinal cord are the *anterior spinal artery*[7,10] and the *vessel of Adamkiewicz.*[7,10,11] The anterior spinal artery is a singular vascular structure, lying in the anterior median (Fig. 4-13) sulcus of the anterior spinal cord. The vessel originates in the calvaria, being derived from the (posterior) basilar artery and vertebral artery portion of the midbrain circulation. From the union of these three vessels comes the anterior spinal artery. Once the vessel reaches the mid-portion of the cervical spinal cord, its source of blood is derived from several vascular sources, including the vertebral arteries (primarily on the right), the ascending cervical artery from the thyrocervical trunk, the deep cervical artery from the costocervical trunk, and from the area of the first rib, the first intercostal artery (a segmental artery arising from the thoracic aorta). Thus, the anterior spinal artery actually is the primary vascular structure supplying the whole of the cervical (central gray matter) spinal cord. To a much lesser degree, the peripheral white matter of the cervical spinal cord is supplied by the two *posterior spinal arteries*, derived superiorly at the level of the brain stem from the posterior communicating arteries arising from the posterior cerebellar arteries in the area of the medulla (Fig. 4-13). As these vessels descend on the posterior surface of the cervical spinal cord, they too receive segmental support from collateral arterioles at various levels, but on a much less consistent basis than the anterior vessels. Thus, the *anterior spinal artery* is the principal blood vessel from the medulla to the spinal level of C7–T1.

Beginning at the level of T1, while the *anterior spinal artery* is still the single identifiable anterior vascular structure, the source of the blood supply within this structure changes. Beginning with the *superior (or first) intercostal artery*, a segmental branch off the thoracic aorta, along with the watershed blood supply derived from the upward flow from the *vessel of Adamkiewicz* (which enters and joins the *anterior spinal artery system* at the level of T10 to L2), the whole of the thoracic and lumbar-conus medullaris-cauda equina portions of the spinal cord is supplied. The lower the entry of the *vessel of Adamkiewicz*, the more its origin will differ. If the vessel enters at T10, it will be a segmental branch off the thoracic aorta. If it enters at L2, it is a branch off of the abdominal aorta or may be derived from one of the vessels entering with a cauda equina (sacral) rootlet and thus a sacral arterial vessel derived from the pelvis.

The venous system is complicated, inconsistent, and vastly more abundant than the arterial system. It plays no major or specific role in the metabolism of the spinal cord. It does provide for a high vascular turnover and thus has a major role in the venous drainage of the spinal cord, the spinal column, and

the pelvis, and it communicates directly with the venous sustem draining the head, chest, and abdomen. It is this interconnection that allows for the metastatic spread of disease or infection from the pelvis to the calvaria, or from the chest to the vertebral column, etc.[22-26]

Appreciating the origin of the spinal cord vasculature does not, by itself, offer clinical assistance in the management of spinal column or spinal cord injuries. It does provide an appreciation of the origin of the vessels that contribute to the health and survival of the spinal cord and provides an awareness of the crucial areas of the vertebral column that require special precaution or attention. It may

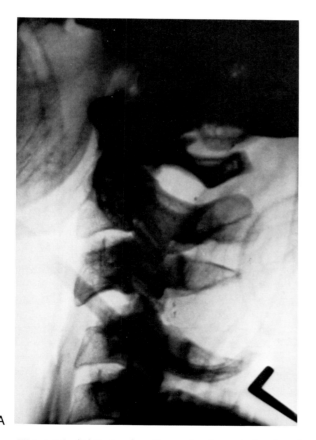
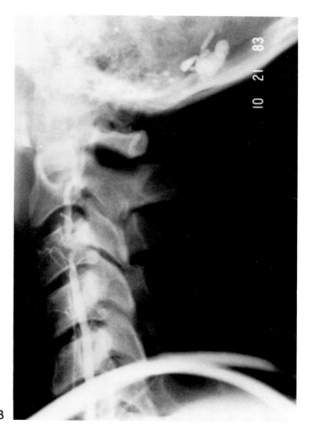

Fig. 4-15. (A) Lateral radiograph of cervical spine demonstrating unilateral facet dislocation and forward subluxation of C3 and C4. Note diastasis between posterior elements of C3 and C4, forward luxation of vertebral body of C3 and C4 (20 percent), and perched facets. (B) Lateral radiograph after reduction. Note arteriogram demonstrating injury to vertebral artery at level of previous dislocation. Patient demonstrated hemiplegic signs secondary to this vascular injury, in addition to neurologic changes secondary to the unilateral facet dislocation.

also explain the appearance of unusual post-traumatic or nontraumatic neurologic patterns. An excellent example of the latter was the appearance of hemiplegia with facial changes (secondary to occlusion of one vertebral artery) in a patient who sustained a unilateral facet dislocation) (Fig. 4-15A). Injury to the vertebral artery was confirmed by arteriogram (Fig. 4-15B). As noted earlier, a second patient, admitted with an hour of injury, demonstrated a compression fracture of the vertebral body (without spinal canal occlusion) at T11. Over the ensuing 36 hours after injury, the neurologic level gradually ascended to the watershed level of T4. A myelogram revealed no obstruction of contrast flow past T11 or any pathologic condition along the entire thoracic spinal column. The explanation was injury to the vessel of Adamkiewicz at its entry point into the neural canal, via the neuroforamen, at the level of either T10–T11 or T11–T12.

REFERENCES

1. Allen AR: Surgery of experimental lesions of spinal cord equivalent to crush injury of fracture dislocation of spinal column. JAMA 57:878, 1911
2. Feeney JF, Watterson RL: The development of the vascular pattern within the walls of the central nervous system of the chick embryo. J Morphol 78:231, 1946
3. Woolam DHM, Millen JW: In discussion on the vascular disease of the spinal cord. Proc R Soc Med 51:540, 1958
4. Meyer PR: Complications of fractures and dislocations of the spine: dorsolumbar spine. In Epps JB (ed): Complications in Orthopaedic Surgery. JB Lippincott, Philadelphia, 1978
5. Schneider RC: Transposition of compressed spinal cord in kyphoscoliosis patients with neurologic deficits. With special reference to vascular supply of the cord. J Bone Joint Surg 42A:1027, 1960
6. White AA, and Panjabi MM: Functional spinal unit and mathematical models. In: Clinical Biomechanics of the Spine. JB Lippincott, Philadelphia, 1978
7. Dommisse GF: The blood supply of the spinal cord. J Bone Joint Surg 56B:225, 1974
8. Winter RB: Congenital kyphoscoliosis with paralysis following hemivertebra excision. Clin Orthop 119:116–125, 1976
9. Dwyer AF, Schafer MF: Anterior approach to scoliosis. J Bone Joint Surg 56B:218, 1974
10. Dommisse GF: The Arteries and Veins of the Human Spinal Cord from Birth. Churchill Livingstone, New York, 1975
11. Adamkiewicz A: Die Blutgefasse des Menschlichen Ruckenmarkes, IL Teil. Die Gefasse der Ruckenmarkoberflache. SB Heidelberg Akad Wiss 85:101, 1882
12. Stagnara P: Scoliosis in adults: surgical treatment of severe forms. Excerpta Medica Foundation International Congress Series no. 192, 1969
13. Stagnara P, Fleury D, Pauchet R, et al; Scolioses majeures de l'adulte superieures a 100°—183 castraites chirurgicalement. Rev Chir Orthop 61:101, 1975
14. Holdsworth FW: Fracture-dislocation and fracture-dislocations of the spine. J Bone Joint Surg 52A:534, 1970
15. Bergan JJ: Vascular Surgery, Department of Surgery, Northwestern University Medical School, personal conversation
16. Thorek P: Anatomy in Surgery. p. 616. JB Lippincott, Philadelphia, 1955
17. Lazorthes G, Gouaze A, Zadeh JO, et al: Arterial vascularization of the spinal cord. J Neurosurg 35:253, 1971
18. Braakman R, Vinken PJ: Unilateral facet interlocking in the lower cervical spine. J Bone Joint Surg 49B:2, 1967
19. Dichiro G, Fried LC Doppman JL: Experimental spinal cord angiography. Br J Radiol 43:19, 1970
20. Lusted LB, Keats TE: Atlas of Roentgenographic Measurement. 4th Ed. p. 123. Year Book Medical Publishers, Chicago, 1978
21. Suh TH, Alexander L: Vascular system of the human spinal cord. Arch Neurol Psychiatry 41:659, 1939
22. Batson OV: The function of the vertebral veins and their role in the spread of metasteses. Ann Surg 112:138, 1940
23. Batson, OV: The vertebral vein system as a mechanism for the spread of metastesis. Am J Roentgenol Radium Ther 48:715, 1942
24. Abrams HL: The vertebral and azygos venous system, and some variations in systemic venous return. Radiology 69:508, 1957
25. Herlihy WF: Revision of venous system: the role of the vertebral veins. Med J Aust 22:661, 1947
26. Stephen RB, Stillwell DL: Arteries and Veins of the Human Brain. Charles C Thomas, Springfield, IL, 1969

5

Neuroanatomy

Paul R. Meyer, Jr.

To fully discuss and describe the nervous system would require a separate text, and yet, not to review this segment of the human system would be unfortunate omission. Thus, an overview of the neuroanatomic system must suffice.

The influence and effect of the nervous system become readily apparent when one examines the acutely injured spinal cord victim. It is easy to recognize and map the affected area of objective motor loss, but it is more difficult to describe the extent and the effect of the loss of the subjective sensory function. Then there is that segment of the nervous system that seemingly functions on its own, self-starting, self-stopping, and revealing an inherent reflex activity. This is the autonomic nervous system, composed of the sympathetic and parasympathetic systems. Although in the intact nervous system this visceral efferent and afferent system appears to operate independently, actually it does not. Rather, it is significantly influenced by the efferent corticobulbar and corticospinal (motor) system and the efferent superficial and deep tactile (sensory) system. The result to the spinal cord-injured patient is altered neurologic reflex patterns that affect the heart, the blood vessels (see Ch. 4), and the pulmonary system (see Ch. 9).

NEUROLOGIC PATTERNS

The mechanism of injury to the spinal cord varies widely, as may the extent of the injury. The determinant appears to be the force of energy dissipated across the spinal column and spinal cord and the effects of that force on the neural tissue which result in spinal cord contusion, compression, or laceration. Although complete anatomic severance or break in spinal cord continuity (anatomic transection regardless of the etiology) is rare, complete loss of neurologic function, on the other hand, is not. More often, a severe injury to the spinal cord results in a *functional* neurologic transection. The effects are the same — complete loss of efferent (cranial-to-caudal direction) motor function below the level of spinal cord injury (Fig. 5-1) and complete loss of afferent (caudal-to-cranial direction) sensory function from the most distal portion of the body upward to the neurologic level of the spinal cord injury. Any lesser injury (not a complete injury) is classified as an incomplete injury.

NEUROLOGIC ANATOMY

Motor Function

The two areas of the central nervous system that contain "motor" cells and fibers are the cerebral cortex and the spinal cord. The pathways through both areas are described.

First, pyramidal fibers, originating from Betz cells (Fig. 5-1K; see also Fig. 5-5A) within the motor cortex, comprise the cerebral cortex "motor strip" (Fig. 5-1K). This area lies along the lateral plane of the cerebral cortex, just anterior to the posterior central gyrus (see Fig. 5-6), and includes the superior, medial, and inferior portions of the anterior central gyrus (Fig. 5-1K). Highest and

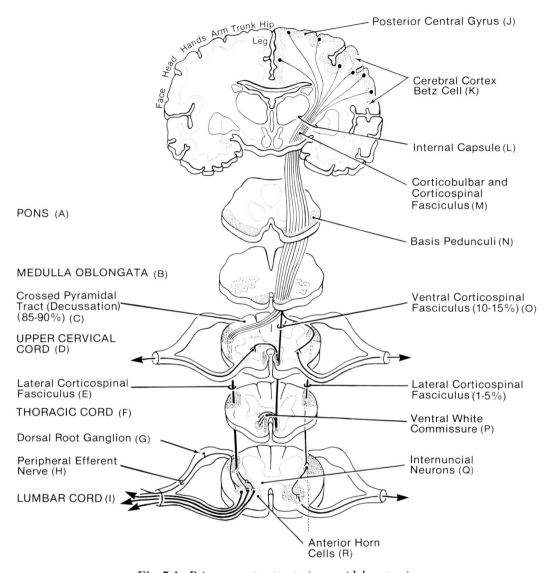

Face Head Hands Arm Trunk Hip Leg

Posterior Central Gyrus (J)

Cerebral Cortex Betz Cell (K)

Internal Capsule (L)

Corticobulbar and Corticospinal Fasciculus (M)

PONS (A)

Basis Pedunculi (N)

MEDULLA OBLONGATA (B)

Crossed Pyramidal Tract (Decussation) (85-90%) (C)

Ventral Corticospinal Fasciculus (10-15%) (O)

UPPER CERVICAL CORD (D)

Lateral Corticospinal Fasciculus (E)

Lateral Corticospinal Fasciculus (1-5%)

THORACIC CORD (F)

Ventral White Commissure (P)

Dorsal Root Ganglion (G)

Peripheral Efferent Nerve (H)

Internuncial Neurons (Q)

LUMBAR CORD (I)

Anterior Horn Cells (R)

Fig. 5-1. Primary motor tracts (pyramidal system).

closet to the posterior central gyrus of the motor cortex, and overlapping into the space along the hemispheric sagittal sinus, is the area representing the foot, leg, and adjacent regions (see Fig. 5-7). Slightly more inferior, along the outer hemispheric cortex, lies the arm region of the motor cortex. Further inferior and lateral lie the regions representing the head. From this same area arise the corticobulbar (respiratory motor function) and corticospinal fasciculus motor tracts (Fig. 5-1M), which course distally through the internal capsule

of the brain (Fig. 5-1M; see also Fig. 5-5F), just lateral to the thalmus, where fibers to the lower extremity, trunk, and upper extremities combine to form a corticospinal tract (Fig. 5-1L). From here they enter the crus cerebri, through the basi pedunculi to the next lower brain level, the anterior lateral aspect of the midbrain or mesencephalon (Fig. 5-5F). From there the fibers spread out again, enter the mid-anterior portion of the pons (Fig. 5-1A), and then reach the most anterior portion of the medulla oblongata (Fig. 5-1N) and the upper cervical spinal cord (Fig. 5-1D), to form respective crossed pyramidal tracts (Fig. 5-1B, C), known as the "pyramid."

The second area to be considered is the separation of the corticospinal fasciculus into three bundles at the lower level of the medulla oblongata (Fig. 5-1C). At this point, fibers of the corticospinal tract begin their crossover, or decussation. An estimated 85 to 90 percent of the fibers decussate, to descend as the lateral corticospinal fasciculus (crossed pyramidal tract) of the spinal cord (Fig. 5-1E). A small number of fibers from the lateral corticospinal fasciculus do not decussate but descend into the lateral corticospinal tract of the same side (Fig. 5-1). The third group of fibers, 10 to 15 percent, continue distally on the same side (Fig. 5-1O) in the vicinity of the ventromedian fissue (Fig. 5-1Q) as the ventral corticospinal fasciculus (also known as the direct pyramidal tract). Interestingly, the fibers in this bundle continually cross to the opposite side via the ventral white commissure. Having reached the segmental mid-portion of the thoracic spinal cord, this unilateral ventral tract (having completely crossed) disappears[1] (Fig. 5-1Q).

Generally, cortical pyramidal tract connections are unilateral and crossed, but exceptions to this rule exist. Double innervation exists for muscles of the eye, the muscles of the upper face (frontalis and orbicularis oculi), the muscles of mastication and deglution (except the tongue), and the muscles of the larynx, the sternomastoid, the upper trapezius, and the diaphragm. There may be sufficient bilateral innervation to prevent noticeable paralysis after a unilateral upper motor neuron lesion. Similarly, trunk muscles may reveal only slight neuromuscular involvement because of this dual innervation. The percentages of corticospinal fibers ending at different levels are estimated at 55 percent in the cervical segments, 20 percent in the throacic spinal segments, and 25 percent in the lumbosacral spinal segments.[2]

Sensory Function

The more easily defined and traced portions of neurologic anatomy, as well as those more relevant to spinal cord injury, are pain, temperature, and light touch (Fig. 5-2) via the lateral spinal thalamic tracts, and deep sensibility or proprioception and tactile discrimination (Fig. 5-3) via the dorsal columns of the spinal cord.

Sensory afferent pathways begin in the periphery of the extremity at the site of stimulation (see Fig. 5-2P). This is true regardless of the type of stimulus or the distribution represented. Therefore, for discussion purposes, both pain and temperature and touch and proprioception originate caudally and pass through the nervous system via separate posterior and posteriorlateral tracts, decussating at the level of entry to the spinal cord (Fig. 5-2G), and passing by way of the thalamus to terminate in the cerebral cortex in specific areas of the postcentral gyrus (Fig. 5-2C), depending on the site of origin of the stimulus.

Pain, Temperature, and Light Touch

Stimuli for pain, temperature, and light touch (Fig. 5-2) enter the nervous system via superficial sensory end organs, from which they pass through the afferent portion of mixed peripheral (sensory [afferent]-motor [efferent]) nerves to enter the lateral division of the dorsal roots of spinal nerves at specific neurologic levels commensurate with the site of origin of the stimulus. From here, stimuli progress via two pathways. Fibers of the first order enter the dorsolateral fasciculus of Lissauer (Fig. 5-2N) in which they ascend to synapse on the same side at a higher level at the tip of the dorsal central gray matter (known as the substantia gelatinosa of Rolandi). There they may progress cephalad by decussating at the level of the medulla oblongata and pons in the medial lemniscus, and, further, to the general somatesthetic sensory center of the cerebral cortex via the medial lemniscus of the mesencephalon (midbrain) and the posterolateral portion of the ventral nucleus of the thalamus.

Fibers of the second order (Fig. 5-2O), most of which reach the dorsal tip of the central gray matter (substantia gelatinosa of Rolandi) (Fig. 5-2F), cross rapidly at that same level through the ventral commissure (Fig. 5-2G) to the opposite lateral funiculus, in which they ascend, forming the lateral spinothalamic fasciculus (Fig. 5-2H). As the lateral spinothalamic fasciculus passes upward, it grows by the addition of fibers to its ventromedial border. Thus, at each given level, fibers from the lower

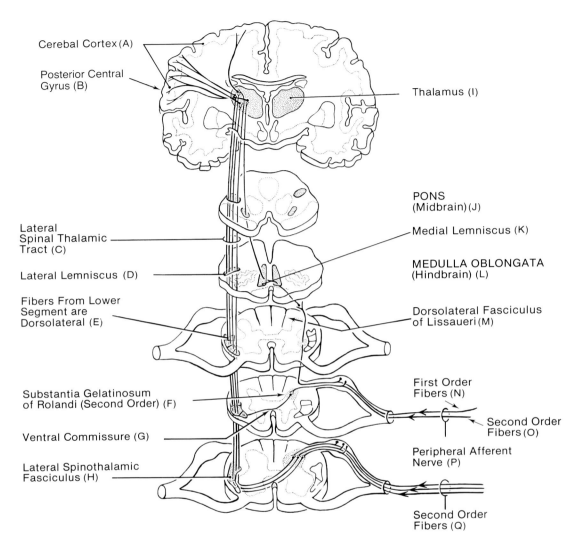

Fig. 5-2. Pain, temperature, and light touch.

segments of the spinal cord are mostly dorsolateral. This characteristic accounts for the sacral symptoms that result from the more superficial involvement of the lateral funiculus at even higher levels of the cord. As the fibers ascend through the lateral spinothalamic tract (Fig. 5-2C), they enter the spinal lemniscus (Fig. 5-2D) of the medulla oblongata (Fig. 5-2L), pons (Fig. 5-2J), or midbrain, passing through and synapsing in the thalamus (Fig. 5-2I). They finally end in the somatesthetic sensory center of the cerebral cortex (Fig. 5-2B).

Neuroanatomists generally agree that minor variations may exist in the ascension of these fibers. Likewise, it is generally believed that the fibers of pain and temperature sensitivity are greatly mixed with each other. Many neurologist regard the spinal thalamic tract as a pathway for pain and temperature and direct light touch (Fig. 5-3J) (to include discriminative touch), which is conducted upward through the posterior funiculus (Fig. 5-3K) by neurons of the first order, synapsing in the nucleus gracilis and cuneatus (Fig. 5-3I) at the level of the

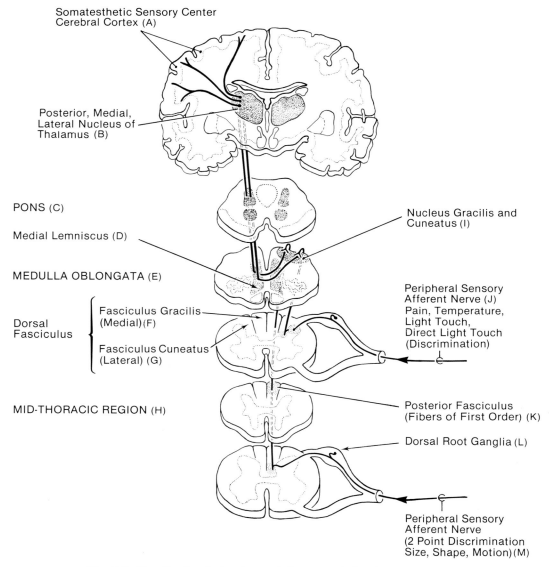

Fig. 5-3. Tactile discrimination and deep sensibility (proprioception).

medulla oblongata (Fig. 5-3E) upon which fibers decussate to the medial lemniscus (Fig. 5-3D) of the opposite side at the same level. From here, the ascension continues via the medial lemniscus of the pons (Fig. 5-3C) and midbrain to the posteromedial and lateral nucleus of the thalamus (Fig. 5-3B), the site of the another synapse and final ascension to the somatesthetic sensory center of the cerebral cortex (Fig. 5-3A).

Tactile Discrimination and Deep Sensibility

That portion of the spinal cord that provides awareness of passive movement, position in space of various segments of the body, two-point discrimination, awareness of size, shape, surface texture, and stereognosis is the dorsal columns (Fig. 5-3M). This dorsally and centrally located area lying between the two posterior horns of the central gray matter is divided bilaterally into two sections, the fasciculus gracilis medially and the fasciculus cuneatus laterally, which together form the dorsal funiculus (Fig. 5-3F). Extending cephalad from the cervical spinal cord into the medulla oblongata (myelencephalon) are the nuclei of the fasciculi gracilis and cuneatus (Fig. 5-3I). Stimuli entering the peripheral nervous system from the deeper portions of the body wall, the muscles, tendons, ligaments, joints, and bones enter the dorsal rami of the root corresponding to the level of the spinal cord to which larger afferent fibers innervate, arising from the large cells of the dorsal root ganglia.

On entering the spinal cord, the ascending branches form the dorsal funiculus (Fig. 5-3F,G). Fibers from the lower spinal nerves are more medial and those from higher levels are more lateral. Actually, fibers entering the spinal cord below the midthoracic segment lie in the fasciculus gracilis and fibers entering above this level lie in the fasciculus cuneatus. Thus, the fasciculus cuneatus does not exist below the midthoracic spinal cord.

The ascending branches of the first-order neurons reach the medulla oblongata, terminating in the nucleus gracilis and cuneatus (Fig. 5-3I). Second-order neurons give origin to the internal fibers, most of which ascend via the medial lemniscus of the opposite side, terminating or synapsing in the posterolateral portion of the ventral nucleus of the thalamus (Fig. 5-3B). From here, fibers pass cephalad to the appropriate representative sensory centers of cerebral cortex. (Fig. 5-3A).

RESPIRATORY SYSTEM

Owing to reflex and referred sensations established by the respiratory organs, both afferent and efferent pathways play a role in this visceral system's innervation.[1] The afferent nerve from the lung parenchyma is principally derived from the vagus, or 10th cranial nerve (Fig. 5-4C). Stimuli arrive from the periphery (the hilus of the lung, the bronchi, trachea, and larynx; Fig. 5-4A) to the fasciculus solitarius in the brain stem portion of the spinal cord (Fig. 5-4M). From here, fibers go im-

mediately to the primary respiratory center (expiratory and inspiratory) in the medulla oblongata (Fig. 5-4L). Here, the secondary respiratory centers from the telencephalon and the upper lateral portion of the pons also discharge into the chief respiratory center. In turn, fibers are distributed to the efferent neurons that innervate the respiratory muscles, such as the diaphragm (C3, C4, and C5 nerve roots) (Fig. 5-4I), the scaleni (Fig. 5-4D), and the abdominals (Fig. 5-4H). Some afferent fibers, principally from the pleura and the hilus of the lung, enter the upper five thoracic nerves (Fig. 5-4B). Whether they enter via the vagus (Fig. 5-4C) or the spinal nerves (Fig. 5-4B) these fibers represent a special interconnection between the upper spinal cord segments.[1] Frequently, with certain diseases of the lung, tone increases in the sternomastoid and trapezius muscles secondary to reflexes passing out through the spinal accessory nerve (11th cranial nerve) (Fig. 5-4D) and phrenic nerve (Fig. 5-4I) to the diaphragm on the same side.

Rasmussen believed that the phrenic nerve, the primary nerve of respiration, arises from the fourth cervical nerve principally, but also from C3 and C5 (Fig. 5-4G), known as the accessory phrenic.[1] He states that accessory phrenics join the main trunk of the phrenic as low as the hilus of the lung. The phrenic nerve is the sole motor supply to the muscle of the diaphragm. The sensory areas of the diaphragm originate from two sources, in the central and posterior regions by fibers from the phrenic nerve (Fig. 5-4B) and anteriorly and laterally by afferent fibers from the lower six thoracic intercostal nerves (Fig. 5-4K). This dual innervation is due to the dual embryonic origin of the respective parts of the diaphragm. The nerve supply to the center portion of the diaphragm arises from the cervical region because as the septum transversum descends through the chest (Fig. 5-4B) it carries its nerve supply with it. The peripheral portion arises from the pleuroperitoneal membranes, and the mesentery portion from the thoracoabdominal region (Fig. 5-4K). As a result, when the central portion of the diaphragm is irritated, pain is felt over the trapezius region (Fig. 5-4H), the surface dermatome of the fourth cervical cutaneous nerve branches. Also, when the margins of the diaphragm are diseased, radicular pain travels over the cutane-

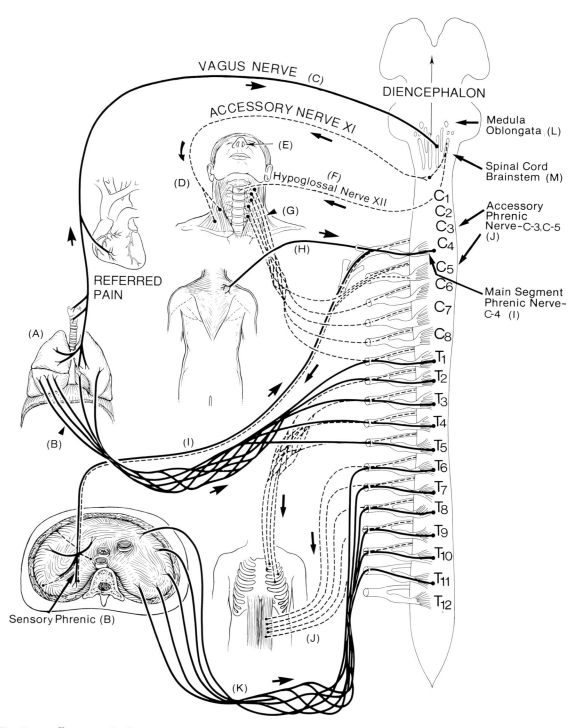

Fig. 5-4. Afferent and efferent innervation of the organs of respiration. Solid lines show afferent (sensory) nerves; broken lines show efferent (motor) nerves.

ous branches of the lower six thoracic nerves and is felt in the lower chest and abdomen. Therefore, the visceral and cutaneous areas are interconnected via afferent fibers having the same spinal cord representation.

Other Clinical Aspects of Neurologic Involvement of Respiration

Paralysis of the intercostal muscles causes compensatory or reflex hyperactivity of the accessory muscles of respiration (Fig. 5-4D,G): the scalenus muscles (C3 to C5), the sternocleidomastoid muscles (C1 to C3), the platysma, the omohyoid (C2 to C3), the sternohyoid (12th cranial nerve and C1 to C4), the levator scapulae (C3 to C5), and the trapezius (11th cranial nerve to C3 and C4) muscles, along with the submental muscles.[3] They serve to stabilize the hyoid bone both upward and anteriorly, allowing the deeper infrahyoid and cervical muscles, along with the more superficial occiput and mental attached muscles, to both stabilize and elevate the upper chest (ribs 1 and 2 and the clavicle) during the simultaneous downward motion of the diaphragm during contraction (inspiration). Two other muscles that contribute to this altered inspiratory effort are the ala nasi muscles of the nose (7th cranial nerve), which hold open the nares, and the vocal cords (12th cranial nerve) (Fig. 5-4F), which allow air to enter the trachea during inspiration. If there is evidence of direct trauma to the anterior neck, attention should be focused on the larynx. Occasionally, the effect of trauma to the larynx, upper trachea, or vocal cords may be subtle and not apparent. However, the injury is evidenced over time by the victim's increasing respiratory effort, which develops into laryngeal stridor and crowing during inspiration. Simultaneously, arterial blood gas ratios will worsen, reflecting deterioration of the respiratory mechanisms. Arterial blood gas values are an important early determinant of injury when other components appear stable and the specific injury has not yet become apparent (see Ch. 9).

Likewise, subclinical evidence of injury to the trachea and esophagus must be considered. With either respiratory mechanism, the anteroposterior

(AP) chest film will show a widening of the mediastinal shadow. Injury to the mediastinal great vessels (aorta or superior vena cava) can also be evidenced by such a widening.

THORACOLUMBAR VISCERAL EFFERENT SYSTEM: SYMPATHETIC AUTONOMIC SYSTEM

Neurologically Altered Vital Signs

Trauma to the cervical and upper thoracic spinal cord resulting in complete neurologic injury disengages the intact proximal central nervous system from the spinal cord below the lesion. The result is a loss of sympathetic motor control to the heart and to the peripheral vascular system.

Loss of Sympathetic Nervous System Function

The loss of the sympathetic nervous system produces a loss in acceleratory influences to the heart and a loss of motor innervation to the peripheral apocrine (sweat) glands. The consequences of this disengagement of the sympathetic nervous system are (1) peripheral vasodilation below the level of the lesion, resulting in venous dilation (producing hypotension); (2) slowing of the heart rate resulting from the loss of the sympathetics (acceleration stimulation) to the heart and an unbalanced vagal nerve (10th cranial nerve) suppression of the heart rate (producing bradycardia); and (3) a loss of body heat regulation below the level of the neurologic lesion due to sympathetic (motor) denervation of the apocrine (sweat) glands. The outcome is inability to perspire and a consequent loss of temperature control. If this physiological event begins shortly after injury, it is due to traumatic sympathetic interruption, and is accompanied by peripheral vascular dilation. Thus, body heat is lost secondary to heat radiation from the dilated superficial vessels (hypothermia). Later, as the peripheral vascular system re-establishes a reflex tone, conservation of body heat resumes, but because autonomic compensation cannot occur via

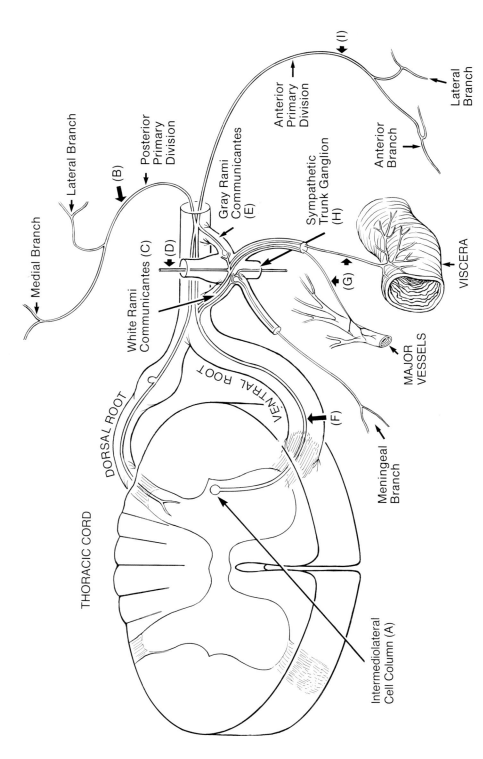

Fig. 5-5. Schematic representation of the thoracic sympathetic nervous system, its motor influence over various organ systems by way of interconnections between the gray and white rami communicantes, and the sensory afferents returning to the dorsal column of the spinal cord by way of a segmental dorsal sensory root.

controlled perspiration, hyperthermia occurs, and compensation (through perspiration) is absent.

The mechanism of this post-traumatic sympathetic nervous system injury triad, which culminates in hypotension, bradycardia, and hypothermia, is a preganglionic fiber injury. Preganglionic fibers (white rami communicantes) (Fig. 5-5C) arise from the intermediolateral cell column (Fig. 5-5A) in the lateral horn of the central gray matter of the entire thoracic and upper two or three lumbar spinal cord segments. These fibers exit the cord via the ventral root into the trunk of a corresponding thoracic or upper spinal nerve (Fig. 5-5F). The preganglionic fibers arising from the upper thoracic sympathetic trunk tend to enter the upper half of the spinal cord and run upward, reaching the superior sympathetic cervical ganglion at the level of C3-4 (the upward passage of the sympathetic trunk lies anterior to and across the sixth cervical transverse process) (Fig. 5-5D). The preganglionic fibers entering the sympathetic trunk at or below T6 descend to lower vertebral ganglia. A few of the white rami communicantes pass directly through the sympathetic trunk to synapse with outlying ganglionic cells near the origin of the blood vessels

of the thoracic viscera (Fig. 5-5G) (i.e., vasoconstrictors of the lung and vasodilator of the coronary arteries); however, the majority of fibers exiting the sympathetic trunk (Fig. 5-5H) are nonmyelinated, postganglionic fibers (gray rami communicantes) (Fig. 5-5E). These fibers synapse with outlying ganglia, providing vasomotor function to blood vessels of the abdominal viscera, motor function to plain muscles of sweat glands and hair follicles, and secretory fibers to the sweat glands via the postganglionic gray rami sympathetic fibers within the regions innervated by their respective spinal nerves (Fig. 5-5I).

Corticospinal (Pyramidal) Motor System

Conscious, purposeful, voluntary, discrete, and skilled motor impulses originate within the cerebral cortex and progress outward (the Bell-Magendie law),[2,3] as opposed to sensory stimuli that reach the cerebral cortex after originating in the more caudal or peripheral areas of the nervous system. Like the sensory cortical representation, the motor cortex lies just anterior to the central sulcus

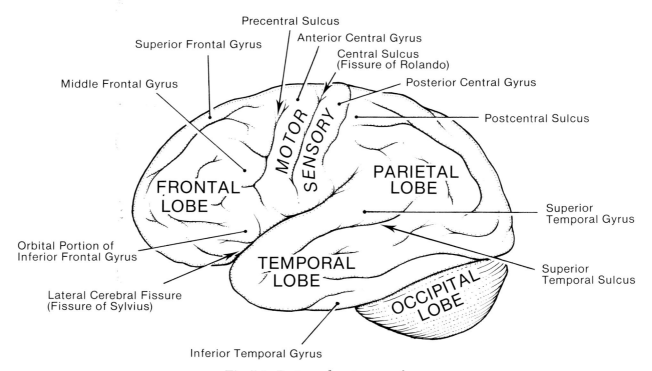

Fig. 5-6. Brain surface topography.

fissure of Rolando (Fig. 5-6), with the leg representation lying more posteriorly and along the superior and medial aspect of each cortical hemisphere within the sagittal sinus (Fig. 5-7). The motor cortex areas of the trunk, arm, and head lie progressively more inferiolateral and anterior to the central sulcus (Fig. 5-6).

It is not known how many, if any, pyramidal fibers connect directly with lower motor cells.[1] Transverse sections through selected levels of the brain, brain stem, and spinal cord illustrate the common familiar motor (pryamidal) pathways (Figs. 5-1 and 5-5).

Spinal Nerve Roots

Fibers arriving at the respective segmental levels of the spinal cord via the lateral corticospinal tract (Fig. 5-1E) synapse with internucial cell neurons

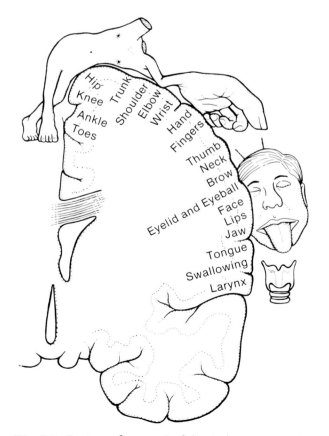

Fig. 5-7. Brain surface cortical (motor) representation through the precentral gyrus.

(Fig. 5-1Q). These internuncial cell neurons synapse with anterior horn cell neurons (Fig. 5-1R), from which mylinated axons pass outward via the ventral root fiber to form the anterior component of the spinal nerve root (Fig. 5-1H). This anterior component of the spinal nerve root is joined posteriorly and external to the spinal cord by the dorsal root (Fig. 5-1G) exiting from the dorsal horn area of the cord, and the two unite to form a segmental nerve (Fig. 5-1H). In the area of the thoracic and upper lumbar spinal cord, branches of the sympathetic nerves arise from the cord (white rami communicantes, (Fig. 5-5D) and unite with the sympathetic trunk (Fig. 5-5G). From here, fibers pass outward to secondary ganglia, innervating smooth muscles, visceral organs, and blood vessels within the chest, abdomen, and extremities. Likewise, mixed motor and sensory branches of the spinal nerves divide into anterior and posterior primary divisions, providing motor innervation to appropriate anterior and posterior striated muscle groups and sensation to associated segmental dermatomes (Fig. 5-5I).

Relative Size of Nerve Root Conduction Fibers

There are three types of nerve fibers which differ in diameter: A, B, and C fibers. The large A fibers are myelinated somatic nerves that conduct electrical impulses most rapidly, according to Sherrington's all-or-none law.[4] If an impulse is strong enough to be propagated, the size of the response and the spread of its conduction will be independent of the size of the stimulus, so that the obtained response is all that the nerve can send (at the moment). The velocity at which a nerve impulse is conducted is independent of the strength of the stimulus. The impulse set up by a strong stimulus travels no faster than that from a weak stimulus.

Nerve Conduction Speeds

The large A fibers also conduct proprioception and somatic motor impulses at a rate of 70 to 120 m/sec; touch and pressure at a rate of 30 to 70 m/sec; motor to muscle spindles at a rate of 15 to 30 m/sec; and pain, temperature, and touch at a rate of 12 to 30 m/sec.

B fibers are smaller, myelinated fibers. They represent the preganglionic sympathetics, and impulse travel at 3 to 15 m/sec.

C fibers convey electrical impulses most slowly. Most are unmyelinated and conduct pain and reflex responses (0.5 to 2 m/sec) and postganglionic sympathetics at (0.7 to 2.3 m/sec).

PARASYMPATHETIC AUTONOMIC SYSTEM: CRANIOSACRAL VISCERAL EFFERENT SYSTEM

This portion of the autonomic nervous system provides efferent (motor) nerves to visceral smooth muscles and glands and supplies inhibitory fibers to the heart via the vagus nerve. The cells of origin of preganglionic fibers are small, myelinated fibers, and like the sympathetic nervous system, the postganglionic fibers are nonmyelinated.

The parasympathetic nervous system preganglionic cells originate in two areas: intracranially within the midbrain, pons, and medulla oblongata; and within the sacral portion of the spinal cord. Intracranially, nuclei arise within the mesencephanon (Fig. 5-1A,N) or midbrain,[1,2] which supplies sphincter activity to the pupil and motor activity to the ciliary muscles of the eye for accommodation. From within the pons and medulla oblongata (Fig. 5-1A,B) nuclei arise for glands of the eye, and palate, the sublingual, maxillary, and parotid glands of the neck, as well as the muscles of the pharynx, esophagus, small and large intestines, and most glands of the alimentary tract. These postganglionic fibers also provide vasoconstrictor effects to the coronary arteries, vasodilatory fibers to the lung, and inhibitory effects to the heart and upper sphincters of the gastrointestinal tract, via the glossopharyngeal nerve (9th cranial nerve). Although this nerve lies proximal (in the upper neck), many of its functions occur in the lower neck, chest, and abdomen. This is possible through the parasympathetic preganglionic and postganglionic synaptic connections, which lie in the prevertebral and terminal ganglia of the neck, thorax, and upper abdomen. Unlike the sympathetics, the parasympathetic nerves have no organized, anatomically visible trunk arising from the thoracic and upper lumbar segment of the cord. The cranial and sacral segments of the parasympathetic nervous system and its ganglionic connections occur within the adventitious connections of the splanchnic or hypogastric nerves, in association with connections from the sympathetic trunk.

As just noted, the second major neurologic area of contribution to the parasympathetic nervous system is in the mid-sacral segment of the spinal cord. Here, the visceral efferent cells are found near the base of the anterior horn, dorsal to the groups of large somatic motor cells. The preganglionic parasympathetic fibers are shunted past the sympathetic trunk, leaving the cord via the efferent ventral rami of the second and third sacral nerves to reach the hypogastric and pelvic plexuses. In the pelvis, the parasympathetics provide motor function to the descending colon, rectum, anus, bladder, and muscles of the external genitalia. They also provide vasodilation to the external genitalia, secretory function to the prostate and Bartholin glands, and inhibitory fibers to internal sphincters of the anus, bladder, and urethra.

CONCLUSION

It is incumbent on the surgeon managing patients with acute spinal cord injuries to focus on the anatomy of the nervous system and the spinal cord. By so doing, the physician is able to appreciate segmental neurology and is thus capable of interpreting peripheral nervous system injuries. Such knowledge enables accurate diagnosing and prognostication of functional return.

Taking a close look at the neuroanatomy of the brain and the central and peripheral nervous systems helps one to understand the multitude of alterations in neurologic vital functions, which are seemingly uncoordinated. The best example of this is Figure 5-3, which shows that alterations and balance in respiration are managed by the vagus nerve (to the lung), the spinal assessory nerve (to the sternocleidomastoid muscle), the hypoglossal nerve (to the muscles of the neck and larynx), the phrenic nerve (to the diaphragm), the T6 to T12 somatic sensory nerve (from the diaphragm), the T1 to T6 motor nerves (to the muscles of the upper chest), and the motor nerves of T6 to T12 (to the abdominal muscles).

Similarly, with the heart, injury to the spinal cord above the sympathetics (T6) results in the loss of sympathetic influence on peripheral vessels (causing vasodilation and hypotension); the loss of sympathetic stimulation of the heart, because only the vagus nerve influence on the heart remains, resulting in bradycardia; and the loss of sympathetic influence on peripheral sweat glands (with inability to perspire), causing loss of temperature control (initially hypothermia, followed later by hyperthermia).

Other notable areas of the nervous system are discussed in Chapters 12, 17, 20, and 22. Each of these chapters relate specifically to the cervical,

thoracic, thoracolumbar, lumbar, and sacral segments of the spine and their accompanying nervous system. Specific changes to the nervous system secondary to injury of the spinal column are also reviewed. Neurologic alterations resulting from vascular injuries to the spinal cord are reviewed in Chs. 4 and 5.

REFERENCES

1. Rasmussen AT: The Principal Nervous Pathways. 4th Ed. MacMillian, New York, 1952
2. Carpenter MB: Core Text of Neuroanatomy. 2nd Ed. Williams & Wilkins, Baltimore, 1978
3. Chusid JG: Correlative Neuroanatomy and Functional Neurology. 17th Ed. Appleton & Lange, 1979
4. Sherrington C: The Integrative Action of the Nervous System. Yale University Press, New Haven, CT, 1947

6

Evaluation of Spinal Cord Function by Means of Evoked Potentials

Tod B. Sloan

J. Richard Toleikis

Antoun Koht

Sensory evoked potentials have been used extensively for the detection and diagnosis of neurologic abnormalities because they are a noninvasive technique for evaluating neural structures that are often otherwise inaccessible. Further, since they may be used to test uncooperative patients or those who have derangements in mental status, they are one of only a few methods for evaluation of patients with a severe head injury or under general anesthesia.

The application of these powerful techniques for the evaluation of the spinal cord-injured patient is the subject of this chapter. After a discussion of the principles of evoked potentials (with special focus on somatosensory evoked potentials), the application of these techniques for the evaluation and prognosis of spinal cord-injured patients is reviewed. A discussion of their use during general anesthesia (intraoperative monitoring) and in the evaluation of patients with head trauma follows. The chapter concludes with a perspective on their current limitations and future applications.

PRINCIPLES OF EVOKED POTENTIALS

Credit for the first measurement of electrical potentials over the brain in response to sensory stimulation usually goes to Caton, whose findings were published in 1875.[1,2] However, in 1947 Dawson was the first to demonstrate these evoked potentials in human subjects using a photographic superimposition technique.[3,4] Four years later, Dawson developed a summation technique that is the forerunner of the present-day averagers. The significant time lag between discovery, application, and the widespread use (not to occur until 20 years after Dawson) of the evoked potential technique is primarily due to the complex nature of the equipment required to accurately measure the small electrical signal in the midst of the larger electrical background activity—of the brain (electroencephalogram, EEG), heart (electrocardiogram, ECG), muscle activity (electromyogram, EMG), and of the electrical noise in hospital rooms. Several excellent reviews of the methodology and technology are available,[5-10] so only the essentials will be presented here.

Figure 6-1 shows the basic schematic of the instrumentation currently used for obtaining evoked potentials. A variety of stimuli are routinely used to elicit these signals. These include visual light flashes or alternating checkerboard patterns (light-emitting diode or strobe visual evoked response and pattern reversal visual evoked response, respectively), auditory clicks or tone bursts (brainstem auditory evoked response [BAER]), and mild electrical stimuli of major sensory nerves or cutaneous dermatomes (somatosensory evoked potentials [SSEP] and dermatomal evoked potentials [DEP], respectively). A variety of other sensory modalities can be used to elicit these responses and are being used on a more limited basis.

Each of these stimuli is associated with an electrical response that occurs at various points along the appropriate sensory pathways. Each occurs at a fixed time interval from the onset of the stimulus (owing to consistent nerve conduction velocity along the sensory paths involved) and is, therefore, time locked to the stimulus. The electrical signal

can be measured by recording electrodes placed over appropriate areas of the sensory pathways. The signal is filtered to remove low- and high-frequency electrical activity and is converted to digital signals for microprocessor manipulation. The signal is analyzed by averaging several hundred recordings taken over a fixed time interval after each trigger impulse. Using this technique, the random fluctuations of EEG and other background noise are averaged, resulting in baseline fluctuations of electrical activity much smaller than the consistently repeatable evoked response.

Figure 6-2 shows typical normal evoked responses to visual pattern reversal, auditory click, and posterior tibial nerve electrical stimulation (VEP, BAER, and SSEP-PTN, respectively). The VEP consists of one major wave at about 100 msec (P_{100}). The short latency (10 msec) BAER consists of seven positive waves probably generated by or near several brain stem structures (wave I, 8th cranial nerve; wave II, medulla cochlear nuclei; wave III, superior olivary complex and trapezoid body; wave IV, medial geniculate body; wave V, inferior colliculus; wave VI, medial geniculate body; wave VII, auditory radiations to cortex). Mixed sensory and motor nerves such as the posterior tibial, median, ulnar, and peroneal nerves are well suited for SSEP measurements since a motor twitch with each stimulus ensures that the nerve trunk is being stimulated.

As shown in Figure 6-3, electrical responses can be recorded at many locations along the afferent tracts. With the exception of the EMG response at the foot, the earliest potential (10 msec) can be recorded over the nerve at the knee (popliteal fossa). Analysis of this peak allows verification of the stimulus when no motor response can be obtained (e.g., anesthetic paralysis) and allows calculation of nerve conduction velocity to document peripheral nerve injuries. Using these recording sites, the H and F reflexes of the monosynaptic and polysynaptic pathways in the spinal cord can also be measured. Similar types of recordings can be made for the upper extremity by using the median or ulnar nerves with recordings of the incoming volley of activity over the brachial plexus at Erb's point.

The next response can be measured over the lumbar spine and typically shows a biphasic re-

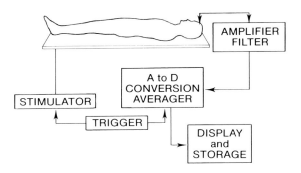

Fig. 6-1. Schematic diagram of system used to measure sensory evoked responses. The trigger device simultaneously sets in motion the stimulator and the averager. The stimulus module delivers the sensory stimulus to the patient (such as mild electrical impulses applied to major nerves to elicit SSEPs). The bioelectrical response is acquired by the amplifier and filtered. It is then converted from analog to digital information. The averager accumulates the results from each stimulation. The resulting averaged response may be stored and/or displayed for evaluation.

sponse consisting of a negative deflection thought to be generated by the dorsal roots of the spinal column followed by a positive potential thought to be the result of synaptic activity in the spinal cord at the level of entry (L4 to S2). These potentials therefore confirm sensory stimulation and evaluate an additional segment of the afferent pathway.

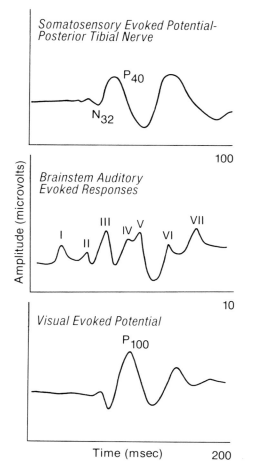

Fig. 6-2. Waveforms of typical evoked responses acquired in normal patients. Somatosensory evoked responses from the posterior tibial nerve (SSEP-PTN) result in consistent deflections at about 32 msec and 40 msec (N_{32} and P_{40}, respectively). Brain stem auditory evoked responses (BAERs) from audible clicks result in seven peaks (I to VII) during the 10 msec after stimulus. Most normal persons will reliably demonstrate peaks I, III, and a IV-V complex. Visual evoked responses (VEPs) to a reversing checkerboard stimulation typically show a strong response at about 100 msec (P_{100}).

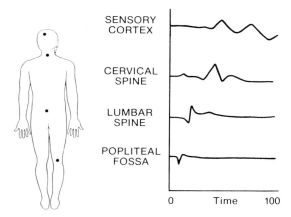

Fig. 6-3. Evoked responses from stimulation of a posterior tibial nerve at the ankle can be recorded at several locations along the somatosensory pathway. Shown here are typical responses as recorded at the knee (popliteal fossa), over the lumbar spine, at the cervical vertebra (seventh vertebra), and over the sensory cortex. Such multiple recording sites allow localization of the abnormality in the sensory tract.

Potentials such as those recorded over the lumbar spine can be recorded at many locations along the spine. Analysis of spinal cord conduction velocity (typically, 57 m/sec) along each segment allows the level of abnormality to be pinpointed for this pathway within the cord. Unfortunately, recording these signals can be difficult owing to the distance of surface electrodes from the spinal cord. Invasive placement of recording electrodes in the epidural space,[11-14] spinal canal,[15-17] or spinous processes[18,19] allows improved recording but adds risks to an otherwise benign examination. Perhaps the most easily obtainable spine potentials are those recorded over C7 and C2 of the cervical spine. These pinpoint abnormalities of nerve conduction below the level of the brain stem.

The next reliable recording location is on the midline of the scalp over the sensory cortex. This places the recording electrode nearest the somatotopic representation of the foot. As shown in Figures 6-2 and 6-3, the signal here is rather complex and represents the culmination of electrical potentials generated at more distal sites and transmitted by volume conduction. This signal includes those signals in the numerous brain stem relay paths along with those produced in the thalamus and cortex. Thus, each peak represents a composite of several generator sites. However, there is reasonable agreement that the peak at about 32 to 45 msec represents the response of the primary sensory cortex (also called the primary specific complex) and that the later large positive wave at about 300 msec represents sensory interaction processed by the cognitive centers.

The response of the scalp and over the cervical spine may be used to evaluate the conduction time through the brain stem (so-called central conduction time[20,21]).

SOMATOSENSORY EVOKED POTENTIALS IN EXPERIMENTAL SPINAL CORD INJURY

To understand fully the evoked potentials that are recorded in patients with spinal cord injury, a large number of recordings have been made in animals during and after experimentally induced injury. It is instructive to review these experiments in animals since the evoked potential response appears similar to that of humans. In these experimental animals, the evoked response can be correlated with the anatomic pathology produced by injury.[22]

There are two frequently used experimental models of injury. The most widely used is the weight drop method initially used by Allen.[23-28] Here, the dura is exposed by laminectomy, a standard weight (in grams) is dropped from a standard height (in centimeters), and the impact is distributed across the width of the cord. The impact is recorded in g·cm. The second method is the production of intradural pressure by the inflation of a Fogarty catheter. The balloon may be placed anterior, posterior, or lateral to the cord. Other methods include the production of an experimental acceleration-deceleration injury by using a special mechanical apparatus.[29]

In general, mild trauma is associated with transient dysfunction of the cord. In impact studies, this is associated with perivascular hemorrhages in the gray matter secondary to disruption of postcapillary venules. This is also associated with high extracellular concentrations of potassium, suggesting a disruption of the electrochemical gradients. This suggests that the mechanical concussion causes a transient disruption of electrical function. This period may last from 1 to 60 minutes. Evoked potentials are lost during this period with eventual return to baseline. If the insult was mild, no further changes occur and the animal returns to full function. Studies of spinal cord blood flow (SCBF) show that the physiology of the spinal cord region is abnormal for about a week,[27,30] during which time a marked hyperemia is seen. SCBF returns to normal after 1 week.

With a more severe impact, the recovery period gives way to eventual neurologic deterioration. Anatomically, the small hemorrhages progress within 2 hours to larger central petechiae with polymorphonuclear and microglial reactions. Hemorrhages appear in the gray matter. This period is associated with the presence of evoked potentials, but neurologic dysfunction occurs at the level of the impact owing to gray matter abnormalities. This injury leaves the animal with a permanent central cord lesion, but the ascending and descending functions of the cord are unimpaired. SCBF studies show only mild hyperemia after injury with return to normal by 1 week.

If the injury is severe, edema occurs within 4 hours and the central gray matter begins undergoing necrosis. Initially, vacuolation and swelling of capillary endothelium is seen, but finally central hemorrhage and necrosis of the spinal cord is noted. Necrosis begins centrally and gradually extends outward. Thus, as injuries of increasing severity cause radially increasing amounts of gray matter injury until the white matter is involved. Very severe trauma can injure the entire cross section (complete cord injury). During this period, the evoked potentials become abnormal and finally absent as the white matter is involved in the degeneration process. Motor dysfunction ranges from normal through paresis to paralysis, depending on the extent of cord involvement. Measurements of SCBF show severe reduction of flow with cord hypoxia. SCBF takes many weeks to return to normal, if it returns at all.

Extremely severe trauma produces immediate and permanent loss of local cord function consistent with severe physical disruption of the entire cord structure. Evoked potentials disappear and never return. The entire process of necrosis ensues, and, as with strong impact, the entire cord is an amorphous mass of necrotic tissue at 24 hours.

Conclusions about evoked potential studies in these animals show that for injuries in the thoracic and cervical regions the prognosis was extremely poor if there was no evoked potential by 4 hours after impact.[31] Further, the presence of any evoked potential between 24 hours and 1 week was associated with residual motor function. The extent of loss of function correlated with the degree of SSEP abnormality.

Other researchers using Fogarty catheters in the epidural space suggest that the sustained mechanical pressure of dislodged vertebral bodies or edematous swelling of the cord.[32-34]

These studies show that slow increase of pressure on the cord maintains dorsal column function and evoked potentials until SCBF approaches zero. Anatomically, the cord shows vacuolization and glial reaction with mild cystic degeneration. It appears that the dorsal column axons may be able to withstand up to 5 minutes of zero blood flow (monkey) before irreversible damage occurs. This period is longer than the tolerance of the gray matter and is consistent with the known relative sensitivity of synapses and axons to ischemia. In some animals, the evoked potentials did not return until 3 hours after the pressure was relieved. In these animals, the evoked response eventually returned, as did ascending and descending cord function.

With more severe balloon pressure, the return of evoked potentials was only transient. Within 12 to 24 hours, the evoked potentials eventually disappeared permanently. In these animals, gliosis and central cystic degeneration were severe and the process of cord necrosis took its toll in neurologic injury. These animals were all ultimately paraplegic.

Finally, with very severe inflation pressures, the evoked response was lost at inflation, never to return. All these animals were ultimately paraplegic.

As in the impact studies, the absence of an evoked potential at 4 hours was associated with no return of function. Further, the presence of any evoked potential after 12 to 24 hours was associated with preserved motor function and incomplete cord injury.

In similar studies,[35] the balloon was acutely inflated. Here, complete irreversible loss occurred if inflation remained longer than 1 minute. The loss here clearly differs from that described above and may represent a slightly different type of injury.

In an attempt to correlate these studies with real injuries, monkeys were subjected to hyperflexion-compression injuries, using a special apparatus to simulate a motor vehicle accident. Here, the animals sustained edema and swelling of the spinal cord for one to two segments in each direction from the level of physical injury. Microscopically, they sustained small hemorrhages in the gray and white matter with associated astrocytic and microglial reactionary changes. The evoked potentials were lost after 30 to 90 seconds and returned by 24 hours.

Although controversy exists as to the contribution of each of the pathologic forces involved (i.e., the contribution of mechanical factors, vascular factors, edema, etc.), all these experimentally induced injuries show a remarkable similarity of events. There may be multiple factors working independently, and some investigators have suggested that the initial dysfunction and the hemorrhagic process have separate etiologies.[36]

Consistently, however, the spinal cord sustains an initial physical concussion with temporary loss of function and evoked potentials. This is associated with mild hemorrhages in the gray matter. The function returns, as do the evoked potentials, only to give way to loss of function and evoked potentials at about 3 to 4 hours if the process of central necrosis extends outward sufficiently. Usually, the residual neurologic function is stable, as are the evoked potentials by 24 hours.

SOMATOSENSORY EVOKED POTENTIALS IN THE EVALUATION AND PROGNOSIS OF HUMAN SPINAL CORD INJURY

Several studies have been conducted of patients who sustained spinal cord injury. In humans, the spinal cord is known to undergo histologic and pathologic sequences similar to those described above[37] for animals. Several researchers have aggressively followed injured patients from arrival at the injury center until discharge. Of note are the studies by Perot,[38-40] Spielholtz et al.,[41] Young,[42] Rowed,[37,43,44] and others.[45-48] Their studies were based on the observation of serial change in the potentials and their correlation with outcome (i.e., prognostic value of early measurement).

Particular interest in using evoked response techniques revolves around two basic problems with the clinical examination. The first is that many patients, such as those who have sustained head trauma, cannot be tested clinically. In these patients, the evoked potentials can be easily elicited since cooperation of the patient is not always necessary to obtain good electrophysiologic responses. The second is that there is often a great degree of individual observer variation in interpreting examinations. The use of evoked potentials introduces a degree of objectivity that can be used for serial comparisons. In these evaluations, patients were evaluated with upper extremity (e.g., median nerve) and lower extremity (e.g., posterior tibial nerve) SSEPs.

All studies showed uniformly excellent correlation with the clinical sensory examination. Although only a sensory test, results correlated closely with the motor examination. However, an occasional patient did have motor and sensory dissociation (anterior cord syndrome).

Of extreme interest is that in patients with complete injuries, SSEPs from nerves that entered the cord below the injury were uniformly absent. Thus, patients with lesions above C6 who had no median nerve SSEP had neurologically complete lesions. Likewise, lesions in the cervical or thoracic cord in patients with no lower extremity SSEP (peroneal or posterior tibial nerve) were found to be complete. Also of note was the curious observation that upper extremity SSEP measurements were often abnormal with injuries in lower segments, suggesting an ascending influence of the injury.[38] This has also been seen in cats with experimental injury.[49]

Patients with incomplete lesions had SSEPs that were present 24 hours to 1 week after their injury. Here, the degree of abnormality of the SSEP correlated with the time and the amount of functional recovery. For these patients, two observers found that the SSEP change was more sensitive than the clinical examination with the SSEP changes antedating clinical improvement or deterioration.[44] Other observers have found a different time correlation.[38,50] Of note is that the SSEP evaluation at 1 week correlated better with the ultimate outcome than a similar examination at 6 weeks. With the possible exception of transient early changes (less than 24 hours), patients with intact spinal cords showed normal responses.

The conclusions for the prognostic significance of these studies on humans are similar to those of the studies in animals. When a nerve is stimulated 24 hours to 1 week postinjury, the presence of an SSEP signal is almost always a favorable prognostic sign of an incomplete injury. However, the consistent absence of any evoked potential from below the level of the lesion is an unfavorable prognostic sign and correlates with a complete injury.

The information gained from major mixed sensory-motor nerve SSEPs is a valuable prognostic indicator. However, a major problem of the traditional SSEP technique is that it does not provide a means for the full evaluation of the spinal cord of the injured patient. For example, it does not delineate the exact level of abnormality or the extent of the injury. Furthermore, it gives no information about abnormalities in areas that are not serviced by the major nerves. This is true in cases of sacral sparing in which the lower extremity major nerve responses are absent. Perot reported on six such patients in one of his studies.[39]

A few observers have attempted to gain further insight into cord injury by attempting more specific evaluations of the cord. One interesting approach is to determine the conduction velocity through the cord (lumbar to cervical spine).[47,48] These investigators found a marked decrease in conduction velocity with more severe injuries. Further, they found a linear correlation of the conduction velocity with a parameter called VA that was calculated as the ratio of leg to arm SSEP amplitudes. Here, all patients with ratios of 10.5 (correlated with conduction velocities of 36 m/sec) or greater were abnormal. This information, however, did not provide any further information about the location or anatomic extent of injury.

A more invasive approach was studied,[48] in which intraspinal stimulation and recording needles were placed at various locations along the cord and conduction blocks or abnormalities were utilized to discern the level of injury. These researchers found abnormalities when descending conduction velocities were less than 32 m/sec or ascending conduction velocities were less than 57 m/sec. However, this approach is more invasive than desired for routine testing.

DERMATOMAL EVOKED POTENTIALS IN SPINAL CORD INJURY

Techniques for producing evoked potentials on a segmental basis have been detailed in both the European and American literature.[51-62] In this technique, segmental evoked potentials are produced for each dermatome distribution in a fashion similar to that described for the posterior tibial nerve. However, the electrical stimulus is introduced by placing the constant current stimulation electrode on the skin surface rather than over a major nerve. These studies can produce excellent responses when recorded over the scalp (Fig. 6-4) and can be used to more carefully delineate areas of spinal cord pathology.

No large studies have been published of the spinal cord-injured patients studied by dermatomal stimulation. However, several studies of patients with various spinal cord abnormalities or nerve root problems have appeared.[51-61]

The power of this evoked potential technique is nicely demonstrated in studies of subtle disc or nerve root problems.[51,53,59,61] In cases of nerve root disease or spinal stenosis, abnormalities in side-to-side latency or amplitude differences correlate well with the clinical examination and myelographic findings. The technique has been helpful for

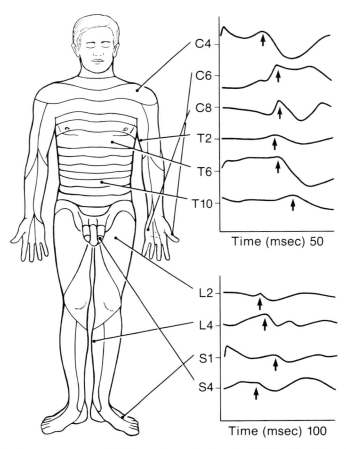

Fig. 6-4. Typical evoked responses recorded over the scalp for stimulation of various dermatomal locations. Responses can be recorded in normal individuals from C4 through S4. Stimulation electrodes should be placed well within the boundaries of the dermatomal distribution to avoid simultaneous stimulation of more than one dermatomal region. Care should be taken to avoid stimulation of underlying major nerves or muscle groups. The level of stimulation should be adjusted so that strong, but not painful, stimuli are felt.

documenting disease when clinical findings were questionable.

However, evaluation of the spinal cord-injured patient is more closely related to the studies of patients with spinal cord abnormalities (from space-occupying or non-space-occupying lesions). These studies showed that the evoked potentials correlated well with the clinical examination and with the pathologic condition found during surgery. They allowed a more detailed delineation of the lesions than conventional SSEPs and allowed the patients to be followed before and after surgery. Although abnormalities were sometimes detectable in conventional SSEP responses, these abnormalities could not be associated with specific levels of injury, thus making the dermatomal studies necessary for a detailed examination.

The logical application of these dermatomal studies to spinal cord-injured patients includes delineation of abnormalities in several regions not testable with conventional major nerve SSEPs. First, abnormalities in the region of injury can be detailed to objectively discern the extent of local injury caudal and cephalad to the anatomic injury. Second, they can be useful in evaluating for sacral sparing in patients with questionable incomplete lesions. Third, in patients with questionable sensory examinations or examinations that are not consistent with the suspected neural injury, they can be used to objectively evaluate specific dermatomal regions.

THE NORTHWESTERN APPROACH TO EVALUATING SPINAL CORD-INJURED PATIENTS WITH EVOKED POTENTIALS

On the basis of the rationale presented above, the Division of Neurophysiologic Monitoring of the Department of Anesthesia of Northwestern University Medical School conducts the following series of evoked potentials for evaluating spinal cord-injured patients 1 day to 1 week after injury.

First, a sensory examination is conducted to familiarize our service with the extent of the sensory deficit and to provide support for the clinical sensory examination done by the managing physicians. This study delineates regions of absent or questionable sensory function.

Second, conventional short-latency SSEP studies are conducted on the upper limbs (typically, median nerves) and on the lower limbs (typically, posterior tibial nerves) to provide objective support for the gross findings of a complete or incomplete lesion as determined by the subjective studies discussed above.

Third, the degree of abnormality of segmental function in the region of the anatomic injury is delineated by dermatomal studies. Several segments caudal and cephalad to the level of injury (extending to include one "normal" region) are studied by this technique.

Fourth, in patients whose lower extremity major nerve SSEPs are absent, at least two sacral dermatomes are studied to evaluate for sacral sparing or a possible incomplete lesion.

Finally, if regions of questionable sensory function exist in an intact patient or unusual regions of sensory function exist well below a suspected complete or incomplete lesion, these areas are also tested.

The results to date reveal that the above protocol is extremely useful for objectively evaluating spinal cord-injured patients. Of note is the finding that many patients may have normal major nerve SSEPs and yet may have abnormal segmental studies. This suggests that dermatomal responses are mediated by different neurologic tracts from the pathways thought to mediate the mixed nerve SSEPs.[63,64] This also suggests that dermatomal studies are more sensitive in detecting abnormalities in these patients.

EVOKED POTENTIALS IN THE EVALUATION OF MULTIPLE TRAUMA AND HEAD INJURY

It is logical to extend these powerful diagnostic tools to the monitoring of nerve tracts in patients during surgery (see Evolved Potentials in Monitoring Surgical Procedures of the Spinal Column, below) or to the diagnosis of central nervous system injury in multiple trauma patients with head injury.[21,65-68]

It has repeatedly been shown that evoked potentials are a valuable tool for the evaluation of comatose patients. By assessing the normality of the responses mediated by these sensory nerve pathways, anatomic regions of injury can be ascertained and the extent of multiple injury locations can be determined. Furthermore, baseline responses can be obtained and repeat studies can be performed to objectively check for changes such as a patient's response to therapy. These studies lend valuable functional information to supplement the anatomic information obtained from such studies as computed tomography (CT) scanning.

SSEPs and DEPs have been evaluated in terms of their usefulness in diagnosing the extent of spinal cord injury. Similarly, multimodality evoked potential testing (MEP) has been evaluated for its prognostic value in patients with head trauma. One study noted that MEP was the best single prognostic indicator of outcome of those studied in 133 patients with severe head injuries (91 percent accuracy). In addition, when these data were correlated with the other diagnostic, clinical, and physiological measurements (i.e., patient age, Glasgow coma scale, CT scan, intracranial pressure measurements, and pupillary response and eye movements), accuracy approaching 100 percent could be obtained.

Thus, as with spinal cord injury, the evoked potential studies provide a valuable adjunct to the clinical, physiological, and other diagnostic measurements that have been found to be useful in the diagnosis and management of head-injured patients.

EVOKED POTENTIALS IN MONITORING SURGICAL PROCEDURES OF THE SPINAL COLUMN

The application of evoked potentials to the assessment and monitoring of patients undergoing spinal corrective or stabilization surgery is a logical extension of the principles of monitoring.[69,70] Since evoked potentials can be measured without the patient's cooperation and when the patient is anesthetized deeply enough to allow surgery, this mode of monitoring is becoming more common.[10,18,71-75]

Techniques for intraoperative monitoring differ somewhat from those used routinely for diagnostic studies. Stimulation sites must be secured to withstand mechanical manipulation of the extremities and to remain stable throughout the operation. Recording electrodes must be attached securely and must remain stable for the duration of surgery as well. Needle electrodes can normally be used, but with some patients it may be more desirable to use disc electrodes secured with collodion.

The recording technique is usually one that employs multiple channel recording sites (e.g., with posterior tibial nerve stimulation, recordings might be taken at the popliteal fossa, on the spine below the surgical site, on the spine above the surgical site, and over the cortex) to help pinpoint the location (and possibly the etiology) of abnormalities as they occur and to have backup channels for recording changes if one channel should malfunction.[73] Further, many recordings are being made with electrodes in the spinal canal[16,76,77] or peridural region (such as paraspinous muscles[72,73] or in the vertebral bone[18,19] where the spinal cord signal can be recorded. These spinal cord signals are usually less susceptible to anesthetics. If introduced via the surgical field, these electrodes are not an invasive technique, but they are subject to noise from nearby surgical manipulation.

The motivation for monitoring these patients is that their spinal cords are at significant risk for a variety of reasons. First, anatomic deformities may narrow the normal spinal canal or impinge on the neural structures, thus reducing the margin of safety for mechanical manipulation or normal surgical swelling. Second, vascular injury sustained with the trauma may place tissues at significant risk for decreased perfusion and delivery of metabolites. Third, the injury itself may cause neurons to function marginally, creating an increased demand for nutrients such as oxygen and therefore reducing the margin of physiologic safety. Fourth, edema and alterations in SCBF are known to accompany injury. These reduce the viability of the spinal cord, increasing its risk to permanent damage. Finally, the physiology of the spinal cord patient is altered by the nature of the injury (i.e., cardiovascular and ventilatory instability), thus increasing the risk of decreased cord perfusion during a surgical procedure.

When the spinal cord-injured patient comes to the operating room, the functional status of the cord can be categorized into three general areas. The first is when the neurons forming the cord are uncompromised and are functioning normally. Here, the risk to injury is the mechanical and vascular effects of normal surgery and anesthesia. The functioning of the cord is monitorable, but is not particularly liable to small insults. The second area is that in which the neurons forming the cord are irreversibly damaged and not functioning. Cord function is, therefore, not monitorable, and no further damage can be done. The third area is that in which the cord has been partially damaged; some neurons are irreversibly damaged and the others are normal, but are usually functioning marginally. These remaining neurons that are functioning marginally are at the greatest risk. Having sustained injury, their margin of safety has been reduced from normal levels, making them more susceptible to physiological and surgical insults. These tracts are usually monitorable (unless they are extremely abnormal). Here, in addition to preserving normal tissue, the surgeon hopes to maintain and possibly improve the chance of survival of these cells.

With a careful and extensive clinical examination and with evoked potential studies done preoperatively, the surgeon knows how tenuous and extensively damaged the spinal cord is in the region of proposed surgery. However, without evoked potential monitoring during the procedure, the normal monitoring of physiological variables does not allow the assessment of neurologic viability of the cord. Further, the anesthesiologist has no means of assessing the effects of positioning or physiological fluctuations during the procedure. The advent of evoked potentials in the operating room makes possible continuous intraoperative assessment of the neurologic function of the testable tracts. Thus, the surgical and anesthetic management could theoretically be tailored to the individual patient to avoid undesired neurologic deterioration. To assess the impact of this testing, we should review the results in animals and then in humans.

Monitoring of Animals Undergoing Experimental Surgery

Two excellent studies of evoked potentials during experimental surgery on animals demonstrate the utility of evoked potential monitoring. In one study,[78] dogs were subjected to various degrees of segmental cord compression. When the cord was compressed to 51 percent of its normal anteroposterior (AP) diameter, the evoked potential showed a significant delay in latency. At 67 percent compression, the waves began to disappear, the earliest waves first. When the compression was immediately relieved, the SSEP returned within 20 minutes. Of interest is that sustained compression at the point of loss of potential demonstrated hemorrhage, neuronal damage, flattened blood vessels, and vacuolization in the gray matter (similar to experimental injury).

When comparing the intraoperative data with postoperative motor recovery, it was noted that as long as the evoked potential was maintained at a level of at least 50 percent of the amplitude before compression, motor recovery was good. This suggests that submaximal compression was well tolerated. Further, at the point of compression at which the evoked potentials were just lost (67 percent), full motor recovery appeared if the compression was maintained less than 2 hours.

This study suggests that motor function could be predicted by neurologic assessment in a topographically related cord region (i.e., the posterior columns) and that the evoked potentials were very sensitive indicators in normal cords of the factors that ultimately lead to motor injury. Of interest is that the evolution of evoked potential deterioration during compression of the cord just to the point of disappearance of the evoked potential mimicked exactly the changes found during asphyxia of the dogs at the conclusion of the experiments. These studies are consistent with the physiological conclusion that during periods of limited nutrients the cells can cease electrical function and maintain viability for at least 2 hours at the threshold level of compression. However, longer periods produced irreversible damage and loss of function. This is similar to the studies of outcome in scoliosis patients, in whom attempts to reverse postoperative paraplegia after instrumentation for scoliosis were increasingly successful as the time from instrumentation to their removal was shortened (i.e., the cord could survive a finite period of time, but beyond this there was an increasing amount of permanent damage).[79]

A second experiment[17] involves monitoring evoked potentials during controlled experimental spine distraction in cats. In these studies, the motor function was assessed intraoperatively by a wake-up test at several degrees of distraction. This allowed simultaneous correlation of evoked potentials with motor function. The results showed that amplitudes as low as 50 percent of the baseline evoked potentials (measured over the spinal cord) were compatible with motor function but that amplitudes of 4 to 26 percent were associated with paralysis. When allowed to recover from distraction, the animals with evoked potentials that had undergone less than a 50 percent reduction had intact motor function. Those with measurable potentials but more than a 50 percent amplitude reduction showed paresis, and those with no recordable potential (distraction beyond that necessary to cause loss of potential) showed minimal or no motor function.

These studies are consistent with the known increased susceptibility of synapses (i.e., the gray matter of motor tracts) as compared with axons (i.e., the white matter of sensory tracts) to ischemia (the presumed pathophysiologic event associated with distraction). Of note is that injury to the motor tracts appeared not to occur if the amplitude of the sensory signal remained greater than 50 percent of baseline during distraction. Further, severe degrees of distraction appeared detrimental and suggested to the investigators that irreversible mechanical injury was also a factor in postoperative paralysis.

These studies demonstrate that intraoperative evoked potentials in animals are predictive of the status of motor function at the moment of mechanical change and are useful prognostic indicators of outcome. (Sensory studies were not conducted, but these indicate that selected sensory tracts can be used as an indicator of global cord function in these experimental settings.)

Surgical Monitoring Studies of Humans with Spinal Surgery

Although it may be argued that the findings in animal studies do not necessarily relate well to human spinal cord injury, controlled experiments in humans cannot ethically be performed. However, several series of observations have been published. The rationale and methods for intraoperative studies have been presented in several articles and differ from diagnostic studies only in priorities and problems; the principles of testing remain the same.

Intraoperative evoked potentials signal when the margin of safety for the cells has been reduced to the point of electrical shutdown. As with critical compression of the spine of cats, a limited time is available for correction before the damage occurs. Variables known to be deleterious usually relate ultimately to decrease in spinal cord blood flow or oxygenation (e.g., hypoxia,[80] hypotension, hypercapnia or hypocapnia, hypovolemia). Other variables probably relate to a combination of ischemia and mechanical effects (e.g., incorrect positioning,[81] blunt trauma). Clearly, when the anesthetic used permits continued monitoring (i.e., avoidance of moderate to deep levels of inhalational agents[10,41,71,82,83]) the anesthesiologist can utilize the evoked potentials as an index of cord viability and can adjust the physiological variables accordingly to optimize the neural integrity.

With respect to surgical manipulation, there appear to be three basic mechanisms producing evoked potential deteriorations. The first is a transient, reversible loss secondary to direct trauma, similar to the transient loss seen with mild impact in experimental injury. In humans, the time for return of response is directly proportional to the degree of trauma. In certain abnormal regions, the cord appears to be very sensitive to even mild manipulation. The second form of mechanical disruption produces a more sustained deterioration of the evoked potential to a fraction of baseline values. This is similar to the studies of compression or distraction, and appears to correlate with eventual cord damage if not reversed. The third form is loss of potentials from severance or sacrifice of the nerves involved.

The published results of monitoring experience demonstrate the following conclusions. When adverse physiological conditions existed, the cord was more sensitive to manipulation.[74] The proper choice of anesthetics clearly improved the ability to monitor. Amplitude changes of up to 50 percent decrease were not associated with poor outcome.[10] The intraoperative loss of evoked potentials without recovery was a poor prognostic sign, whereas maintenance of evoked potentials or reversible loss was a good prognostic sign. All authors indicated that monitoring is a valuable adjunct to patient care.[16,18,74,75,77,83–86]

The experience at Northwestern University agrees with the above conclusions. Of note is that there are no published limits of graded outcome as correlated with graded intraoperative changes. Similar to the Northwestern University experience, this suggests that each patient must be evaluated individually to attempt to determine the acceptable limit of intraoperative variation. Of note is that amplitude changes of greater than 50 percent or latency increases of 10 percent or more usually correlate with a potentially deleterious physiological or surgical change (in the absence of anesthetic or technical changes).

Clearly, as experience grows with this intraoperative technique, our knowledge of the optimal intraoperative care will improve.

PERSPECTIVE

The literature cited above clearly demonstrates the value of evoked potentials in the diagnosis and management of the spinal cord-injured patient. There are, however, several factors that are important to keep in perspective when referring to these studies.

First, evoked potentials are no replacement for the clinical examination in the diagnosis of cord function. The clinical examination has the potential for assessing a wide multitude of cord modalities that are not testable by evoked potentials. As an objective adjunct to the clinical examination, evoked potentials are useful in several situations. They are useful in testing patients who are comatose or who cannot cooperate for a clinical exami-

nation. They are useful in objectively evaluating a patient when the clinical examination is equivocal. They are useful in detecting subtle changes when the gross nature of the sensory examination suggests normality. Finally, evoked potential testing is able to detect the functioning of pathways that appear to be clinically absent. In these cases, the sensory pathway may be of no real value to the patient. However, the above studies suggest that the presence of evoked potentials is a favorable prognostic sign in the first week after injury.

Second, the evoked potential study only evaluates a very selected pathway in the spinal cord. This, coupled with the known greater sensitivity of gray matter synapses than white matter axons to ischemia (shown above in experimental models) and the known anatomic separation of the vascular supply to the anterior cord (anterior spinal artery) from that to the posterior cord (posterior spinal arteries), suggest that problems can be occurring in other cord regions (notably the motor tracts) without an alteration in evoked potentials. However, the experimental studies of cord injury and operations demonstrate that posterior column changes are usually associated with cord insults, thus verifying the clinical usefulness of the technique. However, there are documented rare occurrences of injury (most notably anterior spinal artery syndrome) without evoked potential changes.[83] There clearly may also be more subtle effects in these patients that are to date unappreciated.

In seeking a perspective on the future of evoked potentials, several experimental studies suggest that future applications will allow the routine assessment of motor function. Studies of the potentiation of the H reflex by the Jendrassik's maneuver[31] have met with little success. However, direct testing of motor function would readily become a valuable addition to the diagnostic battery if the technique was developed. At present, the methodology is available but the methods are too invasive or risky. One technique involves electrical stimulation of the brain either over the scalp or via needles through the cranium with concomitant assessment of descending electrical activity.[87–93] Another, perhaps more readily applicable technique is the stimulation of the cord via intraspinal[15,17,76,77] or epidural[11,13,14,16,48,77] electrodes and the use of similar electrodes to record cord potentials at more caudal locations. Of interest is that these techniques can be used to test ascending as well as descending pathways.

These techniques are probably the forerunners of future methods for testing the motor tracts. However, until their value is shown to outweigh their risks, their application will probably remain experimental. To date, the classic methods discussed above (SSEP, BAER, VEP, DEP) remain readily applicable with very little risk and can provide a very meaningful addition to the total diagnosis and management of the spinal cord-injured patient.

REFERENCES

1. Dawson GD: A summation technique for detecting small signals in a large irregular background. J Physiol 115:2P, 1951
2. Dawson GD: A summation technique for the detection of small evoked potentials. Electroencephalogr Clin Neurophysiol 6:65, 1954
3. Caton R: Interim report on investigation of the electric currents of the brain. Br Med J, suppl, 1:62, 1877
4. Caton R: The electric currents of the brain. Br Med J 2:278, 1875
5. Chiappa KH, Ropper AH: Evoked potentials in clinical medicine: part 1. N Engl J Med 306:1140, 1982
6. Chiappa KH, Ropper AH: Evoked potentials in clinical medicine: part 2. N Engl J Med 306:1205, 1982
7. Chiappa KH: Evoked Potentials in Clinical Medicine. Raven Press, New York, 1983
8. Eisen A, Elleker G: Sensory nerve stimulation and evoked cerebral potentials. Neurology 30:1097, 1980
9. Larson SJ, Holst RA, Hemmy DC, Sances A, Jr.: Lateral extracavity approach to traumatic lesions of the thoracic and lumbar spine. J Neurosurg 45:628, 1976
10. Stochard JJ, Sharbrough FW: Unique contributions of short-latency auditory and somatosensory evoked potentials to neurologic diagnosis. Prog Clin Neurophysiol 7:231, 1980
11. Hattori S, Seiki K, Kawai S: Diagnosis of the level and severity of cord lesion in cervical spondylotic myelopathy: spinal evoked potentials. Spine 4:478, 1979
12. Sedgewick EM, El-Negamy E, Frankel H: Spinal cord potentials in traumatic paraplegia and quadriplegia. J Neurol Neurosurg Psychiatry 43:823, 1980
13. Shimoji K, Higashi H, Kano T: Epiduralrecording of spinal electrogram in man. Electroencephalogr Clin Neurophysiol 30:236, 1971
14. Tamaki T: Clinical benefits of ESP. Seikagaku 29:681, 1977
15. Ertekin C, Mutlu R, Sarica Y, Uckardesier L: Electrophysiological evaluation of the afferent spinal roots and nerves in patients with conus medullaris and cauda equina lesions. J Neurol Sci 48:419, 1980
16. Macon JB, Poletti CE: Conducted somatosensory evoked potentials during spinal surgery. Part 1: control conduction velocity measurements. J Neurosurg 57:349, 1982
17. Nordwall A, Axelgaard J, Harado Y, et al.: Spinal cord monitoring using evoked potentials recorded from feline vertebral bone. Spine 4:486, 1979
18. Brown RH, Nash CL, Jr.: Current status of spinal cord monitoring. Spine 4:466, 1979
19. Reger SI, Henry DT, Whitehall R, et al.: Spinal evoked potentials from the cervical spine. Spine 4:495, 1979
20. Hargadine JR, Branston NM, Symon L: Central conduction time in primate brain ischemia — a study in baboons. Stroke 11:637, 1980
21. Hume AL, Cant BR: Central somatosensory conduction after head injury. Ann Neurol 10:411, 1981
22. Cohen AR, Young W, Ransohoff J: Intraspinal localization of the somatosensory evoked potential. Neurosurgery 9:157, 1981
23. Albin MS, White RJ, Acosta-Rua G, Yashor D: Study of functional recovery produced by delayed localized cooling after spinal cord injury in primates. J Neurosurg 29:113, 1968
24. Croft TJ, Brodkey JS, Nulsen FE: Reversible spinal cord trauma: a model for electrical monitoring of spinal cord function. J Neurosurg 36:402, 1972
25. D'Angelo CM, VanGilder JC, Taub A: Evoked cortical potentials in experimental spinal cord trauma. J Neurosurg 38:332, 1973
26. Ducker TB, Saleman M, Perot PL, Jr., Ballentine D: Experimental spinal cord trauma. I. Correlation of blood flow, tissue oxygen and neurologic status in the dog. Surg Neurol 10:60, 1978
27. Ducker TB, Saleman M, Lucas J, et al.: Experimental spinal cord trauma. II. Blood flow, tissue oxygen, evoked potentials in both paretic and plegic monkeys. Surg Neurol 10:64, 1978
28. Osterholm JL: The pathophysiological response to spinal cord injury: the current status of related research. J Neurosurg 40:3, 1974

29. Singer JM, Russell GV, Coe JE: Changes in evoked potentials after experimental cervical spinal cord injury in the monkey. Exp Neurol 29:449, 1970

30. Sentar HJ, Vennes JL: Loss of autoregulation and posttraumatic ischemia following experimental spinal cord trauma. J Neurosurg 50:198, 1979

31. Numoto M, Flanagan M, Wallman L, Donaghy R: Proc Veterans Adm Spinal Cord Inj Conf. 18:227, 1971

32. Bennett MH, McCallum JE: Experimental decompression of spinal cord. Surg Neurol 8:63, 1977

33. Kobrine AI, Evans DE, Rizzoli H: Correlation of spinal cord blood flow and function in experimental compression. Surg Neurol 10:54, 1978

34. Kobrine AL, Evans DE, Rizzoli HV: Experimental acute balloon compression of the spinal cord. J Neurosurg 51:841, 1979

35. Martin SH, Bloedel JR: Evaluation of experimental spinal cord injury using cortical evoked potentials. J Neurosurg 39:75, 1973

36. Young W, Tomasula J, DeCrescito V, et al.: Vestibulospinal monitoring in experimental spinal trauma. J Neurosurg 52:64,1980

37. Tator CH, Rowed DW: Current concepts in the immediate management of acute spinal cord injuries. Can Med Assoc J 121:1453, 1979

38. Perot P: The clinical use of somatosensory evoked potentials in spinal cord injury. Clin Neurosurg 20:367, 1973

39. Perot PL, Jr.: Somatosensory evoked potentials in the evaluation of patients with spinal cord injury. p. 160. In Marley TP (ed): Current Controversies in Neurosurgery. WB Saunders , Philadelphia, 1976

40. Perot PL, Jr., Vera CL: Scalp-recorded somatosensory evoked potentials to stimulation of nerves in the lower extremities and evaluation of patients with spinal cord trauma. Ann NY Acad Sci 388:359, 1982

41. Spielholz NI, Benjamin MV, Engler G, Ransohoff J: Somatosensory evoked potentials and clinical outcome in spinal cord injury. p. 217. In Popp AJ, Bourke RS, Nelson LR, Kimelberg HK (eds): Neural Trauma. Raven Press, New York, 1979

42. Young W: Correlation of somatosensory evoked potentials and neurological findings in spinal cord injury. p. 153. In Tator CH (ed): Early Management of Acute Spinal Cord Injury. Raven Press, New York, 1982

43. Rowed DW, McLean JAG, Taot CH: Somatosensory evoked potentials in acute spinal cord injury: prognostic value. Surg Neurol 9:203, 1978

44. Rowed DW: Value of somatosensory evoked potentials for prognosis in partial cord injuries. p. 167. In Tator CH (ed): Early Management of Acute Spinal Cord Injury. Raven Press, New York, 1982

45. Bohlman HH, Behniuk E, Field G, Raskulinecz G: Spinal cord monitoring of experimental incomplete cervical spinal cord injury. Spine 6:428,1981

46. Chehrazi B, Parkinson J, Bucholz R: Evoked somatosensory potentials to common peroneal nerve stimulation in man. J Neurosurg 55:733, 1981

47. Dorfman LJ, Parkash I, Bosley TM, Cummins KL: Use of cerebral evoked potentials to evaluate spinal somatosensory function in patients with traumatic and surgical myelopathies. J Neurosurg 52:654, 1980

48. Shimoji K, Kano T, Morioka T, Ikezono E: Evoked spinal electrogram in a quadriplegic patient. Electroencephalogr Clin Neurophysiol 35:659, 1973

49. Katz S, Blackburn JG, Perot PL, Lam CF: The effects of low spinal injury on somatosensory evoked potentials from forelimb stimulation. Electroencephalogr Clin Neurophys 44:236, 1978

50. Halliday AM, Wakefield GS: Cerebral evoked potentials in patients with dissociated sensory loss. J Neurol Neurosurg Psychiatry 26:211, 1963

51. Toleikis JR, Scarff TB, Dallmann DE: Dermatomal somatosensory evoked potentials in the diagnosis of lumbosacral root entrapment. p. 16. Nicolet Potentials, Fall, 1982

52. Baust W, Ilsen HW, Jorg W, Wambach G: A neurophysiological method for the localization of transverse lesions of the spinal cord. Acta Neurochir (Wien) 26:352, 1972

53. Green J, Gildemeister R, Hazelwood C: Dermatomally stimulated somatosensory cerebral evoked potentials in the clinical diagnosis of lumbar disc disease. Clin Electroencephalogr 14:152, 1983

54. Jorg J: Die Electrosensible Diagnostik in der Neurologie. Springer-Verlag, Berlin, 1977

55. Jorg J, Dullberg W, Koeppen S: Diagnostic value of segmental somatosensory evoked potentials in cases with chronic progressive para- or tetraspastic syndromes. p. 347. In Courjon J, Manguiere F, Revol M (eds): Clinical Applications of Evoked Potentials in Neurology. Raven Press, New York, 1982

56. Scarff T, Toleikis JR, Bunch W, Parrish S: Dermatomal somatosensory evoked potentials in children with myelomeningocele. Z Kinderchir 28:384, 1980

57. Schramm J, Oettle GJ, Pichert T: Clinical application of segmental somatosensory evoked potentials (SEP) — experience in patients with non-space occupying lesions. p. 455. In Barber C (ed): Evoked Potentials. MTP Press, Leichester, 1980

58. Schramm J, Krause R, Shigeno T, Brock M: Experi-

mental investigation on the spinal cord evoked injury potential. J Neursurg 59:485, 1983.

59. Eisen A, Hoirch M, Moll A: Evaluation of radiculopathies by segmental stimulation and somatosensory evoked potentials. Can J Neurol Sci 10:178, 1983

60. Louis AA, Gupta P, Perkash I: Localization of sensory level in traumatic quadriplegia by segmental somatosensory evoked potentials. Electroencephalgr Clin Neurophysiol 62:313, 1985

61. Scarff TB, Dallmann DE, Toleikis JR, Bunch WH: Dermatomal somatosensory evoked potentials in the diagnosis of lumbar root entrapment. Surg Forum 32:489, 1981

62. Toleikis JR, Sloan TB, Schrader S, Koht A: Scalp distribution of dermatome evoked potentials. p. 59. In Schramm J, Jones SJ (eds): Spinal Cord Monitoring. Springer-Verlag, Berlin, 1985

63. Giblin DR: Somatosensory evoked potentials in healthy subjects and in patients with lesions of the nervous system. Ann NY Acad Sci 112:93, 1964

64. Halliday AM: Changes in the form of cerebral evoked responses in man associated with various lesions of the nervous system. Electroencephalogr Clin Neurophysiol, suppl., 25:178, 1967

65. Greenberg RP, Mayer DJ, Becker DP, Miller JD: Evaluation of brain function in severe human head trauma with multimodality evoked potentials. Part 1: evoked brain-injury potentials and analysis. J Neurosurg 47:150,1977

66. Greenberg RP, Mayer DJ, Becker DP, Miller JD: Evaluation of brain function in severe human head trauma with multimodality evoked potentials. Part 2: localization of brain dysfunction and correlation with posttraumatic neurological conditions. J Neurosurg 47:163, 1977

67. Greenberg RP, Miller JD, Becker DP: Clinical findings associated with brainstem dysfunction: an electrophysiological study in severe human head trauma. p. 229. In Popp AJ, Bourke RS, Nelson AR, Kimelberg HK (eds): Neural Trauma. Raven Press, New York, 1979

68. Newlon PG, Greenberg RP, Hyatt MS, et al.: The dynamics of neuronal dysfunction and recovery following severe head injury assessed with serial multimodality evoked potentials. J Neurosurg 57:168, 1982

69. Grundy BL: Monitoring of sensory evoked potentials during neurosurgical operations: methods and applications. Neurosurgery 11:556, 1982

70. Grundy BL: Intraoperative monitoring of sensory-evoked potentials. Anesthesiology 58:72, 1983

71. Engler GL, Spielholz NI, Bernhard WN, et al.: Somatosensory evoked potentials during Harrington instrumentation for scoliosis. J Bone Joint Surg 60A:528, 1978

72. Hahn JF, Lesser R, Klem G, Leuders H: Simple technique for monitoring intraoperative spinal cord function. Neurosurgery 9:692, 1981

73. Leuders H, Gurd A, Hahn J, et al.: A new technique for intraoperative monitoring of spinal cord function: multichannel recording of spinal cord and subcortical evoked potentials. Spine 7:110, 1982

74. Nash CL, Lorig RA, Schatzinger LR, Brown RH: Spinal cord monitoring during operative treatment of the spine. Clin Orthop 126:100, 1977

75. Raudzens PA: Intraoperative monitoring of evoked potentials. Ann NY Acad Sci 388:308, 1982

76. Levy WJ: Spinal evoked potentials from the motor tracts. J Neurosurg 58:38, 1983

77. Macon JB, Poletti CE, Sweet WH, et al: Conducted somatosensory evoked potentials during spinal surgery. Part 2: clinical applications. J Neurosurg 57:354, 1982

78. Kojima Y, Yamamoto T, Ogino H, et al.: Evoked spinal potentials as a monitor of spinal cord viability. Spine 4:471, 1979

79. MacEwen GD, Bunnell WP, Sriram K: Acute neurological complications in the treatment of scoliosis: a report of the Scoliosis Research Society. J Bone Joint Surg 57A:404, 1975

80. Grundy BL, Heros RC, Tung AS, Doyle E: Intraoperative hypoxia detected by evoked potential monitoring. Anesth Analg 60:437, 1981

81. Grundy BL, Procopio PT, Janetta PJ, Line et al.: Evoked potential changes produced by positioning for retromastoid craniectomy. Neurosurgery 10:766, 1982

82. Clark DL, Rosner BS: Neurophysiologic effects of general anesthetics. I. The electroencephalogram and sensory evoked responses in man. Anesthesiology 38:564, 1973

83. Spielholz NI, Benjamin MV, Engler G, Ransohoff J: Somatosensory evoked potentials during decompression and stabilization of the spine: methods and findings. Spine 4:500, 1979

84. Low MD, Purves S, Purves BL: A critical assessment of the use of evoked potentials in diagnosis of peripheral nerve, spinal cord and cerebral disease. p. 169. In Marley TP (ed): Current Controversies in Neurosurgery. WB Saunders, Philadelphia, 1976

85. McCallum JE, Bennett MH: Electrophysiologic monitoring of spinal cord function during intraspinal surgery. Surg Forum 26:469, 1975

86. Nash CL, Schatzinger LH, Brown RH, Brodkey J: The unstable thoracic compression fracture: its

problems and the use of spinal cord monitoring in the evaluation of treatment. Spine 2:261, 1977

87. Grossman RG, Lindquist C, Feinstein R, Eisenberg HM: Monitoring of the excitability of the cerebral cortex in brain injury with the direct cortical response. p. 237. In Popp AJ, Bourke RS, Nelson AR, Kimelberg HK (eds): Neural Trauma. Raven Press, New York, 1979

88. Levy WJ, York DH, McCaffrey M, Tanzer F: Motor evoked potentials from transcranial stimulation of the motor cortex in humans. Neurosurgery 15:287, 1984

89. Levy WJ, McCaffrey M, York DH, Tanzer F: Motor evoked potentials from transcranial stimulation of the motor cortex in cats. Neurosurgery 15:214, 1984

90. Levy WJ, York DH: Evoked potentials from the motor tracts in humans. Neurosurgery 12:422, 1983

91. Merton PA, Morton HB, Hill DK, Maisen CD: Scope of a technique for electrical stimulation of human brain, spinal cord and muscle. Lancet 2:597, 1982

92. Merton PA, Morton HB: Stimulation of the cerebral cortex in the intact human subject. Nature 285:287, 1980

93. Merton PA, Morton HB: Electrical stimulation of human motor and visual cortex through the scalp. J Physiol (Lond) 355:9, 1980

7

Neurologic Assessment and Management of Head Injuries

Julian E. Bailes

Leonard J. Cerullo

Herbert H. Engelhard

The experience of the Northwestern University Spine Injury Center in treating acute spinal cord injuries between June 1972 and December 1986 demonstrated that multiple trauma is a major factor influencing outcome for spine injured patients. Forty three percent of the patients admitted with acute spine injuries had multiple trauma. Of this population, 26.2 percent had a head injury. In 1979, West et al. reported a study of the outcome for trauma patients admitted to hospitals in Orange County, California, in which the patients were admitted irrespective of the ability of the institution to provide specialized care for head trauma.[1] He concluded that 33 percent of the patients with head trauma who died would have survived had they been admitted to an appropriate institution. The absolute influence of head trauma on the mortality of patients with spinal cord trauma is not known. It is known, however, that in 1986 the mortality rate in the Northwestern University Spine Injury Center was 2.7 percent. For the period from 1972 to 1981, the mortality for the center

varied from 2 percent to 13 percent. The average hospital stay for patients with acute spinal cord injuries is 22 days. The length of stay for patients who also have head trauma is 5 days longer. The median admission time to the Center for 2,710 patients (from a catchment area 200 miles in radius) was 6.2 hours. Were it not for the early arrival of patients and the immediate assessment of the severity index of their injuries, the high incidence of head trauma in spine-injured patients would likely have a much more serious effect on recovery and outcome.

The general term *head injury* covers trauma sustained to the scalp, skull, and brain (Fig. 7-1). In most instances, however, damage to the brain is the matter of clinical importance.[2] *Closed head injury* refers to all nonpenetrating trauma to the head and, in the civilian population, accounts for the majority of injuries. *Cerebral injury* is classically divided into two types: focal and diffuse. Focal injuries are radiographically visible lesions, including contusions and hematomas. Diffuse injuries cause wide-

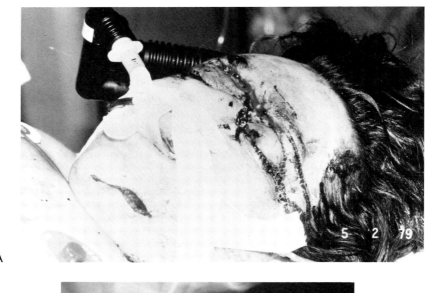

A

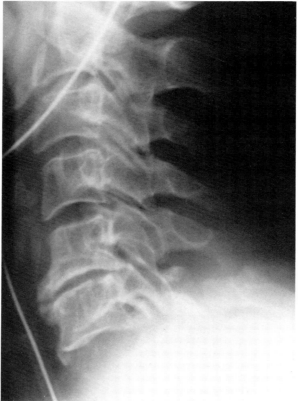

B

Fig. 7-1. Head trauma and spinal cord-injured victim. (A) Operating room view of cervical spine-injured patient who sustained extension injury to the cervical spine (C6–C7), multiple open extremity fractures, and significant face and head trauma. (B) Lateral radiograph of cervical spine showing extension injury to C6–C7 with evidence of avulsion of anterior longitudinal ligament and widening of C6–C7 disc space. Note also fracture of posterior element of C6 and the dislocation of facet joints of C6–C7.

spread cerebral dysfunction without a macroscopically identifiable brain insult.

PRIMARY HEAD INJURY: DEFINITIONS

Fractures

Skull fractures are either linear or depressed, and their incidence varies with the head injury population under study, increasing with the severity of trauma. In a study of 207 patients with post-traumatic intracranial mass lesions, Cooper and Ho found that 76 (37 percent) had a skull fracture.[4] Harwood-Nash et al. found 27 percent of 4,465 children with head injuries to have skull fractures.

Linear skull fractures involve a break in the calvaria in which the bony fragments are not displaced or depressed (Fig. 7-2). Linear fractures are of significance insofar as they reflect the magnitude of the force applied to the head and in terms of their relationship to underlying dural vessels and venous sinuses. If these structures are damaged, an epidural hematoma may form. However, about the same number of patients with and without skull fractures have epidural hematomas.[6] Linear skull fractures may also be of importance if they occur in the skull base, where they may damage cranial nerves at their exit foramina or cause a leak of cerebrospinal fluid (CSF). Triscot and Hallot found seven patients with skull fractures in a series of 270 traumatic paraplegic patients.[7]

A *depressed skull fracture* involves offset of fracture fragments, which may impinge on the brain

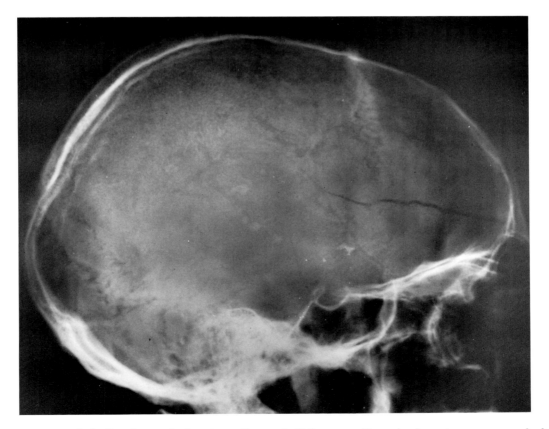

Fig. 7-2. Lateral skull radiograph showing a linear skull fracture. Note the lucent appearance, lack of sclerotic border, and failure to branch.

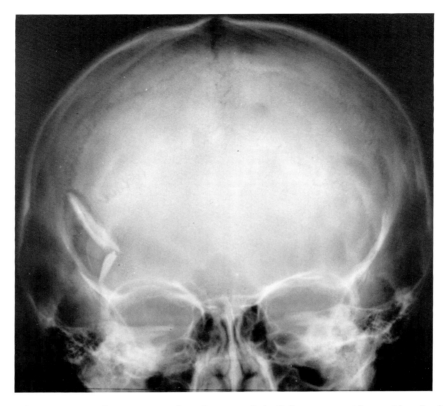

Fig. 7-3. Frontal projection of a patient with a depressed skull fracture, evidenced by the hyperdensity signifying overlapping bone edges.

(Fig. 7-3). Depressed skull fragments may lacerate underlying tissues or form an irritative focus for seizure activity. A *closed* or *simple* skull fracture has no overlying scalp laceration, whereas an *open* or *compound* fracture is located adjacent to or under a communicating scalp laceration.

Brain Injury

Primary brain injury is injury that occurs as a result of direct, immediate cerebral damage. Concussion is a frequent if not invariable concomitant of significant head injury. In practical terms, concussion is defined as physiologic rather than anatomic dysfunction.[3] Clinically, *concussion* covers a spectrum of syndromes which may include disorders of the level of consciousness, retrograde and/or posttraumatic amnesia, and confusion.

Cerebral swelling is due to a temporary loss of vasomotor tone with a resultant diffuse increase in brain blood volume. It occurs mainly in children. Cerebral edema is due to increased brain water secondary to traumatic disruption of the blood-brain barrier with extravasation of fluid into the extravascular spaces with the potential of causing a mass effect.

Contusions are fixed parenchymal injuries characteristically appearing in areas where the brain and skull are in close contact, such as the anterior temporal and frontal lobes. They are heterogeneous and include hemorrhage, edema, and tissue necrosis. They are dynamic and may begin or evolve throughout the early days after injury. An intracerebral hematoma results from extravasation of blood into brain tissue or into a potential space, often after a deceleration or shearing injury. It is a homogeneous, well-delineated collection of blood that usually appears immediately or within hours after injury. Like cerebral contusions, the clinical presentation of intracerebral hematoma is one of a focal or destructive lesion of the area involved, with the potential for subsequent development of edema and further mass effect. Delayed development of an intracerebral hematoma may occur.

Traumatic acute subdural hematoma is caused by bleeding from veins that course from the cerebral surface to the dura, or from contusions that allow bleeding into the subdural space.[8,9] Clinically, the patient may have signs referable to local brain injury, to the amount of extrinsic pressure, or to both. With time, acute subdural hematomas may evolve into subacute and chronic hematomas with a slowly progressive clinical course.

An *extradural hematoma* is caused by bleeding into the potential space between the dura and inner table of the skull, originating from a breach in a meningeal vessel or dural sinus. In children, it may result from diploic oozing from a skull fracture, and in adults, it is usually but not unvariably associated with a fracture of the skull.[10] It may progress to a large size with significant mass effect along with rapid deterioration and death of the patient if the clot is not identified and surgically evacuated.[11-13]

SECONDARY BRAIN INJURY

In addition to the effects of initial direct brain injury, there may be secondary cerebral insults resulting from elevated intracranial pressure (ICP) and/or brain shift.[14] As intracranial volume increases to reach a critical level, the brain's compensatory capacity (i.e., displacement of CSF and blood) is exceeded and there is a sharp rise in ICP (Fig. 7-4). There may be resulting displacement of the brain in a cephalocaudal direction, with the uncus of the temporal lobe being compressed through the tentorial incisura. This displacement leads to an immediate onset of a symptom complex due to regional ischemia of vital midbrain structures, and classically including a depression in the level of consciousness, ipsilateral oculomotor nerve palsy, and contralateral hemiparesis. With global ischemia, a generalized, symmetric central nervous system depression occurs, most characteristically reflected in an alteration of the patient's level of consciousness, and proceeding to coma if severe. If uncontrolled, compression of vital structures is life-threatening (Fig. 7-5). The "Cushing reflex" is a response to an acutely rising ICP and presages uncal herniation. It consists of hypertension, bradycardia, and alterations of the respiratory pattern.

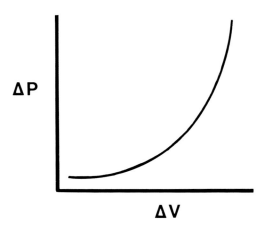

Fig. 7-4. The intracranial pressure-compliance curve demonstrates that initially the cranium can compensate for increases in pressure. As a critical volume is reached (e.g., expanding hematoma), the brain can no longer compensate and there is a rise in the ICP. As ICP increases, and assuming that mean systemic blood pressure remains unchanged, cerebral perfusion will be compromised.

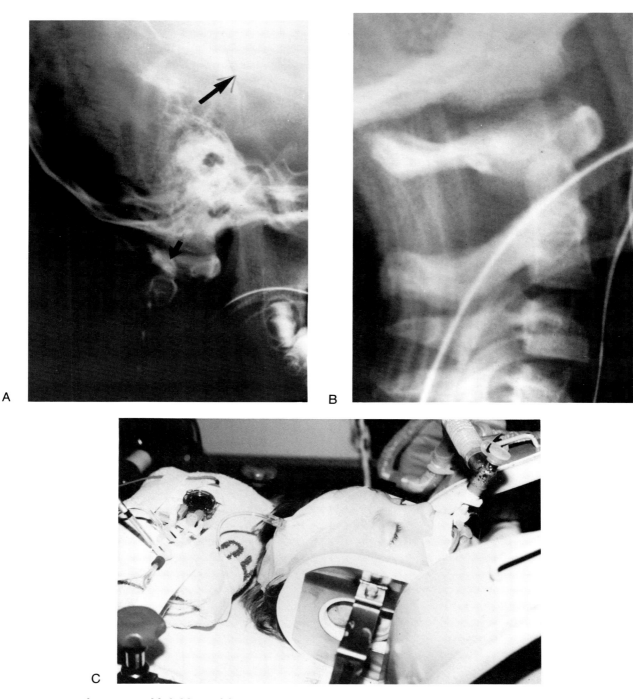

Fig. 7-5. Three-year-old child struck by a car. (**A**) Lateral radiograph of cervical spine shows global dissocia-tion of C1 – C2 ligamentous attachment. Note the linear skull fracture over the temporal area (arrow). (**B**) Lateral radiograph showing further dissociation between C1 and C2 with the application of minimal trac-tion. (**C**) Child in spinal cord intensive care unit with intracranial pressure monitor in place. The child was sustained on a ventilator for 3 days before succumbing to brain and brain stem death.

VASCULAR INJURY MIMICKING HEAD INJURY

Among spinal cord-injured patients, there is a subgroup whose neurologic compromise is secondary to damage to major vascular structures. Blunt or penetrating cervical trauma may cause direct injury to the vertebral or carotid arteries. The patient with a vascular complication of a cervical spine injury may radiologically show a traumatic fracture-dislocation, predisposing chronic subluxation, or a normal spine.[15]

Clinically, the patient sustaining an injury to the internal carotid artery in the neck usually has a discernible pattern of symptoms, though there may be no obvious indication of trauma to the neck. One or more of the following may be found: neck pain, cervical hematoma, fracture (of the spine, mandible, shoulder, thorax, or skull base), or a Horner's syndrome. It is estimated that one-third to one-half of the patients have no external evidence of neck injury.[16-18] Since the carotid artery supplies the anterior circulation to the cerebral hemispheres the most common signs reflect hemispheric dysfunction (hemiplegia, hemianesthesia, homonymous visual field defects). A delay in the appearance of a neurologic deficit is most characteristic, even up until several days.[19-21] Transient ischemic attacks (TIAs) in the territories of the anterior or middle cerebral artery may result from distal embolization of particulate material forming at the point of intimal damage. Regional cerebral ischemia and infarction cause focal neurologic deficit, although the clinical picture depends on the degree of collateral circulation and the presence of associated cerebral trauma.[17,22,23]

Often the most perplexing problem in the acute evaluation of the patient is distinguishing between primary parenchymal cerebral damage (hematoma, contusion, and secondary ischemic insult) and vascular injury. The main differentiating feature is the rapid deterioration of the level of consciousness seen with an intracranial mass, which is often not seem immediately after a limited ischemic insult to the anterior circulation.[15,16,24] One should realize that the patient's original condition may preclude this assessment, that there may be concomitant intracranial and extracranial patho-

logic processes, and that ischemic infarcts may eventually result in edema with mass effect.

The vertebral artery may be damaged by an injury causing a fracture above C6, either by direct compression by bony elements, by stretching of the artery by vertical movement, or by an expanding hematoma within the foramen transversarium.[22,25-27] Considerable evidence indicates that the vertebral arteries are most vulnerable to injury at the level of the first and second cervical vertebral segments and where they enter the foramen magnum (Fig. 7-6). Any compromise of the vertebral artery may lead to structural damage to the vessel wall or to vasospasm, with resultant ascending thrombosis and hindbrain ischemia[17,22] (Fig. 7-7).

Sherman et al. reviewed more than 50 cases of vertebrobasilar insufficiency secondary to nonpenetrating cervical injury. In 80 percent of the patients, ischemic symptoms followed chiropractic or other neck manipulation.[28] Injuries of the vertebrobasilar arterial system have been reported after motor vehicle accidents, exercise, minor falls, and simple turning of the head.[17,29,30] Schneider et al. reported six cases caused by football mishaps.[31]

Injuries to the cervical vertebral artery often are symptomatic immediately after the traumatic insult, and the developing neurologic deficit may be gradual and mild or sudden and severe.[22,32] The resulting clinical picture is one of many possible brain stem or cerebellar syndromes.[17] Signs of vertebrobasilar insufficiency or infarction include dysarthria, ataxia, diplopia, and vertigo. Complete brain stem infarction, albeit rare, may occur. In contrast to compromise of the anterior cerebral circulation, there is a lower incidence of altered level of consciousness and lateralizing signs. In the absence of demonstrated intracranial injury, computed tomography (CT) scanning may be unrevealing or may show typical vascular patterns, depending on time after the onset of symptoms. When the clinical picture includes a negative CT scan along with a significant hindbrain neurologic deficit, one should suspect vascular injury and consider angiography. The demonstration and treatment of arterial injury depends on the expeditious performance of cervical and cerebral angiographic studies. Angiography should be performed immediately on all patients with suspected vascular injury, particularly in those with penetrating neck trauma, unless

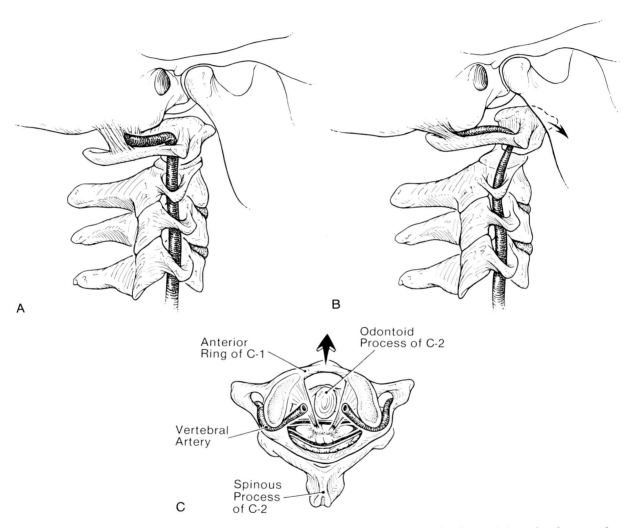

A

B

Anterior
Ring of C-1

Odontoid
Process of C-2

Vertebral
Artery

Spinous
Process
of C-2

C

Fig. 7-6. (**A**) The normal relationship of the vertebral artery to the spinal column. (**B**) With atlantoaxial dislocation, there is impingement on the vertebral artery primarily at two points: as it winds around the lateral border of the atlas and as it pierces the dura to enter the foramen magnum.

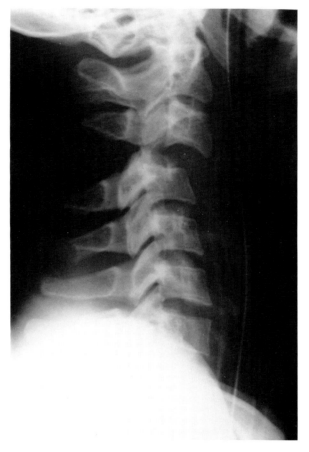
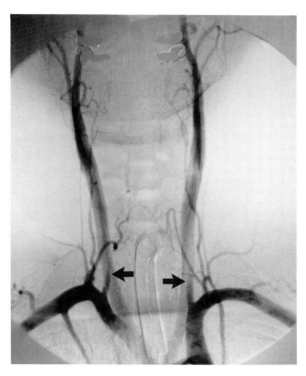

A

B

Fig. 7-7. (**A**) 28-year-old man injured in a diving accident suffered C3–C4 subluxation, complete quadriplegia, and apnea. In the first few days after injury, he progressively lost lower cranial nerve function and had a Dejerine defect of facial sensation. (**B**) An angiogram performed at 1 week shows bilateral occlusion of the vertebral arteries 2 cm from their origin (arrows).

other immediate life-threatening conditions (e.g., airway maintenance, major hemorrhage, shock) supervene.

COINCIDENCE OF HEAD AND SPINAL INJURY

The true incidence of significant head injury has been difficult to assess because of its frequent association with multiple injuries, a paucity of details in recording the cause of death, the non-hospitalization of a percentage of patients with minor injuries

and rapid recovery, and incomplete clinical documentation. According to a study by the National Safety Council, 62 percent of fatalities in motor vehicle accidents are the result of head injuries.[33] Among all victims of automobile accidents, the head was the area of the body injured most commonly, but only 5 percent of all head injuries caused by vehicular accident were fatal. By body area, the percentage of injuries that were fatal in order of increasing incidence were: head (5 percent), chest and thoracic spine (6 percent), and neck and cervical spine (16 percent).[33,34] Seventy percent of motor vehicle injuries involve some form of craniocerebral trauma.[35] About 6 percent of patients with work-related accidents have head injury.[36]

Tonge et al., in an autopsy study of 908 traffic accident victims, found that 48.3 percent had brain injuries; spinal fractures and/or dislocations occurred in the lumbosacral spine in 15.3 percent, in the thoracic spine in 7.7 percent, and in the cervical spine in 2.2 percent.[37] The correlation of the association between spinal injury and head injuries in this report is high. In the total population (2,710), the incidence of multiple trauma was 42.9 percent. Of this group, 26 percent also had head trauma.

The association between head trauma and spinal injury has long been noted. Injury sufficient to damage one will often affect the other. Jefferson first reported that an axial force directed to the top of the skull may be transmitted to fracture the ring of the atlas in a centrifugal manner.[38,39] Davis et al. performed autopsies on 50 patients who died of acute injury to the head and/or neck, and made detailed examinations of the craniospinal region.[40] The cause of injury in 43 cases was a motor vehicle accident, with 33 victims suffering instantaneous death. An additional nine patients died within 3 hours of trauma. Of the cases, 61 percent had both brain lesions and spinal cord damage. Skull damage and cervical spine damage were both present in 25 percent, while in 20 percent, no evidence of simultaneous injury was found despite lethal brain or spinal cord lesions. The authors concluded, "That the head and neck should be considered as a unit in discussing trauma seems to be obvious from this study. Not only are these types of injury in the brain and spinal cord quite similar, but rarely is one structure involved to the exclusion of the other except, when the force is indirect and the heavy head uses a cervical vertebra as a fulcrum."[40]

Alker et al. conducted a radiographic analysis of 312 motor vehicle accident victims who died at the scene of the accident or shortly thereafter.[41] Seventy-six (24.4 percent) had evidence of cervical injury on radiographic examination. Seventy percent of cervical injuries occurred at the atlanto-occipital or C1–C2 level. Of the victims in this study, 35.2 percent had head injury only, 14.4 percent has isolated neck injury, and 9.9 percent sustained both head and neck injury.[41] Shrago studied 50 trauma patients who had radiographic evidence of cervical spine injury and found that 53 percent of those with upper cervical spine injuries had concomitant head trauma. Lesions of the lower cervical spine were associated with head injury in only 9 percent.[42]

Silver et al. reviewed the cases of 100 consecutive patients admitted to a spinal cord unit.[43] Seventy-five percent had associated injuries. Head trauma was seen in 50 percent of the cases. Of the 50 head injuries, 41 were of a minor nature, whereas 9 were more serious (skull fractures, CSF leak, and subdural hematoma). Head injuries were present in 17 patients with cervical lesions, in 28 with thoracic lesions, and in 5 with lumbar lesions. Commenting on the unusual finding that fewer head injuries were seen with cervical lesions than with thoracic lesions, Silver and colleagues postulated that patients with serious head injury may not survive until eventual transfer to the spinal cord unit.[43] Harris found an 8 percent incidence of major head trauma among spinal cord-injured patients.[44]

Porter reviewed 216 autopsies performed on patients with nonfatal spinal cord injury who died 3 to 27 years later.[45] Sixty-two of 216 patients (29 percent) had had significant injury to the brain or skull as determined by clinical history or autopsy findings. Fifty percent of patients with head injuries had cervical spine fractures (C4 to C7). The remainder had fractures from T5 to L4, with a predominance at the thoracolumbar junction. The majority (17 of 28) with fractures of the thoracolumbar junction had basilar skull fractures.[45]

PATIENT ASSESSMENT

The early evaluation of the patient should give the examiner an idea of the seriousness of the injury. When there is little evidence of direct head or body impact, brief or no loss of consciousness, and normal mental status and neurologic examination, there is little likelihood that the patient has sustained a serious brain injury. The patient is then placed in a category of low-probability head injury, but may nonetheless require observation for delayed complications (e.g., intracerebral hematoma), especially if the mechanism of injury was of a severe nature.

History

Once the patient is stable, attention is turned to the evaluation of brain and spinal cord involvement. Quite often the exact nature of the accident can be gleaned from passengers, other witnesses, or paramedics—for example, the patient's location during the accident (e.g., driver, passenger, pedestrian); loss of consciousness, initial motor, sensory, and sensorium status; direct head impact; and any evidence of associated injury (especially to the scalp, face, or neck). Likewise, for a baseline it is important to have documentation of the overall and neurologic condition of the patient at the site of initial evaluation and primary acute care. All available neuroradiologic studies, records, and physician's notes should accompany the patient to the definitive care facility. The presence of modifying factors such as alcohol or drug ingestion, pre-existing medical illness (hypertension, diabetes, neurologic disease including seizure disorder, cardiac or hematologic disease, and medication) must be considered. One should keep in mind that patient hysteria may also play a significant role in emergency situations. The examining physician assesses closed or open head trauma, obvious external injury, the extent of any amnesic period, and the initial level of consciousness and spontaneous activity. If possible, a concise but thorough history concerning the circumstances of the accident should be obtained from the patient, as occurs in any emergency setting.

Neurologic Examination

After medical stabilization and history, attention should be directed to the neurologic examination. As always, and especially in the trauma setting, inspection of the patient is carried out first. Scalp lacerations and contusions, while usually not in themselves of major importance, may provide evidence of underlying injury (e.g., depressed skull fracture). Periorbital ecchymosis (raccoon eyes) and mastoid ecchymosis (Battle's sign) or hemotympanum suggest a basilar skull fracture. In such patients, a CSF leak from the nose (rhinorrhea) or ear (otorrhea) should be sought.

Level of Consciousness

Perhaps the most sensitive and important indication of central nervous system dysfunction is the level of consciousness. The patient's level of consciousness is assessed in a conventional manner, noting state of arousal, orientation, and degree of interaction in following commands. Any alteration should be considered to indicate possible intracranial injury. In addition, the mechanism of injury, a history of loss of consciousness (usually, longer than 5 minutes is considered significant), or signs of external head trauma (e.g., scalp lacerations, facial trauma) may heighten one's index of suspicion.

In Porter's 62 patients with combined spinal and head injuries, at the time of admission 37 had a depressed sensorium of such a degree as to prevent meaningful communication.[45] Commonly, anoxia is the cause of confusion in this patient population.[43] Alterations of consciousness due to ethanol should not occur at blood alcohol levels below 200 mg%, and conversely, coma may be produced by levels greater than 300 mg%.[46,47] In addition, a postictal state may be present if a seizure has occurred. Epileptic patients are more difficult to assess, and detailed knowledge of the past medical history is imperative. Alterations of consciousness or coma secondary to brain stem ischemia may also be seen with high cervical injuries.[48] Because of the frequent relationship between spine injury, head injury, and alcohol or substance abuse, a drug screen should be performed on every acutely injured patient as part of the initial evaluation.

A head injury that produces significant depression of the level of consciousness or coma may simulate or mask a spinal cord injury, and vice versa. This is particularly true with high cervical injuries. Bilateral anterior cerebral artery occlusion may result in paraplegia with decreased sensation in the lower extremities, stimulating a spinal cord lesion.[49] Kline reported the case of a 14-year-old girl who, after a motor vehicle accident, presented with coma, hemiplegia, and midrange dilated pupils, all simulating a head injury. She was subsequently shown to have an atlantoaxial dislocation secondary to odontoid hypoplasia.[50] Absent intercostal muscle function, flaccid extremities, and loss of deep tendon reflexes indicate spinal injury regardless of the mental status of the patient.

In evaluating the level of consciousness of a patient, one of the most helpful parameters is serial assessment. In an effort to quantitate the neurologic status, the Glasgow Coma Scale was developed[51] (Table 7-1). This scale has been found to be accurate in estimating the extent of injury and prognosis. For patients with spinal injury, we use a modified version of the Glasgow Coma Scale to serially assess the neurologic status (Table 7-1).

Table 7-1.   The Glasgow Coma Scale

Eye opening	
Spontaneous	4
To speech	3
To pain	2
None	1
Verbal response	
Oriented	5
Confused conversation	4
Inappropriate words	3
Incomprehensible sounds	2
None	1
Motor response	
Obeys	6
Vocalizes	5
Withdraws	4
Abnormal flexion	3
Extensor response	2
None	1
Total	3–15

Modified Scale for Paralyzed Patients

Motor response	
Obeys	3
Withdraws	2
None	1

(Modified from Teasdale et al.,[51] with permission.)

The Glasgow coma scale is used for a rapid and reproducible clinical assessment of the head-injured patient. If used in serial examinations, it may aid in early detection of a progressive neurologic lesion by quantifying the state of arousal and function of the cerebral cortex. Sum scores of 7 or less define coma.

For paralyzed patients, the modified motor scale is used, which yields a total possible score of 12. For paraplegic patients, arm movements are used for motor assessment.

Cranial Nerve Assessment

Attention is then turned, if time permits, to systematic examination of the cranial nerves. The olfactory nerve is injured in about 7 percent of the cases of head trauma, owing to its frontobasal location.[52] Its integrity may be tested by having the patient smell an aromatic substance with the opposite nostril occluded.

The eyes are frequently injured when facial trauma is involved (see Fig. 7-1). The visual system may be injured at any site from the cornea to the occipital visual cortex. Optic nerve trauma may be intrabulbar, intraorbital, or intracanalicular.[53] If injured by a basilar skull fracture or other osseous injury or pressure phenomena, it may require emergent surgical decompression. Damage to the optic nerve has been variously reported in 0.3 percent to 13 percent of patients with head injuries.[54-57] Indeed, Jennett et al. state that it is the most common cranial nerve injury seen in survivors of head trauma.[58]

The nerves innervating the extraocular muscles are sometimes directly involved in head injury.[59] Schneider and Johnson reported two cases of bilateral 6th nerve palsy.[60] In one case the palsy was associated with an atlantoaxial dislocation, and in the other, with a hangman's fracture. They suggest that in severe hyperextension cervical injuries, the abducens nerve may be avulsed by the rigid petrosphenoid ligament as the brain moves posteriorly and upward.[60]

Oculomotor nerve injury is revealed by pupillary dilation and failure of normal reactivity to light. One must be certain that no medication has been instilled in the eye and that there was no preexisting pupillary defect nor a prosthetic eye. Lesions of the midbrain may cause the pupils to become midpositional and fixed or to exhibit hippus. Hemorrhage in the pontine area may cause pinpoint pupils. Hypothermia, seen in the spinal cord-injured patient when sympathetic tone is lost, may cause fixed pupils. The oculomotor nerve supplies innervation to the superior, inferior, and medial recti and inferior oblique muscles and the eyelid elevators. The function of these muscles is more difficult to evaluate in the unconscious patient, and injury may not be appreciated if pupillary function is spared. Third nerve dysfunction may also occur secondary to increased ICP with uncal herniation.

Pupillary findings must be interpreted in the light of the variety of normal reaction. It should be remembered that local ocular trauma, metabolic disturbance, hypotension, hypothermia, fluctuation in intracranial pressure, anoxia, postictal state, and an inadequate light stimulus may all affect the pupillary response. Injury to the cervicothoracic spinal cord in the brachial plexus region may cause sympathetic denervation of the ipsilateral eye (Horner's syndrome). As in all of such situations, these findings should be interpreted with respect to the overall picture, although bilaterally unreacting pupils for a period of several hours when other causes are absent is evidence for significant brain dysfunction. Injury of the abducens nerve is determined by failure of abduction of the eye. The abducens may be injured along with the 7th and 8th cranial nerves in petrous bone fractures or with distorting, crushing skull trauma.[61] An abducens palsy may be seen with increased ICP and is not of localizing value as the nerve may be compressed anywhere along its intracranial route. Since the palsy does not determine a specific causal anatomic lesion, it is referred to as a "false-localizing sign". The trochlear nerve is most susceptible to major frontal impact, in which the cranium is accelerated and damages the midbrain as it is compressed against the tentorial incisura.[62] Fourth nerve injury produces a vertical diplopia that is worse on downward and inward gaze, but obviously the patient must cooperate to evaluate this function.

Extraocular muscle function is much easier to evaluate in the conscious patient, but if the level of consciousness is depressed, voluntary eye movement may not be present. The functional integrity of the reticular formation in the brain stem is then evaluated by using the oculocephalic and oculovestibular responses. In patients with known or suspected cervical spine injury, only the latter examination is done, using ice water irrigation. In the presence of an interrupted tympanic membrane, this may be accomplished using a small catheter looped several times in the external auditory canal. This test may have limitations if there is injury to the semicircular canal or vestibular nerve or if there is orbital edema. The oculovestibular response and extraocular muscle function allow interpretation of the integrity of the pupillary pathways in the brain.

Injury of the corticobulbar pathways to the trigeminal nerve nucleus may be detected by the corneomandibular response (contralateral deviation of the jaw with corneal stimulation). High cervical cord lesions may involve the descending tract of the trigeminal nerve, which, in the upper cervical region, contains sensory fibers supplying the perimeter of the face. When this portion of the tract is involved, the patient may lose facial sensation in an "onion-peel" pattern from outside in—the so-called Dejerine effect.

Trauma to the 7th and 8th cranial nerves may occur with fractures of the petrous bone. Seventh nerve injury is suspected by asymmetry of the facial structures. An abnormal corneal reflex in comatose patients may be unreliable in determining injury. In the awake patient, the 8th cranial nerve may be evaluated by verbal stimulation, or in the comatose patient, by brain stem auditory evoked potentials. The 9th through 12th cranial nerves may be examined, respectively, by determination of a symmetric palatal elevation, gag reflex, phonation, neck musculature, and tongue function. They are most commonly injured by basilar skull fractures involving their exit foramina. The lower cranial nerves may occasionally be involved by an upper cervical or an ascending cervical lesion or by vascular compromise (e.g., carotid artery dissecting injury).

Respiration
Respiratory dysfunction after head injury may be classified into central and peripheral types.[63] In the former category, a medullary lesion and drugs may cause respiratory depression. Abnormal breathing patterns include periods of apnea at regular intervals, termed Cheyne-Stokes respiration and caused by bilateral dysfunction of the cerebral hemispheres or diencephalon. *Ataxic breathing* is apnea with an irregular pattern of random shallow and deep breathing. It indicates a disruption of the medullary neurons that generate respiratory rhythm. A third abnormal pattern is central neurogenic hyperventilation (CNH), seen with destructive lesions of the rostral brain stem tegmentum. True CNH in humans is believed to be rare.[64]

Peripheral respiratory dysfunction in the trauma patient may have many causes, chiefly aspiration, chest injury, disseminated intravascular coagulation, pulmonary edema, fat embolism, pulmonary embolism, or acute respiratory distress syndrome (ARDS). Of these, chest injury and aspiration are the most common. A third category of respiratory dysfunction is seen in the spinal cord-injured patient who may have lost the use of the intercostal muscles (thoracic or cervical lesion) or in a patient with a high cervical (C5 and above) injury that also involves the cervical innervation of the diaphragm (C3,4,5).

Although the motor system may be damaged anywhere along its descending pathway to the spinal cord, a consistent upper motor neuron lesion usually implies cerebral hemispheric dysfunction. This is most often the result of a supratentorial mass lesion, such as an epidural, subdural, or intracerebral hematoma. When there is hemispheric involvement, often there is a contralateral paresis or paralysis. Aphasia is almost always due to left hemispheric damage. Decorticate posture (flexion of the upper extremity and extension of the lower extremity) is seen with injury to the corticospinal tract in its proximal cerebral portion, whereas decerebrate posture (extension of upper and lower extremities) reflects corticospinal tract dysfunction at the midbrain level. A Babinski sign (dorsiflexion of the great toe upon stroking the sole of the foot) as well as hyperactive deep tendon reflexes are abnormal findings that also indicate corticospinal tract involvement.

Injury to the posterior fossa may produce dysfunction of the brain stem or cerebellum. With the latter, there may be ataxia, incoordination, or nystagmus, but cerebellar signs are, overall, infrequent. More often, patients with posterior fossa mass lesions have nuchal rigidity or corticospinal tract abnormalities. The most common posterior fossa injury is an epidural hematoma.[65]

Hysteria

Not uncommonly, a trauma patient may be hysterical, either because of an underlying personality disorder or because of the emotional trauma of the accident. Alternatively, the physician may declare a patient to be hysterical when, in reality, true pathology exists.

In the former situation, hysterical symptoms usu-

ally take the form of a paresis, paralysis, or sensory loss involving an extremity or one half of the body. These symptoms often conform to what the patient perceives as the midline or boundary of an extremity rather than to patterns of innervation. Repeated examination, observation, and assessment of the reproducibility of the deficit are valuable in managing these patients.

A far more serious situation is when real symptoms or neurologic deficit are ascribed by the physician to a psychological cause. This is the source of much postinjury dispute and litigation. The clinician must realize that head and spinal cord injury may occur simultaneously and that one may mimic the other. Symptoms relating to root lesions or partial spinal cord syndromes commonly cause such confusion. In addition, cerebral cortical injury may present with deficits suggesting spinal cord damage but without vertebral injury.

We recommend that the clinician faced with a patient whose symptoms seem to disagree with objective data, approach the case with extreme diligence. The patient's complaints should be considered valid until adequate confirming tests have been performed and the patient has been observed over time. A CT scan of the head should be performed to identify or exclude a cerebral basis of injury.

Radiologic Evaluation

The most basic neuroradiologic procedure is the plain skull film. In the trauma patient, it is used primarily to identify a skull fracture or intracranial foreign body. In the stable patient with a low probability of a significant intracranial lesion, it is the procedure of choice to diagnose the above-mentioned entities.

The presence of a skull fracture does not per se indicate associated brain damage in either adult or children.[66] In the absence of clinical or radiographic findings of central nervous system abnormalities, recognizing a fracture has little effect on the patient's outcome. The utility and cost effectiveness of the plain skull X-ray series has been the subject of controversy.[67,68] Cooper and Ho found that only one (0.5 percent) head trauma patient would have been managed differently if a plain skull film examination had been performed. They concluded that the presence of a linear skull fracture per se would rarely alter patient care.[4] We likewise adhere to this philosophy.

Computed tomography is now the recommended neuroradiologic procedure when significant brain injury is suspected.[69,70] The high resolution, noninvasiveness, and rapid scanning of CT has radically changed our ability to accurately diagnose and treat intracranial traumatic lesions. In the patient with brain and suspected spinal injury, utmost attention should be directed to adequate vertebral column immobilization during this procedure. The timing of the scan must be in accordance with priorities for associated injuries. However, the patient with evidence of serious brain trauma and neurologic compromise whose respiratory and cardiovascular functions are stable should have immediate CT evaluation.

Cerebral swelling is seen in children on CT scan as bilateral ventricular compression, effacement of

CSF cisterns and cortical sulci, and a normal cerebral density pattern. Cerebral edema appears as a hypodense area that is diffuse or localized, bilateral or unilateral, and with or without mass effect.

Traumatic hematomas are readily detected in the acute stage as a hyperdense lesion on noncontrast CT scan. An epidural hematoma characteristically occurs in the temporal, frontal, and occipital regions and has lentiform or biconvex shape with distinct margination (Fig. 7-8). This is due to dura being adherent to the skull at both ends of the hematoma, preventing the blood collection from spreading diffusely along the convexity.

A subdural hematoma may occur anywhere from the vertex to the skull base and appears crescent-shaped between the inner skull table and cortical surface (Fig. 7-9). It is hyperdense in the acute stage, but with time becomes isodense to hypo-

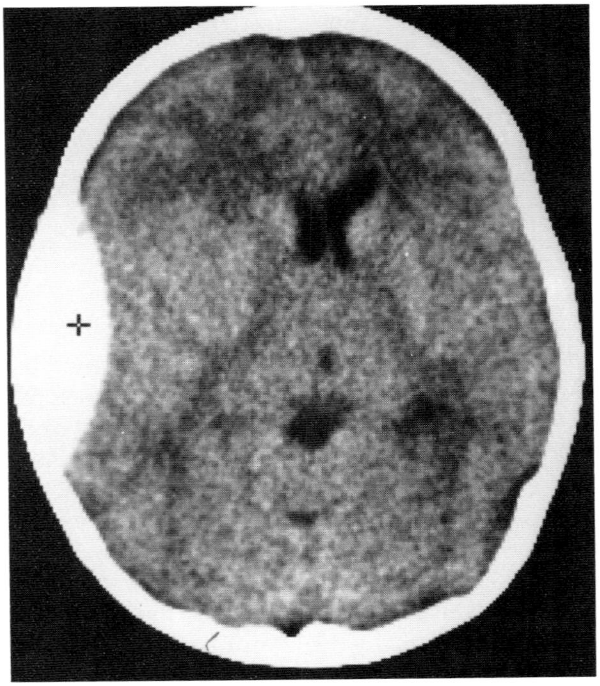

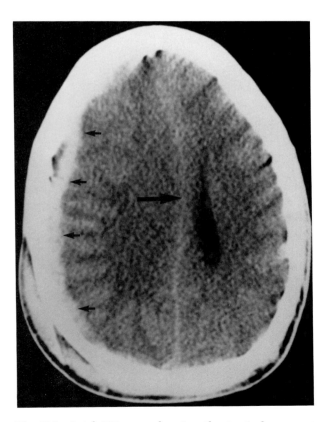

Fig. 7-8. Axial CT scan showing the typical lenticular appearance of an epidural hematoma. There is associated mass effect with effacement of the ipsilateral frontal horn of the lateral ventricle.

Fig. 7-9. Axial CT scan showing the typical crescent shape of an acute subdural hematoma (small arrows). There is associated mass effect with shift of the midline falx cerebri (large arrow).

dense and may be loculated. Occasionally, epidural and subdural hematomas do not show a characteristic shape and are referred to by the more general term *extracerebral hematoma*.

Traumatic intracerebral hematomas are seen as homogeneous, circumscribed, hyperdense lesions, the result of extravasation of blood into brain parenchyma (Fig. 7-10). Most are located superficially in the frontal or temporal lobes, and by 48 hours to 72 hours after injury are associated with a surrounding area of low-density edema. Brain contusions are seen as smaller areas of heterogeneous hyperdense lesions. They are focal areas of laceration that tend to develop directly at the site of impact (coup injury) or directly opposite (contrecoup injury).

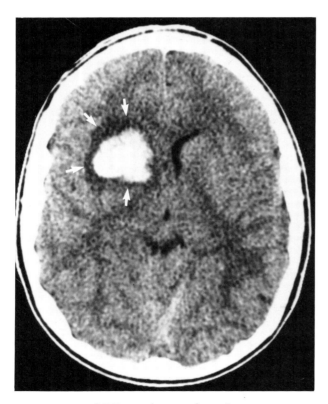

Fig. 7-10. Axial CT scan showing frontal traumatic intracerebral hematoma. Note the surrounding low-density edema (arrows) with obliteration of the ipsilateral frontal horn.

Angiography

Computed tomography has replaced angiography for the diagnostic evaluation of patients with acute brain injury. We have used cerebral angiography to exclude the presence of a mass lesion when a cervical immobilization device (e.g., halo vest), kyphotic deformity, morbid obesity, or other problem has made it impossible to fit the patient into the CT gantry.

If a vascular injury is suspected, angiography is the diagnostic procedure of choice. As discussed in the section on vascular trauma (see Vascular Injury Mimicking Head Injury, above), vertebral and carotid angiography can demonstrate intimal tear, dissection, and partial or complete occlusion resulting from traumatic injury to the cervical region. In some instances, digital subtraction angiography may suffice for evaluation of vascular injury in the neck.[71]

TREATMENT

The treatment of head injuries begins with medical stabilization, adequate immobilization of the spine, and an assessment of the degree and nature of neurologic compromise. Not infrequently, factors such as anemia, hypotension, upper airway obstruction, hypoxia, hypercapnia, or seizure may lead to an early demise in the neurologic patient.[72,73] These potential problems should be addressed and prevented.

A period of loss of consciousness is frequent after even minor head trauma. Loss of consciousness per se does not necessarily indicate significant brain injury, and is usually considered insignificant if it is of short duration. Amnesia for events before the accident (retrograde amnesia) and subsequent to the event (anterograde amnesia) may serve as a clue to the severity of impact. Amnesia of less than 1 hour is considered indicative of mild head injury.[74] For patients with loss of consciousness for less than 5 minutes and/or a brief period of amnesia, and a normal neurologic examination, hospitalization for observation is probably not indicated. Of course, patients with significant spinal or other trauma require hospitalization, as do patients with any new onset of seizures, those with alcohol or drug intoxification that precludes accurate neurologic assessment, a focal neurologic deficit, or any extenuating circumstances.

A linear skull fracture that is not associated with an intracranial lesion requires no specific treatment. Basilar skull fractures are apt to cause CSF leaks. The prophylactic use of antibiotics for a CSF leak is controversial; we do not routinely use it.[75,76] A patient with a depressed skull fracture usually requires hospital admission for observation of neurologic status and for development of a CSF leak.

A depressed skull fracture is considered significant if the outer skull table is depressed below the margin of the inner table. It is best not to attempt to elevate a depressed fracture in the emergency room, since this may lead to unexpected hemorrhage or dural sinus tear. Penetrating wounds (e.g., bone, foreign bodies, bullets, or metallic fragments) should also be debrided in the operating suite.

The detection of an intracranial mass lesion forces a decision concerning surgical evacuation. This decision is based on the patient's neurologic condition and the results of the radiologic investigation. The physician is admonished to recognize a neurologic deficit early in its clinical course so that definitive treatment may be instituted before significant brain compression has occurred.

Both extra-axial and intra-axial hematomas, if of significant size and/or associated with midline shift, are evacuated via craniotomy. Burr hole or trephination explorations are not definitive treatment and, if performed initially, should be expanded to a formal craniotomy as soon as possible to allow for complete clot evacuation. If there is no significant midline shift on CT scan, most patients may be treated conservatively by intracranial pressure monitoring (see Fig. 7-5) and serial CT examinations. One must be aware of the capability of small traumatic hematomas to expand, of delayed hematomas to develop,[77] and of edema to form. Post-traumatic edema characteristically begins in the first 12 hours, may be seen almost immediately,[78] and usually reaches its maximum by 48 to 72 hours.

Treatment of carotid and vertebral arterial injuries has been unrewarding and controversial. In general, if the injury can be diagnosed and is accessible to surgical approach soon after injury (less than 6 hours), patients with a neurologic deficit may benefit from thrombectomy. Anticoagulation and bypass procedures have been attempted, but neither is without significant potential for complication. At present, no one therapy can be recommended, although the conservative approach is the one most often followed.

Treatment of Increased Intracranial Pressure

All patients with significant head trauma are presumed to have increased ICP. The medical management of elevated ICP involves manipulation of the natural cerebral compensatory mechanisms: reduction of blood volume, diminution of extracellular water content, and displacement of CSF.

Blood volume is primarily reduced by elevating the head and placing it in the neutral position. The latter maneuver ensures that cerebral venous return is not impeded by compression of the jugular vein. Head positioning must be done judiciously in the patient with known or suspected cervical spine injury.

Hyperventilation reduces ICP by decreasing PCO_2, which causes vasoconstriction of cerebral vessels and reduction of intracranial vascular volume. This is the most effective method to rapidly reduce ICP; however, long-term use (more than 48 to 72 hours) may result in significant metabolic derangement. We prefer to maintain the PCO_2 in the range of 28 to 34 torr to avoid these potential metabolic abnormalities and to have a margin for rapid decrease in PCO_2 (and thus ICP) in the circumstance of acute intracranial hypertension (e.g., brain herniation syndrome).

Osmotic diuretics have been shown to reduce tissue water content from areas of normal brain. Intravenous mannitol (0.5 to 1.0 g/kg) is administered initially and, thereafter, may be given in a reduced dosage every 4 to 6 hours. Despite attempts to achieve a reduction of brain water content, severe dehydration of the patient by depletion of intravascular volume should be prevented. This is especially important in children and in the critically impaired patient in whom the cardiovascular status is tenuous. The patient is probably best managed by giving slightly less than maintenance fluids, using half normal saline.

Patients with neurologic impairment should be considered for ICP monitoring, regardless of the decision concerning craniotomy for a mass lesion (see Fig. 7-5). Although there are several methods for ongoing measurement of ICP, it is usually accomplished by a subarachnoid bolt or an intraventricular catheter. The latter method has the added advantage that it can be used to vent CSF as the ICP rises.

The use of corticosteroids in head trauma patients has not been unequivocally shown to significantly improve outcome.[79,80] At present it cannot be endorsed from a scientific standpoint. When the patient has maintained persistently high ICP levels despite the conventional therapy mentioned above, barbiturate coma may be induced. This form of treatment involves extensive monitoring in an intensive care unit and a staff experienced in its use.[81,82]

CONCLUSIONS

The salient points of this chapter may be summarized as follows.

1. There is a significant association between cervical spine injury and head injury, particularly when the upper cervical spine is involved.
2. Once medically stable and immobilized, the patient who exhibits alterations of mental status or other cerebral deficits should have immediate neurologic and radiologic evaluation.
3. The work-up of a patient with head injury along with spinal injury is similar to the work-up of other head-injured patients with the exception that the presence of an unstable spine must be considered.
4. The initial evaluation of the spinal cord-injured patient should determine the probability of significant head injury. The subsequent work-up should proceed accordingly, with expeditious

management of patients with intracranial mass lesions and increased ICP.
5. All patients with significant neurologic deficits secondary to cranial trauma are assumed to have increased ICP and should be considered for ICP monitoring.
6. Neurologic deficits may be secondary to concomitant head injury, vascular injury, intoxication, metabolic derangement, or hysteria.

REFERENCES

1. West JG, Trunkey DD, Lim RC: Systems of care. Arch Surg 114:455, 1979
2. Jennett B, Murray A, MacMillan R, et al.: Head injuries in Scottish hospitals. Lancet 2:696, 1977
3. Gennarelli TA: Cervical concussion and diffuse brain injuries. p. 83. In Cooper PR (ed): Head Injuries. Williams & Wilkins, Baltimore, 1982
4. Cooper PR, Ho V: Role of emergency skull X-ray films in the evaluation of the head-injured patient: a retrospective study. Neurosurgery 13:136, 1983
5. Harwood-Nash DC, Hendrick EB, Hudson AR: The significance of skull fractures in children. A study of 1,187 patients. Radiology 101:151, 1971
6. Henry RC, Taylor PH: Cerebrospinal fluid otorrhea and otorhinorrhea following closed head injury. J Laryngol Otolaryngol 92:743, 1978
7. Triscot A, Hallot R: Traumatic paraplegia and associated fractures. Paraplegia 5:211, 1968
8. Richards T, Hoff J: Factors affecting survival from acute subdural hematoma. Surgery 75:253, 1974
9. Rosenbluth PR, Arias B, Quartetti EV, Carney AL: Current management of subdural hematoma. Analysis of 100 consecutive cases. JAMA 179:759, 1962
10. McLaurin RL, Ford LE: Extradural hematoma. Statistical survey of 47 cases. J Neurosurg 21:364, 1964
11. Cordobes F, Lobato R, Rivas JJ: Observations of 82 patients with extradural hematoma. J Neurosurg 54:179, 1981
12. Phonprasert C, Suwanwela C, Hongsaprabhas C et al.: Extradural hematoma: analysis of 138 cases. J Trauma 20:679, 1980
13. Jamieson KG, Yelland JDN: Extradural hematoma. Report of 167 cases. J Neurosurg 129:13, 1968
14. Cerullo LJ, Raimondi AJ: Neurological emergencies. p. 297. In Beal JM (ed): Critical Care for Surgical Patients. MacMillan, New York, 1982
15. Lyness SS, Simcone FA: Vascular complications of

upper cervical spine injuries. Ortho Clin North Am 9:1029, 1978

16. Dragon R, Saranchak H, Lakin P et al.: Blunt injuries to the carotid and vertebral arteries. Am J Surg 141:497, 1981

17. Hart RG, Easton JD: Dissection of cervical and cerebral arteries. Neurol Clin North Am 1:155, 1983

18. Stringer WL, Kelly DJ, Jr.: Traumatic dissection of the extra cranial internal carotid artery. Neurosurgery 6:123, 1980

19. Batzdorf U, Bentson JR, Machleder HI: Blunt trauma to the cervical carotid artery. Neurosurgery 5:195, 1979

20. Woodhurst WB, Robertson WD, Thompson GB: Carotid injury due to intraoral trauma: case report and review of the literature. Neurosurgery 6:559, 1980

21. Schermann BM, Tucker WS: Bilateral traumatic thrombosis of the internal carotid arteries in the neck: a case report with review of the literature. Neurosurgery 10:751, 1982

22. Schneider RC, Crosby EC: Vascular insufficiency of brain stem and spinal cord in spinal trauma. Neurology 9:643, 1969

23. French BN, Cobb CA, Dublin AB: Cranial computed tomography in the diagnosis of symptomatic indirect trauma to the carotid artery. Surg Neurol 15:256, 1981

24. Higazi I: Post-traumatic carotid thrombosis. J Neurosurg 20:354, 1963

25. Carpenter S: Injury of neck as cause of vertebral artery thrombosis. J Neurosurg 18:849, 1961

26. Schneider RC, Schemm GW: Vertebral artery insufficiency in acute and chronic spinal trauma. J Neurosurg 18:348, 1961

27. Murray DS: Post-traumatic thrombosis of the internal carotid and vertebral arteries after nonpenetrating injuries of the neck. Br J Surg 44:556, 1957

28. Sherman DG, Hart RG, Easton JD: Abrupt change in head position and cerebral infarction. Stroke 12:2, 1981

29. Krueger BR, O'Kazaki H: Vertebral-basilar distribution infarction following chiropractic cervical manipulation. Mayo Clin Proc 55:322, 1980

30. Marshall LF, Bruce DA, Bruno L, Langfitt TW: Vertebrobasilar spasm: a significant cause of neurological deficit in head injury. J Neurosurg 48:560, 1978

31. Schneider RG, Gosch HH, Norrell H et al.: Vascular insufficiency and differential distortion of brain and cord caused by cervicomedullary football injuries. J Neurosurg 33:363, 1970

32. Kassel NF, Boarini DJ, Adams HP, Jr.: Intracranial and cervical vascular injuries. p. 275. In Cooper PR (ed): Head Injuries. Williams & Wilkins, Baltimore, 1982

33. National Safety Council: Accident facts. National Safety Council, Chicago, 1978

34. National Safety Council: Body area of motor vehicle occupant injured in motor vehicle accident. National Safety Council, Chicago, 1966

35. Weiss MH: Head trauma and spinal cord injuries: diagnostic and therapeutic criteria. Crit Care Med 2:311, 1974

36. National Safety Council: Part of body injured in work accidents. National Safety Council, Chicago, 1982

37. Tonge JI, O'Reilly MJJ, Davison A, Johnston NG: Traffic crash fatalities: injury patterns and other factors. Med J Aust 2:5, 1972

38. Jefferson G: Fracture of atlas vertebra: report of four cases and review of those previously recorded. Br J Surg 7:407, 1920

39. Jefferson G: Remarks on fractures of first cervical vertebra. Br Med J 2:153, 1927

40. Davis D, Bohlman H, Walker AE et al.: The pathological findings in fatal craniospinal injuries. J Neurosurg 34:603, 1971

41. Alker GJ, Oh YS, Leslie EV: High cervical spine and craniocervical function injuries in fatal traffic accidents: a radiological study. Orthop Clin North Am 9:1003, 1978

42. Shrago GG: Cervical spine injuries: association with head trauma. Radiology 118:670, 1973

43. Silver JR, Morris WR, Ottinowski JS: Associated injuries in patients with spinal injury. Injury 12:219, 1976

44. Harris P: Associated injuries in traumatic paraplegia and tetraplegia. Paraplegia 5:215, 1968

45. Porter RW: Some problems in the management of the spinal cord injury patient with associated head or facial trauma. Proc VA Spinal Cord Injury Conf 19:29, 1973

46. Rutherford WH: Diagnosis of alcohol ingestion in mild head injuries. Lancet 1:1021, 1977

47. Galbraith S, Murray WR, Patel AR, Knill-Jones R: The relationship between alcohol and head injury and its effect on the conscious level. Br J Surg 63:128, 1976

48. Schneider RC, Crosby EC: Vascular insufficiency of brain stem and spinal cord in spinal trauma. Neurology 9:643, 1959

49. Carpenter MB: Core Text of Neuroanatomy. 2nd Ed. p. 324. Williams & Wilkins, Baltimore, 1978

50. Kline DG: Altantoaxial dislocation simulating a head injury: hypoplasia of the odontoid. J Neurosurg 24:1013, 1966

51. Teasdale G, Jennett B: Assessment of coma and impaired consciousness. A practical scale. Lancet 2:81, 1974
52. Sumner D: On testing the sense of smell: Lancet 2:895, 1962
53. Rovit RL, Murali R: Injuries of the cranial nerves. In Cooper PR (ed): Head Injury. p. 99. Williams & Wilkins, Baltimore, 1982
54. Gjerris F: Traumatic lesions of the visual pathways. In Vinken PJ, Bruyn GW (eds): Handbook of Neurology. Vol. 24. p. 27. Elsevier Science Publishing, New York, 1976
55. Crompton MR: Visual lesions in closed head injuries. Brain 93:785, 1970
56. Jefferson A: Ocular complications of head injuries. Trans Ophthalmol Soc UK 81:595, 1961
57. Elisevich KV, Ford RM, Anderson DP et al.: Visual abnormalities with multiple trauma. Surg Neurol 22:565, 1984
58. Jennett B, Snock J, Bond MR, Brooks N: Disability after severe head injury. Observations of the use of the Glasgow Outcome Scale. J Neurol Neurosurg Psychiatry 44:285, 1981
59. Turner JWA: Indirect injuries of the optic nerve. Brain 66:140, 1943
60. Schneider RC, Johnson FC: Bilateral traumatic abducens palsy. A mechanism of injury suggested by the study of associated fractures. J Neurosurg 34:33, 1971
61. Summers CG, Wirthschafter JD: Bilateral trigeminal and abducens neuropathies following low velocity, crushing head injury. J Neurosurg 50:508, 1979
62. Lindenberg R: Significance of the tentorium in head injuries from blunt forces. Clin Neurosurg 12:129, 1966
63. Frost EAM: The physiopathology of respirations in neurosurgical patients. J Neurosurg 50:699, 1979
64. Plum F, Posner JB: The Diagnosis of Stupor and Coma. p. 36. FA Davis, Philadelphia, 1980
65. Wright RL: Traumatic hematomas of the posterior cranial fossa. J Neurosurg 25:402, 1966
66. Royal College of Radiologists: A study of the utilization of skull radiography in 9 accident-and-emergency units in the UK. Lancet 2:1234, 1980
67. Cummins RO: Clinicians' reasons for overuse of skull radiographs. AJNR 1:339, 1980
68. Eyes B, Evans AF: Post-traumatic skull radiography: time for a reappraisal. Lancet 2:85, 1978
69. Koo AH, La Roque RL: Evaluation of head trauma by computed tomography. Radiology 123:345, 1977
70. Robertson FC, Kisheri PRS, Miller JD: The value of serial CT in the management of severe head injury. Surg Neurol 12:161, 1979
71. Christenson PR, Oritt TW, Fisher HD et al.: Intravenous angiography using digital video subtraction: intravenous cervicocerebrovascular angiography. AJNR 1:379, 1980
72. Rose J, Valtonen S, Jennett B: Avoidable factors contributing to death after head injury. Br Med J 2:615, 1977
73. Miller JD, Sweet RC, Narayan R, Becker DP: Early insults to the injured brain. JAMA 240:439, 1978
74. Russell WR, Smith A: Post-traumatic amnesia in closed head injury. Arch Neurol 5:16, 1961
75. Ingelzi RJ, Vander Ark GD: Analysis of the treatment of basilar skull fractures with and without antibiotics. J Neurosurg 43:721, 1975
76. Einhorn A, Mizrahi EM: Basilar skull fractures in children. The incidence of CNS infection and the use of antibiotics. Am J Dis Child 132:1121, 1978
77. Brown FD, Mullan S, Duda EE: Delayed traumatic intracerebral hematomas. J Neurosurg 48:1019, 1978
78. Kobrine AI, Timmins E, Rajjoub RK et al.: Demonstration of massive traumatic brain swelling within 20 minutes after injury. J Neurosurg 46:256, 1977
79. Gudeman SK, Miller JD, Becker D: Failure of high-dose steroid therapy to influence intracranial pressure in patients with severe head injury. J Neurosurg 51:301, 1979
80. Gianotta SL, Weiss MH, Apuzzo MLJ, Martin E: High dose glucocorticoids in the management of severe head injury. Neurosurgery 15:497, 1984
81. Marshall LF, Smith RW, Shapiro HM: Outcome with aggressive treatment in severe head injuries. II. Acute and chronic barbituate administration in the management of head injury. J Neurosurg 50:26, 1979
82. Rockoff MA, Marshall LF, Shapiro HM: High dose barbituate therapy in humans: a clinical review of 60 patients. Ann Neurol 3:83, 1979

8

Anesthesia for Spinal Cord Injury

Antoun Koht
Paul R. Meyer, Jr.

Motor vehicle accidents, falls, and sport-related injuries account for more than half of the 10,000 new spinal cord injuries each year in the United States.[1] Many of these acutely injured patients, as well as the 250,000 existing paraplegics and quadriplegics in this country, during some period in their lifetime will require some type of surgical procedure. The anesthesia considerations related to the spine include airway management (particularly in managing an acute cervical spine injury) and the effects of spine injury on the cardiovascular system, due to either altered neurologic reflexes or aging. Knowledge of the problems allows for appropriate and timely management, helps to minimize the patient's risk during surgery, and improves the survival rate of traumatized neural tissue. This chapter specifically addresses the problems related to the anesthetic management of the spine-injured patient.

PREOPERATIVE EVALUATION

In addition to the general medical preparations of a preoperative patient, specific attention must be directed to the spinal pathology and the planned operative procedure. There are four special considerations which must be addressed: the level of the injury, the patient's age, the spine's stability or instability, and the neurologic completeness or incompleteness of the injury.

Level of Injury

Injuries to the spinal cord present specific problems at each level. Patients with cervical lesions present the widest spectrum of potential problems. Usually, the difficulty lies in management of the airway, owing either to the acute injury or to the limited range of motion from a previous fusion. Ventilation may be inadequate owing to injury to the spinal roots that make up the phrenic nerve, which innervates the diaphragm (C3, C4, C5), along with a loss of innervation of the intercostal and abdominal musculature, which serve as accessory muscles of respiration (see Ch. 5). Cardiovascular performance may be significantly altered as a result of decreased cardiac autonomic (sympathetic) activity (resulting in bradycardia in spinal cord injuries above T4), and/or decreased activity in the peripheral vascular system resulting in vasodilation and hypotension. Finally, in addition to the above conditions, these patients may have problems with temperature control owing to loss of apocrine (sweat) gland innervation and loss of peripheral vascular sympathetic vasomotor tone.

Such patients become poikilothermic, with a body temperature that alters passively with ambient temperature. In patients with long-standing spinal injuries, autonomic control may become hyper-reactive, resulting in uncontrolled muscle movements (spasticity) and autonomic sympathetic hyper-reflexia (discussed below).

In thoracic injuries, the airway is not compromised and airway management is the same as in the non-spinal cord-injured patient. Spinal cord injuries cephalad to T5 are frequently associated with the loss of cardiac (sympathetic) accelerator innervation, manifested by bradycardia. Blood pressure is also affected with injuries above T10, owing to the loss of peripheral sympathetic vasomotor tone. *In general, the lower the spinal cord injury, the less there will be alterations in vasomotor tone, temperature control, blood pressure, and heart rate.*

Patients with injury to the lumbar spinal cord are free of the neurologic complications mentioned above, but may have bowel and bladder dysfunction.

In general, patients with high-level spinal cord injuries are less active owing to their neurologic injury, may be bedridden, and are prone to problems related to the gastrointestinal and urologic systems. In long-standing spinal cord patients with a history of repeated rectal enemas along with the persistent use of an indwelling catheter, urinary tract infections can become a chronic complication.

Age of Injury

Severe spinal cord injury is followed initially by a state of decreased spinal cord activity (spinal shock) below the level of injury.[2,3] This results in immediate flaccid paralysis and a total absence of all spinal reflexes below the level of injury. This state lasts from one to several weeks after injury. During this period, the major cause of morbidity and mortality is impaired alveolar ventilation combined with an inability to protect the airway and to clear bronchial secretions. Aspiration of gastric contents, bronchopneumonia, pulmonary edema, and pulmonary embolism (from acute deep venous thrombosis) occur frequently and complicate the clinical situation.

This period eventually changes into a chronic stage by a gradual return of spinal cord reflexes. This chronic stage is characterized by sympathetic overactivity and involuntary muscle spasm. Sympathetic overactivity occurs because of the loss of cortical control over spinal cord-mediated sympathetic autonomic reflexes. During this stage, the anesthesiologist must address the concerns for cardiovascular instability and impaired alveolar ventilation, while also being alert to the occurrence of abnormal thermoregulation or autonomic hyper-reflexia. Furthermore, the problems and complications of a debilitated patient, such as chronic infections, anemia, and decubitus ulcers, must be considered. Because of the problems related to muscle paralysis, succinylcholine must never be administered within the first year after the onset of spinal cord injury. If used, it will induce a sudden hyperkalemia by release of potassium liberated from the paralyzed muscle, which can induce fatal cardiac arrest. *The drug succinylcholine is contraindicated.*

Stable or Unstable Injury

When an endotracheal tube is inserted as an airway and for administration of general anesthesia, the head is often flexed or extended to help expose the vocal cords. Because patients with unstable cervical fractures are usually in cervical traction, such flexion or extension of the head and neck may jeopardize the reduction of an already present spinal cord injury or, worse, produce an injury where only spinal column instability existed. Therefore, both the intubation and the patient's positioning on the operating table for surgery are matters of specific concern for the anesthesiologist. For patients with thoracic and lumbar spine injuries, the main concern is preventing further injury during the positioning of the patient on the operating table.

Complete or Incomplete Injury

Complete neurologic injury is defined as the absence of all voluntary motor function and all sensory function below the level of spine injury. An *incomplete neurologic injury* is one where there is

Fig. 8-1. Operating room scene showing use of SSEP monitor for spine injury surgery. Patients sustaining spinal cord injury are evaluated by SSEP preoperatively. If found to have an incomplete lesion, they are monitored during surgery. SSEP equipment and monitoring is a function of the anesthesia department.

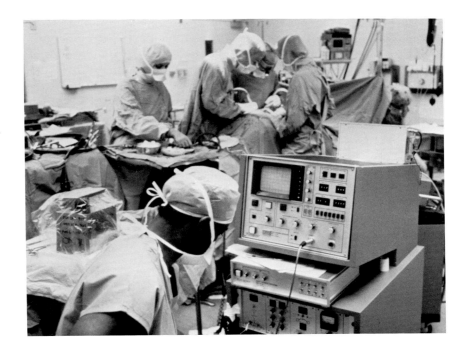

evidence of either sensory or motor function below the level of injury. As anticipated, medical and cardiovascular complications decrease as the degree of neurologic injury lessens.

Complete neurologic injuries present various medical problems, depending on the level of spine injury. Acute incomplete injuries, on the other hand, regardless of the level, require absolute attention during anesthesia induction, to prevent further neurologic injury. For the performance of surgical procedure in the patient with incomplete neurologic injury, somatosensory evoked potentials (SSEPs) have been used as an excellent means of monitoring spinal cord function during surgery[4-6] (Fig. 8-1).

POSITION DURING SURGERY

The anesthetic care required for the spinal cord-injured patient is influenced by the procedure to be performed, the surgical approach, and the patient's position on the operating room table during surgery.[7] Generally, one of four positions is used.

Supine Position

The supine position is used for anterior cervical and anterior transperitoneal lumbar surgical procedures. This position is associated with the fewest anesthesia problems during spinal surgery. Cardiovascular and respiratory functions are easily monitored and well preserved. The supine position is also best for re-establishing an airway, for rapidly replacing blood, and for resuscitation should an unexpected emergency occur.

Lateral Position

The lateral position is utilized for the performance of the combined anterior decompression and posterior spine stabilization procedures, and for the standard anterolateral chest or flank approach to the thoracic or lumbar spine. With either or both approaches, to expose the spine, it is often necessary to incise the diaphragm. This, along with opening the chest, further compromises ventilation both during surgery and postoperatively. A major concern is ventilation/perfusion mismatch, which results in decreased oxygenation.

In any position, undue pressure between body surfaces and the surface of the surgical table may result in skin, vascular, or peripheral nerve compromise or injury. In the lateral position, the brachial plexus and axillary artery are at specific risk and must be protected by a chest roll placed under the upper rib cage. After the patient is placed on the operating table, checking for the radial artery pulse will confirm proper extremity positioning. To protect the sciatic and peroneal nerves, the legs must be cushioned in a neutral position. As noted above, intrathoracic or intra-abdominal procedures expose the patient to the hazards of significant blood loss, owing to the close proximity of the aorta and the vena cava to the operative field.

Prone Position

The prone position is the most common position in both elective spine surgery (e.g., for scoliosis) and acute spinal cord injury surgery. In this position, during anesthesia, ventilation may be affected by the limitation of chest and abdominal wall motion resulting from the weight of the patient against the table. This may result in ventilation/perfusion mismatch as well as decreased lung compliance. Cardiovascular function may be compromised in this position because of pressure against the abdomen, and the impeding of venous return via the inferior vena cava. Numerous areas of the body surface are exposed to pressure, which may result in pressure problems. They are, notably, the breasts in women, the genitalia in men, iliac crests, knees, heels, toes, arms, and face. During the preparation of a patient for a posterior cervical spine procedure, the eyes may receive burns from the antiseptic solution used to prepare the skin. Scrubbing the posterior neck may cause the cleansing agent to run forward, entering the patient's eyes, and producing a chemical conjunctivitis or corneal irritation. This can be prevented by applying ophthalmologic ointment into the eyes and covering them with an occlusive dressing before turning the patient. If the patient becomes inadvertently extubated in the prone position, it is difficult to re-establish the airway. Hypoxia is a serious consequence. Therefore, always ensure the placement and security of the endotracheal tube before turning the patient prone. No patient should be turned prone without an indwelling catheter carefully in place to monitor urinary output. This is particularly important when blood loss could be high. Care must be taken to ensure that the catheter or drainage tube does not become mechanically obstructed.

Sitting Position

The sitting position is an unusual position in spinal cord surgery, but it is occasionally used, and it is of particular concern to the anesthesiologist. It is usually used only for patients requiring a combined anterior and posterior cervical procedure. In this position, the patient is prone to the occurrence of hypotension and venous air embolism. Venous air embolism may occur when the surgical field is sufficiently above the level of the heart and the surgical wound is open. In this situation, open venules in either the soft tissue or the bone are exposed. Because the venous pressure is negative, air can be sucked into the venous vascular system. The effects of air embolism depend on the volume of air aspirated and the speed of aspiration. By obstructing the pulmonary tree and depressing the pumping action of the heart, venous air embolism may effect ventilation, oxygenation, and cardiac function. The potential for air embolism requires a monitoring system designed to detect air embolism. This includes precordial ultrasonic doppler, end-expiratory CO_2, a pulmonary artery catheter, or a central venous pressure monitoring system.[8] If a central venous pressure (CVP) catheter is used, its tip should be located just above the junction of the superior vena cava and the right atrium to allow potential air recovery.[9] The location of the catheter's tip should be confirmed by chest radiographs, by an electrocardiogram (ECG) recorded from the tip of the catheter (i.e., biphasic P wave), or by observing the CVP tracing (identify a ventricular tracing and withdraw to an appropriate position). Characteristic changes in doppler sounds are an early warning of a small amount of air entering the venous system; they are followed by changes in end-expiratory CO_2 or pulmonary artery (PA) pressure. In dogs, the injection of air (0.5 ml/kg of body weight) drops end-expiratory CO_2 and raises the PA pressure.[10]

AIRWAY MANAGEMENT FOR SPINAL CORD-INJURED PATIENTS

Patients with cervical spine injuries may display airway problems as a result of traction or devices used for external stabilization. Further, fear of extending the neurologic injury may limit the use of conventional rigid laryngoscopy and intubation techniques that require flexion or extension of the neck. To avoid the latter, the airway can be secured by one of the following methods: *awake nasal or oral fiberoptic intubation*[11] (Fig. 8-2) or *awake blind nasotracheal or oral intubation.* (Fig. 8-3) Regardless of the approach, it is advisable to document the neurologic function after intubation and before proceeding with surgery. Likewise, it is advisable to positively identify that the endotracheal tube is in the trachea, and not the esophagus, upon insertion.

Awake Fiberoptic Nasotracheal Intubation

Fiberoptic intubation of the awake patient is the method least traumatic to the cervical spine, and the technique most utilized at Northwestern University. Over 500 patients with cervical spine and spinal cord injuries have been safely intubated utilizing this technique, without neurologic extension. The patient is prepared preoperatively with anticholinergic agents to dry the oral and nasal cavity and with sedatives when appropriate. Cocaine or phenylephrine hydrochloride (Neo-Synephrine) is applied to the tips of cotton applicators and placed into both nasal passages (Fig. 8-3D). These agents constrict the nasopharynx vascular membranes and dilate the nasal passages. In addition, cocaine anesthetizes the nostril and spares the use of local anesthetics. Special care is taken to prevent nasal bleeding. Blood as well as secretion may obscure the fiberoptic view and hinder intubation. In the operating room, the patient is sedated with an intravenous injection of narcotics and/or sedatives, in incremental doses, and titrated to prevent excitement, excessive movement, or violent coughing. The trachea and vocal cord are anesthetized

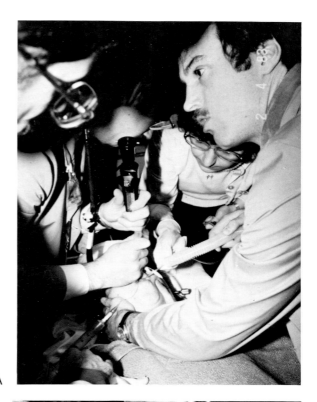

A

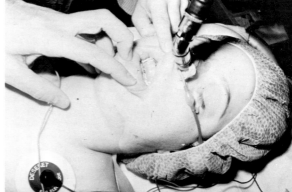

B

Fig. 8-2. (A) Scene of emergency intubation in elderly patient with severe cervical spine fracture dislocation at C4–C5. Note physician in foreground holding head and neck and physician with fiberoptic scope passed through endotracheal tube. Passing fiberoptic scope in trachea allows for easy insertion of endotracheal tube via the nasal tracheal route. Nasal tracheal intubation is preferred in unstable cervical spine injuries. **(B)** Nasal tracheal intubation in patient requiring internal stabilization of thoracic spine injury. Note rubber band-wired position of upper and lower teeth for stabilization of comminuted mandibular fracture.

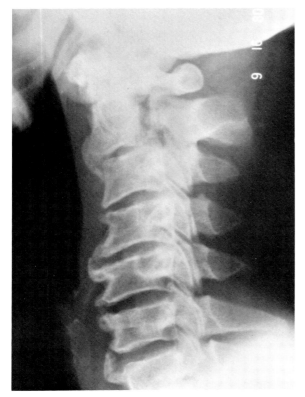

A

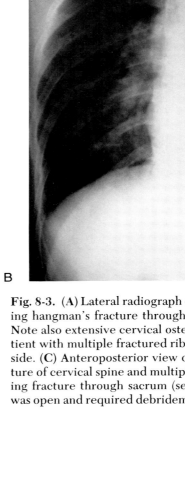

B

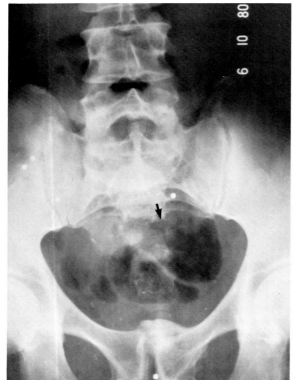

C

Fig. 8-3. (A) Lateral radiograph of cervical spine revealing hangman's fracture through posterior element C2. Note also extensive cervical osteoarthritis. (B) Same patient with multiple fractured ribs (5 through 9) on right side. (C) Anteroposterior view of the patient with fracture of cervical spine and multiple fractured ribs revealing fracture through sacrum (see arrow). This fracture was open and required debridement. *(Figure continues.)*

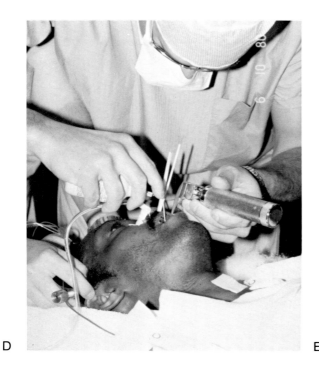

D

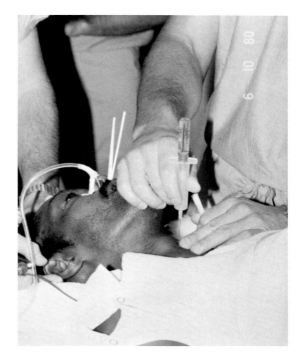

E

Fig. 8-3 *(Continued).* (**D**) Because of the fracture of the cervical spine and need for open debridement of the fractured sacrum, nasotracheal intubation was planned for anesthesia. Note cotton swabs in nasal passage. Swabs are soaked in local anesthetic and placed into posterior nasopharynx. Note also instillation of local anesthetic into posterior oropharynx (in physician's right hand). Patient is in Gardner-Wells tongs with traction on a Stryker frame. (**E**) Local anesthetic injected into upper trachea via percutaneous transtracheal route. Note presence of nasogastric tube to ensure evacuation of abdominal contents. (**F**) Nasotracheal catheter inserted into left nostril and guided across posterior pharynx by careful laryngoscopic visualization. Care is taken to flex and extend cervical spine only under the guidance and control of a physician. *(Figure continues.)*

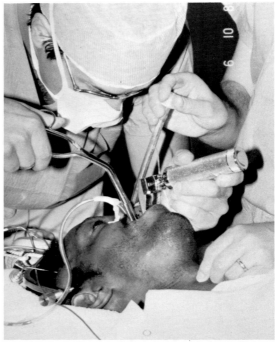

F

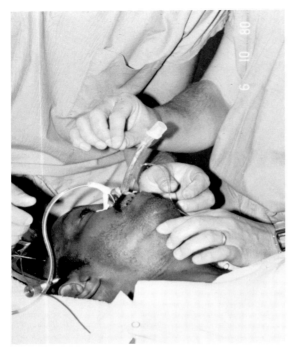

G

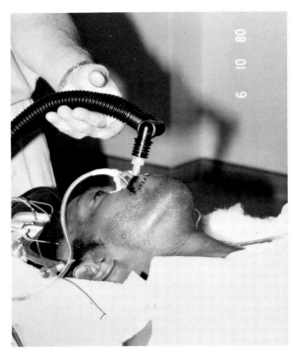

H

Fig. 8-3 *(Continued).* **(G)** Nasotracheal catheter inserted into upper trachea. Verification of placement is made by visual appearance, alternating condensation on catheter wall, and palpable movement of air through catheter at tip. **(H)** Nasotracheal catheter in place and connected to anesthesia machine. Care must be taken to follow this step by stable fixation of endotracheal tube to patient's head to prevent dislodgement while turning or with patient in prone position.

with 2 to 3 ml of 4 percent lidocaine (Xylocaine) either through the fiberoptic scope or by transtracheal injection (avoiding the latter with anterior cervical surgery) (Fig. 8-3D,E). Alternatively, lidocaine can be applied with a nebulizer inhaler. After the topical anesthesia has been applied, a lubricated and warmed endotracheal tube is gently inserted through the nostril into the posterior pharynx. The tube and pharynx are suctioned and then the fiberoptic scope is inserted through a nasal endotracheal tube into the upper pharynx. The vocal cords are identified anteriorly, and the scope is passed through them into the trachea. Once the position is confirmed by seeing tracheal rings through the scope, the endotracheal tube is slid over the scope and tested for location (Fig. 8-2A). The fiberoptic tube is removed, after confirmation of position, and the nasal endotracheal tube is fixed in place.

Awake Blind Nasotracheal Intubation

Awake blind nasotracheal intubation (Fig. 8-3D to H) is an alternative method for ensuring the airway is open. This procedure is done by anesthetizing the nose and the trachea as previously described (Fig. 8-3D,E). In a patient with relatively active spontaneous respiration, the tube is inserted and guided by the sounds of ventilation. This technique may require changing the position of the head, which may be limited by the presence of the injury. Multiple trials may be required to place the tube correctly in the trachea. This can lead to trauma of the posterior nasopharyngeal soft tissues and vocal cords. Again, patient neurologic functions are reassessed to ensure a stable situation. *Nasal intubation is contraindicated in patients with suspected base of the skull fracture or increasing intracranial pressure.*

Rigid Oral Intubation

Rigid oral intubation is used when the other two techniques are not applicable. Oral intubation is better done with the help of a surgeon or other medically knowledgeable person. This person holds the head to prevent excessive head movement during intubation, which could be harmful. Oral fiberoptic intubation is an alternative to rigid endoscopy. Oral fiberoptic intubation requires a higher degree of skill when using the fiberoptic scope. A spray of local anesthesia is applied to the oral cavity (Fig. 8-3D). A special oral airway is placed into the mouth to facilitate the use of the fiberoptic scope. Tracheostomy is not necessary to establish an airway if one follows the above methods for intubation.

VENTILATION IN SPINAL CORD INJURY

Normal inspiration is primarily achieved by contraction of the diaphragm, which is innervated by the phrenic nerve (C3,4,5). Expiration at sea level is entirely passive; that is, with relaxation of the diaphragm, the elastic structure of the lung, chest cage, and the lungs and the tone of the abdominal muscles return each segment to its resting length and force the diaphragm upward. If forceful expiration is required, the diaphragm can be pushed upward to expel air from the lungs by active contraction of the abdominal muscles against the abdominal contents. Thus, the abdominal muscles become a muscle of expiration. This obviously requires active abdominal muscle function. The phrenic nerve, the motor nerve of the diaphragm, which originates at C3, C4, and C5, is the principal nerve of respiration, whereas the intercostal and abdominal wall muscles are innervated by nerves from the thoracic region (see Fig. 5-4). Injuries at C3 or above are life-threatening if ventilation is not provided or supported by mechanical assist. Injuries below C5 usually ensure that the patient has enough reserve for oxygenation and ventilation under normal situations; however, the patient will require assistance during anesthesia, surgery, and

other stressful situations.[2] For these reasons, patients with cervical spine injuries require close attention during surgery and in the postoperative recovery period. The lower the spinal cord injury, the less effect on ventilation. Patients undergoing combined anteroposterior procedures on the chest and spine may have postoperative ventilatory compromise resulting from the chest having been opened (pain, splinting, hemopneumothorax, and the upper diaphragm taken down). Special attention should be directed to these patients during the first 24 hours after the operation, during which time the patient may require intubation and mechanical assistance to meet his ventilation requirements.

CARDIOVASCULAR CONSIDERATIONS IN SPINAL CORD INJURY

Patients with spinal cord injury may display signs of early and late cardiovascular changes.[3] Early cardiovascular changes are the result of sudden *sympathetic loss*. Spinal cord injury above T5 may affect cardiac accelerators, arising from T1 to T4, thus leaving the vagus nerve innervation of the heart unopposed. This results in *bradycardia*. Systemic vascular resistance is decreased by the sympathetic block, leading to a drop in blood pressure *(hypotension)*. The magnitude of this decrease is related to the level of injury and the extent of disruption of the sympathetic system. The higher the spinal cord injury (above T4), the more nerves are affected and the more profound is the effect (hypotension). Vasodilation associated with sympathetic block creates a mismatch between intravascular blood volume and intravascular space, leading to hypotension and *hypothermia*. Hypotension can be corrected by the intravenous infusion of fluids. Cardiovascular responses to trauma are the most intense in the minutes and hours immediately following injury, when effects of the trauma are most identifiable.

A drop in pulse rate will be seen when a supine patient is turned into the prone position (pressure over the carotid arteries). A similar effect occurs during the movement of a tracheostomy tube. The cause is stimulation of the vagus nerve, which in turn slows the heart. The *cardiovascular changes in the chronic stage include hypertension, arrythmia, and bradycardia.* It is important to carefully observe cardiovascular parameters during patient positioning and induction of anesthesia. The *side effects of vagal nerve stimulation* (pulse and blood pressure) *can be blocked by* the intravenous administration of *atropine* and intravascular fluids.

ROLE OF MUSCLE RELAXANTS IN SPINAL CORD INJURY

Chronically denervated muscle tissue, massive burns, and massive trauma are each accompanied by a rise in serum potassium when succinylcholine is administered.[12–15] This rise in potassium starts within 2 minutes and lasts for about 15 minutes. The rapid increase in the extracellular potassium concentration has been documented to be the cause of increased myocardial sensitivity after the injection of succinylcholine. Tobey has shown changes in the ECG pattern associated with a rise in serum potassium.[16] These include an elevation in the P wave and a depression of the R wave. If uncorrected, this effect can lead to ventricular fibrillation and cardiac arrest. This period of increased cardiac sensitivity can occur as early as 24 to 48 hours after injury and peaks within 2 months. It then gradually subsides over the next 4 months. A more cautious approach is to avoid succinylcholine in patients with spinal cord injury (with paralysis) from 1 day to 1 year postinjury. The use of nondepolarizing muscle relaxants (pancuronium, D-tubocuraine, vancuronium, or atracurium) has no effect on serum potassium. D-tubocuraine and atracurium cause histamine release and bradycardia that could intensify the ambiguous hemodynamic status.

AUTONOMIC HYPER-REFLEXIA DURING SPINAL SURGERY

Autonomic hyper-reflexia is an acute syndrome resulting from massive, unchecked sympathetic reflexes that result in response to stimulation of the sympathetic autonomics below the level of injury. This abnormal sympathetic response only occurs in patients with injuries at T7 or higher. It is characterized by hypertension (250/150), anxiety, sweating, pounding headache, and at times bradycardia.[3] Autonomic hyper-reflexia may occur in 85 percent of all patients with cervical spine and spinal cord injuries during their lifetime.[17]

Pathophysiology of Hyper-reflexia

Although there is still discussion about the actual pathophysiology of this process, Kurnick's classical description is still useful.[18] This reflex should be viewed as a disorder of autonomic homeostasis. The essential defect is a failure of the inhibitory supraspinal reflexes to travel down the spinal cord (because of the spinal cord injury) and restore autonomic equilibrium.[19] Bladder distension may cause pelvic and hypogastric nerves to transmit impulses into the dorsal column and spinothalamic tracts. These ascending tracts synapse with sympathetic neurons in the thoracic and upper lumbar intermediolateral cell columns of the lateral horn, inducing generalized sympathetic hyperactivity, self-perpetuation of the disorder, and hypertension. *Sudden hypertension triggers impulses from baroreceptors at the arch of the aorta and within the carotid sinus*, which are transmitted via the glossopharyngeal and vagus nerves to the brain stem. The brain stem, in turn, completes two sets of arc reflexes. One arc enters through the vagus nerve producing *bradycardia*, and the second arc enters the vasomotor center and produces vasodilator activity. *The result is vasodilation above the level of injury,* while below the level of injury, hyperactivity continues to cause vasoconstriction. Vasoconstriction and vasodilation are competing factors for the control of blood pressure. When the injury is above T7, the area with vasoconstriction exceeds that with vasodilation and the patient will display hypertension.

Management of Hyper-reflexia

Only direct-acting agents such as *sodium nitroprusside, nitroglycerine, and trimethaphan* should be used. Central-acting drugs such as methyldopa

(Aldomet) and clonodine have no effect at the site of vasoconstriction and should not be used. Although hydralazine and other similar drugs work, they are of little value in an emergency situation owing to their slow action. *Any treatment must include both the use of drugs and cessation of the stimulating factor.* This prevents further triggering of the reflex. If stimulation is removed without treatment, the signs and symptoms will persist. Therefore, the treatment of choice is a combination of drug therapy and stopping the stimulation. Autonomic hyper-reflexia can be prevented by avoiding the stimulation or by the use of anesthesia, either general or regional. The source of peripheral stimulation, as noted, may be a distended bladder, with kinking of the catheter, or an overdistended rectum. Emptying the bladder (and injecting a local anesthetic into the bladder) or digital extraction of feces from the rectum alleviates the problem.

BLOOD LOSS AND BLOOD TRANSFUSION DURING SPINAL SURGERY

Certain operations are associated with large blood loss. Anterior cervical spine fusions involve only minor blood loss, whereas the chest and thoracic spine anteroposterior procedure may be associated with major blood loss (6,000 ml). Blood loss can be decreased by injecting vasoconstrictor agents into the area of the planned surgical incision, by using a deliberate hypotension technique, and/or by hemodilution. Retrieving blood lost during surgery by means of the Cell Saver (Fig. 8-4) significantly decreases bank blood requirements, recycling the patient's lost blood back to the patient.

Local infiltration. Epinephrine, 1/200,000 to 1/400,000 injected into the skin at the surgical site induces vasoconstriction, thus minimizing blood loss at the skin incision site. The drug can be mixed in a saline base or with lidocaine (Xylocaine), which increases the depth of anesthesia.

Deliberate hypotension. This technique may be used to minimize blood loss during spinal surgery. Lower blood pressure can be achieved by

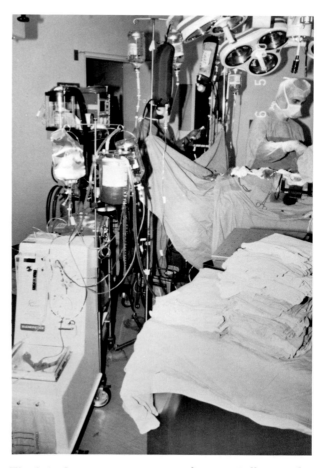

Fig. 8-4. Operating room scene showing Cell Saver device used for capturing and recycling lost blood during operative procedure. Use of this device allows for 87 percent capture of lost red cells during surgery.

deepening anesthesia or using vasodilators. *Deep inhalation anesthesia adversely effects the evoked potential and should not be used when evoked potentials are to be monitored.* Vasodilators such as sodium nitroprusside or nitroglycerine, except in deep hypotension, do not affect evoked potentials.[20] Special attention should be taken to avoid the risk of cyanide toxicity and *deep hypotension, which may affect spinal blood flow.*

Hemodilution. In hemodilution, hemoglobin is lowered from the normal 12 to 15 g/100 ml down to 8 to 10 g/100 ml, while oxygen-delivering capacity stays stable. *Oxygen-delivering capacity is the cardiac output multiplied by the oxygen-carrying capacity.* When hemoglobin is lowered, viscosity decreases, and cardiac output increases to maintain the oxygen-delivering capacity. *The two major compensators for hemodilution are increased cardiac output and increased oxygen extraction by the tissue.* Contraindications for hemodilution are fixed cardiac output and severe anemia, both of which deprive the body of the compensatory mechanisms. Hemodilution can be achieved by using vasodilators and increasing the blood volume (vascular filling) with normal saline or Ringer's solution. Another method for hemodilution is to withdraw 20 to 40 percent of the blood volume and replace it with crystalloid or colloids before surgery. After the surgical procedure, the blood is reinfused into the patient.

The Cell Saver. (Fig. 8-4) Blood is collected from the surgical field and heparin is added. The blood is washed of surgical debris and transfused back into the patient. Clotting factors are vulnerable during the use of the Cell Saver; therefore, a replacement of clotting factors is essential to maintain normal homeostasis.

However, in some spinal operations massive blood loss can occur and an adequate amount of fresh whole blood from the blood bank should be readily available for replacement. Complications of massive blood transfusion include hemolytic reactions, hepatitis, bacterial contamination, circula-

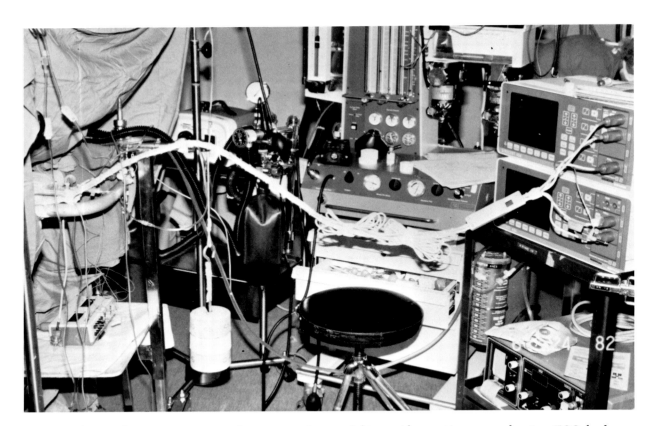

Fig. 8-5. Anesthesia monitoring equipment: monitor on right provides continuous read-out on ECG, body temperature, blood pressure, mean pressure, pulse, and expired CO_2. In center is standard anesthesia unit. On the left is patient undergoing operative procedure for cervical spine fracture. Note weights in place and presence of **SSEP** scalp electrodes entering junction box, at head of Stryker frame.

tory overload, air embolism, fever, allergic reactions, potassium intoxication, citrate intoxication, hypothermia, metabolic acidosis, acute respiratory distress syndrome (ARDS), acquired immune deficiency syndrome (AIDS), and coagulation problems.

MONITORING DURING SPINAL CORD SURGERY

Depending on the surgery to be performed and the position of the patient, different monitors may be needed. The routine monitors used during spinal surgery are ECG, blood pressure, temperature, urine output, pulse, and oxygen concentration (Fig. 8-5). Patients undergoing surgery in the sitting position are at risk of developing venous air embolism, hypotension, and cerebral ischemia. Special monitors are required when the sitting position is used to decrease the risks and alert the team to the entrance of the air embolism. These monitors include precordial Doppler, CVP, end-expiratory CO_2, end-expiratory nitrogen, and pulmonary artery pressure. During surgery, in the anterior cervical spine region, the retractors used to assist in viewing the surgical field may inadvertently occlude one or the other of the carotid arteries and endanger the brain on that side. Checking the temporal pulse before surgery on both sides and rechecking it each time the retractor is repositioned will minimize the risk of carotid artery occlusion and prevent possible permanent brain injury. The most dramatic complication of spinal surgery is spinal cord trauma with loss of neurologic function. Two methods can be used to monitor against cord injury: the wake-up test and somatosensory evoked potentials.

Wake-Up Test

Neurologic injury to the spinal cord during surgery is a recognized complication of spinal surgery. Primarily utilized by the scoliosis service, the wake-up test[5] is a method of evaluating neurologic function during surgery and is a well-recognized

and reliable technique. To perform the test, it is necessary for the anesthesia level to be decreased and the patient briefly lightened and awakened. He is asked to move his legs on command, and his movements are carefully observed. Depending on the patient's performance, the surgeon makes a decision to continue to completion or to alter his attempt at surgical correction. If motor function is decreased or absent, all internal fixation and surgical correction is removed, and the patient is observed for improvement. One of the disadvantages of the wake-up test is the risk of displacing the endotracheal tube during the period of light anesthesia. Also, the value of the wake-up test is limited only to the time of testing and does not ensure the same results at the end of surgery.

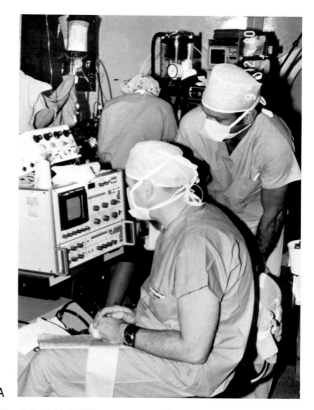

A

Fig. 8-6. (A) SSEP unit, in use during operative procedure. Neurophysiologist and/or anesthesiologist monitors spinal cord function during operative procedure. *(Figure continues.)*

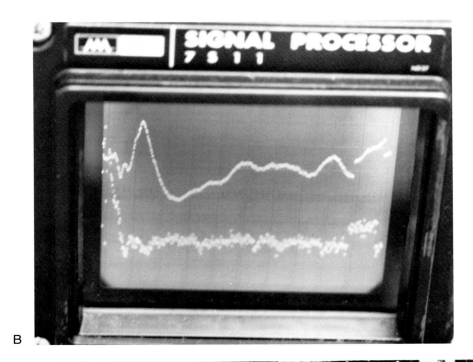

B

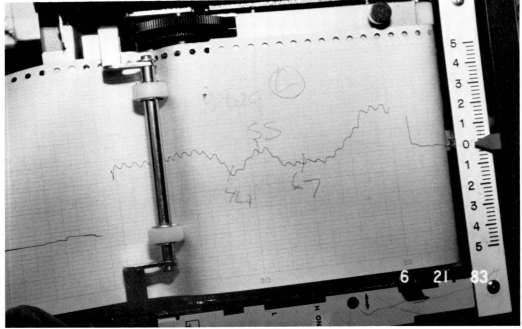

C

Fig. 8-6 *(Continued).* **(B)** Visual somatosensory signal on unit monitor. **(C)** Print-out of SSEP for record keeping.

Evoked Potential Monitor

(Fig. 8-6A – C) In recent years, the technique of somatosensory evoked potentials has been introduced into spinal cord surgery and has been gaining acceptance. As discussed in Chapter 6, SSEP consists of stimulating a peripheral nerve (Fig. 8-7A) and recording the responses over the head and neck (Fig. 8-7B). Changes in the latency (length of time for the impulse to travel from the lower extremity to the head) and in the amplitude (strength of the electrical signal) of the SSEP waveform can be the result of surgical manipulation, technical difficulties, physiologic alterations, or anesthetic effects.[4,6] A smooth anesthesia and stable intraoperative physiology is helpful in shortening the list of possible causes for change in the evoked potentials during surgery.

ANESTHESIA MANAGEMENT FOR SPINAL CORD-INJURED PATIENTS

Few changes in anesthesia technique are required for spinal cord surgery. The use of succinylcholine is contraindicated in patients with neurologic injury and motor loss secondary to spinal cord injury. This is true from 1 day to 1 year posttrauma. Using succinylcholine — a depolarizing (paralyzing) agent — causes a sudden release of potassium from the paralyzed muscles. This sudden increase in serum potassium can cause cardiac arrest in diastole.

The routine use of oral endotracheal intubation with rigid laryngoscopy in the cervical spine-injured patient is limited.

The use of certain inhalation anesthetic agents

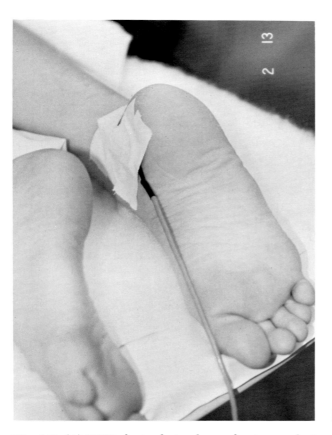

A

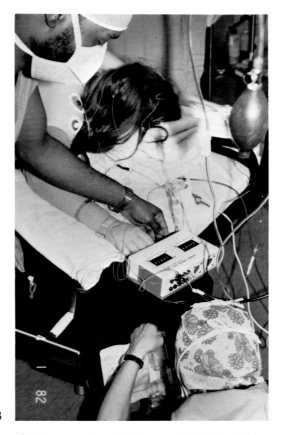

B

Fig. 8-7. (A) SSEP electrode in place subcutaneously in area of right posterior tibial nerve. (B) View of posterior cervical spine and calvaria electrode junction box during set-up period for use of intraoperative SSEP.

(e.g., nitrous oxide) alters the evoked potential response. *Evoked potentials are vulnerable to all inhalation agents and therefore these must be kept to a minimum concentration, since all inhalation agents affect SSEPs in a dose-related fashion.* Bolus doses of intravenous drugs may also have an effect. For this reason, it is suggested inhalation agents be used only in low concentration(less than 0.5 the minimum alveolar concentration [MAC]). Fluctuation in anesthesia levels may alter the evoked potentials responses and interfere with monitoring during a critical period. The anesthesia state should therefore be maintained at a stable and steady level so that evoked potentials can be successfully monitored. At Northwestern University, *a narcotic-base anesthetic course is used.* It consists of *sufentanil, fentanyl, or alfentanyl* and *muscle relaxants* combined with the use of either a low dose of inhalation agent, usually *isoflurane (<0.5 percent)*, or *intravenous infusion of thiopental. Nitrous oxide has a depressant effect on SSEPs;* cortical waves are lowered by more than 50 percent during the use of 50 percent nitrous oxide.[21] Ideally, patients are awake at the end of surgery and breathing spontaneously. If ventilation is still slow, a small dose of narcotic antagonist is used to reverse the respiratory effect of the narcotic used during surgery. *Patients undergoing anteroposterior fusion or with limited ventilatory reserve are managed in the spinal cord intensive care unit, with the endotracheal tube in place and ventilation assisted mechanically.*

In general, an appreciation of the physiologic and pharmacologic effects of anesthetic agents on the spinal cord-injured patient helps the anesthesiologist to safely maintain the anesthetized patient during surgery.

REFERENCES

1. Young JS: Initial hospitalization and rehabilitation costs of spinal cord injury. Orthop Clin North Am 9:263, 1978
2. Quimby CW, Jr., Williams RN, Greifenstein FE: Anesthesia problems of the acute quadriplegic patient. Anesth Analg 52:333, 1973
3. Schonwald G, Fish KJ, Perkash I: Cardiovascular complications during anesthesia in spinal cord injured patients. Anesthesiology 55:550, 1981
4. Koht A, Sloan TB, Ronai AK, Toleikis JR: Intraoperative deterioration of evoked potentials during spinal surgery. p. 161. In Schramm J, Jones SJ (eds): Spinal Cord Monitoring. Springer Verlag, New York, 1985
5. Stagnara P: Scoliosis in adults: surgical treatment of severe forms. Excerpta Med F Int Congr Ser 192, 1969
6. Sloan TB, Ronai AK, Koht A: Reversible loss of somatosensory evoked potentials during cervical spine fusion. Anesth Analg 65:96, 1986
7. Martin J: Positioning in Anesthesia and Surgery. WB Saunders, Philadelphia, 1978
8. Albin MS, Carroll RG, Maroon JC: Clinical consideration concerning detection of venous air embolism. Neurosurgery 3:380, 1978
9. Bunegin L, Albin MS, Helsel PE: Positioning the right atrial catheter: a model for re-appraisal. Anesthesiology 55:343, 1981
10. Adornato DC, Gildenberg PL, Ferraria CM, et al.: Pathophysiology of intravenous air embolism in dogs. Anesthesiology 49:120, 1978
11. Ovassapian A, Land P, Schaefer M, et al.: Anesthetic management for surgical corrections of severe flexion deformity of the cervical spine. Anesthesiology 58:370, 1983
12. Stone WA, Beach TP, Hamelberg W: Succinylcholine: danger in spinal cord injured patient. Anesthesiology 32:168, 1970
13. Cooperman LH, Strobel GE, Kennel EM: Massive hyperkalemia after administration of succinylcholine. Anesthesiology 32:161, 1970
14. Thomas ET: Circulatory collapse following succinylcholine: report of a case. Anesth Analg 48:333, 1969
15. Stone WA, Beach TP, Hamelberg W: Succinylcholine-induced hyperkalemia in dose with transected sciatic nerves or spinal cords. Anesthesiology 32:168, 1970
16. Tobey RE: Paraplegia, succinylcholine and cardiac arrest. Anesthesiology 32:359, 1970
17. Basta JW, Niedjalik K, Pallares V: Autonomic hyperreflexia: intraoperative control with pentolinium tartarate. J Anesth 49:1087, 1977
18. Kurnick NB: Autonomic hyperreflexia and its control in patients with spinal cord lesions. Ann Intern Med 44:678, 1956
19. Erickson RP: Autonomic hyperreflexia: pathophysiology and medical management. Arch Phys Med Rehab 61:431, 1980
20. Grundy B, Nash CL, Jr., Brown RH: Arterial pressure manipulation alters spinal cord function during correction of scoliosis. Anesthesiology 54:249, 1981
21. Sloan TB, Koht A: Depression of cortical somatosensory evoked potentials by nitrous oxide. Br J Anesth Analg 57:849, 1985

9

Pulmonary Effects of Acute Spinal Cord Injury: Assessment and Management

Roy D. Cane
Barry A. Shapiro

The alteration in pulmonary function caused by spinal cord trauma varies with the level of injury. Denervation below the level of L1 seldom produces significant respiratory compromise, whereas thoracic-level injuries often result in significantly limited pulmonary function. Cervical spinal cord injury resulting in quadriplegia always produces respiratory pathophysiology affecting morbidity, mortality, and the ultimate potential for rehabilitation. With better understanding of the impact of spinal cord injury on pulmonary function, more comprehensive respiratory management has evolved. Although significant reductions in respiratory-related morbidity and mortality have been accomplished in traumatic quadriplegia, pulmonary complications still account for as many as half of the deaths associated with cervical spinal cord trauma.

Pulmonary function is determined by three major components: central ventilatory drive, ventilatory muscle function, and lung parenchyma. Spinal cord injury does not alter central ventilatory drive or lung parenchyma directly; rather, the primary effect is alteration of neuromuscular components with consequent changes in pulmonary mechanics.

PULMONARY MECHANICS

Consideration of pulmonary mechanics requires an understanding of static and dynamic lung volumes and capacities.

Lung Volumes and Capacities

The total lung capacity (TLC) is defined as the maximum volume of gas the lungs can contain. In clinical practice, this is defined as the volume of gas contained within the lungs at the end of a maximal inspiratory effort. The TLC comprises four lung volumes: inspiratory reserve volume (IRV), tidal volume (V_T), expiratory reserve volume (ERV), and residual volume (RV) (Fig. 9-1).

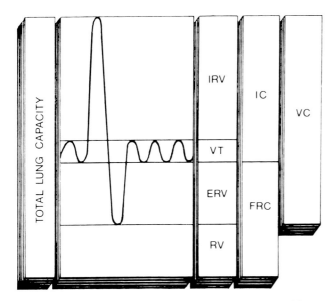

Fig. 9-1. The divisions of total lung capacity. Total lung capacity (TLC) is the maximum amount of air the lungs can hold. The TLC is divided into four primary volumes: inspiratory reserve volume (IRV); tidal volume (V_T); expiratory reserve volume (ERV); and residual volume (RV). Capacities are combinations of two or more lung volumes. They are inspiratory capacity (IC), functional residual capacity (FRC), and vital capacity (VC). (From Shapiro et al.,[1] with permission.)

When the thorax is intact, the lungs contain gas even after a maximal expiratory effort. The gas remaining after a maximal expiratory effort is defined as residual volume (RV). All individuals manifest a basal ventilatory pattern at rest. This ventilatory pattern occurs at a volume significantly above the residual volume. The amount of gas expired during normal resting ventilation is the tidal volume (V_T). The gas volume between V_T and RV is the expiratory reserve volume (ERV). The ERV represents a volume of gas available for increasing V_T that is not utilized during normal resting ventilation. The volume of gas between the tidal volume and the upper limit of the total lung capacity is the inspiratory reserve volume (IRV). It represents a volume of gas available for increasing V_T that is also not utilized in normal resting ventilation.

Assuming a normal man has a total lung capacity of 6 liters, the V_T is ideally 0.5 liter, the IRV is 3.1 liters, the ERV is l.2 liters, and the RV is 1.2 liters. A

rule of thumb in the normal adult lung is that the IRV is as large or larger than the other three volumes combined and that ERV and RV are close to equal.

Lung capacities are combinations of two or more lung volumes. There are two lung capacities that are especially important in acute respiratory care: vital capacity and functional residual capacity.

Functional Residual Capacity

The functional residual capacity (FRC) is defined as the combination of the RV and the ERV:

$$FRC = RV + ERV$$

In essence, this measurement represents the content of gas remaining in the lungs at the end of a normal expiration. Over the past 20 years it has become apparent that arterial blood oxygenation and lung compliance are affected by changes in FRC. Although FRC cannot be readily measured in acutely ill patients, the concept of FRC and its effect on gas exchange and work of breathing in the acutely injured patient is important.

Vital Capacity

The vital capacity (VC) is defined as the combination of the IRV, V_T, and ERV:

$$VC = IRV + V_T + ERV$$

In other words, the vital capacity is the total lung capacity minus the residual volume. The VC represents the patient's maximum breathing ability. It is simple to measure since it requires the patient only to take the deepest inspiration possible and then expire as completely as possible. The amount of exhaled air is the vital capacity.

Vital capacities can be measured with the patient forcing or not forcing his expiration. Using a recording spirometer, one can measure the forced vital capacity and obtain what is called the forced expiratory spirogram (Fig. 9-2). This is an extremely important measurement in respiratory care because numerous measurements can be obtained from this one simple maneuver. In addition, the forced expiratory spirogram can be obtained at the bedside; that is, reliable measurements do not require moving the patient to a pulmonary function laboratory.

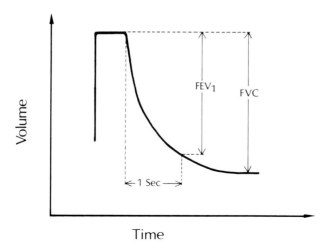

Fig. 9-2. Schematic representation of a forced expiratory spirogram. Moving from left to right, a maximum inspiration is depicted by the rapid increase in volume (representing inspiratory capacity). The patient holds his breath at maximum inspiration and then forces the air out as fast as possible. The total air expelled is the forced vital capacity (FVC); the volume expelled in the first second is FEV_1. (From Shapiro et al.,[1] with permission.)

The measurement of a forced vital capacity (FVC) makes two important measurements readily available: the actual vital capacity under stress and the volume expired in the first second (FEV_1).

The FVC is a useful measurement in acute respiratory care because it represents the maximum ventilatory volume available to the patient under conditions of stress. The patient's measurement is then compared with the predicted normal based on sex, height, and age. The percent of forced vital capacity (FVC%) reflects the patient's present capability for exchanging air in relation to his theoretical normal capability.

The forced expiratory volume in 1 second (FEV_1) is the measurement of the volume of air forcefully expired in the first second of an FVC maneuver. Normally, at least 75 percent of the total VC will be expired in the first second. The FEV_1 may be compared with the actual FVC and referred to as $FEV_1\%$. The greatest use of the FEV_1 in respiratory care is as an indication of the potential effects of airway resistance on the work of breathing.

Muscles of Ventilation

The lungs function as a to-and-fro valveless pump. This mechanically inefficient system is powered by muscles that are anatomically and functionally separate from the lungs. The ventilatory muscles are commonly considered as three distinct groups: the diaphragm, intercostal muscles, and accessory muscles.

The diaphragm is composed of both a membranous and a muscular portion. The muscle fibers originate and insert on the inferior surface of the lower ribs. The two muscular hemidiaphragms are connected by a membranous midline portion. Motor innervation originates from the spinal cord at the third through fifth cervical roots, which combine to form the phrenic nerve. Although the diaphragm is the major muscle of ventilation and performs all the work associated with normal breathing, the other inspiratory muscles provide great reserve.

The intercostal muscles form two layers of fibers connecting the ribs and are innervated by spinal nerves from T1 through T11. The external intercostal muscles elevate the anterior chest wall and facilitate inspiration, whereas the internal intercostals act in the opposite direction and are believed to play a role in forceful expiration.

The accessory muscles of ventilation serve to elevate and stabilize the chest wall in its greatest diameters and thereby improve the efficiency of diaphragmatic excursion. The major accessory muscles are the scalene, sternocleidomastoid, trapezius, and pectoralis muscles, whose innervation is derived from the upper cervical roots. They are not normally active during resting ventilation.

Inspiration is always an active muscular event, whereas expiration is normally passive, elastic recoil of the lung and chest wall providing the expiratory energy.

Abdominal muscles (external oblique, rectus abdominis, internal oblique, and transverse abdominis) play a major part in active expiration. Innervation of the abdominal muscles is via spinal nerves from T6 through L1.

Acute spinal cord injuries at levels higher than T11 adversely affect pulmonary mechanics by decreasing ventilatory muscle innervation. This re-

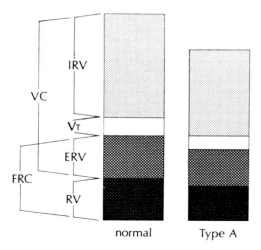

Fig. 9-3. Bar graph of acute restrictive pathology. RV, residual volume; ERV, expiratory reserve volume; V_T, tidal volume; IRV, inspiratory reserve volume; FRC, functional residual capacity; VC, vital capacity. Type A is the diminishment of all lung volumes commonly seen with neuromuscular disease, e.g., acute spinal cord injury. (Modified from Shapiro et al.,[1] with permission.)

sults in a diminished TLC with a major diminishment of VC (Fig. 9-3).

Relationships of the Lung and Thorax

The mechanics of ventilation depend in large part on the elastic forces of the lung parenchyma and chest wall. These elastic forces tend to passively return chest wall and lung parenchyma to their resting state after active inspiration. At the end of a normal expiration, the elastic forces of the chest wall (including the resting muscle tone) tend to expand the intrathoracic volume, whereas the elastic forces of the lung tend to reduce the intrathoracic volume (Fig. 9-4). Thus, the end-expiratory lung volume (FRC) is the resultant of these opposing forces. Spinal cord injuries initially diminish the chest wall elastic forces, leaving the elastic forces of the lung tissue relatively unopposed. Therefore, patients with acute spinal cord injuries will have a reduced FRC, mostly at the expense of ERV (Fig. 9-3).

Lung Elastic Forces

The elastic forces of the lung are primarily generated by interstitial elastic fibers and alveolar fluid surface tension. The elasticity of the alveoli may be approximated by the behavior of elastic spheres that obey LaPlace's Law. The distending pressure necessary to expand an alveolus is determined by both the surface tension and radius. If surface tension forces remain constant, the smaller the radius, the greater the elastic force tending to collapse the alveolus and hence the greater the distending pressure required to maintain a given alveolar volume. However, alveolar surface tension normally decreases as alveolar size decreases because of the

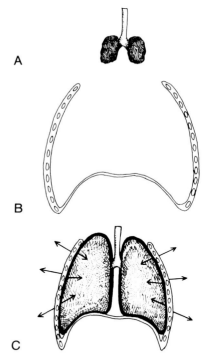

Fig. 9-4. (A) Resting state of normal lungs when removed from the chest cavity; i.e., elasticity causes total collapse. **(B)** Resting state of normal chest wall and diaphragm when apex is open to atmosphere and the thoracic contents are removed. **(C)** End expiration in the normal, intact thorax. Note that elastic forces of lung and chest wall are in opposite directions. The pleural surfaces link these two opposing forces. (From Shapiro et al.,[1] with permission.)

presence of surfactants, substances that reduce the surface tension forces as alveoli become smaller. Spinal cord injuries do not affect surfactant production; however, the reduction in functional residual capacity due to the loss of chest wall tone results in alveoli of smaller diameters. Hence, more work is required to expand the lungs.

When the TLC is significantly diminished for several days, the smaller alveoli have a critical volume below which the elastic forces become overwhelming despite surfactant action and lead to collapse. Since spinal cord injuries predispose to a reduction in thoracic gas volume, they result in a situation in which alveoli are more likely to collapse. Hence, atelectasis of the dependent lung is a common complication of acute spinal cord injury.

Compliance

Compliance is best conceived of as the reciprocal of elastance.[1] Low pulmonary compliance is associated with increased elastic forces such that greater degrees of work must be performed to expand the lung. In acute spinal cord injury, since the chest wall forces that ordinarily act to minimize the lung elastic forces are diminished, lower lung compliance occurs (Fig. 9-5).

Work of Breathing

The work of breathing is the energy required to overcome pulmonary resistance and compliance. Acute spinal cord injuries do not usually produce

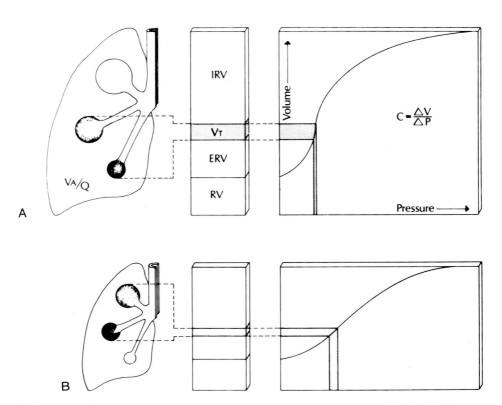

Fig. 9-5. (A) The normal relationships between lung volumes, compliance, and VA/Q. (B) The changes that may occur in patients with acute high-level spinal cord injuries. IRV, inspiratory reserve volume; V_T, tidal volume; ERV, expiratory reserve volume; RV, residual volume. (Modified from Shapiro et al.,[1] with permission.)

significant changes in airway resistance, but compliance is decreased and therefore work of breathing will be increased.

Normally, the work of breathing consumes 5 percent of total oxygen consumption. However, when the work of breathing is increased, the energy expenditure for breathing increases exponentially. The relationship of minute volume to oxygen consumption for work of breathing can be graphically depicted (Fig. 9-6A); a similar relationship can be derived relating oxygen consumed by the work of breathing to tidal ventilation represented as a percentage of vital capacity (see Fig. 9-6B). Measurement of V_T and VC allows for assessment of the work of breathing and VC becomes a reflection of ventilatory reserve.[2] The more of the VC a patient uses for tidal ventilation, the less he can increase tidal ventilation to meet a stressful situation, i.e., the less the ventilatory reserve.

For a more detailed discussion of pulmonary anatomy and mechanics, the reader is referred to other texts.[3,4]

Ventilatory Muscle Fatigue

The function of the ventilatory pump depends on the ability of the ventilatory muscles to achieve the required work loads. Inability of the muscles to do so is *fatigue*. Muscular work consumes energy. The amount of energy is determined to a large degree by the work load and the efficiency of the musculoskeletal system in question. When subjected to high work loads for prolonged periods, skeletal muscles may fatigue. Muscle fatigue may be generally defined as the energy demands exceeding the energy supply.

The energy demands on ventilatory muscles are determined by the work load in relation to the efficiency. The work load is determined mainly by the minute ventilation, airway resistance, and lung compliance, whereas efficiency is determined by factors such as stability of the chest wall, the freedom of movement of the chest wall and abdomen, the intrathoracic gas volume, the nutritional status, and energy storage within the muscles. The energy supply commonly is conceptualized in terms of blood flow, arterial oxygen content, blood substrate concentration, and energy stores. Ventilatory muscle fatigue may lead to acute ventilatory failure.

Patients with high spinal cord lesions have an increased ventilatory work load because of decreased compliance, and a reduced ventilatory efficiency because loss of chest wall tone impairs

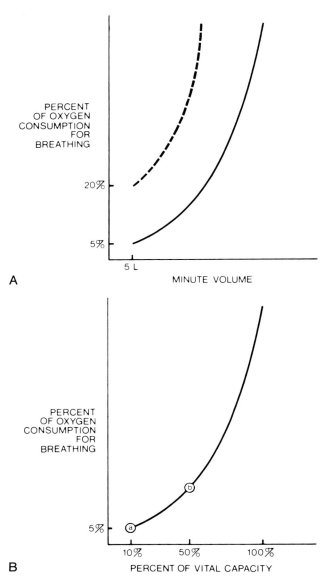

A

B

Fig. 9-6. (A) The work of breathing in relation to minute ventilation. In (B) point *a* represents a V_T of 500 ml with a VC to 5 liters; point *b* represents a V_T of 500 ml with a VC of 1 liter. (From Shapiro et al.,[1] with permission.)

chest wall stability. These factors in conjunction with weakness of the inspiratory muscle because of partial denervation make the spinal cord-injured patient particularly susceptible to development of ventilatory muscle fatigue.

It has been demonstrated that patients breathing against fatiguing work loads intermittently switch inspiratory work between the diaphragm and the intercostal muscles.[5] It has been suggested that this is an adaptive mechanism that helps conserve energy when breathing against a fatiguing work load. The patient with a cervical spinal cord injury cannot use this adaptive mechanism because of denervation of the intercostal muscles. For more detail on ventilatory muscle fatigue, the reader is referred to recent reviews.[6,7]

SPINAL CORD INJURY AND PULMONARY FUNCTION

Acute spinal cord injuries, particularly ones involving the upper thoracic and cervical segments of the cord, will result in predictable changes in pulmonary function. Restrictive pulmonary disease is manifested as reduced lung volumes and capacities as well as decreased pulmonary compliance. Such acute restrictive pathology results in increased work of breathing and a propensity for alveolar collapse (atelectasis) because of the general reduction in alveolar size.

Static Lung Volumes and Capacities

In stable patients with chronic spinal cord injuries, Fuglmeyer found total lung capacities ranging from 69 percent of predicted normal in patients with low cervical lesions to 99 percent of normal in patients with lumbar lesions.[8,9] A similar pattern was observed in the vital capacity, which ranged from 42 percent of normal for cervical lesions at C4 through C8 to 95 percent of normal for lumbar spinal cord lesions. The FRC was reduced to l0 percent to 25 percent of normal. The ERV was reduced by as much as 75 percent in the patients with cervical lesions and 20 percent in patients with lumbar lesions, whereas RV was barely reduced.

Similar findings have been reported in stabilized chronic patients by McMichan et al.,[10] Ohry et al.,[11] and Ledsome and Sharp.[12] In the acute phase of spinal cord injury, even greater reductions in VC, which subsequently improved in the initial period after injury, have been reported. McMichan's patients had vital capacities of 1.5 liters on admission; these improved to 2.7 liters by 18 weeks after injury.[10] Ohry and colleagues reported similar findings, with VCs increasing from 31 percent of predicted normal to 40 percent of predicted normal in the first 6 months of injury for patients with cervical lesions and 69 percent improving to 92 percent of predicted normal in patients with lumbar lesions.[11] Our own experience in the Midwest Spinal Cord Injury Center confirm these findings: initial VCs are greatly reduced, and the level of lesion correlates with the degree of reduction. For all levels of lesion, vital capacity improves during the first 7 days after injury.

Dynamic Lung Volumes

Expiratory flow rates measured as the FEV_1 expressed as a percentage of the actual FVC were essentially normal in the population studied by Ohry et al.[11] and Ledsome and Sharp;[12] however, peak expiratory flow rates were decreased by 50 to 40 percent, as were maximal expiratory flows at 50 percent of VC. Maximum voluntary ventilation measured by Fuglmeyer was markedly reduced, averaging 34 percent of predicted normal in quadriplegic patients.[9] Measured changes in forced inspiratory volumes in 1 second correlated with the degree of reduction in vital capacity, and in those patients studied, the forced inspiratory flow rates were higher than the forced expiratory flow rates. Fuglmeyer measured static and dynamic compliance and found static lung compliance in a stable group of quadriplegic patients to range from 0.15 to 0.22 L/cmH_2O. Dynamic compliance was lower than static compliance.[9]

Hypoxemia

In addition to the changes in ventilation, spinal cord injuries are frequently associated with hypoxemia.[12,13] In many instances, this hypoxemia can be explained on the basis of associated injuries such as pulmonary contusion. In the absence of pulmonary parenchymal injury, hypoxemia presumably results from an increase in areas of the lung with low ventilation/perfusion (V/Q) ratios owing to the reduction in FRC and hence alveolar size, particularly in dependent parts of the lung[14,15] and possibly resulting from changes in distribution of pulmonary perfusion secondary to the acute sympathectomy associated with many cervical and upper thoracic spinal cord injuries.

Bronchial Hygiene

The reduction in vital capacity secondary to cervical or high thoracic spinal cord injury dramatically affects the patient's ability to maintain normal bronchial hygiene. To generate the high alveolar-to-mouth pressure gradient required for an effective cough, a patient needs a vital capacity of at least 15 ml/kg body weight. Thus, the ability to cough must be diminished by high spinal cord lesions. In quadriplegic patients, Fuglmeyer demonstrated reduced maximal esophageal pressures during forced expiratory vital capacity and coughing maneuvers.[9] This reduced efficacy of coughing predisposes to retention of secretions with associated pneumonia and atelectasis. Ciliary action, a component of the normal mucociliary escalator that aids in bronchial hygiene, may be impaired after adrenergic denervation, which may further contribute to retained secretions.[16]

SPINAL CORD INJURY AND PULMONARY COMPLICATIONS

Two elements contribute to the high incidence of pulmonary morbidity in patients with acute spinal cord injuries: restrictive effect of spinal cord injury on pulmonary function, and morbidity associated with the immobilization required in the management of these injuries. Retained secretions, atelectasis, and pneumonia are the common complications.

Acute ventilatory failure occurs when the pa-

tient's level of ventilation (minute volume) is insufficient to excrete metabolically produced carbon dioxide, and is manifested as an elevation of arterial PCO_2 (>50 mmHg) and a consequent fall in arterial pH (<7.30). Acute ventilatory failure secondary to ventilatory muscle weakness, discoordinate activity, and fatigue is a not uncommon problem in the early phases of cervical spinal cord injuries. Respiratory failure is reported as the most common cause of mortality in patients with spinal cord injuries with incidences ranging from 15 percent to 40 percent.[10,17–19] The high mortality rates reported in earlier series of patients have been reduced by application of modern respiratory care techniques.[10]

Table 9-1 shows the relationship between level of neurologic injury and incidence of pneumonia, acute ventilatory failure developing after hospital admission, and mortality in a series of 1,698 patients with acute spinal cord injuries admitted to the Midwest Regional Spinal Cord Injury Center. The higher the level of neurologic deficit, the greater the incidence of complications.

RESPIRATORY MANAGEMENT OF SPINAL CORD-INJURED PATIENTS

The underlying principle of pulmonary management of spinal cord injuries is the identification of spared musculoskeletal function in the ventilatory muscle groups, and the maximal development of this muscle function. Every attempt should be made to develop the patient's pulmonary function to the point that bronchial hygiene is effective and the patient can be as independent of mechanical ventilatory aids as possible. This allows the patient to be mobilized and hence reduces potential complications. It also enhances the potential for rehabilitation.

For reasons of clarity, management will be considered in two sections: first, management of patients who are ventilating spontaneously on admission after spinal cord injury, and second, management of patients who require mechanical ventilatory support immediately or shortly after their injuries.

Table 9-1. Relationship Between Pulmonary Complications, Mortality, and Level of Neurologic Injury[a]

Pathology	Level of Neurologic Injury (% of Patients)							
	C1–C2	C3–C5	C6–C8	T1–T6	T7–T12	L1–L5	S1–S5	Total (N = 1,698)
Pneumonia	37.5	16.7	8.9	13.2	7.1	4.2	0.0	8.2
Acute ventilatory failure	25.0	15.1	7.3	5.5	1.9	1.6	0.0	5.9
Death	37.5	7.1	4.7	7.1	2.6	1.6	0.0	4.4

[a] Data pertain to 1,698 patients admitted to Midwest Regional Spinal Cord Injury Center.

Spontaneously Ventilating Patient

The initial assessment of spontaneously ventilating patients must determine the degree of impairment of pulmonary function and the pulmonary reserve. It is important also to seek for evidence of chest wall or lung trauma, as these may affect the patient's first few days of therapy. Initial pulmonary assessment includes at least measurements of vital capacity, tidal ventilation, respiratory rate, as well as a chest roentgenogram and an arterial blood gas analysis.

In our experience, a patient with a vital capacity of 15 ml/kg or more requires no specific supportive intervention in the acute phase. When there is no chest wall or pulmonary trauma, these patients invariably have adequate arterial oxygenation in room air. However, if the patient is hypoxemic (arterial PO_2 less than 80 mmHg), oxygen therapy (24 to 35 percent) via a mask or nasal catheter is usually sufficient.

These patients should be started on a program designed to improve the coordination of diaphragmatic contractions and to increase the strength and endurance of the functioning ventilatory muscles. We have had good results with a program of breathing and coughing exercises and incentive spirometry. Electromyographic feedback for the breathing and coughing exercises is useful in some patients as it replaces the patient's lost proprioceptive sense.[20]

Several techniques are available to increase ventilatory muscle strength and endurance, including isocapnic hyperpnea,[21] inspiratory resistive breathing exercises,[6] and breathing against graded weights placed on the abdomen. In our experience, inspiratory resistive breathing exercises are the preferred technique as they require only inexpensive disposable devices and minimal patient cooperation, and progress can be easily monitored. Patients should be instructed to breathe with an appropriate inspiratory resistance for 10 minutes to 15 minutes two to three times per day.

Several techniques to determine the desired level of inspiratory resistance have been described. We have found the measurement of mouth pressures to be a simple, inexpensive, and effective technique.[6] Response to this therapy should result in an increase in vital capacity, which will plateau when maximal benefit has been reached.[22] Our experience before the use of inspiratory resistive breathing exercises showed that a plateau was reached after 10 to 14 days of intensive physical therapy. To date, our experience with graded inspiratory resistive breathing exercises is that a higher vital capacity is achieved over a similar time period.

Spontaneously ventilating spinal cord-injured patients with vital capacities less than 15 ml/kg frequently require additional support beyond the regimens of breathing and coughing exercises outlined above. Intubation is often necessary to facilitate tracheobronchial toilet. Given that the pulmonary reserve will in most instances increase with physical therapy and, further, that the level of neurologic injury may recede as cord edema resolves, it is reasonable to establish a nasotracheal or endotracheal airway at this stage. If an airway is still indicated after 7 days, tracheostomy should probably be performed. In view of the restrictive effects of acute spinal cord injuries on pulmonary function, once an artifical airway has been established it is advisable to maintain low levels of positive pressure on the airway (continuous positive airway pressure [CPAP] of +5 to +10 cmH$_2$O). This minimizes further reduction in functional residual capacity and may improve pulmonary compliance and consequently decrease the work of breathing.[23] The bronchial hygiene techniques found to be most effective in intubated patients include frequent endotracheal suctioning with intermittent positive pressure ventilation and inflation hold. In the event that the patients develop retention of secretions and/or atelectasis, postural drainage with chest wall percussion and vibration should be added.[24]

The simplest and most reliable way to monitor the reserves of the spontaneously ventilating patient is by serial measurement of vital capacity. Vital capacities of less than 10 ml/kg are associated with impending ventilatory failure, and these patients should be closely followed. It is important to serially monitor all the spontaneously ventilating patients with cervical spinal cord injuries, as the level of injury may ascend in the first few days owing to increasing edema of the spinal cord. Development of pulmonary complications such as atelectasis, retention of secretions, pneumonia, or onset of ventilatory muscle fatigue result in a similar decrement in vital capacity.

The onset of ventilatory muscle fatigue is also heralded by signs of increasing work of breathing, specifically increasing respiratory rate, heart rate, and systolic blood pressure, onset of diaphoresis, and complaints of increasing dyspnea.

Patient with Ventilatory Failure

C1–C2 Neurologic Injury
Patients with cervical cord injuries higher than C3 will have apnea. They require mechanical ventilation, and a pattern of slow rate (8 to 10/min), deep volume (12 to 15 ml/kg body weight) ventilation with 5 cmH_2O positive end-expiratory pressure (PEEP) is probably optimal. Ventilation should be maintained until it is unlikely that there will be further change in the patient's neurologic level. At this time, if the patient still manifests a level of neurologic deficit higher than C3, plans for alternate forms of chronic mechanical ventilation should be formulated. The ideal in patients with C1 or C2 lesions is phrenic nerve pacing because it enables greater rehabilitation of the patient and some degree of mobility.[25-27] Long-term survival

of patients on positive-pressure ventilators is not good, as they are exposed to the additional complications of mechanical ventilation and prolonged immobilization in bed.[28]

C3–C5 Neurologic Injury
Lesions at the level of C3 through C5 result in partial loss of diaphragmatic innervation. Patients in ventilatory failure with C3–C5 neurologic deficit may well recover sufficient ventilatory function to breathe spontaneously. Strengthening the innervated diaphragm by means of graded inspiratory resistance exercises may allow the patient to return to spontaneous ventilation. Once the patient has been stabilized and the acute phase of the injury has passed, it is necessary to decrease the amount of mechanical ventilatory support for short periods by use of the intermittent mandatory ventilation technique, and to work at diaphragmatic coordinated contractions in much the same way as outlined for the spontaneously ventilating patients. Meticulous tracheobronchial toilet and the use of positive airway pressure to maintain the functional residual capacity and compliance of these patients is of paramount importance.

Ventilatory assist devices such as rocking electric beds or pneumobelt have a role in the management of these patients since they can be used to augment existing ventilatory function. Strengthening of the cervical muscles can augment ventilatory muscle function and enable weaning from a mechanical ventilatory in some instances. Programs in which patients are kept off ventilators during the day and then ventilated at night to rest them are feasible.

REFERENCES

1. Shapiro BA, Harrison RA, Kacmarek RM, Cane RD: Clinical Application of Respiratory Care. 3rd Ed. Ch. 2. p. 34. Year Book Medical Publishers, Chicago, 1985
2. Shapiro BA, Harrison RA, Walton JR: Clinical Application of Blood Gases. 3rd Ed. Ch. 11. p. 111. Year Book Medical Publishers, Chicago, 1982
3. Shapiro BA, Harrison RA, Kacmarek RM, Cane RD: Clinical Application of Respiratory Care. 3rd Ed. Ch. 1–3. p. 1-61. Year Book Medical Publishers, Chicago, 1985

4. Nunn JF: Applied Respiratory Physiology. 2nd Ed. Ch. 3–5. p. 63. Butterworth, London, 1977
5. Macklem PT: Respiratory muscles: the vital pump. Chest 78:753, 1980
6. Pardy RL, Leigh DE: Ventilatory muscle training. Respir Care 29:278, 1984
7. Derenne H, Macklem PT, Roussos CH: The respiratory muscles: mechanics, control and pathophysiology, Part III. Am Rev Respir Dis 118:581, 1978
8. Fuglmeyer AR: Effects of respiratory muscle paralysis in tetraplegic and paraplegic patients. Scand J Rehab Med 3:141, 1971
9. Fuglmeyer AR: Ventilatory function in tetraplegic patients. Scand J Rehab Med 3:151, 1971
10. McMichan JC, Michel L, Westbrook PR: Pulmonary dysfunction following traumatic quadriplegia. JAMA 243:528, 1980
11. Ohry A, Molho M, Rozin R: Alterations of pulmonary function in spinal cord injured patients. Paraplegia 13:101, 1975
12. Ledsome JR, Sharp JM: Pulmonary function in acute cervical cord injury. Am Rev Respir Dis 124:44, 1981
13. Simha RP, Ducker TB, Perot PL: Arterial oxygenation. Findings and its significance in central nervous system trauma patients. JAMA 224:1258, 1973
14. Bergofsky EH: Respiratory failure in disorders of the thoracic cage. Am Rev Respir Dis 119:643, 1979
15. Bergofsky EH: Mechanism for respiratory insufficiency after cervical cord injury. A source of alveolar hypoventilation. Ann Intern Med 61:435, 1964
16. Foster WM, Bergofsky EH, Bohning DE, et al.: Effect of adrenergic agents and their mode of action on mucociliary clearance in man. J Appl Physiol 41:146, 1976
17. Cheshire DJE: Respiratory management in acute traumatic tetraplegia. Paraplegia 1:252, 1964
18. Silver JR, Gibbon NOK: Prognosis in tetraplegia. Br Med J 4:79, 1968
19. Bellamy R, Pitts FW, Stauffer ES: Respiratory complications in traumatic quadriplegia: analysis of 20 years' experience. J Neurosurg 39:596, 1973
20. Sadowski HS, Geyer JR, Harman PO, Cane RD: Use of myoelectric and volume-linked feedback for breathing training in a patient with spinal cord injuries. Respir Care 26:130, 1981
21. Leigh DE, Bradley M: Ventilatory muscle strength and endurance training. J Appl Physiol 41:508, 1976
22. Gross D, Ladd HW, Riley EJ, et al.: The effect of training on strength and endurance of the diaphragm in quadriplegia. Am J Med 68:27, 1980
23. Shapiro BA, Cane RD, Harrison RA: Positive end-expiratory pressure therapy in adults with special reference to acute lung injury: a review of the literature and suggested clinical correlations. Crit Care Med 12:127, 1984
24. Shapiro BA, Harrison RA, Kacmarek RM, Cane RD: Clinical Application of Respiratory Care. 3rd Ed. Ch. 9 and 10. p. 133. Year Book Medical Publishers, Chicago, 1985
25. Glenn WWL, Holcomb WG, McLaughlin AJ, et al.: Total ventilatory support in a quadriplegic patient with radiofrequency electrophrenic respiration. N Engl J Med 286:513, 1972
26. McMichan JC, Piepgras DG, Gracey DR, et al.: Electrophrenic respiration. Mayo Clin Proc 54:662, 1979
27. Glenn WWL, Hogan JF, Loke JSO, et al.: Ventilatory support by pacing of the conditioned diaphragm in quadriplegia. N Engl J Med 310:1150, 1984
28. Wicks AB, Menter RR: Long-term outlook in quadriplegic patients with initial ventilator dependency. Chest 90:406, 1986

10

Radiologic Assessment of Acute Neurologic and Vertebral Injuries

Lee F. Rogers

The role of radiography in the assessment of spinal injuries is three-fold: first, to establish the diagnosis; second, to fully evaluate and categorize the injury; and third, to assess healing and document surgical treatment. Radiographic examinations should not be obtained as a matter of routine, but rather to answer specific questions concerning the care of the patient. Is there a fracture or dislocation? How extensive is the injury? Are there other areas of involvement? Has the fracture or dislocation been reduced? Have the fixation devices maintained their position? Is there evidence of healing? The type of radiographic examination and the number of radiographic views obtained are tailored to answer these specific concerns.

When dealing with actual or potential injuries of the spine, the primary consideration under any circumstance must be the proper handling of the patient. All personnel responsible for patient care, transportation, and performance of various examinations must be adequately trained and constantly aware of the requirements for judicious handling and movement of the patient. It is essential that movement of the patient be sharply curtailed until the possibility of spinal injury has been excluded. Before this, the patient should not be moved from stretcher to bed to examining table by any less than three trained individuals (Fig. 10-1). Often, the x-ray technologist is left to perform radiographic

examination on these critically injured patients without assistance. This is true not only in the emergency room, but in the patient's hospital room and within the radiology department. It is imperative that enough assistance be readily available so that manipulation of the patient does not result in the onset or progression of neurologic injury. Everyone involved must recognize this possibility and manipulate a patient judiciously to ensure that it does not occur.

Most spinal cord injuries occur immediately at the time of trauma and are obvious when first seen by medical or paramedical personnel. Five percent to 10 percent are late complications, and the remaining 5 percent to 10 percent occur in the immediate postinjury period after the patient has come under the care of medical or paramedical personnel.[1] These patients have usually sustained an unrecognized unstable injury of the spine, which comes to light only when the patient experiences a sudden neurologic deficit, frequently precipitated by movement of the patient (Fig. 10-2). Such tragedies can only be averted by maintaining diagnostic vigilance. Every seriously injured patient must be considered to have a spinal injury until proven otherwise. The first line of defense is an adequate initial physical examination. The cervical spine is the most easily examined area of the spine, but that is because the thoracic and lumbar spine are less

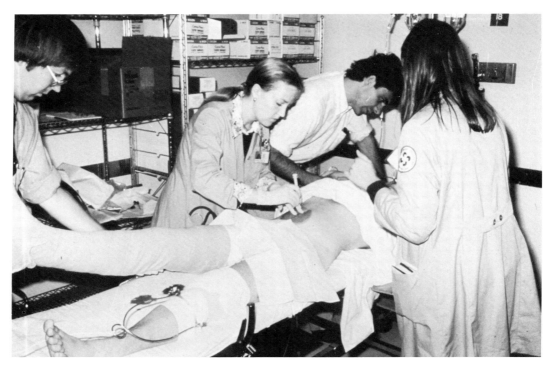

Fig. 10-1. Patients with either proven or potential spinal injuries should be transferred or moved by no less than three attendants. All personnel involved in their care should be trained in the proper techniques of patient handling.

accessible with the patient in the supine position. Fractures involving the thoracic spine and the cervicothoracic and thoracolumbar junctions are the most frequently overlooked injuries. Most oversights could be prevented by proper physical examination and careful scrutiny of the radiographs with these possibilities in mind.

The radiographic examination must be tailored to the needs of the patient. There are three principal settings: the examination of the obviously injured, the examination of the questionably injured, and the examination of an individual who has persistent pain or other symptomatology after a previous episode of trauma, but whose initial radiographic examination failed to disclose any evidence of abnormalities. As one progresses through these stages, the radiographic findings are usually less obvious and the need for additional views or projections to establish the diagnosis is greater.

The initial examination of a patient with an obvious injury of the spine, with or without a neurologic deficit, requires an anteroposterior (**AP**) and lateral projection in the area of interest (Fig. 10-3). The lateral view is obtained with a horizontal beam, which allows the patient to remain in the supine position. When there is an obvious injury, the patient need not, and should not, be moved to obtain a radiograph in the lateral projection. There is a common misconception that if the cross-table lateral projection reveals no evidence of fracture or dislocation, all gross and significant abnormalities are excluded, and it is quite safe to maneuver the patient to obtain additional radiographs. This is not true. Significant displacements may not be obvious on the lateral projection. Before the patient is manipulated, an examination in both the **AP** and lateral projections should be obtained and reviewed by the physicians in attendance. If there is no obvi-

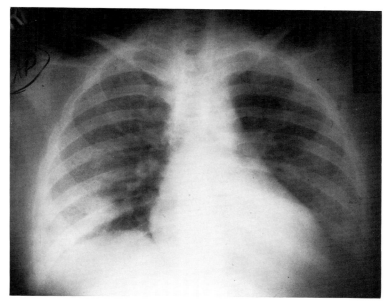

A

Fig. 10-2. A 30-year-old man who sustained a fracture-dislocation at T7 – T8 with delayed spinal cord injury as a result of an automobile accident. **(A)** The initial portable chest radiograph obtained in the emergency room. The underexposure does not allow visualization of the spine. Note that there does appear to be a slight angulation in the mid-dorsal area. The patient was taken from his hospital room to the radiology department for a repeat examination. During the transfer from the stretcher to the patient's hospital bed upon returning from the radiology department, he felt a heavy sensation in the lower extremities and became immediately and totally paraplegic. *(Figure continues.)*

ous injury to be seen on these two projections, it is safe to assume that there is no gross instability and that no severe fracture or dislocation is present. If the injury is obvious, no additional views may be required at this time. If there is no obvious injury, it is safe to proceed with the radiographic examination and obtain additional views.

The use of fixed instead of portable radiographic equipment is to be encouraged since this facilitates the examination by allowing the use of a moving grid and short exposure times, both of which greatly improve the diagnostic quality of the radiographic image. Vertical moving grids are of particular value in obtaining cross-table lateral examinations.

In general, the posterior elements of the spinal column are not well visualized on the cross-table lateral radiograph. However, the posterior elements are visualized on the AP projection, and many, if not the majority, of fractures involving the posterior elements can be discovered on the AP projection. Furthermore, it must be realized that isolated fractures of the posterior elements may not be as significant as fractures involving the vertebral bodies. The cross-table lateral examination does allow visualization of abnormalities of alignment, and when subluxations or dislocations are present as manifested by malalignments of the vertebral bodies, it can be assumed that injuries are present in the posterior elements.

The most significant problem in obtaining cross-table lateral radiographs is including the entire area of interest on the radiograph. This is particularly true for the cervical spine. Be certain that the radiograph includes all seven cervical vertebra (Fig. 10-4). This is not as easy as it might be assumed.

A similar problem exists at the thoracolumbar

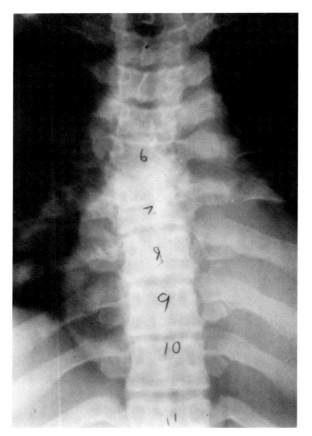

B

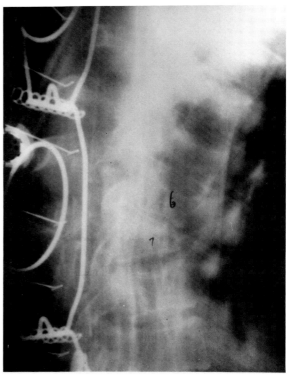

C

Fig. 10-2 *(Continued).* **(B) AP** view of the dorsal spine. This film was obtained after the onset of neurologic symptoms. Note the paraspinous mass and fracture of the body at T7. **(C)** Lateral view of the dorsal spine. There is an anterior dislocation of T7 on T8 with a compression fracture of T8 and a small anterior superior fragment of T8 displaced anteriorly.

junction. When the lower back is traumatized, an examination of the lumbar spine is ordered. The examination should then extend proximally to include at least the tenth and preferably the eighth dorsal vertebral. The thoracolumbar junction must be included to safely exclude the presence of a fracture or dislocation.

It is extremely difficult to visualize the cervicothoracic junction and upper dorsal spine on the cross-table lateral radiograph because of the overlying pectoral girdle. These injuries are usually best visualized on the AP projection, although the radiographic findings are often subtle (see Fig.

10-32). Usually, displacements are minimal, and it is difficult to visualize the vertebrae because of the overlying mediastinal soft tissues. Particular attention must be paid to widening of the mediastinum as this is a common manifestation of upper dorsal spine vertebral injury. Widening of the mediastinum in a traumatized patient may be due to mediastinal hemorrhage from aortic rupture, venous laceration, or dorsal spinal fracture. Aortic rupture and dorsal spinal fractures are two of the most commonly overlooked injuries in the multiply injured patient. To avoid oversight, always examine the radiograph closely for evidence of mediastinal wid-

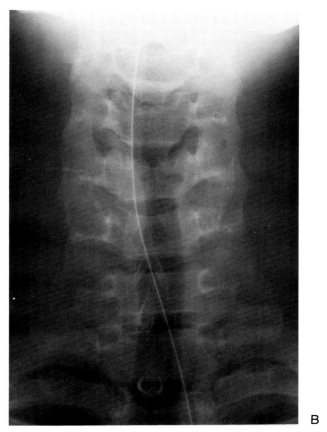
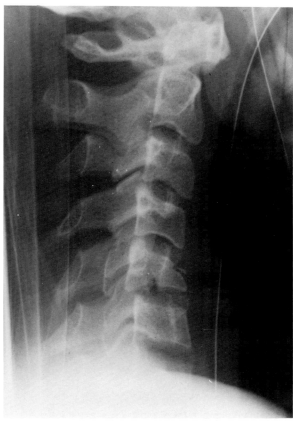

A

B

Fig. 10-3. Teardrop fracture in a 19-year-old man as a result of a driving accident. (**A**) AP view. There is a loss of height of the fifth vertebral body. A nasogastric tube is in place. (**B**) Cross-table lateral view. A teardrop fracture of C5 is visible, with characteristic posterior displacement of the involved vertebra compromising the spinal canal. The finding of a retropulsed superior vertebral body indicates the presence of a bilateral laminar fracture. This is a very unstable fracture. The patient was quadriplegic. Note that the associated hemorrhage has increased the width of the retropharyngeal soft tissues.

ening and always consider the possibility of an aortic rupture or a dorsal spinal fracture (see Fig. 9-1C).

Approximately 20 percent of patients with spinal injury will have associated injuries of the extremities and a similar percentage an associated injury of the skull or face.[2] The Midwest Regional Spinal Cord Injury Care System (**MRSCICS**) statistics reveal an incidence of 8.5 percent injuries to the extremities and 26.2 percent injuries to the head and face. When the patient is comatose or there is gross distortion of the extremities, attention is easily diverted from the spine, thus neurologic injuries may be overlooked. Care must be taken to exclude the presence of the spinal injury in every patient who has sustained multiple injuries or is comatose.

The radiographic examination of the ambulatory, questionably injured patient can proceed in an entirely different fashion than in those who are obviously injured. The cervical spine is best examined with the patient in the upright position, and

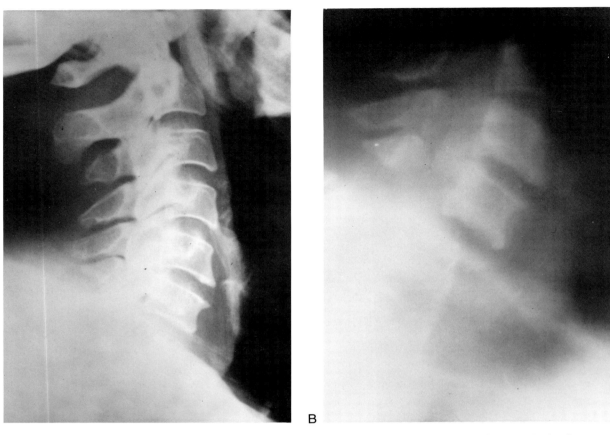

Fig. 10-4. Fracture-dislocation of C7–T1 in a 40-year-old man. **(A)** Initial lateral view shows only the first six cervical segments. **(B)** Lateral tomogram of the cervicothoracic junction demonstrates a fracture-dislocation with anterior displacement of C7 on T1. Note the fracture at the spinous process of C7. Tomography was necessary because standard views including the swimmer's view had failed to demonstrate the abnormality.

this should be done whenever the patient's condition allows. When not possible, the examination of the thoracic and lumbar spine is done with the patient in the horizontal position.

ROUTINE RADIOGRAPHIC EXAMINATION

The routine examination of the cervical spine consists of an **AP** view of the spine and an **AP** open mouth view of C1–C2, a lateral view to include C7, and a right and a left 45-degree oblique projection.

Routine views of the thoracic spine are an **AP** and lateral view of the entire spine and a "swimmer's view" of the cervicothoracic junction. The swimmer's view is made with one of the patient's arms extended over the head and the other held behind the back so that the shoulders are rotated to allow visualization of the cervicothoracic junction. In the straight lateral view, the shoulders overlie this area, and it is impossible to visualize. Oblique views of the dorsal spine are of little value and may be omitted.

The routine radiographic examination of the lumbar spine should consist of an **AP**, lateral, and when possible, right and left 45-degree oblique

Fig. 10-5. Patient is in position for a lateral tomogram of the cervical spine. The patient is maintained in position by a band across the torso and foam rubber bolsters. Cranial traction is maintained by suspending the weights over the end of the table. Positive end-expiratory pressure (PEEP) therapy is also maintained through the tracheostomy tube.

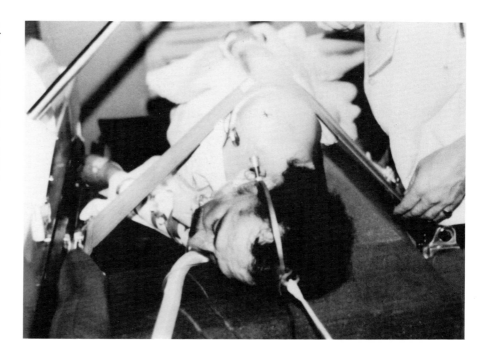

views extending from the level of the tenth dorsal vertebra to at least the first three segments of the sacrum.

If these standard views fail to demonstrate any abnormalities, it is safe to assume that in most cases no fracture or dislocation exists. If there is a question, additional views or tomography should be obtained before the patient is discharged.

The third category of patients are those who continue to experience symptoms despite a normal radiographic examination at the time of the initial injury. These individuals will require a repeat examination and possibly additional special oblique views, flexion-extension views of the area in question, and/or tomography. Multiple angled views are often used in the cervical spine. It is common to proceed directly to tomography in the thoracic and lumbar spine. Such extended examinations can be safely reserved for those patients who have persistent symptoms after trauma and need not be employed routinely in the exclusion of injuries.

The patient who has experienced a fracture or dislocation with an associated spinal cord injury should have an examination of the entire length of the spine in the AP and lateral projections as soon as possible after their condition is stabilized and all life-threatening injuries have been treated.[3] This examination is necessary since approximately 5 percent of all spinal cord-injured patients have a second level of injury remote from the primary fracture or dislocation that resulted in the spinal cord injury.[3] By identifying and stabilizing such fractures, the potential of proximal extension of the neurologic injury and subsequent deformities and other problems arising in the rehabilitation process can be averted.

TOMOGRAPHY

Tomography or laminagraphy is a method of obtaining a radiographic view limited to a plane of the body. This method is accomplished by simultaneous movement of the x-ray tube and film through a fulcrum at the level of interest. The motion of the tube may be linear, circular, ovoid, spiral, or hypocycloidal. The latter is a complex motion mimicking a clover leaf. Such complex-motion projections are known as polytomograms. The sharpness of the image and the clarity of the detail are increased as the motion becomes more complex.[4,5] However, in most situations complex-motion tomography and fine detail are not absolutely necessary to disclose fractures and fully evaluate the traumatized spine. Under most conditions, when polytomograms are not available, simple linear tomography is satisfactory.

The indications for tomography are to evaluate questionable findings on the radiograph, to disclose otherwise inapparent injury[4] (see Fig. 10-4), and to fully evaluate a known fracture or fracture-dislocation to assist in the decisions regarding surgical management. The advantage of tomography over plain films is that all segments or anatomic parts of the spine can be clearly visualized. The disadvantages are that multiple exposures are required, increasing the radiation dose to the patient, and for obtaining a tomogram in the lateral projection, the patient must be turned on his side. This problem is not an insurmountable one in the severely injured patient. By judicious handling of the patient, proper use of bolsters and restraints, and with simultaneous rotation of all body segments, the patient can be safely turned without incurring or extending a neurologic injury (Fig. 10-5). Furthermore, life support systems and traction[7] may be maintained during the examination.

COMPUTED TOMOGRAPHY

Because of the cross-sectional display, computed tomography (CT) (Fig. 10-6) offers a unique opportunity to evaluate fractures by precisely localizing fragments in relation to the spinal canal and demonstrating otherwise obscure fractures of the posterior elements.[8-11] There is also a distinct advantage in that it is not necessary to move the patient to the lateral projection. Life support and traction may be maintained during the examination. While it is easy to visualize a single vertebra, it is harder to visualize the relationships between adjacent vertebrae. This relationship is best and most easily appreciated on either plain film radiographs or tomograms. The reconstruction of images in the sagittal and coronal plane is available (see Fig. 10-6G,H,I) and improves the information obtainable by CT scans by allowing visualization of adjacent segments. The anatomic detail, however, is

much less than that demonstrated by standard tomography. Although CT has essentially the same information content and is usually sufficient for establishing the diagnosis and making therapeutic decisions, it is esthetically less pleasing.

The principal indications for CT should be to establish the presence and relationship of fracture fragments to the spinal canal and to evaluate the degree of compromise of the canal. Some authorities now would prefer to perform CT instead of standard tomography in the initial evaluation of spinal injuries. This is particularly true in centers in which reconstruction of CT images is possible.

INCIDENCE AND DISTRIBUTION OF INJURIES

Jefferson[12] found that the incidence of injury peaked for three areas of the spinal cord: C1 to C2, C5 to C7, and T12 to L2 (Fig. 10-7). Meyer (MRSCICS, 1972 to 1986) has identified in 2,710 patients the following areas of peak incidence (trimodal distribution): C2 (9.7 percent), C5 (19.1 percent), and T12 and L1 (6.3 percent and 7.6 percent, respectively). In children, fractures of the cervical spine are less frequent, but an increased incidence is found between the midthoracic and upper lumbar spine.[13,14] In the Northwestern University series, 55.8 percent of pediatric injuries are cervical (121 of 217 patients). The distribution of fractures in patients with spinal cord injuries differs to some extent from the general distribution of spinal fractures (Fig. 10-7). There are three areas of peak incidence: the lower cervical spine, the thoracolumbar junction, and the midthoracic spine.[3]

Fractures involving adjacent vertebrae are relatively common, particularly in children.[13,15,16] Fractures of widely dispersed segments are uncommon, and when encountered, are a manifestation of severe trauma and often are accompanied by spinal cord injury.[3,17,18]

Spinal cord injuries occur in 10 percent to 14 percent of spinal fractures and fracture-dislocations.[19] The incidence of spinal cord injury is increasing.[20] Injuries of the cervical spine produce neurologic damage in approximately 40 percent of

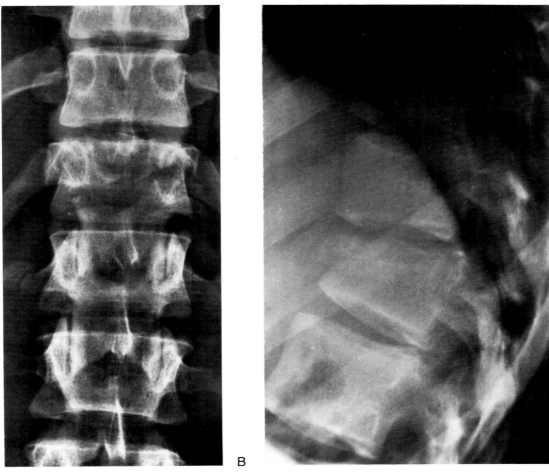

A   B

Fig. 10-6. (A) AP view demonstrates compression fracture of T12 with fractures of the left pedicle and lamina. (B) Lateral view demonstrates anterior dislocation of T11 on T12 with anterior wedging of T12 vertebral body. The posterior elements are not visualized. *(Figure continues.)*

cases[21] (at Northwestern University from 1972 to 1986, the incidence was 86 percent), whereas injuries to the thoracolumbar junction involve the spinal cord at an incidence of 4 percent (Northwestern 1972 to 1986, 70.4 percent), and those of the thoracic spine, at an incidence of approximately 10 percent (Northwestern 1972 to 1986, 88 percent). However, in patients sustaining fractures of the vertebral bodies and posterior elements with some degree of malalignment of the spine, the incidence of neurologic deficit is approximately 60 percent.[22]

Approximately 10 percent of traumatic cord injuries have no overt radiographic evidence of ver-

tebral injury[19,23,24] (Northwestern 1972 to 1986, 12.8 percent). These cases are generally the result of hyperextension injuries in either older patients with degenerative arthritis of the spine or younger patients with narrow spinal canals.[25] The injuries occur in the cervical or upper dorsal spine. As the spine is hyperextended, the cord becomes compressed in older individuals between the osteophytic spurs on the posterior margin of the vertebral bodies and the hypertrophied ligamentum flavum posteriorly, resulting in hematomyelia and associated neurologic deficits.[26] In the younger individual, the cord is similarly compressed between

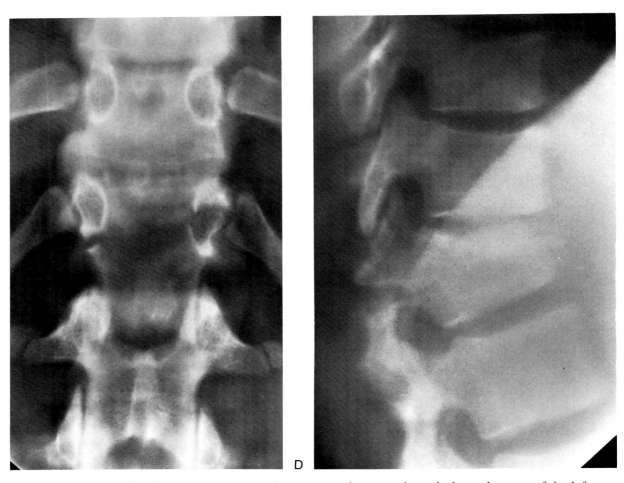

C   D

Fig. 10-6 *(Continued).* **(C)** AP polytomogram demonstrates fractures through the midportion of the left pedicle and at the base of the right pedicle of T12. **(D)** Lateral tomogram demonstrates the fracture through the base of right pedicle and the anterior wedge compression of the vertebral body. *(Figure continues.)*

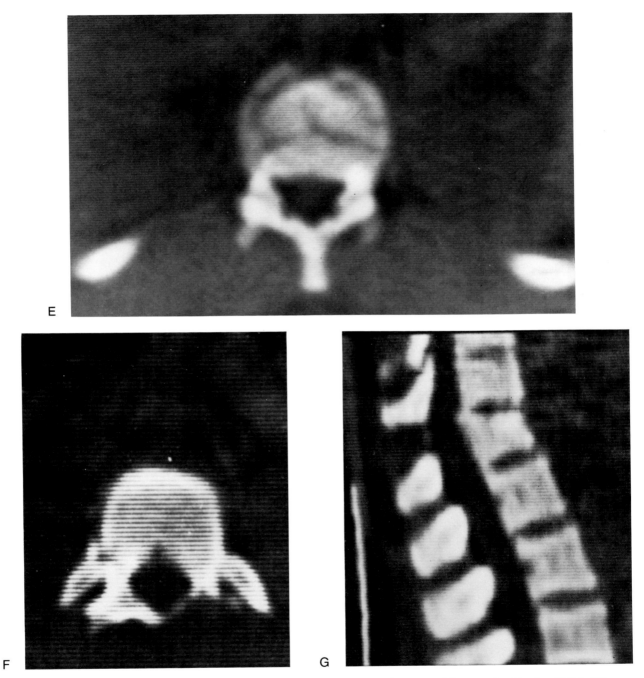

E

F

G

Fig. 10-6 *(Continued).* **(E)** CT scan demonstrates the comminuted fracture of the vertebral body of T12. **(F)** CT scan at slightly lower level demonstrates a fracture through the left pedicle. **(G)** The lateral reconstruction of the CT scan demonstrates the separation of the spinous processes of T11 and T12 with an anterior wedge compression of T12. *(Figure continues.)*

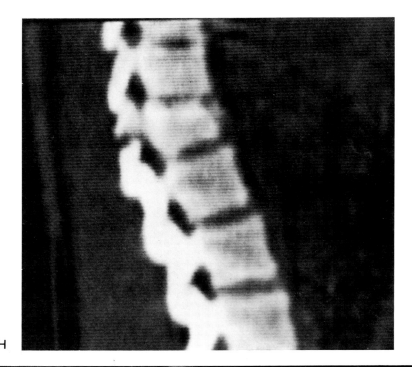

H

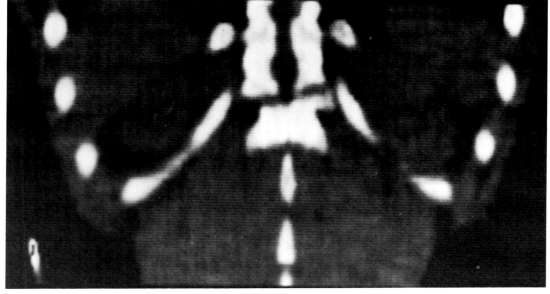

I

Fig. 10-6 *(Continued).* **(H)** A lateral reconstruction through the right pedicles demonstrates the fracture at the base of the right pedicle at T12 and the anterior wedge compression of the 12th vertebral body. Note the slight posterior displacement of the superior posterior portion of the T12 vertebral body. **(I)** Coronal reconstruction through the level of the pedicles and lamina demonstrates the fracture involving the pedicles and lamina of T12. (From O'Callaghan JP, Ullrich CG, Yuan HA, Kieffer SA: CT of facet distraction in flexion injuries of the thoracolumbar spine: The "naked facet." AJNR 1:97, 1980, with permission.)

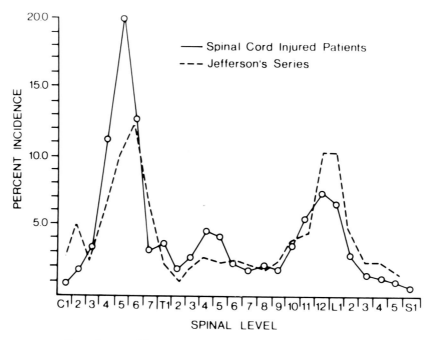

Fig. 10-7. Comparison of incidence of fractures of the spine in 2,006 cases of Jefferson's series with 710 spinal cord-injured patients at the MRSCIS as reported by Calenoff et al.[3] (From Rogers LF: Radiology of Skeletal Trauma. Churchill Livingstone, New York, 1982, p. 273.)

normal structures of the spine owing to the narrowness of the spinal canal.[27]

MULTIPLE-LEVEL SPINAL INJURIES

Injuries to the vertebral column occasionally occur at more than one site, with each site being separated by an area of normal spine.[3,17,18] These have been defined as multiple noncontiguous vertebral injuries. Although uncommon, they are clinically important in those patients with spinal injury. An unrecognized second level of injury may lead to extension of neurologic deficit or subsequently cause pain, instability, or deformity.[3] The largest series of such injuries was reported by Calenoff et al. based on 710 patients admitted to the Midwest Regional Spinal Cord Injury Care System Northwestern University, Chicago, IL.[3] An incidence of 4.5 percent of multiple-level spinal injuries was found. This is in agreement with the few other investigations and reports of this problem

published in the literature.[28-32] Generally, the incidence reported is between 3 percent and 5 percent. The presence of such injuries is a manifestation of severe trauma, thus the association with spinal cord injury. It is quite rare for multiple noncontiguous injury to occur in the absence of spinal cord injury in our experience.

In our series of 710 patients,[3] 4.5 percent had multiple-level spinal injuries. Of these patients, 80 percent had sustained a fracture at two levels and 20 percent had three or more levels of injury. The injury thought to account for the spinal cord deficit was called the primary injury, and additional fractures or dislocations were called secondary or tertiary. Of the primary injuries, 83 percent were fracture-dislocations and 5 percent were compression fractures. Of the nonprimary lesions, 64 percent were compression fractures and 17 percent were fracture-dislocations. Thirteen percent were isolated neural arch fractures, and 4 percent were isolated vertebral body avulsions. Forty percent of the secondary lesions occurred above and 60 percent below the primary lesion. The majority, 77 percent, occurred in three major patterns and one minor subpattern (Fig. 10-8). In pattern A, six of seven primary lesions occurred at C5 to C7 and were associated with secondary injuries at T12 or in the lumbar spine; in pattern B, six of eight primary injuries at T2 to T4 were associated with secondary injuries of the cervical spine; and in pattern C, five of seven primary injuries at C12 to L2 were associated with secondary injuries at L4 to L5. There was a cluster of six primary injuries at T5 to T7 in which the pattern of secondary involvement was not clearly defined; three secondary lesions were proximal within the cervical spine and three were distal at the thorocolumbar junction.

There was significant peak of incidence of primary fractures at T2 to T7 in patients with multiple-level injuries (Figs. 10-9 and 10-10). Although these levels account for 46.7 percent of all primary fractures in the multiple-injured group, they ac-

count for only 9.1 percent of vertebral injuries in the patient population at the Midwest Regional Spinal Cord Injury Care System consisting of patients with spinal cord injuries.[3] Thus, in patients with multiple-level, noncontiguous fractures, there are a disproportionate number of primary vertebral injuries in the mid- and upper dorsal spine.[18,33,34] A primary injury at this level should alert the physician to the possibility of a second vertebral injury elsewhere.

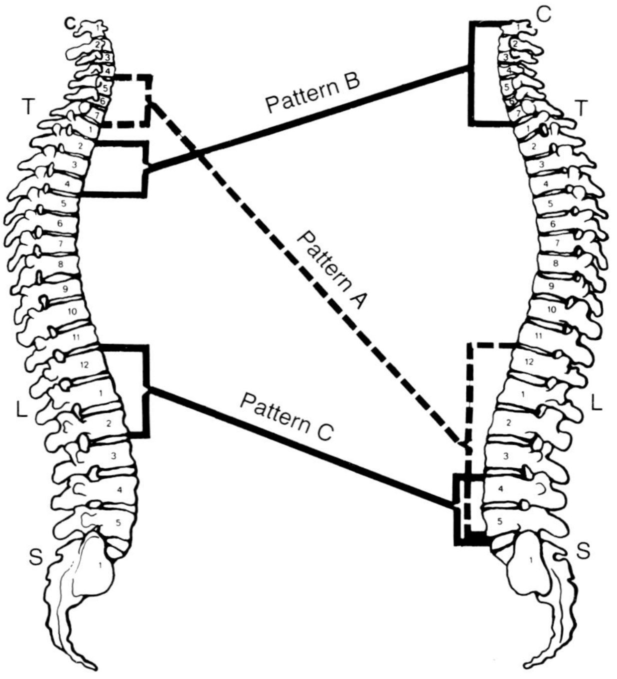

In multiple-level noncontiguous fractures, the secondary lesions are disproportionally numerous at L4-L5, accounting for 28.6 percent (Fig. 10-11). There is also a peak of secondary injuries at C1-C2 (14.2 percent) (see Fig. 10-10). Thus, 42.9 percent of secondary injuries in multiple-level spinal fractures occur at the extremes of the spine.[3] These areas might easily escape radiographic evaluation because of the lack of neurologic findings and the fact that these areas are somewhat remote from the primary injury.

These identifiable patterns of noncontiguous fractures should serve as an aid in directing attention to the probable area of secondary fracture and give reason to insist that radiographs be obtained of these areas as soon as possible.[3,18] The early recognition of second and third levels of fractures is important because of their clinical significance. An unrecognized secondary lesion proximal to a primary lesion may result in pain or extension of the neurologic deficit proximally. Distal secondary lesions can result in instability, progressive scoliosis, and problems with skin maintenance caused by abnormal stress from altered body mechanics. In an apparent upper motor neuron paraplegic or quadriplegic patient, conversion of bladder, bowel, and sexual functions to those associated with a lower motor neuron lesion may result from a distal secondary fracture. Decisions regarding bowel and bladder care, sexual counseling, and possible surgical intervention may be influenced.

PRIMARY LESION   SECONDARY LESION

Fig. 10-8. Three patterns of multiple-level injury. There is also a significant subpattern not illustrated that consists of primary injuries in the mid-dorsal spine with the secondary injury in either the cervical spine or thoracolumbar junction. (From Calenoff,[3] with permission.)

MECHANISM OF INJURY

Injuries to the spine are the result of indirect forces generated by movement of the head and trunk. They are rarely the result of direct blows to

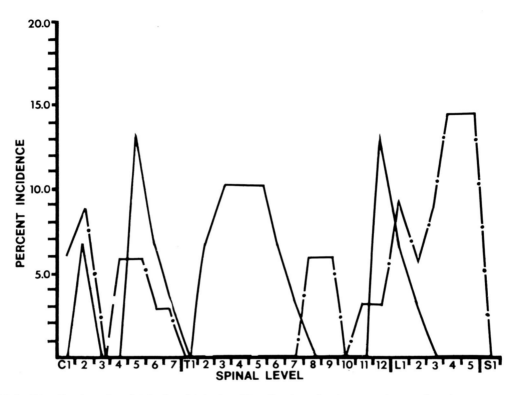

Fig. 10-9. Distribution of multiple-level injuries. Distribution of primary and secondary lesions in patients with multiple noncontiguous fractures. Note the high incidence of secondary lesions at the ends of the spinal column and the high incidence of primary lesions within the dorsal spine. (From Calenoff,[3] with permission.)

the vertebrae. An appreciation of the forces involved in the creation of spinal fractures is a great aid in the assessment of patients who had sustained an injury of the spine.[35,36] Admittedly, this is an abstraction. The forces that created the injury are never observed and are rarely recalled by the individual who sustained the injury. If these are only theoretical, it is reasonable to ask "Why bother?" Each force appears to be associated with a relatively specific pattern of injury of some vertebral element. The identification of this characteristic fracture allows the prediction and guides the search for associated injuries of the vertebrae and elsewhere. Almost everyone who acquires an understanding of spinal fractures and fracture-dislocations has first studied and learned to appreciate

the mechanisms of injury. These forces are thoroughly discussed elsewhere in the text.

The forces involved in any injury are probably multiple and complex. The combination of flexion, compression, rotation, and shearing is particularly common.[31,37-39] It is of value, however, to consider the potential forces separately since each is associated with a relatively specific pattern of injury. In general, it is difficult to state categorically that compression, flexion, and extension forces create one kind of injury and that rotational and shearing forces create another. Possibly there is a preponderance of fractures with the former, and of ligamentous injuries with the latter.

Fractures of the spine occur in repetitive patterns like fractures of the extremities. Each pattern

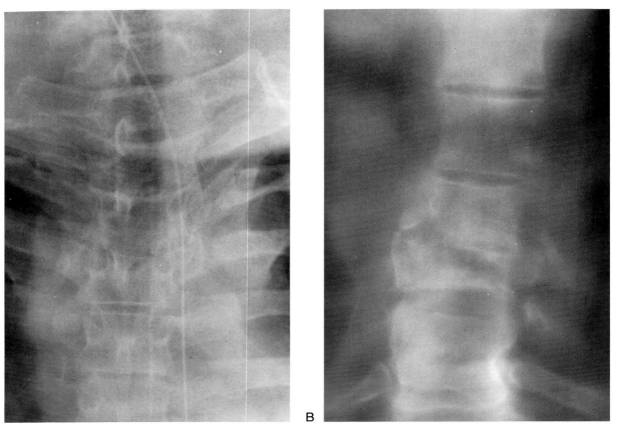

A   B

Fig. 10-10. Fracture dislocation at T3–T4 associated with fracture of neural arch of C1. This 34-year-old man was involved in an automobile accident. **(A)** The fracture-dislocation is difficult to visualize. Note the lateral offset of T3 on T4 and the associated mediastinal hematoma that extends over the apex of both lungs. **(B)** Frontal tomogram clearly demonstrating the fracture of T3 with lateral offset of T3 on T4. *(Figure continues.)*

is based on a characteristic fracture of the vertebral body or posterior elements. The fracture of the vertebral body is usually the most obvious and serves as a key to recognize the type of injury the patient has incurred. The recognition of the pattern is important since it reveals the mechanism of injury and allows the prediction of commonly associated injuries that should be searched for, identified, or excluded. Furthermore, each pattern or type of injury is frequently associated with a rather specific neurologic deficit in a certain percentage of patients. For example, a tear-drop fracture of the cervical spine is associated with complete quadriplegia in 75 percent of cases. A hangman's fracture of the second cervical vertebra is rarely associated

with a permanent neurologic deficit but often presents with a transient quadriparesis.[40] Total motor and sensory loss below the level of injury are usually associated with a bilateral facet lock or severe bursting fractures of the vertebral bodies such as the teardrop fracture or a fracture with vertebral displacement in the thoracic spine. The central spinal cord injury syndrome[23] consists of disproportionally more motor impairment of the upper than of the lower extremity, bladder dysfunction and usually urinary retention, and varying degrees of sensory loss below the level of the lesion. This syndrome is associated with hyperextension injuries, including those without obvious fractures. The anterior spinal cord injury syndrome[41] is character-

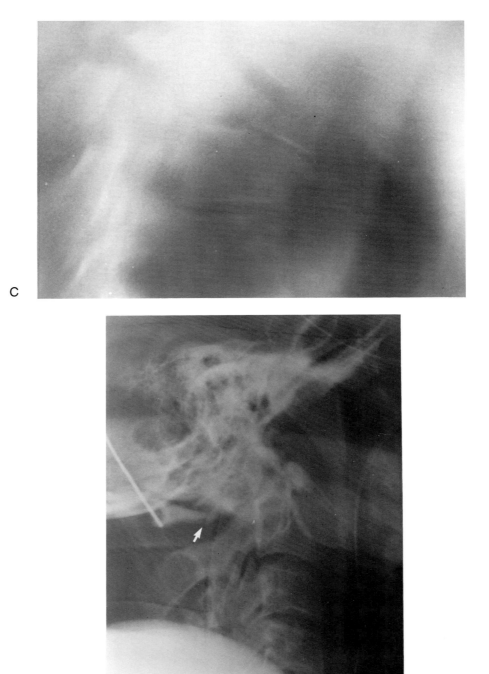

Fig. 10-10 *(Continued).* (**C**) Lateral tomogram. The fracture-dislocation of T3 on T4 is demonstrated, as well as the associated fracture through the lamina of T3. (**D**) Lateral view of the cervical spine reveals fracture of the neural arch at C1 (arrow). Note also the soft tissue swelling within the nasopharynx.

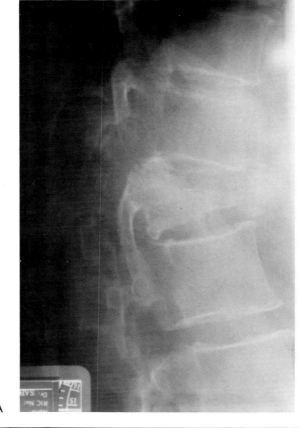

A

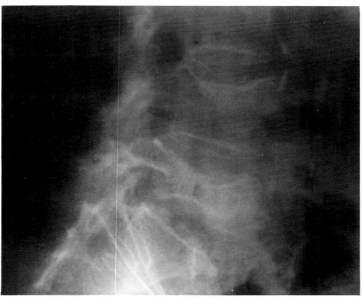

B

Fig. 10-11. Double level of fracture in a 59-year-old woman who fell from a third-floor window. (A) Comminuted fracture of T12. (B) Compression fracture of the vertebral body of L5 and of the superior end plate of L4.

ized by immediate complete motor paralysis with hypesthesia and hypalgesia to the level of the lesion with the preservation of motion, position, and vibratory senses. This syndrome is usually associated with bursting and tear-drop fractures of the vertebral body. Motor weakness or paresis either in all four limbs or confined to the upper extremity without sensory loss is often associated with fractures of the axis (C2) — a hangman's fracture or a fracture of the dens or unilateral facet lock of the lower cervical spine. The deficit is usually transient. The Brown-Séquard syndrome consists of unilateral motor paralysis and contralateral loss of pain and temperature sense. It is commonly associated with unilateral facet locks or bursting fractures and may occasionally be seen as a result of hyperextension injury. It is also seen in lesions resulting from gunshot or stab wounds.

Spinal cord injuries are usually associated with fracture-dislocations of the spine.[2,19,42-44] Spinal cord injury accompanies 85 percent of bilateral facet locks, 75 percent of teardrop and severe crush fractures, and 30 percent of unilateral facet locks. Ten percent of spinal cord injuries have no evidence of fracture or dislocation.[19,23,45] The MRSCICS experience reveals that in the cervical spine, spinal cord injury accompanies 85 percent of vertebral body fractures, 84.7 percent of axial compression fractures, 77.6 percent of facet dislocations and fractures, and 96.1 percent of gunshot wounds. The recognition and use of the neurologic and radiographic patterns of injury is a great aid in the assessment of the spinal cord-injured patient. The diagnostic evaluations made on the basis of knowledge of these patterns can proceed with confidence and result in an accurate and thorough description of the injuries encountered. The therapeutic decisions can then be made on a sound basis, and the prognosis can be predicted with reasonable certitude.

PRINCIPLES OF RADIOGRAPHIC INTERPRETATION

When presented with a potential injury of the spine, there are two principal considerations: Is there a fracture or fracture-dislocation? Is the in-

jury stable or unstable? When the lesion is obvious, these questions are easily answered, but in the absence of displacement and gross fracture, the injury may not be immediately apparent. To observe the more subtle injuries, one must be aware of the normal radiographic appearance of the spine, the statistical frequency of injury at various sites, the radiographic appearance of specific injuries, and signs within the soft tissue indicating a hematoma pointing to the presence of an underlying fracture.

It goes without saying that to recognize the abnormal, one must be familiar with the normal appearance of structures. This is certainly true of the spine. The better acquainted one is with normal radiographic anatomy, the easier it is to identify abnormalities.

Knowledge of the statistical frequency of injury aids in the search by directing attention to common sites of injury. It is more productive to look at these sites to exclude an injury than simply to look at the radiograph expecting to identify the abnormality without specific questions in mind. By knowing the sites and appearance of common injuries, the search can be directed specifically to exclude those injuries. The interpretation is then performed with confidence.

Soft tissue signs indicating a hematoma and pointing to an underlying fracture are readily visualized in the cervical spine[46] and to a lesser extent the dorsal spine[34] (see Fig. 10-10). Hemorrhage associated with injuries of the vertebral bodies of the first two lumbar segments may extend proximally into the lower dorsal spine, but this is neither as common nor as reliable as demonstrating the presence or absence of hematomas in the cervical and dorsal area. Demonstration of hematomas associated with fractures of the lower lumbar spine requires sufficient hemorrhage to obliterate or displace the fascial planes of the psoas muscle. This is uncommon and cannot be relied on to point to underlying fracture. Certainly when these signs are present an injury to the retroperioneal structures must be considered, but a fracture can exist without these signs.

By using a disciplined approach to the interpretation of radiographs, the diagnosis of an injury is facilitated and the confidence of the interpretation, either in the identification or exclusion of injuries, is greatly enhanced.

The stability of the spinal column is maintained by the combination of bony elements, the vertebra and their associated soft tissue structures, the ligaments, the apophyseal joint capsules, and the intervertebral discs.[47] The degree of stability or instability is dependent on the extent of the disruption of these structures and the relative strengths of the structures remaining intact.[37,38,48] The spine is often described as consisting of two columns, an anterior column and a posterior column. If an injury involves both components, the injury is by definition unstable. However, if one of the two columns remains intact, it is likely that the injury is stable. The anterior column is composed of the vertebral bodies, the intervertebral disc, and the anterior and posterior longitudinal ligaments. The anterior longitudinal ligament is a tough structure closely applied to the anterior vertebral body and the anulus of the intervertebral disc. The posterior longitudinal ligament is considerably weaker and less important. It is applied to the posterior surface of the vertebral bodies and the anulus of the intervertebral disc lining the ventral surface of the spinal canal. The posterior column is formed by the facets, apophyseal joints, pedicles, laminae, spinous process, and all intervening ligaments.[37]

Disruption through bone or soft tissue is equally important in the determination of stability. Since there is no direct radiographic evidence of soft tissue injury the presence of such injuries must be implied by variations in the alignment of or distance between the bony elements joined by the soft tissue structure in question.[45,49-52] Therefore, an important clue to the presence of a significant injury is a variation in the distance, either an increase or decrease, between the apposing surfaces of adjacent vertebrae, particularly the intervertebral discs, the apophyseal joints, and the spinous processes (see Fig. 10-30). Offsetting of parallel apposing adjacent vertebral surfaces is equally important. Such offsetting, narrowing, or widening of the distance between parallel apposing vertebral elements indicates disruption of the intervening soft tissue structures, the intervertebral disc, the apophyseal joints, and/or the interspinous ligaments. It is as important to determine the presence or absence of alignment and the distances between various portions of the vertebral bodies as it is to identify fractures of the vertebrae themselves. It

should be realized at the time of the radiographic examination that only residual displacement between vertebral elements is visualized. At the time of injury there may have been gross displacements that have spontaneously reduced, partially or completely, leaving minimal deformities. Certainly, the displacement encountered at the time of the radiographic evaluation is, in most cases, much less than that which occurred during the creation of the injury.

The standard radiographic examination of the cervical spine (Fig. 10-12) consists of five projections: an AP, an AP open mouth view of the upper cervical spine, lateral, and right and left oblique.

The initial lateral spine radiograph should be obtained with the patient in supine position with a horizontally directed beam. The patient should not be manipulated or turned from this position until it has been established that the spine is intact. It is mandatory that this view include all seven cervical vertebra.[53-56] Injuries of C6 and C7 are common but may be easily overlooked when these vertebrae are not included on the lateral radiograph. The appearance of the lateral radiograph can be very deceiving when it includes only the first five or six cervical vertebra. It is surprising how easy it is to be mislead and assume that the entire cervical spine is included on the radiograph. To be safe, it is necessary to count the vertebral bodies to make sure that all seven cervical vertebra are visualized.

The lower vertebrae are frequently obscured by the overlying shoulders. By pulling down on the patient's arms while holding the wrists, the visualization may be improved. If this should fail, a "swimmer's" projection should be obtained. This may be accomplished by extending one arm of the patient over the head while the other arm remains by the side (Fig. 10-13). This places the upper torso in a slightly oblique projection and allows visualization of the cervicothoracic junction. At times, it is necessary to resort to tomography to demonstrate the lower cervical vertebral bodies.

An AP view of the entire spine and an open mouth view of the atlas and axis (C1–C2) should also be performed at the time of the initial examination. All three of these radiographs must be reviewed to exclude an obvious injury before the patient is moved to obtain oblique projections or other additional radiographs as required. Serious

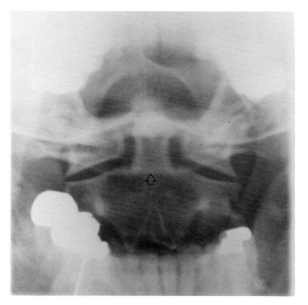

A

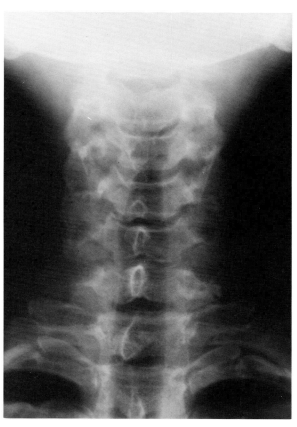

B

Fig. 10-12. Normal cervical spine in a 46-year-old woman. **(A)** Open mouth view of C1 and C2. Note that the lateral margins of C1 are exactly opposite the lateral margin of C2 and that the distance between the medial margin of the vertebral body of C1 and the lateral margins of the dens is equal bilaterally. The notches at the base of the dens are normal. The posterior arch of C1 (arrow) crosses at the base of the dens. This is at times associated with a Mach band which may be mistaken for a fracture. **(B)** AP view of the cervical spine. The vertebral body heights of the midcervical spine can be evaluated because both the superior and inferior end plates are visualized. The undulating smooth margins of the facets are seen, but the apophyseal joints are not visualized since they lie at an angle with the central beam. The spinous processes of the lower cervical spine are nicely visualized by their ovoid cortical margins. The spinous processes of the upper cervical spine are bifid and not seen as clearly. The spinous processes should lie in the midline in the absence of rotation. *(Figure continues.)*

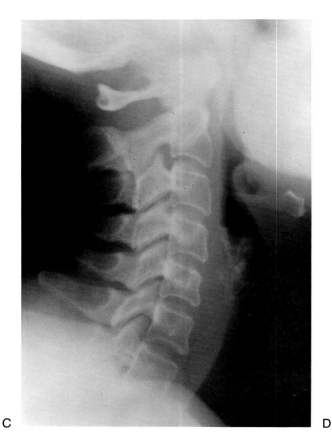

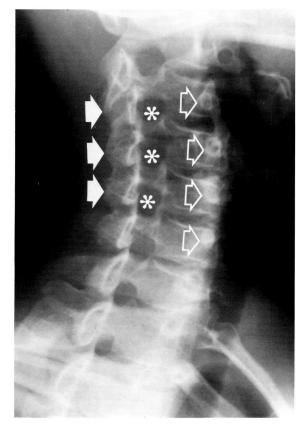

C

D

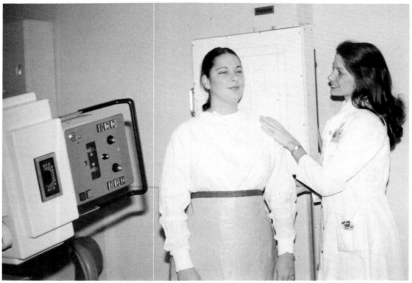

E

Fig. 10-12 *(Continued).* (**C**) Lateral view. It is most important that all seven cervical vertebrae be visualized. The alignment of the vertebral bodies, the heights of the vertebrae, and the intervertebral disc space should be determined, and the soft tissues anterior to the spine should be evaluated. (**D**) Oblique view of the spine. This is a left posterior oblique view which demonstrates the right intervertebral foramina (asterisk). Note the left pedicles (open arrows). The lateral margins of the facets are undulating and smooth as seen in the frontal projection (arrows). (**E**) Patient in position for a left posterior oblique view of the cervical spine. Note that the right side of the neck is brought forward and the right lateral mass and intervertebral foramina are visualized. Compare with Fig. B.

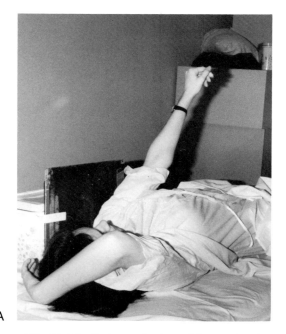

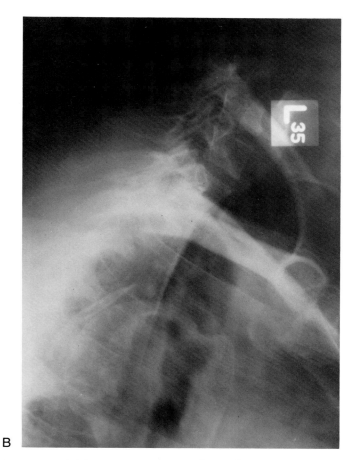

A B

Fig. 10-13. Swimmer's view of the cervicothoracic junction. (**A**) Patient in position to obtain this projection. Note the position of the arm. (**B**) The resulting radiograph allows the visualization of the upper thoracic vertebral bodies and the cervicothoracic junction.

injuries cannot be excluded on the basis of a lateral view alone. At times, significant lateral dislocations are encountered that are not evident on the lateral view.

It is possible to obtain oblique radiographs while the patient is in the supine position[57] by angling the tube 30 degrees from the horizontal plane and placing a nongrid cassette flat on the table adjacent to the patient's neck on the side opposite the tube.

Flexion and extension views are often necessary to confirm instability or subluxation of the cervical spine (Fig. 10-14). The radiographic findings on the standard projections in these injuries may be quite subtle, and these views are necessary to substantiate the injury. Flexion and extension views do not need to be obtained routinely and should never be performed without the immediate assistance of the radiologist or attending physician. The performance of flexion and extension in an unstable spine could potentially lead to a neurologic injury. The physician in attendance should assist the patient with flexion and extension to prevent this from occurring.

Interpretation

The foremost consideration is the identification of fractures and dislocations. After the identification of an obvious fracture, it is necessary to identify all of the associated injuries. This is when knowledge of patterns of injury and of specific fractures is most helpful.

If a fracture is not immediately obvious, look at specific sites of frequent injury to identify specific types of fracture. This is when information regarding the statistical frequency of injury is most useful. There are sites that are more likely to be injured, and time is better spent looking at these areas than in a general survey of the spine. If fractures have been excluded, then attention may be brought to the possibility of subluxation or dislocations. Very serious injuries may be manifested by minor degrees of malalignment. On the lateral view, four separate anteriorly convex lines (Fig. 10-15) may be formed by joining the anterior margins of the vertebral bodies, the posterior margins of the vertebral bodies, and the anterior margin of the spinous processes at their junction with the laminae and finally at the posterior tip of the spinous processes.[53-55] Any abrupt reversal or angulation or disruption of these lines indicates the presence of an underlying dislocation or subluxation. The word *abrupt* must be emphasized. The cervical spine may be straightened or the normal cervical curve reversed by positioning or muscle spasm. In the latter, there is a gradual transition in alignment as apposed to the abrupt angulation or offset encountered as a result of a subluxation or dislocation (see Figs. 10-14 and 10-30).

The width of the intervertebral disc spaces should be evaluated.[52] Trauma to the intervertebral disc is manifested by a change in the height of the disc space, usually a decrease, but rarely an increase. More commonly, the injury is manifested by a lack of parallelism between the apposing end plates of the adjoining vertebral bodies. Normally, the anterior and posterior heights of the intervertebral disc are quite similar. In the presence of a disruption of the disc, this distance may be increased or decreased, resulting in a loss of parallelism of the end plates (Fig. 10-14). The disc space becomes wedge shaped. These changes may be subtle. Recognition depends on observing that the involved disc space is narrower or wider or different in some way than the intervertebral disc space above and below the space in question. Disruption of the disc is often associated with a minimal degree of subluxation, on the order of 1 to 3 mm.

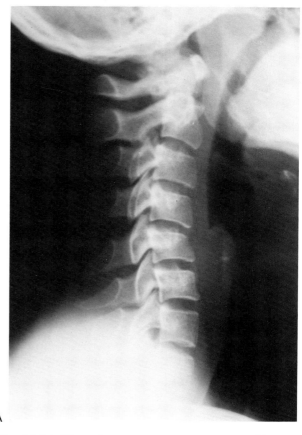

A

Fig. 10-14. Hyperflexion strain in a 26-year-old man. (A) Neutral lateral view of the cervical spine demonstrates a reversal of the normal lordotic angulation of the cervical spine with an abrupt change in the alignment at the C4–C5 interspace. Note that there is slight decrease in the height of the interspace at this level and a distinct offset of the apposing surfaces of the apophyseal joints and a widening of the interspinous distance. Compare with Fig. 10-30. *(Figure continues.)*

Similarly, on the lateral view the facet joints at C2 through C6 should be evaluated. Here again the apposing joint surfaces should be parallel and apposed. Subluxation is manifested by an offset and loss of parallelism of the apposing joint surfaces of the facets.

The distance between the spinous processes, the interspinous distance, should also be evaluated to determine the status of the interspinous ligaments. Widening of an interspinous distance when compared with the adjacent vertebrae above and below

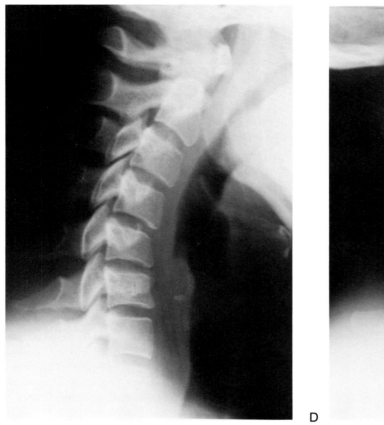
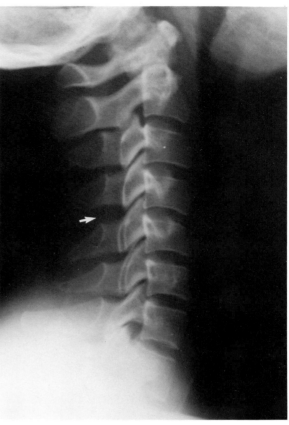

C

D

Fig. 10-14 *(Continued).* **(B)** Flexion accentuates the changes seen in Fig. A. **(C)** Extension view. This view practically eliminates the radiographic findings. However, there is a persistent widening of the interspinous distance at C4–C5 (arrow).

the level in question suggests the presence of a disruption of the interspinous ligaments (Fig. 10-14). Rotational displacement of vertebrae is often best visualized on the AP projection. Normally, the spinous processes should be projected in the midline of the vertebral bodies. With rotational displacement, the spinous processes are displaced toward the side of the rotated or dislocated facet (see Figs. 10-28 and 9-12B).

If neither fracture nor dislocation or subluxation is evident, the retropharyngeal soft tissue should be examined closely since it serves as an important clue to underlying injury of the cervical spine[46,53,58] (Fig. 10-14). The retropharyngeal soft tissues consist of the anterior longitudinal ligament, the posterior wall of the pharynx, and the intervening fascia. When an increase in the retropharyngeal soft tissue is identified following trauma, it indicates the presence of retropharyngeal hemorrhage and undoubtedly indicates that there has been a serious injury of the underlying cervical spine. The fracture or dislocation itself may have been overlooked on the initial viewing, but the identification of the increase in the retropharyngeal soft tissue should heighten suspension and direct the observer to review the examination for more subtle evidence of fractures or dislocation overlooked on the initial viewing. The normal width of the soft tissue between the air column within the pharynx and the anterior margin of the vertebral body measures approximately 4 mm anterior to the third and fourth cervical vertebral

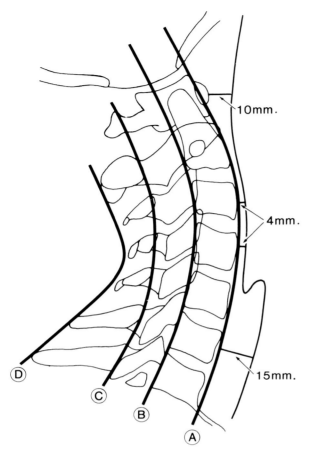

10mm.

4mm.

15mm.

(D)

(C)

(B)

(A)

Fig. 10-15. Lateral view of normal alignment of the cervical spine showing four convex lines: *A*, anterior vertebral bodies; *B*, posterior vertebral bodies; *C*, lamina junctional line; *D*, posterior tip of spinous processes. Normal width of retropharyngeal soft tissue is also shown.

bodies (Fig. 10-15). The width of the soft tissue anterior to C6 (the retrotracheal space) should not exceed approximately 15 mm in children and 20 mm in adults. The changes in the width of the retropharyngeal soft tissue at C3–C4 are a much more sensitive index than at the more inferior level. Swelling of the nasopharyngeal soft tissues is an important clue to underlying injuries at the craniovertebral junction. There is a wide variation in the measurement at this location, but normally the width of the soft tissue anterior to the anterior arch of C1 does not exceed 10 mm. The presence of

adenoidal tissue makes this determination less reliable in the child than in the adult. Furthermore, hemorrhage associated with fractures of the facial skeleton often extends into the nasopharynx.

Fractures involving the posterior elements and those fractures of the vertebral body in which the anterior longitudinal ligament remains intact may be associated with little or no retropharyngeal hemorrhage. Generally, compression fractures of the vertebra are associated with a moderate retropharyngeal hemorrhage. Hyperextension injuries resulting in tears of the anterior longitudinal ligament consistently result in the most extensive retropharyngeal hemorrhage. The radiographic signs of such injuries are otherwise quite subtle, at times even inapparent. Therefore, the presence of retropharyngeal hematoma serves as an important clue to the possibility of an underlying hyperextension injury.

Hemorrhage manifested by an increased width of the retropharyngeal soft tissue may not be demonstrated on the initial radiograph if it is obtained shortly after the injury, but should be readily apparent within three hours.[46] It usually remains obvious for at least 2 to 3 days, but thereafter hemorrhage begins to resorb and the width of the retropharyngeal soft tissues returns to normal within 1 week to 2 weeks.

CRANIOVERTEBRAL JUNCTION

The craniovertebral junction consists of atlas and axis and the adjacent occipital condyles at the margins of the foramen magnum. The atlas and axis differ considerably in structure from the remaining cervical vertebra.[59]

The atlas or C1 is a ringlike structure consisting of two lateral articular masses joined by thin anterior and posterior arches. The lateral articular masses contain the superior and inferior articular facets. The superior facets articulate with the occipital condyles, and the inferior facets articulate with the superior facets of the axis.

The axis or C2 consists of a vertebral body on the superolateral margins of which are broad, sloping surfaces, the superior articular facets (see Fig.

10-12A). A bony protrusion, the dens, extends superiorly in the sagittal plane. The anterior aspects of the dens articulate with the posterior surface of the anterior arch of the axis. The pedicles of the axis are pierced by the foramina transversaria superiorly and posteriorly, which divide the pedicles into two short segments. The pedicles are contiguous with the laminae that complete the neural canal. The laminae are broadened on their inferior margins to form the inferior articular facets. The superior and inferior articular facets of C2 are not superimposed but are separated by the pedicles. A prominent spinous process extends posteriorly from the junction of the laminae.

Broad, tough ligaments extend from the margin of the spinal canal formed by the ring of C1 and C2 to the margins of the foramen magnum. The dens is attached to the anterior margin of the foramen magnum by three distinct ligaments, the apical and paired alar ligaments, each extending from the right and left lateral surfaces of the dens. A very substantial ligament, the ligamentum transversarium, extends between the lateral articular masses of C1. The dens lies between this ligament and the anterior arch of the atlas.

The fulcrum of flexion and extension of the cranium on the neck lies at the second cervical vertebra. The weight of the cranium is transmitted through the occipital condyles and atlas to the superior articular facets of the axis. The weight is then divided into three portions and transmitted inferiorly: anteriorly through the vertebral bodies and intervertebral discs and posteriorly through the pedicles onto the inferior articular facet and from there to the apophyseal joints and facets of the remainder of the cervical spine.

In a properly positioned radiograph in the neutral position, C1 sits squarely on C2 without offset, that is, the lateral margin of the lateral articular mass of C1 lies exactly opposite of the apposing largeral margin of C2[53,60-62] (Fig. 10-12A). The distance between the medial margin of the lateral articular masses of C1 and the dens is symmetric. With rotation or abduction of the head, C1 moves the unit toward the side to which the head is rotated or abducted. The lateral articular mass of C1 is then offset laterally toward the side of this motion, and the distance between the medial margin of the lateral mass and the dens increases on this side. On the opposite side, there is a corresponding medial offset of the lateral articular mass of C1 and a decrease in the distance between the medial borders of the lateral mass and the dens. Thus, rotation or abduction of the head produces a unilateral offset of C1 on C2. Usually, this is of a magnitude of 1 to 2 mm and rarely as much as 4 mm.

The important radiographs in the evaluation of craniovertebral injuries are the AP open mouth projection and the lateral view of the cervical spine. Tomography is frequently required for full clarification of abnormalities. Before all injuries can be safely excluded, it may be necessary to obtain tomograms in both the AP and lateral projections. Many injuries of the craniovertebral junction are only minimally displaced and therefore may be overlooked if the examination is not done in both projections. The injuries are frequently associated with soft tissue swelling of the nasopharynx. The identification of soft tissue swelling in this area should increase suspicion of an underlying injury at the craniovertebral junction. Computed tomography is an excellent means of identifying vertical fractures in the ring of either the atlas or axis or fractures involving the occipital condyle. Because of volume averaging, transverse or horizontal fractures are not demonstrated unless they are significantly displaced. Thus, fractures of the dens, which are almost invariably transverse, and horizontal fractures of the anterior arch of C1 are likely to be overlooked by computed tomography.

Fractures of the craniovertebral junction occur as a result of forces transmitted through the cranium and its contents, that is, movements of the head relative to the neck. The nature of the resultant injury depends on the amount and direction of the force and the relative position of the head and neck at the time of injury.

From the clinical standpoint, fractures and dislocations of the craniovertebral junction are rarely associated with permanent neurologic deficits, although transient paresis may occur. However, postmortem examination of individuals who die in automobile and other accidents have demonstrated an appreciable incidence of such injuries.[63] There is no discrepancy between these two statements, since a severe injury to the cord at this level leads to immediate death and the victim is taken directly to the morgue. With immediate resucitation, it is possible that an occasional patient with a high spinal cord transection may survive the initial injury and be brought to the emergency room.

Fractures and dislocations of the craniovertebral junction may occur without the patient sustaining a neurologic injury since the spinal cord occupies only 50 percent of the spinal canal at this level. This affords an appreciable margin for safety. It is possible to reduce the dimensions of the spinal canal by 50 percent without necessarily injuring the spinal cord. At C1, approximately one-third of the spinal canal is occupied by the dens and its associated ligaments, one-third by the spinal cord, and the remaining one-third by the subarachnoid space, meninges, and epidural fat. Despite the presence of the dens, there is still a 50 percent margin of safety at C1. Therefore, when a dislocation occurs, provided there is no more than a 50 percent reduction in the dimension of the spinal canal, no neurologic injury need occur. Fractures of the ring of the atlas practically always increase the width of the spinal canal by centripetal displacement of the fragments. This, in effect, decompresses the canal by increasing its dimensions. Thus, neurologic injury is avoided.

THE ATLAS

Fractures of the Neural Arch

The most common fracture of C1 is a bilateral vertical fracture through the neural arch.[64,65] This is caused by hyperextension of the head on the neck, which compresses the neural arch at C1 between the occiput and the neural arch of C2. This is best demonstrated on the lateral view (Fig. 10-10D). Characteristically, there is minimal displacement and angulation because of the ligamentous attachments. There is no risk of neurologic injury. This fracture should be differentiated from a Jefferson fracture, a comminuted fracture of the atlas described below that involves the anterior arch and lateral masses in addition to the neural arch. It is often difficult to visualize the fracture component in the neural arch of a Jefferson fracture. The distinction is best made on the AP open mouth view. In a Jefferson fracture, the normal

relationship between the atlas and axis is disrupted by lateral displacement of one or both lateral masses of the atlas relative to the superior facets of the axis. With an isolated fracture of the neural arch of the atlas, the normal relationship is maintained. If there is any serious question, a tomogram or computed tomogram should be obtained. The fracture must also be distinguished from developmental defects that vary from a complete absence of the posterior neural arch to short segmental defects, which might be mistaken for fractures. The margins of these defects are characteristically rounded or pointed and covered completely by cortical bone. There is often a separation or gap in the arch in association with these congenital defects.

Horizontal Fractures of the Anterior Arch

The anterior longitudinal ligament and the longus colli muscle are attached to the anterior tubercle of the anterior arch of C1. With hyperextension of the head on the neck, there may be sufficient tension within the muscle and ligament to result in an avulsion at the site of attachment, creating a horizontal fracture of the anterior arch (Fig. 10-16). Horizontal fractures of the anterior arch are characteristically minimally displaced and best visualized on the lateral view. They may be associated with fractures of the dens.

Jefferson Fracture

A Jefferson fracture is a comminuted fracture of the ring, involving both the anterior and posterior arches.[64,66,67] This allows centripetal displacement of the fragments. Sir Geoffrey Jefferson, a British neurosurgeon, described the mechanism of injury in 1919.[12] The fracture is created by blows on the vertex, the force being transmitted from the cranium to the cervical spine through the occipital condyles. The lateral articular masses of the atlas become compressed between the condyles and the superior articular facets of the axis. Since the lateral articular masses of C1 are wedged shaped, as the occipital condyles are driven towards the axis, the lateral articular masses are displaced laterally.

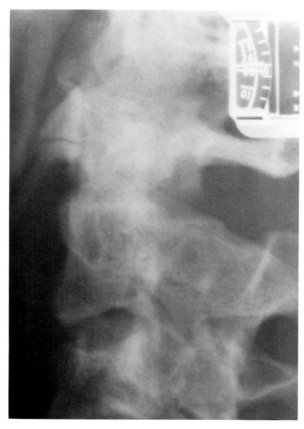

Fig. 10-16. Fifty-six-year-old man who sustained a hyperextension injury that resulted in a quadriplegia at C5–C6 and an associated transverse fracture of the anterior arch at C1. This type of injury is caused by hyperextension of the cervical spine with the avulsion occurring at the site of the attachment of the longus colli muscle.

The weaker segments of the atlas, the anterior and posterior arches, are stressed and finally broken, which disrupts the ring and spreads the articular masses apart. The most significant radiographic findings are on the frontal projections of the atlas and axis (Fig. 10-17). The crucial observation is the offset or spreading of the lateral articular masses of C1 in relation to the apposing articular surfaces of C2. This is usually bilateral. Frontal tomograms or CT scans may confirm this diagnosis. It is often difficult to visualize the lines of fracture on plain films, but their presence can be inferred from the lateral displacement of the lateral masses relative to the peripheral margins of the superior facet of

C2 as seen on the frontal projection. The demonstration of the fractures themselves is not an absolute necessity; the displacements suffice to make the diagnosis. The displacement of the fractures is then very well demonstrated by computed tomography.[11]

THE AXIS

Fractures of the axis are frequently undisplaced and may be difficult to visualize on the standard radiographic examinations. Tomography is often necessary.

Hangman's Fracture

The hangman's fracture is a fracture of the neural arch of the axis and is one of the most common injuries of the cervical spine.[40,68–70] It is the result of an acute hyperextension of the head and neck and is commonly sustained in an automobile accident as the chin or forehead encounters the steering wheel or dashboard, forcing the head into hyperextension. The injury is identical to that created by judicial hanging, thus the designation the hangman's fracture. As the head is hyperextended on the neck, the stress is focused within the pedicles of the neural arch of C2 between the superior and inferior articular facet (Fig. 10-18). The fracture is usually an oblique fracture from superior and posterior to anterior and inferior. When the fracture involves both sides in a symmetric fashion, there is a slight distraction of the fracture and is readily identified on the lateral radiograph. However, the fracture may occur in different locations within the neural arch on each side, and in the absence of distraction it may be obscure. The fracture is usually associated with an anterior subluxation of C2 on C3. This may be difficult to identify on the radiograph. Normally, the superior portion of the cervical curve points slightly posteriorly. Often, the subluxation of C2 is such that it simply straightens the curve or slightly reverses it at the C2–C3 interspace. When the head is placed in hyperextension, the anterior longitudinal ligament is placed under tension and disrupted. This may be

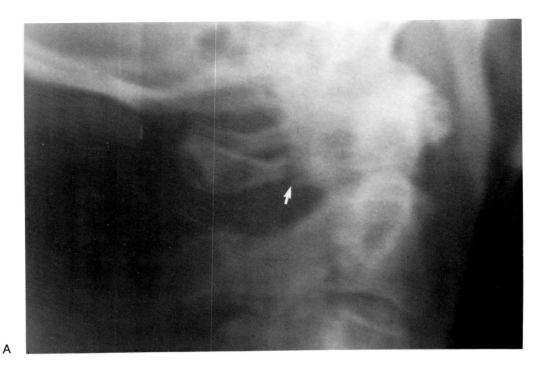

A

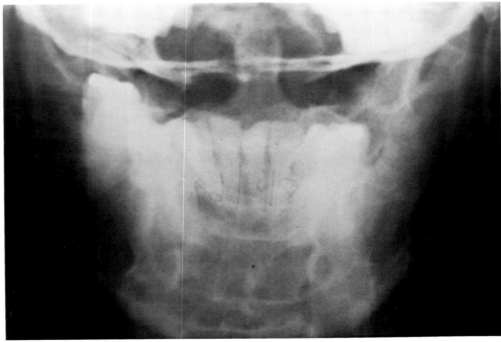

B

Fig. 10-17. Jefferson fracture in a 42-year-old man. (A) Lateral view of the cervical spine shows a fracture through the neural arch at C1 (arrow) and an increase in the width of the soft tissue anterior to the craniovertebral junction. (B) Open mouth view. The lateral masses at C1 are widely separated from the dens. *(Figure continues.)*

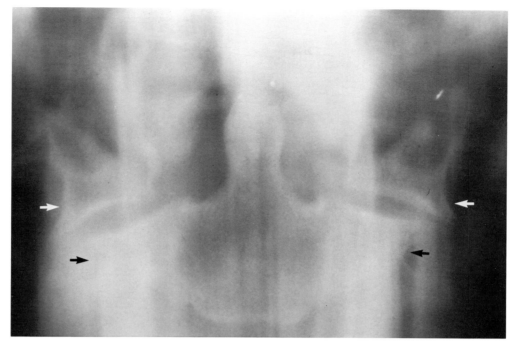

C

Fig. 10-17 *(Continued).* (**C**) Linear tomogram demonstrates the bilateral offset of the lateral masses at C1 relative to C2 (arrows). This injury requires that there be at least two fractures, one in the anterior arch and the other in the posterior arch. They are frequently difficult to visualize.

associated with an avulsion fracture of the anterior inferior margin of C2 or anterior superior margin of C3. The intervertebral disc is disrupted. Occasionally, there is an accompanying fracture of the neural arch at C1. Normally, the frontal projections reveal no evidence of the fracture. Oblique views may demonstrate the fracture of the neural arch. Tomograms may be necessary to confirm the injury in questionable cases. In postmortem studies of head and neck injuries of fatal traffic accident victims, Alker and co-workers found that this was the most frequent fracture of the cervical spine.[63] However, in clinical situations there is often no neurologic finding in association with this fracture. When present, the findings are usually that of a quadriparesis that proves to be transient. This paradox is explained by the duration of the hyperextending force.[40] If the hyperextension is transient, fracture may occur without neurologic injury. However, when the force is sustained as in a judicial hanging, the spinal cord is transsected, resulting in death.

Fractures of the Dens

Fracture of the dens or odontoid process is most frequently transverse and located at its junction with the body[32,71-73] (Fig. 10-19). On occasion, fractures of the tip of the odontoid process occur. The latter are avulsion fractures mediated through the attached apical or alar ligaments. Oblique fractures may occur that extend into the body of the axis, either anteriorly or posteriorly. The dens is most frequently displaced anteriorly, less commonly posteriorly, but may be displaced in any direction. The fracture fragments are rarely separated by more than 2 to 3 mm. Fractures of the dens are often difficult to visualize because of this minimal displacement. The diagnosis depends primarily on the radiographic findings in the AP projection. On the lateral projection, the minimal displacement usually precludes identification of the fracture with certainty. Tomography is usually required and should be performed in both the AP and lateral projections.

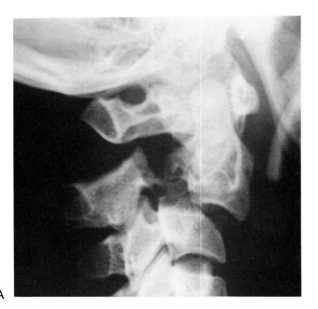

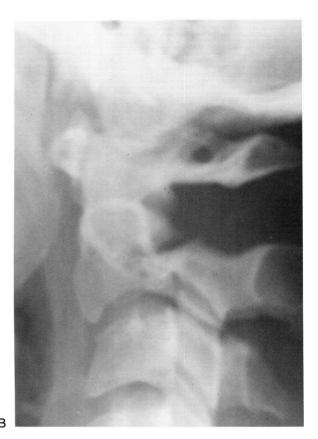

A

B

Fig. 10-18. Hangman's fracture. Bilateral fractures of the neural arch of C2. (A) A fatal hangman's fracture with anterior dislocation of C2 on C3. (Case courtesy of Justin Elliott, Garberville, CA.) (B) Fracture of the neural arch at C2 with minimal subluxation of C2 on C3. This 18-year-old man experienced no neurologic deficit.

The transverse fracture at the base of the dens must be differentiated from the os odontoideum, a developmental abnormality. The os is rounded, has cortical bone around its entire surface, and is usually more widely separated from the base of the odontoid process than is a fracture. At times, however, the distinction is difficult. A nonunion of a fracture of the dens is frequent in the adult. When the os is close apposition with the base of the odontoid process and is more normal in shape with a smooth inferior cortical margin, it may be impossible to distinguish an os odontoideum from an old nonunited fracture. Fractures of the dens are occasionally associated with atlantoaxial dislocations[40] and fractures of C1[74] (Fig. 10-19).

Apophyseal Separations of the Dens

Fractures of the dens are infrequent in children,[75] but occasionally an apophyseal separation is encountered that involves the synchondrosis between the ossification centers of the dens and body. The normal synchondrosis should not be mistaken for a fracture.

Hyperextension Fractures

An isolated avulsion fracture of the anterior inferior margin of C2 occurs as a result of hyperextension (Fig. 10-20). The avulsion occurs because of

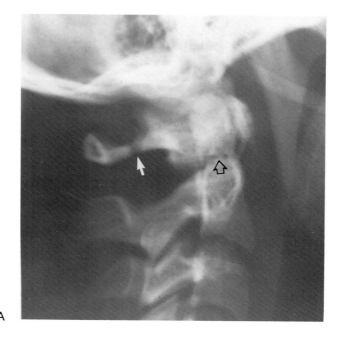

A

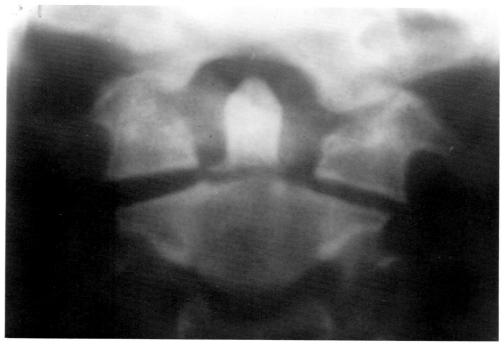

B

Fig. 10-19. Fractures of the dens in an 18-year-old man. (**A**) Lateral view demonstrates fracture at the base of the dens (open arrow), soft tissue swelling anterior to the craniovertebral junction, and fracture of the neural arch of C1 (white arrow). (**B**) Frontal polytomogram clearly demonstrates the transverse fracture at the base of the dens.

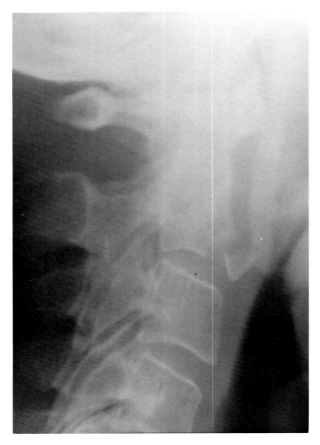

Fig. 10-20. A so-called "hyperextension teardrop fracture" at the anteroinferior margin of C2. This is a result of a hyperextension injury. At times, this type of fracture is associated with a hangman's fracture, so when this fragment is visualized, the neural arch of C2 should be scrutinized. The neural arches are intact in this case.

tension in the attachment of the anterior longitudinal ligament. Since this fracture is frequently a component of the hangman's fracture it is important to look for a neural arch fracture at C2 when such a fracture is identified.[40]

Fractures of the Body of the Axis

Occasionally, fractures occur through the superior articular facets as a result of lateral compressive forces. These are best demonstrated on the frontal projections as a disruption in the superior articular facet.

DISLOCATION AND SUBLUXATION INVOLVING THE CRANIOVERTEBRAL JUNCTION

Atlanto-occipital Dislocation

Atlanto-occipital dislocations are almost invariably fatal[63] (Fig. 10-21). The spine is usually displaced posteriorly, which results in a disruption of the medulla oblongata and immediate death. Survivals have been reported, however.[76,77]

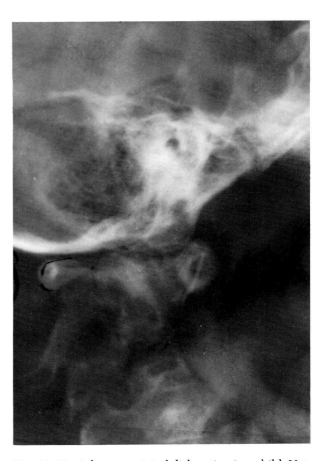

Fig. 10-21. Atlanto-occipital dislocation in a child. Note that the atlas is displaced posterior in relation to the occipital condyle. This is associated with an atlantoaxial dislocation as well. Note the wide separation between the anterior margin of the dens and the posterior margin of the anterior arch of C1. (Case courtesy of James Martin, Winston-Salem, NC.)

Atlantoaxial Dislocation and Subluxation

Traumatic disruption of the ligamentum transversarium occurs as a result of hyperflexion forces on the occiput. This is an unusual traumatic injury (Fig. 10-22). The atlantoaxial subluxation is more commonly found in association with rheumatoid arthritis or rheumatoid variants and is rarely caused by trauma. Nontraumatic subluxation also occurs in Down's syndrome. Normally, the distance between the anterior cortex of the dens and the posterior cortex of the anterior arch of the atlas is 2.5 mm in adults and 5 mm in children. Measurements in

excess of these dimensions are indicative of an atlantoaxial subluxation. This is demonstrated on the lateral projection and may not be evident with the spine in neutral position or in extension.[78,79] Flexion stress views may be necessary to disclose the subluxation. Posterior dislocation of the atlas on the axis has been reported.[60] In this rare injury, the anterior arch of the atlas comes to rest against the posterior surface of the dens. This is most likely a result of hyperextension with disruption of most, if not all, of the ligaments between C1 and C2 on the dens and the foramen magnum. The abnormality should be easily demonstrated on the lateral projection.

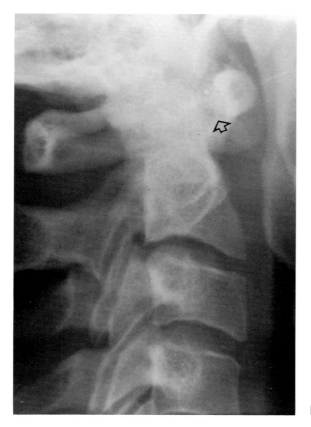

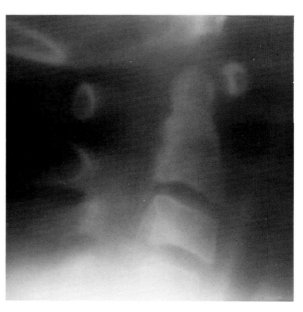

A   B

Fig. 10-22. Traumatic rupture of the transverse ligament of C1 in a 38-year-old man. **(A)** Lateral view of the cervical spine. There is soft tissue swelling anterior to the craniovertebral junction. The atlantoaxial distance measured 7 mm (arrow). **(B)** Lateral tomogram demonstrates the separation of the anterior arch of C1 and dens to better advantage. The normal atlantoaxial distance in adults should not exceed 2.5 mm.

THE LOWER CERVICAL SPINE

Fractures of the Vertebral Body

Anteriorly Wedged Compression Fractures

The anterior wedge compression fracture is a common fracture of the vertebral body. It is due to a mechanical flexion moment that results in a varying degree of anterior wedging of the vetebral body.[36,80,81] The wedge is formed predominantly by depression of the superior end plate. The degree of depression is dependent on the severity of the forces involved. The anterior wedging may be accompanied by a small triangular fragment from the anterosuperior surface of the vertebral body (Fig. 10-23).

The fourth or fifth vertebral body, or both, may normally be shorter than the adjacent third and sixth vertebral bodies. In the absence of significant associated wedging, this is a normal variant. If the anterior height of a vertebral body is 3 mm or more less than the posterior vertebral body height, a wedge fracture of the vertebral body is highly suspect. When the anterior wedging is minimal, there may be no distinct disruption of the cortex, yet a distortion in the profile of the vertebral body can be best visualized in the lateral projection.

Burst Fractures

When marked anterior wedging of the vertebral bodies is present, it is important to realize that the fragments are driven centripetally and that often a fragment from the posterior superior surface is driven into the spinal canal (Fig. 10-24). This may result in spinal cord injury. The fragment may not be obvious on the plain radiograph. When faced with a severely comminuted or markedly compressed vertebra, tomography should be obtained to exclude or identify a posteriorly displaced fragment within the spinal canal.

The Teardrop Fracture The teardrop fracture is a specific form of burst fracture described by Schneider and Kahn.[48] The injury is a fracture-dislocation consisting of a comminuted fracture of a vertebral body with a characteristic triangular or quadrilateral fragment from the anteroinferior margin of the vertebral body and posterior dislocation of the spine at the level of the fractured vertebral body (Figs. 10-3, 10-25). The fracture is usually accompanied by a spinal cord injury, and because of this and the appearance of this anteroinferior vertebral fragment, the authors coined the term *teardrop fracture.* When associated posterior displacement of the superior vertebra on the lower vertebra occurs, tomography will usually demonstrate a bilaminal fracture posteriorly at this level. This is a very unstable fracture.

There are often associated fractures of the spinous processes or disruptions of the interspinous ligaments. There may also be a vertical sagittal split in the affected vertebra, and at times there is a similar fracture in the vertebral bodies above the primary fracture (Fig. 10-25B).

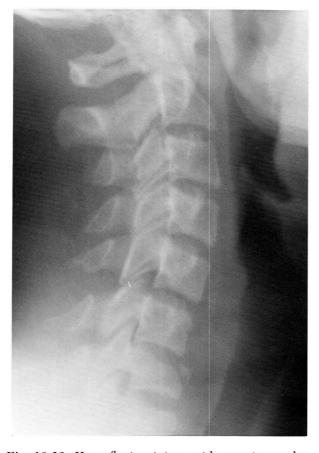

Fig. 10-23. Hyperflexion injury with anterior wedge compression fracture of C7 in a 17-year-old boy. Note the small triangular fragment from the anterosuperior surface of C7.

Fig. 10-24. Severe compression of C7 in an 18-year-old man. (**A**) Cross-table lateral view demonstrates a severe compression of the vertebral body with anterior displacement of the anterior portion of the vertebral body. The posterior portion of the vertebral body is not visualized. (**B**) Lateral tomogram demonstrates displacement of the superoposterior portion of the vertebral body into the spinal canal. This is a common finding in association with severely compressed vertebral bodies.

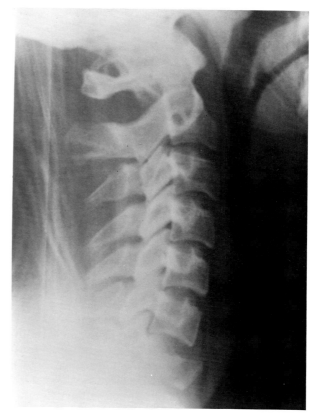

A

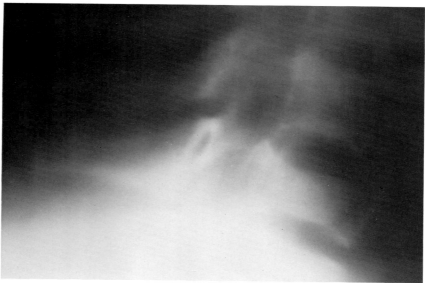

B

Sagittal Split of the Vertebral Body

On occasion, a vertical split may be encountered within the vertebral body without other associated fractures of the vertebral body[82-84] (Fig. 10-25). This is created by predominantly compressive forces in the sagittal plane. The mechanism is thought to be an acute herniation of the intervertebral disc into the vertebral body. The vertebra splits into almost equal halves in the sagittal plane. Characteristically, there is very little separation. The fracture line is only apparent on the frontal projection and may be easily mistaken for air in the larynx or obscured by an endotracheal or nasogastric tube. It is difficult to create a single fracture in a ring of bone. Therefore, it is not surprising that a similar vertical fracture may be identified within the lamina of the involved vertebra. Thus, this injury is similar to the Jefferson fractures of the atlas.

Hyperextension Teardrop Fractures

Isolated avulsion fractures of the anteroinferior margins of the vertebral bodies may occur without associated compression of the vertebra. These are due to hyperextension, are most commonly identified at C2 (Fig. 10-20), and are due to avulsions by the attached anterior longitudinal ligament. In patients with spondylosis or degenerative arthritis of the spine, the equivalent injury is a fracture of an anterior osteophytic spur.[19,23,45] These fractures may be the only direct radiographic evidence of injury in patients who have sustained hyperextension injuries of the spinal cord. Hyperextension injuries in the elderly, rigid, spondylitic spine most frequently occur at the C6 to C7 level. Frequently associated with this injury is a central cord neurologic injury.

FRACTURES OF THE POSTERIOR ELEMENTS

Fractures of the vertebral body and posterior elements often occur in combinations. These combinations are variable, depending on the forces involved. While fractures of any of the posterior elements may occur in isolation, they more often occur in combination with fractures of the vertebral body. In large measure fractures of the poste-

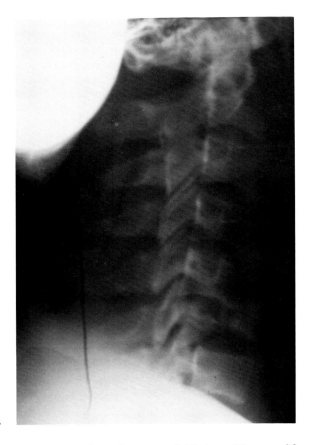

A

Fig. 10-25. Teardrop fracture of C6 in a 25-year-old man. Patient was quadriplegic. (A) Initial cross-table lateral radiograph demonstrating severely comminuted fracture of C6 with a typical anteroinferior triangular fragment and posterior displacement of the vertebra at the level of the injury that compromises the spinal canal. *(Figure continues.)*

rior elements can be predicted based on the pattern of fracture of the vertebral bodies. The fractures are more likely to result from pure hyperextension or combinations of axial load and extension than from pure flexion forces alone.

Isolated Fractures of the Spinous Process — Clay Shoveler's Fracture

The spinous processes of the upper cervical spine are bifid and have a slightly irregular, chevron appearance. The lower cervical and upper

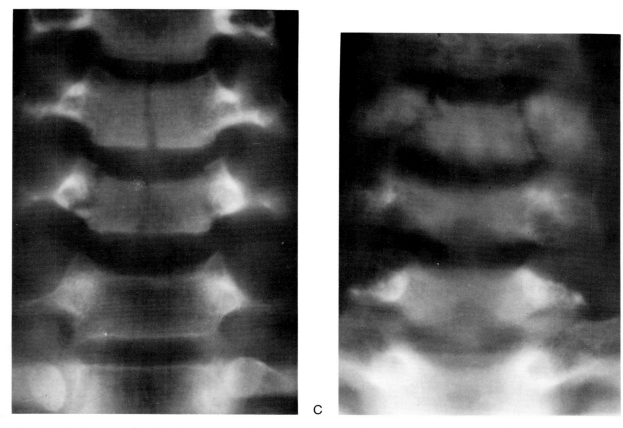

B   C

Fig. 10-25 *(Continued)*. **(B)** AP tomogram demonstrates vertical sagittal fractures (through the vertebral bodies) of both C5 and C6. The compression of C6 is demonstrated. **(C)** AP tomogram through the posterior elements reveals bilateral fractures of the laminae of C6.

dorsal spinous processes are oval in contour when viewed en face in the frontal projection.

Isolated fractures of the spinous process of the lower cervical and upper thoracic spine occur as a result of rotation of the trunk relative to the head and neck.[85] These are known as "clay shoveler's fractures" since they were first described in men involved in that activity. Fractures of the spinous process may also occur as a result of hyperextension resulting in compression of one spinous process against another[86] (Fig. 10-26). The fractures are best visualized in the lateral projection. Displacement is minimal. In some cases, the fractures may be visualized on the frontal projection. When there is slight offset of the fragment, it results in a double projection of the cortical margin. There-

fore, instead of seeing a single oval outline of the cortex of the spinous process, a double cortical outline is visualized, one representing the fragments attached to the neural arch and the other the displaced posterior fragment of the spinous process.

Fractures of the Articular Pillars and Facets

Fractures of the articular pillars and facets occur as a result of either compression or shearing.[57,80] Pure hyperextension results in bilateral fractures, whereas bending to one side or the other may produce unilateral fractures.[36,85] Avulsion fractures at the margins of a facet occur as a result of shearing as

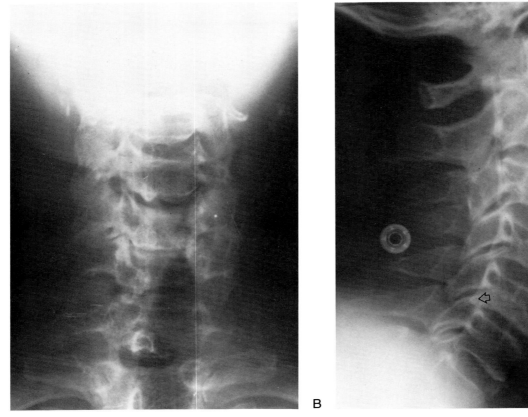

A   B

Fig. 10-26. Hyperextension injury resulting in a C5 quadriplegia in a 66-year-old man with spondylosis of the cervical spine. **(A)** AP view. There is narrowing of the C5–C6 interspace with osteophytic spur formation at the joints of Luschka. No other abnormalities are demonstrated. **(B)** Lateral view demonstrates posterior spur formation at C5 (arrow) and narrowing of the C5–C6 interspace. *(Figure continues.)*

one vertebra is displaced anteriorly on the other. These may be bilateral or unilateral.

On both the AP and oblique projections, the lateral margin of the articular pillar presents a smooth undulating surface (Fig. 10-12). Any cortical disruption or break in this line indicates a fracture. The pillars normally lie at a 25 to 30 degree angle with the horizontal plane, and therefore the articular surfaces of the facets cannot be visualized in profile on a routine AP projection utilizing a perpendicular central ray. To visualize the articular facets in the frontal and oblique projection, it is necessary to angle the central beam 20 to 30 degrees caudally. These are known as *pillar views*. They allow a profile view of the articular pillars and

more readily reveal fractures involving these structures. Tomography is often necessary to demonstrate them with certainty.

Fractures of the Laminae

Fractures of the laminae may be either vertical or horizontal. Occasionally they occur in isolation, but usually are components of more complex fractures involving the vertebral body and other posterior elements. They are difficult, if not impossible, to identify on the plain radiographs and are best seen on either tomography or computed tomography (Fig. 10-25C).

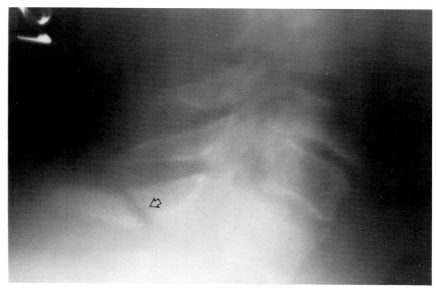

C

Fig. 10-26 *(Continued).* **(C)** Lateral tomogram demonstrates the changes at the C5–C6 interspace with posterior spur formation and a fracture of the spinous process of C7 (arrow). The latter is a clay shoveler's fracture.

DISLOCATIONS AND FRACTURE-DISLOCATIONS OF THE LOWER CERVICAL SPINE

Dislocations may occur as a result of either hyperextension or hyperflexion. The combination of hyperflexion and axial loading is far more common than either hyperextension or hyperflexion or axial loading alone. Dislocation is usually the result of either flexion or extension forces associated with varying amounts of rotational shearing and distraction. The resultant injury is dependent on the relative degree of distraction or compression. Tensile forces are usually combined with some degree of rotation and result in disruption of the intervertebral discs and interspinous ligaments with fewer and less extensive fractures of the vertebrae. Compressive (axial loading) forces generated either in flexion or in extension result in fractures of the vertebra. Flexion forces focus on the vertebral body, and extension forces focus on the posterior elements. Shearing forces tend to affect the apposing surfaces of the articular facets since the facets are oriented 50 to 60 degrees from the horizontal plane.

The underlying injuries in large measure can be predicted on the direction and degree of displacement of one vertebral body relative to the other. Anterior displacement of 50 percent or more of the width of the vertebral body is associated with bilateral facet locking[87,88] (Fig. 10-27); 25 percent anterior displacement is associated with unilateral locking and hyperextension sprain fractures[87–89] (Fig. 10-28); minimal anterior displacements of 1 to 2 mm are associated with hyperflexion and hyperextension strains, whereas posterior displacement irrespective of the degree is usually a result of a tear-drop fracture-dislocation (Figs. 10-3, 10-25).

Bilateral Facet Locking

Bilateral facet locking injuries are the result of flexion combined with distraction forces that disrupt the interspinous ligaments and interverte-

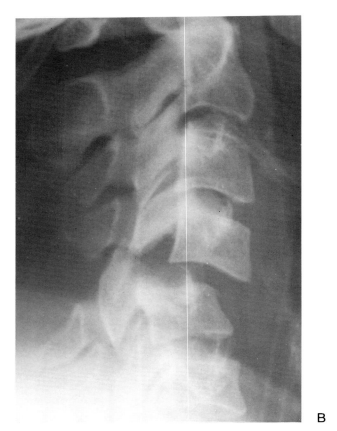
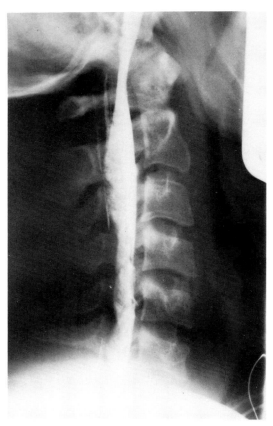

A   B

Fig. 10-27. Bilateral facet lock in a 26-year-old man with quadriplegia. (A) C4 is displaced anteriorly on C5 by approximately 50 percent of the width of the vertebral body. The apophyseal joints at this level are completely disrupted, and the posteroinferior margin of the facets of C4 lie anterior to the anterior margin of the facets of C5; the facets are locked in this position. The patient had sustained a complete quadriplegia. (B) A myelogram was performed after reduction. It demonstrates a diffuse displacement of the subarachnoid space from the posterior margin of the vertebral bodies. This is due to an epidural collection of blood.

bral disc.[36,87,88] The apophyseal joints are completely disrupted, which allows the superiorly located vertebra to displace anteriorly to such a degree that the facets become locked in a position anterior to the facets of the vertebral bodies below (Fig. 10-27). This requires at least a 50 percent displacement of one vertebral body on the other. There may be small fractures of the facets and slight anterior wedging of the vertebral body below the level of dislocation. The spinal canal is severely compromised by this displacement, and significant spinal cord injuries are frequent.

Unilateral Facet Locking

Unilateral locking of the facet is caused by a combination of flexion, distraction, and rotation resulting in a unilateral displacement and locking of the facet joints.[36,87–89] The anterior displacement is usually approximately 25 percent of the width of the vertebral body (Fig. 10-28). The degree of anterior displacement may be decreased by associated fractures of the affected facet. These fractures usually involve the posterior margin of the anteriorly displaced facet (Fig. 10-29). On the AP

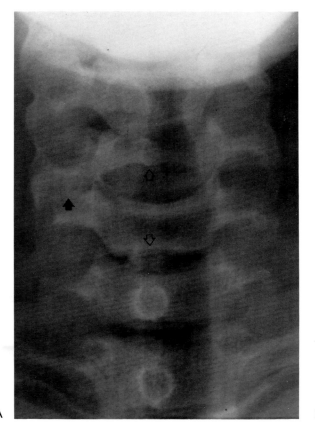
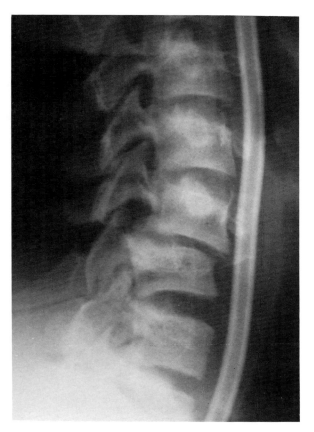

A B

Fig. 10-28. Unilateral facet lock at C5–C6 in a 16-year-old boy. **(A)** There is a separation of the spinous processes of C5 and C6 (open arrows). The upper spinous processes are rotated to the right. There is an increased density (solid arrow) at the facet joint of C5–C6 on the right owing to overlap of the facets. **(B)** C5 is displaced anterior on C6 by approximately 25 percent of the width of the vertebral body. The facet joint at C5–C6 is disrupted. The vertebral bodies above the level of dislocation are seen in the oblique position. Note the pedicles. The vertebral bodies below the dislocation are seen in the lateral profile. This indicates a rotary subluxation. *(Figure continues.)*

view, the spinous processes are displaced toward the affected side at the level of the injury. On the lateral view, the articular pillars are visualized on the true lateral profile below the injury but are usually identified in the oblique profile above the injury.

If there is an anterior subluxation of 25 percent or more, the facets should be examined closely at this level to determine whether the apophyseal joints are intact. Are the apposing surfaces aligned? It is not always easy to recognize that the spine is

rotated. Identify the posterior cortical margin of the facets. Are they aligned? With rotation, the circular cortical outline of the pedicle is often visualized. It should not be seen on the lateral projection and indicates rotation of the vertebra. It is often stated that with rotation you can see both facets of one vertebrae adjacent to one another giving a "butterfly" or "bow tie" appearance.[53,54] This depends on the degree of rotation and is not always evident. It may be more obvious after the placement of cranial traction.

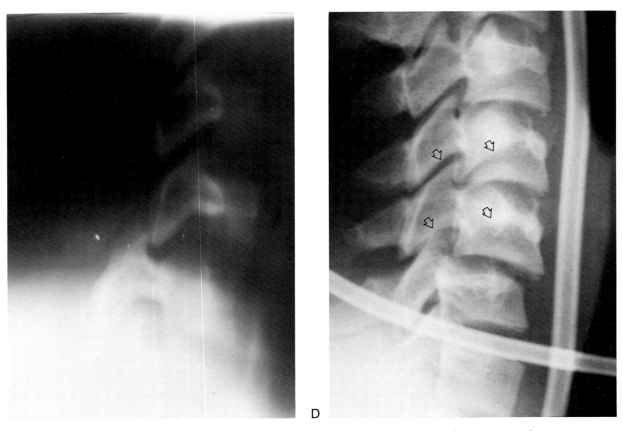

C   D

Fig. 10-28 *(Continued).* **(C)** Lateral tomogram through the right pedicles clearly demonstrates the anterior displacement of C5 on C6 with locking of the facets. The opposite side was intact. **(D)** Repeat lateral view after traction. With traction, the opposite facets are well seen and have a typical bow-tie or butterfly appearance (arrows). The obliquity of the vertebral body is more easily appreciated after the initiation of traction.

Hyperflexion Strain

Flexion and distraction forces may disrupt the facet joints and result in a subluxation with minimal displacement without locking. This is best identified on the lateral view[36,54,55] (Fig. 10-30). The articular pillars are not properly seated but are offset. This is usually accompanied by an anterior angulation of the spine at the involved interspace. The interspaces become wedge shaped, narrower anteriorly than posteriorly. The interspinous distance, that is, the distance between the spinous processes, is increased between the affected vertebrae. There is often minimal anterior subluxation of the verte-

bral body at the affected interspace. This rarely exceeds 1 to 2 mm and at times there may be no displacement whatsoever. These injuries are unstable, and often the deformity will progress and become much more evident on follow-up examinations.

In older patients with spondylosis or degenerative arthritis of the cervical spine, spondylolisthesis occurs, which must be differentiated from an anterior subluxation resulting from hyperflexion strain. Spondylolisthesis with minimal to moderate anterior subluxation characteristically occurs at C4–C5, one level above a markedly degenerated intervertebral disc at C5–C6. It is presumed that this

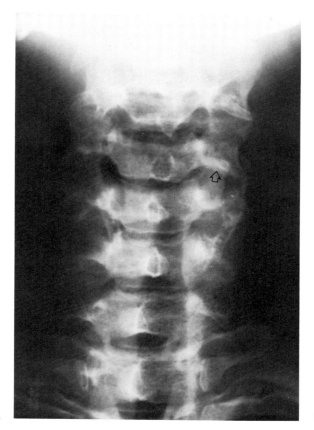
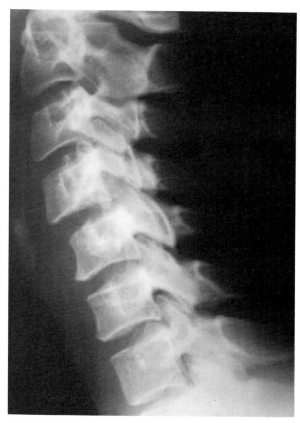

A

B

Fig. 10-29. Unilateral facet lock with facet fracture at C4 on the left in a 30-year old woman. **(A)** AP view. The spinous processes at C4 is slightly displaced to the left, and there is increased density in the region of the C4–C5 facet joint on the left (arrow), which suggests a facet lock. **(B)** Lateral view. C4 is displaced anteriorly by approximately 25 percent of the width of the vertebral body in relation to C5. Note the soft tissue swelling. It is difficult to appreciate any degree of rotation in this projection. *(Figure continues.)*

may also occur at other levels. The subluxation is due to degenerative changes in the C4–C5 apophyseal joints and occurs in the absence of a fracture or defect in the neural arch similiar to spondylolisthesis occurring in the lumbar spine in association with degenerative arthritis without associated defects in the pars interarticularis. If the patient has a history of recent trauma, the distinction between a hyperflexion strain and spondylolisthesis associated with degenerative arthritis or spondylosis may not be an easy one to establish and accept with certainty. The absence of retropharyngeal soft tissue swelling and the presence of a fixed deformity, persistent subluxation, on flexion and

extension views above the level of a degenerated narrow intervertebral disc space are in keeping with spondylolisthesis secondary to spondylosis of the cervical spine.

When all the ligamentous structures between two adjacent vertebra are disrupted without associated bony injury, the radiographic findings may be subtle and easily overlooked. Gross instability is often demonstrated after the patient is placed in cranial tongs and the vertebrae become widely separated despite the use of only 10 to 15 lb of traction. The only way to avoid error is to be suspicious of seemingly minor variations in alignment. The phrase "delayed traumatic dislocation of the cervi-

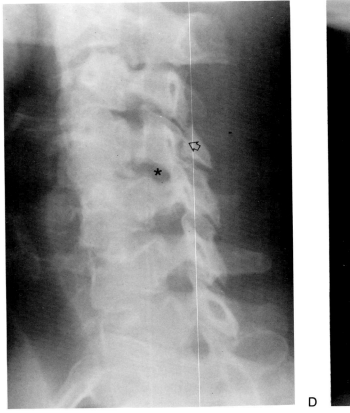

C

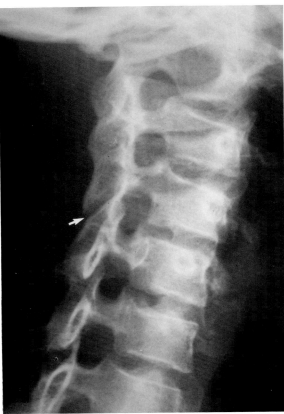

D

Fig. 10-29 *(Continued).* **(C)** A right posterior oblique view demonstrates the fracture of the facet at C4 (arrow) with anterior displacement of the facet and compromise of the C4–C5 intervertebral foramina (asterisk). **(D)** Left posterior oblique view demonstrates the slight separation of the C4–C5 facet joint (arrow) without compromise of the C4–C5 intervertebral foramina.

cal spine" has been utilized to describe cases in which the initial radiographs are normal but some degree of subluxation is identified on the subsequent examinations.[30] In fact, these are nothing more than ligamentous disruptions of the cervical spine that were either not demonstrated or not recognized on the initial radiograph. Later, the spine is either intentionally or inadvertently displaced and the abnormality is recognized.

Hyperextension Strain

Hyperextension and distraction forces may disrupt the intervertebral disc and anterior spinous ligament without associated fractures.[35,36] The radiographic findings are often subtle because of the absence of significant displacement and fractures. There is usually an increase in the retropharyngeal soft tissues secondary to hemorrhage associated with a disruption of the anterior longitudinal ligament[46] (Fig. 10-31). The affected interspace may be slightly widened or wedged shaped, with greater height anteriorly than posteriorly. It may be necessary to obtain flexion and extension views to demonstrate this with assurance. The hyperextension teardrop fractures are unusual, except at the second cervical vertebra (Fig. 10-20), encountered do serve as important clues to this form of injury. Spinal cord injuries are frequent, particularly in older patients with spondylosis. In such circumstances, the only radiographic finding may be retropharyngeal soft tissue swelling or an avulsion fracture of an osteophytic spur on the anterior

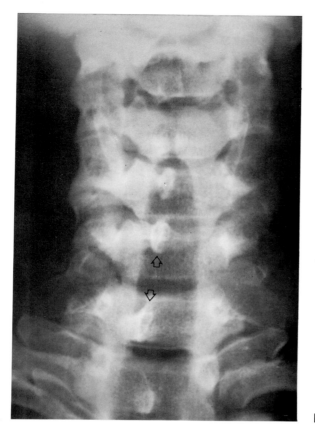
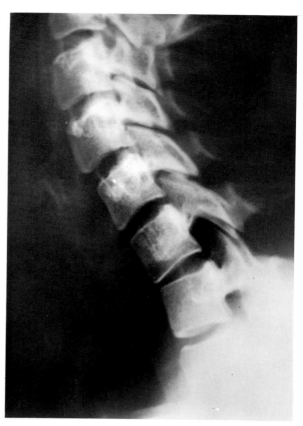

A   B

Fig. 10-30. Hyperflexion strain at C6–C7 sustained by a 28-year-old woman in a diving accident. **(A)** AP view demonstrates only separation of the spinous processes at C6–C7 (arrows). **(B)** Lateral view clearly demonstrates a separation between the spinous processes of C6–C7, a subluxation at the apophyseal joints, and an angulation of the spine at C6–C7 with narrowing of the anterior portion of the disc space. There is no associated fracture. The findings are characteristic of a hyperflexion strain. Compare with Fig. 10-14.

margin of a vertebral body.[25,26] At times there are fractures of the posterior elements, which should serve as another important clue to the mechanism of injury. Carefully observe for widening of the intervertebral disc space anteriorly. Hyperextension injuries occur frequently at C6–C7.

Hyperextension Fracture Dislocation

If the forces that create a hyperextension strain are severe, there may be an anterior dislocation of vertebra above the affected intervertebral disc.[90] These are associated with compression fractures of the apposing surfaces of the apophyseal joints at this level. The displacement of the vertebra is ap-

proximately 25 percent and therefore mimics unilateral facet locking. The distinction is made by recognizing that the displacement is due to comminuted fractures of the apposing margins of the articular facets and the absence of facet locking. This is often best determined by tomography.

FRACTURES OF THE UPPER DORSAL SPINE (T1 to T8)

The upper dorsal spine (T1 to T8) is considered separately from the remainder of the spine because it is subject to its own peculiar forms of injury and

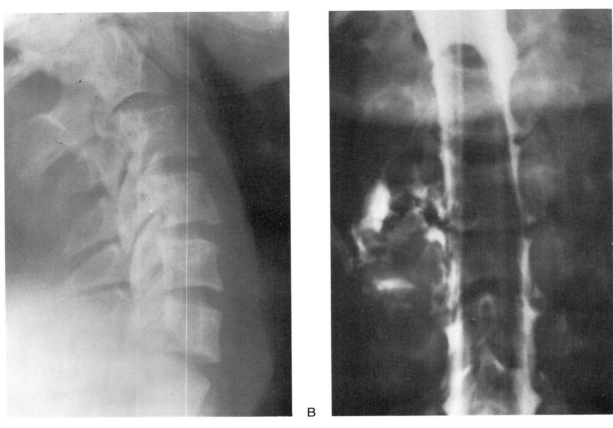

A   B

Fig. 10-31. Hyperextension injury with quadriplegia in a 23-year-old man. The injury was sustained in an auto accident. (**A**) Lateral view demonstrates considerable hemorrhage in the retropharyngeal soft tissues. There was a very subtle subluxation of C4 on C5 that is better appreciated by viewing the spine with the patient in the horizontal position. (**B**) AP view of a myelogram demonstrates a widening of the cord indicative of a hematomyelia. Note also the dural tear revealed by the extravasation of the Pantopaque on the right.

because there are unique problems in the radiographic demonstration of its anatomic components. The lower dorsal spine functions as a component of the thoracolumbar junction and is subject to stresses that differ considerably from those encountered in the upper dorsal spine. Fractures of the mid- and upper dorsal spine are relatively uncommon in adults (Fig. 10-7) except for those resulting from convulsions caused by either electroshock therapy or tetany. The relative incidence of fractures in this segment of the spine is greater in children than adults.[13,16] Fractures involving adjacent vertebrae are relatively common throughout the dorsal and lumbar spine, particularly in chil-

dren, in whom multiple contiguous fractures are the rule rather than the exception.

Isolated fractures of the posterior elements of the upper dorsal spine are distinctly unusual and would undoubtedly require computed tomography or standard tomography to identify with certainty.

Radiologic Examination

The initial examination should be properly exposed and positioned AP and lateral views. The cervicothoracic junction, including the first four or five segments of the dorsal spine, is impossible to visualize in the normal lateral projection because of the overlying pectoral girdle. A swimmer's view is required to adequately visualize the upper thoracic spine and the cervicothoracic junction (Fig. 10-13). This may be obtained while the patient lies supine with one arm held fully extended over the head and the other held at the side. It is helpful to have the patient grasp an IV pole with the extended arm to maintain this position.

Paraspinous masses and mediastinal hematomas (Fig. 10-32) serve as indirect clues to the presence of fracture or fracture-dislocation. The paraspinous masses represent hematomas that accumulate beneath and dissect along the paraspinous ligaments. These are easily demonstrated along the lateral margins of the spine on the AP projection. They are usually bilateral, often asymmetric, and may extend considerably beyond the fracture site.

Fractures of the first four or five thoracic vertebra may result in mediastinal hematomas (Fig. 10-32A) that widen the superior mediastinum and may extend over the apex of the lung. Such fractures are often difficult to visualize because there is displacement on the AP projection and they are obscured by the overlying pectoral girdle on the lateral projection.

The paraspinous hematomas are encountered in association with more severe fractures and fracture-dislocations of the upper thoracic vertebra and are quite similar in appearance to mediastinal hematomas associated with aortic transection or other vascular disruptions in the mediastinum. In the severely injured patient, it is also difficult to obtain the swimmer's view. In multiply injured patients, one should always be suspicious of upper thoracic spinal fractures and the possibility of aortic rupture when a widened mediastinum is identified. The upper dorsal spine should be closely evaluated and consideration given to the performance of an aortogram to exclude the possibility of an aortic rupture.

Tomography (Fig. 10-32B) is almost mandatory to clarify injuries of the upper thoracic spine, to determine the status of the posterior elements, and to verify the presence or absence of suspected fractures. Computed tomography (Fig. 10-32C) is helpful in the precise localization of fracture fragments in relation to the spinal canal and in the demonstration of fractures of the posterior elements.

Compression Fractures

Compression fractures are the result of the combination of truncal flexion and axial compression. They are by far the most common fractures encountered in both the thoracic and lumbar spine. The characteristic features are either an anterior wedging or a depression of the superior end plate of the vertebral body. Less commonly, the force of compression is focused at the inferior instead of the superior end plate and results in a deformity that is the mirror image of one resulting from involve-

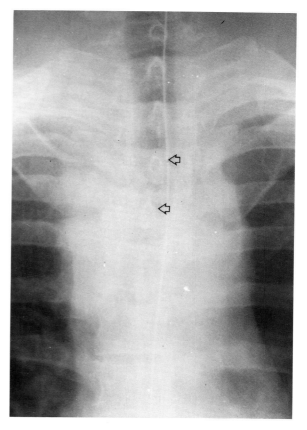

A

Fig. 10-32. Fracture dislocation at T3–T4 with paraplegia in a 35-year-old man. **(A)** AP view demonstrating the widening of the mediastinum and a slight lateral offset of T3 on T4 (arrows). Note the mediastinal hematoma extending over the apices of both lungs. A nasogastric tube is in place and lies in the normal position. *(Figure continues.)*

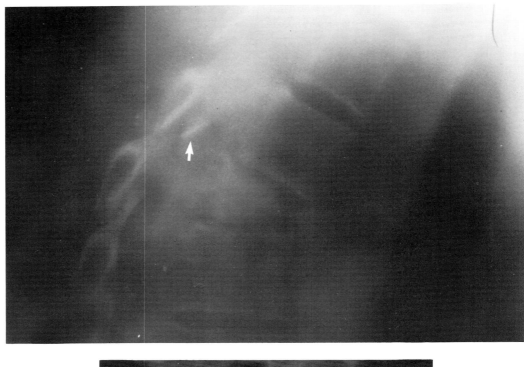

B

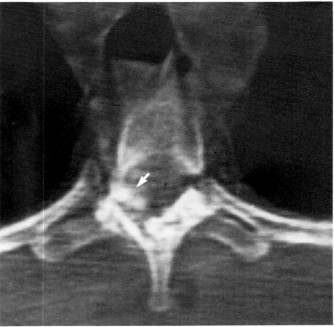

C

Fig. 10-32 *(Continued)*. **(B)** A lateral tomogram demonstrates the fracture-dislocation of T3 on T4. The fourth vertebral body is crushed with a characteristic anterosuperior triangular fragment. There is a fracture of the superior facet of T4 (arrow). **(C)** CT scan at T4 demonstrates the fracture of the superior facet (arrow). This is more easily appreciated on the standard tomogram.

ment of the superior end plate. The extent of vertebral compression and degree of comminution depends on the severity of the force and the relative strength of the vertebra. These fractures are more fully described under the discussion of the thoracolumbar spine.

Fracture-Dislocations of the Dorsal Spine

Fracture-dislocations are the result of the combination of flexion, axial compression, and rotational shearing forces. Most often there are fractures of both the posterior elements and vertebral bodies with anterior and lateral displacement of the vertebral bodies above the level of dislocation[34,91] (Figs. 10-32, 10-33). Most are unstable because of disruptions through the anterior and posterior column. They are partially reduced by simply placing the patient's shoulder in line with the pelvis. It is quite likely that the amount of displacement demonstrated on the radiographic examination is considerably less than that which existed at the time of injury. The residual displacement may be so minimal that it is difficult to appreciate.

Fracture-dislocations of the first through the eighth thoracic vertebrae are almost invariably associated with neurologic deficit. The most common site for fracture-dislocation of the upper thoracic spine is at the level of T4–T5 and T5–T6.[34] The MRSCICS series data concur. Mid- and upper dorsal fracture-dislocations are difficult to visualize on the AP projection because of minimal lateral displacement and rotation.

The typical fracture-dislocation of the upper dorsal spine consists of an anteriorly displaced vertebra associated with a wedged compression fracture of the subjacent vertebral body[34] (Fig. 10-33A). A small triangular fragment of bone is found anterior to the vertebra. The facet joints are frequently disrupted (Fig. 10-33B), with the fracture of the superior facet of the vertebra below the dislocation or fracture through the lamina of the vertebra above the dislocation. Alternatively, there may be locking or perching of the facets of the two affected vertebra. Frequently, there is a

burst fracture of the anterior displaced vertebral body in addition to the compression fracture of the vertebral body below the dislocation. Characteristically, a large posterior superior fragment of the crushed vertebral body remains attached to the pedicles. At times there are additional compression fractures of vertebrae below the level of dislocation.

Complex fracture-dislocations with either anterior or posterior dislocation also occur that are difficult to classify. The basic components are combined fractures of both the posterior elements and vertebral bodies in association with a dislocation.

Minimal anterior or posterior subluxations may occur without associated fractures but with spinal cord injury. Traumatic paraplegia with injury levels of the upper dorsal spine may occur in the absence of fracture-dislocation in the manner similar to that encountered in the cervical spine; a hyperextension injury may result in a compression of the cord between the ligamentum flavum posteriorly and the apposing margins of the vertebral bodies and intervertebral disc anteriorly, producing a hematomyelia. Fractures of the facets or other posterior elements may be identified that attest to the hyperextension mechanism but will almost always require tomography for visualization. Fractures and fracture-dislocations associated with spinal cord injury accounted for 37.5 percent of all thoracic spine fractures in the MRSCICS series; they accounted for 46.7 percent of all multiple levels of spinal injuries[3,34] (Fig. 10-9). That is, almost half of the patients had an associated discontiguous fracture of the spine. In view of this disproportionate number, when a primary injury is encountered at this level, the possibility of a second vertebral injury must be given strong consideration. Injuries of T2 to T4 are associated with secondary injuries in the cervical spine (Fig. 10-10). Injuries of T5 to T8 are associated with injuries either proximally within the cervical spine or distal in the thorocolumbar junction. The associated injuries of the cervical spine are often hyperextension (C2) teardrop fractures, fractures of the spinous process, and hangman's fractures, strongly suggesting that the cervical spine is commonly, if not always, in hyperextension as a fracture-dislocation of the upper cervical spine is created (Fig. 10-10).

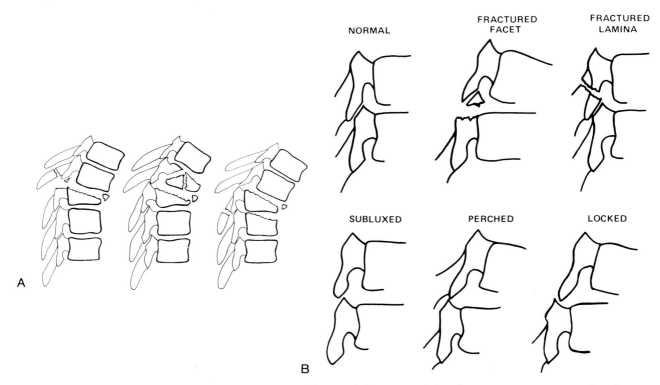

Fig. 10-33. (A) Diagrammatic representation of typical fractures of the thoracic spine associated with paraplegia. On the left is a fracture-dislocation with compression of the vertebral body below and a typical small triangular fragment displaced anteriorly from the compressed vertebra. In the center the vertebral body above the dislocation has sustained a burst fracture of the large posterosuperior fragment that is attached to the pedicle. On the right there is a fracture-dislocation associated with additional compression fractures below the level of dislocation. There are a variety of fractures of posterior elements and dislocation of the apophyseal joint demonstrated in this diagram above the level of dislocation. These are highly variable and not characteristic of any particular injury. (B) Variety of abnormalities found in apophyseal joints in association with fracture-dislocations of the thoracolumbar spine. Note perched facets in which the inferior tip of the superior facet becomes perched on the superior aspect of the inferior facet after disruption of the apophyseal joint. Facets may also become locked, as is more typical of the cervical spine. (From Rogers et al.,[34] with permission.)

FRACTURES OF THE THORACOLUMBAR JUNCTION AND LUMBAR SPINE

Two-thirds of all fractures involving the thoracolumbar spine occur at T12–L1 and L2, 90 percent between T11 and L4 (Fig. 10-7). Approximately 20 percent of thoracolumbar spine fractures are associated with other skeletal injuries.[2,37,92] The association of compression fractures of the thoracolumbar junction with fractures of the calcaneus is frequently reported, as are fractures of the tibia (Fig. 10-34).

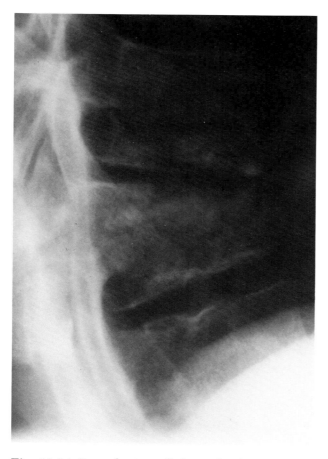

Fig. 10-34. Lateral view of thoracolumbar junction, showing compression fracture of T12 associated with fracture of the calcaneus in a 42-year-old individual who fell from a height. There is an anterior wedge compression fracture at T12 without associated dislocation.

Radiographic Examination

The initial examination should be AP and lateral views of the thoracolumbar junction and lumbar spine. In the severely injured patient, the initial lateral view may be obtained by utilizing a horizontal cross-table beam. If the initial AP and lateral projections fail to disclose any abnormalities, oblique projections may then be obtained. If a significant fracture or dislocation is demonstrated, however, oblique views may not be necessary. In the lower dorsal spine, hematomas may be present beneath the paraspinous ligament as a paraspinous mass. There are no dependable indirect signs of injury in the lumbar spine. It takes a considerable hemorrhage from a fractured vertebral body to obliterate the margins of the psoas muscle. However, the psoas margins are at times obliterated by isolated fractures of the transverse processes.

Tomography is used chiefly to clarify the status of the posterior elements, to verify the presence or absence of suspected fractures, and to determine the position of fragments.[4,6] This is very useful in the evaluation of bursting fractures of the vertebral bodies to locate the position of fragments displaced into the spinal canal and for clarification of the abnormalities associated with fracture-dislocations. Computed tomography allows a percise localization of fracture-fragments in relation to the spinal canal and may demonstrate additional fractures.

Classification

Approximately 75 percent of thoracolumbar fractures are compression fractures with the posterior elements remaining intact (MRSCICS series, 29.1 percent); 20 percent are fracture dislocations that usually involve both the posterior elements and the vertebral body (MRSCICS series, 42 percent); and 5 percent involve only the posterior elements (MRSCICS series, 3 percent). The latter are usually stable.[37,92,93]

Compression Fractures

As in the thoracic spine, compression fractures are the result of a combination of truncal flexion and axial compression and are by far the most com-

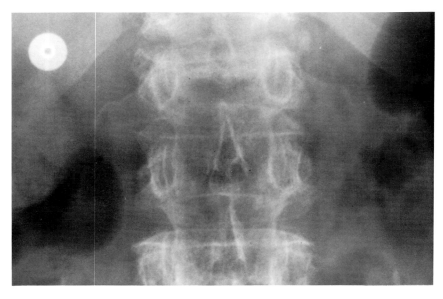

A

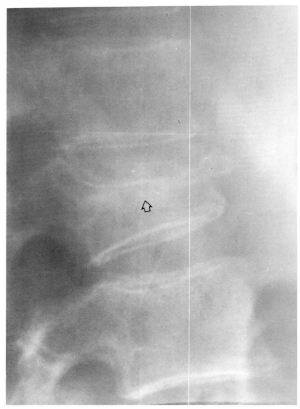

B

Fig. 10-35. Compression of L1 in a 77-year-old osteoporotic woman. **(A)** AP view. The loss of vertebral body height is obvious. The posterior elements appear to be intact. **(B)** Lateral view. The anterior wedge compression involves the superior end plate. Note the small fragment from the anterior superior margin of the vertebral body, the disruption of the end plate, and the impaction of the fracture demonstrated by the zone of increased density (arrow).

mon type of fracture encountered. Usually, the compression or wedging involves the superior end plate; however, on occasion the injury is localized instead to the inferior end plate and inferior surface of the vertebral body. This is of no real significance. It does not denote the presence of pathology within the involved vertebra.

These fractures are best identified in the lateral projection. The vertebral body is wedged shaped with a greater decrease in the height of the vertebral body anteriorly than posteriorly (Fig. 10-34). The posterior portion of the vertebral body may not even be affected, and its height then remains normal. The superior end plate is depressed and forms a concavity in the superior portion of the vertebra (Fig. 10-35). Beneath the concave depression there is a band of poorly marginated sclerosis indicative of impaction of bony trabeculae. The anterior superior margin of the wedged vertebra usually projects as an irregular beak from the anterior border of the vertebral body. This often has a sharp point that projects inferiorly. The anterior cortical margin of the vertebral body is irregular, and although a distinct break in the cortex is usually identified, this is not always the case. The distortion of the anterior rim of the vertebra is confirmed by comparing its profile with that of adjacent vertebrae. At times, the anterior superior margin of the vertebral body may be displaced anteriorly as a separate small triangular fragment. When such a fragment is identified, the alignment of the spine should be examined closely since this frequently heralds a fracture-dislocation. If the inferior end plate is affected, the same findings are identified, although in mirror image.

In children, the bone is resilient and frequently toruslike fractures of the vertebral bodies occur that give rise to a beaklike projection on the anterior margins of the vertebra.[13,16] These are usually on the superior margin but may be found inferiorly, in the middle, or both superiorly and inferiorly. There may be no distinct break in the cortical margin of the vertebra. Comparison with adjacent vertebrae is helpful, although it should be realized that fractures of adjacent vertebrae are quite common.

In older osteoporotic individuals, fractures often occur in the absence of trauma. These are in a sense insufficiency fractures, arising in weakened bone.

They are manifest on the radiograph by various degrees of depression of the superior end plate associated with an underlying band of poorly marginated sclerosis owing to impaction of bony trabeculae (Fig. 10-35). It may be difficult to identify distinct disruption of the cortex of the superior end plate. The anterior superior margin of the involved vertebra is irregular, and it may be difficult to identify distinct disruptions of the cortex. It is often necessary, particularly in an osteoporotic individual, to make the distinction between an old and a new fracture. In contradistinction to acute fractures, an old, healed fracture reveals a fine thin margin of cortical bone at the end plate that is usually concave, there is no underlying increased density of bone, and the anterior margin of the vertebra does not have an irregular beak, but commonly has an osteophytic spur.

Burst Fractures

More severe compressive forces drive the nucleus pulposus into the vertebral body, resulting in a virtual explosion of the vertebral body displacing the fragments centripetally.[37,93] These are termed burst fractures. Frequently, the posterior superior fragment is driven into the spinal canal (Figs. 10-36 and 10-37) which may result in spinal cord, cauda equina, or nerve root injury.[6] These fragments may not be identified on the standard projection, and tomography (Fig. 10-37C), or computed tomography (Fig. 10-37D,E) should be obtained to exclude their presence when faced with a severely comminuted fracture of the vertebral body (Fig. 10-6). These fractures also commonly have a vertical sagittal component within the vertebral body. Burst fractures are very uncommon in the upper dorsal spine, but are common in both the cervical spine and thoracolumbar junction.

Fractures of the posterior elements often accompany the more severe compression fractures of the vertebral body. These consist of either vertebral or horizontal fractures involving the lamina, spinous process, pedicles, facets, and transverse processes.[93] The combination of a severe compression fracture of the vertebral body and fractures of the posterior elements is unstable and frequently accompanied by a dislocation (Fig. 10-37).

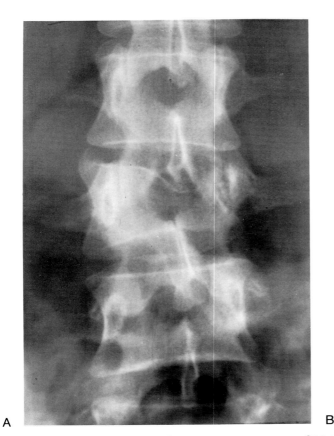
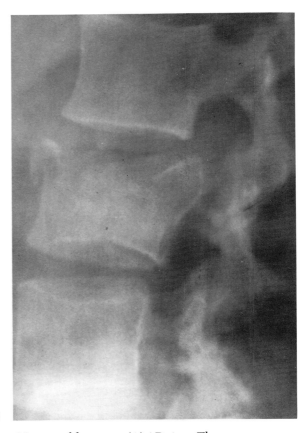

A   B

Fig. 10-36. Explosion or burst-type compression of L3 in a 33-year-old woman. (A) AP view. The compression of the vertebra is more marked on the left than on the right. (B) Lateral projection. The posterosuperior margin of the severely compressed vertebra is displaced posteriorly into the spinal canal. This is typical of severe compression or burst fractures of the vertebral bodies.

Fractures of the posterior elements are frequently obscure on standard radiographs because of the complexity of overlying shadows and lack of displacement of fracture fragments. On frontal projections, there are two clues to the recognition of disruption of the posterior elements.[94] With either a transverse fracture of the posterior elements or disruption of the ligaments, there may be sufficient angulation of the superior fragment of the vertebra so that a portion of the vertebral body is no longer overlaid by the posterior elements. This separation and elevation give rise to an empty or vacant appearance of the vertebral body. Another key is the recognition of the break in the continuity of the cortical margins of the posterior elements, particularly the oval cortex of the pedicles or the tear-shaped cortex of the spinous processes. The fracture line may also be visualized within the lamina or articular processes. Tomography is often required to confirm and fully evaluate these fractures.

The importance of identifying a dislocation or loss of vertebral body height indicating the presence of a compression fracture is readily appreciated. However, it is also important to determine the status of the posterior elements.[93] Disruption of the posterior elements is an important clue to the possibility of an unstable fracture. Fractures involving only the vertebral body are more than likely stable, whereas those involving both the vertebral body and the posterior elements are likely unstable.

It is quite likely that a greater number would be demonstrated by obtaining routine tomographic examinations of the spine in the presence of compression fractures of the vertebral body.[4] It would seem judicious to obtain a tomographic examination when presented with a severe or markedly compressed vertebral body.

Post-Traumatic Collapse — The Kümmell Phenomenon

Kümmel described a post-traumatic collapse in the vertebral body leading to the gibbus deformity. Others have noted a delayed progressive angular deformity after otherwise routine compression fractures or even inapparent or minimal fractures of the vertebral bodies.[95] These deformities are more likely to occur in the thoracolumbar spine. The etiology is thought to be secondary to vascular damage and therefore aseptic necrosis, although this is not proven. The collapse generally occurs within 8 weeks of the initial injury. The extent of the collapse and the degree of the deformity may worsen over a 3 to 6 month period following its initial recognition. Because of this pathologic process, fractures of the vertebral body resulting in greater than 25 to 35 percent compression should be considered for internal fixation. Without internal fixation, the vertebral body will continue to collapse. This phenomenon should not be misconstrued as evidence of a pathologic fracture. Slight progression of vertebral collapse is common after an anterior wedged compression fracture. This is rarely of clinical significance and should probably not be considered as examples of the Kümmel phenomenon. Progressive kyphosis has been identified after unstable fractures of the thoracolumbar spine and is particularly common if a laminectomy is performed to treat the original injury.[35] The more unstable the injury, the more likely the progressive kyphosis. This can be prevented by open reduction with internal infixation and anterior and/or posterior spinal fusions.

Fracture-Dislocation of the Thoracolumbar Spine

Fracture-dislocations are the result of combinations of a flexion, axial compression, and rotational shearing forces[37,38,96,97] similar to those described above for the upper dorsal spine. The predominant features are fractures of both the posterior elements and the vertebral bodies with anterior displacement of vertebral bodies above the level of dislocation.[6,91] Most are grossly unstable because of the disruption through both the anterior and posterior columns. Once again, as described for the upper dorsal spine, the typical fracture-dislocation consists of an anterior displaced vertebra asso-

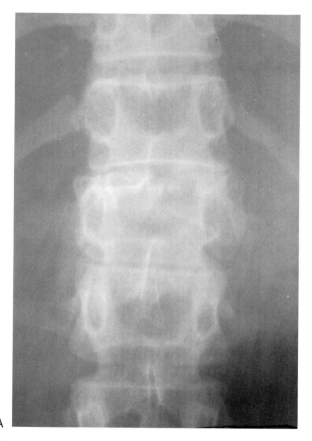

A

Fig. 10-37. Burst fracture of L1 in a 20-year-old woman. (A) AP view. The distortion of L1 is evident. The posterior elements appear to be intact. *(Figure continues.)*

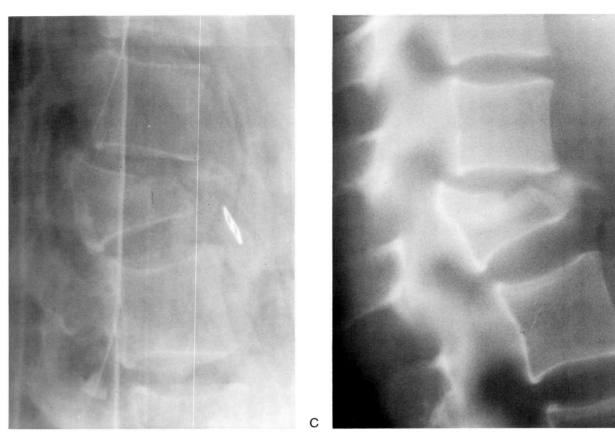

B   C

Fig. 10-37 *(Continued)*. **(B)** Lateral view. A cross-table lateral view demonstrates the severe compression fracture of L1 with an anterior dislocation of T12 on L1. The posterior elements are not well visualized. **(C)** Lateral tomogram demonstrates the severe compression fracture with posterior displacement of the superoposterior margin of the vertebral body. *(Figure continues.)*

ciated with a wedged compression fracture of the subjacent vertebral body. The compressed vertebral body is usually accompanied by a small triangular fragment of bone anterior to the wedged vertebra. Holdsworth described a fracture involving the superior portion of the vertebra in fracture-dislocations which he termed a sliced fracture[37,38] (Fig. 10-38). This consisted of a thin fragment of the superior end plate of the vertebral body at the level of dislocation. In our experience, this type of fracture occurs infrequently. More often, the fragment is small and triangular (Fig. 10-39B).

In fracture-dislocations of the thoracolumbar junction, the intervening facet joints are disrupted with either fractures of the superior facets of the vertebral body below the dislocation or locking or perching of facets similar to that described for the dorsal spine.[34,92,98] At times, the facets on one side are disrupted, whereas the fracture line on the opposite proceeds through the pedicle or pars interarticularis.[99] In general, the fractures found in association with a fracture-dislocation at the thoracolumbar junction tend to be confined to the two vertebrae adjacent to the dislocation, whereas in the upper dorsal spine fractures tend to involve several adjacent vertebrae.

The degree of vertebral body compression is dependent on the degree of compressive force opera-

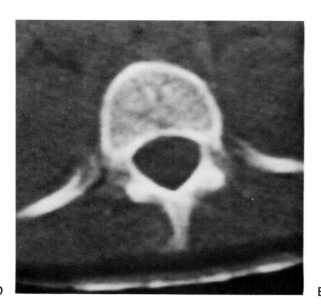
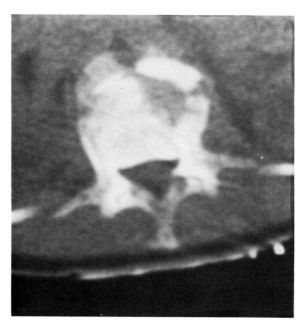

D   E

Fig. 10-37 *(Continued)*. **(D)** Computed tomogram at T12. There is no evidence of fracture. Note the normal configuration of the spinal canal. **(E)** Computed tomogram through L1 demonstrating a comminuted fracture of the vertebral body with posterior displacement of the fragment which compromises the spinal canal. Compare this configuration with the spinal canal in Fig. D.

tive at the time of injury. Under some circumstances, there may be a predominantly distracting force that allows disruption of the intervertebral disc and ligaments without resulting in sufficient compression to create fractures of the vertebral bodies.[100]

On occasion, a dislocation occurs at the thoracolumbar junction with little or no fracture of the involved vertebral bodies. There may be associated fractures of the pedicles, the pars interarticularis, or the laminae. Even less commonly, there is a total ligamentous disruption posteriorly without any identifiable fractures of the adjacent vertebrae.

Fractures of the Posterior Elements

Fractures limited to the posterior elements of the thoracolumbar spine are unusual except for fractures of the transverse processes, which are quite common and are frequently multiple. They may occur from either direct blows or indirectly by

being avulsed by contraction of the paraspinous muscles. The fracture is usually vertical or obliquely oriented. Nonunited transverse process ossification centers mimic fractures. These are more likely to appear in the first two lumbar vertebrae. The distinction can be made by recognizing that the bony margins at the apposing surfaces are sharply defined by cortical bone.

Fractures limited to the pars interarticularis[56,101-103] or articular facets are occasionally encountered. Characteristically, there is very little displacement and the fracture line is obscure. They are rarely evident on the AP or lateral projection but may be identified on oblique views. The fractures may be transverse across the pars or a single facet or may be more vertically oriented, involving one or both superior and inferior facets. The injury is most likely caused by an acute hyperextension.

Isolated fractures of the spinous processes and lamina may be seen occasionally but are very difficult to visualize without tomography.[4]

In a patient who has persistent back pain after

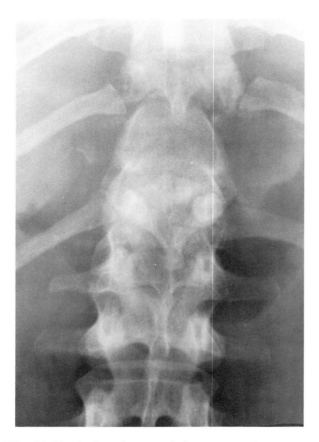

Fig. 10-38. A slice fracture-dislocation at T11–T12. These injuries are due to predominant rotation and shearing forces. AP projection. There is obvious distortion and separation at T11–T12.

trauma, the possibility of a fracture of the posterior elements should be considered and the original radiographs reviewed with this in mind. If no fracture is identified, then it is of value to obtain a tomogram (Fig. 10-40) of the posterior elements in at least the AP and lateral projections in an attempt to visualize an otherwise obscure isolated fracture in one of the posterior elements.

Transverse or Horizontal Fractures of the Spine

Pure transverse fractures of the lumbar spine were first described by G.Q. Chance and are known as "Chance fractures." [94,104] The dominant feature is a horizontal fracture involving the posterior elements with little or no compression of the vertebral body. The injuries are caused by flexion and distraction. The classic example is caused by the wearing of a lap-type seat belt. Smith and Kaufer noted that with hyperflexion of the trunk the fulcrum of the flexion movement is at the anterior margin of the vertebral body.[105] In contradistinction, when the victim is wearing a lap-type seat belt, the fulcrum of flexion is displaced anteriorly to the belt and the entire spine is subjected to distraction without compression (tension stresses). This results in a disruption of the posterior ligaments or, alternatively, transverse or fission-type fractures of the posterior elements (Fig. 10-41). The same injury can be encountered when an individual falls or is thrown forward so that the anterior abdominal wall comes in contact with some object such as a tree limb or fence railing. The object serves as a fulcrum in a manner similar to the seat belt, forces the body into acute flexion, and results in the same type of injury as that seen with the wearing of the seat belt.

There are three basic patterns of injury from these distracting forces[95] (Fig. 10-42). The first pattern is a transverse fracture involving the posterior elements with or without extension into the posterior superior or posterior inferior aspect of the vertebral body. The fracture line may involve one or both pedicles, transverse processes, and articular facets, as well as the lamina and spinous process. This is the classic Chance fracture. The second pattern involves a transverse fracture of the posterior elements with an associated transverse fracture of the vertebral body. This fracture involves the vertebral body as well as the spinous process, lamina, pedicles, and usually the transverse processes. This is the fulcrum fracture of the lumbar spine as described by Howland et al.[94a] The third pattern involves the disruption of the posterior interspinous ligaments, articular facets, and intervertebral disc. The pedicles and spinous and transverse processes remain intact. There may be an associated avulsion of the articular facet or a small fracture of the vertebral body, but the majority of the injury is confined to soft tissues. In this type, there may be a dislocation of the adjacent vertebrae. When it is present, an injury of the spinal cord or cauda equina is likely.

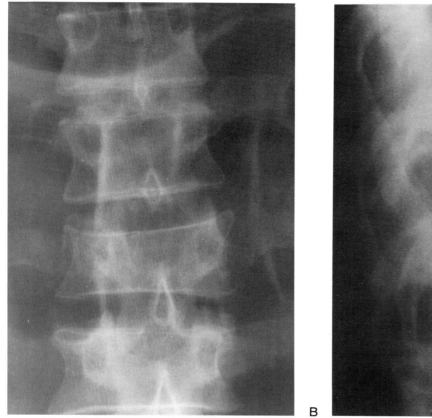
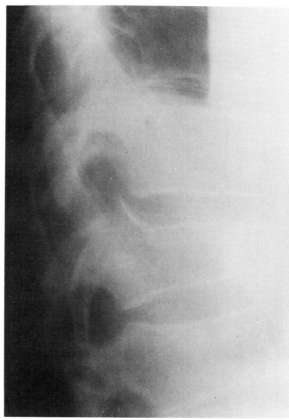

A   B

Fig. 10-39. Fracture-dislocation at T11–T12 with locking of the facets. **(A)** AP view. There is an obvious compression fracture of T12. **(B)** Lateral view. The anterior wedge compression fracture of T12 is demonstrated with minimal anterior displacement of T11. The posterior elements are not clearly visualized.

Characteristically, in any of the three types there is minimal compression of the vertebral body (Fig. 10-41). Significant lateral displacement or rotation of the fracture fragments is also uncommon. How much compression of the vertebral body is allowed before the fracture should no longer be considered a true Chance fracture? Anterior wedge compression fractures of the vertebrae are often associated with horizontal fractures of the posterior elements. This is understandable when one considers the forces at play during the creation of a compression fracture. The fulcrum of flexion is at the anterior margin of the vertebral body, resulting in the compression fracture of the vertebral body. Simultaneously, there is tension in the posterior elements that distracts them and can create horizontal frac-

tures, particularly in the spinous process and lamina. In the fulcrum type of fracture, there should be no significant compression of the vertebra. What is meant by significant compression? The question will remain and arguments will occur because there is no easy definition allowing a sharp distinction between a compression fracture and Chance fracture when associated with transverse fractures of the posterior elements.

Transverse fractures of the lumbar vertebrae are associated with significant visceral injuries in approximately 15 percent of cases. Neurologic injury also occurs in approximately 15 percent of cases. Garrett and Braunstein coined the term "seatbelt syndrome" to describe those injuries frequently encountered in individuals who were injured by

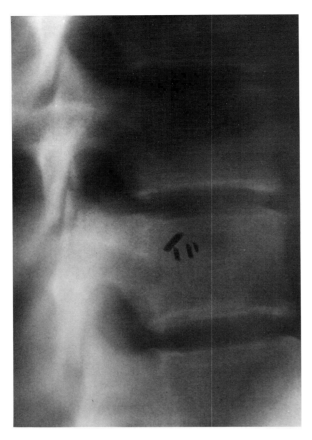

Fig. 10-40. Isolated fracture of the superior facet of T11 without associated dislocation. This 23-year-old woman had persistent back pain after a fall. The plain radiographs were normal, and this tomogram was then obtained, which demonstrates an undisplaced fracture of the left superior facet of the 11th thoracic vertebra.

wearing a lap-type seatbelt.[94,104] Typically, the affected individual is a passenger involved in a head-on collision that resulted in a sudden deceleration at impact. The syndrome consists of one or more of the following injuries:[94,104] transverse abrasions of the lower anterior abdominal wall outlining the position of the seatbelt; ruptures of the anterior abdominal wall musculature; longitudinal lacerations of the small bowel, particularly on the antimesenteric border of the jejunum and ileum; tears of the mesentery; ruptures of the second or third portion of the duodenum, spleen, or pancreas; injuries to the cauda equina or spinal cord; and transverse fractures of the lumbar spine. These injuries may

be both clinically and radiologically obscure, and therefore when a transverse fracture is identified, everyone should be alerted to the potential for associated abdominal visceral injury.

OPEN AND PENETRATING INJURIES: MISSILE AND STAB WOUNDS OF THE SPINE AND SPINAL CORD

Approximately 15 percent of civilian spinal cord injuries are due to open penetrating injuries by bullets or knife wounds.[106] Of the 2,710 patients admitted to the acute spine trauma center at Northwestern University between 1972 and 1986, 275 had gunshot wounds (10.2 percent). This is the third major admission etiologic factor. The caliber and velocity of a missile determine the nature of the spinal fracture and the spinal cord injury.[107,108] Civilian injuries tend to involve lower velocity and smaller caliber than military injuries. The bullet may penetrate and remain within the spinal canal and may be identified within the canal on both the AP and lateral projections (Fig. 10-43). The missile may transit the spine (Fig. 10-44) and come to rest in another portion of the body or pass out of the body through a wound of exit. Small bullet fragments (in low-velocity-missile injuries) may then be identified along the course of the missile (see Fig. 10-44). The missiles may ricochet after encountering some portion of the spine and come to rest elsewhere. The site of impact is identified by multiple small fragments of the bullet and fragmentation of the underlying bone. The degree of fragmentation is dependent on the velocity and caliber of the missile. It is possible to sustain a spinal cord injury without an associated fracture of the spine. The passage of a high-velocity missile close to the spinal canal may cause sufficient blast and concussion to injure the spinal cord without producing radiographically identifiable fractures or more likely without passage of the bullet through the spinal canal.

Stab wounds (Fig. 10-45) are usually located in the dorsal spine and may be associated with fractures of the lamina or other posterior elements at

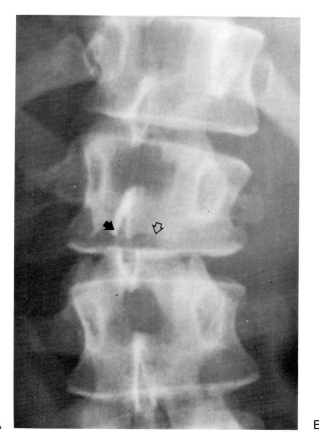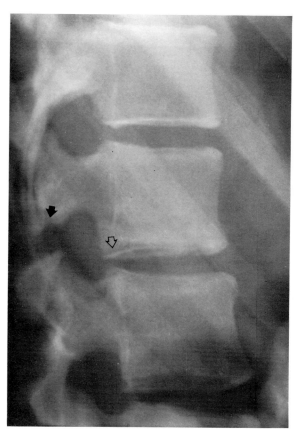

A   B

Fig. 10-41. Chance fracture of L1 in a 17-year-old boy involved in an auto accident. (**A**) AP view. There is minimal compression of the lateral margin at L1. Closer inspection demonstrates fracture through the lamina (open arrow) and the spinous process (solid arrow). (**B**) Lateral view. The fracture of the lamina is demonstrated (solid arrow). There is also a slight avulsion involving the inferior ring apophysis of L1 (open arrow).

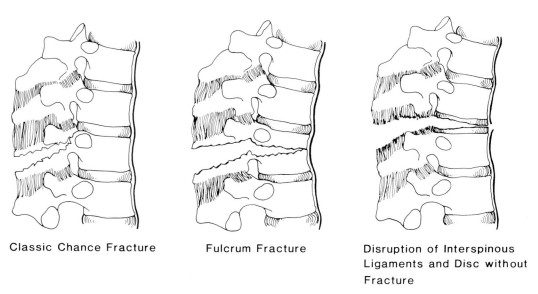

Classic Chance Fracture   Fulcrum Fracture   Disruption of Interspinous Ligaments and Disc without Fracture

Fig. 10-42. Diagram of Chance-type fractures (distraction injuries of the lumbar spine).

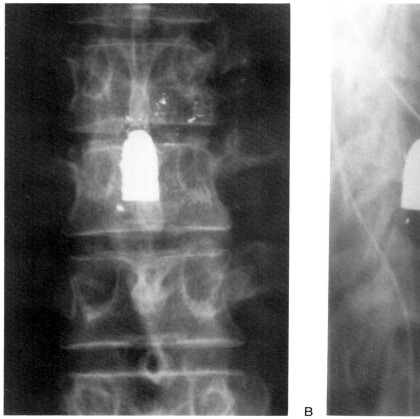
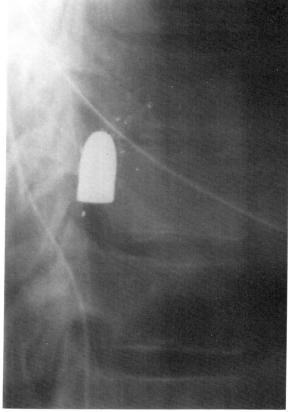

A   B

Fig. 10-43. Gunshot wound sustained by a 39-year-old man with a 38-caliber bullet coming to rest in the spinal canal. The wound of entrance was in the left thorax. **(A)** AP view shows the bullet within the canal. Note the small fragments to the left that outline the course of the bullet. **(B)** Lateral view confirming the presence of the bullet within the spinal canal. The patient was, of course, paraplegic.

the site of injury.[107] Missile injuries are usually associated with complete neurologic deficits, but deficits associated with stab wounds are often incomplete. The Brown-Séquard syndrome is particularly common as a result of stab wounds.

PATHOLOGIC FRACTURES

Metastatic disease to the spine commonly presents with a pathologic fracture, almost invariably a compression fracture of the vertebral body.

The radiographic feature that distinguishes pathologic from other fractures is the presence of an associated bony destruction, particularly involving the cortex of the vertebra (Fig. 10-46). Although the cortex of the pedicle is always mentioned in this context, the recognition of cortical destruction of any component of the vertebra is equally significant. The pedicles may not be involved by the malignant process and in fact are frequently spared in multiple myeloma. The history, of course, is strongly suggestive in that the injury may have been trivial. This does not, however, allow discrimination between an insufficiency fracture of osteoporosis and a pathologic fracture associated with

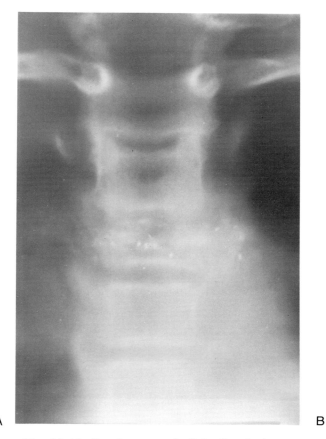
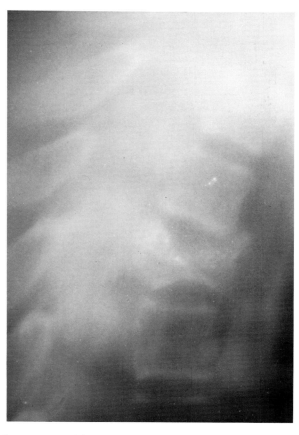

A   B

Fig. 10-44. Gunshot wound of the fourth thoracic vertebra sustained by a 6-year-old child. The bullet transited the vertebra. (**A**) AP tomogram. There is comminution of the involved vertebral body. The small metal fragments outline the course of the bullet. (**B**) Lateral tomogram. The section through the midportion of the vertebra demonstrates the comminution of the vertebra and a few small metallic fragments. The patient was paraplegic.

metastatic disease. The presence of a surrounding soft tissue mass is also suggestive of metastatic disease but could be due to a hematoma, particularly if the mass is small.

Pathologic fractures associated with metastatic disease may also present with depression of the superior end plate without overt evidence of destruction of the vertebral body or pedicles. Diffuse foci of metastatic disease throughout the vertebra may occur without causing cortical disruption, but weaken the vertebra sufficiently to result in a fracture. It is important to consider the possibility of a pathologic fracture in older individuals and to search for evidence of bone destruction, particularly when fractures are multiple or discontinuous.

Spinal cord deficits associated with metastatic deposits in the spine may occur abruptly owing to a sudden fracture and the formation of hematoma with compression of the spinal cord or cauda equina, or may occur more gradually by the growth of the tumor within the spinal canal. Tumors may grow in the epidural space without involvement of the surrounding bone. The degree and exact site of an extradural compression is identified by myelography.

Other forms of pathologic fracture occur but are rare. Vertebra plana is a distinctive form of compression associated with eosinophilic granuloma. A similar deformity may also occur in adults as a result of multiple myeloma.

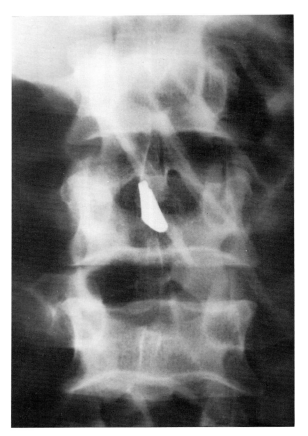 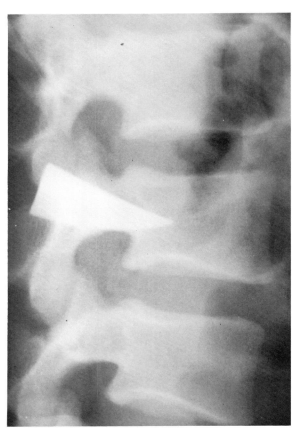

A   B

Fig. 10-45. Stab wound resulting in the severence of the L4–L5 nerve roots on the right in this 28-year-old man. (**A**) AP view. A metallic density projects through the third lumbar vertebral body. (**B**) Lateral view. This reveals that the metallic object is actually the tip of a knife blade. The patient was stabbed, and the knife blade broke during the struggle.

SPINAL FRACTURES IN ANKYLOSING SPONDYLITIS

Fractures of the spine in ankylosing spondylitis have a peculiar pattern owing to the rigidity of the spine and the associated osteoporosis of the vertebral bodies.[24,109–111] They are common in the cervical spine and are often related to trivial trauma, usually hyperextension forces.[42,110,112] The fracture characteristically involves the posterior elements and an associated intervertebral disc of the lower cervical spine, sparing the vertebral body. Similar fractures may occur any place within the spinal column, but are less common. The fracture traverses the syndesmophytes at the involved interspace and characteristically spares the vertebral body. Fracture-dislocations may also occur with the fracture line located in the same position.[42,110,113,114] The degree of displacement and resultant spinal cord injury are variable and depend on the degree of compromise of the spinal canal.

MYELOGRAPHY

The principal reason for obtaining a myelogram in the evaluation of spinal trauma is to identify a lesion that may be surgically attacked with the in-

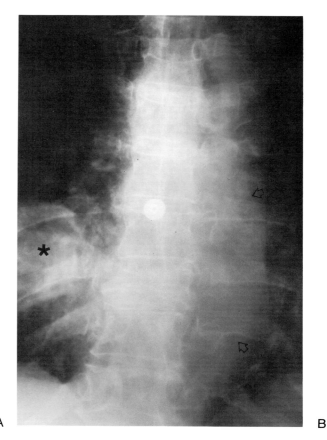

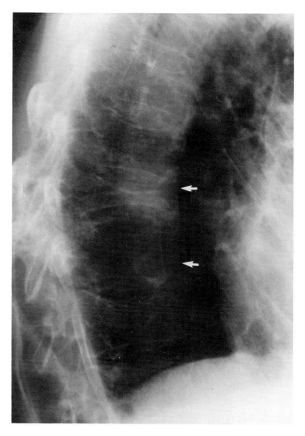

A

B

Fig. 10-46. Pathologic fracture of T9 from metastatic carcinoma of the lung in a 76-year-old man. (A) Compression fracture of T9 is evident, with destruction of a portion of the superior and inferior end plates. The pedicles, however, remain intact. There is a large paraspinous mass, particularly on the left (arrows). The primary tumor is in the lower lobe (asterisk). (B) The severely compressed vertebra is identified. There is cortical destruction at the anterior margin of the vertebral body and a soft tissue mass anterior to the spine (arrows).

tent of preventing, improving, or relieving a neurologic injury. Certainly, there is no basis for performing it routinely. There are risks involved in the use of myelography, not in the least of which is that it requires considerable manipulation of the patient. The examination is usually performed early in the immediate postinjury period and interferes with the initial stabilization of the patient. The use of contrast medium, either oily such as iophendylate (Pantopaque) or water-soluble such as metrizamide (Amipaque), is not without inherent risk. Pantopaque can lead to arachnoiditis, particularly if there is blood in the spinal fluid. Water-soluble contrast media may cause injury or insult as they are absorbed by the central nervous system tissues. These reactions include severe headaches, vomiting, meningismus, and infrequently a seizure. The arachnoiditis associated with the use of Pantopaque is much more commonly encountered if the spinal fluid is bloody or Pantopaque is left within the subarachnoid space. Every attempt should be made to withdraw all of the Pantopaque upon completion of the examination.

Gas myelography has had its proponents for use in the traumatized patient.[115] Gas myelography avoids the potential complications of the use of io-

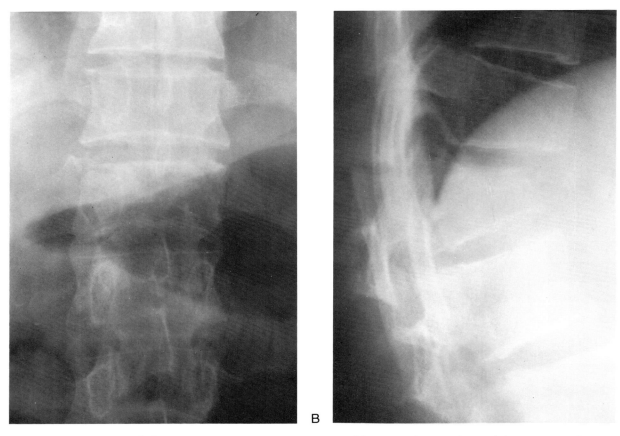

Fig. 10-47. Fracture-dislocation at T11–T12 in a 26-year-old man with paraplegia. **(A)** AP view. The compression fracture of T12 is evident. **(B)** Lateral view. A typical fracture-dislocation is demonstrated. *(Figure continues.)*

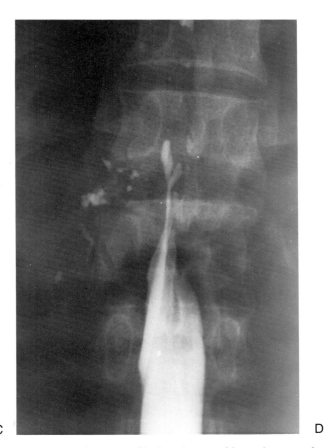

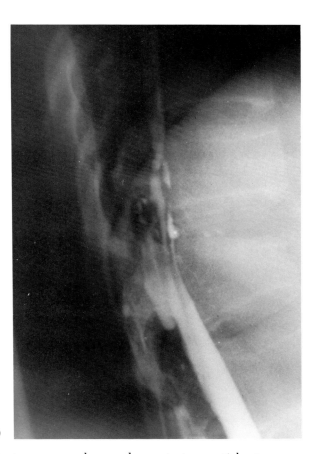

C

D

Fig. 10-47 *(Continued).* **(C,D)** AP and lateral views of Pantopaque myelogram demonstrate a partial extradural obstruction at the level of the fracture dislocation. Small amount of contrast medium is seen to flow proximally anteriorly in the right lateral aspect of the subarachnoid space. There is a dural tear manifested by extravasation of the contrast medium on the right.

dinated contrast materials, but the examination is more complicated, requiring tomography and considerable manipulation of the patient.

Myelography is indicated in the evaluation of suspected spinal injury to identify an operable lesion. It should be performed immediately after the patient has been evaluated clinically and has stabilized and when surgery is considered of value in alleviating or improving a patient's condition. The principal indications from myelography are as follows. (1) The presence of a spinal cord injury with a normal radiographic examination that has failed to disclose either fracture or dislocation. Under these conditions, the examination should reveal the cause of the spinal cord injury, be it a cord swelling from hematomyelia, hematoma, or possibly acute herniation of an intervertebral disc. (2) A neurologic deficit that is not explained by the abnormal findings on the standard radiographic examination. (3) A deterioration in the neurologic status or progression of neurologic injury that is unexplained by standard radiographic examinations.

The possible abnormal radiologic findings identified on myelography in spinal injury are the following.

Complete spinal block. The contrast medium will not flow beyond the level of injury because of obstruction of the spinal canal. This is usually associated with a fracture-dislocation and is caused by a compromise of the spinal canal related to the presence of displacement of the vertebral bodies, fracture fragments, and associated hematoma, both within the cord and in the surrounding extramedulary and extradural spaces. Most blocks encountered in the presence of a fracture-dislocation can be relieved by reducing the fracture-dislocation.

Partial spinal block. The causes of a partial spinal block (Fig. 10-47) are the same as those of a complete spinal blockage. Many complete blocks are converted to partial spinal blocks by reducing the associated fracture-dislocation.

Extradural defects without blockage. These indentations on the column of contrast medium are associated with extradural hematomas (Fig. 10-27B), fracture fragments, and, less commonly, herniated disc fragments (Fig. 10-48).

Avulsions of the nerve roots. These are particularly common in the upper extremity in association with trauma to the shoulder. The outpouchings develop at the site of the traumatized nerve roots. When the examination is performed early, after the injury, the contrast medium may extravasate freely through the side of avulsion, but later the contrast medium is confined to an irreg-

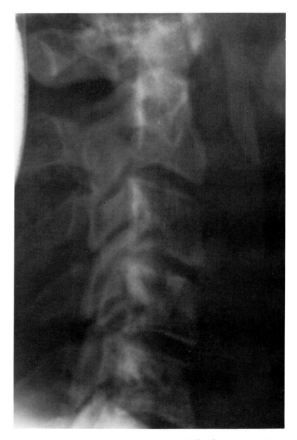

A

Fig. 10-48. Hyperextension injury with disc extrusion demonstrated by myelography in a 30-year-old man. (**A**) Cross-table lateral view demonstrates no evidence of fracture or abnormalities of alignment. The soft tissues anterior to the spine are considerably increased in width, indicating the presence of hemorrhage and suggesting a hyperextension injury. *(Figure continues.)*

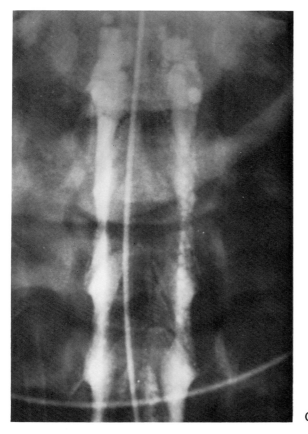

B

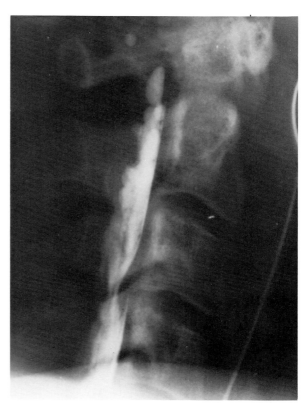

C

Fig. 10-48 *(Continued).* **(B,C)** AP and lateral views of Pantopaque myelogram. The **AP** view demonstrates no obvious abnormalities. On the lateral projection, there is an extradural defect anteriorly at the column of the level of the T3–T4 interspace that proved to be an extruded intervertebral disc.

ular pocket that extends laterally from the subarachnoid space. Avulsions in the lumbosacral nerves are less common but may be associated with fractures of the sacrum and dislocations of the sacroiliac joint.

Dural tears. Traumatic tears of the meninges, the dura mater, and the arachnoid may occur with both closed and penetrating injuries of the spine. The meninges are lacerated, allowing extravasation of the contrast medium out into the spinal canal and beyond (Fig. 10-31). The laceration may occur by puncture from bony fragments or by simply overstretching the membranes. The sinus tracks extend into the surrounding soft tis-

sues and may extend into the pleura or mediastinum.

Swelling of the spinal cord. The combination of hemorrhage and edema (hematomyelia) may cause the cord to expand over a length of several vertebral bodies gradually decreasing to its normal dimensions. The cord is expanded in both the sagittal and coronal plane, thinning the contrast column in both projections at myelography (Fig. 10-49). Extradural compression may also expand the cord but does so only over a short length and only in one plane. The distinction is readily made by viewing the myelogram in both the **AP** and lateral projections.

ANGIOGRAPHY

Angiography has a limited role in the evaluation of spinal trauma.[116] The demonstration of the spinal arterial tree has not been shown to be of any value in the care of the spinal cord-injured patient. While it is possible to demonstrate the anterior spinal artery in approximately 90 percent of cases, the posterior spinal arteries and in particular the delicate intraspinal network cannot be visualized. Furthermore, the examination is tedious and time consuming. To demonstrate the anterior spinal artery, it is necessary to perform a selective catherization of several arteries. In the cervical region, separate selected catherization of the vertebral arteries and the costocervical and thyrocervical trunks on both sides must be performed. The selective catherizations in the thoracic and lumbar regions are done on the intercostal arteries, the subcostal arteries, and the first two lumbar arteries on both sides to visualize the artery of Adamkiewicz. Two to 3 ml of contrast material are utilized in each artery. This amount is normally well tolerated. However, neurologic deficits have been reported after the injection of the artery of Adamkiewicz. To prevent this possibility, it is necessary to flush the catheter with normal saline immediately after the injection of

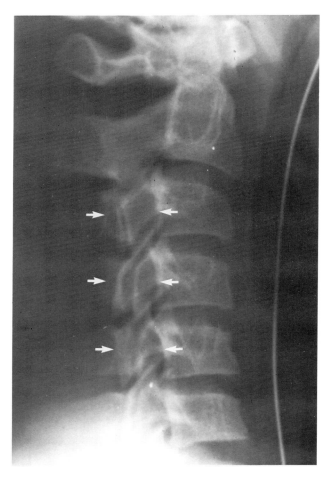

A

Fig. 10-49. Sixteen-year-old boy who sustained a hematomyelia without evidence of fracture or dislocation. (A) Lateral view of the cervical spine. There is a slight reversal of the curvature of the spine without evidence of fracture dislocation or dislocation. Note, however, that the depth of the spinal canal is narrowed as measured from the posterior margin of the vertebral body to the junction of the lamina (arrows). *(Figure continues.)*

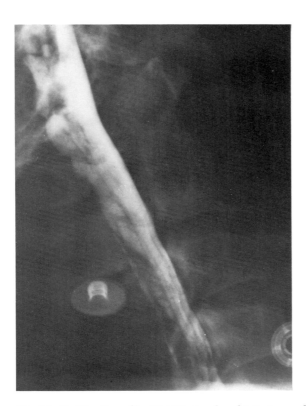

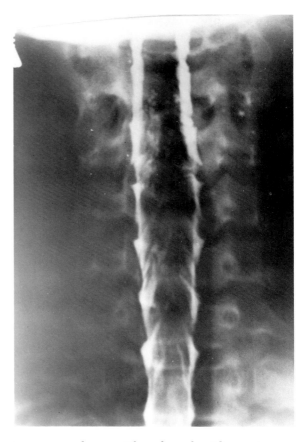

B

C

Fig. 10-49 *(Continued).* **(B,C)** Lateral and AP views of a Pantopaque myelogram. The subarachnoid space is in close apposition to the posterior margins of the vertebral bodies. On the AP view, the cord is diffusely widened over a long segment from C4 through T1. Findings are indicative of an intramedullary process, in this case a hematomyelia.

contrast medium into this artery. In any event, there is little or nothing to be gained by such examinations in the evaluation of the spinal cord-injured patient, and they are rarely, if ever, indicated.

On the other hand, there are occasions when examination of extraspinal vessels may be required. This is more commonly the case in penetrating injuries, particularly gunshot wounds. The missile that injured the spine may also injure surrounding arterial structures. This is often true in the cervical spine. The injury may result in hemorrhage with or without pseudoaneurysm formation or occlusion. The hemorrhage presents as a soft tissue mass, and occluded vessels present (Fig. 10-50) with signs of a cerebrovascular accident. These signs may be evident immediately upon admission but are often de-

layed in appearance for up to 72 hours. On occasion, torsion of the neck, particularly extreme flexion or extension, may result in a simultaneous injury of the spine and the carotid or vertebral arteries. Stretching tears the intima, which may lead to partial or complete thrombosis of the artery. An aortogram may be required to diagnose or exclude an aortic rupture in the presence of a widened superior mediastinum.

Although examination of the extraspinal vessels also requires selected catherization, it is much simpler to perform than spinal cord angiography since the clinical signs usually point to the artery in question and the vessles are of large size and readily visualized. Usually, only one or two arteries must be catherized to accomplish the examination.

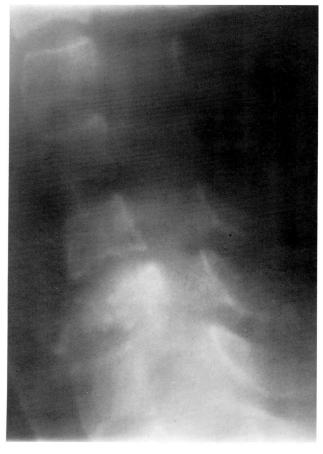

A

Fig. 10-50. A 26-year-old woman who sustained a gunshot wound to the neck. **(A)** Lateral tomogram showing comminuted fracture of the seventh cervical vertebra with posterior displacement of the spine. *(Figure continues.)*

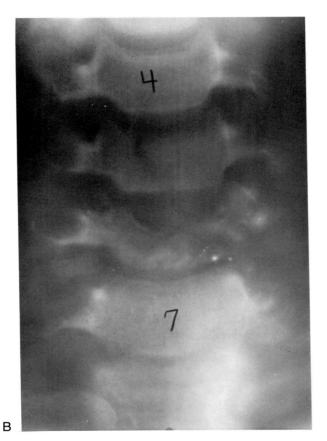

B

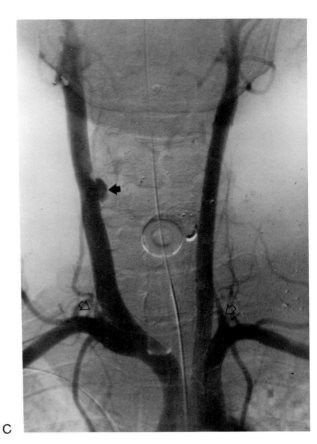

C

Fig. 10-50 *(Continued).* **(B)** AP tomogram. In addition to the comminuted fracture of the vertebral body, there is also a more or less vertical fracture of C5. Multiple small metallic fragments outline the course of the bullet. **(C)** An aortic arch arteriogram demonstrates bilateral occlusions of the vertebral arteries (open arrows) and a pseudoaneurysm (closed arrow) of the right common carotid artery. These vascular injuries occurred simultaneously with the neurologic injury owing to passage of the bullet. Numerous metallic fragments are demonstrated in the soft tissues on this subtraction view.

It is possible to demonstrate vascular injury by a simple venous injection alone, using digital subtraction angiography. This does not require a significant manipulation of the patient, is essentially noninterventional, and is as readily performed as an intravenous pyelogram. Ultimately, this may become the procedure of choice for the evaluation of vascular injuries in the traumatized patient.

REFERENCES

1. Rogers WA: Fractures and dislocations of the cervical spine: an end-result study. J Bone Joint Surg 39A:341, 1957
2. Stauffer ES, Kaufer H, Kling TF: Fractures and dislocations of the spine. p. 987. In Rockwood CA, Jr., Green DP (eds): Fractures. 2nd Ed, Vol. 2. JB Lippincott, Philadelphia, 1984
3. Calenoff L, Chessare JW, Rogers LF, et al.: Multiple level spinal injuries: importance of early recognition. AJR 130:665, 1978
4. Casey BM, Eaton SB, Du Bois JJ, et al.: Thoracolumbar neural arch fractures. JAM 224:1263, 1973
5. Russin LD, Guinto FC, Jr.: Multidirectional tomography in cervical spine injury. J Neurosurg 45:9, 1976
6. Laasonen EM, Riska EB: Preoperative radiological assessment of fractures of the thoracolumbar spine causing traumatic paraplegia. Skeletal Radiol 1:231, 1977
7. Deeb ZL, Martin TA, Kerber CW: Traction device for use with polytame table. Am J Roentgenol 131:732, 1978
8. Colley DP, Dunsker SB: Traumatic narrowing of the dorsolumbar spinal canal demonstrated by computed tomography. Radiology 129:95, 1978
9. Dershner MS, Goodman GA, Perlmutter GS: Computed tomography in the diagnosis of an atlas fracture. Am J Roentgenol 128:688, 1977
10. Sheldon JJ, Sersland T, Leborgne J: Computed tomography of the lower lumbar vertebral column. Radiology 124:113, 1977
11. Tadmor R, Davis KR, Roberson GH, et al.: Computed tomographic evaluation of traumatic spinal injuries. Radiology 127:825, 1978
12. Jefferson G: Discussion on spinal injuries. Proc R Soc Med 21:625, 1927–28
13. Hegenbarth R, Ebel KD: Roentgen findings in fractures of the vertebral column in childhood: examination of 35 patients and its results. Pediatr Radiol 5:34, 1976
14. Hubbard DD: Injuries of the spine in children and adolescents. Clin Orthop 100:56, 1974
15. Henrys P, Lyne ED, Lifton C, Scalciccioli G: Clinical review of cervical spine injuries in children. Clin Orthop 129:172, 1977
16. Horal J, Nachemson A, Scjeller S: Clinical and radiological long term follow-up vertebral fractures in children. Acta Orthop Scand 43:491, 1972
17. Kewalramani LS, Taylor RG: Multiple non-contiguous injuries to the spine. Acta Orthop Scand 47:52, 1976
18. Scher AT: Double fractures of the spine — an indication for routine radiographic examination of the entire spine after injury. S Afr Med J 53:411, 1978
19. Riggins RS, Kraus JF: The risk of neurologic damage with fractures of the vertebrae. J Trauma 17:12, 1977
20. Gehrig R, Michaelis LS: Statistics of acute paraplegia and tetraplegia on a national scale: Switzerland 1960–77. Paraplegia 6:93, 1968
21. Castellano V, Bocconi FL: Injuries of the cervical spine with spinal cord involvement (myelic fractures): statistical considerations. Bull Hosp Joint Dis 31:188, 1970
22. Burke DC: Spinal cord trauma in children. Paraplegia 9:1, 1971
23. Schneider RC, Cherry G, Pantek H: The syndrome of acute central cervical spinal cord injury. J Neurosurg 11:546, 1954
24. Wilkinson M, Bywaters EGL: Clinical features and course of ankylosing spondylitis. Ann Rheum Dis 17:209, 1958
25. Olsson O: Fractures of the upper thoracic and cervical vertebral bodies. Acta Chir Scand 102:87, 1951
26. Marar BC: Hyperextension injuries of the cervical spine. J Bone Joint Surg 56A:1655, 1974
27. Burke DC: Hyperextension injuries of the spine. J Bone Joint Surg 53B:3, 1971
28. Bentley G, McSweeney T: Multiple spinal injuries. Br J Surg 55:565, 1968
29. Gosch HH, Gooking E, Schneider RC: An experimental study of cervical spine and cord injuries. J Trauma 12:570, 1972
30. Kessler LA: Delayed, traumatic dislocation of the cervical spine. JAMA 224:124, 1973
31. Roaf R: A study of the mechanics of spinal injuries. J Bone Joint Surg 42B:810, 1960
32. Schatzker J: Fractures of the dens (odontoid process): an analysis of thirty-seven cases. J Bone Joint Surg 53B:392, 1971

33. Griffith HB, Gleave JRW, Taylor RG: Changing patterns of fracture in the dorsal and lumbar spine. Br Med J 1:891, 1966

34. Rogers LF, Thayer C, Weinberg PE, Kim KS: Acute injuries of the upper thoracic spine associated with paraplegia. Am J Roentgenol 134:67, 1980

35. Macnab I: Acceleration injuries of the cervical spine. J Bone Joint Surg 56A:1797, 1964

36. Whitley JE, Forsyth HF: The classification of cervical spine injuries. Am J Roentgenol 83:633, 1960

37. Holdsworth F: Fractures, dislocations, and fracture-dislocations of the spine. J Bone Joint Surg 52A:1534, 1970

38. Holdsworth FW: Fractures, dislocations, and fracture-dislocations of the spine. J Bone Joint Surg 45B:6, 1963

39. Howorth MB: Fracture of the spine. Am J Surg 92:573, 1956

40. Elliott JM, Rogers LF, Wissinger JP, Lee JF: The hangman's fracture. Radiology 104:303, 1972

41. Schneider RC: The syndrome of acute anterior spinal cord injury. J Neurosurg 12:95, 1955

42. Good AE: Nontraumatic fracture of the thoracic spine in ankylosing spondylitis. Arthritis Rheum 10:467, 1967

43. King DM: Fractures and dislocations of the cervical part of the spine. Aust NZ J Surg 37:57, 1967

44. Marar BD: The pattern of neurological damage as an aid to the diagnosis of the mechanism in cervical-spine injuries. J Bone Joint Surg 56A:1648, 1974

45. Taylor AR, Blackwood W: Paraplegia in hyperextension cervical injuries with normal radiographic appearances. J Bone Joint Surg 30B:245, 1948

46. Penning L: Prevertebral hematoma in cervical spine injury: incidence and etiologic significance. AJR 136:553, 1981

47. White AA, Hirsch C: The significance of the vertebral posterior elements in the mechanics of the thoracic spine. Clin Orthop 81:2, 1971

48. Schneider RC, Kahn EA: Chronic neurologic sequelae of acute trauma to the spine and spinal cord. J Bone Joint Surg (AM) 38:985, 1956

49. Penning L: Diagnostic clues by x-ray injuries of the lower cervical spine. Acta Neurohir (Wien) 22:234, 1970

50. Quesada RS, Greenbaum EI, Hertl A, Zoda F: Widened interpedicular distance secondary to trauma. J Trauma 15:167, 1975

51. Selecki BR: Cervical spine and cord injuries: mechanisms and surgical implications. Med J Aust 1:838, 1970

52. Zatzkin HR, Kveton FW: Evaluation of the cervical spine in whiplash injuries. Radiology 75:577, 1960

53. Gerlock AJ, Kischner SG, Heller RM, Kay JJ: The Cervical Spine in Trauma. WB Saunders, Philadelphia, 1978

54. Harris JH, Jr.: The Radiology of Acute Cervical Spine Trauma. Williams & Wilkins, Baltimore, 1978

55. Harris JH, Jr.: Acute injuries of the spine. Semin Roentgenol 13:53, 1978

56. Jacobs B: Cervical fracture and dislocation (C3–7). Clin Orthop 109:18, 1975

57. Abel MS: Occult Traumatic Lesions of the Cervical Vertebrae. Green, St. Louis, 1970

58. Hanafee W, Crandall P: Trauma of the spine and its contents. Radiol Clin North Am 4:365, 1966

59. Hohl M, Baker HR: The atlanto-axial joint. J Bone Joint Surg 46A:1739, 1964

60. Haralson RH, III, Boyd HB: Posterior dislocation of the atlas on the axis without fracture. J Bone Joint Surg 51A:561, 1969

61. Jacobson G, Adler DC: Examination of the atlanto-axial joint following injury. Am J Roentgenol 76:1081, 1956

62. Jacobson G, Adler DC: An evaluation of lateral atlanto-axial displacement in injuries of the cervical spine. Radiology 61:355, 1953

63. Alker GJ, Young SO, Leslie EV, et al.: Postmortem radiology of head and neck injuries in fatal traffic accidents. Radiology 114:611, 1975

64. Shapiro R, Youngberg AS, Rothman SL: The differential diagnosis of traumatic lesions of the occipito-atlanto-axial segment. Radiol Clin North Am 11:505, 1973

65. Sherk HH, Nicholson JT: Fractures of the atlas. J Bone Joint Surg 52A:1017, 1970

66. O'Brien JJ, Butterfield WL, Gossling HR: Jefferson fracture with disruption of the transverse ligament. Clin Orthop 126:135, 1977

67. Schlicke LH, Callahan RA: A rational approach to burst fractures of the atlas. Clin Orthop 154:18, 1981

68. Buckholz RW: Unstable hangman's fractures. Clin Orthop 154:119, 1981

69. Pepin JW, Hawkins RJ: Traumatic spondylolisthesis of the axis: hangman's fracture. Clin Orthop 157:133, 1981

70. Seljeskog EL, Chou SN: Spectrum of the hangman's fracture. J Neurosurg 45:3, 1976

71. Anderson LD, d'Alonzo RT: Fractures of the odon-

toid process of the axis. J Bone Joint Surg 56A:1663, 1974

72. Apuzzo MLJ, Heiden JS, Weiss MH, et al.: Acute fractures of the odontoid process. J Neurosurg 48:85, 1978

73. Southwick WO: Management of fractures of the dens (odontoid process). J Bone Joint Surg 62A:482, 1980

74. Lipson SJ: Fractures of the atlas associated with fractures of the odontoid process and transverse ligament ruptures. J Bone Joint Surg 59A:940, 1977

75. Seimon LP: Fracture of the odontoid process in young children. J Bone Joint Surg 59A:943, 1977

76. Fox JL, Jerez A: An unusual atlanto-axial dislocation: case report. J Neurosurg 47:115, 1977

77. Woodring JH, Selke AC, Jr.: Traumatic atlantooccipital dislocation with survival. AJNR 2:251, 1981

78. Kattan KR: Backward "displacement" of the spinolaminal line at C2: normal variation. AJR 129:289, 1977

79. Swischuk LE: Anterior displacement of C2 in children: physiologic or pathologic? Radiology 122:759, 1977

80. Babcock JL: Cervical spine injuries: diagnosis and classification. Arch Surg 3:646, 1976

81. Dolan KD: Cervical spine injuries below the axis. Radiol Clin North Am 15:247, 1977

82. McCoy SH, Johnson KA: Sagittal fracture of the cervical spine. J Trauma 16:310, 1976

83. Skold G: Sagittal fractures of the cervical spine. Injury 9:294, 1978

84. Richman S, Friedman RL: Vertical fracture of cervical vertebral bodies. Radiology 62:536, 1954

85. Miller MD, Gehweiler JA, Martinez S, et al.: Significant new observations on cervical spine trauma. AJR 130:659, 1978

86. Forsyth HF: Extension injuries of the cervical spine. J Bone Joint Surg 46A:1792, 1964

87. Beatson TR: Fractures and dislocations of the cervical spine. J Bone Joint Surg 45B:21, 1963

88. Harviainen S, Lahti P, Davidsson L: On cervical spine injuries. Acta Chir Scand 138:349, 1972

89. Braakman R, Vinken PJ: Unilateral facet interlocking in the lower cervical spine. J Bone Joint Surg 49B:249, 1967

90. Gehweiler JA, Jr., Osborne RL, Jr., Becker RF: The Radiology of Vertebral Trauma. WB Saunders, Philadelphia, 1980

91. Jonas JG: Fracture-dislocation of the dorsal spine. South Med J 69:1502, 1976

92. Nicoll EA: Fractures of the dorso-lumbar spine. J Bone Joint Surg 31B:376, 1949

93. Smith GR, Northrop CH, Loop JW: Jumper's fractures: patterns of thoracolumbar spine injuries associated with vertical plunges. Radiology 122:657, 1977

94. Rogers LF: The roentgenographic appearance of transverse or Chance fractures of the spine: the seat belt fracture. AJR 111:844, 1971

94a. Howland WJ, Curry JL, Buffington CB: Fulcrum fractures of the lumbar spine. JAMA, 200:167, 1965

95. Rigler LG: Kümmell's disease with report of a roentgenologically proved case. AJR 15:749, 1931

96. Das De S, McCreath SW: Lumbosacral fracture-dislocations. J Bone Joint Surg 63B:58, 1981

97. Drew R, McClelland RR, Fischer RF: The dominance of vertebral column fractures associated with neurologic deficits among survivors of light-plane accidents. J Trauma 17:574, 1977

98. Kaufer H, Hayes JT: Lumbar fracture-dislocation. J Bone Joint Surg 48A:712, 1966

99. Jacobs RR: Bilateral fracture of the pedicles through the fourth and fifth lumbar vertebrae with anterior displacement of the vertebral bodies; case report. J Bone Joint Surg 59A:409, 1977

100. Rennie W, Mitchell N: Flexion distraction fractures of the thoracolumbar spine. J Bone Joint Surg 55A:386, 1973

101. Fullenlove TM, Wilson JG: Traumatic defects of the pars interarticularis of the lumbar vertebrae. AJR 122:634, 1974

102. Melamed A: Fracture of pars interarticularis of lumbar vertebra. AJR 94:584, 1965

103. Wiltse LL, Widell EH, Jackson DW: Fatigue fracture: the basic lesion in isthmic spondylolisthesis. J Bone Joint Surg 57A:17, 1975

104. Dehner JR: Seatbelt injuries of the spine and abdomen. AJR 111:833, 1971

105. Smith WS, Kaufer H: Patterns and mechanisms of lumbar injuries associated with lap seat belts. J Bone Joint Surg 51A:239, 1969

106. Norrell HA: Fractures and dislocations of the spine. In Rothman RH, Simeone FA (eds), The Spine. Vol 2. WB Saunders, Philadelphia, 1975

107. Black P: Injuries of the vertebral column and spinal cord: mechanisms and management in the acute phase. Ch. 6. In Ballinger WF, Rutherford RB, Zuidema GD (eds), The Management of Trauma. WB Saunders, Philadelphia, 1973

108. Yashon D, Jane JA, White RJ: Prognosis and management of spinal cord and cauda equina bullet injuries in sixty-five civilians. J Neurosurg 32:163, 1979

109. Bergmann EW: Fractures of the ankylosed spine. J Bone Joint Surg 31A:669, 1949

110. Woodruff F, Dwing SB: Fractures of the cervical spine in patients with ankylosing spondylitis. Radiology 80:17, 1963

111. Yau ACMC, Chan RNW: Stress fracture of the fused lumbo-dorsal spine in ankylosing spondylitis. J Bone Joint Surg 56B:681, 1974

112. Rapp GG, Kernek CB: Spontaneous fracture of the lumbar spine with correction of deformity in ankylosing spondylitis. J Bone Joint Surg 56A:1277, 1974

113. Grisolia A, Bell RL, Peltier LF: Fractures and dislocations of the spine complicating ankylosing spondylitis. J Bone Joint Surg 49A:339, 1967

114. Hansen ST, Taylor TKF, Honet JC, Lewis FR: Fracture-dislocations of the ankylosed thoracic spine in rheumatoid spondylitis. J Trauma 7:827, 1967

115. Pay NT, George AE, Benjamin MV, et al.: Positive and negative contrast myelography in spinal trauma. Radiology 123:103, 1977

116. Bussat P, Rossier AB, Djindjian R, et al.: Spinal cord angiography in dorsolumbar vertebral fractures with neurological involvement. Radiology 109:617, 1973

11

Anticipated Urologic-Sexual Dysfunction

John B. Nanninga

Throughout history, the prognosis for neurological recovery has in some manner been based on some aspect of urologic function. The Edwin Smith Surgical Papyrus,[1] written between 2500 and 3000 BC, states that the patient with priapism and incontinence of urine has ". . . an ailment not to be treated." After World War I, statistics revealed that patients sustaining injuries to the spine that resulted in neurologic injury failed to survive the first year after trauma. After World War II, survival was only up to 10 years after injury. The causes for this high mortality rate were: chronic urinary tract infection (with the development of amyloidosis and renal failure) and respiratory tract disease. With increased study, research, and understanding of the clinical-pathologic process, and improved bacteriologic management, both of these causes have since been dramatically reduced.

Today, with advances seen in many areas of medicine, a great effort is being made to normalize the urinary tract function in the neurologically traumatized patient. This implies the early removal or non-use of indwelling urologic catheter systems, the prevention of urologic tract infections, the development of better urinary systems for women, the enhancement of male genital function, and the hope that neurologically impaired fertility of men can be improved. This chapter provides a historical and clinical–neurologic discussion of micturition. It also describes types of bladder dysfunction, bladder management systems, and sexual function in both the male and female.

BACKGROUND ON URINARY BLADDER FUNCTION

Normal micturition depends on three sets of nerves that innervate the urinary bladder.[2,3] The pelvic nerve is the main motor and sensory nerve for the detrusor muscle of the urinary bladder. The motor component originates in the intermediolateral column of the sacral spinal cord between the S2 and S4 levels. (Fig. 11-1). These preganglionic fibers travel to parasympathetic ganglia located near or on the surface of the blader or in the superficial layer of the detrusor muscle. Postganglionic fibers travel a relatively short distance to the smooth muscle fibers of the bladder. The sensory nerves arise from receptors in the bladder smooth muscle and enter the spinal cord at the S2 to S4 level. The sensation of bladder distention is most likely carried by the dorsal columns to higher centers. Pain and temperature travel in the lateral spinothalamic tract of the spinal cord. The sensation of urinating and of urine actually passing through the urethra seems, in part, to be carried by pudendal innervation. The sympathetic nerves to the bladder originate in the lower thoracic and upper lumbar segments of the cord. The preganglionic nerves travel to the hypogastric ganglia. The postganglionic nerves then course to the bladder, bladder neck, and proximal urethra. Experimental evidence suggests that some preganglionic sympathetic nerves actually innervate some parasympa-

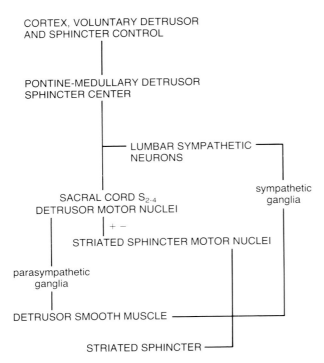

CORTEX, VOLUNTARY DETRUSOR
AND SPHINCTER CONTROL

PONTINE-MEDULLARY DETRUSOR
SPHINCTER CENTER

LUMBAR SYMPATHETIC
NEURONS

sympathetic
ganglia

SACRAL CORD S$_{2-4}$
DETRUSOR MOTOR NUCLEI

$+ -$

STRIATED SPHINCTER MOTOR NUCLEI

parasympathetic
ganglia

DETRUSOR SMOOTH MUSCLE

STRIATED SPHINCTER

Fig. 11-1. Diagram of the levels of the nervous system that control the urinary bladder. The cortex suppresses urination until the sensation of bladder fullness becomes overriding. Then the cortex activates the micturition center in the pontine-mesencephalic region, which in turn sends impulses down the cord to the sacral detrusor motor nuclei, which are activated (+), and the striated sphincter nuclei, which are inhibited (−). This produces a sustained bladder contraction and the passage of urine through an open sphincter. The voluntary interruption of the urine stream is accomplished by the detrusor area of the motor cortex sending impulses down the cord to the striated sphincter motor nuclei and then to the sphincter.

thetic ganglia. Their effect is to inhibit impulses that would otherwise be transmitted to the parasympathetic ganglia and parasympathetic postganglionic nerves.[2]

The pudendal nerve is a somatic (motor) nerve to the periurethral striated sphincter muscle, which surrounds the membranous urethra. It also has a sensory component that provides sensation from the urethra and genitalia. The sensation of urine passing through the urethra probably helps maintain the bladder contraction until no more urine is

passed. Impulses from the detrusor center in the brain stem also suppress activity in the pudendal nerve motor nuclei so that the striated sphincter muscle relaxes.[2] There also seems to be suppression of sympathetic activity.

An important part of storage and expulsion of urine is the function derived by the so-called external striated (periurethral) sphincter. This sphincter surrounds the membranous urethra and extends proximally and anteriorly toward the bladder neck.[4-7] This muscle maintains a certain amount of tone even at rest. Without conscious effort, its activity increases as the bladder fills, and thus it prevents leakage of urine. The striated sphincter tightens when a person assumes the upright position or coughs. When a person wishes to hold the urine voluntarily or interrupt the urinary stream, the external striated sphincter contracts. As the urinary bladder fills and reaches capacity and the person wishes to urinate, the striated sphincter relaxes just before the detrusor muscle contraction.[2,8] This sphincter relaxation allows the unobstructed flow of urine through the urethra, and the bladder neck assumes a funnel shape. An electromyogram (EMG) of the striated sphincter obtained during micturition indicates electrical silence.[8] At the end of urination, electrical activity in the striated sphincter returns. This relaxation of the striated sphincter has been shown to be a reflex that travels to and from the brain stem, near the location of the detrusor center.[2,3] The efferent limb is probably in the reticulospinal tract. The voluntary contraction of the striated sphincter seems to be part of the corticospinal system. Finally, evidence suggests that a certain amount of tension in the region of the striated sphincter (membranous urethra) may be due to sympathetic nerve activity, possibly through local innervation or from catecholamines via blood vessels.[9-12]

The role of the sympathetic nervous system on bladder function is somewhat less well defined. The sympathetic nervous system promotes storage and inhibits micturition. Laboratory data and clinical evidence suggest that sympathetic fibers, through a β-receptor function, inhibit the detrusor muscle contraction.[2] While an α-receptor function of the bladder neck and proximal urethra seems to cause the bladder neck to tighten and prevent incontinence, the sympathetic innervation of the proximal urethra also prevents the retrograde movement of semen into the bladder with emission and ejaculation.[13] Finally, as mentioned earlier, the sympathetic system inhibits transmission of nerve activity through parasympathetic ganglia.

BLADDER DYSFUNCTION

The destructive effect of spinal cord injury produces two types of urinary bladder dysfunction. Neither become immediately apparent after a spinal cord injury because of the period of spinal shock and the loss of detrusor reflex. As seen in Figure 11-1, when injury occurs above the sacral spinal cord, bladder function is expected to return because the local reflex from the detrusor to the sacral cord and back evolves. Usually several weeks to months elapse before bladder activity begins to return.

When the injury is above the sacral cord, the activity within the striated sphincter does not seem to be lost during the acute injury period.[14-16] The persistence of this sphincter activity thus prevents the bladder from expelling urine with external pressure. Later, when detrusor muscle activity returns, normal bladder and sphincter activity may or may not ensue.

Because the spinal injury interrupts the inhibitory activity of the higher nervous system centers, bladder capacity decreases. The patient also experiences loss of or altered sensation of bladder filling. Thus, the patient will not be certain when the bladder is about to discharge its contents, and incontinence occurs. A more serious result of the spinal cord injury is the interruption of tracts in the cord that bring about the reciprocal relaxation of the striated sphincter when the bladder contracts.[3,17,18] Thus, even though the bladder may develop a forceful contraction, it is working against a resisting force from the striated sphincter. To summarize, spinal injury above the sacral outflow spares the sacral parasympathetic motor neurons as well as the striated sphincter motor neurons. Although the bladder will contract, usually at less than normal capacity, it will do so against a sphincter that is not relaxing and that may be contracting. This condition has been referred to as vesicosphincteric dyssynergy. The result is decreased storage capacity and, to some degree, inadequate emptying because of the failure of the detrusor and sphincter to act in a coordinated manner.

The second type of bladder dysfunction is caused by injury to the sacral cord itself. In this case, the parasympathetic motor nuclei are destroyed and perhaps part of the peripheral nerves also. The result is detrusor areflexia. It may take up to 1 year to determine whether the loss of detrusor function is permanent. The areflexic bladder will, over time, develop increased tone and not be completely flaccid; however, it does not regain a true detrusor reflex.[17,18] The motor nuclei of the pudendal nerve may also be damaged from an injury to the sacral cord. The ability to contract the striated sphincter voluntarily will be lost, and the muscle will demonstrate EMG activity compatible with denervation.[19] However, the sphincter seems to maintain tension around the urethra, as evidenced by urethral pressure profile studies.[20,21] Based on the observation that sympathetic antagonists reduce resistance in the bladder neck and membranous urethra, the use of sympathetic antagonists has also been shown to improve voiding, particularly in patients with a low-level injury.[22,23]

Assessment of Bladder and Sphincter Dysfunction

Thus far, the discussion has centered on the expected alteration of function of the bladder after spinal cord injury. The tests that reveal the abnormalities are an important part of the overall evaluation and care of the patient with spinal injury.

Bladder function can be evaluated simply by having the patient, if possible, voluntarily urinate, followed by measurement of the amount of residual urine in the bladder, usually by catheterization.

A cystometrogram, in which the bladder is filled and pressure is monitored, will demonstrate whether the bladder contracts. To perform the study, the patient's bladder is filled with sterile fluid (50 to 60 ml/min) and the catheter is connected to a pressure-measuring device or instrument. In the acutely injured patient in spinal shock, the bladder will not show a contraction. Weeks or months later, the bladder reflex may return if the sacral cord and pelvic nerves are intact.

Along with this measurement, the activity in the striated sphincter can be recorded by inserting a needle electrode into the region of the sphincter.[8,24] In males, the needle is inserted through the perineum up to the membranous urethra area. In females, the periurethral striated muscle is more difficult to locate and the anal sphincter may be substituted because its activity tends to parallel that of the urethral sphincter.[25,26] Surface electrodes on the perineum or perianal region may be substituted for the needle electrode, but the signal is not as precise. The purpose of recording the sphincter EMG is to determine whether it is innervated and whether the sphincter increases activity as the bladder fills and then becomes silent when the bladder contracts. This combined study of cystometrogram and sphincter EMG (Fig. 11-2) is valuable during the recovery period. It provides an

opportunity to observe bladder function as it returns, and to document coordination between the bladder and sphincter function.[17,18,26] This assessment of the sphincter is really a more sophisticated method of determining the pudendal innervation to the pelvic floor than the bulbocavernosus reflex. This reflex will persist in patients who have the spinal injury above the sacral cord and is present shortly after injury. In fact, it may not disappear at all. In patients who have suffered an injury to the conus or cauda equina, the bulbocavernosus reflex is absent unless the injury is incomplete. A return of the reflex when it has been absent probably indicates some improvement in neurologic function. However, a more detailed study of the reflex is provided by the sacral latency.

A profile of urethral pressure also helps to determine the extent of function. The pressure in the urethra can be measured by withdrawing a catheter through which fluid is being perfused at about 2 to 5 ml/min and recording pressure change.[27] The withdrawal rate should be about 1 mm/sec. This study can also be performed with a transducer-tipped pressure-recording catheter, although it is somewhat difficult in males because of the curve of the urethra. Some investigators have used a multichannel catheter with membranes at various intervals from the tip.[28] This device allows the documentation of pressure changes in the urethra when the bladder fills and then contracts. Personal bias suggests relying more on the cystometrogram, sphincter EMG studies, and roentgenogram for documentation of urethral sphincter activity.

The bladder and sphincter can be studied by radiographic techniques.[29,30] A voiding cystourethrogram aids in documenting opening of the bladder neck or sphincter, along with the presence or absence of reflux of the contrast medium up the ureter (Fig. 11-3).

Another technique by which damage to the sacral cord can be determined is to stimulate the penis or clitoris and record the action potential in the striated sphincter with a needle electrode.[31–33] The normal value is about 30 to 40 msec (Fig. 11-4). Although this study does not define actual bladder innervation, it does record activity in the pudendal axis and helps to determine the extent of cord damage.

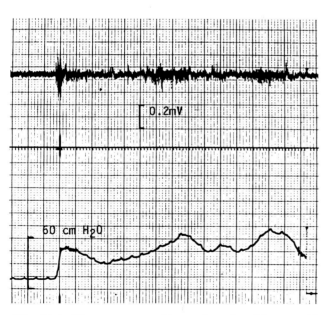

Fig. 11-2. Electromyographic tracing of an 18-year-old paraplegic man with an incomplete spinal cord injury at T10. The sphincter EMG (top line) shows sporadic activity during the bladder contraction (bottom line). This patient has minimal residual urine and has not shown any upper urinary tract deterioration in 3 years.

Fig. 11-3. (A) Normal voiding cystourethrogram, demonstrating the normal appearance of the bladder and urethra; both bladder neck and sphincter are open. (B) Voiding cystourethrogram was obtained from a T7 paraplegic male and demonstrates marked narrowing in the area of the striated sphincter. The bladder neck and prostatic urethra have been opened by the bladder contraction.

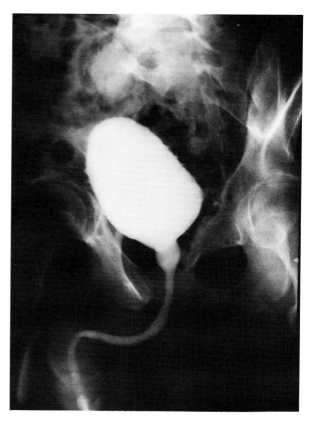

A

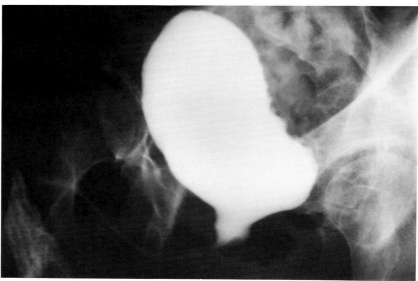

B

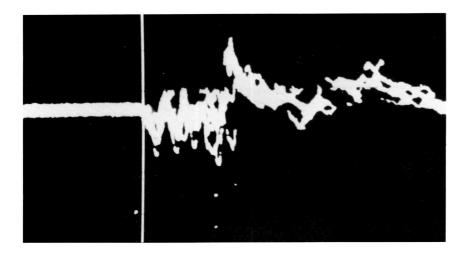

Fig. 11-4. Evaluation of the sacral cord performed by stimulating the dorsal aspect of the penis and recording through an electrode inserted in the perineum. This sacral latency was 31.5 msec.

MANAGEMENT OF THE NEUROLOGICALLY ALTERED BLADDER

Management of the bladder in a patient with spinal cord injury will depend ultimately on the recovery of bladder function and striated sphincter activity. During the period of spinal shock, some means to drain the paralyzed bladder must be provided because of detrusor areflexia. During the first few days after the injury, an indwelling catheter is used to provide continuous urinary drainage and monitor urine output. When the patient's condition has stabilized, the indwelling catheter is removed and the patient is started on intermittent catheterization.[34] This technique consists of passing the catheter under sterile conditions every 4 to 6 hours so that the bladder volume does not exceed 500 ml. The acute spinal injury service uses a sterile technique during the recovery period. If the return of bladder function is delayed for several months, the patient may then be on the clean catheterization technique, which is nonsterile.[35]

Alternatively, we have devised a system in which a catheter is carried in a latex tubing with both ends capped.[36] Inside the tubing is an antiseptic solution such as povidone-iodine or hydrogen peroxide. When the catheter is to be used, the patient uncaps the tubing, grasps the latex tubing, and exposes the catheter tip. Then the patient passes the catheter into the bladder, drains the bladder, and retracts the catheter back into the latex tube, adds antiseptic, and caps the ends. Such a system, while not perfectly sterile, has been very effective in keeping the urine sterile in the hospital setting. The incidence of urinary infection seems to be reduced by catheterizing the patient every 4 hours rather than every 8 to 12 hours.[37] Bacteriuria, however, has been reported as occurring in about 70 to 80 percent of patients during intermittent catheterization.[38,39] Urine culture should be done periodically or whenever clinical signs indicate infection. Prophylactic antibiotics are not recommended because of the risk of antibiotic-resistant bacteria. Infections are treated when they are detected.

According to the literature, the number of patients subjected to intermittent catheterization in whom satisfactory urination is achieved varies considerably. Somewhere between 26 and 95 percent of patients are reported as being catheter free.[40,41] But the catheter-free state often comes with complications. As detrusor function returns, the patient will begin to void small amounts of urine. If the injury is relatively incomplete, normal voiding usually begins within a few days to several weeks. For patients with a complete injury, the bladder is usually working against an obstructing sphincter (Fig. 11-5A, B).[17-19] I am skeptical of so-called bladder training in this situation. As the bladder regains function, the residual urine decreases and it appears that a balanced bladder is being achieved.

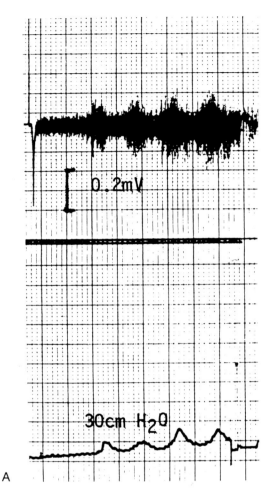

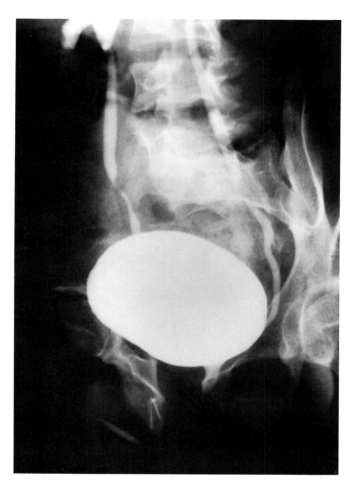

Fig. 11-5. Study of a 20-year old male quadriplegic about 6 weeks after injury. Note the beginning of the return of bladder activity as shown by the series of detrusor contractions (lower line). Coinciding with the bladder filling is a progressive buildup of sphincter activity with sudden bursts of activity as the bladder contractions occur. In our experience, most, if not all, patients demonstrating these findings will be prone to reflux or hydronephrotic changes unless some form of bladder drainage is instituted.

The bladder, however, is still working against an obstruction in many instances, and the patient is in danger of developing hydronephrosis months or years later.[42-44]

A total of 663 spinal cord injury patients have been analyzed by Y. Wu (Rehabilitation Institute of Chicago) during the past seven years. Like O'Flynn,[45] we found that approximately 20 percent of the patients had an incomplete injury in which the detrusor and sphincter functioned in a relatively normal manner. These patients have at least some sensation of bladder distention and a detrusor reflex. The sphincter functioned in a relatively normal manner (documented by the above-mentioned techniques), yet with occasional episodes of incontinence. Two patients in this group seemed to have a nearly complete spinal cord injury, yet had relatively normal bladder and sphincter function. Apparently, those tracts that bring about reciprocal relaxation of the striated sphincter muscle function during micturition had been spared.

In a second group of patients, 25 percent were able to manage the bladder with an external collector or diaper. This group exhibited loss of normal bladder and sphincter function. These patients usually experience detrusor hyper-reflexia and some loss of bladder sensation. The sphincter EMG displayed varying amounts of activity during a detrusor contraction (Fig. 11-6). These patients usually had residual urine below 100 ml, and 1 year later, had no evidence of hydroureteronephrosis. However, about 85 percent of this group are at risk in the future because of some degree of sphincter obstruction. Because of this, follow-up roentgenograms or renal ultrasound are advised.

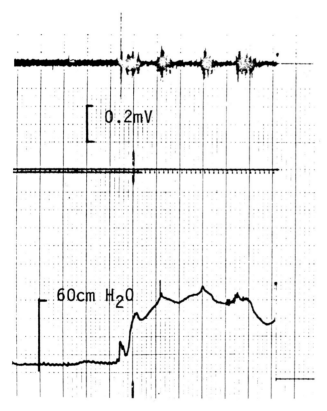

Fig. 11-6. Study of a 42-year-old male quadriplegic with a nearly complete injury who voided in spurts. The bladder pressure (lower line) demonstrates the episodic contractions, coinciding with the bladder contractions are bursts of striated sphincter activity followed by electrical silence. This sphincter activity accompanying the bladder contractions represents a form of vesicosphincter dyssynergy.

MANAGEMENT TECHNIQUES

When evaluation of the patient during the recovery phase or later points to definite sphincter dyssynergy, most patients are continued on long-term intermittent catheterization. Even this technique has hazards. In an analysis of 85 Northwestern patients who had long-term intermittent catheterization, approximately one-third developed reflux or hydronephrotic change on intravenous pyelogram (IVP).[48] To eliminate this condition, I found that patients must be catheterized every 4 to 6 hours, so that the bladder cannot become distended. In those patients with relatively high-pressure filling and detrusor hyper-reflexia, anticholinergic medication was necessary to lower detrusor pressure.[49]

Pharmacologic agents have been reported to reduce urethral resistance.[22,23,46] Northwestern University colleagues have used skeletal muscle-relaxing medication (baclofen) to reduce striated sphincter activity. I have not been impressed with the improvement. In patients with sacral cord injuries, some success results from giving α-sympathetic blocking agents such as phenoxybenzamine.[22,23]

The technique of anal stretch has also been reported as decreasing urethral sphincter activity.[47] This technique requires that mild force be exerted over the bladder so that the bladder contents can be forced through the urethra while the anal sphincter is stretched. Little experience has been obtained with this technique, except in the occasional paraplegic patient.

For patients with marked sphincter dyssynergy who do not wish to continue with intermittent catheterization, or who cannot perform this technique, sphincterotomy by the transurethral route is recommended for the male patient. Several centers have reported success with sphincterotomy and the removal of the indwelling catheter.[50-52] Initially, in my experience, 20 percent of male patients with spinal cord injury underwent sphincterotomy.[53] This percentage has decreased somewhat as more patients have been placed on long-term intermittent self-catheterization. Transurethral sphincterotomy consists of incising the periurethral (external) striated urethral sphincter in the anterior (12 o'clock) position.[55] This technique reduces sphincter resistance and decreases the incidence of impotence, which had been reported after sphincterotomy in the lateral positions.[54-56]

Sphincterotomy

The operation is performed with a standard resectoscope so that the tissue can be examined by the pathologist to confirm the presence of striated skeletal muscle and to confirm that the striated sphincter is incised. There has been little need for repeat sphincterotomy with this technique. The bladder neck is not routinely resected unless there is evidence of bladder neck hypertrophy or prostatic obstruction. Leaving the bladder neck intact seems to enhance the possibility of fertility in the patient's future. Vigorous bleeding may occur during the procedure and may necessitate coagulation of the bleeding points. After the resection of the sphincter, a 24 F catheter is inserted for bladder drainage and is left in place for 5 to 7 days. To avoid traumatizing the sphincterotomy site, a check for residual urine is not performed for at least 2 weeks. Assuming that the patient is voiding satisfactorily, a repeat excretory urogram is performed in 6 months to evaluate the kidneys. Urine culture should be obtained because of the relatively high infection rate after sphincterotomy.[57]

The importance of achieving a catheter-free state has been further emphasized by the finding of an increased incidence of bladder cancer in patients in whom an indwelling catheter has been used for many years.[58-60] Whether it is the presence of the catheter itself or the presence of infection that is responsible for neoplastic change is not clear. Although there may be other risk factors, it seems prudent to perform cystoscopy and biopsy on patients having a long history of indwelling catheter use.

Approximately 30 percent of our spinal cord injury patients eventually wear an indwelling urethral or suprapubic catheter. Slightly more than half of this group are high quadriplegics, while the remainder includes female patients who wear a catheter for convenience and patients of both sexes who have failed to adapt to other means of management. Generally speaking, these patients have not demonstrated any marked deterioration of renal function during the period of follow-up (8 to 10 years). Bladder calculi have been the most common complication.

The use of urinary diversion into a bowel conduit has decreased in frequency in recent years because of the success of other means of managing the urinary tract. The long-term complications from this procedure include stomal stenosis, calculus formation, ureteroenteric stenosis, and urinary infection. In some patients, however, urinary diversion offers a satisfactory means of renal preservation when other methods of treatment have been unsuccessful.[61] The recently developed technique of augmenting the bladder with bowel offers a chance for catheter removal.

URINARY TRACT CALCULI

Urinary calculi have been reported to occur in 5 to 25 percent of patients with spinal cord injury.[58] Several factors predispose the patient to stone formation: the presence of urea-splitting bacteria, an elevated urinary calcium level after injury, and immobilization and obstruction. Any one factor or combination can lead to calculus formation. Management that includes effective bladder drainage, early mobilization, and treatment of infection should reduce the incidence of calculi.

Upper tract calculi have occurred in about 2 percent of the patients on the spinal cord injury service. In the past few years, percutaneous stone removal and extracorporeal shock wave lithotripsy have provided a safe and effective means of removing kidney stones. For large branched or fragmented calculi, the technique of coagulum pyelolithotomy is helpful in removing multiple calculi.[62] For larger branched calculi, the technique of anatrophic nephrotomy may be necessary for removal of the stones.[63] This technique requires occluding the vascular supply to the kidney and using local hypothermia to reduce ischemic damage. With the above mentioned methods, the urological surgeon can remove all calculi. At at later date, predisposing causes of the calculi should be eliminated as much as possible.

Bladder calculi are most likely to be found in patients with indwelling catheters, but patients having intermittent catheterization have also developed bladder stones. Removal of the stones is usually performed by cystoscopy and litholapaxy or electrohydraulic lithotripsy.

Despite the various efforts and techniques to promote bladder drainage, an overview of the incidence of renal failure in the spinal cord injury population indicates that 20 to 40 percent of deaths are of renal etiology.[58,64] Factors other than infection, however, may cause renal damage. These include calculi, untreated reflux or hydronephrosis, analgesic overuse, and recurrent pressure sores, which are associated with renal amyloidosis. Interestingly, the study of Price et al., did not show any one method of treatment to be clearly superior to another.[65]

SEXUAL FUNCTION

The mechanism of penile erection involves the shunting of blood into the corpora of the penis. Evidence suggests that efferent impulses from the sacral cord, S2 to S4, through the pelvic nerve bring about filling of the three corpora through arteriovenous anastomoses.[66-68] It is not clear whether sympathetic innervation is absolutely necessary for erection. It is known, however, that interference with the sympathetic innervation does produce slower detumesence and retrograde ejaculation. The persistence of the erection requires maintaining a stimulus by the psychic mechanism (the erection is mediated through the sacral outflow).[66,67] It follows that if the sacral cord has been damaged, the patient will experience great difficulty obtaining an erection by local tactile stimulation. Conversely, if the injury spares the sacral cord but involves the sympathetic thoracolumbar outflow, then the psychic stimulation will be interrupted. Thus, the patient with sacral injury may obtain an erection by the psychic mechanism and the patient with a lesion above the sacral cord may obtain an erection by local means. About 90 percent of patients with lesions above the sacral cord will have erections; however, only about 25 percent of patients with a lesion of the sacral cord will have erections, although this number increases as the injury is less complete.[69] In patients in whom psychic erections would seem possible, psy-

chologic barriers after spinal cord injury may have to be overcome for the patient to function sexually. Evaluating the recovery of erectile function may take many months. In the patient with an incomplete injury, it may take up to a year to determine the extent of residual sexual function.

Emission and Ejaculation in the Spine Injured Patient

The phenomena of emission and ejaculation involve a coordinated action between (1) the sympathetic innervation to the vas deferens, seminal vesicles, and prostate to produe an emission of seminal fluid into the urethra and (2) the clonic ejaculatory function of the bulbocavernosus, and ischiocavernosus muscles.[5,13,67,70] With an intact sympathetic system to the genitalia, the patient may be able to produce a small emission of seminal fluid during sexual activity. However, there is a loss of the normal propulsive activity from the striated muscles of the perineum. If sympathetic outflow has been damaged, but the sacral cord has been spared, retrograde ejaculation of the semen into the bladder will occur because of the failure of the bladder neck to close. Electroejaculation has been used in an attempt to produce semen with adequate sperm counts for insemination and fertility.[71,72] The results of this technique have documented a deficiency of volume and number of sperm, although repeated stimulation has produced increasing counts.

The ability of a patient to sense orgasm depends on the degree of sensory intactness. Some patients have reported experiencing a vague sensation of orgasm at the level of injury.[69] Again, the amount would seem related to the extent of the injury.

The unilateral loss of a sacral nerve does not produce any marked loss of function except for anesthesia on the side of the injury.[70] Electromyography has documented the normal clonic activity of the perineal muscles during ejaculation in patients with unilateral nerve loss.[70]

Sperm counts seem to be low after spinal cord injury. One study indicates that the levels of follicle-stimulating hormone (FSH), luteinizing hormone (LH), and testosterone in serum are decreased at 2 weeks postinjury.[73] At 6 weeks, the values return to normal in paraplegic patients, but the testosterone level remains depressed for 4 months (in quadriplegics). In addition, a higher-than-normal percentage of abnormal sperm morphology has been noted in spinal cord-injured patients.[74] The mechanisms for this condition are not clear, but it would seem to be related to more than the gonadotropins and testosterone. Further studies are required to elucidate the abnormalities.

Female patients usually lose the normal menstrual cycle for several months.[75] With time or recovery from the injury, the usual menstrual cycle will resume. Complications resulting from spinal injury may delay menstruation even longer. Depending on the level of the injury, the patient may lose sensation over the area of the genitalia. The sensation on the perineum is thought to be at the S2 level. In females loss of sensation does not preclude sexual activity, and pregnancy can occur with the resumption of normal menstruation and the ovulatory cycle. During pregnancy, the patient should be observed for evidence of urinary tract dysfunction. If necessary, a limited IVP or ultrasound may be performed to determine the status of the kidneys. Near the end of the pregnancy, patients with automatic dysreflexia should be followed closely. Delivery may require an anesthetic, but drugs should also be available for blood pressure control.

CONCLUSIONS

Persons who have suffered a spinal cord injury will have alteration of urinary function unless the injury is incomplete enough so that the sacral micturition reflex is spared and the centers in the brain stem and cortex can send the normal signals to the bladder and its sphincter. If the spinal injury is complete and above the sacral outflow, a bladder reflex should return but the normal sphincter relaxation will be absent. If the sacral cord is damaged, the bladder reflex is lost and sphincter contraction is absent. Several treatments are available for patients depending in part on the presence or absence of the bladder reflex.

In complete spinal cord injury, the complex reflex system controlling erection and ejaculation is lost. Patients with an incomplete injury may have

partial function. The sacral cord controls the erection, and the sympathetic (thoracolumbar) system provides for seminal emission.

REFERENCES

1. Elsberg CA: The Edwin Smith Surgical Papyrus, and the diagnosis and the treatment of injuries to the skull and spine 5000 years ago. Am Med Hist 3:271, 1931
2. DeGroat WC, Booth AM: Physiology of the urinary bladder and urethra. Ann Intern Med 92:312, 1980
3. Bradley WE, Rockswold G, Timm G, Scott FB: Neurology of micturition. J Urol 115:481, 1976
4. Hutch JA: Anatomy and Physiology of the Bladder, Trigone and Urethra. Appleton & Lange, New York, 1972
5. Schroder HD: Anatomical and pathoanatomical studies on the spinal efferent systems innervating pelvic structures. J Auto Nerv Syst 14:23, 1985
6. Gosling J, Dixon J, Critchley H, Thompson S: A comparative study of the human external sphincter and periurethral levator ani muscles. Br J Urol 53:35, 1981
7. Lawson JON: The functional anatomy of the pelvic floor muscles and associated sphincters. p. 58. In Wilkinson AW (ed): Recent Advances in Pediatric Surgery. Grune & Stratton, Orlando, 1969
8. Hutch JA, Elliott H: Electromyographic study of electrical activity in the paraurethral muscles prior to and during voiding. J Urol 99:759, 1968
9. Bowman WC, Nott MW: Actions of sympathomimetic amines and their antagonists on skeletal muscle. Pharmacol Rev 21:27, 1969
10. Nordling J, Meyhoff H, Hald T: Neuromuscular dysfunction of the lower urinary tract with special reference to the influence of the sympathetic nervous system. Scand J Urol Nephrol 15:7, 1981
11. Clarke S, Thomas DG: Characteristics of the urethral pressure profile in flaccid male paraplegics. Br J Urol 53:157, 1981
12. Gibbon N, Parsons K, Woolfenden K: The neuropathic urethra. Lancet 2:129, 1974
13. Owman C, Sjoberg NO: The importance of short adrenergic neurons in the seminal emission mechanism of rat, guinea-pig and man. J Reprod Fertil 28:379, 1972
14. Gibbon N: Management of the bladder in acute and chronic disorders of the nervous system. Acta Neurol Scand 42:suppl. 20, 133, 1966

15. Rossier A, Ott R: Bladder and urethral recordings in acute and chronic spinal cord injury patients. Urol Int 31:49, 1976

16. Nanninga J, Meyer PR: Urethral sphincter activity following acute spinal cord injury. J Urol 123:528, 1980

17. Thomas DG, Smallwood R, Graham D: Urodynamic observations following spinal trauma. Br J Urol 47:161, 1975

18. Butler MR: Patterns of bladder recovery in spinal cord injury evaluated by serial urodynamic observations. Urology 11:308, 1978

19. Abel B, Gibbon N, Jameson R, Krishnan K: The neuropathic urethra. Lancet 2:1229, 1974

20. McGuire EJ, Wagner FC: The effects of sacral denervation on bladder and urethral function. Surg Gynecol Obstet 144:343, 1977

21. Sunder GS, Parsons KF, Gibbon N: Outflow obstruction in neuropathic bladder dysfunction: the neuropathic urethra. Br J Urol 50:190, 1978

22. Krane RJ, Olsson CA: Phenoxybenzamine in neurogenic bladder dysfunction. J Urol 110:653, 1973

23. Hachen HJ: Clinical and urodynamic assessment of alpha-adrenolytic therapy in patients with neurogenic bladder function. Paraplegia 18:229, 1980

24. Pedersen E: Electromyography of the sphincter muscles. p. 405. In Cobb WA, Van Duijn H (eds): Contemporary Clinical Neurophysiology. Elsevier Science Publishing, Amsterdam, 1978

25. Pedersen E, Harving H, Klemar B, Toring J: Human anal reflexes. J Neurol Neurosurg Psychiatry 41:813, 1978

26. Girard B, Minaire P, Casteran J, et al.: Anal and urethral sphincter electromyography in spinal cord injured patients. Parplegia 16:244, 1979

27. Abrams PH: Perfusion urethral profilometry. Urol Clin North Am 6:103, 1979

28. Tango EA: Membrane and microtransducer catheters: their effectiveness for profilometry of the lower urinary tract. Urol Clin North Am 6:110, 1979

29. Calenoff L: Radiologic assessment of the urinary system. p. 327. In Calenoff L (ed): Radiology of Spinal Cord Injury. CV Mosby, St. Louis, 1981

30. Thomas D: Clinical urodynamics in neurogenic bladder dysfunction. Urol Clin North Am 6:237, 1979

31. Ertekin C, Reel F: Bulbocavernosus reflex in normal men and in patients with neurogenic bladder and/or impotence. J Neurol Sci 28:1, 1976

32. Krane R, Siroky M: Studies on sacral-evoked potentials. J Urol 124:872, 1980

33. Nordling J, Anderson JT, Walter S, et al.: Evoked response of the bulbocavernosus reflex. Eur Urol 5:36, 1979

34. Guttmann L, Frankel H: The value of intermittent catheterization in the early management of traumatic paraplegia and tetraplegia. Paraplegia 4:63, 1966

35. Lapides J, Diokno AC, Gould F, Lowe B: Further observations on self-catheterization. J Urol 116:169, 1979

36. Wu Y, Hamilton B, Boyink M, Nanninga J: Reusable catheter for longterm sterile intermittent catheterization. Arch Phys Med Rehabil 62:39, 1981

37. Anderson RU: Nonsterile intermittent catheterization with antibiotic prophylaxis in the acute spinal cord injured male patient. J Urol 124:392, 1980

38. Ott R, Rossier AB: Intermittent catheterization in bladder rehabilitation in traumatic acute spinal cord lesions. Urol Int 27:51, 1972

39. Donovan W, Stolov W, Clowers D, Clowers M: Bacteriuria during intermittent catheterization following spinal cord injury. Arch Phys Med Rehabil 59:351, 1978

40. Gjone R, Ween E: Results of bladder training 1966-74. Paraplegia 15:47, 1977

41. Vivian J, Bors E: Experience with intermittent catheterization in the Southwest regional system for treatment of spinal injury. Paraplegia 12:158, 1974

42. Stover S, Lloyd LK, Nepomuceno C, Gale L: Intermittent catheterization: follow-up studies. Paraplegia 15:38, 1977

43. Sher AT: Changes in the upper urinary tract as demonstrated on intravenous pyelography and micturating cystourethrography in patients with spinal cord injury. Paraplegia 13:157, 1975

44. Rosen JS, Nanninga J, O'Connor VJ, Jr.: Silent hydronephrosis: a hazard revisited. Paraplegia 14:124, 1976

45. O'Flynn JD: Neurogenic bladder in spinal cord injury. Urol Clin North Am 1:155, 1974

46. Hachen HJ, Krucker V: Clinical and laboratory assessment of the efficacy of baclofen on urethral sphincter spasticity in patients with traumatic paraplegia. Eur Urol 3:237, 1977

47. Donovan WH, Clowers DE, Kiviat M, Macri D: Anal sphincter stretch: a technique to overcome detrusor-sphincter spasticity dyssynergia. Arch Phys Med Rehabil 58:320, 1977

48. Nanninga JB, Wu Y, Hamilton B: Long-term intermittent catheterization in the spinal cord injury patient. J Urol 128:760, 1982

49. Diokno A, Kass E, Lapides J: New approach to myelodysplasia. J Urol 116:771, 1976

50. Ross JC, Gibbon N, Sunder G: Division of the exter-

nal urethral sphincter in the neuropathic bladder: a twenty year review. Br J Urol 48:649, 1976

51. Schellhammer P, Hackler RH, Bunts RC: External sphincterotomy: rationale for the procedure and experience with 150 patients. Paraplegia 12:5, 1974

52. O'Flynn JD: An assessment of surgical treatment of vesical outlet obstruction in spinal cord injury: a review of 471 cases. Br J Urol 48:657, 1976

53. Nanninga J, Rosen J, O'Connor VJ, Jr.: Experience with transurethral external sphincterotomy in patients with spinal cord injury. J Urol 112:72, 1974

54. Kiviat M: Transurethral sphincterotomy: relationship of site of incision to postoperative potency and delayed hemorrhage. J Urol 114:339, 1975

55. Madersbacher H, Scott FB: The twelve o'clock sphincterotomy: technique, indications, results. Paraplegia 13:261, 1976

56. Schoenfeld L, Carrion H, Politano V: Erectile impotence. Urology 4:681, 1974

57. Hachen HJ, Ott R: Late results of bilateral endoscopic sphincterotomy in patients with upper motor neuron lesions. Paraplegia 13:268, 1976

58. Bors E, Comarr AE: Neurological Urology. University Park Press, Baltimore, 1971

59. Kaufman JM, Fam B, Jacobs S, et al.: Bladder cancer and squamous metaplasia in spinal cord patients. J Urol 125:196, 1981

60. Broecker B, Klein F, Hackler R: Cancer of the bladder in spinal cord patients. J Urol 125:196, 1981

61. Lieskovsky G, Skinner DG: Use of intestinal segments in the urinary tract. p. 2620. In: Campbell's Urology, W.B. Saunders, Philadelphia, 1986

62. Fischer C, Sonda L, Dickno A: Use of cryoprecipitate coagulum in extracting renal calculi. Urology 15:6, 1980

63. Boyce W, Elkins I: Reconstructive renal surgery fol-lowing anatrophic nephrolithotomy: follow-up of 100 consecutive cases. J Urol 111:307, 1974

64. Warren J, Muncie H, Bergquist E, Hoopes J: Sequelae and management of urinary infection in the patient requiring chronic catheterization. J Urol 125:1, 1981

65. Price M, Kottke F, Olson M: Renal function in patients with spinal cord injury: the eighth year of a ten year continuing study. Arch Phys Med Rehabil 56:76, 1975

66. Weiss HD: Physiology of penile erection. Ann Intern Med 76:793, 1972

67. Newman H, Northrup J: Mechanism of human penile erection; an overview. Urology 17:399, 1981

68. DeGroat WC, Booth A: Phsyiology of male sexual function. Ann Intern Med 92:329, 1980

69. Comarr AE: Sexual function among patients with spinal cord injury. Urol Int 25:134, 1970

70. Gunterberg B, Petersen I: Sexual function after major resections of the sacrum with bilateral or unilateral sacrifice of sacral nerves. Fertil Steril 27:1146, 1976

71. Brindley GS: Electroejaculation: its technique, neurological implications and uses. J Neurol Neurosurg Psychiatry 44:9, 1981

72. Francois N, Maury M, Jovannet D, et al.: Electroejaculation of a complete paraplegic followed by pregnancy. Paraplegia 16:248, 1978

73. Naftchi NE, Viao A, Sell GH, Lowman EW: Pituitary-testicular axis dysfunction in spinal cord injury. Arch Phys Med Rehabil 61:402, 1980

74. David A, Ohry A, Rozin R: Spinal cord injuries: male infertility aspects. Paraplegia 15:11, 1977

75. Bedrook GW: The Care and Management of Spinal Cord Injuries. Springer-Verlag, New York, 1981

12

Orthotic Management of the Spine

Mark L. Harlow   James C. Russ
Terrie L. Nolinske   Paul R. Meyer, Jr.

Since before the time of Hippocrates, external supports have been used in the treatment of spinal pain or deformity. Although the methods of management have changed considerably since that time, the goals of management have remained essentially the same. The protection and immobilization of the painful or unstable vertebral column are the keys to effective healing.

This protection and immobilization in most cases is more easily attempted than attained. The spinal column is composed of 24 presacral vertebral units that collectively allow substantial mobility. It possesses both intrinsic stability, provided by the intervertebral discs and ligaments, and extrinsic stability, provided by the attached musculature. With the extrinsic stability removed, it has been shown that a compressive force of only 4.5 lb is sufficient to topple the intrinsically supported thoracolumbar spine.[1,2] If a segment of this flexible rod is somehow damaged or disrupted, it is imperative that the end points be adequately controlled to ensure effective immobilization. Owing to the superficial inaccessibility of the spine, this can be achieved only by applying forces to interposed soft tissues or to contiguous bony structures.

The variations in type or design of spinal orthoses are as numerous as the disabilities they are used to treat, and their implementation is based largely on individual regional philosophy. Despite the multitude of alternatives available, the biomechanical

end results are often nearly the same. In an attempt to curtail the confusion over use of eponyms, the Committee on Orthotics and Prosthetics of the American Academy of Orthopaedic Surgeons (AAOS) developed a technical analysis form (TAF) that standardizes the nomenclature and provides an easily reproducible assessment of the biomechanics of the spine. This new nomenclature requires only the designation of the spinal segments to be encompassed and the types of controls that will be required. Thus, the contols needed, and not the specific components, are the foundation of the orthotic recommendation. In this scheme, a Knight orthosis becomes a lumbosacral orthosis with anterior, posterior, and lateral controls (LSO: APL control). This eliminates the need for the prescribing physician to have an extensive knowledge of orthotic components, and effectively utilizes the expertise of the orthotist.

The spinal TAF consists of four pages that provide a systematic and diagrammatic evaluation of the spine. The first page includes general patient information and a summary of muscular, sensory, and skeletal impairments (Fig. 12-1A). The second page contains a legend to be used in conjunction with the skeletal outline found on page three (Fig. 12-1B,C). Page 4 summarizes functional disability and identifies the treatment objectives (Fig. 12-1D). When this is completed, the orthotic recommendation may be undertaken and any special

TECHNICAL ANALYSIS FORM   SPINE   May

Name _____ No. _____ Age _____ Sex _____ Weight _____ Height _____

Diagnosis _____ Occupation _____

Present Orthotic Equipment _____

_____

    Ambulatory ☐   Non Ambulatory ☐   Wheelchair ☐

Standing Balance: Normal ☐   Impaired ☐   Walking Aid _____

Sitting Position: Stable ☐   Unstable ☐   Reclined ☐   Upright ☐

Sitting Tolerance: Normal ☐   Limited ☐

MAJOR IMPAIRMENTS

A. Structural: No Impairment ☐

    1. Bone: Osteoporosis ☐   Fracture ☐   Level _____

            Other _____

    2. Disc Space: (Describe) _____

    _____

    3. Alignment: Scoliosis ☐   Kyphosis ☐   Lordosis ☐

B. Sensory: No Impairment ☐

    1. Anesthesia ☐   Location _____

    2. Pain ☐   Location _____

C. Upper Limb: No Impairment ☐

    1. Amputation ☐ _____

    2. Other _____

D. Lower Limb: No Impairment ☐

    1. Limb Shortening: Right ☐   Left ☐   Amount _____

    2. Hip Contracture ☐   Ankylosis ☐   Flexion ☐   Degree _____

        Adduction ☐   Degree _____;   Abduction ☐   Degree _____;

        Extension ☐   Degree _____

    3. Major Motor Loss ☐   Location _____

    4. Sensation: Anesthesia ☐   Location _____;

        Hypesthesia ☐   Location _____

        Pain ☐   Location _____

E. Associated Impairments: _____

A   _____

Fig. 12-1. Spinal Technical Analysis Form. (A) Page 1. *(Figure continues.)*

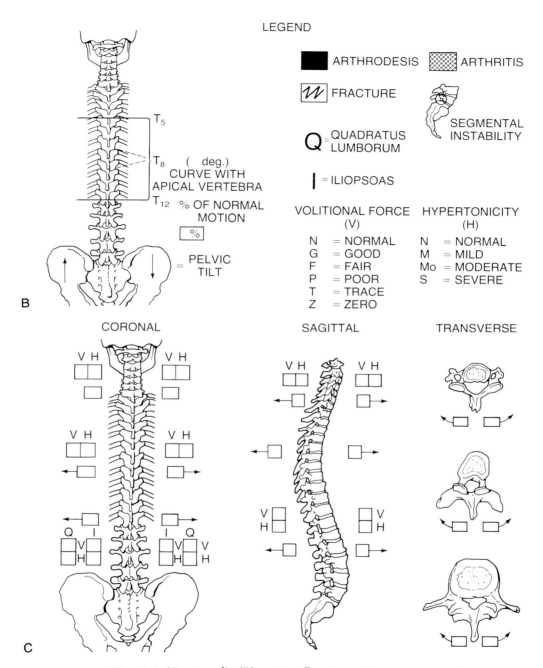

LEGEND

ARTHRODESIS   ARTHRITIS

FRACTURE   SEGMENTAL INSTABILITY

Q = QUADRATUS LUMBORUM

I = ILIOPSOAS

T₅

T₈ (deg.) CURVE WITH APICAL VERTEBRA

T₁₂ % OF NORMAL MOTION

%

= PELVIC TILT

VOLITIONAL FORCE (V)		HYPERTONICITY (H)	
N	= NORMAL	N	= NORMAL
G	= GOOD	M	= MILD
F	= FAIR	Mo	= MODERATE
P	= POOR	S	= SEVERE
T	= TRACE		
Z	= ZERO		

B

CORONAL   SAGITTAL   TRANSVERSE

C

Fig. 12-1 *(Continued).* **(B) (C)**   Page 2.   *(Figure continues.)*

Summary of Functional Disability _____

_____

_____

Treatment Objectives:

                   Spinal Alignment ☐   Motion Control ☐

                   Axial Unloading ☐   Other _____

ORTHOTIC RECOMMENDATION

SPINE		FLEX	EXT	LATERAL FLEXION R	LATERAL FLEXION L	ROTATION R	ROTATION L	AXIAL LOAD
CTLSO	Cervical							
TLSO	Thoracic							
LSO	Lumbar							
	(Lumbo sacral)							
SIO	Sacroiliac	▓▓▓▓▓▓▓▓▓▓▓▓▓▓▓▓▓▓▓						

REMARKS:

_____

KEY: Use the following symbols to indicate desired control of designated function:

    F = FREE   - Free motion.

    A = ASSIST - Application of an external force for the purpose of increasing the range, velocity, or force of a motion.

    R = RESIST - Application of an external force for the purpose of decreasing the velocity or force of a motion.

    S = STOP   - Inclusion of a static unit to deter an undesired motion in one direction.

    v = Variable - A unit that can be adjusted without making a structural change.

    H =   - Elimination of all motion in prescribed plane (verify position).

    L =   - Device includes an optional lock.

_____

Signature

_____

Date

Fig. 12-1 *(Continued).* **(D)** Page 3.

considerations regarding fabrication or component selection may be recorded under the section concerning remarks.

The role of the orthotist is an important one in the team-oriented approach to patient management. However, it should be pointed out that almost all spinal orthoses are interim measures to be used during the post-traumatic or postoperative healing phase. With few exceptions, a spinal orthosis should not be implemented without the intention that it will eventually be eliminated. In addition to the orthosis, a coordinated therapeutic regimen, which includes an exercise program and instruction in protective body mechanics, must be carried out to avoid the undesirable end result of a psychologic dependency on the orthosis. From the patient's point of view, the best orthosis is one that is invisible, weighs nothing, costs nothing, and lasts forever. In other words, the best orthosis is none at all!

This chapter focuses on the orthotic management of soft tissue and bony injuries to the cervical, thoracic, and lumbosacral regions of the spinal column. For each segmental level a plan for management will be suggested, and the advantages and disadvantages of several alternative treatment modalities will be discussed. Particular attention will be paid to pathomechanical considerations and their relation to orthotic design and usage.

CERVICAL SPINE

Acute Care

No discussion of orthotic management of the cervical spine would be complete without a brief mention of the acute care phase of treatment, which is addressed in greater detail in Chapters 1 and 2 of this book. If, at the accident scene (see Ch. 1), the victim has a suspected or confirmed spinal injury, an orthosis or some improvised form of support should be used for extrication and transportation to the hospital. A survey of ambulance and paramedical personnel in the Chicago area reveals that 50 percent use soft collars at the accident scene, 30 percent use a semirigid or rigid metal support, and the remainder use sandbags, air-

splints, or various personal designs. Although all orthoses serve the same purpose, some, most notably the soft collar, do not adequately limit the potentially deleterious rotary or flexion motions that may occur. As mentioned earlier, it is imperative that the end points of the highly mobile cervical spine (i.e., cranium and thorax) be encompassed if truly effective immobilization is to be attained. For this reason, the Meyer cervical orthosis, designed and developed by Dr. Meyer, is becoming increasingly popular (Fig. 12-2A,B,C). It is particularly useful in situations involving fractures or dislocations of the neck. It allows constant cervical spine immobilization or traction while permitting resuscitation or turning of the patient should emesis occur. Stabilization of the cranium and the cervical and thoracic spinal segments is accomplished with a gutter head support with forehead strap, straps over the shoulders and across the chest, a head halter, and traction straps. Moderate adjustable traction may be applied to allow maintenance of linear alignment during the extrication and subsequent manipulation of the patient. The orthosis is also very useful for interhospital transfers of patients with confirmed spine and spinal cord injury.

Soft Tissue Injuries

"Whiplash" is a term used to describe a hyperextension injury to the cervical spine, commonly identified after a motor vehicle accident. In the usual case, a stationary or slowly moving car is struck from behind. This sudden acceleration of the car and victim thrusts the head violently backward, stretching or tearing muscles and ligaments along the anterior aspect of the neck. This hyperextension motion of the calvaria on the cervical spine is followed by an immediate recoil into hyperflexion. This latter motion is rarely clinically significant, as the chin is usually stopped by the chest or steering wheel before damage is done to the extensor muscles or posterior vertebral elements. If there are no significant radiographic or neurologic findings, this injury is conventionally managed by some physicians with a *soft collar cervical orthosis* (CO), local heat treatments, and oral analgesics (Fig. 12-3). The soft collar offers little mechanical restriction to cranial or cervical mo-

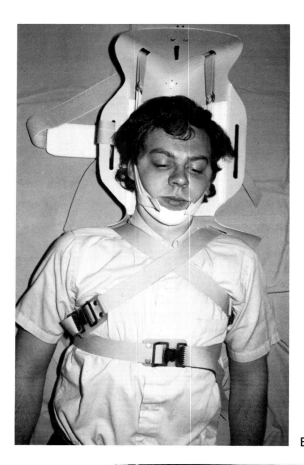

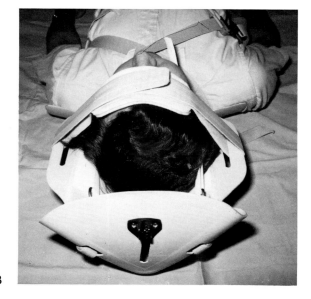

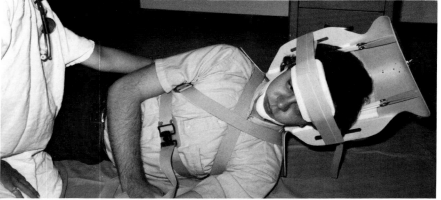

Fig. 12-2. (**A**) Anterior view of Meyer cervical orthosis (Zimmer USA, Inc.). Molded high-strength plastic cushioned V-shaped head rest and posterior extension to level of T12. Note 3-point suspension of posterior thoracic spine support to chest and head halter beneath chin and occiput. Head halter is under mild cervical traction by means of elastic straps visible superiorly. (**B**) Superior view showing position of head and neck in V-shaped support, head rest, and anterior forehead strap. (**C**) Patient in lateral decubitus position in Meyer cervical orthosis. Note that head-neck-thorax relationship is maintained during turning (for example, in case of emesis).

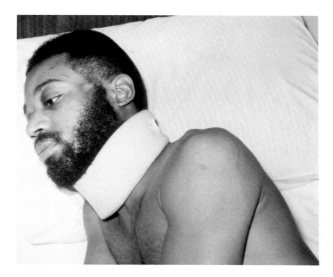

Fig. 12-3. Patient who suffered a motor vehicle accident. A cervical fracture was ruled out. Soft collar was applied for temporary neck support and kinesthetic reminder.

tion, but functions as a kinesthetic reminder. The collar may be fastened either anteriorly or posteriorly without any apparent detrimental effect to its clinical utility. This indicates the lack of stability gained by using this device.

Soft tissue injury may also occur as the result of a direct blow to the cervical region. In addition to contusions, neurologic findings may also be present. The latter are often exacerbated by the osteophytic lipping frequently seen in degenerative cervical osteoarthritis. This process is more common in the older patient. If treatment requires moderate restriction of motion, one of the *semirigid cervical orthoses* may be recommended. This category would include supports such as the *Philadelphia collar* (Fig. 12-4A), the *Thomas collar* (Fig. 12-4B), the *wire frame* (Fig. 12-4C), and the *Camp polyethylene collar* (Fig. 12-4D). Although studies have been conducted,[3] using radiologic and subjective measures to assess their efficacy, it is difficult to say unequivocally which form is the best. All have advantages. The prescribing physician must decide which best fit the needs of the particular patient. If strict limitation of motion is the primary

focus of treatment, these would not be the orthoses of choice.

If symptoms are severe or unusually persistent, a *cervicothoracic orthosis* (CTO) may be required. The extension of the orthosis to the thorax provides a much longer lever arm with which to restrict motion. Orthoses in this category include the extended Philadelphia collar, the sternal occipital mandibular immobilizer (SOMI), the four-poster, and the Guilford two-poster.

The *extended Philadelphia collar* is made of Plastazote with a Kydex superstructure that can be easily heat molded to provide an intimate fit (Fig. 12-5). It affords good mandibular and occipital containment to limit rotation and has long anterior and posterior projections to maintain flexion and extension control. Velcro straps at the neck and around the thorax serve to anchor the orthosis. When properly trimmed and adjusted, it is quite comfortable and is well tolerated by patients for both sleeping and daily activities. Since it is composed of a closed-cell material that does not breathe, the patient may chose to wear a T-shirt or body stocking under the orthosis for comfort.

The extended Philadelphia collar may be considered to be the Plastazote alternative to the Minerva and Queen Anne plaster casts (Fig. 12-6). The use of plaster is rarely indicated today owing to difficulty in hygienic care and excessive weight; however, it may be very useful on an interim basis for the disoriented or uncooperative patient. Plaster bandages may also, at times, be wrapped around the cervical portion of the extended Philadelphia collar to ensure that it remains in place. This may result in skin problems owing to the tendency of the material not to breathe.

The *SOMI* is so named for its points of contact with the body. It consists of a rigid metal anterior portion that serves as the point of attachment for the mandibular support, occipital support, and the crossed strapping arrangement (Fig. 12-7A,B,C). It is very effective in restricting flexion by virtue of the solid strut connecting the mandibular support to the sternal plate, but it is less effective in limiting extension owing to the long lever arm of the occipital support. A major advantage of this orthosis is that it may be applied in its entirety while the patient is supine with no need for logrolling. In addi-

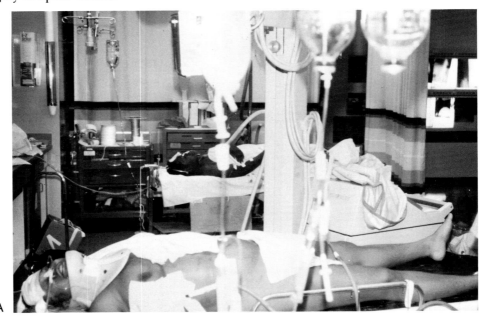

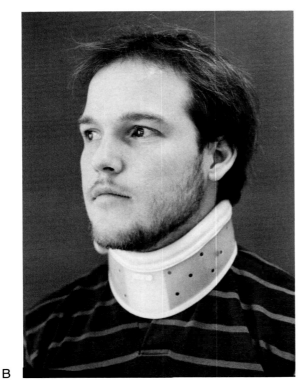

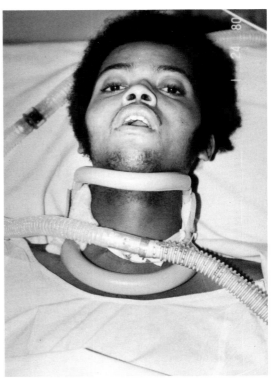

Fig. 12-4. (**A**) Emergency room scene with two cervical spine injury patients arriving simultaneously. Note in foreground patient with a Philadelphia cervical collar in place. This orthosis is used as a temporary cervical supporting orthosis by paramedics. (**B**) The Thomas collar, a nonrigid cervical orthosis. (**C**) Patient with a cervical spine fracture resulting in C5 quadriplegia. Patient required tracheostomy after cervical spine surgery. The ring orthosis shown was used for postoperative cervical spine stabilization because of the tracheostomy. *(Figure continues.)*

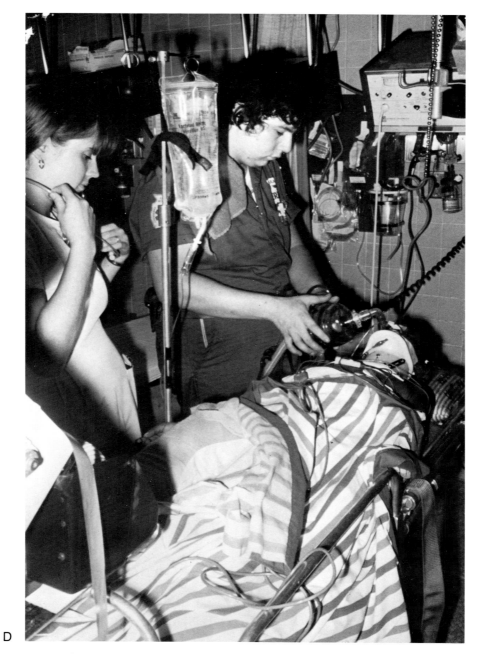

D

Fig. 12-4 *(Continued).* **(D)** Emergency room scene of a child requiring pulmonary resuscitation after occiput-C1 disassociation secondary to motor vehicle-pedestrian accident. Note adjustable rigid polyethylene collar about neck for temporary immobilization. Paramedics stabilized the spine and intubated the patient at the scene of accident.

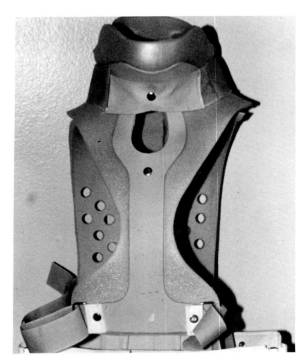

Fig. 12-5. The extended Philadelphia collar, made of Plastazote reinforced with Kydex, limits motion in all planes.

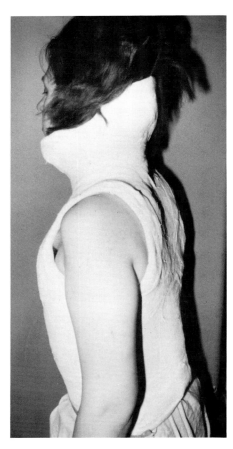

Fig. 12-6. Lateral view of patient who suffered a cervical spine fracture (C5–C6) managed conservatively in a Queen Anne collar cast. This method of immobilization is recommended over other light-weight orthoses when managing patients of questionable reliability.

tion, the optional forehead strap may be used when the mandibular support is removed for eating or shaving (Fig. 12-8). The **SOMI** is versatile and well tolerated.

The *four-poster* consists of anterior and posterior plates that give rise to four supporting rods that are connected to mandibular and occipital supports, which are in turn connected by straps (Fig. 12-9). It is capable of good flexion and extension control but not of control of rotation because it is suspended solely by straps that pass over the shoulders and lacks a circumferential thoracic strap. Thus, as the patient depresses the shoulder girdle, the entire orthosis may migrate inferiorly and will provide little if any encumbrance to rotation of the cervical spine. Experience has shown that it is not comfortable for sleeping and presents difficulties for eating.

The *Guilford two-poster* has both anterior and posterior plates to which are attached the mandib-

ular and occipital supports respectively. The fact that this orthosis has only two connecting rods, whereas the four-poster has four, is of no importance. The two plates are connected by thoracic and shoulder straps, while the mandibular piece slides into locking channels on the occipital piece (Fig. 12-10). This creates a rigid ring that is effective in controlling motion in all anatomic planes. Patients frequently report discomfort when wearing the orthosis while sleeping as well as some difficulty while eating.

None of the orthoses mentioned above are capable of supplying a constant distractive force, owing

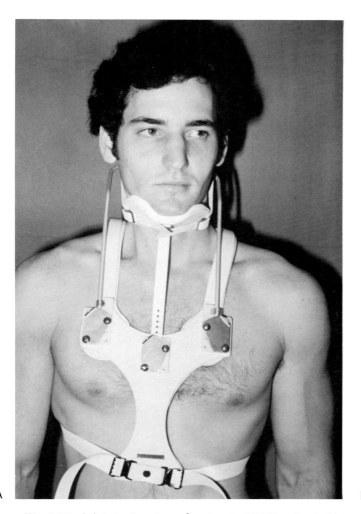

A

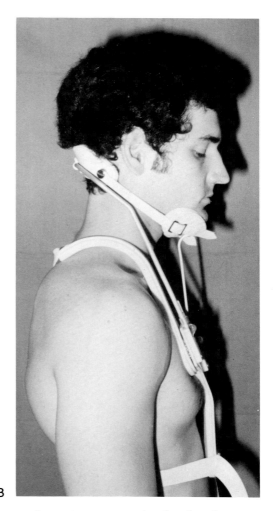

B

Fig. 12-7. (A) Anterior view of patient in SOMI orthosis. Note attempt by patient to rotate head and neck to the left. Stabilization can be improved by proper molding of chin piece and appropriate height of posterior upright. (B) Lateral view of patient in SOMI orthosis. Note position of posterior pad in close contact with posteroinferior surface of occiput. Because of wide range of adjustments possible with this orthosis, the head and neck may be placed in various positions of flexion or extension. *(Figure continues.)*

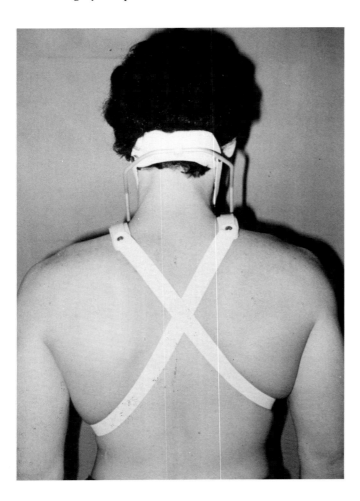

Fig. 12-7 *(Continued).* **(C)** Posterior view of patient in **SOMI** orthosis. Note crossing of straps posteriorly providing more stable orthotic extension.

to the obvious problems of ischemia in the area of the occiput and chin. For this reason, intermittent traction with a head halter may be used to augment the treatment regimen. Also, soft collars may be recommended for night wear for patients who have difficulty sleeping in more rigid orthoses and when rigidity is not a prerequisite, as it is in all injuries resulting in fracture, instability, and neurologic injury.

Bony Injuries

Quadriplegia, resulting from a fractured or dislocated cervical spine, is a most psychologically devastating injury. Owing to the catastrophic con-

sequences of neurologic complications, the cervical region requires management with the utmost care. Any skeletal disruption, no matter how minor, must be considered a serious injury.

Conventionally, bony and ligamentous injuries of the cervical spine are classified as being stable or unstable. Stable injuries, such as a mild anterior compression fracture, may be managed conservatively in a CTO after an appropriate period of bed care with reduction by either skeletal traction or surgery as indicated. The orthosis is worn for 10 to 12 weeks after injury (or surgery), or until there is radiographic confirmation of healing. The choice of a CTO should be based on the desired motion controls as dictated by the extent of the injury and the therapeutic objective, reliable immobilization.

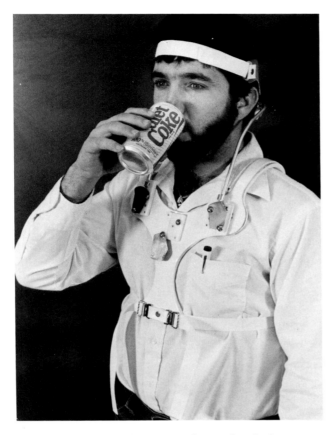

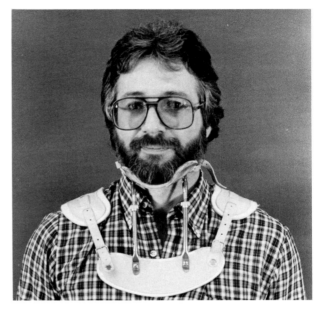

Fig. 12-9. The four-poster orthosis provides rigid flexion-extension control both preoperatively and postoperatively.

Fig. 12-8. A forehead strap may be used with the SOMI for continued rigid fixation while eating, drinking, or shaving.

Unstable injuries are initially managed in Gardner-Wells traction. In many instances this is a preoperative measure to obtain optimal reduction of cervical segments or fragments before operative intervention. If, after surgery, the spine is considered stable, a CTO may be used to protect and stabilize the operative site. The extended Philadelphia collar and the SOMI are perhaps best suited for this purpose as they are well tolerated by recumbent patients and will accomodate a tracheostomy. The Philadelphia collar has an anterior opening provided by the manufacturer, and the SOMI may be easily modified to provide this opening (Fig. 12-11). Although these orthoses are usually worn for approximately 8 weeks to 12 weeks,

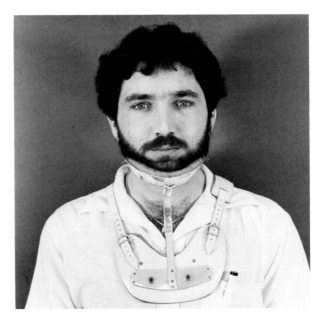

Fig. 12-10. The two-poster orthosis is a custom-made postfusion cervical orthosis.

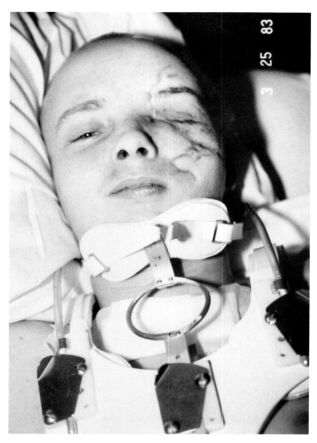

Fig. 12-11. SOMI orthosis with modification to accommodate a tracheostomy (O ring in anterior upright). Injury to face is typical of unbelted motor vehicle accidents. Face, head, and neck injury was secondary to dashboard-windshield impact. (Orthosis modifications by Superior Orthopedic Inc., Chicago, IL.)

the determining factor for term of wear is radiographic confirmation of bony fusion.

If the injury remains unstable after surgery, or if the patient was not a surgical candidate, the orthosis of choice would be the low-profile halo vest (Fig. 12-12A,B). The superior end point control provided by invasive cranial fixation makes it the most effective orthosis in the orthotic armamentarium for immobilizing the cervical spine. The sheepskin-lined pastic vest is preferred over the plaster cast alternative owing to cosmesis and concerns of skin breakdown in the patient without sen-

sation. The halo should be worn optimally for 12 weeks or, if there is no problem with cranial fixation, until there is radiographic demonstration of sufficient healing. Upon removal, the patient usually will not require a "step down" orthosis, but if this is so, the patient may be placed in a CTO for protection until it is determined that healing is complete.

Initial traction may also be achieved with Gardner-Wells tong traction (see Fig. 12-11A). Application of the ring at this time obviates the need for two additional pin sites. Regardless of when it is applied, it is of paramount importance that it be properly located and aligned. If the ring is askew, it is difficult to attach the superstructure and still maintain correct skeletal positioning in all anatomic planes.

When properly applied and maintained, the halo can be worn comfortably for as long as 1 year. If improperly aligned, it may be a constant source of discomfort for the patient and, ultimately, the surgeon as well. One of the most common causes of rejection is placement of the anterior pins in the temporal fossae. Ostensibly, this is done to place the small resultant scar within the hairline for cosmesis. This perforation of the temporalis muscle results in painful chewing and places the pin in relatively thin bone. Similarly, with constant motion of the skin and muscle over the pins, infections around this area are not uncommon. A more appropriate location would be in the lateral third of the frontal bone, which is thicker and provides a more durable fixation. Another frequent reason for rejection is the elderly patient who complains of the pins being too tight. To avoid this condition, the pins should be inserted with a torque value of 4 inch-pounds rather than the customary 5.25 inch-pounds.

As noted at the beginning of this chapter, a spine devoid of musculature possesses little inherent stability. For this reason, the patient with a cervical injury resulting in quadriplegia may need an external support to prevent or retard the progression of a kyphotic or scoliotic deformity. To achieve this support, a total contact, *bivalved thoracolumbosacral orthosis* (TLSO), commonly called a body jacket, may be indicated (Fig. 12-13A,B). The total contact provision ensures that the forces required for postural maintenance are distributed over a

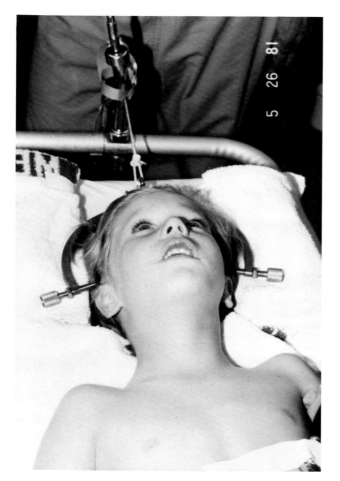

Fig. 12-12. (A) Three-year-old child after motor vehicle-pedestrian injury with fracture through epiphysis at base of odontoid. Child is in 2 lb of Gardner-Wells skeletal traction. (B) Postanesthesia view of same patient after application of low-profile halo vest orthosis. This device was worn for 3 months.

A

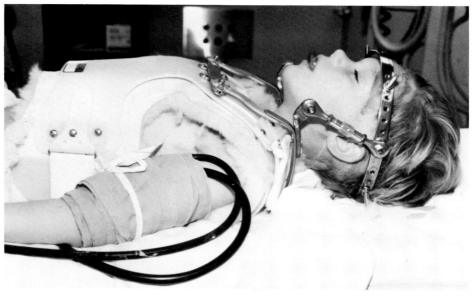

B

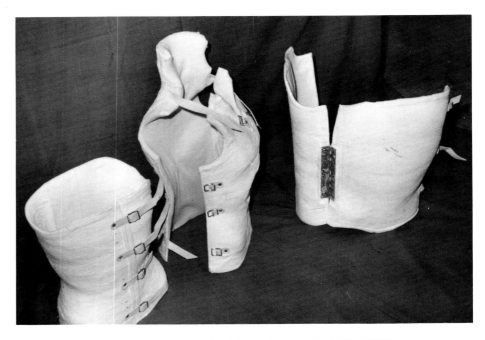

A

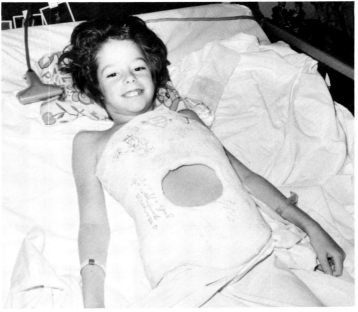

B

Fig. 12-13. (**A**) Three plaster jackets of various designs demonstrating the versatility of plaster for spine immobilization. Note moleskin lining (foreground) and stockinette sheet cotton lining (middle); and application of straps by brads with attachment of anteroposterior shelves through hinges. (**B**) Child with fracture dislocation of T10 – T11 requiring open reduction and internal stabilization. Patient was managed in hyperextension plaster body cast for 3 months. Orthosis extends from symphysis to sternal notch.

broad area, and the bivalved design facilitates donning and doffing. This orthosis, which aligns the thorax over the stable pelvis, provides the wheelchair-bound patient with sitting balance and thereby frees the upper extremities for other activities. If surgical stabilization is not undertaken, the body jacket becomes one of the few definitive spinal orthoses encountered.

THORACIC SPINE

The goals of acute-phase management of injuries to the remainder of the vertebral column are essentially the same as those discussed for the cervical spine. The primary concern is to prevent any secondary mechanical disruption of bony fragments that may result in either mechanical or vascular compromise of the spinal cord. Of the paramedics and ambulance personnel surveyed, they indicated that each vehicle was equipped with spinal stabilization-traction boards that were used if a bony or neural injury was even remotely suspected. Inclusion of the lower extremities on this support is important, as pelvic motion may affect spinal alignment.

The thoracic spine has several unique biomechanical features that may influence the nature of the injury and the subsequent course of treatment. These vertebrae, particularly the first seven, have the advantage of circumferential reinforcing members in the form of ribs that serve to minimize segmental displacement should a fracture or dislocation occur. However, even moderate displacement may result in spinal cord damage, as the vertebral column is relatively narrow in this region. The ribs may also be used to transmit peripheral orthotic forces to the thoracic vertebral column either directly, as with the thoracic pad of a Milwaukee brace, or indirectly via the sternum, as with a body jacket. The articular facets are oriented to allow the greatest freedom of motion in the transverse plane and as such do not easily accomodate flexion, extension, and lateral bending stresses. Furthermore, the seventh thoracic vertebrae is the transitional level for rotation of the vertebral column. During ambulation, the vertebrae above T7 follow

the shoulder girdle.[4] These factors must be taken into account when choosing a treatment regimen.

Perhaps the most commonly seen stable injury is the anteriorly wedged compression fracture of the vertebral body. After an appropriate period of bed rest, the patient with this injury is conventionally managed for approximately 6 weeks to 12 weeks in an anterior hyperextension TLSO, commonly known as a *Jewett orthosis* (Fig. 12-14). Anterior

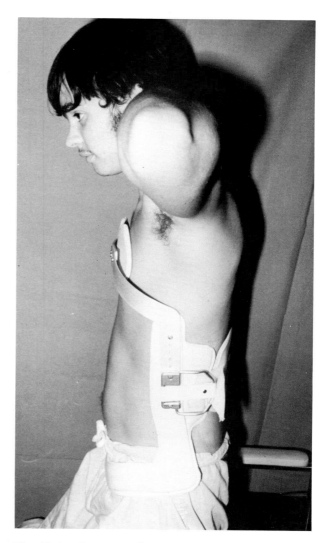

Fig. 12-14. Patient with 20 percent compression fracture of L1 managed in Jewett three-point hyperextension orthosis.

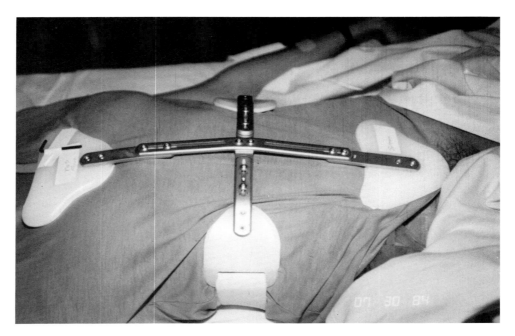

Fig. 12-15. Patient with burst fracture of L2 and incomplete neurologic injury with associated traumatic colon injury requiring emergency colostomy. The patient's spine injury was managed conservatively with a CASH orthosis. This orthosis is lightweight and has adjustable thoracic and symphysis pubis uprights.

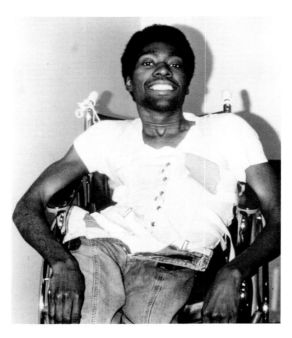

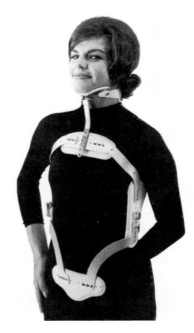

Fig. 12-16. Thoracolumbar corsets are lightweight and are less restrictive in providing thoracic immobilization.

Fig. 12-17. The Jewett anterior hyperextension orthosis with cervical extension is best used with lesions between T1 and T6.

pressures are exerted on the suprapubic region and the sternum, while a posterior counterpressure is applied at, or immediately below, the involved vertebral level. This three-point pressure system maintains spinal extension and prevents potentially damaging flexion postures during the healing period. The design of the Jewett orthosis makes it difficult in some cases to provide adequate breast and axillary relief and still maintain the desired control. For this reason, the *cruciform anterior spinal hyperextension* (CASH) orthosis is becoming increasingly popular (Fig. 12-15). It is lightweight, cosmetic, and well tolerated by most patients.

The anterior wedge compression fracture is frequently seen in the osteoporotic spines of the elderly. Generally, these patients do not tolerate an orthosis that is unduly restricting or uncomfortable. Therefore, a *thoracolumbar corset* is used (Fig. 12-16). Its biomechanical effectiveness may be less than optimal, but it is well tolerated and restricts the patient's activity sufficiently to serve as a protective reminder. The inclusion of rigid paraspinal stays increases flexion control and may help redirect bending and lifting activities.

The TLSOs described are effective for treating injuries that occur between T7 and T12. If the trauma occurs between T1 and T6, a cervical extension must be attatched to the TLSO to ensure adequate cephalad and point control, thus making the orthosis a CTLSO (Fig. 12-17). This concept is generally held to be true for all categories of fractures and dislocations of the thoracic spine.

The management of stable injuries generally requires the limitation of gross motion in only one plane, whereas unstable injuries require three-dimensional control. The total contact bivalved TLSO offers a virtually infinite number of three-point force systems to restrict motion. When extended to the level of the manubrium, it is particularly effective in controlling the rotational strains that may dislodge the Harrington rod hooks during the healing phase. In addition, it may serve as an excellent vehicle for the attachment of a cervical extension. The patient wearing a CTLSO should also be given a CTO for night wear until healing is complete. Should the trauma result in paralysis, this orthosis has the option of being used nondefinitively.

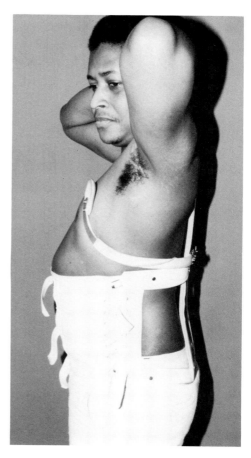

Fig. 12-18. Lateral view of Knight-Taylor orthosis with pectoral horns on a patient with a compression fracture of L1 requiring internal stabilization and fusion. Note abdominal apron to maintain stable fixation between abdomen and thoracolumbar area of spine against posterior metal uprights. Pectoral horns help to maintain extension of upper thoracic spine and to prevent kyphosis with axial loading.

An alternative to this orthosis is the *Knight-Taylor TLSO with pectoral extensions* (Fig. 12-18). This orthosis consists of pelvic and thoracic bands connected posteriorly by rigid paraspinal bars and anteriorly by an abdominal apron or corset. The thoracic band is extended anteriorly and superiorly to the infraclavicular region to provide rotary control. It will also accommodate a cervical extension when necessary (Fig. 12-19A,B,C). These two thoraco-

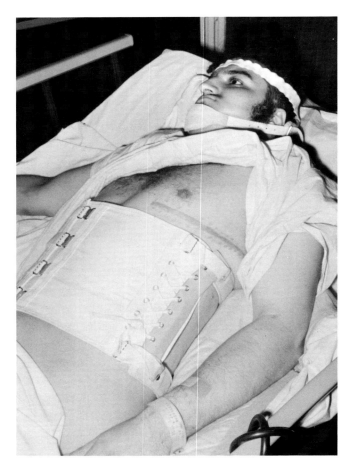

A

B

Fig. 12-19. (A) Patient with postoperative fracture dislocation of C3–C4 and fracture dislocation of T5–T6 with T5 complete paraplegia. Note abdominal apron attached to Knight-Taylor frame and anterior forehead and chin strap attached to cervical upright. (B) Posterior view. Note cervical extension attached to midportion of Knight-Taylor frame. *(Figure continues.)*

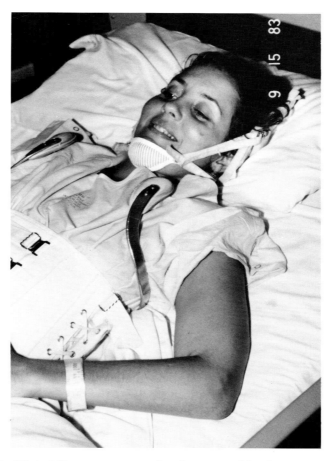

Fig. 12-19 *(Continued).* (C) A different patient with a flexion axial load compression fracture of T5 with associated hemopneumothorax from multiple fractured ribs. She is neurologically normal. Note addition of pectoral horns to Knight-Taylor orthosis with cervical extension. Pectoral horns further ensure maintenance of extension of upper thoracic segment.

lumbar orthoses, the Knight-Taylor TLSO with pectoral horns and the Knight-Taylor TLSO with cervical extension (Figs. 12-18 and 19), along with the SOMI orthosis (Fig. 12-7A,B) for fractures of the cervical spine, are the three most frequently prescribed orthoses on the acute spinal injury unit at Northwestern University. The Knight-Taylor TLSO with pectoral horns is less effective than the *total contact TLSO* in controlling alignment (Fig. 12-20), but many patients prefer it because it is cooler and less bulky. Another advantage is that it is easily adjusted if the patient loses weight during

the course of rehabilitation. Length of wear is approximately 8 weeks to 12 weeks but is contingent upon radiographic confirmation of healing.

A final note on thoracic orthoses pertains to the use of axillary straps. The shoulder girdle is attached to the axial skeleton only at the sternoclavicular joint and is highly mobile on the thorax. Axillary straps serve to retract the shoulders and have very little direct effect on the thoracic spine. In selected cases, they may provide an inductive effect, but they should be used judiciously. If a more substantial application of force through the

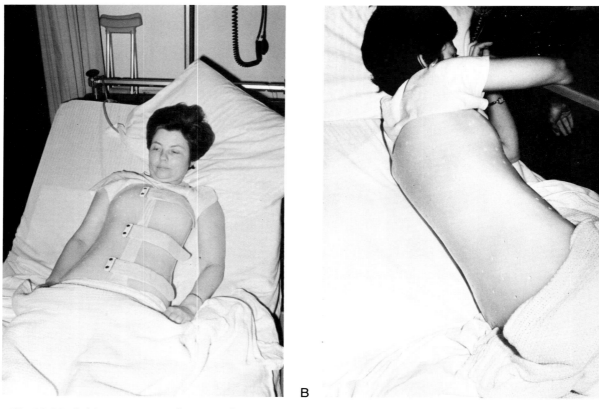

A   B

Fig. 12-20. (A) Anterior view of patient after compression fracture dislocation of vertebral body at T12–L1 requiring operative stabilization. Molded plastic orthosis with cushioned lining extending from sternal notch to pubic symphysis was used for external immobilization. (B) Lateral view of molded plastic jacket. Note uniform placement of holes in jacket to improve breathing.

ribs to the spinal column is required, either a sternal pad or two infraclavicular (pectoral) pads should be prescribed.

LUMBOSACRAL SPINE

Undoubtably, the most difficult portion of the spine to manage orthotically is the lumbosacral region. Effective immobilization of this area requires fixation of the pelvis and is exceedingly difficult to achieve by noninvasive methods. The use of orthoses for low-back injuries is a controversial subject; however, if used within the context of a compre-

hensive management plan, they may be valuable adjuncts to treatment.

Soft tissue injuries without fractures, such as strains and sprains, are usually managed by bed rest, medication, and admonitions to use proper body mechanics. If symptoms are persistent, a *lumbosacral orthosis* (LSO) may be recommended. Prolonged use of the LSO will weaken the abdominal musculature. Therefore, the orthosis should not be prescribed without a concomitant plan of exercise. The LSO corset is frequently used to treat this type of patient (Fig. 12-21). It offers moderate restriction of motion and can partially unload the spinal column. It achieves this latter effect by increasing the pressure within the abdominal and thoracic cavities. It has been shown that during daily activi-

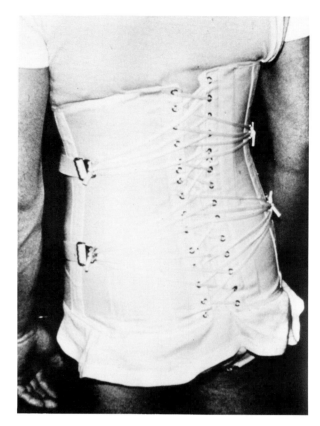

Fig. 12-21. A lumbosacral corset offers support for soft tissue injuries.

ties, this elevation of pressure reduces the load borne by the intervertebral discs by 30 percent in the lumbar spine and by as much as 50 percent in the thoracic spine.[4] Furthermore, if rigid paraspinal stays are incorporated into the corset, it can reduce lumbar lordosis and thereby relieve pressure on the posterior vertebral elements.

If more substantial restriction of motion is required, a Knight or chairback LSO may be applied. The Knight LSO consists of pelvic and thoracic bands connected by paraspinal and lateral bars (Fig. 12-22). The chairback LSO differs only in that it lacks lateral supports and should therefore not be used when strict control of side bending is needed. The paraspinal bars are contoured to allow the reduction of lordosis, and the orthosis is held in its proper position either by an abdominal apron or by wrapping a corset entirely around it. To be effec-

tive, it must be worn as tightly as comfort will allow. It cannot be emphasized enough that these orthoses should be worn only until symptoms subside. If necessary, a brief weaning period may be allowed.

As in the cervical and thoracic regions, fractures and dislocations of the lumbar and sacral spine are categorized as stable or unstable, and the goals of management remain fundamentally the same as outlined above for the cervical and thoracic regions. Immobilization and protection remain the essential ingredients for expeditious and effective healing.

For the patient with a stable fracture, such as an unstable fracture that has been surgically stabilized, a rigid TLSO is usually prescribed (Fig. 12-18), preferred, and conventionally recommended, although the reliable patient may require only the LSO. The point to appreciate is that regardless any TLSO or LSO will perform the desired function if it meets the following criteria: (1) ab-

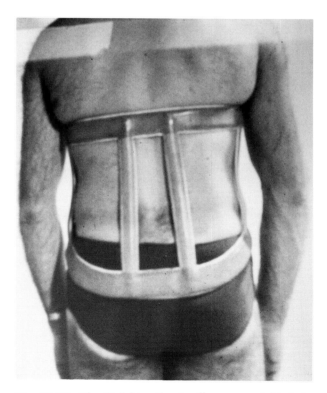

Fig. 12-22. The Knight orthosis offers more rigid skeletal immobilization than a corset.

dominal compression must be supplied to elevate intracavitary pressure and provide the necessary component of axial unloading; (2) the orthosis must provide reasonable caudad end point control; (3) if the pelvic band or strap is inappropriately located or insufficiently tightened, it may in fact increase the motion at the lumbosacral junction;[5] and (4) it must encompass the upper thoracic spine (as high as T6) for the TLSO and the lower thoracic spine to obtain adequate cephalad end point control. It must include rigid paraspinal or lateral controls or both to maintain upright postures. If these criteria are met, the TSO and LSO will serve their purpose as a supportive measure in healing and alleviating symptoms.

The patient with an unstable fracture in the upper lumbar region or one who is considered unstable after a surgical procedure is managed only in a TLSO. Both the body jacket and the Knight-Taylor TLSO with pectoral extensions have given excellent results. A plaster body cast may occasionally be used for the unreliable patient, but a concern is covering insensitive skin for long periods. Great care must be taken.

If an unstable fracture occurs within the lower lumbar spine, or a fusion is required across the lumbosacral joint, and if more pelvic stability is required than is offered by an LSO or TLSO, then a thoracolumbar and sacropelvic orthosis should be prescribed. This orthosis includes a body jacket that is carefully padded and molded around the pelvis and extends proximally to the sternal notch and distally, unilaterally to the knee. This orthosis is the *body cast-unilateral hip spica* (Fig. 12-23). Although this cast or "orthosis" is bulky, hot, and makes bowel and bladder care more difficult, it does provide optimal three-dimensional stabilization. Another L5 orthosis that has been constructed for the spine-injured patient with a fracture involving the lower lumbar spine and lumbosacral joint is the molded plastic lumbosacral jacket, with a molded plastic thigh corset connected by a hinged "drop lock" locking device across the hip joint on one side (Fig. 12-24A,B). This device allows the patient with insensitive skin while bedfast, to be taken out of the orthoses to receive skin care. When the patient is out of the bed, the hip joint is maintained in the locked position. Considering the high rate of spinal deformity after fracture and high

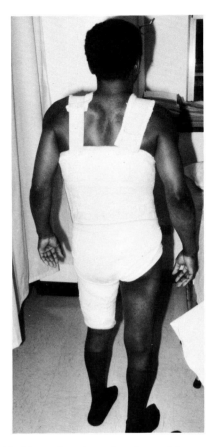

Fig. 12-23. Posterior view of patient with postoperative open reduction internal fixation and fusion fracture-dislocation of L5–S1. To ensure stability across the lumbosacral joint, a body cast was carried from the sternal notch anteriorly to the pubic symphysis, and carried across the hip joint to the level of the supracondylar region of the left thigh. Adjustable straps were applied across shoulders bilaterally to assist in suspension.

failure rate of fusion at the L4–L5 and L5–S1 levels, this method of immobilization seems reasonable despite disadvantages. For ease of application, plaster remains the material of choice in this case.

CONCLUSION

This brief review has presented representative orthotic alternatives for the management of traumatic injuries to the vertebral column. The choice

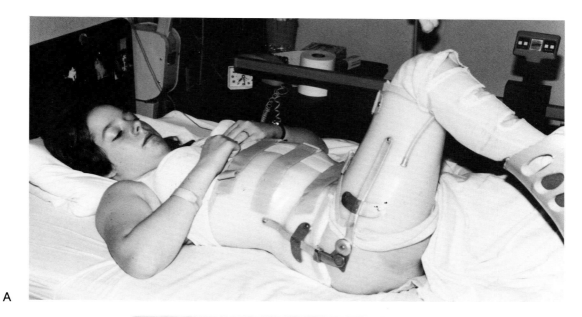

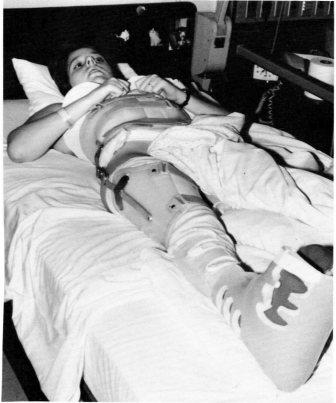

Fig. 12-24. (A) Molded plastic lumbosacral orthosis with molded plastic thigh corset, attached by lateral drop-lock metal hinge centered at the greater trochanter. Note alternating air compression stockings used for prevention of deep venous thrombosis while patient is at bed rest. (B) View with hip joint in straightaway locked position. Orthosis used in reliable patients in place of unilateral body cast-spica cast.

of one orthosis over another is based on the patho-mechanical problems induced into the spine by injury (stable versus unstable) and the therapeutic goals that must be achieved. Effective orthotic management requires a very close and cooperative participation between the physician, the orthotist, and the remainder of the rehabilitation team.

The usual period required for fracture healing is 3 months. Therefore, it can be anticipated that orthotic support of the area of the vertebral column under acute care will be required for a similar period. Weight loss is a reality during the initial post-injury period, and therefore it is necessary for frequent orthotic evaluations to be made, either by the physician or by the orthotist.

Finally, the type of orthotic device ordered for the patient should be such that fracture immobilization and healing proceed unimpeded. The orthotist must have full knowledge and appreciation that the patient's rehabilitation process includes and requires mat and floor activities, transfer activities, and maximum mobility to overcome any neurologic disability.

REFERENCES

1. Lucas DB, Bresler B: Stability of the Ligamentous Spine. Technical Report 40. Biomechanics Laboratory, University of California, San Francisco, 1961
2. White AA, Panjabi MM: Functional spinal unit and mathematical models. p. 35. In: Clinical Biomechanics of the Spine. JB Lippincott, Philadelphia, 1978
3. Hartman JT, Palumbo F, Hill BJ: Cineradiography of the braced normal cervical spine: a comparative study of five commonly used cervical orthoses. Clin Orthop 109:97, 1975
4. Morris JM, Lucas DB, Bresler B: Role of the trunk in the stability of the spine. J Bone Joint Surg 43A:327, 1961
5. Norton PL, Brown T: The immobilizing effect of back braces: their effect on the posture and motion of the lumbosacral spine. J Bone Joint Surg 39A:111, 1957

13

Orthotic Management of the Neurologically Involved Upper and Lower Limb

Terrie L. Nolinske
Mark L. Harlow
James C. Russ

The anatomic level of spinal cord lesions should reflect the patient's ultimate function. Nevertheless, owing to anatomical variation, exact segmental innervation may vary by as much as one spinal cord level when function is assessed. It may be more realistic to evaluate the patient's functional abilities rather than rely on the lesion level per se — that is, what can the patient's residual musculature actually do?

In addition to the obvious loss of motor power, there are other factors preventing attainment of maximum function. These include loss of sensation, decubitus ulcers, loss of bowel and bladder control with related infections, impaired respiratory function, spasticity, disturbances in the autonomic nervous system, and decalcification of the skeletal system. The patient may be anxious, depressed, and even apathetic. Attention to psychological aspects of loss and adjustment to disability should play an important role in rehabilitation.

All of these factors necessitate involvement of many members of the rehabilitation team, including the orthotist. In conjunction with the physician and occupational and physical therapists, the orthotist must evaluate the patient's range of motion (ROM), coordination, muscle strength, hypertonicity, sensation, motivation, and personal goals to determine the patient's functional ability. Then the most appropriate orthoses or adaptive aids may be recommended for each patient to achieve a maximum level of function.

This chapter focuses on the orthotist's role in managing the spinal cord-injured patient. Quadriplegic levels are discussed first, followed by paraplegic spinal cord lesion levels. Each discussion includes the following: patient evaluation using the technical analysis form, principles of various orthotic systems, application of specific biomechanical principles, and orthotic rationale for both upper and lower limb spinal cord lesion levels.

PRINCIPLES OF UPPER LIMB ORTHOTICS

The ultimate goal of upper limb orthotics is to provide the patient with a functional hand. This begins by ensuring proximal stability through positioning of the trunk, shoulder, arm, elbow, forearm, wrist, metacarpophalangeal (MP) and interphalangeal (IP) joints, because the hand's versatility of motion depends on the amount of motion in every joint proximal to it. The resting position of the hand is said by Bunnell to be the mid-position of the ROM at each joint, the position that creates equal tension among all musculature (Fig. 13-1).[1] That is, with the forearm midway between pronation and supination, the wrist should be extended to about 20 degrees, the longitudinal and transverse arches should be supported, the digital phalanges should be slightly flexed, and the thumb pad should be opposed to the pads of digits two and three. This differs from the functional hand position, in which the wrist is extended to 30 degrees, the transverse and longitudinal palmar arches are supported, the MP joints are flexed to 55 degrees, the IP joints are flexed to 45 degrees, and the thumb pad is opposed to the pads of digits two and three. Metacarpophalangeal joint motion is the key to major excursion of the fingertips, bringing both IP joints and fingertips to the center of the palm for fine grasp and pinch patterns. In addition, the longitudinal and transverse arches must be maintained, for they allow adaptation of the hand to objects of various sizes. The longitudinal and transverse arches may be reversed by poor orthotic positioning, intrinsic musculature paralysis, edema, and scarring of the dorsal skin on the hand. In both the resting and functional positions, the thumb must be stabilized to oppose the second and third digits. While the thumb must be stable to ensure adequate grasp-release and prehensile patterns, it must also retract to allow flat-handed activities, including transfers and activities of daily living.

It is extremely important to maintain the upper limb resting position immediately after a spinal cord injury to minimize the development of contractures. The most common contracture resembles a cadaver hand and is typified by wrist extension, MP hyperextension, and IP flexion (Fig. 13-2). The key to positioning any limb is a three-point force system, that is, pressure is exerted at three primary points to maintain the desired position. Although each orthosis includes at least one primary three-point system, most use an infinite

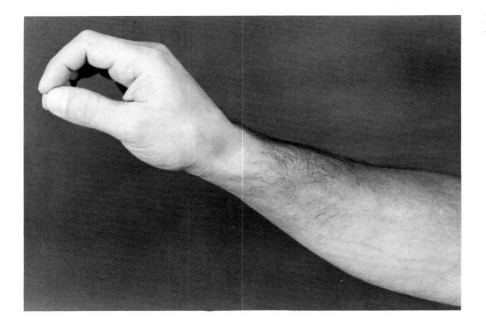

Fig. 13-1. Resting position of the wrist and hand.

Fig. 13-2. Common cadaver contracture of a quadriplegic hand.

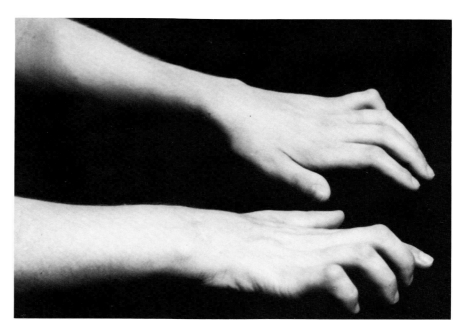

number. For example, the primary three-point force system used to prevent wrist flexion uses a dorsally directed force at midforearm, a volarly directed force at the wrist, and a dorsally directed force at the metacarpals and phalanges. Between these three primary points lie an infinite combination of other force systems, also controlling wrist flexion. Regardless of the limb position desired, it will be achieved through the application of one primary three-point force system assisted by many secondary force systems. This will ensure that muscles and tissues retain their normal effective lengths so that, as function returns, the muscles will not be stretched and muscle re-education may progress without delay.

Just as orthoses have multiple force systems, they often have multiple purposes as well.[2] Orthoses may selectively assist or resist motion, prevent muscular imbalance, stabilize and protect weak muscles, correct deformity, substitute for a permanently paralyzed muscle, aid in the transfer of power from one muscle to another, as well as be applied preoperatively and postoperatively. Orthoses are often limited in their ability to provide strength only to certain gross motions and muscle groups and may provide either mobility or stability

to any joint at any given time. It is difficult, if not impossible, to provide both simultaneously.

An orthosis can do virtually nothing to improve sensation and, because of its design, often hinders what residual sensation the patient does have. Poor cosmesis is another limitation, and the orthosis wearer must often settle for poor cosmesis to gain adequate function. This is especially true for upper limb orthoses, for, as the patient gains strength within a movement pattern, substitution patterns may develop that negate using orthoses altogether.

Many factors must be taken into consideration when making an orthotic recommendation so that it functions to achieve the patient's goals.[2] These include the patient's motivation, age, height, weight, general health, secondary problems, resources available for orthotic training and follow-up, social history, and financial obligations. Achieving these goals demands an immense armamentarium of orthotic designs, systems, and materials so the patient receives the most cosmetic and functional orthotic management possible.[3] Those systems most commonly used for upper and lower limb orthotic management are the Rancho, Lehneis, Engen, and low-temperature-plastic systems.

Materials

The Rancho system was developed by Jack Conry of Warm Springs, GA, and Roy Snelson of Rancho Los Amigos Hospital in Downey, CA. It is an aluminum system and may be lined with either white felt or flesh-colored Plastazote[3] (Fig. 13-3A). Some advantages of using this system are that it is easily fabricated to either measurements or a cast, may be easily modified, and is relatively inexpensive. For these reasons, it is perhaps the most widely used, although the least cosmetic, of all the systems.

Hans Lehneis at the Institute of Rehabilitation Medicine in New York developed a system employing yellow Nyloplex (Fig. 13-3B). Using a series of spirals, he designed the orthoses to self-suspend on a patient's limb to eliminate the need for straps.[4] Lehneis stresses the importance of locating the orthosis over fixed skeletal components of the hand rather than mobile segments to avoid inhibiting motion. Therefore, the palmar bar lies proximal to the second and third metacarpal heads, yet ends between the third and fourth metacarpals to allow full MP flexion and full fourth and fifth metacarpal movement. Nyloplex is a high-temperature material and must be formed to a cast after appropriate cast modifications have been made. Minor modifications to the orthosis may be made with a heat gun, but discoloration and brittleness result with repeated attempts. The new, clearer Plexidure is quite cosmetic, and has the added advantage of being able to effectively and accurately monitor pressure areas.

Thorkild Engen of the Texas Institute of Rehabilitation and Research, Houston, TX, utilizes a thermosetting polyester resin and laminated system that makes the system extremely cosmetic (see Fig. 13-3C).[5] With a full dorsal opening, the hand orthosis holds the thumb posted opposite digits two and three while generously supporting the palmar arch. The prefabricated hand shell is available in small, medium, medium-large, and large sizes, ordered according to the width of MP joints two through five. Owing to the fact that the orthosis is prefabricated by using casts taken of normal hands as a frame of reference, the orthosis does not readily accommodate a tight or small web space. Modi-fications may become difficult, for too much heating and reshaping tends to break down the lamination.

Low-temperature plastics, while most often used by occupational therapists, may also be used by orthotists. Low-temperature materials require about 155°F of heat before becoming malleable enough to form either directly to a patient or to a cast. Orthoplast, Polyform, and Kaysplint are but a few of the choices available in various colors including white, beige, and pink (Fig. 13-3D). Although low-temperature materials may be used on either a definitive or interim basis, it must be emphasized that these materials will lose their shape when exposed to temperature extremes and may be less cosmetic than previously described systems.[6]

EVALUATION OF PATIENT WITH UPPER LIMB INJURY

To determine what orthotic system and materials would best benefit the patient, the orthotist must thoroughly and accurately assess the patient's functional abilities and disabilities. The Upper Limb Technical Analysis Form (TAF) was developed by the Committee on Orthotics and Prosthetics of the American Academy of Orthopaedic Surgeons for this purpose.[2] Designed as a means of communication among the rehabilitation team, the TAF provides a biomechanical analysis of the patient's functional abilities and disabilities. The first page provides information on patient history with a summary of major impairments (Fig. 13-4A). Page 2 gives a diagrammatic representation in the sagittal, coronal, and transverse planes, with shaded circles at each joint indicating normal ROM in 30-degree increments (Fig. 13-4B). Muscle strength, hypertonicity, and proprioception are recorded in boxes beside each joint representation, while sensation may be recorded in the box provided. Page 3 provides detailed information on the hand including active and passive ROM, muscle strength, hypertonicity, proprioception, grasp, and pinch strength (Fig. 13-4C).

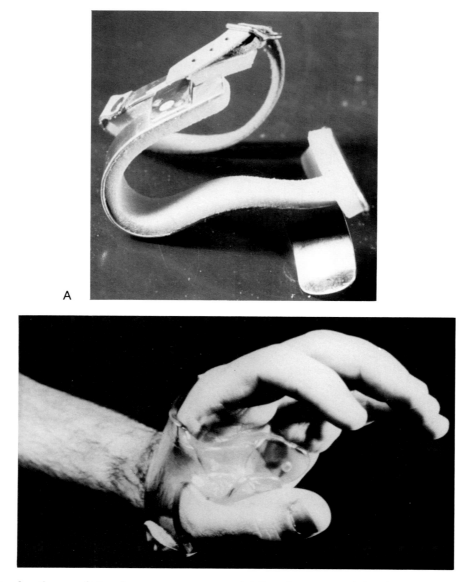

Fig. 13-3. Hand orthoses of the short opponens type. **(A)** Rancho system. **(B)** Lehneis system. *(Figure continues.)*

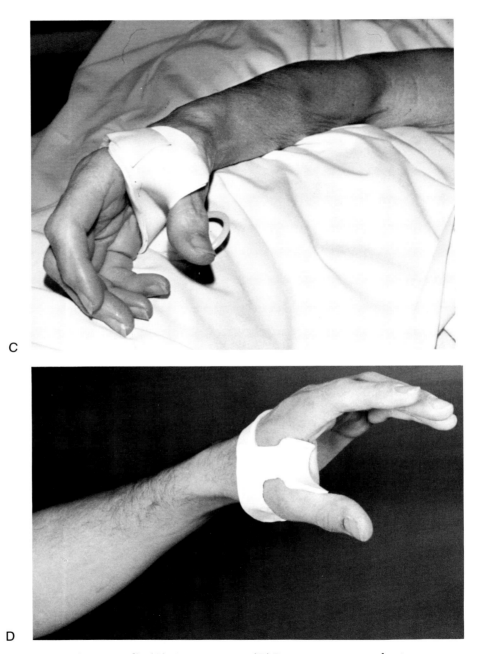

C

D

Fig. 13-3 *(Continued).* **(C)** Engen system. **(D)** Low-temperature plastic system.

TECHNICAL ANALYSIS FORM   RIGHT UPPER LIMB   Revised March

Name _____ No. _____ Age _____ Sex _____

Date of Onset _____ Cause _____

Occupation _____ Present Upper Limb Equipment _____

Diagnosis _____

Hand Dominance: Right ☐   Left ☐

Status of other upper limb: Normal ☐   Impaired ☐

1. Ambulatory status: Normal ☐   Impaired ☐   Walking Aid ☐

2. Wheelchair ☐   Sitting Position: Stable ☐   Unstable ☐   Reclined ☐   Upright ☐
    Sitting Tolerance: Normal ☐   Limited ☐   Duration _____
    Propulsion: Manual ☐   Motor ☐   Dependent ☐

3. Cognition: Normal ☐   Impaired ☐

4. Endurance: Normal ☐   Impaired ☐

5. Skin: Normal ☐   Impaired ☐

6. Pain ☐   Location _____

7. Vision: Normal ☐   Impaired ☐

8. Coordination: Normal ☐   Impaired ☐   Function: Normal ☐   Compromised ☐
                                                                                   Prevented ☐

9. Motivation: Good ☐   Fair ☐   Poor ☐

10. Associated impairments: _____

_____ LEGEND _____

⊕ ↓ = Direction of Translatory
        Motion
        (Grade 1, 2 or 3)

⊕   = Abnormal Degree of
 60°   Rotary Motion

⊕   = Fixed Position
 30°

∿∿/   = Fracture

Volitional Force (V)
N = Normal
G = Good
F = Fair
P = Poor
T = Trace
Z = Zero

Hypertonic Muscle (H)
N   = Normal
M   = Mild
Mo = Moderate
S   = Severe

Sensation
☐ = Normal
▨ = Hypesthesia
▧ = Paresthesia
■ = Anesthesia

Proprioception (P)
N = Normal
I = Impaired
A = Absent
D = Distension or
       Enlargement

A

Fig. 13-4. Upper limb TAF. **(A)** Page 1. *(Figure continues.)*

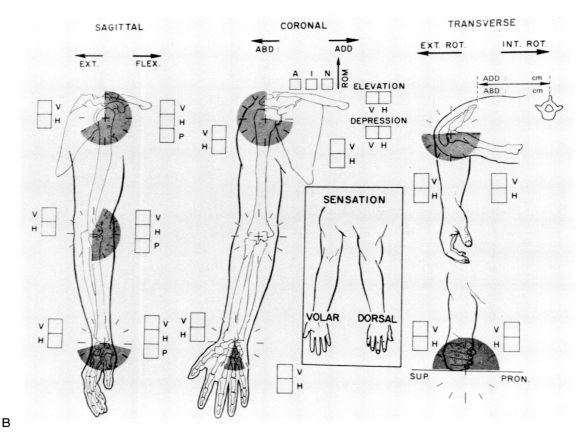

Fig. 13-4 *(Continued).* **(B)** Page 2. *(Figure continues.)*

With these data, the orthotist must determine what the patient's capabilities are as well as postulate what may be accomplished mechanically to enhance function. A summary of functional disability is recorded on page 4 before orthotic goals are identified (Fig. 13-4D). The orthotic recommendation is then determined, and only that portion of the matrix corresponding to the desired orthotic management need be completed, depending on whether the motion needs to be assisted, resisted, limited, held, or stopped. Motions not applicable to respective joints are deleted. The orthosis that results from this biomechanical analysis should provide the patient with more efficient function as well as enhance motion gained in occupational and physical therapies.

ORTHOTIC MANAGEMENT OF THE QUADRIPLEGIC PATIENT

Orthotic treatment goals for patients with a spinal cord injury are relatively standard per lesion level, although the degree of goal achievement is proportionate to the completeness of the lesion and patient motivation. Again, ROM, muscle strength, hypertonicity, psychological acceptance, and social history are among some of the factors influencing orthotic goal achievement.

The patient with a lesion at Cl, C2, or C3 has relative degrees of function in the sternocleidomastoid, levator scapulae, and upper trapezius muscles. Neck control is important to this patient,

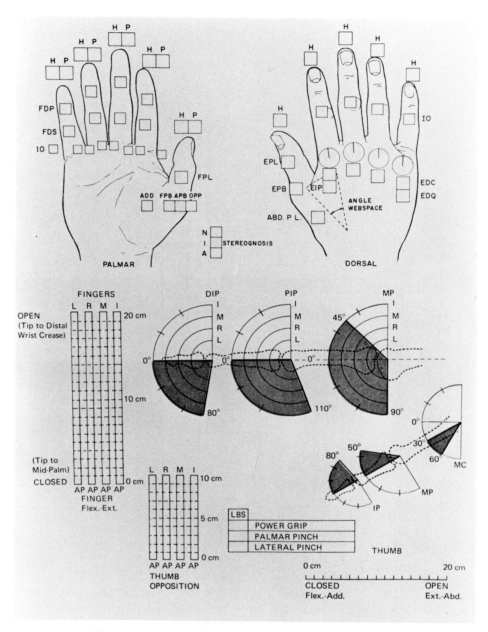

Fig. 13-4 *(Continued).* **(C)** Page 3. *(Figure continues.)*

Summary of Functional Disability _____

_____

_____

_____

_____

Treatment Objective: Prevent/Correct Deformity ☐   Improve Function ☐
                         Relieve Pain ☐   Other _____

ORTHOTIC RECOMMENDATION

UPPER LIMB		FLEX	EXT	ABD	ADD	ROTATION Int.	ROTATION Ext.	AXIAL LOAD
SEWHO	Shoulder							
EWHO	*Humerus*	███	███	███	███	███	███	
	Elbow			███	███	███	███	
	Forearm	███	███	███	███	(Pron.)	(Sup.)	
WHO	Wrist			(RD)	(UD)			
HO	Hand							
	MP							
Fingers 2-5	PIP			███	███	███	███	
	DIP			███	███	███	███	
	CM					(Opposition)		
Thumb	MP							
	IP			███	███	███	███	

REMARKS:

_____   _____
Signature   Date

KEY: Use the following symbols to indicate desired control of designated function:
F = FREE   - *Free* motion.
A = ASSIST - Application of an external force for the purpose of increasing the range, velocity, or force of a motion.
R = RESIST - Application of an external force for the purpose of decreasing the velocity or force of a motion.
S = STOP   - Inclusion of a static unit to deter an undesired motion in one direction.
v = Variable - A unit that can be adjusted without making a structural change.
H = HOLD   - Elimination of all motion in prescribed plane (verify position).
L = LOCK   - Device includes an optional lock.

D

Fig. 13-4 *(Continued).* **(D)** Page 4. (From McCollough,[2] with permission.)

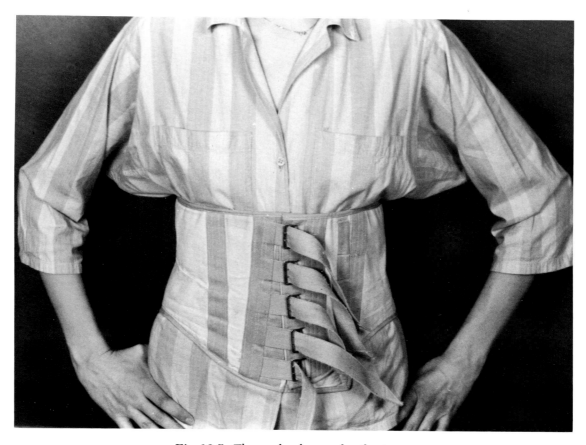

Fig. 13-5. Thoracolumbosacral orthosis.

and often head, neck, and trunk supports are necessary to provide proximal trunk stability within the wheelchair. Owing to the fact that the diaphragm is innervated by spinal nerves C3, C4, and C5, patients with lesions at this level may require respiratory support. Physical endurance is very low, so that any adaptive aids and orthoses must be designed and used accordingly.

The C1, C2, or C3 patient may wear an abdominal binder to aid respiratory functions, maintain visceral position, and afford proximal stability (Fig. 13-5). Static wrist-hand orthoses (WHOs) must be worn at night and intermittently during the day to prevent formation of the cadaver hand so often seen in high-level quadriplegics (Fig. 13-6A). Adaptive aids and utensil channels may be added to the static WHOs or utilized on another orthosis

(see Fig. 13-6B). Although a fully reclining electric wheelchair with chin or breath control may be preferable, a standard reclining wheelchair can also be used (Fig. 13-7). Advantages of the standard wheelchair include ease in transferring both patient and wheelchair in or out of a car. Electric mouth, head, and joystick controls may be used to operate many things including electric typewriters, tape recorders, and pushbutton/speaker telephones or to turn pages in a book (Fig. 13-8). Environmental control systems with a variety of centralized control switches for various appliances may afford the patient the most independence within a prescribed area at the lowest energy expenditure (Fig. 13-9). Regardless of what is used, a lap or wheelchair board is ideal for keeping items within easy reach for both patient and his full-time

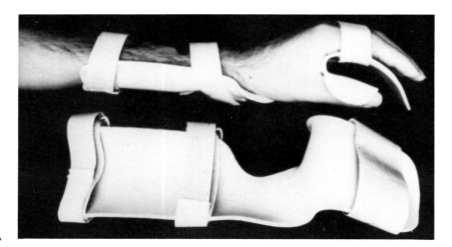

A

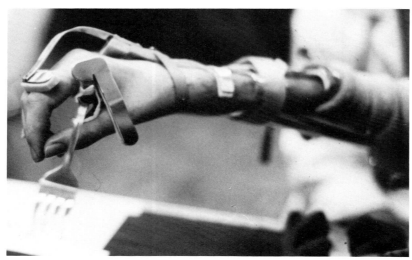

B

Fig. 13-6. WHOs may provide static positioning of function. **(A)** Resting type maintains the balance of musculature. **(B)** Long opponens type provides a functional utensil channel in addition to positioning the wrist and hand.

attendant. Although many mechanical aids may be used at this level, the patient's own "gadget tolerance" plays a large role in whether he will accept or reject adaptive aids and orthoses provided.

The patient with a lesion at C4 has full innervation of the sternocleidomastoid and trapezius muscles with partial innervation of the diaphragm and levator scapulae muscles, enabling him to elevate, depress and retract the shoulder girdle. This patient may inevitably need such specialized equipment as balanced forearm orthoses (BFO), suspension slings, or counterbalanced pulleys to assist in arm raising and gross hand placement (Fig. 13-10). He may also need bilateral WHOs for static posi-

tioning and attachment of adaptive aids, all of which may be used in conjunction with slings and BFOs. A mouthstick might enable the patient to type, turn pages, and manipulate objects at tabletop level. A reclining electric wheelchair may be controlled with a mouthstick or hand controls. A standard wheelchair may be used, as it is lighter in weight and may be folded to fit into a car trunk or back seat. Also available are electric feeders, page turners, environmental control systems, and externally powered shoulder-elbow-wrist-hand orthoses with battery packs and carbon dioxide (Fig. 13-11). An upper limb orthotic system employing functional electrical stimulation of paralyzed mus-

Fig. 13-7. Electric, fully reclining chair with hand controls affords high-level quadriplegic mobility with low energy expenditure.

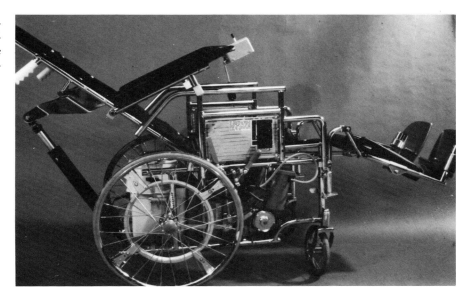

Fig. 13-8. A variety of switches and controls allows easy access and independence in daily activities.

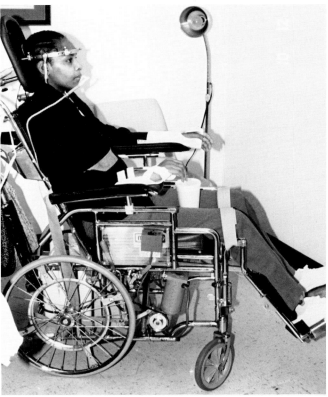

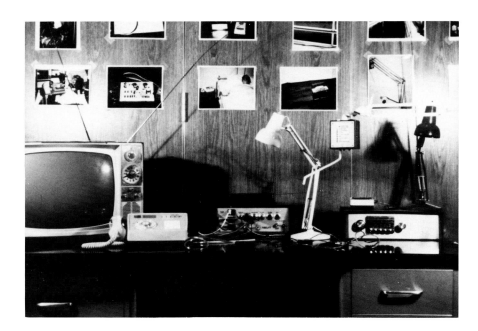

Fig. 13-9. Environmental control systems allow maximum function for high-level quadriplegic patients.

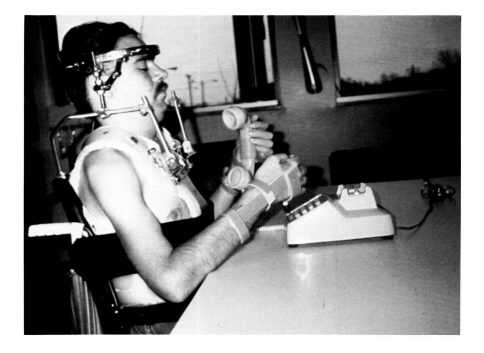

Fig. 13-10. BFOs facilitate forward hand placement and minimize fatigue.

Fig. 13-11. Externally powered carbon dioxide tenodesis orthosis provides patients with three-point prehension.

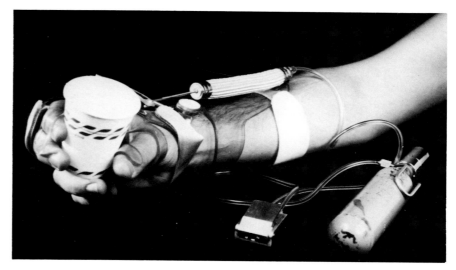

cles to achieve grasp-release is being evaluated at Case Western Reserve University and other facilities. By electrically exciting muscles in the forearm and hand, either palmar prehension-release or lateral pinch-release may be achieved.[7] It is important to remember that the C4 quadriplegic still has a very low vital capacity and thus has low endurance for most activities.

The patient with a lesion at C5 is able to elevate, depress, protract, retract, and externally rotate his neck. Weak scapular adduction, glenohumeral abduction, internal and external rotation, flexion and extension, forearm supination, and elbow flexion are present. This musculature may be prevented from becoming functional by the absence of prime shoulder extensors, horizontal adductors, and scapular abductors plus incomplete innervation of shoulder stabilizers.

It is important to note the acquisition of forward hand placement at the C5 level. Use of suspension slings and BFOs may be necessary in early activities to minimize fatigue because proximal strength in these patients is still only fair. Part-time setup and standby assistance may be needed as the patient performs many activities of daily living including eating, shaving, brushing teeth, washing the face, combing hair, applying makeup, typing, telephoning, and dressing the upper limbs. Sliding board transfers may need assistance, but the patient can

usually propel a wheelchair for short distances on level ground using wheelrim projections and wheelchair gloves (Fig. 13-12). A WHO of the long opponens type may be used as is or modified to increase function and wrist stability.

Because of the absence of wrist extensors, the C5 quadriplegic may accomplish these and other activities by using a universal cuff, a WHO with attachments, adaptive aids with built-up and lengthened or adaptive handles, or externally powered or harnessed orthoses (Fig. 13-13). The WHO of the ratchet type requires passive positioning of the wrist and fingers to achieve three-point prehension and is an excellent choice for patients performing sustained tasks, as the utensil being used is held in place by the mechanical orthosis rather than the patient's active musculature (Fig. 13-14).

The patient with a lesion at C6 has good shoulder rotation, abduction, adduction, flexion, extension, and scapular protraction with a noted increase in proximal stability. Elbow flexors and pronators are good, with radial wrist extensors initiating development of wrist tenodesis action to facilitate light active grasp in the hand.

The C6 quadriplegic may dress the upper limb and lower limb with minimal assistance, eat, write, perform hygienic care, transfer with a sliding board, propel a standard or lightweight wheelchair using vertical or oblique wheelrim projections, and

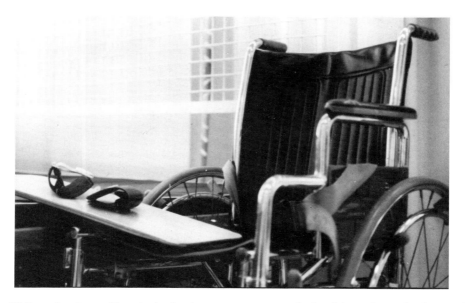

Fig. 13-12. Oblique/horizontal/vertical wheelrim projections and wheelchair gloves facilitate self-propulsion.

drive a car equipped with hand controls. An electric wheelchair with hand controls may still be the most efficient for prolonged use, although a standard wheelchair is easiest to get in and out of cars. Using either a natural tenodesis or the wrist-driven flexor hinge orthosis for stronger, more efficient grasp-release, the patient may also use universal cuffs for activities needing increased leverage, including dressing and cutting meat (Fig. 13-15). Balanced forearm orthoses are still utilized to facilitate foward hand placement and minimize fatigue. In general, this patient performs most activities more efficiently using less equipment than the patient with a C5 lesion.

In addition to those movements already described, the patient with a lesion at C7 is able to extend the elbow as well as flex and extend the wrist and fingers. A claw-hand deformity may develop owing to the unopposed action of the long extensors at the MP joint and may be orthotically managed with an MP extension stop attached to either a hand orthosis (HO) or a WHO, depending on wrist stability. Stopping MP extension in 15 degrees of flexion may enable the long extensors to extend the IP joints. Other components that may

be used with either an HO or WHO include an IP extension assist, a thumb adduction stop to maintain the web space, or a spring swivel thumb if enough thumb flexion is present to overcome the force into extension and abduction (Fig. 13-16).

The **WHO** of the wrist-driven flexor hinge type may be used to achieve a three-jaw chuck prehension through wrist extension and a parallelogram tenodesis system. The Rehabilitation Institute of Chicago (RIC) orthosis uses no mechanical joints, simply harnessing the patient's volitional motion into a patterned three-point prehension. The RIC orthosis is most efficiently used by a patient with good muscle strength, ROM, and endurance (Fig. 13-17).

Wheelchair transfers by a C7 quadriplegic are more efficient, and wheelchair propulsion may or may not require projections on a standard or lightweight chair. Although a part-time attendant may be required, the C7 patient is usually independent in activities of daily living although adaptive aids and/or orthoses may be used to minimize fatigue. Again, if driving is to be undertaken, it must be with hand controls.

At the C8 level, patients acquire MP flexion, MP

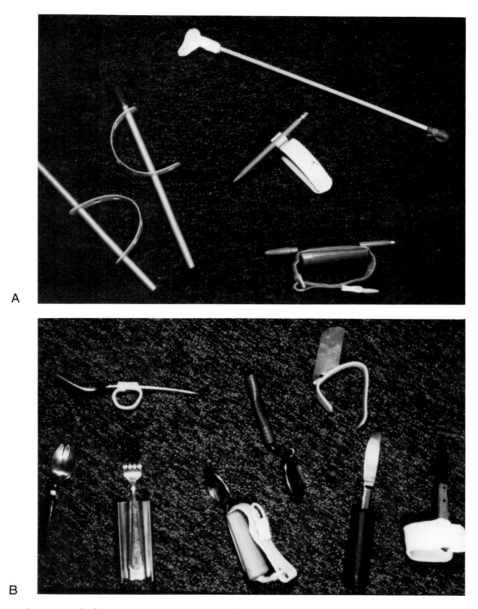

Fig. 13-13. Adaptive aids for (**A**) communication and (**B**) eating contribute greatly to functional independence.

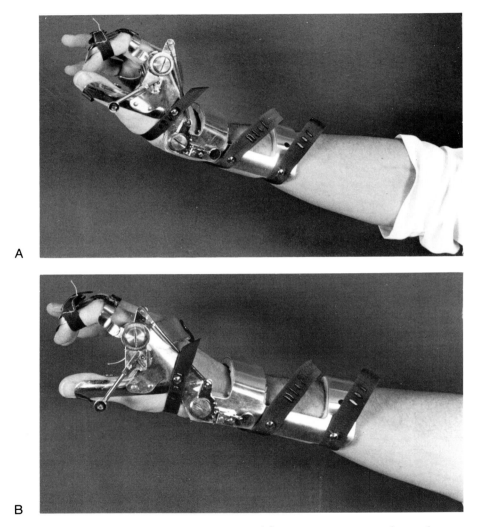

Fig. 13-14. Rachet-type WHO requires passive wrist and finger positioning to achieve three-point prehension, seen here in both (**A**) open and (**B**) closed positions.

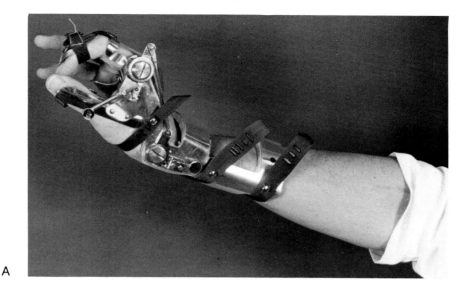

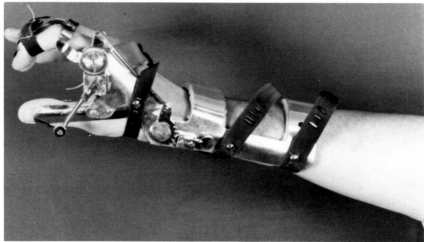

Fig. 13-15. Wrist-driven flexor hinge-type WHO uses radial wrist extensors to achieve three-point prehension: **(A)** grasp, **(B)** release.

abduction, adduction, and thumb movements. An HO with an MP extension stop may be used to balance hand intrinsic musculature while assists and positioning attachments are added and deleted as necessary. Obtaining the desired function is largely dependent on the degree of voluntary ROM and muscle strength. This patient should ultimately be regarded as independent in self care, transfers, standard wheelchair propulsion, driving with hand controls, and wheelchair transfers in and out of the car.[8] This patient should also be a strong candidate for participation in both indoor and outdoor wheelchair sports.

As evidenced by the cervical spinal cord lesion levels, the quadriplegic patient must overcome many physical, psychological, and environmental problems to achieve even a relative degree of independence. In collaboration with the rehabilitation team, the orthotist plays a key role in contributing to the quadriplegic patient's functional indepen-

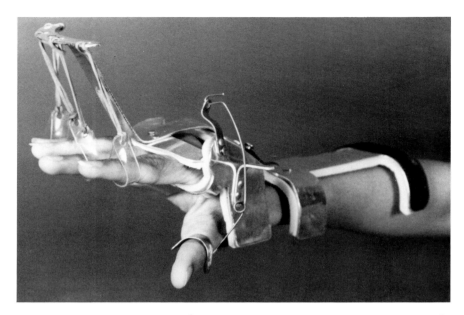

Fig. 13-16. Long opponens-type WHO with MP extension stop, IP extension assist, and spring swivel thumb.

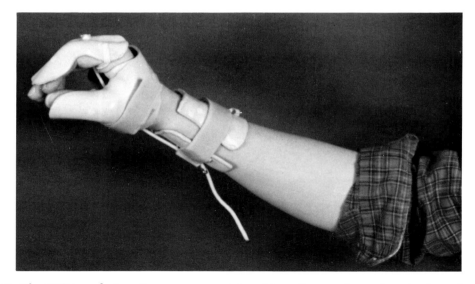

Fig. 13-17. The RIC tenodesis patterns movement to achieve three-point prehension by using anatomic rather than mechanical joints.

Table 13–1. Summary of Quadriplegic Lesion Levels

Lesion Level	Key Musculature	Orthoses/Adaptive Aids
C1–C3	Sternocleidomastoid Levator scapulae Upper trapezius	Positioning Environmental control systems Electric/standard wheelchairs
C4	Trapezius Diaphragm	Positioning WHOs, BFOs Adaptive aids
C5	Deltoid Biceps Supinator	WHO: rachet Adaptive aids
C6	Extensor carpi radialis longus and brevis	WHO: wrist-driven flexor hinge WHO: long opponens Hand controls for driving
C7	Flexor carpi radialis Triceps Latissimus dorsi	WHO: RIC WHO: long opponens with MP extension stop
C8	Long flexors/extensors Partial hand intrinsics	HO: short opponens with assists

dence by evaluating the patient and applying biomechanical principles to ensure the most appropriate selection of orthoses and adaptive aids for that patient (Table 13-1).

LOWER LIMB ORTHOTIC CONSIDERATIONS

While management of the quadriplegic upper limb is concerned with re-education of hand placement, grasp-release, and fine sensorimotor coordinative activities, the functional goal with the paraplegic lower limb is to activate general muscle groups for standing, balance, and ambulation. Although some will not achieve ambulatory status because of the high energy expenditure, most may at least be orthotically stabilized to control motion, compensate for weakness, and maintain alignment, thus minimizing further deformity. The orthotic systems used to achieve these and other goals may include those previously discussed, with emphasis on the Rancho and high-temperature polymer systems such as polypropylene, polyethylene, and copolymer. These materials are available in various thicknesses, with polypropylene considered to be the most rigid and the polyethylene the most flexible regardless of the thickness used. Copolymer lies somewhere in between, containing primarily polypropylene with enough polyethylene to lend flexibility. These materials are most readily available in white. When used, they must be heated at a high temperature and either vacuum formed or hand draped over a cast of the patient's limb.

Orthotic designs and systems used may be influenced by a variety of factors. The level and completeness of the lesion may be the most critical, whereas the length of time after onset may dictate whether the orthosis will be considered interim or definitive in nature. In many cases, both the physician and the therapist are hesitant to change from one system to another during the patient's rehabilitation process, for they think that changing from plastic to metal or vice versa might be considered a step backwards. Hence, patients often get locked into a system and are not re-evaluated, but as their muscle strength, ROM, sensation, hypertonicity, and proprioception change, so should their program of orthotic management. Another orthosis or system may well be more functional, more cosmetic, and less expensive in the long run than continuing with the system presently being used.

Although many orthotic systems offer stability, none can address the sensory loss incurred unless the orthosis extends to a sensate area of the limb in an attempt to regain a small portion of proprioceptive input. Loss of sensation, especially proprioceptive feedback, immediately puts whatever residual volitional movement the patient does have on a cortical level. It requires conscious thought and concentration to do a task that requires more energy and time to execute.

Hypertonicity may influence the orthotic design to be used or it may negate orthotic management altogether. Mild hypertonicity can assist the patient in dressing, transfers, and standing activities, providing just enough rigidity to stabilize the lower limbs. It may also help prevent muscle atrophy in the lower limbs. Moderate to severe hypertonicity may contraindicate orthotic management and necessitate medical attention.

A patient's age and premorbid height and weight may affect the most efficient orthotic system. The higher the center of gravity from the floor, the more difficult it becomes to orthotically balance the residual musculature and ligaments for standing and ambulation. Hence, a 5-year-old child with a complete lesion at T4 might ambulate, whereas a 20-year-old patient with a lesion at that same level might not because of the increase in both body weight and height of the center of gravity.

LOWER LIMB ALIGNMENT

Stability in standing is normally achieved by passive alignment, with the anatomic weight line lying posterior to the hip joint and anterior to both knee and ankle joints. If this alignment relationship between hip, knee, and ankle is not considered when discussing orthotic management, the orthosis may serve to augment rather than diminish the patient's problem.

Owing to natural tibial torsion, the medial malleolus is usually more anterior and proximal than the lateral malleolus. That is, the ankle axis is rotated externally 20 to 30 degrees with respect to the knee axis. The axes of rotation at both knee and ankle are perpendicular to the midsagittal line so that if the orthosis is fabricated in relation to that

line, the bands and joint axes will also be perpendicular and the joint surfaces parallel to the midsagittal line. Since most orthoses do not provide motion corresponding to the subtalar joint, the correct location of the mechanical ankle axis at the distal tip of the medial malleolus, in accordance with the concept of external rotation, is important in allowing free ankle motion. Toe-out must also be accounted for and may be defined as the relationship of the long axis of the foot to the line of progression, usually an angle of 15 degrees. Although toe-out does not bear a constant relationship to external rotation, it may be affected by many things, including the amount of forefoot abduction or adduction, varus or valgus of the ankle, and rotation in the hip and knee.[9]

Effects of incorrect anatomic and mechanical alignment are varied. If the mechanical joints are not perpendicular to the midsagittal line, there may be uneven shoe-floor contact, instability resulting from uneven weight distribution, increased sheer stress, and uneven wear of the joint surfaces. If the mechanical ankle joint is internally rotated with respect to the anatomic joint, there may be excessive pressure concentrating on the lateral surface of the foot during ambulation that in turn may lead to a valgus or pronated forefoot condition. Consequently, there will be an increase in the wear of the mechanical joints secondary to torque and an increase in both patient energy exertion and patient fatigue owing to binding between anatomic and mechanical joints.[9]

Inadequate compensation for toe-out may result in an increase of varus at the foot as well as cause the orthosis to externally rotate on sitting. If the mechanical ankle or knee joint is located too proximally or distally, pistoning between the orthosis and the leg will occur during movement in the sagittal plane. This relative motion may cause discomfort and pressure sores, increasing with the amount of ankle and knee joint movement.[9]

Patient Evaluation

The first step in ensuring optimum lower limb alignment is a thorough and accurate evaluation of the paraplegic lower limb. As in the evaluation of the quadriplegic upper limb, use of the TAF ensures that the rehabilitation team will collect the

TECHNICAL ANALYSIS FORM   LOWER LIMB   Revised March 1973

Name _____ No. _____ Age _____ Sex _____

Date of Onset _____ Cause _____

Occupation _____ Present Lower Limb Equipment _____

Diagnosis _____
_____
_____

Ambulatory ☐   Non-Ambulatory ☐

MAJOR IMPAIRMENTS:
A Skeletal
   1. Bone and Joints: Normal ☐   Abnormal _____
   2. Ligaments: Normal ☐   Abnormal ☐   Knee: AC ☐   PC ☐   MC ☐   LC ☐
                                           Ankle: MC ☐   LC ☐
   3. Extremity Shortening: None ☐   Left ☐   Right ☐
      Amount of Discrepancy: A.S.S.-Heel _____   A.S.S.-MTP _____   MTP-Heel _____

B Sensation: Normal ☐   Abnormal ☐
   1. Anesthesia ☐   Hypesthesia ☐   Location _____
      Protective Sensation: Retained ☐   Lost ☐
   2. Pain ☐   Location _____

C Skin: Normal ☐   Abnormal: _____

D Vascular: Normal ☐   Abnormal ☐   Right ☐   Left ☐

E Balance: Normal ☐   Impaired ☐   Support _____

F Gait Deviations _____
_____

G Other Impairments _____
_____

LEGEND

⊕↑ = Direction of Translatory Motion

⊕ 60° = Abnormal Degree of Rotary Motion

⊕ 30° = Fixed Position
1 cm

∿ = Fracture

Volitional Force (V)
N = Normal
G = Good
F = Fair
P = Poor
T = Trace
Z = Zero

Hypertonic Muscle (H)
N = Normal
M = Mild
Mo = Moderate
S = Severe

Proprioception (P)
N = Normal
I = Impaired
A = Absent
D = Local Distension or Enlargement

⊔⊓ = Pseudarthrosis

= Absence of Segment

A

Fig. 13-18. Lower limb TAF. (A) Page 1. *(Figure continues.)*

most pertinent information. Developed by the Committee on Orthotics and Prosthetics of the American Academy of Orthopaedic Surgeons, the lower limb TAF consists of four pages.[2] The first includes patient history, skeletal impairments such as bone or joint and ligamentous laxity or tightness, limb shortening with length discrepancy noted, sensation, balance, gait deviations, and skin conditions (Fig. 13-18A). Page 2 provides a diagrammatic representation of the right lower limb in the sagittal, coronal, and transverse planes (Fig. 13-18B). Normal ROM is indicated by the shaded

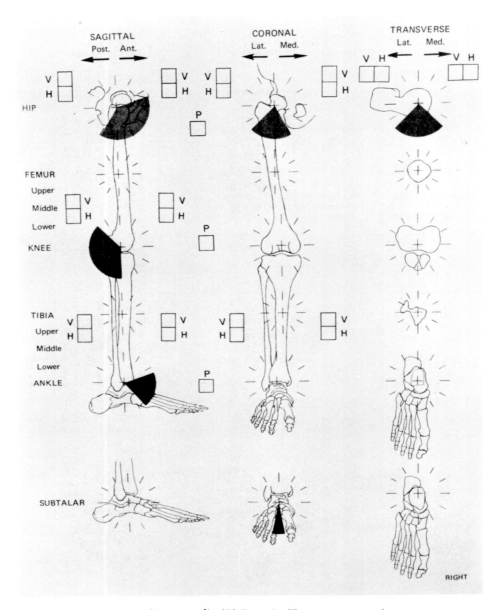

Fig. 13-18 *(Continued).* **(B)** Page 2. *(Figure continues.)*

arcs within the limb, with muscle strength, hypertonicity, and proprioception recorded in the box appropriate to the joint. Page 3 provides identical base information for the left lower limb (Fig. 13-18C). Page 4 provides space for a summary of functional disability, the orthotist's treatment objectives, and the matrix to be completed in accordance with the biomechanical evaluation and orthotic recommendation (Fig. 13-18D).

LOWER LIMB BIOMECHANICS

In general, the biomechanical management of the paraplegic patient may be broken down into several categories, grouped by the pathomechanical problem seen at each joint. It then becomes a matter of orthotically applying three-point force systems to stabilize the limb biomechanically. Pa-

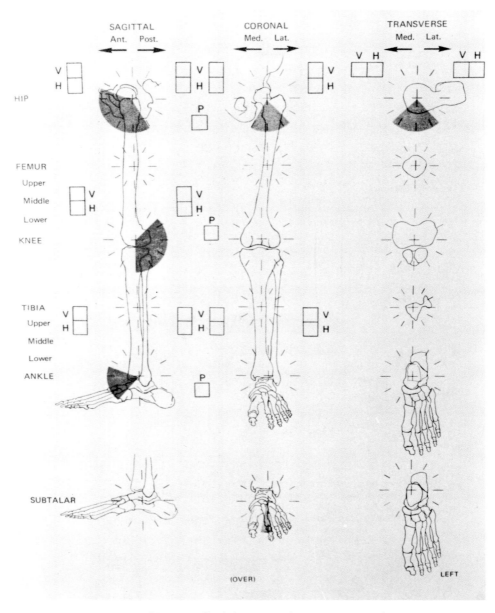

C

Fig. 13-18 *(Continued)*. **(C)** Page 3. *(Figure continues.)*

tients with proximal paraplegic lesions will have virtually no lower limb musculature, so that control of the lower limb will necessitate use of one of a variety of hip-knee-ankle-foot orthoses (HKAFOs) (Fig. 13-19A). A pelvic band may be used initially for hip abduction and rotary control, thus aiding the patient in maintaining balance. To ambulate,

the patient must manipulate the center of gravity to effect a swivel type of gait with the aid of crutches. An abduction bar, usually connected to the plantar surface of the shoes, may be used in conjunction with the knee-ankle-foot orthosis (KAFO) (Fig. 13-19B). The abduction bar was originally designed to replace the pelvic band as a hip abduction

Summary of Functional Disability _____

_____

_____

_____

_____

_____

Treatment Objectives:

Prevent/Correct Deformity ☐		Improve Ambulation ☐	
Reduce Axial Load ☐		Fracture Treatment ☐	
Protect Joint ☐		Other _____	

ORTHOTIC RECOMMENDATION

LOWER LIMB			FLEX	EXT	ABD	ADD	ROTATION Int.	ROTATION Ext.	AXIAL LOAD
HKAO	Hip								
KAO	*Thigh*		███	███	███	███	███	███	
	Knee								
AFO	*Leg*		███	███	███	███	███	███	
	Ankle		(Dorsal)	(Plantar)					
		Subtalar					(Inver.)	(Ever.)	
FO	Foot	Midtarsal			███	███	███	███	
		Met. phal.					███	███	

REMARKS:

_____   _____
          Signature   Date

KEY: Use the following symbols to indicate desired control of designated function:

F = FREE   - *Free* motion.
A = ASSIST - Application of an external force for the purpose of increasing the range, velocity, or force of a motion.
R = RESIST - Application of an external force for the purpose of decreasing the velocity or force of a motion.
S = STOP   - Inclusion of a static unit to deter an undesired motion in one direction.
v = Variable - A unit that can be adjusted without making a structural change.
H = HOLD   - Elimination of all motion in prescribed plane (verify position).
L = LOCK   - Device includes an optional lock.

D

Fig. 13-18 *(Continued).* **(D)** Page 4. (From McCullough,[2] with permission.)

and rotary stop to facilitate donning and doffing the orthosis.

A paraplegic exhibiting knee hyperextension may be biomechanically managed by raising the heel height of the involved limb. This dorsiflexion assist may be accomplished orthotically by trimming a polymer ankle-foot orthosis (AFO) posteriorly to both malleoli, through use of the Lehneis spiral system[10] or a double-action ankle joint on a conventional metal system (Fig. 13-20). If more

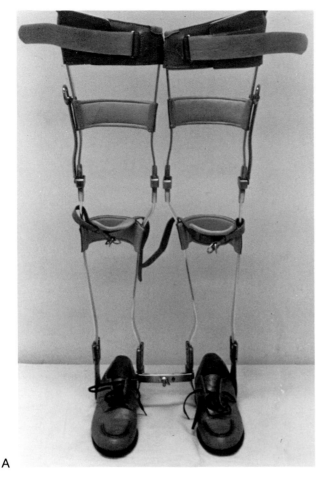
A

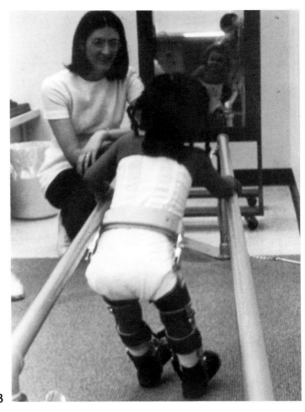
B

Fig. 13-19. (A) HKAFO with pelvic band to minimize hip abduction and rotation. (B) Standard KAFO with abduction bar to minimize hip abduction and rotation.

knee control is needed, a KAFO with a shallow distal thigh band is used to move the tibia anteriorly in relation to the foot.

If excessive knee flexion is present, it is wise to promote Achilles tendon tightness through physical therapy to achieve intrinsic balance. The paraplegic with fair-grade musculature may benefit from either a metal or polymer AFO set in plantar flexion. This will create an extension moment at the knee at heel strike. If more control is required and the patient can passively achieve full knee extension, a KAFO with ring drop locks or spring-loaded or cam locks may be used to lock the knee (Fig. 13-21A). Dial control locks, knee pads, or polymer

extensions are ideal for those patients who cannot achieve full knee extension (Fig. 13-21B). Genu valgum and varum are best controlled with a KAFO and dial pads at the knee, with extended polymer medially to control genu valgum or laterally to control genu varum (Fig. 13-21C).

If the foot cannot be dorsiflexed and is fixed in relative plantar flexion, the heel height could be raised with a wedge to accomodate the deformity. A paraplegic exhibiting flaccid equinus affecting both the anterior and posterior leg compartments might benefit from an AFO with a solid ankle trimline. A solid ankle trimline necessitates use of either a cushioned wedge added to the heel or a

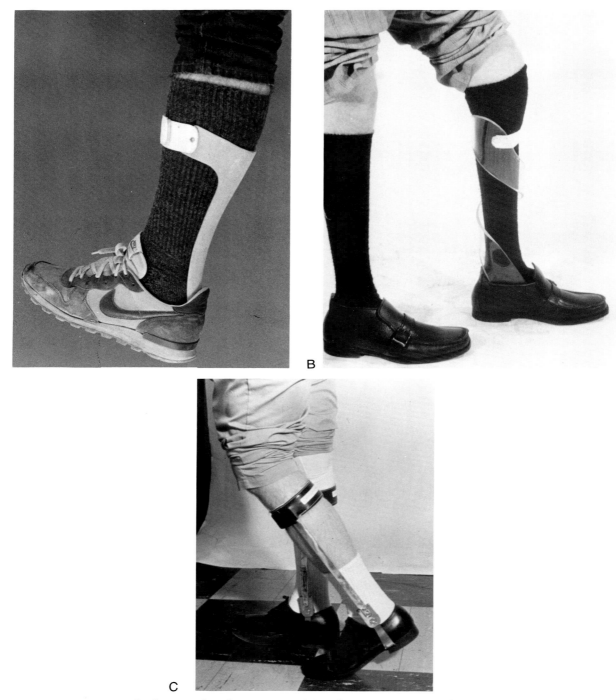

Fig. 13-20. Means of achieving dorsiflexion assist. (**A**) Polymer AFO trimmed posterior to malleoli. (**B**) Lehneis spiral AFO. (**C**) Conventional AFO with double-action ankle joints and springs in the posterior channel.

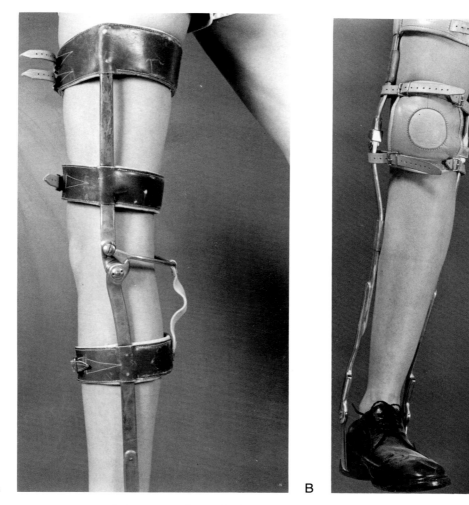

Fig. 13-21. (A) KAFO with cam lock. (B) KAFO with knee pad. *(Figure continues.)*

rocker sole to facilitate smooth rollover at heel strike (Fig. 13-22). An orthosis with a solid ankle might also be well-suited for those patients exhibiting pain, spasticity, or clonus.

It must be understood that there is no unequivocal orthotic recommendation and management for any particular lesion level. The components and orthotic applications suggested thus far are only a frame of reference from which to work. This will become more apparent as the paraplegic lesion levels are examined to determine residual function and subsequent orthotic management.

ORTHOTIC MANAGEMENT OF THE PARAPLEGIC

As in management of the quadriplegic, orthotic treatment goals for the paraplegic patient[11] are relatively standard per lesion level, with the degree of goal achievement proportionate to the completeness of the lesion and patient motivation. As before, ROM, muscle strength, hypertonicity, psychological acceptance, and social history are among some of the factors considered in orthotic goal achieve-

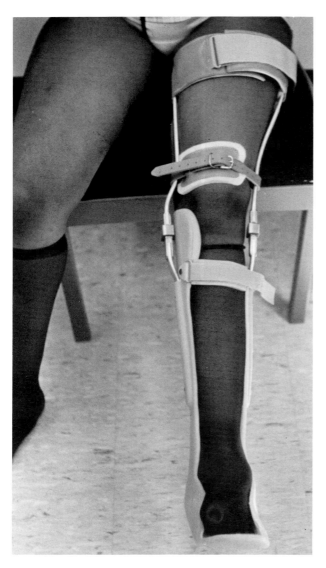

Fig. 13-21 *(continued).* **(C)** KAFO with medial valgus pad to control genu valgum.

ment at each paraplegic level. Because of their functional similarity, the lesion levels will be grouped to simplify the following discussion.

The patient with a lesion between T1 and T5, inclusive, has full innervation of the upper limb, including hand intrinsics. This provides both strength in grasp-release and manual dexterity. Poor trunk control still exists, so that most patients with injuries superior to and inclusive of T6 require an abdominal binder to increase intra-abdominal pressure and aid respiration. This patient is independent in activities of daily living, most transfers, and may perform wheelchair wheelies over curbs and inclines. Hand controls may still be necessary for driving a car.

Wearing a thoracic support and bilateral HKAFOs, the T1 to T5 paraplegic could conceivably use crutches and the good strength of the upper limbs to achieve a "drag to" gait pattern. The HKAFOs must be locked into hip and knee extension for stabilization and ankle dorsiflexion to clear the toes during ambulation.

In addition to the more conventional HKAFOs available, the paraplegic individual might also benefit from use of Louisiana State University's reciprocating gait orthosis (RGO).[12] Using a combination of pelvic band/mold, reciprocating hip joints, cable system, plastic KAFOs with posteriorly offset knee joints, and a solid ankle, the system should be balanced for hand-free standing and reciprocal gait (Fig. 13-23).[13]

While physically possible, ambulation is not functional for the patient with a T1 to T5 injury owing to limited respiratory reserve, limited endurance, and the exorbitant amount of energy demanded by this task. In a series of energy studies conducted by Tom Lunsford, at Rancho Los Amigos Hospital, one of the conclusions drawn was that of 813 paraplegics with complete lesions at the more distal level of T12–L1, only 2 became successful community ambulators, owing to the energy expenditure required.[11]

A study on the follow-up and use of orthoses by paraplegics 7 to 10 years postinjury was conducted by Stauffer in 1978.[14] After reviewing 100 paraplegic patients, Stauffer found that of 44 patients with complete lesions between T1 and T11, not one was a community ambulator, whereas 11 of 12 paraplegics with incomplete lesions at the same level did well with community ambulation. The study also discussed patients with more distal paraplegic levels and their functional abilities.[14]

This only serves to underscore the fact that a paraplegic with a T1 to T5 lesion will probably not be a functional ambulator. It is important, however, for this patient to engage in standing and weight-bearing activities to promote circulation

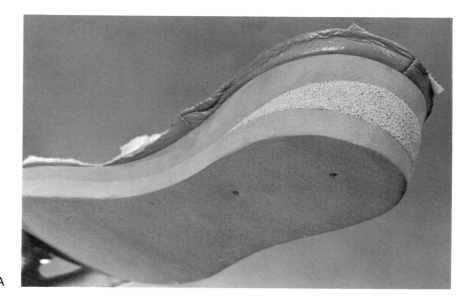

A

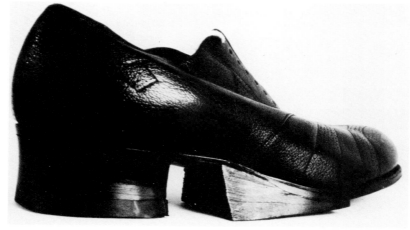

B

Fig. 13-22. Shoe modifications. Use of a solid ankle AFO requires addition of (A) a cushioned heel or (B) a rocker sole to smooth out ambulation.

and minimize osteoporotic changes (Fig. 13-24).

Paraplegics with a lesion between T6 and T11, inclusive, have strong upper limbs. Full innervation of thoracic musculature becomes helpful for achieving stability in heavy lifting. This patient will achieve independence in activities of daily living, transfers, donning and doffing orthoses used, and driving with hand controls. Such aids as grab rails and door bars are often helpful to facilitate transfers and mobility. Physiological standing for

exercise purposes may be achieved with a standing table as well as bilateral polymer KAFOs with locked knee and ankle joints set in several degrees of dorsiflexion.

The Craig-Scott KAFO is often successfully used by patients with paraplegic levels distal to T5, providing the patient has minimal spasticity, 5 degrees to 10 degrees of hip hyperextension available, and is relatively free of contractures (Fig. 13-25).[15]

The aforementioned HKAFOs may also be used

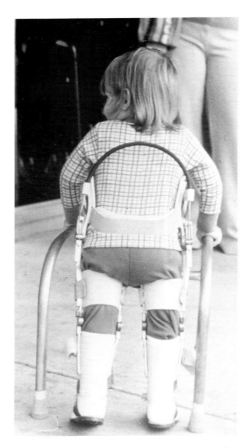

Fig. 13-23. LSU reciprocating gait orthosis (posterior view).

gained. The lower back is still weakened due to partial lumbar innervation. Partial innervation of the hip adductors, secondary elevators, and knee extensors allows the patient to become independent in activities of daily living, transfers, and wheelchair mobility. Independence in ambulation may be influenced by many factors including peer pressure, cardiac and vital capacities, motivation, and completeness of lesion. Wearing bilateral KAFOs with an optional abduction bar to keep the legs together, patients may ambulate indoors and outdoors, negotiating various terrain levels. Ambulating might take the form of two-point alter-

for those patients needing increased hip stability. These patients encounter the difficulty of not having hip hikers to elevate the pelvis and therefore must rely on their shoulder girdle to elevate the lower limbs to clear the floor should ambulation be attempted. Whether using HKAFOs or KAFOs with an abduction bar, the T6 to T11 paraplegic is physically capable of achieving a "swing-through" gait, although a "swing to" pattern may be more stable. But, with the Rancho study[14] in mind, both patterns still require so much energy that, again, ambulation may be considered nonfunctional at these levels.

From the level of T12 to L3, the paraplegic acquires full innervation of the hip flexors while maintaining the thoracic strength previously

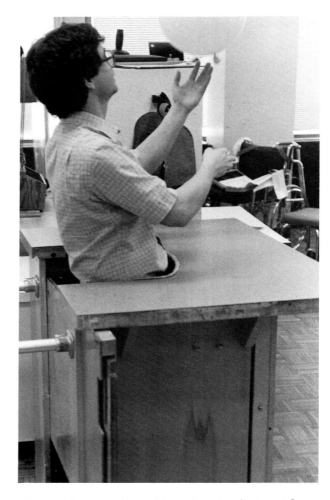

Fig. 13-24. A standing table assists circulation and promotes a more positive body image.

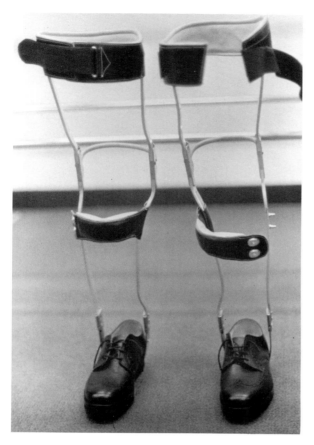

Fig. 13-25. The Craig-Scott KAFO combines several shoe modifications with an altered KAFO design.

A third option is a dorsiflexion stop to prevent tibial collapse while allowing free plantar flexion. Ankle joints allowing limited motion may be necessary to effect a smoother gait pattern because of muscular imbalance in both the anterior and posterior leg compartments. Without crutches, this patient exhibits a bilateral gluteus maximus-medius gait that exerts deforming forces on residual musculature as well as demanding energy.[14] The gluteus medius lurch causes the trunk to shift toward the affected gluteus medius side and over the leg during stance, thus reducing the stress on the hip abductors. The gluteus maximus lurch consists of hip hyperextension during the stance phase, thus stabilizing the hip by shifting the center of gravity posterior to the hip joint. Crutches and/or canes are usually suggested to minimize lateral and posterior pelvic deviations. Although this patient is a very functional ambulator, a wheelchair may still be useful on the job, at home, at school, or for long distances.

A paraplegic with an injury between S1 and S4, inclusive, progresses from full innervation of the hip extensors and knee flexors with partial use of plantar flexors and an intrinsic minus foot to full innervation of all the above. Orthoses might include bilateral AFOs to aid in maintaining endurance while balancing out any residual weakened musculature. A dorsiflexion assist may still be needed because of various degrees of paralytic equinus. Shoe inserts such as those developed at the University of California, Berkeley, Laboratories (UCBL)[16] or New York University[17] in conjunction with UCBL may be utilized to support the transverse and longitudinal arches of the foot. A soft tissue supplement may be utilized independently or in conjunction with any of the above (Fig. 13-26).

As evidenced from this overview of thoracic, lumbar, and sacral spinal cord lesion levels, the paraplegic patient must overcome many physical, psychological, and environmental factors. The orthotist, as a valuable member of the rehabilitation team, may provide the paraplegic with shoe inserts, AFOs, KAFOs, HKAFOs, and mobility and adaptive aids to contribute to the paraplegic's functional independence and feelings of self-worth (Table 13-2). In managing the spinal cord-injured patient, the orthotist must take into account not only the cause and location of the lesion, but the

nate, four-point, or swing through pattern, depending on the individual's muscle strength, activity involved, and terrain. Although axillary crutches may be used most often, Lofstrand crutches may also provide the support necessary to navigate. A standard wheelchair is still considered to be the most efficient means of mobility.

The L4-L5 paraplegic possesses full innervation of the knee extensors, medial knee flexors, and ankle dorsiflexors and partial innervation of the hip abductors and subtalar invertors. Owing to the stability offered by the knee extensors, this patient may effectively use bilateral AFOs. A solid ankle might guard against tibial collapse, while a solid ankle set in slight plantar flexion might serve to stabilize the knees by using ground reaction forces.

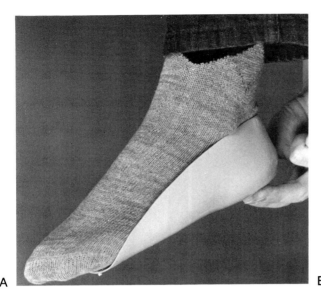
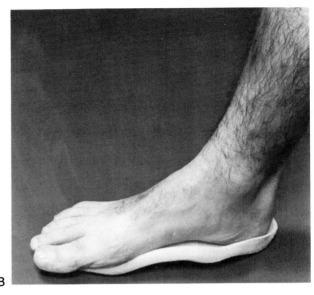

A   B

Fig. 13-26. Foot orthoses help balance out the foot. **(A)** UCBLs may be laminated or vacuum formed to fit inside the shoe to control the forefoot and subtalar joints. **(B)** Soft tissue supplements made of combinations of high- and low-density foams support the arches and metatarsal heads.

Table 13-2. Summary of Paraplegic Lesion Levels

Lesion Level	Key Musculature	Orthoses/ Adaptive Aids
T1–T5	Full upper limb	Wheelchair Hand controls for driving Standing table HKAFOs
T6–T11	Full thoracic Partial abdominals	Wheelchair Standing table Crutches HKAFOs KAFOs
T12–L3	Full abdominals Hip flexors	KAFOs Crutches
L4–L5	Knee extensors Dorsiflexors	AFOs Crutches
S1–S4	Hip extensors Knee flexors Plantar flexors	AFOs UCBL NYU-UCBL Arch supports

patient's age, sex, height, weight, residual muscle strength and ROM, sensation, hypertonicity, psychological acceptance, and motivational goals.

By integrating this with results from the orthotic evaluation and any other information from the rehabilitation team, the orthotist is able to provide the best orthotic management possible. Re-evaluations to monitor patient progress and institute changes must be scheduled to ensure that orthoses and aids still meet patient needs. Only if this is done can the patient feel that he or she has received the best orthotic care possible. In short, the orthotist, in collaboration with the rest of the team, must look to see and listen to hear.

REFERENCES

1. Bunnell S: Surgery of the Hand. 3rd Ed. JB Lippincott, Philadelphia, 1956
2. American Academy of Orthopaedic Surgeons (ed):

Atlas of Orthotics, Biomechanical Principles and Applications. CV Mosby, St. Louis, 1975

3. Anderson MH: Upper Extremities Orthotics. Charles C Thomas, Springfield, 1965

4. Lehneis HR: Upper Extremity Monograph. New York University, New York, 1976

5. Engen T: Engen Upper Limb Orthotic System. Texas Rehabilitation Institute, Baylor University, Houston, 1976

6. Malick MH: Manual on Static Hand Splinting. Vol. 1. Revised Ed. Harmarville Rehabilitation Center, Pittsburgh, 1972

7. Peckham PH: Development of upper extremity orthoses, employing electrical stimulation. p. 57. In Bulletin of Prosthetic Research Rehabilitative Engineering Research and Development. Vol. 18, No. 2. BPR 10-36. 1981

8. Malick MH, Meyer CM: Manual on Management of the Quadriplegic Upper Extremity. Harmarville Rehabilitation Center, Pittsburgh, 1978

9. Lehneis HR: Principles of Orthotic Alignment in the Lower Extremity. p. 131. A.A.O.A. Instructional Course Letters.

10. Lehneis HR: Spiral Monograph. Institute of Rehabilitative Medicine, New York University, New York, 1976

11. Lunsford T: Metal vs. Plastic AFO Comparison on the Basis of Energy Cost and Velocity. Unpublished.

12. Douglas R, et al.: The LSU reciprocation-gait orthosis. Orthopaedics 6:834, 1983

13. Durr Fillauer Medical, Inc.: LSU Reciprocating Gait Orthosis. A Pictoral Description and Application Manual. 1983

14. Stauffer ES, Hoffer ES, Nickel ZL: Ambulation in thoracic paraplegia. J Bone Joint Surg 60A:823, 1978

15. Lehmann JF, Warren CG, Hertling D, et al.: Craig-Scott orthosis: a biomechanical and functional evaluation, Arch Phys Med Rehabil 57:438, 1976

16. Campbell-Inman: UCB insert. Prosthet J 1976

17. Orthotic Prosthetic Department, New York University, New York.

14

Cervical Spine: Overview and Conservative Management

Paul R. Meyer, Jr.

The cervical vertebral column, owing to its construction, its exposure, and the presence of a centrally located and fragile spinal cord, is vulnerable and susceptible to injury. Atop a cervical vertebral column of seven segments, whose facet joint articulations allow "four degrees of motion" including flexion, extension, lateral bending, and rotation, sits the calvaria, weighing approximately 9 pounds. The application of unsuspected high-force loads causes the cervical spine to undergo ranges of motion past its normal limits, setting the stage for injury. The single force that consistently results in or is most capable of producing neurologic injury is flexion. Because of the alignment or "facing" of the facet joints (anteroposterior, superoinferior, and side to side; (Fig. 15-43), flexion forces applied to the cervical spine frequently result in subluxations or dislocations of one or both facets with greater ease than other injuries resulting from other directional forces. The latter include, in order of their frequency of occurrence: axial (or vertical) compression injuries, lateral bending injuries, rotatory injuries, and extension injuries. A combination of one or more of these forces generally results in a serious neurologic injury.

INTRODUCTION TO CONSERVATIVE CARE

Conservative management of cervical spine fracture actually begins with notification of the patient's injury or upon admission to the hospital emergency area. Experience has repeatedly demonstrated that the best patient care immediately post-trauma occurs when the managing team follows a prearranged and in-place trauma protocol. This specialty-oriented "guideline" to spinal cord emergency room care should be in place and followed identically with each admission. The use of this scheme reduces the incidence of management oversights and allows care to proceed from task to task, with adjustments made based on the dynamics of the patient's condition and the physical and neurologic findings.

General Considerations

The suspicion or finding of a fracture of the cervical spine requires the identical initial assessment. As noted above, regardless of the referring history

341

or the patient's own account of the injury, initial patient care should be performed as though a fracture is present. With the patient in a supine position on a stretcher (usually on a spine board), two areas require simultaneous evaluation (and stabilization): the cervical spine and the cardiorespiratory system. When the staff is satisfied that both are stable, the patient can be transferred to either an emergency room cart or fracture bed frame. This transfer is suggested early for several reasons:

1. Frequently, the patient, when transferred over long distances, particularly in the presence of a major neurologic injury, will have been motionless on his back (and on a spine board) for varying periods of time, often long. It is well recognized that the insensate spine injured patient will, within a short period of time (3 to 4 hours), undergo significant skin pressure injury. Many times these early skin "blemishes" will result in decubitus ulcers or pressure sores. The areas of the body where this is more likely to occur are the sacrum, the skin over the scapulas, the heels, and the occiput area of the head.

2. Moving the patient to an emergency room cart allows the patient to be managed in the Trendelenburg position (should shock or emesis occur) if required and to be transported (to radiology, surgery, etc.) as indicated.

3. It frees up the ambulance attendants' equipment and allows them to leave the emergency department.

The most appropriate means of transferring a patient between an ambulance cart and an emergency room cart or Stryker frame is to pick the patient up by means of the long spine board often utilized at the scene of the accident. One person maintains control of the head and neck position and two additional individuals, one at each end, lift the patient. When a board is not available, the transfer requires a minimum of three individuals along one side and a fourth individual at the head to manage the victim's head and neck. After placement on an appropriate cart or frame (I prefer the first transfer in the emergency room be to a Stryker wedge frame), the patient may then be transported to radiology if adequate portable facilities are not available. When portable equipment is available, cervical spine "scout" films (lateral cervical spine and an open

mouth view) should be obtained in the emergency room. This arrangement[1] allows for early fracture recognition and management and often eliminates the need for an additional patient transfer onto a radiology table, without the patient having been placed in traction. Delay in injury identification results in prolongation of potential neurologic embarrassment. As stated earlier, experience dictates that factors that influence neurologic preservation or recovery after injury are (1) immediate and appropriate accident scene care; (2) prevention of additional vertebral column injury (by adequate spine splinting); (3) early arrival at an appropriately predesignated spine trauma facility; and (4) early injury reduction and stabilization in traction. It therefore becomes imperative that decompression of the compromised neural canal by means of traction (gaining closed reduction) be attained as soon as possible after injury recognition. Seldom does this require immediate operative intervention. Once traction has been applied and the head and neck are stabilized, follow-up radiographs of the cervical spine should be obtained to observe the effects of traction. At this same time, other evaluative radiographs may be obtained. It is important to note that because of the rather high incidence of multiple trauma in the spine-injured victim (50.1 percent),[2] total vertebral column radiographic evaluation is recommended, particularly in the presence of neurologic deficits or an altered level of consciousness, when an accurate assessment is difficult to obtain and subject to error.

Other investigators have emphasized the importance of a complete radiographic assessment of the spine after trauma. Calenoff et al.,[3] in discussing multiple-level (noncontiguous) spinal column fractures in 30 multilevel spine fracture patients, noted that 24 percent had as a primary fracture (defined as the injury thought to have produced the spinal cord injury) an injury between C5 and C7. Also noted was the 14.3 percent incidence of a secondary cervical spine fracture at C1–C2 in patients having a primary fracture in the upper thoracic vertebral column. Similarly, when a primary fracture was found in the cervical spine between C2 and C7, the principal secondary area of injury was often at T12 or the lumbar spine. Calenoff's review of 710 spine-injured patients admitted to the Midwest Regional Spinal Cord Injury Care System between 1972 and 1979 revealed a multilevel noncontiguous fracture incidence of 4.5 percent. He also noted that 80 percent sustained fractures at two levels and that 20 percent had fractures at three or more levels, and that when looking at secondary lesions alone, 40 percent occurred above and 60 percent occurred below the level of the primary lesion.

Sources of Pathology

The most common cause of injury to the cervical spine is trauma. Trauma most frequently occurs in the youthful patient. Within the United States, motor vehicle accidents are the most common source of injury (48 percent).[4] Data from the Northwestern University Spine Center[2] reveal that of 1,484 patients with cervical spine injuries admitted between 1972 and 1986, 36.3 percent of the injuries followed a motor vehicle accident, 23.8 percent followed falls (second), 15.6 percent resulted from diving accidents (third), and 5.5 percent were gunshot wounds. Pedestrian accidents resulting in injury to the cervical spine in the adult

Table 14-1. Etiology of Spine Injury (Northwestern University Acute Spine Injury Center, 1972 to 1986)

Etiology	No.	Percent
Auto	538	36.3
Fall	353	23.8
Diving	231	15.6
Other traumatic[a]	98	6.6
Gunshot	81	5.5
Other sports	73	4.9
Motorcycle	46	3.1
Pedestrian	39	2.6
Other medical	22	1.5
Missing[b]	3	0.2
Total	1,484	100.0

[a]Other traumatic includes those with multiple etiologies.
[b]Etiology is unavailable.

population are few in number. Of 1,484 injuries, 39 were results of pedestrian accidents (2.6 percent). Four of the 39 patients (10 percent) were below the age of 5 years. No pediatric patient was older than 5 years in this group (Table 14-1). Asso-

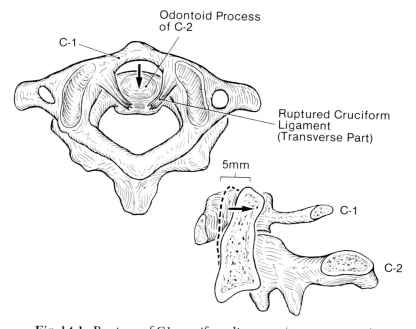

Fig. 14-1. Rupture of C1 cruciform ligament (transverse part).

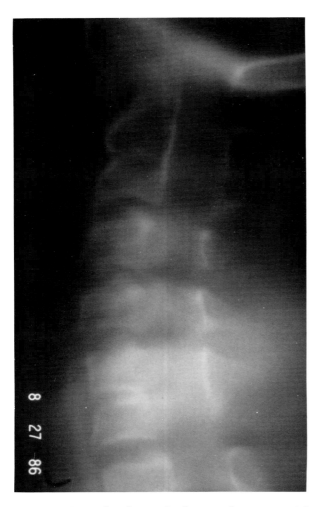

Fig. 14-2. Lateral radiograph of cervical spine in a 16-year-old boy showing numerous congenital abnormalities, include failure of the C1 vertebra to develop, and failure of segmentation of C1–C2.

posterosuperior aspect of the cervical spine[5-7] associated with an abnormal rotary position of the head and neck (the face facing opposite the side of the neck pain) and a loss in cervical spine rotary mobility.[8-10] When it occurs at the C1–C2 level, seldom does either fracture or neurologic injury follow. According to Calenoff and co-workers,[3,11] patients sustaining cervical spine injuries should be carefully observed for the presence of multiple sequential level injuries as well as noncontiguous injuries (4.5 percent; see Ch. 10).

Recognizing that trauma is the primary cause of injury to the cervical spine, the second major condition contributing to problems related to the cervical spine is cervical osteoarthritis and spondylosis. Other subtle and unsuspected pathologies must be considered. They include primary or metastatic tumors and pannus-forming diseases such as rheumatoid arthritis. The principal radiologic defect arising in the rheumatoid cervical spine (at the C1–C2 interval) is erosion of the odontoid process (or dens) of C2, or narrowing of the height of the joint space between the lateral mass of the occiput and C1 or the facet joints between C1 and C2. This process follows the occurrence of bone or, more frequently, cartilage erosion by the highly vascularized rheumatoid pannus or granulation tissue lying either within the synovial joint between the ring of C1 and the odontoid process or between the odontoid process and the posterior transverse alar (suspensory) ligaments of the dens (odontoid process). With the latter, subluxation between the odontoid process and the ring of C1 occurs (Fig. 14-1). With erosion of the articular joints between both the occiput and C1 and C1 and C2, upward protrusion of the odontoid process into the foramen magnum may occur.[12,13] The diagnosis of rheumatoid arthritis is particularly suspect when there is a history of multiple joint involvement.

An additional and incidental finding that occasionally contributes to the causes of injury to the cervical spine arises from congenital or developmental variations in the spine anatomy.[14] Their presence and finding are usually coincidental and are noted only during a trauma evaluation. The more common variations include failure of union of vertebral segments (such as pedicle, resulting in spondylolysis or spondylolisthesis) or, in the cervical spine, failure of segmentation of vertebral

ciated head-cervical spine trauma in the adult population occurs at a rate of 38.3 percent. In the pediatric pedestrian-motor vehicle accident group (under 16 years of age) the rate is higher owing to the victims' low silhouette height.

Trauma to the upper cervical spine, if coupled with rotational forces, can along with other injuries produce a rotatory subluxation type injury at the C1–C2 junction. This injury often follows a seemingly uneventful episode of horseplay or tumbling. The first indication of potential injury is pain in the

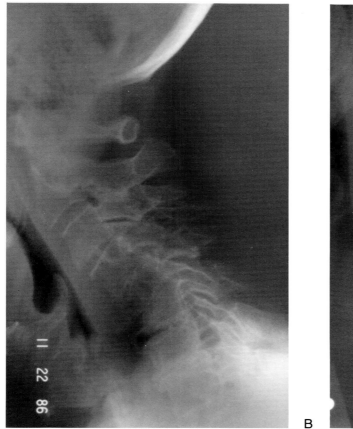 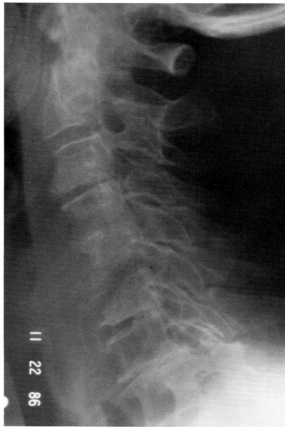

Fig. 14-3. (A) Lateral radiograph of the cervical spine in a 92-year-old man after the onset of weakness involving both upper extremities and spastic hyper-reflexia in the lower extremities. The patient's initial complaint was shoulder pain. Radiographs demonstrated loss of disc space at C5–C6. (**B**) Lateral radiograph of same patient in cervical traction. Note loss of disc space and adjacent vertebral bodies at C6–C7 interval. Also note widening of prevertebral soft tissue space opposite C5–C6. Anterior decompression revealed the presence of *Staphylococcus aureus* osteomyelitis with an epidural abscess.

bodies of elements or failure of segments to congeal (to form such structures as the odontoid process). No positive evidence exists whether an os odontoideum is the result of trauma or failure of segments to congeal, although there is evidence for the latter.[15-18] Other developmental failures include failure of union between the posterior ring of C1 and its lateral masses and a total failure in the development of the posterior C1 ring,[19] etc. (Fig. 14-2).

Last, a less frequent cause today, are infectious processes that involve the spine.[20] Infectious pro-

cesses involving the spine may be either primary or metastatic (Fig. 14-3). The latter should be suspect in patients who are living under adverse conditions, nutritionally deprived, or chronically ill (diabetes mellitus, renal disease). Two groups fall victim to the above: the poor and the elderly. Though not as prevalent, tuberculosis is again on the rise in many metropolitan cities and continues to be highly suspect.

Also noted is the occurrence of metastatic disc space and vertebral body infections affecting the cervical spine in patients known to be intravenous

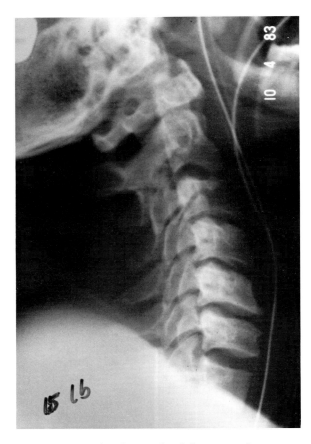

Fig. 14-4. Lateral radiograph of the cervical spine in a 67-year-old man after a fall that resulted in extension injury to the cervical spine. The lateral radiograph failed to demonstrate a fracture. Note significant posterior osteoarthritic changes of C4 and C5. Neurologic examination revealed a C5 central cord lesion.

drug abusers.[21,22] The most common bacterial offender is *Pseudomonas aeruginosa* appearing alone or in combination *Staphylococcus aureus*. Both infections involve the vertebral body as well as the adjacent disc spaces.[21,23,24] The organism spreads to the cervical vertebra most likely by way of Batson's plexus of veins.[25,26] Stone and Bonfiglio[27] suggested that the spread may also be by way of the anterior longitudinal ligament. However, although it may, infection seldom spreads directly to vertebrae.

In the pediatric patient, acute tonsillitis and otitis media were once worrisome infectious processes,

capable of producing infections in and around the upper cervical spine. This is less likely to occur today owing to the early administration of antibiotics. In the past, however, prevertebral (retropharyngeal) abscesses or an inflammatory process involving the articular facets of C2-C3 were not unusual. Such infections resulted in ligamentous laxity and capsular distention resulting in either subluxation or dislocation of the affected facet joints. With the latter, there often followed a torticollis (or "wry neck" deformity), the result of cervical joint pathology and "protective" muscle spasm.

Patients, otherwise healthy, who present with a history of cervical spine pain of subtle onset in the absence of trauma must have the presence of pathology ruled out. The most commonly encountered (benign) process is cervical degenerative spondylosis with associated disc pathology, resulting in nerve root irritation (Fig. 14-4). The concern, however, is the presence of hidden pathology, that is, either a primary or metastatic vertebral column tumor producing neurologic compromise (Fig. 14-5). This is particularly true when neurological symptoms include radicular pain into one or both upper extremities or the posteromedial scapular region, along with motor or sensory dysfunction or both in either upper extremity. It is absolutely necessary to keep in the back of one's mind esoteric processes, such as an epidural abscess, etc. (Fig. 14-6). Over 6 months, this unusual pathologic process was identified (by tomography and myelography) in two elderly patients. Thus, any time there is an unusual history with overt neurologic symptoms, a thorough and carefully performed evaluation is required.

Anatomic variations within the vertebral column represent developmental aberrations. They are usually asymptomatic and are often identified during the process of evaluating complaints referrable to other causes. An example of such is the identification of an os odontoideum (Fig. 14-7). Although this anomaly could represent the presence of previous trauma,[28-30] it can indicate a failure of fusion of the occipitocervical mesenchymal condensation segments (or secondary centers of ossification).[14-18,31] These centers normally coalesce by adolescence, though some may persist into adulthood. Thus, many and varied vertebral

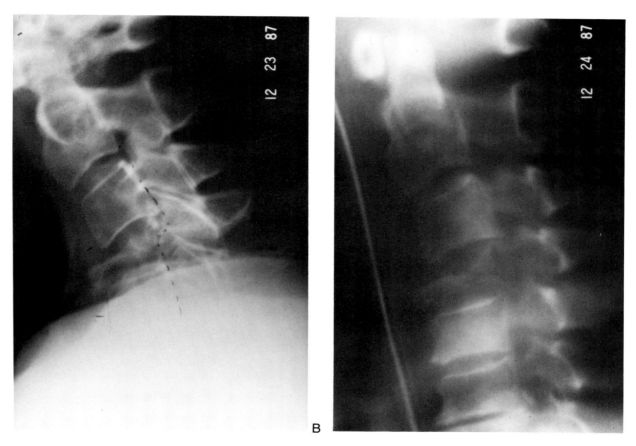

Fig. 14-5. (A) Lateral radiograph of the cervical spine in a 53-year-old woman. The patient's complaints were limited to pain in the midcervical spine. Radiograph demonstrates destruction of the C4 vertebral body, cervical kyphosis with retropulsion of C3, and a diastasis between the C4 and C5 spinous processes. (B) Lateral radiograph with the patient in Gardner-Wells skeletal traction. Note improved alignment. *(Figure continues.)*

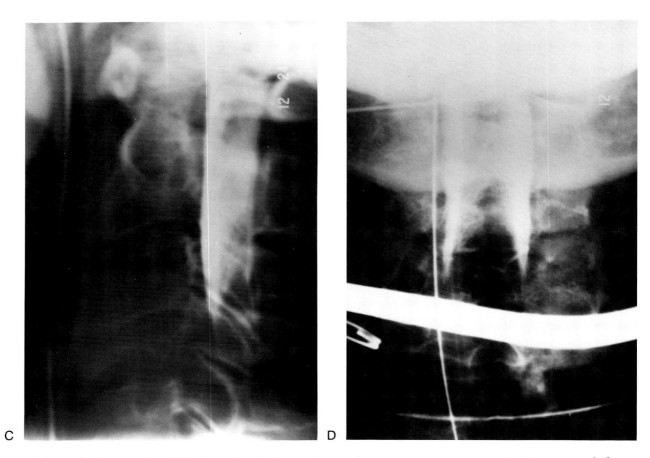

Fig. 14-5 *(Continued).* **(C,D)** Lateral and AP myelogram shows a mass posterior to C4. Biopsy revealed metastatic carcinoma of the breast.

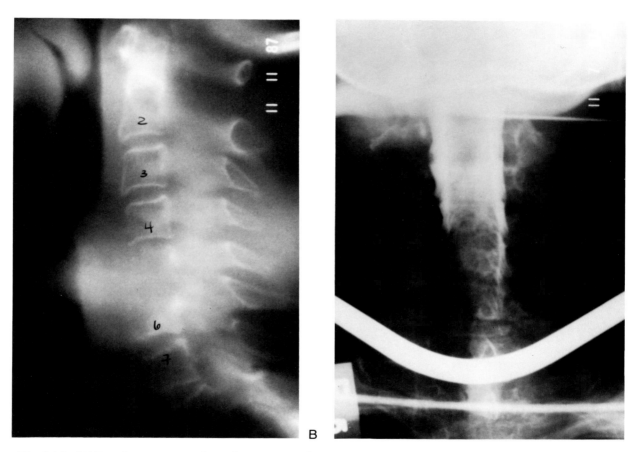

A   B

Fig. 14-6. (A) Initial preoperative lateral tomogram of cervical spine of the patient in Figure 14-3, showing osseous destruction of C5 and C6 as a result of *Staphylococcus aureus* osteomyelitis. This radiograph was obtained following emergency decompression. (B) AP myelogram showing obstruction of contrast flow at the level of the abscess. *(Figure continues).*

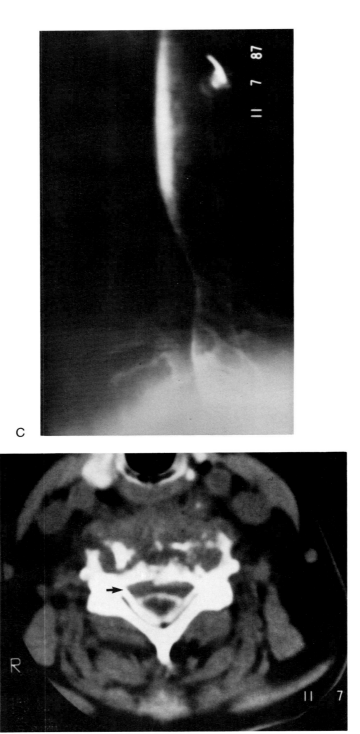

C

D

Fig. 14-6 *(Continued)*. **(C)** Lateral myelogram demonstrating the epidural abscess at C5–C6. **(D)** CAT scan showing destruction of the C5 vertebral body and the presence of the epidural abscess (arrow).

Relationship of Cervical Spine Trauma to Neurologic Trauma

Numerous investigators have attempted to classify fractures of the cervical spine to associate the fracture with both the resulting vertebral column instability and the resulting neurologic injury. While there is little question that the greater the displacement of bony elements, the greater the neurologic injury will be, a direct injury-neurologic disability correlation cannot be attained. Likewise, it is very difficult to classify fractures of

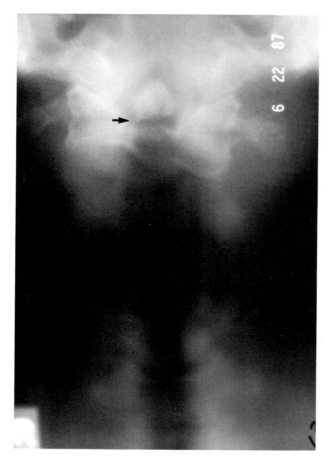

Fig. 14-7. AP radiograph showing the presence of os odontoideum (C2). Patient gave no history of trauma.

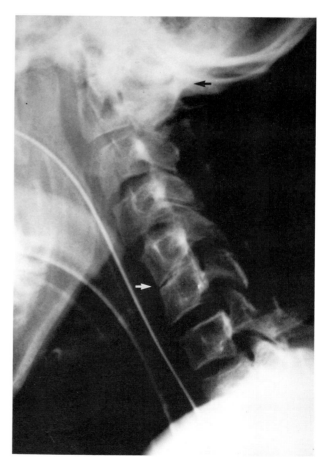

Fig. 14-8. Lateral radiograph of cervical spine in a 23-year-old man with numerous congenital abnormalities, including a basilar impression between the occiput and C2 and failure of segmentation of C5 and C6.

element alterations in architecture may be identified. A rather common one is the failure of segmentation, and thus the fusion of one or more cervical vertebral bodies, not infrequently identified at the C3–C4, C4–C5, or C5–C6 level (Fig. 14-8). Others include the absence of the posterior ring of C1 and the presence of a cervical hemivertebra (Klippel-Feil syndrome) (Fig. 14-9). When one hemivertebra is identified, a second will frequently exist at another level. When this occurs on the opposite side, a "balanced" defect results, and the spine appears straight, though short.

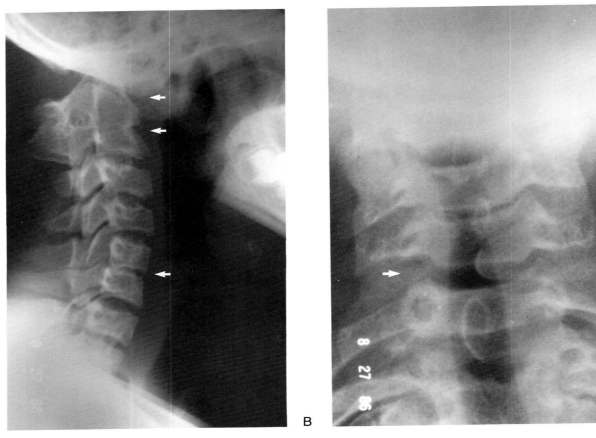

A   B

Fig. 14-9. (A) Lateral radiograph of cervical spine in a 16-year-old boy with absence of ring of C1, basilar impression (with extension of the odontoid into the foramen magnum), failure of segmentation of C2–C3, and abnormal articulation of vertebral elements C6–C7 (Klippel-Feil syndrome). (B) AP tomogram demonstrating abnormal lateral mass development of C6–C7. *(Figure continues.)*

the cervical vertebral column and to affix to each a prescribed fracture management scheme. Generalities can be drawn, such as "the more significant the fracture, the greater the displacement, the more obvious the instability," but the final decision rests on numerous factors. These include the extent of the neurologic injury, the need for anterior versus posterior surgery for neurologic decompression, etc.

The problem is, some cervical spine injuries result in neurologic injury without fracture, defying classification. These neurologic injuries are more than likely the result of a vascular injury. Although Bedbrook suggests that neural canal enchroach-

ment up to 50 percent can occur without overt neurologic compromise,[32] there does seem to be some correlation between injury and the extent of neural enchroachment between C1 and C7, and throughout the thoracic spinal canal as well. (Fig. 14-10). For example, the space within the neural canal posterior to C1 and C2 falls within the "rule of thirds." One-third of the space posterior to the anterior ring of C1 is taken up by the odontoid process. The middle one-third of the neural canal within the ring of C1 is taken up by the spinal cord, and the posterior one-third of the canal is free. Thus, the neural canal, measuring from the posterior border of the odontoid process to the anterior

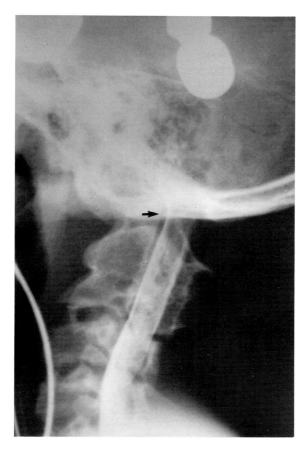

Fig. 14-9. *(Continued).* **(C)** Lateral myelogram of cervical spine demonstrating narrowness of the neural canal between the odontoid process and the posterior foramen magnum. This space should measure approximately 2 cm.

surface of the posterior ring of C1, measures 2.1 cm, whereas the spinal cord at this level is only 1 cm thick (Fig. 14-10.) It is this 1-cm "grace" distance that offers the upper cervical spinal cord immunity from injury and allows for the low incidence of neurologic injury after fractures of the odontoid (type II) (8.9 percent complete neurologic injury, 19 percent incomplete, and 70 percent intact).[2] The luxury of neural canal space does not exist below the level of C2. Beginning here, the canal rapidly narrows, and it reaches its most narrow point between C4 and C6. Although injury to the cervical vertebral column is most frequent at this

level, again it is noted that greater than 50 percent compromise may be required before neural injury is likely to occur.[32] This correlation was verified by Alker et al.[7] in a postmortem study of fatal traffic accident head and neck injuries. Coincidentally, it was found that a fracture of C1 was the most frequently identified injury in his series.

Generally, injuries to the lower cervical spine (C3-C7) result in some form of spinal cord injury with varying residuals of neurologic injury. In my experience, when a unilateral facet dislocation (or lock condition) occurred, 30 percent of the patients demonstrated neurologic injury (usually in the form of a Brown-Séquard neurologic injury) with a unilateral loss of motor function and contralateral loss of pain and temperature perception. This type of facet joint displacement follows a combination of flexion, distraction, and rotary forces.

From a biomechanical viewpoint, I found that 831 (56 percent) of the 1,484 cervical spine injured patients sustained either an axial load or a flexion load injury, resulting in either a "wedge" compression fracture or a "teardrop" fracture involving the anteroinferior aspect of the superior vertebra. The result, in terms of producing a neurologic injury, was that of the 831, 675 (81 percent) sustained either an incomplete or a complete neurologic injury, with only 19 percent remaining neurologically intact (Table 14-2). The type of injury most often occurring was that of a complete (motor-sensory) cord injury or an anterior cord syndrome with loss of motor function and preservation of the posterior column (proprioception and light touch) sensory tracts. When bilateral facet dislocation or a vertebral body burst fracture occurs, with greater than 50 percent of the neural canal in the midportion of the cervical spine compromised, 85 percent resulted in complete loss of motor and sensory function. Here the mechanism of injury is either flexion-distraction (bilateral locked and often fractured facets with significant vertebral element displacement) or axial load (burst fracture).

Allen et al.[8] in their classification of cervical spine fractures noted that the highest incidence of injury occurred with forces on the cervical spine resulting from compression-flexion injuries (22 percent), distraction-flexion injuries (37 percent), and compression extension injuries (24 percent).

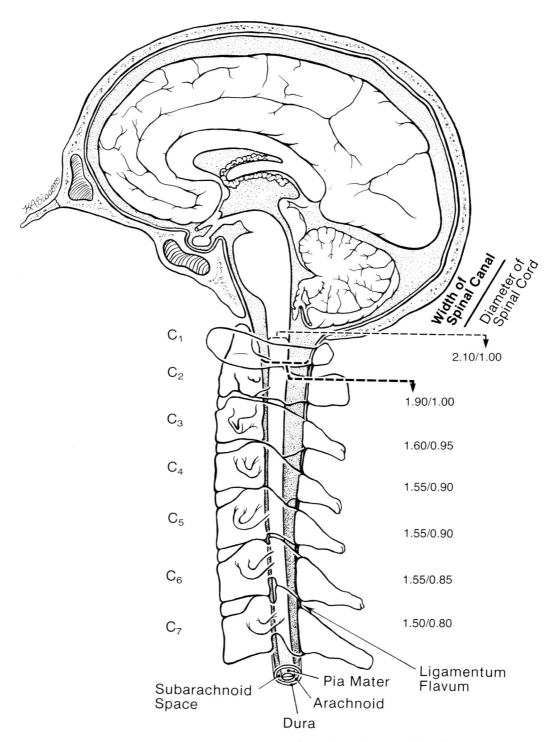

Fig. 14-10. Measurement ratio of spinal canal to spinal cord.

Table 14-2. Biomechanical Force by Extent (Northwestern University Acute Spine Injury Center 1972 to 1986)

Biomechanical Force	Total	Intact		Incomplete		Complete		Missing[b]	
		No.	Percent	No.	Percent	No.	Percent	No.	Percent
Axial	292	56	19.2	129	44.1	104	35.6	3	1.0
Flexion	547	100	18.3	232	42.4	210	38.4	5	0.9
Rotation	187	40	21.4	88	47.1	56	30.0	3	1.6
Direct	2	2	100.0	0	0.0	0	0.0	0	0.0
Extension	71	23	32.4	36	50.7	11	15.5	1	1.4
Odontoid	112	83	74.1	19	17.0	8	7.1	2	1.8
Other	163	42	25.8	67	41.1	51	31.3	3	1.8
Missing[a]	110	3	2.7	66	60.0	38	34.5	3	2.7
Total	1,484	349	23.5	637	42.9	478	32.2	20	1.3

[a]Biomechanical force is unavailable.
[b]Extent is unavailable.

The least number of neurological injuries followed distraction-extension (0.05), lateral bending-flexion injuries. (0.03 percent), and vertical-compression injuries (0.08 percent). Other researchers have described compression-flexion injuries of the spine,[33] distraction-flexion injuries,[34] distraction-extension injuries,[35,36] and compression-distraction injuries.[37]

Finally, while they occur with less frequency, hyperextension injuries of the cervical spine do occur and so one must be on the lookout for them (Fig. 14-11). This injury at the C2 level may result in an anteroinferior avulsion teardrop fracture, with rupture or loss of the attachment of the anterior longitudinal ligament. As already noted, at the C2 level, with acute hyperflexion and axial loading, a fracture of the posterior ring of C1 and C2 is possible. Neurologic injury at this level, however, is rare, because fracture of the posterior elements of C1 and C2 further widens the neural canal rather than decreases it, as occurs below these levels. If neurologic injury does occur, it is usually transient.

On the other hand, with a hyperextension injury to the midportion of the cervical spine with an associated anteroinferior teardrop fracture of the vertebral body and fracture of a posterior element, or when no fracture of the vertebral column can be identified, neurologic injury can still result. In the latter case, when no fracture can be identified, the occurrence of a central cord syndrome-type neurologic injury (with loss of motor and sensory function in the upper extremities and preservation of both in the lower extremities) can result from compression of the spinal cord between osteophytic spurs along the posterior border of the midcervical vertebral bodies (anterior to the spinal cord) and the hypertrophied and often calcified ligamentum flavum along the posterior neural canal, adjacent to the posteriorly located lamina (Fig. 14-12). This neurologic picture occurs in approximately 10 percent of the cases in which no fracture is identified. Usually this occurs in the older adult and not infrequently may be followed by an extension of the neurologic injury. This event is probably due to further embarrassment of an already fragile spinal cord vascular supply.

Emergency Room Management

The admission of a patient to a spinal trauma center mandates, in the victim's interest, that the receiving facility be notified of the patient's impending arrival before it occurs. Such notification allows for staff anticipation and preparation before, and not after, the patient's arrival. Such a plan implies that the physicians to whom total patient care responsibilities will fall have been informed. Al-

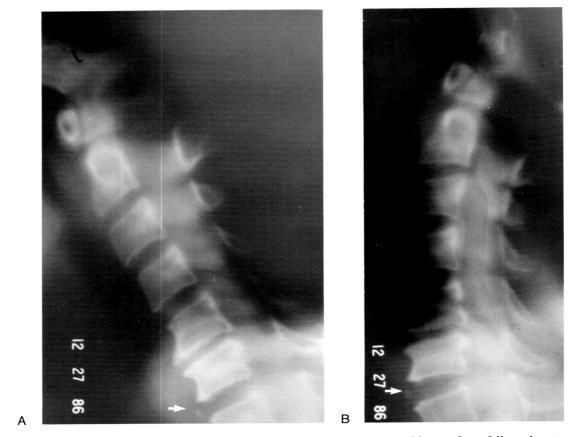

A   B

Fig. 14-11. (**A**) Lateral flexion tomogram of the cervical spine in a 70-year-old man after a fall resulting in a hyperextension injury to the cervical spine. The radiograph shows an increased C6–C7 intervertebral space. (**B**) Lateral tomogram with the head and neck extended. Note avulsion fracture and increased intervertebral disc space at C6–C7.

though physician notification seems obvious, it is in fact a relatively new management procedure, drawn from trauma team management concepts and protocols developed by the emergency medical service programs.[1] These concepts suggest that improved patient care occurs when a physician anticipates a patient's arrival, rather than finds out after the fact. When the physician on whom the responsibility for the patient care will fall is neither available nor informed, the patient's initial assessment and management are often delayed, disjointed, and confused. It may even be too late! Critical care procedures that normally are instituted under certain situations may be either delayed or omitted. When the admitting physician (or team manager) is well informed, the system is more likely to ensure that the normal procedures will be performed.[38-40] Such a system also provides quality assurance (see Emergency Room Protocol, Radiographic Protocol). The members of the medical management team that should be prenotified and available upon arrival of the patient in the emergency room are the emergency room physician, the assigned orthopaedic surgeon and neurosurgeon (or their assigned senior residents), a respiratory therapist or anesthesiologist, and in the case of mass trauma, a general surgeon (or the house staff's senior general surgery resident), who becomes the "team captain" until the attending physicians arrive.

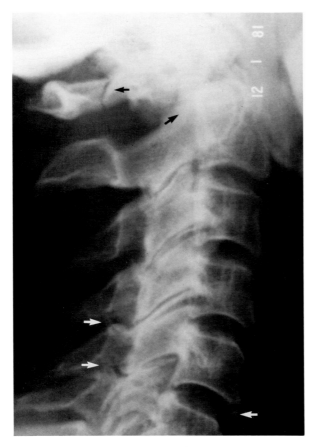

Fig. 14-12. Lateral radiograph of the cervical spine in an elderly patient who sustained a hyperextension injury resulting in a fracture of the posterior ring of C1, a type III fracture of the odontoid (C2), and an avulsion injury to the anterior longitudinal ligament at C5–C6. Note the widening of the intervertebral space anteriorly at C5–C6, and the evidence of ligamentum flavum calcification at C4–C5, C5–C6.

The first patient assessment procedure carried out on any acute trauma patient, and certainly on the suspected cervical spine-injured victim, is evaluation of the respiratory system. Crucial observations include the patient's color and respiratory rate, the presence of labored respiration (secondary to either neurologic injury or a hidden chest injury e.g., (hemothorax, pneumothorax, flail chest, etc.), the nature of the respiration (diaphragmatic and unaccompanied by chest expansion), the use of accessory muscles of respiration, including the strap muscles of the neck (sternocleidomastoid,

sternohyoid, omohyoid), and associated flaring of the ala nares. These latter two observations frequently serve as the initial indicators of a deteriorating voluntary respiratory system. To substantiate these observations, serial arterial blood gas values should be obtained. The initial signs of ventilatory deterioration can be found within the admission blood gas values: (1) a low arterial pH, (2) a hemoglobin saturation of less than 95 percent, and (3) an elevation in the arterial $PaCO_2$ are early indicators (see Ch. 13, Influences of Neurologic Injury on Respiration). One of the benefits of being aware of the patient's injury and impending arrival is that arterial blood gas studies can be ordered and obtained before patient transfer, and treatment measures can be instituted before and during transit to the tertiary care spine facility. A prerequisite during the preadmission (transfer) period of all cervical spine-injured patients is that nasal oxygen (5 liters/min) (see the discussion of preadmission protocol in Chapter 1) be administered during patient transfer. This supplemental oxygen must be taken into consideration when assessing the first postadmission blood gas readings.

A second evaluation procedure to be done is a cursory but carefully performed neurologic examination. This first neurologic examination, regardless by whom it is performed, becomes the all-important neurologic examination. Upon these findings, with reference to the spine and its neurologic injury, all future care, conservative or surgical, will be based. Having performed this task, scout radiographs (lateral or the cervical spine and an anteroposterior open mouth view of the odontoid process at C1–C2) should be obtained if not already available from the referring institution. If the patient is conscious, alert, and able to provide a history, it is much simpler to obtain an appropriate emergency room-area portable radiologic examination. If on the other hand, the neurologic examination is complicated by the presence of symptoms secondary to severe head trauma, the suspected area of spinal trauma may be hidden. Generally speaking, in the unconscious victim, when respiration is abdominal, the upper extremities are in a flexed position, and a priaprism is present, the level of injury is highly suspect to be in the cervical spine.[41,42] Nonetheless, in this particular situation, the entire spine must be radiographically evalu-

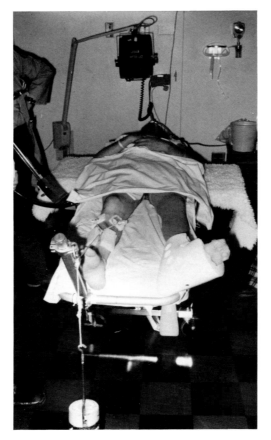

A

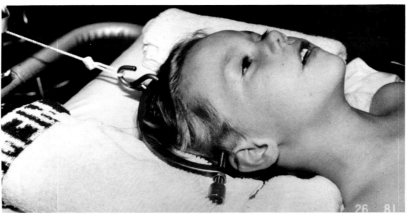

B

Fig. 14-13. (A) Bedside view of cervical spine injured (odontoid type II) patient on a Stryker wedge frame. The patient also sustained a posterior fracture dislocation of the right hip. The patient is being managed in skeletal traction. (B) Lateral photograph of a child in Gardner-Wells cervical tong traction. Note the position of the cervical tong pins approximately 1 cm above the pinna and aligned with the external auditory canal.

ated. The first two films to be obtained are the standard anteroposterior view (open mouth view of the odontoid and anterior cervical spine) and a lateral view of the cervical spine (always including C7). Careful attention must be paid to visualize all seven segments of the cervical spine. If the patient is large or has a short neck, it may be necessary to pull down on both arms toward the feet (thus lowering the shoulders) while taking the lateral view. It is emphasized that these two views, the initial anteroposterior and lateral radiographs, are only for "first knowledge." A more careful radiologic evaluation of the cervical spine should follow later, with the patient's assessment performed on a standard radiology table on which quality films can be obtained and, depending on the requirements of the managing physician, other films can be obtained (see Ch. 10).

Application of Cervical Traction

Should the spine-injured patient arrive at the emergency room without initial scout radiographs of the cervical spine or other areas of major concern, it is probably advisable to leave the patient on the ambulance stretcher until the injuries present are identified. Once these are known, the patient can, with appropriate assistance, be carefully moved to a fracture bed or frame. The frame that I routinely use is the Stryker wedge frame. The Stryker wedge frame eliminates the necessity of applying a special traction apparatus to the head of a standard bed. When the patient is transferred to the Stryker frame, he can be rapidly placed in skeletal tongs traction (Gardner-Wells tongs) (Fig. 14-13) The application of the Gardner-Wells tongs is uncomplicated. It requires only the preparation of the skin over each ear by shaving, and scrubbing with a cleansing agent such as Betadine (povidone-iodine). The skin over the top of the ear (just above the pinna) is infiltrated with 1 percent Xylocaine (lidocaine) and the tongs are applied. This usually requires less than 1 minute. The only determinant as to position placement of the tongs is whether to place the tong directly superior to the pinna of the ear (1 to 1.5 cm) to allow for straightaway traction or, if a slight amount of flexion is required (as when managing an extension injury to the spine), to in-

sert the tongs in line with the posterior border of the ear. If, as when treating an acute flexion injury, an extension movement of the head and neck is preferred, the tongs are inserted in line with the anterior border of the pinna of the ear (Fig. 14-14). The Gardner-Wells tongs do not require predrilling of the outer table of the skull. The tips of the tongs are very sharp and penetrate the skin easily with tightening, to engage the outer table firmly. The tongs have a self-contained spring-loaded indicator in one of the two points, providing a visual indication when the correct amount of counter pin pressure is present. My rule is to maintain appropriate pin tightness (at the same pressure) by observing the visual indicator daily.

The amount of initial traction used varies with the type and location of the cervical spine injury. As a rule, it is suggested that 5 lbs of weight be used per level of injury. Obviously, it is vitally important not to produce significant overdistraction. To prevent this condition, serial radiographs should be obtained during the early post-traction management hours to provide evidence whether additional weights are required for reduction or whether excess weight exists, necessitating some weight removal. For example, if a patient sustains a bilateral facet dislocation at C5–C6, the planned initial amount of weight to be utilized is 25 to 30 lbs. Every effort must be made to obtain an early spinal reduction. Most authorities agree that the most effective method of spinal cord decompression is obtaining a reduction and an improvement in the cervical vertebral columns alignment. This is easily identified in the presence of a bilateral facet dislocation. Here the superior vertebra is displaced anterior to the adjacent inferior vertebra by at least 50 percent of the vertebral body's width. Keeping in mind that the width of the neural canal at C5–C6 is approximately 1.55 cm (from the posterior vertebral body border of C5 to the anterior border of the laminar cortex posteriorly at C5) (Fig. 14-10), the canal width becomes reduced to 0.78 mm. With the spinal cord at this level measuring 0.9 mm thick, spinal cord compression with vascular compromise occurs. I have found that the spinal cord cannot undergo the slightest compression (even controlled and carefully applied retraction on the dura and its contents) without neurologic changes resulting. Thus, anterior pressure against

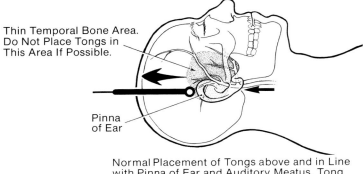

Thin Temporal Bone Area.
Do Not Place Tongs in
This Area If Possible.

Pinna
of Ear

Normal Placement of Tongs above and in Line
with Pinna of Ear and Auditory Meatus. Tong
Placement to Produce "Straight-Away" Traction.

A

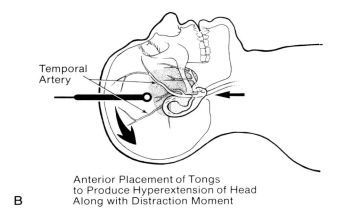

Temporal
Artery

Anterior Placement of Tongs
to Produce Hyperextension of Head
Along with Distraction Moment

B

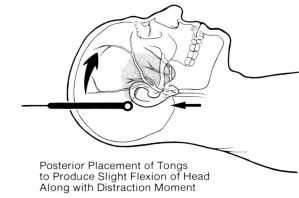

Posterior Placement of Tongs
to Produce Slight Flexion of Head
Along with Distraction Moment

C

Fig. 14-14. Correct insertion of Gardner-Wells tongs.

the spinal cord greatly compromises the anterior spinal artery. This structure in the normal state is very small, often less than a millimeter wide, yet it provides the principal arterial blood supply to the spinal cord and all of the central gray matter[43] (see Ch. 4).

Normally, with cervical traction applied, the angular deformity quickly straightens. To reduce a facet dislocation, additional weights will be required. Experience has demonstrated that even in the presence of a bilateral facet dislocation, the extent of ligamentous injury cannot be immediately determined. Therefore, follow-up lateral radiographs must be obtained within 30 to 45 min-

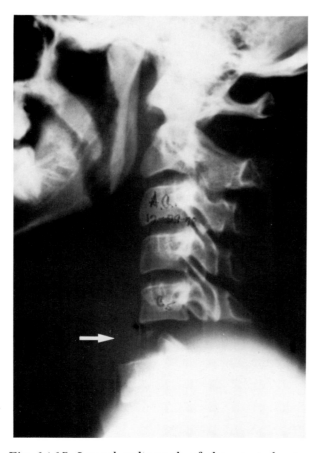

Fig. 14-15. Lateral radiograph of the cervical spine showing gross malalignment at C5–C6. The patient is in 20 lbs of Gardner-Wells cervical traction. Note three-column ligamentous instability with distraction between C5 and C6.

utes of the application of traction and the addition of each additional weight. In the case shown in Figure 14-15, even with the addition of what was believed to be appropriate weight (based on the rule of 5 lbs per level of injury), extensive ligamentous injury existed, allowing an abnormal amount of distraction to occur. An additional reason for obtaining early follow-up radiographs is that frequently a second level of injury will be identified (approximately 4 percent).

FIRST 24 HOURS

Monitoring and Limiting Neurologic Injury Extension

Once the cervical spine-injured patient (particularly in the presence of a neurologic injury) has been evaluated in the emergency area, cervical traction has been applied, and all other immediately required aspects of the clinical and radiologic evaluation have been completed, the patient should be admitted to and observed in an intensive care unit[1] for at least the first 24 hours. Clinically, any patient who sustains a cervical spine injury between C3 and C6 is a candidate for extension of the resulting neurologic injury. Often, the first indication of this condition will be a very slow and almost imperceptible decrease in pulmonary compliance, unfortunately on occasion identified by the sudden onset of respiratory failure and the calling of an "arrest." Although this is more likely to happen to the patient with a C4–C5 neurologic injury, it may also occur in the patient with a lower cervical spinal cord injury. We do not actually know what pathologic process leads to ascension of the neurologic deficit, but experience suggests that within the spinal cord, further hemorrhage or edema occurs, interrupting the spinal cord's microvascular blood supply, thus allowing for the occurrence of extension of the neurologic deficit.

One rule that has been found to be repeatedly true is that a patient who demonstrates a subtle loss of neurologic function usually, with time, will demonstrate a return of that function to the predeterioration (not to be confused with the pretrauma neurologic state) stage. This finding has repeatedly proved itself to be the case in those patients who on admission had voluntary ventilation, but within hours required intubation and ventilator assistance. It is supposed that edema and vascular compromise result in a proximal extension of this neurologic dysfunctional process, affecting the central gray matter and the anterior horn cells that provide motor function to the diaphragm via the phrenic (C3–C4–C5) nerve, principally by way of the C4 nerve root.[44] In an attempt to prevent cord edema and the subsequent loss of spinal cord capillary blood flow, drugs such as Decadron (dexamethasone) are administered during the early hours after spinal cord injury.[3,45–49] No conclusive evidence has been presented that steroids prevent or reduce spinal cord edema or convert a complete neurologic injury into an incomplete injury. Isolated case reports of the benefits of steroids exist,[11,50] but it is difficult to attribute neurologic stabilization or improvement solely to steroids, in light of the possibility of previously unrecognized or subclinically present incomplete neurologic function, or pure "chance" recovery. Similarly, while obvious beneficial effects of spinal cord cooling have been identified in the research laboratory, such benefits have not been reliably transcribed to the clinical setting. Kuchner et al.[50] noted that the combined effects of hypothermia and dexamethasone (steroids), when administered to laboratory animals immediately after induced neurologic injury, were superior to either therapy alone. Because the use of hypothermia requires the immediate application of this mode of therapy to be effective, and because considerable surgical dissection is required to derive the beneficial effects of hypothermia, this technique is not utilized. Recently, naloxone hydrochloride (Narcan) has been discussed as a drug to be used in the immediate postinjury period.[51,52] At present, I am not aware of direct evidence that this drug reduces neural tissue's responses to trauma or improves the traumatized spinal cord's vascular supply; however, the latter appears to be the most plausible.

During this initial evaluation period, I strongly recommend, at a minimum, (1) the continuous electrocardiogram monitoring of the ECG; (2) continuous arterial pressure monitoring; (3) the obtaining of frequent arterial blood gas values via an arterial catheter; (4) continuous urine output measurement; (5) intermittent gastric pH measurement; and (6) neurologic reassessment and documentation every 2 hours.

Because the two major complications that may occur in the acute cervical spine-injured patient during the early hours after injury are a decreasing ventilatory function and generalized neurologic deterioration, and because the two are related, the spinal cord intensive care unit should be administered by a "medical intensivist" such as a respiratory critical care physician. This ensures that the patient is carefully supported and observed by a service acutely involved in the initial phase of care.

Prevention of Neurologic Shock

In my opinion, the most effective means of preventing further neurologic deterioration after injury to the spinal column (and spinal cord) is to prevent one of the primary and initial effects of cervical spinal cord injury, that of peripheral vascular dilation (with resulting hypotension) secondary to the traumatic interruption of the sympathetic autonomic nervous system (see Ch. 5). To assist in counteracting this reflexogenic rather than blood-loss state of hypotension, the administration of intravenous fluids (0.9 normal saline or lactated Ringer's solution) immediately post-trauma reduces the effects of peripheral vasodilation resulting from a loss of autonomic (sympathetic) function[1] (see Chapter 1). Neurologic tissue does not tolerate even short periods of hypoxemia or hypotension. Some factor of care has contributed to the improved neurologic statistics now being witnessed in the major spinal cord injury centers within the United States.[4] For example, data derived from the center at Northwestern University reveal a continued decrease in the number of complete spinal cord injuries between 1972 and 1986. Whether the decrease from 70 percent complete neurologic injuries (1972) to 44 percent complete neurologic injuries (1986) is cumulative or the singular effect of any of the following is not yet appreciated: improved, immediate response, accident scene care; careful extraction and splinting; the early referral of the suspected spinal cord-injured victim to an appropriate care facility; the early administration of steroids; the early administration of intravenous fluids (or blood) for the prevention of shock; or the early reduction of a spine dislocation. More than likely, each factor has contributed, with the culmination being a dramatic improvement in the preservation of residual neurologic function.

Ancillary Evaluative Procedures

Multitrauma patients sustaining both a spine and a neurologic injury requires a disciplined evaluation of their injuries. After an initial ABC (airway, breathing, and circulation) assessment, the observed level of neurologic function serves as the indicator of additional evaluation responses to be obtained. In the presence of a complete neurologic injury, in which no function exists below the level of injury, attention can be directed strictly to the state of spinal alignment. An incomplete neurologic injury, on the other hand, requires a determination as to whether the findings can be influenced or altered by the performance of some procedure or technique (i.e., cervical traction with improved spinal alignment, myelogram, tomogram, computed axial tomography [CAT] scan, magnetic resonance imaging [MRI], surgical intervention, etc.). Once the patient's condition has been stabilized, further assessment should proceed along a prescribed course, varying only upon the specifics relating to each patient.

Myelography

The use of the water-soluble contrast material metrizamide for myelographic evaluation of neural canal compromise is a very valuable assessment tool. Its use in the acutely injured spinal cord patient is based on criteria arrived at over many years by neurosurgeons and orthopaedic surgeons (see Ch. 15, p. 412). Appreciating that the procedure is not without complication, particularly in the recently traumatized cervical spine injured patient, it is not performed without specific indication. For example, should a spine-injured patient be admitted with a unilateral facet dislocation, and evidence of either a Brown-Séquard or central cord incom-

plete neurologic injury, the most logical explanation for the neurologic injury would be the presence of the facet dislocation. The first order of management therefore would be attaining a reduction of the facet dislocation. This having been accomplished, the neurologic status would be anticipated to improve without further intervention, other than the probable administration of steroids at the time of the patient's admission. Should, in this initial phase of management, the patient's dislocation not be reducible, and an incomplete neurological injury be present, surgery may be contemplated, necessitating obtaining a preoperative myelogram. If spine reduction can be accomplished and neurologic function within a prescribed period of time does not demonstrate improvement, a myelogram is indicated. Similarly, should there occur a sudden deterioration in neurologic function, a myelogram becomes indicated.

Each of the above situations calls for a varied response on the part of the evaluator. To assist in determining the need for obtaining a myelogram, the following indications have been arrived at:

1. The occurrence of a rapidly progressive and otherwise unanticipated neurologic deterioration.
2. The presence of neurologic injury in the absence of radiologic evidence of bone or ligamentous injury.
3. When a patient exhibits post-traumatic neurologic recovery with an abrupt neurologic plateau.
4. When an elective spinal stabilization procedure is planned on a patient with an incomplete neurologic injury. (This is considered the only prophylactic reason for myelography.)
5. When the clinical neurologic level does not coincide with the somatosensory evoked potential (SSEP) neurologic level.

There is little indication for obtaining a myelography in a patient that already has a complete neurologic injury. An exception might be further neurologic deterioration in the patient who already has a complete neurologic injury. However, from careful evaluation of greater than 2,700 acute spinal cord injuries, this is very rare.

Standard and Nonstandard Radiographs

When a patient presents with a history of injury to the cervical spine, with or without neurologic injury, but without visual evidence of vertebral column trauma, the question always exists, "How do you confirm the presence or absence of a recent injury?" The patient who has sustained an associated neurologic injury is managed as described in the spinal cord protocol, with skeletal tong traction. This provides the patient protection and suggests to those caring for the patient that a spine injury is suspected. Following this, an evaluative technique found most helpful is flexion-extension radiographs, in the lateral projection, with the patient in light cervical traction on a Stryker wedge frame. If skeletal tongs are in place, the weights may require being reduced. This procedure should be performed by a physician trained to recognize potential problems as they may arise. The patient may have to be turned into the prone position to obtain the extensive view. This is one reason for placing such patients on a Stryker frame on admission.

Again, using the hypothetical patient who has sustained a neurologic injury in the absence of a recognized vertebral column injury, a procedure found diagnostically helpful is the standard technetium-99 bone scan. This procedure is very sensitive to increased blood flow or the presence of localized hemorrhage. Should this study return as negative and the patient have no associated neurologic injury, the patient can be discharged, using a semirigid cervical collar as a splint, depending on the patient's complaints. When the radiographic evaluation, in the presence of a recognized neurologic injury, fails to reveal any evidence of vertebral column or ligamentous instability, a myelogram becomes indicated. If this too is negative, the patient should continue to be managed conservatively in traction for a variable period, providing continued protection to the cervical spine while awaiting subsidence of the neurologic injury.

Additional radiographs beneficial for evaluation of the cervical spine during the initial evaluative process include the standard open mouth view of the odontoid process (C2), the "swimmer's" (lateral) view of C6–C7–T1 area of the spine, particu-larly in the patient with a short neck and broad shoulders in whom C7 fails to appear in the standard lateral radiograph (Fig. 14-16). Right and left oblique radiographs of the cervical spine (for the visualization of the facet joints) may be helpful for some physicians and therefore can be obtained. Care must always be taken to instruct the radiology technician not to move the neck to obtain a radiograph, rather to move the x-ray tube to the position required.

Polytomography and Computed Axial Tomography

Although there may be some controversy as to which is the more valuable as an evaluative tool, CAT or polytomography, both have their place. Polytomography provides a "macroscopic" longitudinal view of the spine over multiple levels simultaneously, in either the anteroposterior or lateral plane. This is important in determining the extent of bony injury over multiple levels and assists the managing physician in determining the number of levels over which internal fixation may be required. It also provides better visualization and localization of fracture fragments in a lateral projection, demonstrating the extent of existing spinal malalignment resulting from injury.

Conventional tomography, in my opinion, is the best technique available for the evaluation of upper cervical spine injuries (C1 and C2). In the presence of an odontoid process, facet, or lateral mass fracture, the plane of injury may coincide with the horizontal (CAT scan) level above or below the level of injury, thus failing to reveal the extent of the injury. The same fracture, however, can be readily identified by two-plane tomography.

Computed axial tomography (CAT scan) is extremely valuable in assessing the vertebral column in a horizontal plane. This procedure provides for both soft tissue and bone anatomy evaluation and provides the best method of assessing the extent of vertebral canal compromise. As noted, it also allows for the identification of soft tissue (intervertebral disc) injuries. Combining this procedure with the use of a metrizamide contrast myelogram,

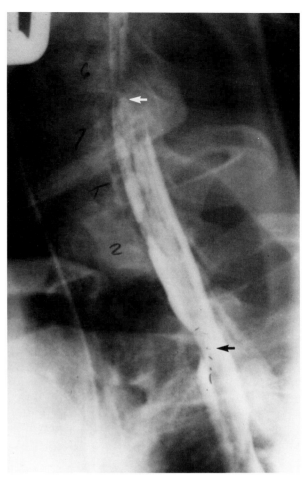

Fig. 14-16. Lateral radiograph of the cervicothoracic junction obtained by the "swimmer's view" technique, which allows for evaluation of the cervicothoracic junction. Note myelographic defect at C6–C7, posterior subluxation at C6–C7 and myelographic defect at T4–T5.

any compression of the neural canal and the dural column can be ascertained (Fig. 14-5D).

My institution obtains both evaluative procedures on each patient during the postadmission evaluation process. The procedures are often complementary to each other in terms of the presence of fractures, alterations in bone and soft tissue anatomy, displacement of fragments, spinal alignment, and neural canal integrity.

Magnetic Resonance Imaging

Magnetic resonance imaging (MRI) is the newest and most recent radiologic technique being used for the evaluation of the spine- and spinal cord-injured patient. Two of the most valuable aspects of this procedure are that it is neither x-ray producing nor invasive. The physics of the procedure involves the placement of a patient into a superconducting magnet-computer imaging unit, which by virtue of the lines of magnetic flux aligns cellular structure protons (of various tissues: bone, muscle, hematoma) into a position in which they parallel the magnetic field. With the intermittent addition of a variable radio frequency applied across the magnetic field, the protons within the structures under evaluation emit a signal (with a signal intensity) generated from within the body. This signal varies in accordance with the radio frequency, the level of the body under evaluation, the tissue (bone or soft tissue) response, and the "normalcy" of the tissue. There are two signals utilized: T1, which is basically described as the "relaxation time, in relation to the environment of the proton," and T2, which is defined as "the relaxation time in relation to other nearby protons, and relates to the proton attempting to tilt back to its normal position, thus is out of alignment." The difference between these two "signals" provides the variations seen in pictorial representation, allowing for the identification of specific structures or processes, normal anatomy, or structural changes, best seen in T1 (spinal cord, intervertebral disc, vertebral bodies, paravertebral muscle, etc.) or in T2 where pathologic processes (hematoma, tumor) in the above structures are best identified (Fig. 14-17).

The use of this evaluative tool has been slow in coming for the acute spinal cord-injured patient, particularly during the evaluation of the patient with an unstable spine injury requiring maintenance in skeletal traction (e.g., the cervical spine) or careful transfer in the presence of an unstable thoracolumbar injury. For the cervical spine-injured patient, the presence of ferrous (iron-containing) materials used on the patient (as with skeletal tongs) made evaluation by this means prohibitive. This is now changing, as alternative nonferrous materials become available for patient

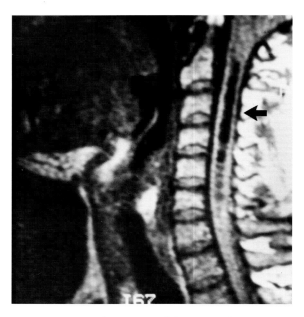

Fig. 14-17. Lateral MR view of the cervical spine revealing a syrinx or cyst involving the central spinal cord (dark area within spinal cord).

management. Unquestionably, the information obtained by this technique alone is often superior to that obtained by the numerous other procedures, even when used in combination. This is particularly the case for spinal (bone or neural tissue) tumors and for determining the presence of a spinal cord syrinx (Fig. 14-17).

According to Kulkarni et al,[53] three magnetic resonance (MR) patterns have been identified in spinal cord injury. The type I pattern reveals the T1 weighted image (WI) to be "inhomogeneous", and the T2 WI is hypointense in the central area with "a thin rim of hyperintensity in the periphery." These images coincided with spinal cord hemorrhage and a clinical finding of poor neurologic recovery. In the second (II) and third (III) MR patterns, the T1 WIs were normal, while the T2 WI in the central area revealed hyperintensity and small areas of hypointensity, while in the periphery, the type II MR demonstrated hyperintensity and the type III MR demonstrated a thin rim of hyperintensity. In the latter two MR types (II, III), significant neurologic recovery occured. These investigators found that the optimum time for the obtaining of the MRI was within 24 to 72 hours postinjury.

Somatosensory and Cortical Evoked Potential Monitoring

Somatosensory and cortical evoked potential monitoring has become a very reliable evaluative tool for determining the electrical presence or absence of neurologic function below the level of injury. Not only has this technique enabled the accurate functional mapping of the peripheral sensory dermatomes, but it has also been effectively utilized to ascertain the presence or altered function of the dorsal (sensory) columns, and for the determination of the all-important presence (or absence) of perianal "sacral sparing." On the motor side, the use of the SSEP has been increasingly helpful in the prognostic assessment of motor function return. By recording the H reflex by means of electrodes placed over the sural nerve and the tibialis anterior muscle groups, special attention is placed on the muscle groups' excitability as measured by maximal H-to-M response ratio, the threshold of its appearance, and its "recovery" period. This tool provides data on the preservation of the cortical spinal tracts. A complete lesion in this pathway is indicated by a marked increase in the excitability of the H reflex and a drastic shortening of its recovery period. In doubtful cases, additional information can be provided by changes of the H reflex amplitude when the patient attempts to perform a requested voluntary activity in the above-named muscle group. Significant changes in the H reflex amplitude will occur in this condition, even in the absence of voluntary movement. The electromyogram (EMG) will usually indicate significant sparing of the long descending pathways.

The use of the SSEP as a neurologic evaluative tool has increased significantly over the past several years as the technique became refined and better interpreted. The procedure is now utilized for preoperative neurologic assessment and, in the neurologically incomplete patient, as an intraoperative neurologic "monitoring" device. Alterations in the intraoperative SSEP can result from a number of events, including ambient room temperature (lowering of the patient's body temperature), the administration of cold fluids (saline, blood, etc.), various anesthetic agents (Flurane) injury to the nervous system resulting from the surgery, etc. The most concerning alteration is a change or lengthing of the SSEP's "latency period," or the period of time it takes for an induced electrical stimulus applied to the median nerve (at the wrist) to reach the posterior cervical spine or the cerebral cortex. This procedure is now utilized on any patient undergoing spinal surgery who demonstrated preoperatively the presence of either normal neurologic function or an incomplete neurologic injury.

A new and exciting area of research presently under way at Northwestern University, by Richard Katz of the Rehabilitation Institute, on spinal cord patients is the use of the Cadwell MES model 10 magnetic stimulator for the production of peripheral motor activity by evoking a cerebral cortical response with an externally applied, noninvasive stimulus. The signal, induced transcortically by means of an electrical wire coil external to but in proximity to the vertex of the skull, emits a stimulus intensity of 350 volt root mean square (RMS), over 100 microseconds, resulting in a 0.25 weber (RMS) magnetic flux or flow of energy (Fig. 14-18). The result of this stimulus is the production of an "elec-

trodeless electrical stimulus" (magnetic electrical stimulus), causing a localized depolarization of cortical and subcortical tissue that results in peripheral motor activity in either the upper or lower extremities. Both the latency and the amplitude of the induced stimulus can be measured, similar to that observed with somatosensory cortical evoked responses. Both studies, motor and sensory evoked responses, will enable monitoring of the central nervous system (cerebral cortex and spinal cord), providing information relevant to alterations in neurologic function secondary to trauma, disease, or tumor.

Isotope Scanning Techniques

It is not unusual for a patient who has sustained known trauma to the spine to have the injury go undetected on either standard or flexion-extension radiographs. Under these circumstances, a procedure found very helpful in the evaluative process is the use of the technetium-99 (^{99}Tc) bone scanning or imaging technique. The rationale for the use of this scanning technique in a trauma patient is the fact that the procedure is very sensitive to any process resulting in increased vascularity (trauma, infection, or a cellulitis).[54] Using technetium-99 (^{99}Tc diphosphonate) alone to accurately differentiate between trauma and infection is not possible. For this reason, additional isotope techniques are required. They include the gallium-67 and the indium-111 studies. The latter study requires the injection of labeled autologous leukocytes and is very specific for the identification of infectious processes resulting from an accumulation of white cell debris (musculoskeletal sepsis). For example, in the presence of a known pseudoarthrosis, in which a gallium scan may demonstrate a positive signal even in the absence of an infection, under similar circumstances a ^{111}In-labeled leukocyte scan will be negative in the absence of an infection and positive in the presence of an infection when associated with a pseudoarthrosis. Thus, fracture evaluation by isotope scanning (^{99}Tc diphosphonate) can be utilized, knowing the patient's pretrauma condition. When questions exist, more careful assessment of the etiology of increased isotope uptake can be performed by using gallium-67 or the se-

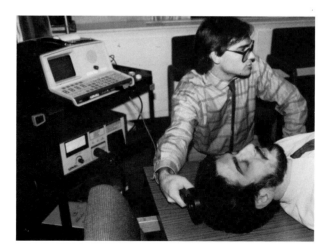

Fig. 14-18. Photograph demonstrating the use of a hand-held magnetic coil over the vertex of the skull, used to emit magnetic flux or flow of energy. This noninvasive electrical stimulation of the cerebral cortex allows for direct motor (pyramidal) tract stimulation.

quential technetium/gallium or the indium-111 scanning techniques.

CLASSIFICATION OF CERVICAL SPINE INJURIES

Cheshire[55] and Burke and Tiong,[56] in their effort to determine the success or failure of conservative management of cervical spine and spinal cord injuries, defined spinal stability as "the absence of abnormal mobility between any pair of vertebrae, without pain or other clinical manifestation, when lateral flexion and extension radiographs of the cervical spine were obtained at the conclusion of conservative treatment for a fracture or fracture-dislocation." Both reported a very low incidence of instability (7.5 and 4.2 percent, respectively). The classification of cervical spine injuries utilized by Cheshire and Burke included the following major categories:

1. Atlantoaxial injuries
2. Flexion-rotation injuries that include subluxation, unilateral facet dislocation or fracture-dislocation, bilateral dislocation or fracture-dislocation
3. Extension injuries:
    a. Extension disruption of a normal spine, or a spine affected by cervical spondylosis
    b. Extension disruption of a spine affected by ankylosing spondylitis
    c. Extension injury of a normal spine, or a spine affected by cervical spondylosis, without bony injury or ligamentous disruption
    d. Complete instability in apparent extension injuries
    e. Extension injuries leading to fracture-dislocation
4. Compression or axial load injuries
5. Cervical spinal cord concussion (a temporary neurologic injury, normally recoverable within the first 24 hours)
6. Miscellaneous

In Burke and Tiong's review, categories 3a, 3c, 5, and 6 were eliminated from the classification, since they seemed to contribute little. Allen et al.[8]

in 1982 suggested the use of a more anatomically detailed classification of cervical spine fractures. To do so is more cumbersome, though it allows, like the Frankel scale, a uniform and clearly defined method of comparing types of cervical spine injuries and a more objective method of comparing conservative versus surgical management of specific injury types. Other researchers contributing to the development of a cervical spine fracture classification were Whitley and Forsyth[57] and Gschweiler et al.[14] Included in their classifications were hyperflexion and extension rotational injuries. Most authors agreed that there must be certain anatomic structures, or combinations of structures, considered when comparing alternate management schemes (Table 14-3). These included the type of vertebral body fracture; the presence or absence of fractures of the pedicles; whether the articular processes were involved; fracture or disruption of the posterior elements (lamina, spinous process or intervening ligaments); and the state of neurologic function in each (see Table 15-1). As noted elsewhere in the chapter, the correlation between the "state of neurologic function" and the fracture type is difficult to ascertain and often unrelated, therefore of little benefit.

Another area of general agreement in the definition and evaluation of cervical spine stability is a common awareness of structures forming the "columns" of the cervical spine. Before 1983, when Denis presented the "three-column" theory relating to the thoracolumbar spine (Fig. 18-9),[58] only the two-column theory existed. Rogers in Chapter 10 of this book defined the columns as follows. The "anterior column" included the anterior longitudinal ligament, the vertebral body, the intervertebral disc, and the posterior longitudinal ligament (Fig. 10-14). Of the two longitudinal ligaments, the stronger and more important is the anterior ligament. The "posterior column" is composed of the facet apophyseal joints, the pedicles, the lamina, the spinous process, and the intervening ligaments. An area of some minor disagreement is whether or not, if one of the two columns remains intact, the entire vertebral column could be considered stable. A consensus exists that when both remain intact, stability is ensured.

Inasmuch as injury to the soft tissue supporting structures of the anterior cervical spine cannot be

Table 14-3. Fracture Type by Treatment (Northwestern University
Acute Spine Injury Center, 1972 to 1986)

Fracture Type	Total	Conservative		Surgical	
		No.	Percent	No.	Percent
Body	359	232	64.6	127	35.4
Axial body compression-burst	185	104	56.2	81	43.8
Subluxation	97	52	53.6	45	46.4
Body compression	87	40	45.9	47	54.1
Bilateral facet lock and dislocation	77	28	36.4	49	63.6
Facet	77	42	54.5	35	45.5
Unilateral facet lock	69	15	21.7	54	78.3
Type II odontoid	56	36	64.3	20	35.7
Bullet fragments	54	53	98.1	1	1.9
Hangman's	41	36	87.8	5	12.2
Avulsed chip	39	18	46.2	21	53.8
Spinous process	34	30	88.2	4	11.8
Lamina	34	20	58.8	14	41.2
Pedicle	19	11	57.9	8	42.1
Posterior ligament disruption	19	11	57.9	8	42.1
Jefferson	15	12	80.0	3	20.0
Type III odontoid	15	11	73.3	4	26.7
Type I odontoid	10	6	60.0	4	40.0
Spondylolisthesis	8	8	100.0	0	0.0
Bilateral lamina	7	3	42.9	4	57.1
Anterior ligament disruption	5	2	40.0	3	60.0
Atlantoaxial subluxation	2	2	100.0	0	0.0
Transverse process	2	1	50.0	1	50.0
Bilateral pedicle	1	1	100.0	0	0.0
Other	62	44	71.0	18	29.0
None	110	104	94.5	6	5.5
Total	1,484	922	62.1	562	37.9

directly visualized by radiographic evaluation, the presence of such pathology should be suspected when flexion-extension radiographs of the cervical spine reveals abnormal motion and widening anteriorly, and when there is abnormal tissue swelling within the retropharyngeal space anteriorly, between C4 and C7. Though swelling in the retropharyngeal space can result from direct trauma to the anterior neck, more often it is the result of a hyperextension force resulting in injury to the anterior longitudinal ligament. With bleeding into this space, various degrees of a prevertebral soft tissue shadow will occur. While difficult to equate absolutely to the presence of pathology, a widened retropharyngeal space, greater than seven-eighths the width of the vertebral body (or 15 mm), opposite or below the C4-C5 interspace is suggestive of pathology. Likewise, a prevertebral shadow greater than 10 mm (at C1) or 4 mm (at C3-C4) requires careful evaluation (Fig. 10-14).

Another subtle finding representing evidence of posterior column instability is the finding of a wedge-shaped intervertebral disc at the suspected level of injury (see Ch. 10). The anterior intervertebral disc will be slightly decreased in height, while the posterior disc border will be slightly increased. Often accompanying this will be a minimal anterior subluxation (up to 1 to 2 mm) of the upper vertebral body, referred to as "sagging." A disruption of the disc alone is often associated with this minimal degree of subluxation. This subtle shift in position should be taken into consideration when reviewing spine films. In this same area, normally the anterior alignment of the cervical spine will reveal a clean, smooth, convex anterior vertebral body alignment. The only normal deviation from this is anticipated anterior displacement of the ring of C1, anterior to the odontoid process.

The anatomic region of the spine known as the craniovertebral angle (cranioatlantoaxial joints) requires separate consideration. It has been reported[3,57] that the most likely site of vertebral column injury in motor vehicle and pedestrian victims succumbing at the scene of the accident is injury to the craniovertebral area. The rationale for this is based on two facts: autopsy[3] and the anatomic finding that the space available for the brain stem and the spinal cord at the foramen magnum and C1 and C2 neural canal levels is two times wider than the spinal cord[59,60] at these levels. Injury to the brain stem or spinal cord above the level of the nerves to the diaphragm (C3 – C4 – C5) will result in immediate death, unless the patient is immediately ventilated by some means. When death does not result, only a minor or transient neurologic injury, or no neurologic injury at all, will occur. Admittedly, with improvement of paramedical care at the accident scene, it is conceivable that increasing numbers of victims with such injuries could survive with early resuscitation.

The important anatomic structures providing stability to the cranioatlantoaxial articulation include the broad ligamentous structures connecting the anteroposterior surfaces of the spinal canal between the foramen magnum and C1. From the apical tip of the odontoid process extending proximally to the anterior margin of the foramen magnum is the cruciform ligament (superior longitudinal crus) (Fig. 15-27), and extending from either side of the dens to either side of the foramen magnum are the alar ligaments. Between the two lateral articular masses of C1, just posterior to the odontoid process of C2, lies the transverse liga-

ment, also known as the ligamentum transversum. Thus, the dens (or odontoid process) lies between the anterior arch of the atlas, held in place by the transverse ligament, and separated from both by a true joint anteriorly and a synovial joint posteriorly.[61] It is for this reason that the C1-C2 bony processes are so often involved in the rheumatoid arthritic patient with widespread disease (see Fig. 15-21). When that occurs, the result is an insidious and progressive dissolution of the odontoid process by rheumatoid pannus. Eventually, atlantoaxial instability develops. The findings are often subtle, making the diagnosis difficult or leaving the examiner with questions. When no obvious instability is noted, the patient should be splinted by a cervical collar (rigid or soft) until no longer symptomatic.

ANATOMY: NORMAL CERVICAL SPINE MOTION

In place of a vertebral body at C1 (the atlas), an upward extension to the body of the C2 (axis) develops, resulting in a flucrum-rotatory joint between the residual anterior arch of the atlas and the upward extension of the body of C2 known as the odontoid process, the dens, or the epistropheus. Between the odontoid process and the anterior arch of the atlas lies a synovial joint. The atlantoaxial relationship is maintained by major ligamentous structures, which include (Fig. 15-27) the anterior longitudinal ligament that extends cephalad to the anterior tubercle of C1; the posterior longitudinal ligament that extends upward posterior to the cervical vertebral bodies to attach on the basilar portion of the occipital bone; the strong transverse ligament that passes transversely posterior to the odontoid process, is separated from it by a synovial joint, and attaches to either side along the inner side of the lateral mass of the atlas. It provides the primary stability between the atlas and the odontoid process of the axis.

Coutts[62] noted that a single ligamentous deficiency, that of the transverse odontoid ligament, could allow for the displacement of the atlas on the axis by as much as 5 mm and, at 45 degrees of flexion, could lead to a dislocation between C1 and C2. With ligamentous instability, displacement is possible, there being only short muscles connecting the axis to the cranium to prevent it. The extent of motion that exists at the occipital-C1 level is 15 degrees of flexion and extension. Widening of more than 2 to 3 mm between the odontoid process and the rig of C1 indicates transverse ligament instability. The extent of rotation between C1 and C2 is approximately 45 degrees of motion in either direction.[63]

On the other hand, flexion, extension, and rotary motion that occurs between C2 and C7 vertebrae is shared at each of the five intervening vertebral levels by their respective facet or apophyseal joints. A wide range of motion occurs at each of these levels as a result of the configuration and angular relationship of the articular processes. Thus, independent motion is not possible. Complete dislocation of the lateral articular masses between the atlas and the axis occurs at approximately 65 degrees of rotation. At this position, the canal is reduced to 7 mm (Fig. 15-41C). The spinal cord at this level measures approximately 0.95 cm in width. Thus, such displacement would result in significant cord compression.

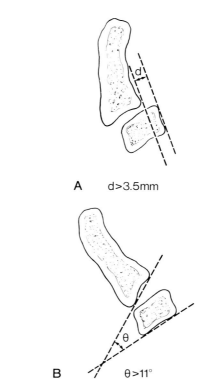

Fig. 14-19. Instability at the C2–C3 interval is indicated by translation (**A**) or angular (**B**) deformities at C2–C3.

MEASURING EXTENT OF INSTABILITY

Levine and Edwards,[64] in their review of traumatic spondylolisthesis involving the axis (C2), noted two criteria for classifying fractures involving the posterior arch of C2. One is the classification of White and Panjabi,[65] as used by Francis and associates,[66] the limits of instability as measured between C2-C3 relative to the forward displacement of the body of C2 on C3 (greater than 3.5 mm), and the flexion-angular tilt between the body of C2 and C3 (greater than 11 degrees) (Fig. 14-19). The second classification was that of Effendi et al,[67] in which the fracture types include types I, II, IIa, and III associated with bilateral facet dislocation (the most unstable).

There are other important measurements or "in-

nuendos" of cervical pathology that have been or will be described in other areas of this chapter. Because it was believed that together they represent important diagnostic measurements, it was thought appropriate to include them into one area.

Fractures or congenital failure of fusion between multiple apophyseal growth centers in the proximal third of the odontoid process (os odontoideum) may result in significant narrowing between the posterior body of C2 and the inner aspect of the posterior ring of C1, particularly with flexion of the neck. Spierings and Braakman[68] refer to this as being abnormal when there exists a "D_{min}" (a minimal sagittal diameter less than 13 mm). This narrowness can be correlated with an increased risk of permanent or progressive spinal cord neurologic signs. When either are present, a occipitocervical or atlantoaxial fusion is indicated.

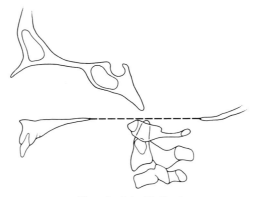

Chamberlain Method
Position of Odontoid Is Abnormal if Odontoid
Extends 6.6mm above Chamberlain's Line

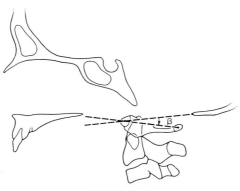

Bull Method
Position of Odontoid Is Abnormal if β >13°

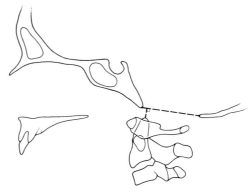

McRae Method
Position of Odontoid Is Abnormal if Odontoid
Extends above McRae's Line

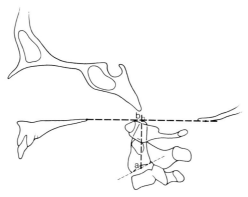

Redlund-Johnell Method
Position of Odontoid Is Abnormal if ab ≤ 33mm

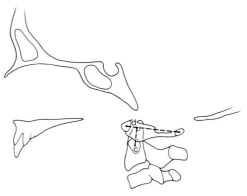

Ranawat Method
Position of Odontoid Is Abnormal if cd ≤ 13mm

Fig. 14-20. Measurement of the base of the skull for basilar invagination based on normal anatomy.

The extent of "normal" horizontal motion between the occipitoatlantal joint in flexion-extension is 1 mm[69] of translation. In the presence of such congenital deformities as failure of segmentation or developmental multisegmental fusions within the upper cervical spine, a compensatory hypermobility may exist.

Radiographs of the cervical spine always require careful visualization of the upper cervical spine (occiput, C1, C2 relationship) for the presence of pathology. For fractures of the ring of C1 (Jefferson fracture), spreading or "overhanging" of the lateral mass of C1 on C2 can best be identified on an anterioposterior view. Fractures of the odontoid can best be visualized on the lateral radiograph. Also best seen in the lateral projection is the presence of abnormal upper migration of the odontoid process into the foramen magnum (basilar impression). Several radiographic lines have been established to serve as indicators of the presence of this pathologic process. They include Chamberlain's line,[70] McRae's line,[105] and the method of Bull[72] (Fig. 14-20). An extension of the odontoid process above Chamberlain's line by more than 6.6 mm indicates the presence of pathology (Fig. 14-21).

Rheumatoid arthritis produces alterations in the anatomic relationship between C1 and C2 as a result of pannus or vascular erosion of either ligamentous or osseous structures, in those areas where synovial tissue exists. These areas include the space between the anterior ring of C1 and the odontoid process. A space greater than 5 mm indicates the presence of instability, though not necessarily a need for stabilization. In the presence of trauma, a measurement of greater than 5 mm indicates instability and a need for surgical stabilization (Fig. 14-21).

Rheumatoid arthritis also results in loss of the C1-C2 articular joint space resulting in the upward (pathologic) migration of the odontoid process in the direction of the foramen magnum. Two lines have been devised to account for the presence of this pathologic process: Redlund-Johnell (line a–b less than 33 mm being abnormal) and Ranawat (where the line c–d being 13 mm or less is abnormal) (Fig. 14-20).[86,87]

Appreciating that 60 percent of all cervical spine rotation occurs at the C1–C2 level, it is important to recognize that the further loss of facet joint rotation and flexion-extension motion below this level after the performance of a multilevel cervical spine fusion can result in a disabling loss of cervical range of motion.

With lateral gliding of C1 on C2, the odontoid process will appear as lying asymmetrically between

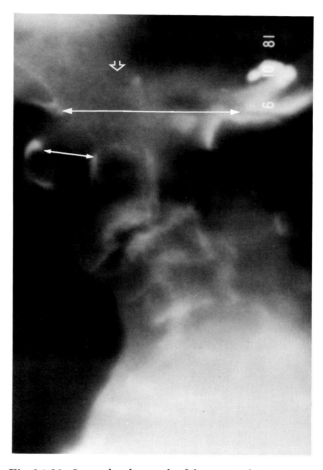

Fig. 14-21. Lateral radiograph of the cervical spine in an elderly patient with rheumatoid arthritis. The long arrow represents McRae's line, marking the foramen magnum space between the clivus and the posterior foramen magnum. The open arrow indicates the tip of the odontoid process and demonstrates significant protrusion of this structure into the foramen magnum. The shorter thin arrow reveals significant C1–C2 instability (greater than 5 mm). Note distraction and loss of intervertebral space at C2–C3 and loss of the occiput–C1 space.

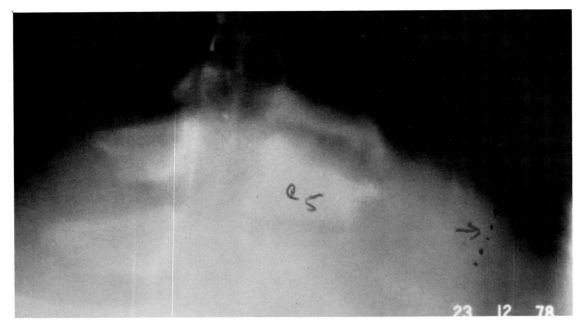

Fig. 14-22. Lateral tomogram of the cervical spine demonstrating an infectious process at C4–C5 and C5–C6. Note excessive widening of the prevertebral space (greater than 15 mm). Surgical debridement revealed a *Pseudomonas* abscess. The patient was a known drug abuser.

the lateral masses of the atlas. The offset can be as much as 2 to 4 mm. Though it is sometimes difficult to differentiate between normal gliding and subluxation, asymmetric positioning (or centering) of the odontoid along with some degree of

lateral articular offset, in the absence of a fracture, does not indicate subluxation.

Loss of motion at the atlantoaxial joint rarely results in a decrease in rotation of more than 15 to 25 degrees in either direction. Depending on the

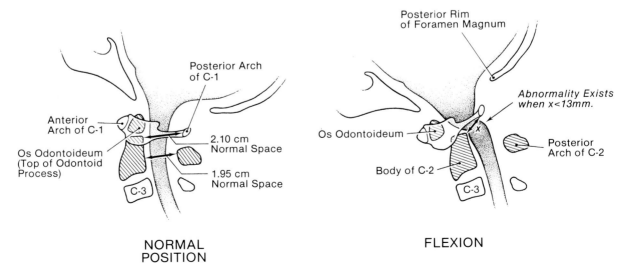

Fig. 14-23. Abnormal relationship of C1 and C2 in the presence of an os odontoideum.

age of the patient, facet joints between C2 and C7 compensate for this lost motion. The patient with a degenerative spine, however, can be anticipated to loose a greater degree of rotary as well as flexion-extension motion.

A subtle finding representing evidence of posterior column instability is the presence of a wedge-shaped intervertebral disc at the suspected level of injury (see Fig. 10-4). The anterior intervertebral disc will be slightly decreased in height, and the posterior disc border will be slightly increased. Frequently accompanying this will be minimal anterior subluxation (up to 1 to 2 mm) of the upper vertebral body, referred to as "sagging." A disruption of the disc alone can result in some minimal degree of anterosuperior vertebral subluxation.

Although it is difficult to absolutely equate to the presence of pathology, a widened retropharyngeal space measuring greater than seven-eighths the width of the adjacent vertebral body (15 mm), opposite or below the C4–5 interspace, is suggestive of pathology (Fig. 14-22). A prevertebral shadow greater than 10 mm (at C1) or 4 mm (at C3–C4) also requires careful evaluation (Fig. 10-15).

The presence of a D_{min} of less than 13 mm between the posterior border of the body of C2 and the posterior atlantal (C1) arch, in the presence of an os odontoideum, becomes the primary indication for surgery. Pain, cerebral symptoms, and gross instability also serve as surgical indicators (Fig. 14-23).

INJURIES AND FRACTURES INVOLVING THE CERVICAL SPINE

Occipital Condyle Fractures

Fractures of the occipital condyle are either exceedingly rare or they are missed during the assessment of patients with lethal head and cervical spine injuries. According to Harding-Smith et al.,[15] up until 1981, only eight cases of this fracture had been recorded in the English literature since 1817.[73,74] Certainly, this injury is but one of many injuries to occur to the base of the skull with trauma.[75] The actual mechanism of injury, the

symptoms, or the suggested management have not been duly recorded by investigators. Harding-Smith and colleagues[15] noted in a personal case resulting from a motor vehicle accident that the patient was unconscious on admission. Roentgenographic evaluation revealed an associated fracture through the right squamous temporal bone, a thickening of the prevertebral soft tissue from C1 to C4, and an asymmetry of the dens. Tomograms showed, by virtue of bony displacement, the presence of severe ligamentous injuries to the atlanto-occipital joints, the joint capsules, and the intervertebral disc spaces between C2 and C3 along with fractures. Bolender and colleagues[74] reported a hematoma anterior to the brain stem on CAT scans in one patient, and nerve palsy accompanying a fracture through the jugular foramen and hypoglossal canal at the base of the skull. Harding-Smith et al.[15], reported that substantial prevertebral and local extradural hematoma was inevitable when accompanied by a fracture through one or both occipital condyles. The two patients reported by Bolender et al.[74] and the one reported by Harding-Smith and co-workers[15] recovered with conservative care.

Management begins with fracture recognition. Paramount is rigid immobilization between the head and neck. When fractures are identified in the vicinity of the petrous and squamous portions of the temporal bone, it should be determined whether there might be a fracture or ligamentous injury involving the occipitoatlantal articulations. Evaluation techniques follow the judicious insertion of skeletal tongs. Radiological studies suggested include standard anteroposterior and lateral views of the occipital-vertebral junction; anteroposterior and lateral radiographs of the entire cervical spine; and open mouth odontoid views.

When there is difficulty in visualizing the fracture and developing an appropriate management plan, the following studies should be done: anteroposterior and lateral tomograms of the upper cervical spine and CAT of the occipital-C1–C2 area; a myelography (lumbar) may be indicated in the presence of an incomplete neurologic injury involving either the lower cranial or upper cervical neurologic plexus.

When fracture and, more specifically, ligamentous injury is identified, strict bed care with cervical traction for a period of 4 to 6 weeks is recommended, followed by an orthosis (halo vest) for an additional 6 to 8 weeks. Upon removal of the orthosis (after 3 months), flexion-extension radiographs should be obtained to rule out instability. If instability is noted, a posterior occiput-to-C2 fusion is indicated.

Injuries at the Occipitoatlantal Junction

Davis et al.[51] report that most injuries at the occipitoatlantal junction are fatal, though there are reports of patients surviving injuries to the cervical spine at this level.[76–80] This injury most often is the result of a distraction force, as might occur with a automobile-child pedestrian accident, or from an impact injury to the head-neck junction by a falling object. The result is usually the immediate onset of brain stem injury (with coma), followed by death. Roentgenograms reveal disassociation between the articular processes of the occiput and C1, with the skull dislocated anteriorly. The normal horizontal motion at the occipitatlantal joint with flexion-extension motion is 1 mm.[69] In the presence of congenital deformities within the area of the upper cervical spine, particularly when a failure of segmentation of developmental fusion exists, there may be a compensatory hypermobility.

Bohlman,[44] in a series of 300 cervical spine fractures, reports two injuries at the occiput-C1 level (0.1%). I found an equally low occurrence of occipitoatlantal disassociation injuries in my series of 1,484 injuries to the cervical spine. Autopsies of both of Bohlmann's patients revealed a spinal cord transection at the occipitoatlantal level and a total disruption of all ligamentous attachments between the occiput, the atlas, and the axis.[44]

Increasing numbers of patients sustaining injury at the occipitoatlantal junction, though unconscious and unable to ventilate voluntarily immediately after injury, survive the accident and arrive alive in the emergency room, owing to improved accident scene care, prompt ventilatory and circulatory resuscitation, and expeditious transfer to an appropriate medical facility. Despite the fact that patients with this type of an injury seldom survive and, while alive, require permanent passive ventilatory assistance, still, emergency spinal cord in-

jury care is indicated. Placing the patient in very light Gardner-Wells cervical tong traction does not result in either fracture reduction or saving the victim's life (Fig. 14-24) (see Fig. 15-21C) when significant neurologic injury is present. Patients sustaining injury at this level of the vertebral column, if injury to the medullary portion of the brain stem has not occurred, should be able to demonstrate only cranial nerve function to the level of cranial nerve XII (the hypoglossal nerve).

Wiesel and Rothman[69] cite two cases with normal neurologic examinations. They performed occipital-to-C2 fusion posteriorly with successful fusion in both.

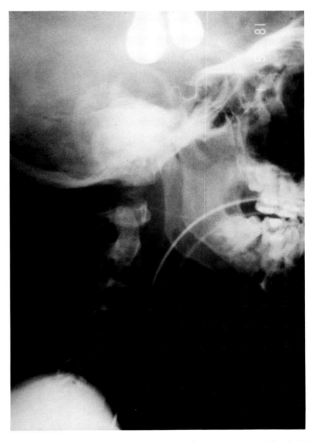

Fig. 14-24. Lateral radiograph of a 13-year-old child struck by a motor vehicle, showing distraction dislocation of the occiput from C1. The patient died of this injury within six hours following trauma.

Ring of the Atlas Fracture (Jefferson Fracture)

Fracture of the ring of the atlas was first described by Sir Geoffrey Jefferson in 1920,[81] and the description was expanded by Garber[82] in 1961. Bohlman[44] reported on 69 patients (in a series of 300 fractures) of whom 58 had no neurologic deficit. Ten patients sustained a fracture of the atlas (eight were managed conservatively).

The most common etiology of a fracture occurring at C1 is a direct extension-axial load across the atlanto-occipital joint, after a fall or a direct injury to the crown of the head.[83] A load so applied results in a splitting apart of the lateral masses of C1, with fracture of either or both of the anterior or posterior arches. This force, similar in manner to the occurrence of a break on opposite sides of a doughnut, will result in a fracture in two areas across the C1 ring (Fig. 14-25).

Although it is conceivable that a flexion injury to the cervical spine could result in an "avulsion"-type injury to the posterior ring of C1, it is rare. I have only seen this occur once in a series of 1,484 fractures of the cervical spine (see Fig. 15-16E). It is not uncommon, however, for a pure hyperextension injury to the head-neck region to result in a bilateral fracture through the posterior ring of C1. This fracture is frequently associated with a fracture involving the posterior element of C2, a hangman's fracture, which also results from a hyperextension injury (see Fig. 15-25B). When this occurs, the head and neck are driven into extreme hyperextension, with the posterior ring of C1 becoming entrapped between the occiput above and the posterior element of C2 below.

As borne out elsewhere in this chapter, considering only fractures involving C1 and C2, of 101 fractures of the ring of C1, 41 (41 percent) occurred at C1 only, while 60 (60 percent) occurred in conjunction with a fracture at C2. This association occurs at other levels of the cervical spine. Calenoff et al.[3] noted that fractures of C1 are frequently seen as a secondary fracture in the presence of a primary fracture in the upper thoracic spine.

Vertebral element displacement at the occipitoatlantal junction is uncommon because of the inherent stability of the convex and concave articulations of the atlanto-occipital joint; the joint capsules; and the superior extension of the strong anterior longitudinal ligament connecting the anterior arch of C1 and C2, with the upward extension of the apical odontoid ligament, between the odontoid apex and the anterior margin of the foramen magnum (the clivus). These ligaments serve as check reins. Because the vertebral neural canal is anatomically at its maximum at the C1-C2 level (2.1 cm, Fig. 14-10), neurologic injury seldom follows injuries at either the occipitoatlantal or C1-C2 levels (odontoid or hangman's).[83] The exception to this rule is the uncommon child pedestrian injury in which a distraction-type occipitoatlantal injury more frequently occurs, resulting in either a brain stem or upper cervical cord injury. When the latter occurs, death usually ensues.

Because stability is not a problem, the patient can be managed with cervical Gardner-Wells tong traction initially (until concern for neurologic injury dissipates after 1 to 2 weeks) followed by a halo vest for 8 to 10 weeks or cervical skeletal traction for 3 to 4 weeks followed by a sternal occipital mandibular immobilizing (SOMI) orthosis or Philadelphia collar for 6 weeks (Fig. 14-26). Day and co-workers[52] report an instance in which a Jefferson fracture went untreated and the patient developed neurologic symptoms resulting from the presence of a unilateral displacement of one lateral articular mass. Kahanovitz et al.[84] report a fracture of the posterior ring of C1 in a 54-year-old woman who sustained blunt trauma to the left occiput with the occurrence of a subdural hematoma. This hematoma was promptly evacuated. The fracture of C1 was initially undiagnosed and untreated and became entrapped within the foramen magnum, resulting in neural compromise. Surgical decompression failed to result in improved neurologic function. (Normal measurements of the foramen magnum are 3.2 to 3.6 cm in the sagittal plane, and 2.5 to 3.4 cm in the transverse plane.)

Other concerns relevant to fractures or injuries within the occipitoatlantoaxial region of the upper cervical spinal column include basilar impression or abnormal development of the cerebellar portion of the brain and the calvaria, and basilar invagination or impression of the odontoid process of C2 through the ring of C1 into the foramen magnum

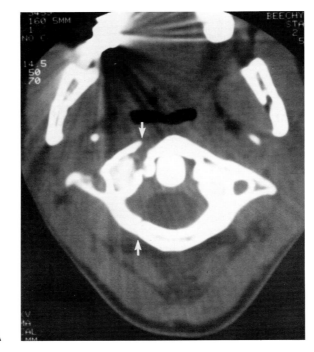

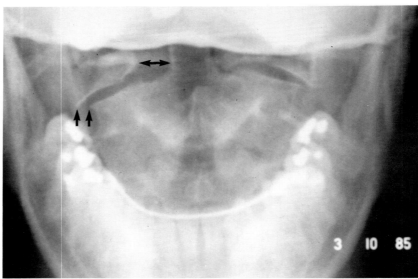

Fig. 14-25. (**A**) Horizontal CAT scan of C1 demonstrating anterior and posterior ring fracture (Jefferson fracture) (arrows). Note normal approximation between the anterior arch of C1 and the odontoid process (C2). (**B**) AP ''open mouth'' view of the C1–C2 interspace. Note lateral displacement of the lateral mass of C1 (short perpendicular arrows) and wide displacement of the lateral mass from the odontoid process. These findings are typical of a Jefferson ring fracture of C1.

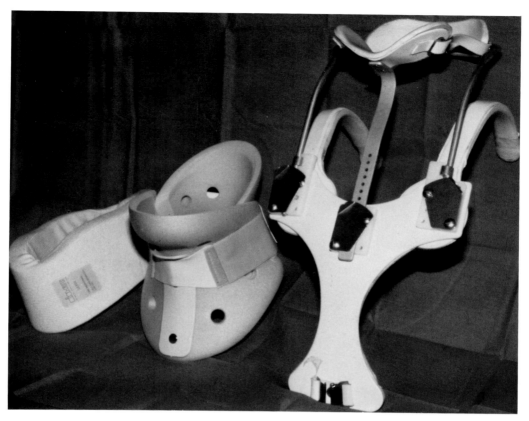

Fig. 14-26. Cervical orthotic devices. Only the Philadelphia collar (center) and SOMI (right) orthosis provide adequate postoperative immobilization. A soft cervical collar (left) is not recommended for injuries to the cervical spine requiring hospital admission.

(Fig. 14-27; see also Fig. 15-51). This anatomic abnormality can and does occur with rheumatoid arthritis,[12,13,85] and is particularly indicative of deterioration of the C1-C2 articular joints along with involvement of the odontoid process (erosion) by the presence of rheumatoid pannus.[86] The result is upward migration of the odontoid process into the foramen magnum with medullary compression of the brain stem and spinal cord vascular compromise (anterior spinal artery syndrome). Bernini and colleagues[43] report a high incidence of vascular anomalies with occipital-cervical deformities. Deaths have been recorded.[87]

It is also important to be as alert to a victim of a motor vehicle accident who gives a history of wearing a three-point lap-sash belt as to one injured without the wearing of a belt. Epstein et al[88] and

Taylor et al.[89] report injuries occurring in victims of a motor vehicle accident in which, apparently by means of a lateral flexion-compression load (over the shoulder strap), fracture of the arch and pedicle of C1 occurred with anterior dislocation, without neurologic consequences. Kewalramani and Krauss[90] reported 12 cases, in a series of 46 patients with injuries caused by collision sports, in which 14 neural arch fractures occurred. In each, the arch fracture was accompanied by a vertebral body or spinous process fracture, with associated vertebral element subluxation.

These latter examples underscore the need for careful evaluation of the occipital–C1–C2 area in either victims surviving potentially lethal injury or those who have sustained multiple trauma, including trauma to the head.

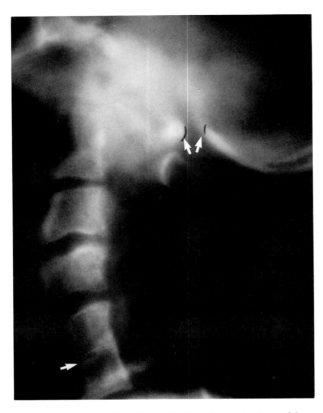

Fig. 14-27. Lateral radiograph showing anterior subluxation of the posterior ring of C1 inside the foramen magnum (see Fig. 15-51). Note the patient also has failure of segmentation of C5 and C6.

Injuries Involving the Atlantoaxial Joint

Atlantoaxial (or atlantoepistropheal) subluxation was first recorded in 1908.[91] Another reference to this injury was reported by Coutts in 1934,[62] but the most accurate and descriptive paper on this subject is that by Fielding and Hawkins[61] in 1977. The etiology is described as a distraction-rotary subluxation injury of the atlas about the odontoid process of C2. The result is a partial dislocation of the lateral articular mass of C1 on C2. The injury often follows trivial injury and, as a result, goes unrecognized. It occurs in young patients after a fall, episodes of horseplay, or wrestling or after an episode of upper respiratory infection resulting in an unknown positional injury. Alone, the injury

seldom results in neurologic injury despite the fact that the neural canal can be significantly reduced in size during the period of subluxation.

Depending on how long the pathology may have been present or unrecognized, the patient may present with a history of a persistent and sometimes painful torticollis. This condition is occasionally accompanied by a failure in the development in one side of the face (when it occurs in the very young child), with a resulting facial asymmetry, and a decreased and painful range of cervical spine motion. Adults normally present with a history of significant trauma in which multiple injuries may have occurred, but the neck symptoms fail to manifest attention. An adult man presented himself to me, describing a motorcycle accident two years before. His presenting complaints were persistent suboccipital pain and unequal rotation of the neck to one side. A second patient, an 8-year-old girl, was referred to the spine center with a 2-day history of a minor injury, persistent neck pain, and an acute decrease in head and neck rotation in one direction and a fixed rotation and tilt toward the side opposite the pathology.

The most appropriate radiographic techniques for evaluation of the atlantoaxial joints are (1) 15-degree rotation, open mouth views to the right and left; (2) lateral views; (3) carefully obtained flexion-extension lateral views to determine possible incompetence of the transverse ligament and atlantoaxial (odontoid) instability; (4) polytomograms; (5) CAT; and (6) if available, cineradiography, which is the most accurate method of making the diagnosis in the patient with longstanding disability. With lateral gliding of C1 on C2, the odontoid process will appear asymmetric between the lateral masses of the atlas and can be offset as much as 2 to 4 mm. Sometimes it is difficult to differentiate between normal lateral gliding and subluxation. Without the presence of a fracture, asymmetric positioning of the odontoid with lateral offset of the articular surfaces does not indicate subluxation. Similarly, in the older patients, in the presence of osteoarthritis involving the atlantoaxial joint, degenerative spurs may asymmetrically narrow the space between the lateral masses and the odontoid process, along with a decrease in the vertical height of the joint space between the lateral masses of the atlas and the axis. Though often difficult to identify, on the standard anteroposterior open mouth radiograph, with the head in the midline, it may be possible to note the presence of lateral displacement of the spinous process of C2 away from the midline when rotary subluxation is present. As noted earlier, the presence of the pathology is determined by the decrease in combined vertical height of the atlas and the axis. A decrease normally occurs with rotation. It is related to the biconvex nature of the joint surfaces. According to Hohl,[63] the low points of each joint surface come in contact when head rotation is maximized. When the head is in the neutral position, the highest points are in contact. Thus, the articular joint spaces are then at their widest.

In the patients with a longstanding atlantoaxial rotary subluxation (several months duration), pain is moderate to severe, and malposition of vertebral elements occurs in various degrees.[85] Neurologic symptoms, if present, are of either recent or late occurrence,[31,44,55,56,61,62,92–97] and when present suggest the need for surgical considerations. Although manipulation is a helpful technique in the acute injury, it is not in the late injury. Indications for surgical intervention include[61] correction of spinal malalignment and restoring stability, whether associated with neurologic injury or not; when on the anteroposterior open mouth radiograph, the displacement between the lateral mass of C1 and the side of the dens of C2 is greater than 2 to 4 mm; and when previous conservative management has failed. Initial care often includes preoperative cervical traction (10 to 15 lbs) for 1 to 2 weeks to regain positional correction. The age of the patient determines the amount of weight to be initially applied: for the young child, 2 to 3 lbs; for an older child or adult, between 5 and 7 lbs. It is always advisable to begin with low weights, adding more as required. After confirmation of the diagnosis, often a reduction can be achieved with a gentle and nonforced rotational manipulative procedure (with weights in place) as though one were manipulating a "perched" facet present at one of the lower cervical vertebral levels.

If conservative management fails and atlantoaxial subluxation recurs, arthrodesis by the Gallie[98] or the Garber-Meyer posterior C1–C2 fusion technique is appropriate to prevent dislocation-subluxation recurrences.

After surgery, because of the likelihood of losing position, it is suggested by Fielding and Hawkins[61] that the patient remain in traction for 6 weeks postoperatively, allowing undisturbed early union to occur. Variables including the reduction, the anticipated stability, and the neurologic finding present dictate the type of orthosis required postoperatively (SOMI or halo vest). When early mobilization is advantageous and stability of the reduction is a concern, the use of a halo vest is most indicated.

Loss of motion at the atlantoaxial joint rarely results in a decrease in rotation of more than 15 to 25 degrees in either direction. Depending on the age of the patient, the lower facet joints greatly compensate for lost motion. In the degenerative spine, however, one should anticipate a greater degree of lost motion.

Dislocation: Atlantoaxial Junction (C1 – C2)

Pure dislocations involving the C1–C2 articulation are fortunately rare. Most result in either immediate death or death within the first 48 hours after injury. A good percentage of the injuries follow a pedestrian accident. On admission to the emergency room, the patient will be unresponsive and unable to ventilate spontaneously. Neurologically, the patient will have sensation only from the level of the ear upward. The pathologic finding at autopsy is disruption of the spinal cord at the occipitovertebral junction.

The only management indicated is the careful application of cervical traction (stabilization of the head-neck complex) by means of Gardner-Wells tongs. Great care must be taken to monitor radiographically the amount of weight applied to the traction apparatus (including the weight holder) to prevent overdistraction. The anticipated amount of weight in the adult would be 2 to 3 lbs at the most. Even this may be too great. Should the patient survive, stabilization of C1 to C2 would be required. Bohlman[44] reports three patients having no neurologic injury after atlantoaxial dislocation who required a fusion and two (with neural injury) requiring fusion. I have seen only three atlantoaxial dislocations in a population of 1,484 cervical spine-injured patients (0.2 percent). Each of the patients required the use of a ventilator upon admission and none survived more than 72 hours after injury.

Fracture: Ring of the Axis (C2 Hangman's Fracture)

While fracture of the ring of the axis is not the most common fracture in the cervical spine, it is also not uncommon (2.7 percent). Likewise, it is not unusual to find it in association with another fracture of the cervical spine. Effendi[67] noted that of 131 pedicle or pars interarticularis fractures involving the arch of C2, 19 other fractures of the cervical spine were identified. These included eight arch fractures of the atlas (6 percent), two nondisplaced odontoid fractures, four fractures of C3, and six fractures involving the lower four cervical vertebrae. A similar finding was noted by Francis et al.[66] In a report of 123 fractures of the arch of the axis, an even higher association with other cervical spine fractures was noted (39 [32 percent]). Of these, 10 (8.1 percent) were fractures involving the arch of the atlas (C1), 4 were fractures of the odontoid, 6 were fractures of the arch of C3, and 5 were compression fractures of C3.

Calenoff et al.,[3] in their discussion of traumatic primary and secondary fractures of the spine, noted two interesting fracture associations. Of 30 multiple-level noncontiguous fractures, the fracture considered as secondary was disproportionately located at two levels: L4 and L5 in 28.6 percent and C1 and C2 in 14.3 percent. Calenoff's statistics also pointed out the need for careful observation of the entire spine, particularly when the primary lesion exists in the upper thoracic spine. They noted that of 710 patients with acute spine injuries admitted to the Midwest Regional Spinal Cord Injury Care System (1972 to 1979), 16 percent sustained a primary fracture at T2 to T7. In my experience, of 1,485 patients with acute cervical spine fractures admitted (1972 to 1986) to the same Midwest Regional Spinal Cord Injury Care System, 41 fractures (2.7 percent) occurred through the arch of the axis (C2).

Fractures of the arch of C2 have been recognized as an entity since their description by Haughton[99] in 1866. He recorded the pathologic findings noted after criminals were executed by hanging. But it was Wood-Jones[91,100] who noted the relationship of fatal fracture-dislocations of the axis and the position of the submental knot. Grogono[101] in 1954 noted the similarity of the C2 arch fracture recorded by Wood-Jones (from hanging) and those resulting from motor vehicle accidents. Garber[82] termed the fracture "traumatic spondylolisthesis" of the axis. Schneider et al.[102] are credited with the euphemism "hangman's fracture" and first called attention to the dissimilarity between the fracture produced by hanging and that produced by axial load and hyperextension (as with motor vehicle accidents). Roy-Camille et al.[103] in 1975 described the fracture as "la fractue du pendu."

The mechanism of injury that produces the hangman's fracture is still only supposed. Most researchers agree that the direction of injury is extension.[91,100,103] The question is, what other directional forces contribute to the fracture? Effendi and colleagues' type III injury classification[67] seems to indicate extension as the mechanism of injury, though some continue to suggest flexion also. The vertebral body of C2 is displaced anterior to the body of C3 (with disruption of both the anterior and posterior longitudinal ligaments), and this is occasionally accompanied by the presence of dislocated facet joints and posterior arch fracture (Fig. 14-28, type III). Because of the numerous questions raised concerning stability with this single injury entity, investigators disagreed on the state of stability and the method of management. Francis et al.[66] believed the fracture to be stable. Cornish[104] believed the fracture to be unstable and to require operative stabilization.

Fractures involving the posterior arch of C2, the hangman's fracture, have encouraged many investigators to review their own, and collaborative, series to arrive at a management scheme. Whether the most correct or not, Effendi and associates'[67] classification of fractures seems most plausible. These researchers subdivided the fracture of the pedicle-pars interarticularis region of C2, with occasional involvement of a portion of the posterior wall of the body of C2, into three types (Fig. 14-28). Generally, Francis and associates[66] agree. The difference between the two was the extent of the hyperextension force applied across the C2 posterior elements, in addition to the extent of axial

TYPE I

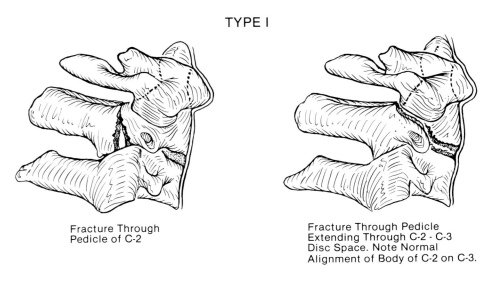

Fracture Through
Pedicle of C-2

Fracture Through Pedicle
Extending Through C-2 - C-3
Disc Space. Note Normal
Alignment of Body of C-2 on C-3.

TYPE II

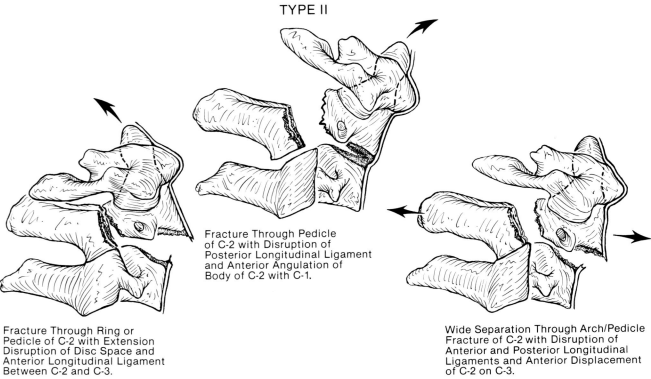

Fracture Through Pedicle
of C-2 with Disruption of
Posterior Longitudinal Ligament
and Anterior Angulation of
Body of C-2 with C-1.

Fracture Through Ring or
Pedicle of C-2 with Extension
Disruption of Disc Space and
Anterior Longitudinal Ligament
Between C-2 and C-3.

Wide Separation Through Arch/Pedicle
Fracture of C-2 with Disruption of
Anterior and Posterior Longitudinal
Ligaments and Anterior Displacement
of C-2 on C-3.

Fig. 14-28. Effendi classification of hangman's fractures types I, II, and III. *(Figure continues.)*

TYPE III

Fracture Through Arch/Pedicle
of C-2 with Dislocated Facets C-2,
Disruption of Anterior and Posterior
Longitudinal Ligaments, and
Anterior Dislocation of C-2 on C-3.

Fig. 14-28 *(Continued).*

loading that occurs during the course of the hyperextension load. It is believed by both that with maximum extension and axial load, the combination is the most likely cause for extension of the fracture line into the posteroinferior aspect of the body of C2. Logically then, with maximum load with both force vectors, the body of C2 is likely to be displaced forward on the body of C3 (type III). As stated above, it is this single finding that leads some investigators to believe that the mechanism of injury is flexion.

Effendi's classification follows:

Type I. Type I fractures are the result of an extension force on the face and head. Francis et al.[66] noted a high incidence of associated head injury (79 percent). This results in a nondisplaced hyperextension-induced fracture through the ring of the axis, along with minimal displacement of the body of C2[67] (Fig. 14-28). While the fracture line may extend into the posteroinferior aspect of the body of C2, the disc space between C2 and C3 remains normal and is stable.

Type II. The fracture line through the posterior element is wide and the disc space below C2 is abnormal. The body of C2 may be slightly displaced forward, either in extension or flexion.

Type III. The body of C2 is definitely displaced forward on C3 and lies in a flexed position. The fracture through the posterior element is widely separated, and the facet joints of C2 are dislocated and locked forward on the facets of C3.

The stability of fractures involving the arch of the C2 has been a controversial subject. Most, if not all, of the recent articles agree that the type I fractures by themselves are inherently stable by virtue of the sustained continuity of both the anterior and posterior longitudinal ligaments. For type II and III fractures, however, although experience has demonstrated that these also are relatively stable, greater observation and care are required because of the disruption of both the anterior and posterior longitudinal ligaments, the disc, and occasionally the facet joints. It is for this reason that each of these fractures is usually managed in traction for a period of 4 to 6 weeks before placing the patient into an orthosis (halo vest or SOMI). If one considers the advantages of surgical stabilization of fractures of C2 when there is a fracture involving the posterior element, it is necessary to appreciate that surgical stability might not be anticipated when there is also a fracture of the posterior element of C1. This occurrence is not rare. To point this out, of 250 patients sustaining fractures at C2, 60 patients (24 percent) also sustained a fracture at C1. This could be an additional reason for considering conservative management of hangman's fractures.

I, as well as Francis et al.[66] and Effendi et al.,[67] have noted that although neurologic injury is possible with fracture of the posterior ring of the axis, it is usually an incomplete neurologic injury with an excellent chance for complete recovery. When significant neurologic injury occurs, it usually accompanies an associated injury at a lower level of the cervical spine where occlusion of the vertebral artery has been identified by arteriography or is found in a patient with multiple trauma. Effendi et al.[67] reported an overall mortality rate of 6.8 percent. Francis and associates[66] found that 46 percent of patients in his series had multiple trauma. While 8 of 181 patients demonstrated neurologic loss (6.5 percent), all but two recovered.

Management of the Os Odontoideum

Controversy exists as to the origin of os odontoideum. The management of it depends on one's philosophy as to the development of this bony ossicle, which lies proximal to the main body of the odontoid process. One etiology is congenital (or developmental) and relates to a failure of fusion or proper segmentation of the occipitocervical mesenchymal condensation segments (or secondary centers of ossification) between the occiput-C1-C2 somites during the embryonic development of the ring of C1 and the odontoid process.[14,18,31] These centers normally coalesce by adolescence, though some may persist into adulthood. When os odontoideum is found in association with other congenital anomalies of the cervical spine, the likelihood of a congenital origin is greater. A rather common one is a failure of segmentation resulting in the fusion of one or more cervical vertebral bodies. Other abnormalities include the absence of the posterior ring of C1 or the presence of a cervical hemivertebra (Klippel-Feil syndrome) (Fig. 14-9). When one hemivertebra is identified, a second frequently exists at another level. When this occurs on opposite sides, a "balanced" defect results, with the spine appearing straight, though short.

The second, and somewhat more plausible, etiology is that of unrecognized trauma during childhood. Here the process probably arises from a fracture of the odontoid process. Some patients have been found to have documented normal odontoid processes followed by the development of an os odontoideum.[28-30] Fielding et al.[29] described "the dystopic position of the os odontoideum as a result of the upward pull of the broken-off tip of the odontoid process by the alar ligaments."

Because the presence of an os odontoideum can lead to instability at the atlantoaxial joint and can, under certain circumstances, when present and allowed to persist, carry a grave prognosis resulting in neurologic deficit, considerable attention has been directed to this area of the spine when this malady is present. An excellent review of this topic has been presented by Spierings and Braakman.[68] Their patient population consisted of 37 cases, the average age at the time of diagnosis being 38. Initially, it was the authors' belief that the presence of an os odontoideum gives notice of the presence of an unstable condition requiring surgical fusion. Because of the anticipated instability associated with the condition, surgical fusion was thought to be indicated. After two surgical complications, both resulting in patient deaths, management became more conservative and fell into four management

categories: those having no neurologic (cord) symptoms who are managed conservatively (16 patients); those with neurologic (cord) symptoms who are managed conservatively (4 patients); those having no neurologic (cord) symptoms who are managed surgically (9 patients); and those with neurologic (cord) symptoms who are managed surgically (8 patients).

Conservative care has been advocated in a few patients having such neurologic symptoms as dizziness, headaches, transient myelopathy, and mild degrees of instability. These same symptoms served as surgical indications (cervical fusion) in the series of patients reported by McRae,[105] Dastur et al.,[106] Dijck,[16] Fielding et al.,[29] and others.

Spierings and Braakman[68] noted in their os odontoideum series "a 10 to 1 chance of a patient developing permanent spinal cord changes in the presence of a D_{min} (distance between the posterior border of the body of C2 and the posterior atlantal (C1) arch of less than 13 mm.)" (Fig. 14-23). This single measurement became their primary indication for surgery. Most surgeons managing similar problems include constant cervical spine pain, and instability less than 13 millimeters, and intermittent neurologic symptoms that include dysarthra, dysphagia, dizziness, hypertonicity in both upper and lower extremities, etc.

Conservative Management of Fractures of the Odontoid Process

Because of the concern over instability at the fracture site (between the body of C2 and a type II odontoid process fracture), cervical traction must be carefully observed by serial radiographs. When radiographs reveal that the vertebral segments are not grossly unstable and an angular deformity persists, additional weight may be added, but at this level, not in excess of 10 lbs.

I reviewed 29 patients with consecutive and separate fractures of C1 and C2 admitted within 72 hours of injury to the acute spine center in 1981. Eight patients were eliminated from the study because of death, young age, or extreme confusion. The remaining 21 were managed in an identical manner. The patient sample included those with fractures of the ring of C1, hangman's fractures, type I, II, and III fractures of the odontoid, and one rotary subluxation (reduced by traction) of C1 on C2. Each patient, regardless of the presence or absence of neurologic injury (24 normal, 3 complete, 2 incomplete), was placed initially in Gardner-Wells skeletal traction for a period varying from 1.5 weeks to 5 weeks. Each patient was then immobilized in a SOMI (Fig. 14-29) orthosis for 3-months. All fractures (including type II and III odontoid fractures) were healed after 3 months and were without evidence of instability as diagnosed by flexion-extension films obtained at 3 months. No patient required the use of either a halo vest or an operative stabilization procedure.

Similar results were obtained by Effendi and associates,[67] Francis and associates,[66] and Seljeskog

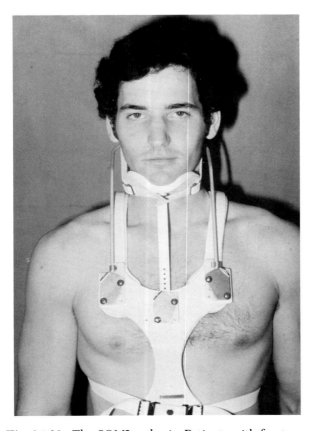

Fig. 14-29. The SOMI orthosis. Patients with fractures of the odontoid process without evidence of gross malposition or instability can be initially managed in cervical tong traction (1½ to 5 weeks) followed by immobilization in a SOMI orthosis.

and Chou.[107] All fractures were managed conservatively at first because of a propensity for spontaneous healing despite less than perfect reduction. Each author agreed that type I fractures require the shortest period of total immobilization (1 to 3 weeks traction followed by halo vest and immediate ambulation, or by the immediate application of a cervicothoracic brace, bypassing any period of cervical traction). Type II and III fractures should be maintained in cervical traction for 3 to 6 weeks before placing in an orthotic device and allowing ambulation. While in Effendi's series[67] of 131 patients, 32 were fused posteriorly (24 percent) and 10 anteriorly (8 percent), Francis et al.[66] noted that 94 percent healed by 16 weeks when managed conservatively. The authors suggest that conservative care be conducted for a minimum of 8 to 12 weeks. If, at 3 months, an obvious fracture line persists or, with flexion-extension radiographs, motion or pain in the area of trauma persists, a fusion should be entertained. Where the patient already has limited cervical spine motion (see Fig. 15-48), an anterior fusion is appropriate to further reduce loss of rotary motion of the cervical spine. Francis and associates[66] concur.

MANAGEMENT OF CERVICAL INJURIES BETWEEN C3 and C7

Fractures of the cervical spine between C3 and C7 can be divided into three categories: fractures occurring at more than one vertebral level, either contiguous or noncontiguous; flexion injuries; and extension injuries.

Dislocations without Fracture

Any injuries to the cervical spine resulting in ligamentous disruption involving all three columns are grossly unstable and require surgical stabilization (Fig. 14-30). Uniformly, a severe and nonrecoverable neurologic injury will accompany the dislocation.

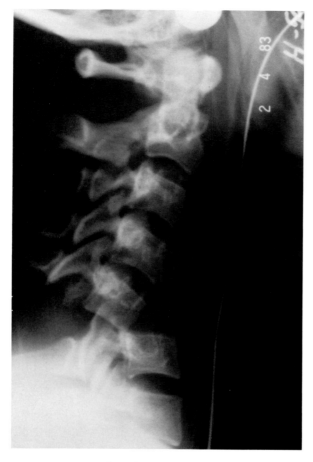

Fig. 14-30. Lateral radiograph of the cervical spine showing complete dislocation at C5–C6. This injury represents a three-column ligamentous injury and is grossly unstable. Operative stabilization and fusion is required.

Fractures at Multiple Levels

As a rule, when fractures at more than one vertebral level are present simultaneously between C3 and C7, consecutive (nonoperative) management is recommended. The rationale for this management decision is based on two consistent findings. First, the identified fractures are frequently more extensive, and numerous, than initially anticipated (Fig. 14-31). Second, were one to attempt to gain operative stability under such conditions, at least one surgical level above the highest fracture and one surgical level below the lowest fracture would have to be incorporated to gain "fracture stability." The result, with a fusion, would be a severely restricted cervical spine, with very limited motion. Since 60 percent of all cervical spine rotation occurs at the C1-C2 level, rotation may not be severely limited, but flexion, extension, and bending below C2 would be very restricted. Therefore, to maintain the maximum available motion, in the presence of more than one vertebral level fracture, it is suggested that the spine be managed conservatively in a halo vest for 12 weeks, or in the elderly, managed in Gardner-Wells skeletal traction for 3 to 5 weeks, followed by either a SOMI orthosis or a halo vest for the remaining 8 weeks.

A variation from this theme is the occurrence of a very comminuted cervical vertebral fracture with involvement of any two of the three columns of stability. Under this circumstance, loss of position or collapse of the vertebral column across this segment can be anticipated. Two management courses exist: (1) surgical stabilization (and anteriorly placed bone graft along with the insertion of an anterior three-level AO plate) or (2) prolonged cervical tong traction for 6 to 8 weeks, followed by a cervical orthosis for 4 weeks. This latter choice often follows in the multiple trauma patient, when ambulation or out-of-bed mobilization is not an immediate consideration.

Flexion Injuries: C3–C7

The most common mechanical force resulting in injury to the cervical spine is flexion. Should this mechanical force be associated with distraction, either incomplete dislocation (subluxation) or pure dislocation of the facet joints, tearing or disruption of the posterior interspinous ligaments, and rupture of the posterior longitudinal ligament and posterior fibers of the anulus fibrosus, gross spinal column instability results. Attempts at conservative management of this injury commonly fail, particularly in the absence of any fracture (Fig. 14-30). The reason is failure of ligamentous healing sufficient to provide a ligamentous "scar" strong enough to maintain good spinal alignment. For this reason, injuries, usually flexion induced, without fracture frequently require surgical stabilization.

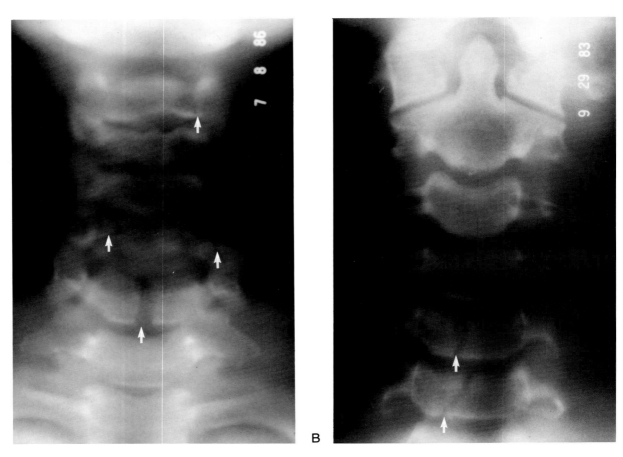

Fig. 14-31.   (A) AP tomogram showing widely displaced fractures over multiple levels (C2, C5, C6). The patient was neurologically normal. The fracture was managed conservatively in a halo vest. (B) AP tomogram showing an axial load compression fracture involving C5 and C6. The fracture was managed conservatively in a SOMI orthosis.

On the other hand, when elements of the vertebral column do fracture, spinal stability can be obtained on many occasions by conservative care alone.

The initial management of fractures or dislocations of the cervical spine includes the placement of the patient into Gardner-Wells skeletal long traction (5 lbs of weight per level of injury) for an initial evaluation period. During this time, all pertinent studies required for injury evaluation should be done, including flexion-extension films for the presence of instability (if this is a question), a myelogram, tomograms, MRI, CAT scan, etc. These studies, and the neurologic injury present, dictate the management scheme to be followed. Normally,

the patient remains in cervical traction for an initial 9 to 14 days, during which time the neurologic injury (edema) subsides. The neurologic injury is carefully monitored for any evidence of extension or sudden deterioration. Should this happen (as might occur with a loss of cervical spine alignment), immediate surgical decompression (anteriorly) or surgical stabilization (anteriorly or posteriorly) is indicated. When the patient remains stable, and the patient's condition is not conducive to surgery, or the injury is not in need of surgical stabilization, the patient should be maintained in cervical traction for 4 to 6 weeks, followed by the use of a SOMI-type orthosis for the remaining 6 weeks.

Extension Fractures: C3-C7

Extension injuries to the cervical spine, as noted earlier, frequently occur in the elderly patient. The history usually includes a fall face forward onto either the pavement or down stairs. Either way, in the presence of extensive cervical osteoarthritis or a restricted range of cervical spine motion, it is not uncommon with forced extension for either a fracture of the odontoid process (type II extension, with posterior displacement of the odontoid process on the body of C2) (Fig. 14-32) or an extension

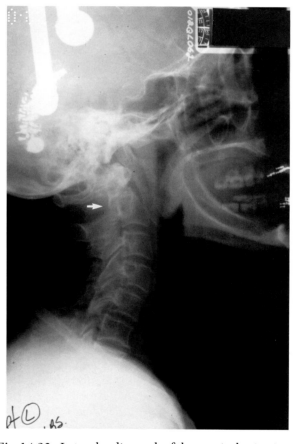

Fig. 14-32. Lateral radiograph of the cervical spine in an 81-year-old woman who sustained a hyperextension injury to the cervical spine from a fall. Note the oblique extension fracture through the base of the odontoid process and posterior aspect of C2. The patient was managed conservatively in cervical traction (flexion) followed by SOMI orthosis.

fracture of the cervical spine between C6 and C7 (Fig. 14-11) to occur. Because the size of the neural canal is less likely to be compromised with a hyperextension injury, neurologic injury is less likely to occur. In my experience, when a hyperextension injury does not result in a vertebral element fracture, but rather a ligamentous or soft tissue-disc space disruption, an anterior surgical stabilization is indicated. Conservative management can be attempted, but is likely to fail. The technique presently used for fixation is either a one- or two-level anterior AO plate and screw stabilization, along with the use of a "tricortical" intervertebral body bone graft between each disc space crossed by the plate.

Unexplained Ear Pain with Injuries to the Cervical Spine

For unexplained reasons, patients sustaining bony injury to the midportion of the cervical spine may, after admission, may begin to complain of pain in one or both external auditory canals. Several possible etiologies for this exist.

Trauma sufficient to fracture the cervical spine can also result in trauma to the face, the zygomatic arch, the temporal bone, the base of the skull, or direct trauma to the ear. A patient who complains of pain deep within the external auditory canal requires evaluation of the canal for the presence of either a foreign body or an infection. Another possible source of concern is the presence of a subclinical infection resulting from the insertion of Gardner-Wells tongs. When each potential source has been evaluated and found negative, it is still not uncommon for the patient to continue to complain of external auditory canal pain. A possible explanation lies with involvement of the auricular branch (nerve of Arnold) of the jugular ganglion in the jugular foramen, which receives a branch from the petrosal ganglion of the glossopharyngeal nerve, which enters the petrous portion of the temporal bone through a foramen in the lateral wall of the jugular fossa. There, the nerve either communicates directly or lies in contact with the facial nerve. The nerve leaves the temporal bone by the stylomastoid foramen behind the auricle and divides into two branches. One joins the posterior auricular branch of the facial nerve. The other supplies sensory fibers to the posterior and inferior parts of the external auditory meatus and the back of the auricle. This latter branch also supplies twigs to the osseous part of the external auditory meatus and the lower outer surface of the tympanic membrane. The innervation of the tympanic membrane may result in vomiting and coughing associated with an infection of the meatus, or the pain experienced by the patient may be the result of trauma to the nerve as it passes through the petrosal portion of the temporal bone, or with injury to the glossopharyngeal nerve, trauma to the nerve may have resulted from injury (direct trauma) or surgery (anterior surgical fusion) in the upper neck or submandibular region.

Medical Complications

Upon review of the complication most frequently identified during the management of patients having sustained fractures of the cervical spine, a group of complications was found to occur most often (Table 14-4). These included the following.

The most common complication was that of urinary tract infection (41 percent). While every attempt has been made to observe good nursing and urinary management techniques, the problem persists. One reason given is the frequent (some say too frequent) use of an indwelling catheter. While this criticism has some validity, nonetheless, the management of the patient with an acutely injured spinal cord more often requires the careful monitoring of fluid administration and urinary function than does management of the long-term and stable spinal cord patient.

Because of the nature of the neurologic disability resulting from injuries to the cervical spinal cord, it is not surprising to find that pneumonia and respiratory failure are equally prevalent (10.7 and 10.3 percent, respectively). This not only relates to the extent of neurologic involvement affecting ventilation, but to the pre-existence of pulmonary disease, the age of the patient, and the occurrence of the "drown" syndrome in many patients sustaining a cervical spine fracture.

Deep venous thrombosis (9.5 percent) and pul-

Table 14-4. Medical Complications (Northwestern University Acute Spine Injury Center, 1972 to 1986)

Type of Medical Complication	No.	Percent[a]
Urinary tract infection	609	41.0
Pneumonia	159	10.7
Respiratory failure	153	10.3
Deep venous thrombosis	141	9.5
Bradycardia	137	9.2
Pressure sore	128	8.6
Hyperthermic	105	7.1
Hypotensive	83	5.6
Gastrointestinal bleed	57	3.8
Hypothermic	25	1.7
Pulmonary embolism	19	1.3
Died	84	5.7
Other	279	18.8

[a]Summed percentages do not equal 100% because of multiple or no complications.

monary embolism (1.3 percent) are discussed below. Both complications attract a great deal of prophylactic attention in the acute cervical spinal cord-injured patient.

The occurrence of a significant neurologic injury to the cervical spinal cord in which there is a loss of both motor and sensory function produces, as a result of alterations in the autonomic nervous system, the following vital sign changes: bradycardia (9.2 percent) owing to the over-riding influence of the vagus nerve on the heart; hypotension (5.6 percent) as a result of loss of peripheral vasomotor tone and vascular dilatation; and hypothermia (1.7 percent) because as the peripheral vessels dilate, blood reaches the surface of the skin and cools.

There are a group of complications that follow prolonged, debilitating bed care. They include pressure decubiti occurring over areas of insensitive skin (heels, scapula, sacrum, etc.) and hyperthermia secondary to urinary tract infections and to a phenomenon seen in cervical spinal cord patients with neurologic injury as a result of which the patient loses the ability to perspire. The result is an inability of the body to compensate for elevations in body temperature brought on by such changes as rises in ambient temperature, too many covers, infection, etc.

In the total cervical spinal cord population (1,484) cared for at Northwestern University between 1972 and 1986, 84 deaths have occurred (5.7 percent). The primary cause for these deaths was acute respiratory failure or secondary effects of that failure (pneumonia), resulting from the loss of voluntary ventilatory function in the patient with a high cervical spine neurologic injury with a lesion at or above C4. Though it is possible, and does occasionally occur, it is rare for a spinal cord patient to expire as a result of associated musculoskeletal injuries. When it does occur, the most common causes are associated head trauma, multiple organ injury, or pulmonary embolism.

Prophylactic Management of Gastric Ulceration

Other medical management procedures used during the initial care process are the administering of antacids (Riopan [magaldrate] and cimetidine) to reduce gastric hydrochloric acid production and gastric activity.[1] Some investigators have implicated the use of steroids during the acute injury phase as contributing to the occurrence of gastric hemorrhage.[46] This theory has not been proven in a controlled series. In my experience, no difference in the neurologically injured patient (managed with steroids) and the neurologically normal patient (not receiving steroids) has been seen.

During the immediate post-trauma period (1 to 2 weeks postadmission), the use of a nasogastric tube is recommended, along with the daily administration of cimetidine (Tagamet), 300 mg. This drug is utilized to reduce the release of gastric hydrochloric acid. Also used alternately every 2 hours (to reduce the occurrence of diarrhea or constipation by the two drugs) are Riopan (30 ml) and Maalox (30 ml). These drugs are administered through the in-place nasogastric tube.

An additional benefit of having the nasogastric tube in place is the reduction of abdominal distention resulting from the occurrence of a neurologically induced ileus. This frequently follows a neurologic injury. Until reflex bowel activity returns, emesis can be a major concern, particularly in the cervical spine-injured quadriplegic patient.

Prevention of Deep Venous Thrombosis

The development of deep venous thrombosis (see Ch. 15) is an inherent complication in the patient placed at forced recumbency for prolonged periods and is more likely to occur in the patient rendered paralyzed. It is recommended that sodium heparin be used preoperatively, postoperatively, and prophylactically for the prevention of deep venous thrombosis. Various drugs and techniques have been utilized to prevent deep venous thrombosis. These include the use of aspirin (Harris),[108] dextran, alternating above-the-knee "ripple" pressure stockings, elevation, and above-the-knee thigh-high T.E.D. hose. The most effective method of prevention is the use of "adjusted dose heparin" (which requires repeated evaluation of blood-clotting factors), in which in the clotting time is kept at approximately one and one-half to two times normal. A more simplified method of utilizing heparin is the administration of subcutaneous heparin (5,000 units bid). This routine can be maintained for either 6 weeks or until the patient is placed on longer-term therapy. For long-term prophylaxis against the occurrence of deep venous thrombosis or its complication pulmonary embolism, Coumadin (sodium warfarin) (2.5 to 5 mg) is administered each day. Levels of this drug are adjusted by monitoring the prothrombin time (PTT), which is kept at one and one-half to two times normal for 3 to 6 months or until the threat of venous thrombosis is gone. This usually occurs when the patient returns to a preinjury level of activity. The incidence of deep venous thrombosis in the cervical spine-injured patient was 9.5 percent in a population of 1,484 patients. The incidence of pulmonary embolism was 1.3 percent. Others have found a higher incidence.[67,77]

Selection of Surgical Stabilization Procedure

Simply stated, not all injuries occurring to the cervical vertebral column, whether with or without an associated neurologic injury, can always be managed conservatively. A great deal depends on the type of neurologic injury present. Likewise, not all fractures of the cervical spine judged unstable, despite a wide variety of surgical procedures, can be made stable just by surgery. Specific operative procedures vary greatly in their indications and approach (anterior or posterior). The surgeon may use (according to his experience, teaching, or philosophy), a combination of wires and bone grafts,[82,109,110] bone grafts alone,[109,111] screws,[112-114] or in some instances (usually in the presence of tumor) methyl methacrylate.[115-117] Also variable, depending on the selection of the method of internal fixation, will be the direction of the surgical approach (anterior[118-121] or posterior, or both) (see Ch. 15).

REFERENCES

1. Beal J (ed): Critical Care for Surgical Patients. Macmillan, New York, 1982
2. Meyer PR, Yarkony G: Annual Progress Report of the "Midwest Regional Spinal Cord Injury Care System." Grant G008535129. Department of Education, Washington, DC, 1987.
3. Calenoff L, Chessare J, Rogers LF et al.: Multiple levels, spine injuries: importance of early recognition. AJR 130:665, 1979
4. Stover S, Fine R (eds): Spinal Cord Injury, The Facts and Figures. University of Alabama at Birmingham, National SCI Data Center, Birmingham, AL, 1986
5. Abel MS: Occult traumatic lesions of the cervical vertebra. WH Green, St. Louis, 1971
6. Ackerson TT, Patzakis MJ, Moore TM, et al.: Fractures of the odontoid: a ten year retrospective study. Cont Orthop. 4:54, 1981
7. Alker GJ, Young SO, Leslie EV, et al: Postmortem radiology of head and neck injuries in fatal traffic accidents. Radiology 114:611, 1975
8. Allen GL, Ferguson RL, Lehmann TR, O'Brien RP: A mechanistic classification of closed, indirect fractures and dislocations of the lower cervical spine. Spine 7:1, 1982
9. Arey LB: Developmental Anatomy. 6th Ed. WB Saunders, Philadelphia, 1965
10. Black P: Injuries of the vertebral column and spinal cord: mechanisms and management in the acute phase. In The Management of Trauma. WB Saunders, Philadelphia, 1973
11. Calenoff L. (ed): Radiology in Spinal Cord Injury. CV Mosby, St. Louis, 1981
12. Morizono Y, Sakou T, Kawaidi H: Upper cervical involvement in rheumatoid arthritis. Spine 12:721, 1987
13. Rana NA, Taylor AR: Upward migration of the odontoid peg in rheumatoid arthritis. Proc R Soc Med 64:717, 1971
14. Gschweiler JA, Osborne RL, Becker RF: The radiology of vertebral trauma. Monographs in Clinical Radiology. Vol. 16. WB Saunders, Philadelphia, 1980
15. Harding-Smith J, MacIntosh PK, Sherbon KJ: Fracture of the occipital condyle. J Bone Joint Surg 63A:1170, 1981
16. Dijck P: Os odontoideum in children: neurological manifestations and surgical management. J Neurol 2:93, 1978
17. Minderhoud JM, Braakman R, Penning L: Os odontoideum: clinical, radiological and therapeutic aspects. J Neurol Sci 8:521, 1969
18. Sherk HH, Dawoud S: Congenital os odontoideum with Klippel-Feil anomaly and fatal atlanto-axial instability. Spine 6:42, 1981
19. Key, A.: Cervical spine dislocation with unilateral facet interlocking. Paraplegia 13:208–215, 1975.
20. Eismont FJ, Bohlman HH, Prasanna LS, et al.: Pyogenic and fungal vertebral osteomyelitis with paralysis. J Bone Joint Surg 65A:19, 1983
21. Wiesseman GJ, Wood VE, Kroll LL: Pseudomonas vertebral osteomyelitis in heroin addicts. J Bone Joint Surg 55A:1416, 1973
22. Lewis RL, Gorbach S, Attner P: Spinal pseudomonas chondro-osteomyelitis in heroin users. N Engl J Med 286:1301, 1972
23. Cloward RB: Metastatic disc infection and osteomyelitis of the cervical spine. Spine 3:194, 1978
24. Roca RP, Yoshikawa TT: Primary skeletal infections in heroin users: a clinical characterization, diagnosis and therapy. Clin Orthop 144:238, 1979
25. Batson OV: The function of the vertebral veins and their role in the spread of metastases. Ann Surg 112:138, 1940
26. Schaeffer JP (ed): Morris' Human Anatomy: A Complete Systematic Treatise. 11th Ed. Blakiston, New York, 1953
27. Stone DB, Bonfiglio M: Pyogenic vertebral osteomyelitis. A diagnostic pitfall for the internist. Arch Intern Med 112:491, 1963
28. Fielding JW, Griffin PP: Os odontoideum: an acquired lesion. J Bone Joint Surg 56A:187, 1974
29. Fielding JW, Hinsinger RN, Hawkins RJ: Os odontoideum. J Bone Joint Surg 62A:376, 1980
30. Freiberger RJ, Wilson PD, Jr., Nicholas JA: Acquired absence of the odontoid process. J Bone Joint Surg 47A:1231, 1965

31. Garber JN: Abnormalities of the atlas and axis vertebra—congenital and traumatic. J Bone Joint Surg 46A:1782, 1964

32. Bedbrook GM: Some pertinent observations on the pathology of traumatic spinal paralysis. Paraplegia 1:215, 1963

33. Schneider, RC, Kahn, EA: Chronic neurological sequelae of acute trauma to the spine and spinal cord. Part II. The syndrome of chronic anterior spinal cord injury or compression. Herniated intervertebral discs. J Bone Joint Surg 41A:449, 1959

34. Beatson, TR: Fractures and dislocations of the cervical spine. J Bone Joint Surg 45B:21, 1963

35. Taylor, AR, Blackwood, W: Paraplegia in hyperextension cervical injuries with normal radiographic appearances. J Bone Joint Surg 30B:245, 1948

36. Forsyth HF: Extension injuries of the cervical spine. J Bone Joint Surg 46A:1792, 1964

37. Forsyth HF, Alexander E, Davis C, Underdal R: The advantages of early spine fusion in the treatment of fracture-dislocations of the cervical spine. J Bone Joint Surg 41A:17, 1959

38. Meyer, PR, Rosen JS, Hamilton BB, Hall W: Fracture dislocation of the cervical spine: transportation, assessment and immediate management. p. 171. Instructional Course Lectures, American Academy of Orthopaedic Surgeons. Vol. XXV. CV Mosby, St. Louis, 1976

39. Meyer PR: Systems Approach to the Care of the Spinal Cord Injured, Systems Approach to Emergency Medical Care. p. 404. Appleton-Century-Crofts, East Norwalk, CT, 1983

40. Meyer PR, Raffensberger JG: Special centers for the care of the injured. J Trauma 13:308, 1973

41. Holdsworth FW: Review article: fracture, fracture-dislocations of the spine. J Bone Joint Surg 52A:1534, 1970

42. Elsberg CA: The Edwin Smith surgical papyrus, and the diagnosis and the treatment of injuries to the skull and spine 5,000 years ago. Am Med Hist 3:271, 1931

43. Bernini FP, Elefante R, Smaltino F, Tedeschi G: Angiographic study on the vertebral artery in cases of deformities of the occipital joint. AJR 107:526, 1969

44. Bohlman HH: Acute fractures and dislocations of the cervical spine. J Bone Joint Surg 61A:1119, 1979

45. Brachken MB, Collins WF, Freeman DF, et al.: Efficacy of methylprednisolone in acute spinal cord injury. JAMA 251:45, 1984

46. Ducker TB, Hamit HF: Experimental treatments of acute spinal cord injury. J Neurosurg 30:693, 1969

47. De la Torre, JC, Johnson, CM, Goode, DJ, et al: Pharmacologic treatment and evaluation of permanent experimental spinal cord trauma. Neurology 25:508, 1975

48. Miller, JD, Sakalas, R, Ward, JD, et al.: Methylprednisolone treatment in the patient with brain tumors. Neurosurgery 1:114, 1977

49. Hall, ED, Braughler, JM: Glucocoriticoid mechanisms in the acute spinal cord injury. A review and therapeutic rationale. Surg Neurol 18:320, 1982

50. Kuchner EF, Hansebout RR: Combined steroid and hyperthermia treatment of experimental spinal cord injury. Surg Neurol 6:371, 1976

51. Davis D, Bohlman HH, Walker AE, Fischer R., et al: The pathological findings in fatal craniospinal injuries. J Neurosurg 34:603, 1971

52. Day GL, Jacoby CG, Dolan KD: Basilar invagination resulting from untreated Jefferson's fracture. AJR 133:9, 1979

53. Kulkari MV, McArdle CB, Kopaniky DR, et al: Acute spinal cord injury: MR imaging at 1.5 T. Radiology 164:3, 837, 1987

54. Merkel KD, Brown ML, Dewanjee MK, Fitzgerald RH: Comparison of indium-labeled-leukocyte imaging with sequential technetium-gallium scanning in the diagnosis of low grade musculoskeletal sepsis. A prospective study. J Bone Joint Surg 76A:465, 1985

55. Cheshire, DJE: The stability of the cervical spine following the conservative treatment of fractures and fracture-dislocations. Paraplegia 7:193, 1969

56. Burke DC, Tiong TS: Stability of the cervical spine after conservative treatment. Paraplegia 13:191, 1975

57. Whitley JE, Forsyth HF: The classification of cervical spine injury. AJR 83:633, 1960

58. Denis F: The three column spine and its significance in the classification of acute thoracolumbar spine injuries. Spine 8:817, 1983

59. Wollin DG: The os odontoideum. Separate odontoid process. J Bone Joint Surg 45A:1459, 1963

60. Wortzman G, Dewar FP: Rotary fixation of the atlantoaxial joint: rotational atlantoaxial subluxation. Radiology 90:479, 1968

61. Fielding WJ, Hawkins RJ: Atlanto-axial rotary fixation. J Bone Joint Surg 59A:37, 1977

62. Coutts MD: Atlanto-epistropheal subluxations. Arch Surg 29:297, 1934.

63. Hohl M: Normal motions in the upper portion of the cervical spine. J Bone Joint Surg 46A:1777, 1964

64. Levine AM, Edwards CC: The management of

traumatic spondylolisthesis of the axis. J Bone Joint Surg 67:217, 1985

65. White AA, Panjabi MM: Functional spinal unit and mathematical models. p. 35. In: Clinical Biomechanics of the Spine. JB Lippincott, Philadelphia, 1978

66. Francis WR, Fielding JW, Hawkins RJ et al.: Traumatic spondylolisthesis of the axis. J Bone Joint Surg 63B:313, 1981

67. Effendi B, Roy D, Cornish B, et al: Fractures of the ring of the axis. J Bone Joint Surg 63B:319, 1981

68. Spierings ELH, Braakman R: The management of os odontoideum. J Bone Joint Surg 64B:4, 422, 1982

69. Wiesel SW, Rothman RH: Atlanto-occipital hypermobility. Orthop Trans 3:283, 1979

70. Chamberlain WE: Basilar impression (platybasia). Yale J Biol Med 11:487, 1939

71. Hinck VC, Hopkins CE, Savara BS: Diagnostic criteria of basilar impression. Radiology 76:572, 1961

72. Bull JWD, Nixon WLB, Pratt RTC: The radiological criteria and familial occurrence of primary basilar impression. Brain 78:229, 1955

73. Bell C: Surgical observations. Middlesex Hosp J 4:469, 1817

74. Bolender N, Cromwell LD, Wendling L: Fractures of the occipital condyle. AJR 131:729, 1978

75. Jacoby CG: Fractures of the occipital condyle. AJR 132:500, 1979

76. Grisolia A, Bell RL, Peltier LF: Fractures and dislocations of the spine complicating ankylosing spondylitis. J Bone Joint Surg 49A:339, 1967

77. Eismont FJ, Bohlman HH: Posterior atlanto-occipital dislocation with fractures of the atlas and odontoid process. Report of a case with survival. J Bone Joint Surg 60A:397, 1978

78. Evarts CM: Traumatic occipito-atlantal dislocation. J Bone Joint Surg 52A:1653, 1970

79. Farthing JW: Atlantocranial dislocation with survival. A case report. NC Med J 9:34, 1948

80. Gabrielsen TO, Maxwell JA: Traumatic atlanto-occipital dislocation. With case report of a patient who survived. AJR 97:624, 1966

81. Jefferson G: Fracture of the atlas vertebra. Br J Surg 7:407, 1920

82. Garber JN: Fracture and fracture-dislocation of the cervical spine. p. 18. Instructional Course Lectures, CV Mosby, St. Louis, 1961

83. Eismont FJ, Bohlman HH: Posterior atlanto-occipital dislocation with fractures of the atlas and odontoid process. Report of a case with survival. J Bone Joint Surg 60A:379, 1978

84. Kahanovitz N, Mehringer M, Johanson P: Intracranial entrapment of the atlas — complicating an untreated fracture of the posterior arch of the atlas. J Bone Joint Surg 63A:831, 1981

85. Rana NA: Atlanto-axial subluxation in rheumatoid arthritis. J Bone Joint Surg 55B:458, 1973

86. Ranawat CS, et al.: Cervical spine fusion in rheumatoid arthritis. J Bone Joint Surg 61A:1003, 1979

87. Smith HP, et al.: Odontoid compression of the brain in a patient with rheumatoid arthritis: case report. J Neurosurg 53:841, 1980

88. Epstein BS, Epstein JA, Jones MD: Lap-sash three-point seat belt fractures of the cervical spine. Spine 3:189, 1978

89. Taylor TKF, Nade S, Bannister JH: Seat belt fractures of the cervical spine. J Bone Joint Surg 58B:328, 1976

90. Kewalramani L, Krauss J: Cervical spine injuries resulting from collision sports. Paraplegia 19:303, 1981

91. Wood-Jones F: The examination of the bodies of 100 men executed in Nubia in Roman times. Br Med J 1:736, 1908

92. Braakman R, Vinken PJ: Unilateral facet interlocking in the lower cervical spine. J Bone Joint Surg 49B:249, 1967

93. Burke DC, Berryman D: The place of closed manipulation in the management of flexion-rotation dislocations of the cervical spine. J Bone Joint Surg 53B:165, 1971

94. Davis AT: Proposed research project. "Pilot of Multidisciplinary Team Assessment as A Tool in Etiologic Analysis of Childhood Pedestrian Injury." Northwestern University, Northwestern University Medical School, Children's Memorial Hospital, Chicago, IL, 1982

95. Evans DK: Anterior cervical subluxation. J Bone Joint Surg 58B:318, 1976

96. Funk FJ, Wells RE,: Injuries of the cervical spine in football. Clin Orthop 109:50, 1975.

97. Frankel HL, Hancock DO, Hystop G, Melzak J, et al.: The value of postural reduction in the initial management of closed injuries of the spine with paraplegia and tetraplegia. Part 1. Paraplegia 7:179, 1969

98. Gallie WE: Fractures and dislocations of the cervical spine. Am J Surg 46:495, 1939

99. Haughton S: On hanging, considered from a mechanical and physiological point of view. London, Edinburgh, and Dublin. Philosophical Magazine and Journal of Science, 4th series. p. 22, 1866

100. Wood-Jones F: The ideal lesion produced by judicial hanging. Lancet 1:53, 1913

101. Grogono BJS: Injuries of the atlas and axis. J Bone Joint Surg (Br) 36B:397, 1954

102. Schneider RC, Livingstone KE, Cave AJE, Hamilton G: "Hangman's fracture" of the cervical spine. J Neurosurg 22:141, 1965

103. Roy-Camille R, Saillant G, Sagnet P: Lesions traumatiques durachis cervical sans complication neurologique. Encycl Med Chir A-10:15825, 1975

104. Cornish BL: Traumatic spondylolisthesis of the axis. J Bone Joint Surg (Br) 50-B:31, 1968

105. McRae DL: The significance of abnormalities of the cervical spine. AJR 84:3, 1960

106. Dastur DK, Wadia NH, Desai AD, Singh G: Medullospinal compression due to atlanto-axial dislocation and sudden haematomyelia during decompression. Brain 88:897, 1965

107. Seljeskog EL, Chou SN: Spectrum of the hangman's fracture. J Neurosurg 45:308, 1976

108. Harris WH, Salzman EW, Desanctis RW: The prevention of thromboembolic disease by prophylactic anticoagulants. J Bone Joint Surg 49-A:81, 1967.

109. Robinson RA: Anterior and posterior cervical spine fusion. Clin Orthop 35:34, 1964

110. Edwards CC: Results using oblique wiring for rotational instability of the cervical spine. J Bone Joint Surg Orthop Trans 9:142, 1985

111. Cloward RB: Treatment of acute fractures and fracture-dislocations by vertebral body fusion. Report of eleven cases. J Neurosurg 18:201, 1961

112. Baker LD, Hoyt WA, Jr.: The use of interfacet vitallium screws in the Hibbs fusion. South Med J 41:419, 1948

113. Magerl FP: Stabilization of the lower thoracic and lumbar spine with external skeletal fixation. Clin Orthop 189:125, 1984

114. Magerl FP: Stabilization of the cervical spine using the Magerl hook-plate. 45th AO-ASIF Spine Course. Davos, Switzerland, December 16, 1986

115. Housebout RR, Blomquist GA: Acrylic spine fusion. A 20-year clinical series and technical note. J Neurosurg 53:606, 1980

116. Herron LD, Dawson EG: Methylmethacrylate as an adjunct in spinal instrumentation. J Bone Joint Surg 59A:866, 1977

117. Bernhang AM, Rosen H, Leivy D: Internal methyl methacrylate splint provides rapid mobilization in treatment of grossly unstable fractures of cervical spine. Orthop Rev VII:25, 1978

118. Fielding W, Pyle RN, Fietti VG: Anterior cervical body resection and bone-grafting for benign and malignant tumors. J Bone Joint Surg 61A:251, 1979

119. Bloom MH, Raney FL: Anterior intervertebral fusion of the cervical spine, a technical note. J Bone Joint Surg 63-A:842, 1981

120. Robinson RA, Smith GW: Anterior lateral cervical disc removal and interbody fusion for cervical disc syndrome (abstract). Bull Johns Hopkins Hosp 96:223, 1955

121. Robinson RA: Anterior and posterior cervical spine fusion. Clin Orthop, 35:34, 1964

122. Roy-Camille R, de la Caffiniere JY, Saillant G: Traumatismes du rochis cervical superieur C1-C2. Masson, Paris, 1973

15

Surgical Stabilization of the Cervical Spine

Paul R. Meyer, Jr.
Steven Heim

Surgery of the cervical spine is demanding and requires a thorough understanding of vertebral column and neurologic anatomy. For the most part, surgery of the cervical spine is reasonably straightforward, and the results depend on careful interpretation of the injury or pathology present. There are exceptions when the management technique utilized will fail, for example, grossly unstable spine injuries not recognizable solely from bony injury; vertebral column instability resulting from failed previous surgery; turmor involvement of both anterior and posterior osseous structures, etc., simultaneously associated with a deteriorating neurologic status.

Injuries to the cervical spine fall into two categories: those managed conservatively by means of traction, bed care, and orthotic immobilization, and those managed surgically. In the latter category, various surgical techniques can be utilized depending on the osseous or ligamentous structures injured or the structures that remain intact. Together these dictate the approach to be taken: anterior, posterior, or both, bone graft, wire or plate fixation, or a combination of several of these choices.

With reasonable attention to the preoperative physiologic status of the patient, anesthesia, and the performance of operative procedures, complications arising directly from the surgical procedure are infrequent. New internal fixation techniques are being added to the operative armamentarium. Until they are more frequently utilized, they will bring with them unanticipated and unrecognized problems. One such technique that appears to offer promise is a plate-screw combination (the lower end is a hook, and the superior end is a screw hole) to be used as a means of providing rigid fixation between adjacent lamina and facets. The developer, Fritz Magerl (St. Gallen, Switzerland) (Fig. 15-1) reported its use at the 45th AO-ASIF Spine Surgery Course (Davos, Switzerland) in 1986.[1] The procedure is technically demanding and requires that the user have a good working knowledge of cervical vertebral column anatomy. As with all new procedures, unanticipated complications may occur. For example, the hazard of concern with this procedure is injury of the vertebral artery during screw insertion into the lateral mass of the adjacent facet (Fig. 15-2).

397

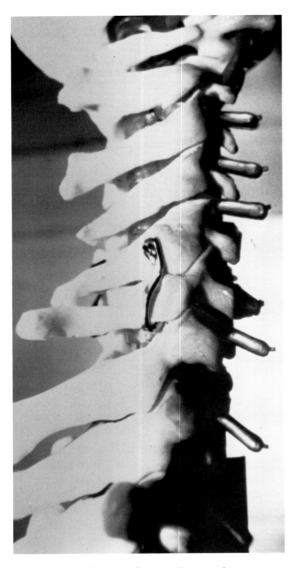

Fig. 15-1. Lateral view of cervical spine showing posterior element stabilization by means of the "Magerl" laminar hook-plate (see Fig. 15-2).

INITIAL MANAGEMENT

It is of cardinal importance that all patients with a history of injury to the cervical spine, regardless of the injury mechanism or type of injury, receive the same initial management. This involves placing the patient on a Stryker wedge frame or bed, from which cervical skeletal traction can be applied with Gardner-Wells tongs. This is indicated for the following reasons. Most important, the true extent of the suspected or known injury cannot be accurately determined until a complete evaluation has been performed. In addition to the standard anteroposterior and lateral radiographs, tomographic evaluation is the study most likely to reveal the greatest evidence of injury or fracture, beyond that initially recognized on the preliminary films. The second reason why constant and similar care must be provided during the evaluative process is determination of the presence or absence of vertebral column instability. Occasionally, the mere application of skeletal traction will identify this problem on follow-up films. In those situations after initial emergency room and radiologic evaluation in which no evidence of injury or instability is found, changes in interlaminar or interdiscal space can and should be obtained by flexion-extension films (with the traction removed), under the observation of a trained physician. It is always appropriate to admit the patient until all studies thought necessary to complete the spinal evaluation are completed.

A second general rule in the management of cervical spine injuries is that when a facet joint (unilateral or bilateral) subluxation or dislocation exists, every effort should be made to obtain an immediate reduction by Gardner-Wells cervical tong traction. As noted in Chapter 14 (see p. 359), the "rule of thumb" for the initial application of weights is 5 lbs per level of injury. Additional weights beyond this are frequently required, as is the use of muscle relaxants and analgesics such as Valium (diazepam; 5 to 10 mg intravenously (IV) slowly) or a newer drug, Versed (midazolam hydrochloride, 1 to 1.5 mg IV over a 2- to 3-minute period if accompanying narcotics are utilized, otherwise 2 to 3.5 mg). This latter drug is used for conscious sedation and is given just before the procedure to induce sleepiness, drowsiness, and relief of apprehension and to impair perioperative memory. Versed, if given in bolus form, can result in respiratory depression. It should not be utilized in patients demonstrating acute alcoholic intoxication. Either Demerol (meperidine hydrochloride) or morphine (in the absence of a history of head injury with loss of con-

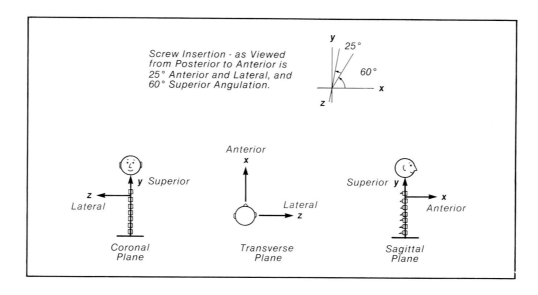

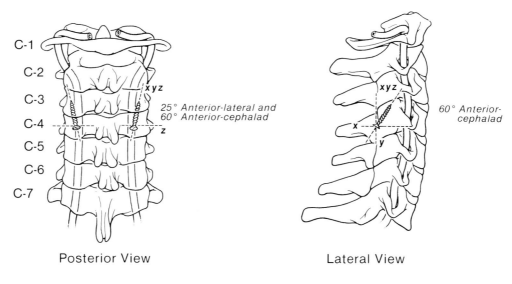

Posterior View   Lateral View

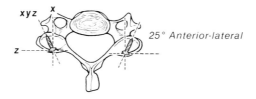

Transverse View

Fig. 15-2. Schematic representation of the angular position of a cervical spine facet internal fixation visualized in the coronal, sagittal, and transverse planes. Screws used for this purpose should be no longer than 18 mm.

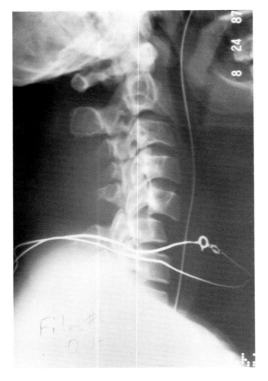

A

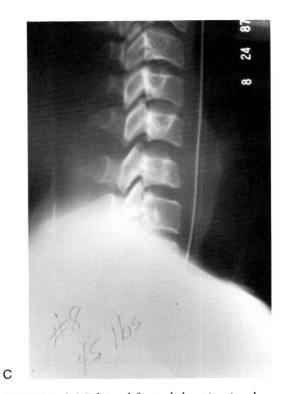

C

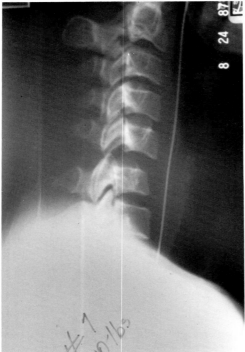

B

Fig. 15-3. (A) Bilateral facet dislocation involving the cervical spine at C5–C6. Patient had an incomplete central cord syndrome. (B) Reduction of fracture after application of 40 lb of cervical tong traction. Note incomplete reduction of one facet. (C) Complete reduction with 45 lb traction. *(Figure continues.)*

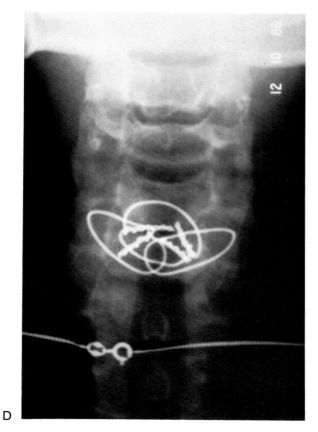

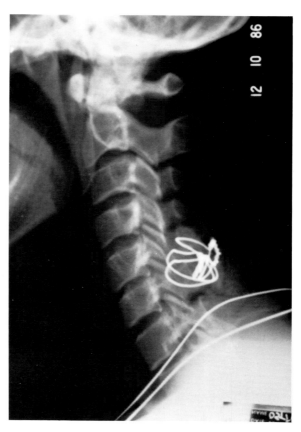

Fig. 15-3 *(Continued).* **(D,E)** AP and lateral radiographs showing bilateral facet and interspinous wiring used to maintain reduction.

sciousness of more than 3 to 5 minutes) can be simultaneously utilized to further induce muscle relaxation and facilitate early facet joint reduction. The reduction of facet joint dislocation, along with the restoration of vertebral column alignment, is the primary means of reducing spinal cord compression.

In cases where excellent muscle relaxation and more than adequate cervical traction (40 to 85 lbs) do not result in reduction of the dislocated facet or facets, in our experience, a facet joint fracture exists (Fig. 15-3). Under such conditions, no further attempt should be made to obtain reduction (particularly in the presence of either an intact or incomplete neurologic injury), the weights should be reduced to a maintenance level of 15 lbs, and plans should be made for an early surgical reduction (by the posterior approach). If the patient

demonstrated neurologic deterioration, immediate surgical reduction would be indicated.

The only two indications for emergent or urgent surgical intervention in a cervical spine-injured patient are incomplete neurologic injury with evidence of progressive neurologic loss, and incomplete neurologic injury with persistent cervical spine dislocation.

CERVICAL SPINE MANIPULATION

Manipulation of the cervical spine should never be performed on the completely anesthetized patient. It is more successful when the patient has been verbally prepared for the manipulation and

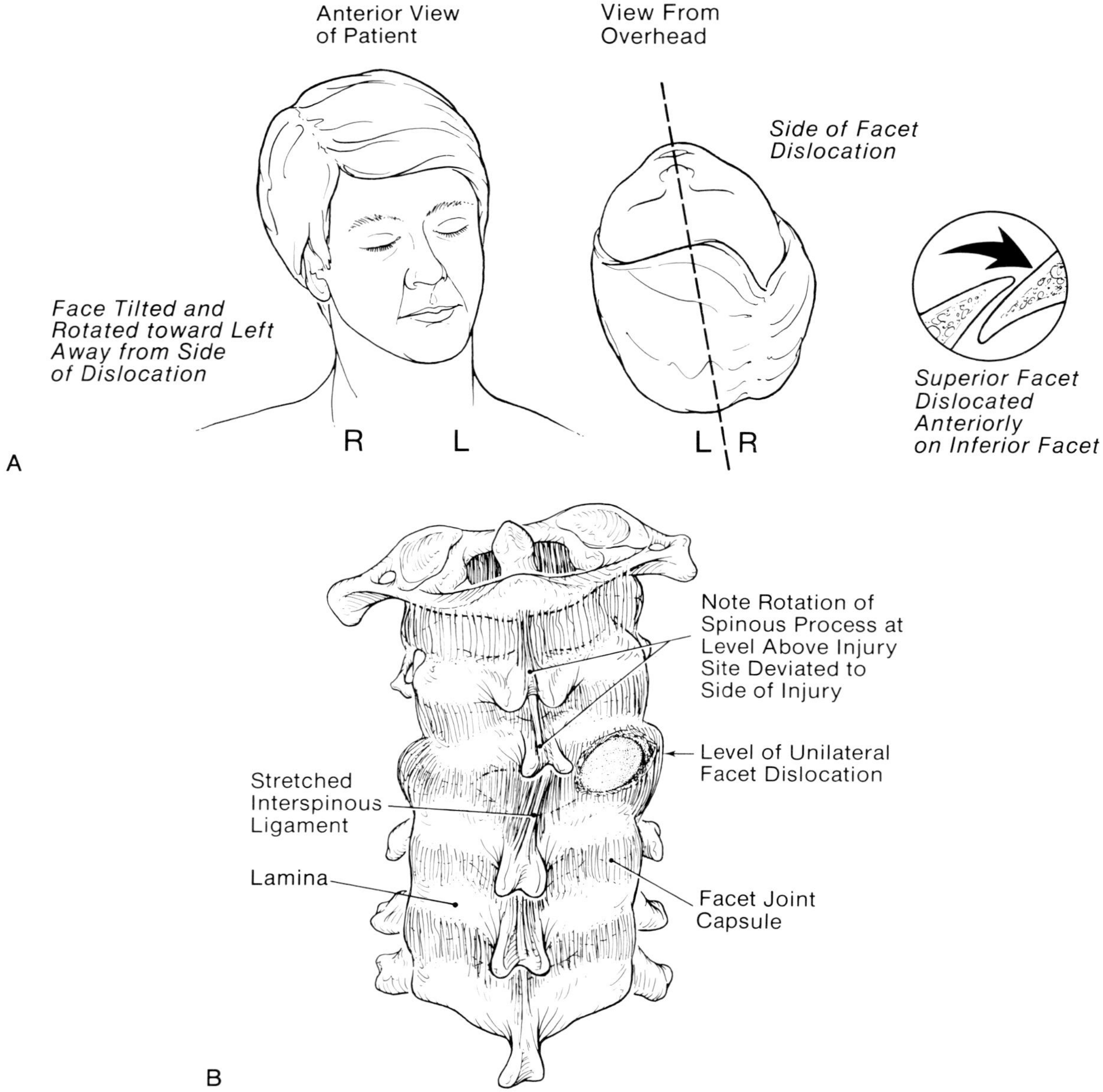

Anterior View
of Patient

View From
Overhead

*Side of Facet
Dislocation*

*Face Tilted and
Rotated toward Left
Away from Side
of Dislocation*

R   L

L   R

*Superior Facet
Dislocated
Anteriorly
on Inferior Facet*

A

Note Rotation of
Spinous Process at
Level Above Injury
Site Deviated to
Side of Injury

Level of Unilateral
Facet Dislocation

Stretched
Interspinous
Ligament

Lamina

Facet Joint
Capsule

B

Fig. 15-4. Anatomic consequences of unilateral facet dislocation. (A) Characteristic tilt of head. (B) Posterior view of spine showing lamina and spinous process prior to reduction. These anatomic findings may be identified on a prereduction AP radiograph or at surgery.

subsequently supported by the administration of analgesic and muscle relaxants as described above (i.e., Valium).

Once the patient's standard and tomographic radiographs reveal the presence and side of a unilat-

eral facet dislocation with locking of the facet, or the presence of an unreducible perched facet, closed reduction can be attempted with little concern of producing or extending a neurologic injury. Physical examination of the patient with a unilateral facet dislocation will reveal tilting of the head and neck to the *side* of injury, and facing of the patient's head and neck to the side *opposite* the side of injury. Careful observation of the anteroposterior radiograph will reveal that the spinous process of the affected vertebra is off the midline, toward the dislocated side.

After determining that the Gardner-Wells tongs are appropriately tightened, the physician slowly rotates the patient's head and neck in the direction opposite the facing of the chin, along with simultaneous lateral bending of the head and neck to the opposite side of the dislocation (Fig. 15-4). This is performed by the application of pressure via the Gardner-Wells tongs. This procedure is usually rewarding. Reduction often can be appreciated by both the patient and the physician by a muffled "pop" and a sudden relief of restricted motion. The patient will often be the first to report the reduction, as is often the case when no manipulation is conducted, but only weights applied. It is therefore appropriate to query the patient and to suggest that he or she report not only any unusual sensations or radiating symptoms, but the sensation of loss of tension and restricted range of motion in the neck, particularly if associated with a "snapping" sensation. With the report of loss of neck pain, a reduction in cervical muscle tension or obstruction to rotation of the head and neck, along with a palpable sensation reported by the patient, the reduction should be immediately confirmed radiographically. When reduction is confirmed on the lateral radiograph, the weights should be immediately reduced to 10 lbs (a maximum of 15 lbs) for maintenance of cervical spine alignment. After the weights are reduced, radiographs should be repeated during the next 24 hours.

In approximately 10 to 15 percent of patients in whom a dislocated facet is reduced by traction, redislocation will occur when the weights are appropriately reduced. This is indicative of several things: incomplete reduction obtained the first time; the presence of an unrecognized facet fracture; or greater ligamentous instability at the injury site than recognized on radiographs.

When there is ease of displacement of the offending facet into recurrent subluxation or dislocation, along with increased widening of the interfacet or interspinous space between the offending element and the adjacent element below, surgical stabilization is indicated. On the other hand, when the spinal reduction remains and no evidence exists of abnormal subluxation or widening of the posterior processes, the spine may, at the surgeon's choice, be managed conservatively. The type of immobilization is also the surgeon's choice. For maximum immobilization, the halo vest is suggested. For the patient with no apparent gross instability, a sternal occipital mandibular immobilization (SOMI) orthosis may be used; however, even when worn by the most reliable patient, this orthosis may fail (see Fig. 15-71).

INDICATIONS FOR EARLY SURGERY AND PREOPERATIVE CONSIDERATIONS

One of the most pressing questions after the admission of a cervical spine-injured patient who shows a significant neurologic injury is whether emergency is indicated. *Emegency surgery is rarely indicated.*

The patient who has sustained a complete (irreversible) neurological injury, who on physical evaluation demonstrates stability both physiologically and neurologically in the presence of a reduced cervical vertebral column fracture or dislocation, cannot attain neurologic improvement by the performance of emergent surgery. The two most frequent procedures erroneously performed (using the rigid criterion of complete neurologic injury as the basis) are anterior vertebral body corporectomy and the insertion of a bone graft, or posterior laminectomy. Both are contraindicated in the immediate post-trauma period. Neurologic recovery will not be enhanced.

The two single indications for emergent or early surgery are the patient who upon repeated neurologic examinations demonstrates deterioration greater than that found on the initial neurologic assessment; and the patient who reveals the presence of an unreducible unilateral or bilateral facet or spine dislocation, in the presence of an incompletely injured neurologic system (Fig. 15-5). If an

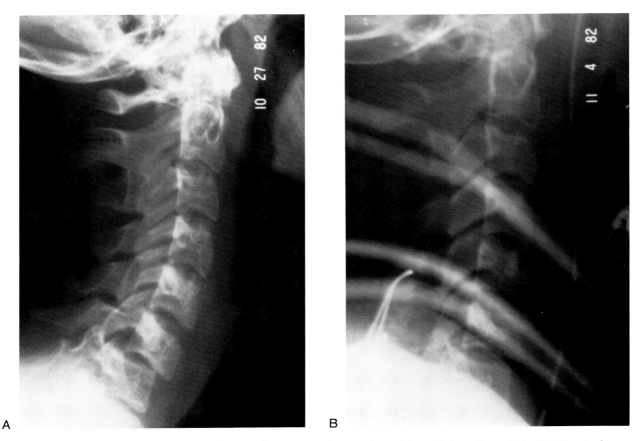

A   B

Fig. 15-5. (**A**) Lateral radiograph of cervical spine revealing unilateral facet dislocation at C6–C7. Cervical spine was reduced by the technique shown in Figure 15-3. Because the patient was neurologically normal and was reliable, a **SOMI** orthosis was used after 2 weeks of cervical traction. Facet dislocation was recurrent, necessitating surgical reduction and stabilization. (**B**) Lateral radiograph showing reduction with posterior interspinous wiring fixation.

unreducible dislocation exists in the neurologically intact patient, the patient should be initially managed conservatively and operated on electively.

There are five major considerations that must be taken into account and made an integral part of the preoperative decision-making and operative management process. (1) Can the planned operative procedure be justified, taking all factors and potential complications into consideration? This includes those unanticipated complications that can and do accompany major (and minor) operative procedures. Paramount under this category are two very serious complications: loss of existing neurologic function resulting from the planned op-

erative procedure or its approach (as with hoarseness resulting from injury to the recurrent laryngeal nerve); or death of the patient from either anesthesia or hemorrhage. (2) Can a stable spine reduction be attained? (3) Can the reduction be maintained until fusion occurs? (4) Will an additional operative procedure be required? (5) Has the family and/or the patient been duly informed of each of the above, either in conversation, with qualified witnesses, or in a thorough, descriptive consent form?

Although many fractures are radiographically similar, they often vary in stability. The same is true of the patient's physiology. Youthful patients are usually in prime physical condition at the time of injury. Elderly patients, however (those above 50 years of age), are more fragile. They are either unaware of existing conditions or exhibit varying degrees of medical illness including cardiovascular (with hypertension), pulmonary, cerebral, vascular, renal, or diabetic disease. With the occurrence of injury, the health balance in which the patient lives is likely to be lost as a result of injury or the performance of surgery. Thus, with cervical spinal cord injury, loss of the normal compensatory cardiac, pulmonary, or peripheral vascular reflexes can and does result in unforeseen physiological consequences that are likely to alter the patient's outcome.

Collectively, those considerations that must be taken under review before performing a cervical spine procedure include the following:

1. A determination of the components of instability.
2. How can stability be restored? By which surgical approach: anterior or posterior?
3. Because of injury-induced instability, is there potential for the worsening of the neurologic injury during prone positioning of the patient on the operating table (or Stryker wedge frame)? This hazard does exist, has occurred, and should be carefully monitored. It is more likely to occur in the patient with extensive cervical spine degenerative disease, spondylosis, or a concomitant herniated disc. Thus, a preoperative myelogram is mandated in the patient with a neurologically incomplete injury (see Indications for Myelography, below). It occurs secondary to extrinsic (extradural) pressure against the anterior spinal cord, arising from accentuation of the hyperextended position of the neck while in the prone position. The hazard exists of "pinching" the spinal cord between osteophytes (along the posterior border of the cervical vertebra) and the calcified ligamentum flavum between the lamina posteriorly (Fig. 15-6). This results in vascular embarrassment to the spinal cord secondary to encroachment on the anterior spinal artery (see Ch. 4). Appreciation of this hazard speaks to the need for evoked potential monitoring of spinal cord function during surgery.

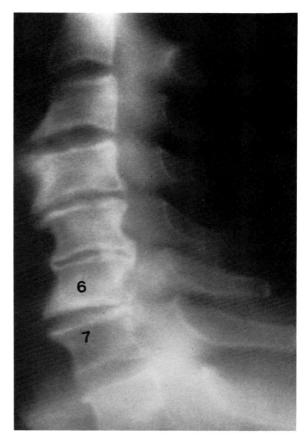

Fig. 15-6. Lateral radiograph of cervical spine showing marked cervical spondylosis and abnormal widening of interspace at C6–C7. Note calcified posterior longitudinal ligament posterior to C6–C7, associated narrowness of the cervical canal at C5–C6, and widening of the disc interspace anteriorly at C6–C7. Patient sustained extension injury resulting in C6–C7 central cord neurologic injury.

4. How many vertebral levels require stabilization and fusion?
5. The internal fixation device most indicated depends on the surgical approach: with an anterior approach, interbody inlay bone graft after vertebral body decompression (Fig. 15-7) or plate and screws with a bone graft (Figs. 15-8 though 15-10); with a posterior approach, spinous process wiring (Fig. 15-11, and see Fig. 15-60) with a corticocancellous bone graft procedure (Fig. 15-12).

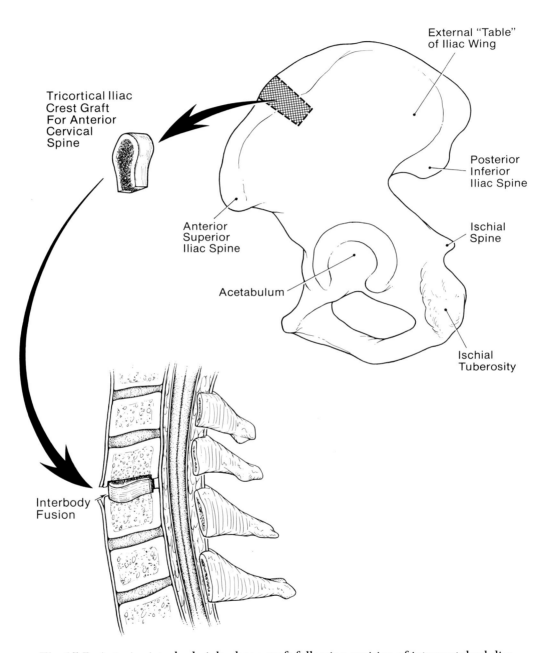

Fig. 15-7. Anterior interbody inlay bone graft following excision of intervertebral disc.

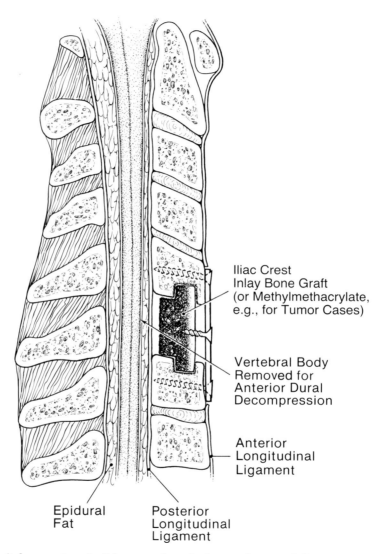

Iliac Crest
Inlay Bone Graft
(or Methylmethacrylate,
e.g., for Tumor Cases)

Vertebral Body
Removed for
Anterior Dural
Decompression

Anterior
Longitudinal
Ligament

Epidural
Fat

Posterior
Longitudinal
Ligament

Fig. 15-8. Anterior (inlay or tricortical) bone graft with plate and screws following vertebral body corporectomy for neural canal decompression. Cortical screws are usually 18 to 20 mm long.

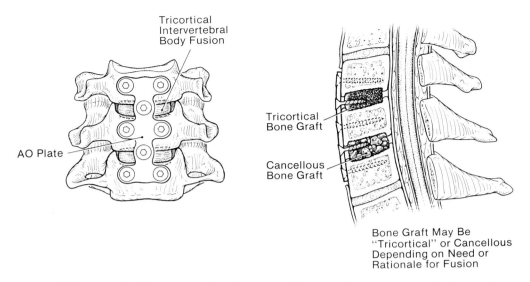

Fig. 15-9. Modification of Robinson-Southwick anterior fusion technique using AO plate and screws for internal stabilization.

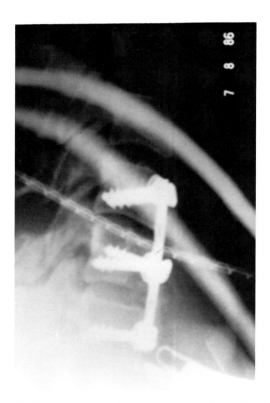

Fig. 15-10. Anterior stabilization using the A-O plate-screw fixation. Anterior surgery is most often used when there is incomplete neurologic injury with evidence of spinal cord or spinal canal encroachment (requiring debridement) by either bone or disc material.

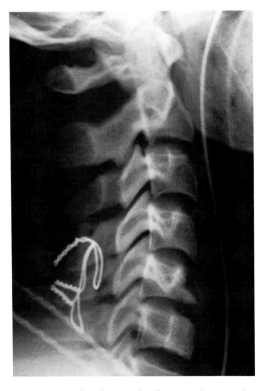

Fig. 15-11. Lateral radiograph of cervical spine showing use of posterior "two-wire" interspinous process wire fixation and bone grafting. Posterior fixation is used when the primary site of spine instability is posterior.

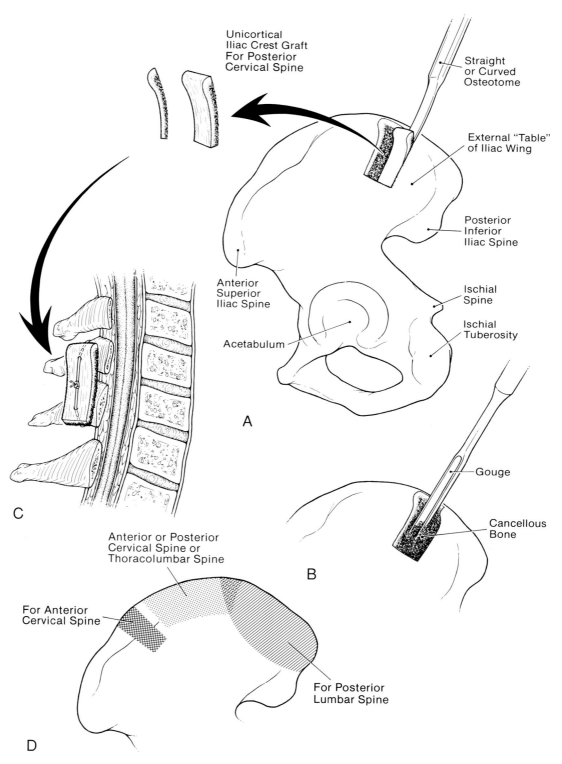

Unicortical
Iliac Crest Graft
For Posterior
Cervical Spine

Straight
or Curved
Osteotome

External "Table"
of Iliac Wing

Posterior
Inferior
Iliac Spine

Ischial
Spine

Ischial
Tuberosity

Anterior
Superior
Iliac Spine

Acetabulum

A

Gouge

Cancellous
Bone

B

C

Anterior or Posterior
Cervical Spine or
Thoracolumbar Spine

For Anterior
Cervical Spine

For Posterior
Lumbar Spine

D

Fig. 15-12. (A–C) Technique for obtaining cortical-cancellous bone graft for use in posterior spinous wiring-fusion technique. **(D)** Areas of pelvic rim from which bone grafts are harvested.

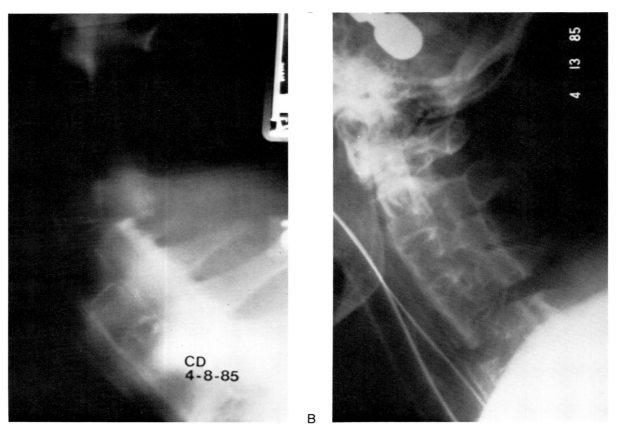

A   B

Fig. 15-13. (A) Lateral radiograph of 58-year-old man with Marie-Strümpell rheumatoid spondylitis who sustained a hyperextension injury to the cervical spine at C4–C5. Note complete fracture through vertebral body and calcified ligaments. Patient sustained immediate complete C4–C5 neurologic injury. (B) To reestablish appropriate cervical reduction, the patient required flexion of the head-neck position, reconstituting the pre-injury existing cervical spine spondylitic deformity.

6. What special considerations might influence the surgical approach? Examples are the presence of a tracheostomy; the level or levels of the cervical spine to be stabilized; surgery at several vertebral levels (limited by a transverse incision); multiple-level procedure (requiring a long oblique sternocleidomastoid muscle approach). Another consideration is the patient's preoperative posture (a patient with rheumatoid spondylitis, with marked cervical kyphosis, would have limited exposure anteriorly were the deformity reconstituted) (Fig. 15-13).

7. Will additional skeletal traction be required during the performance of a procedure (i.e., by anesthesia, by additional weights)?

8. Airway concerns, for example, presence of facial fractures; will a tracheostomy impede the performance of a planned anterior approach?

9. During an anterior approach, can pressure be safely applied to anatomical structures, for example, carotid vessels. (This is a concern in the elderly patient [stroke]; the vessels' patency can be monitored during anesthesia by palpation of the temporal artery. This vessel requires monitoring with each change in retractor position. Concern over stretching of the recurrent laryngeal nerve[2] or pressure (erosion) or perforation injury to the esophagus, trachea, and cervical vessels must be taken with retractor instruments.

10. Whether the taking down of anterior structures during the insertion of an anterior bone graft (longus colli muscles, anterior longitudinal ligament) will result in more extensive anterior (and overall) vertebral column instability (an anterior and a posterior stabilizing procedure). The finding of such may require the use of an alternate management scheme (Fig. 15-14).

11. Will the insertion of an anterior bone graft provide stability, neuroforamen distraction, and nerve root decompression? Determine graft position by intraoperative radiographs (Fig. 15-15).

12. Will spinal cord monitoring (somatosensory evoked potentials [SSEP]) be available during the performance of the surgical procedure? If not, a "wake-up" test must be performed. If planned, the procedure must be explained to the patient preoperatively.

13. Is the required postoperative orthosis available preoperatively?

14. Will the surgical procedure, when completed, provide sufficient skeletal stability to allow the patient to rapidly enter rehabilitation? Sitting lateral radiographs of the patient in the orthosis should be obtained to evaluate postoperative stability. If no change with axial loading (sitting) occurs, rehabilitation can begin.

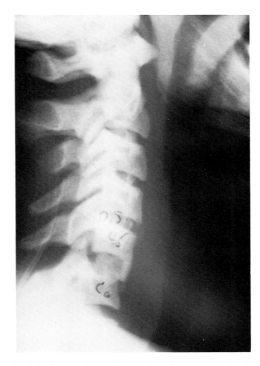

Fig. 15-14. Lateral radiograph of the cervical spine showing postoperative loss of cervical spine alignment, cervical spine fixation, and displacement of intervertebral C5–C6 bone graft. These complications frequently follow inappropriate use of an anterior bone graft approach when the primary site of preoperative instability is posterior. Note widening of space between spinous processes of C5 and C6 indicating site of instability.

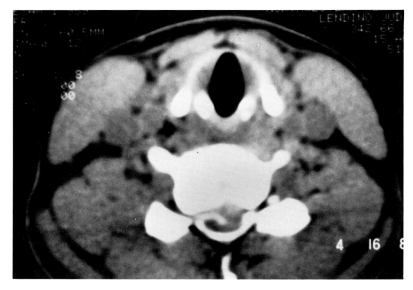

A

Fig. 15-15. (A) Horizontal view of metrizamide CAT scan C5–C6 demonstrating encroachment on the neural canal by herniation of interdiscal material. Patient showed incomplete central cord neurologic injury. *(Figure continues.)*

INDICATIONS FOR MYELOGRAPHY

Patients with complete neurologic injuries do not require preoperative myelographic evaluation unless there is evidence of neurologic injury proximal to the level of spinal cord injury, or the suspicion that multiple-level injuries may exist.

Despite other, more sophisticated methods of spinal column evaluation being available (magnetic resonance imaging [MRI], computed axial tomography [CAT], etc.), the myelogram remains consistently a very reliable procedure, providing the surgeon with a direct correlation between alterations in the contrast medium column and the presence of vertebral column injury.

Experience has revealed unexplained changes in patient neurologic function after admission and the application of standardized spinal cord injury management techniques. In an attempt to anticipate potential pathologic processes that might account for these unsuspected neurologic changes, the following general rules for obtaining a myelogram have been determined. Experience has also demonstrated that using these five criteria for obtaining a myelogram — either immediately after admission

or before surgery — has been successful in identifying pathologic processes that in the past have unsuspectingly produced changes in neurologic function.

The occurrence of a rapidly progressive and otherwise unanticipated neurologic deterioration.

The finding of extensive neurologic injury in the absence of radiologic evidence of bone or ligamentous injury.

When a patient exhibits post-traumatic neurologic recovery with an abrupt neurologic plateau.

When an elective spine stabilization procedure is planned on a patient with an incomplete neurologic injury. (This is considered the only prophylactic reason for myelography.)

When the clinical neurologic examination does not coincide with the SSEP neurologic assessment.

INJURIES TO THE CERVICAL SPINE: STABLE AND UNSTABLE

Positive identification of the extent of any post-traumatic pathology in the cervical spine requires a knowledge of what is "normal" and a sense of de-

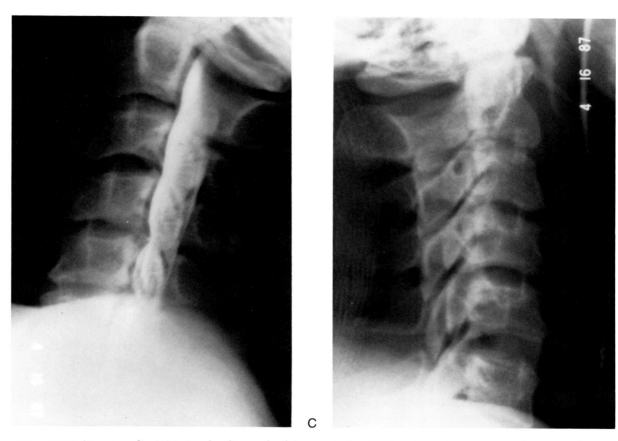

B   C

Fig. 15-15 *(Continued).* **(B)** Lateral radiograph of the cervical spine showing primary encroachment on the neural canal and attenuation of contrast at C5–C6. **(C)** Lateral radiograph after removal of herniated disc and insertion of interdiscal bone graft. Radiograph was obtained before wound closure to ensure proper level of fixation, adequate insertion of the bone graft, and adequate positioning of the bone graft in the interdiscal space. The patient's neurologic status was carefully monitored during surgery by SSEP.

viation from that point. Always required is a high index of suspicion. The actual determination of the existence of pathology follows an initial assessment, a period of observation, and the obtaining of appropriate evaluative procedures including: serial lateral radiographs of the patient, while spinal reduction and realignment are attempted by means of skeletal traction; and when indicated, tomograms, myelography, CAT scans, and contrast medium enhancement CAT scans. in the absence of bone (fracture) pathology, flexion-extension radiographs, under the supervision of a physician, should be obtained to assess ligamentous stability.

Recently, with the advent of MRI, the analysis of such problems as tumor or infection has been greatly enhanced. Occasionally, one or more of these procedures will require repeating for more careful analysis of a specific area. Regardless, on admission, all patients with a history of injury to the head and cervical spine area, require management as though a fracture is present, or until this is ruled out, management on a Stryker wedge frame or horizontal bed, cervical skeletal traction, and a careful and often repeated neurologic assessment.

STABLE POSTERIOR FLEXION INJURIES

In general, fractures of the posterior spinous processes result from either a hyperextension injury (producing a vertical fracture through the posterior element) or a hyperflexion injury (Fig. 15-16). In extension, fracture of the spinous process results from the "prying" of one process against its adjacent member. In flexion, fractures occur as a result of forceful avulsion of the spinous process by the posterior erector spinae muscles ("clay shoveler's fracture") (Fig. 15-16A). The fracture can be recognized as an avulsion fracture by obliqueness of the fracture line (Fig. 15-16B). Fractures of the spinous process may also result from direct trauma. In this instance, the fracture tends to be comminuted. These fractures may be accompanied by stretching or tearing of the interspinous ligament and some widening or subluxation of the adjacent facet joints, but only to a minor degree. Both injuries, flexion and extension, are considered stable and are managed accordingly. To determine accurately the extent of spinal stability, moderate flexion-extension lateral radiographs should be obtained. Without abnormal alignment or widening in either direction, spinal stability is verified and the injury is managed conservatively in an orthosis for 3 to 6 weeks. The type of orthosis normally recommended is a SOMI orthosis or a Philadelphia collar. Repeat flexion-extension radiographs are obtained at 8 to 12 weeks after injury. By this time, the status of cervical spine stability should be known. When the spinous process has healed, athletic endeavors may be resumed (competitive impact sports) within 8 to 12 additional weeks (3 to 4 months postinjury), allowing time for the return of normal cervical spine motion.[3] If the spinous process has not healed, though no abnormal motion or change in alignment is noted on either flexion or extension radiographs, and the patient is asymptomatic, normal (nonimpact) competitive athletic activities may be resumed. At 6 months, the patient can be re-evaluated. With no abnormalities, the patient may resume previous normal activities. *When degenerative changes are noted at the injury site, it is prudent not to allow the patient to re-enter competitive athletics.*

UNSTABLE FLEXION INJURIES

When primary or follow-up evaluation of a cervical spine injury demonstrates the presence of an angular (kyphotic) deformity of greater than 11 degrees at the site of injury, instability exists and posterior spine stabilization is indicated.[1] When only the posterior ligamentous structures are involved (diagnosed by the presence of widening between the two adjacent lamina-facet-interspinous structures), a two-level posterior fusion (Garber-Meyer technique) is indicated (Fig. 15-17). When an anterior vertebral body wedge compression fracture, involving greater than 25 percent of the affected vertebra, results in cervical kyphosis of greater than 11 degrees, a three-level fusion (Meyer-type posterior fusion) procedure (one above and one below the level of injury) is indicated (see Fig. 15-60).

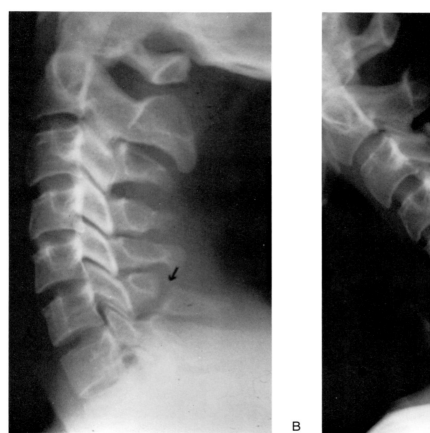 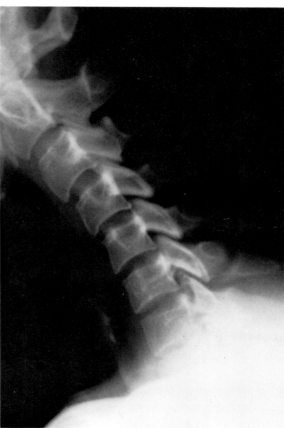

A   B

Fig. 15-16. (A) Lateral radiograph of the cervical spine revealing flexion avulsion (clay shoveler's) fracture of spinous process at C6. No neurologic injury accompanied this injury. (B) Lateral flexion radiograph was obtained to evaluate the presence or absence of posterior cervical spine instability. The spine was found to be stable. *(Figure continues).*

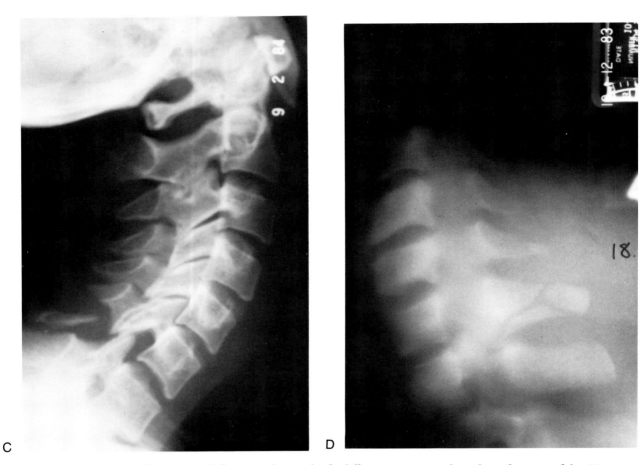

C   D

Fig. 15-16 *(Continued)*. **(C)** Lateral flexion radiograph of a different patient with avulsion fracture of the C6 spinous process. Radiograph demonstrates instability of posterior longitudinal ligament, facet joints, and interspinous ligament requiring cervical spine stabilization. **(D)** Lateral cervical spine radiograph of another patient revealing comminuted fracture of C6 posterior spinous process following extension injury to the cervical spine. Cervical spine was found to be stable on flexion-extension films, and was therefore managed conservatively. *(Figure continues.)*

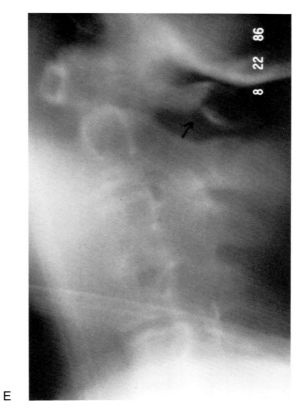

E

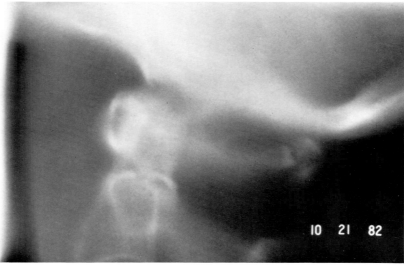

F

Fig. 15-16 *(Continued)*. **(E)** Lateral radiograph of another patient showing avulsion fracture of posterior ring of C1. Patient's neurologic status was normal, and management was conservative. **(F)** Lateral radiograph of cervical spine of another patient demonstrating fracture of the posterior ring of C1 and an extension-induced oblique fracture (type II) of the base of the odontoid. Patient was neurologically normal and was stabilized in a halo vest.

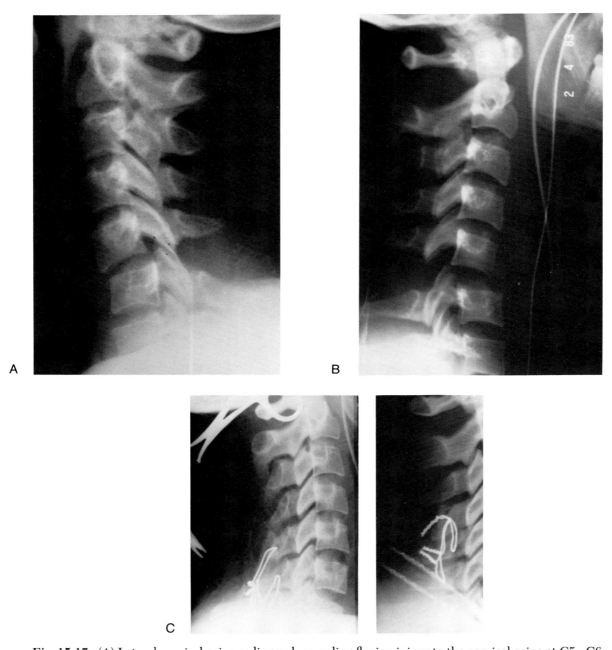

Fig. 15-17. **(A)** Lateral cervical spine radiograph revealing flexion injury to the cervical spine at C5–C6. Note bilateral facet subluxation and widening of interspinous space (indicative of instability) at C5–C6. **(B)** Lateral cervical spine radiograph showing gross instability anteriorly and posteriorly. Note distraction and posterior displacement of C5 vertebral body on C6 along with widening of interdiscal space and gross separation of all posterior elements (facets and spinous processes). **(C)** Lateral cervical spine radiographs showing the Garber-Meyer (posterior interspinous) double wire technique. The difference between the right and left examples is the use of one level of wire fixation (between two spinous processes) when there is associated interspinous ligament widening either above or below the level of primary vertebral column injury. Using the rule of "one level above and one level below," a standard three-level (base of the spinous process) wire and bone graft procedure accompanies the one-level wire fixation.

UNSTABLE FLEXION-AXIAL LOAD-INDUCED BILAMINAR VERTEBRAL BODY INJURIES

An injury that appears initially innocuous, but is not, is the posterior (flexion-axial load) injury of the cervical spine that results in widening of the interspinous process space, with an associated vertebral body compression fracture that is innocently noted to be retrodisplaced 1 to 2 mm. This finding — retrodisplacement of the vertebral body — is indicative of a very unstable cervical spine injury and requires special attention. The presence of a retrodisplaced vertebral body (above) on the vertebral body (below), with either a compression fracture of the involved vertebral body or a small triangular fracture off of the anteroinferior aspect of the involved vertebra, is the *sine qua non* of the presence of an associated posterior finding of a posterior bilaminar fracture (best identified on tomography or CAT scan). Initially, because the primary area of injury was thought to lie posteriorly, the fracture was managed posteriorly. This posterior approach failed (Fig. 15-18). As a result, in our opinion, this became the first flexion-induced fracture with indications requiring an anterior stabilization procedure (Fig. 15-19). The reason the posterior approach failed is conjectured, but it is believed to have occurred because the fracture of the anteroinferior vertebral body disrupts the anterior logitudinal ligament and the anterior anulus fibrosus; the retropulsion of the vertebral body results from an interruption in the continuity of the posterior logitudinal ligament and anulus fibrosus; and the presence of the bilaminar fracture of the posterior element (lamina or pedicles) results in further loss of all posterior stability.

The vertebral column injury described here is now always approached via the anterior approach and has been found to be reliably managed by the insertion of an anteriorly placed anterior cervical spine (AO) plate across three levels.[4] The use of the plate for fixation will allow, depending on the indications, the removal of an involved disc anteriorly, or the removal of a retropulsed fractured vertebral body (a partial corporectomy) with a tricortical interbody fusion (Fig. 15-20) (see p. 479). Postoperatively, the patient can usually be immobilized in a SOMI orthosis. If gross instability persists, a halo vest should be used for a minimum of 3 months.

MULTIPLE-LEVEL FRACTURES

Calenoff and colleagues at Northwestern University reported the occurrence of multiple-level fractures in the spine injury population as 4.5 percent.[5] A similar percentage was noted by Kewalramani and Taylor.[6] In Calenoff's series, 83 percent of the primary fractures (the injury producing neurologic injury) were fracture-dislocations and 5 percent were compression fractures. In the nonprimary fracture group (the injury not producing spinal cord injury), 64 percent were compression fractures and 17 percent were fracture-dislocations. Thirteen percent were isolated neural arch fractures, and 4 percent were avulsion fractures. One nonprimary fracture occurred in the odontoid process, while many primary and secondary fractures occurred between C5 and C7. Of secondary lesions, 40 percent occurred above and 60 percent occurred below the primary lesion.

STABLE AND UNSTABLE EXTENSION INJURIES TO THE CERVICAL SPINE

With the exception of injuries to the cervical spine in patients whose range of motion is markedly restricted, extension injuries to this area of the vertebral column are less likely to result in gross vertebral column instability and neurologic injury than are flexion injuries.[7] As noted, the primary exception to this rule are those extension injuries that occur in patients having Marie-Strümpell rheumatoid spondylitis (Fig. 15-21) or DISH syndrome (disseminated interstitial spinal hyperostosis) (Fig. 15-22).[8-12] In either situation, the resulting ligamentous and bony injury is extensive and, in most series, is associated with the occurrence of a significant neurologic (complete) injury.

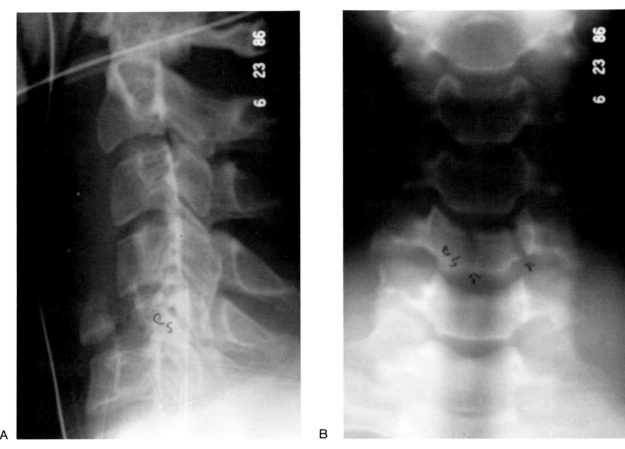

A   B

Fig. 15-18. (A) Lateral cervical spine radiograph following flexion axial load injury. This injury routinely results in a complete neurologic injury. The presence of posterior displacement of the superior vertebral body (C5) on the inferior vertebral body (C6) is the sine qua non of gross cervical spine instability. This finding is frequently evidence of a posterior element laminar fracture and accompanying posterior bilaminar fractures. Note also the typical flexion-induced triangular fracture of the C5 anterior vertebral body. **(B)** Anteroposterior view. Note central and lateral fractures demonstrating presence of bilateral anterior and posterior element fractures. *(Figure continues.)*

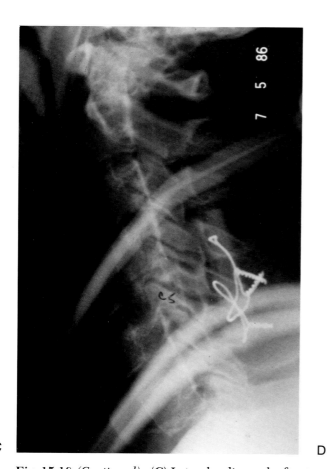 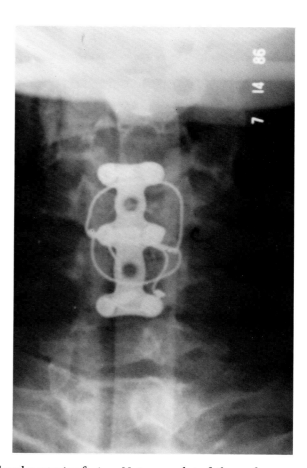

C   D

Fig. 15-18 *(Continued).* **(C)** Lateral radiograph after two-level posterior fusion. Note complete failure of cervical spine alignment with posterior fusion attempt. The patient is in a SOMI orthosis. Similar loss of fixation has occurred when using halo vest fixation. **(D)** AP radiograph showing the posterior wire stabilization supplemented by a three-level anterior A-O plate and screw procedure.

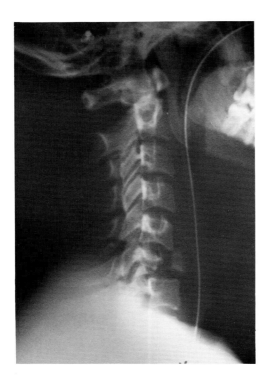

A

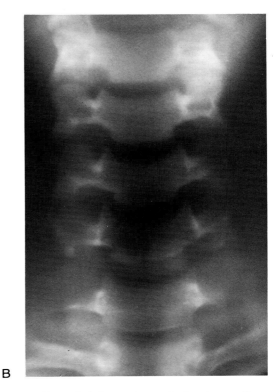

B

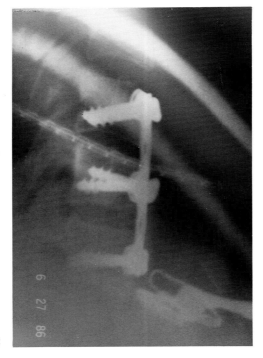

C

Fig. 15-19. (**A**) Lateral cervical spine radiograph of patient with axial load flexion injury resulting in gross spine instability due to loss of three-column stabilization. Note vertical fracture of vertebral body in the sagittal plane, posterior displacement of vertebral body on the next lower vertebral body, and fracture of posterior elements. (**B**) AP radiograph reveals fractures at two sites. (**C**) Lateral radiograph showing stabilization and improved alignment with AO plate and screw apparatus. Patient was managed postoperatively in a SOMI orthosis.

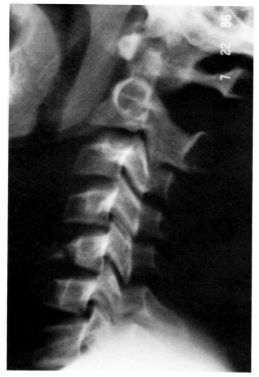

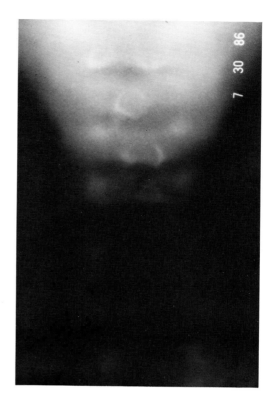

A

B

Fig. 15-20. (A) Lateral cervical spine radiograph revealing flexion injury at C5–C6 resulting in compression fracture of the vertebral body, mild retropulsion of the vertebral body of C5, and diastasis between the posterior spinous processes of C5 and C6. (B) AP tomogram revealing two posterior element fractures at C5. (C) Lateral radiograph after anterior stabilization with AO plate and screw apparatus in conjunction with intervertebral body tricortical bone graft. Patient was immobilized in a SOMI orthosis post-operatively.

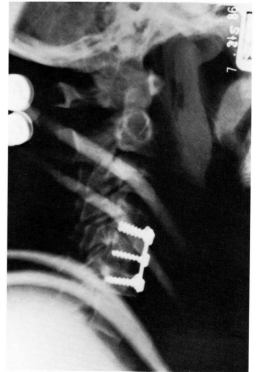

C

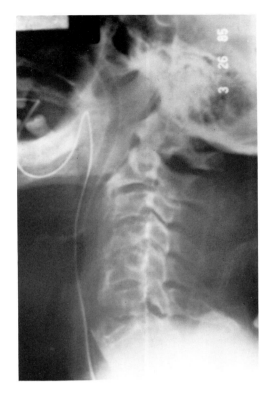

A

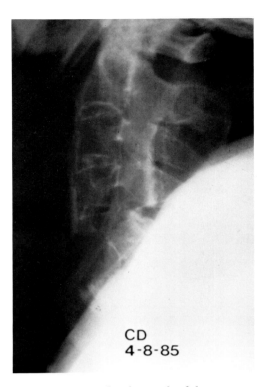

B

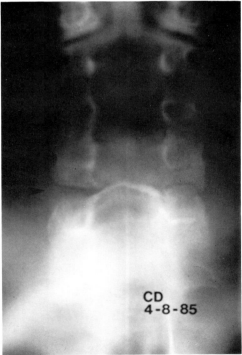

C

Fig. 15-21. (A) Lateral radiograph of the cervical spine in a 63-year-old man who sustained an extension injury. Radiographic examination revealed disseminated interstitial spinal hyperostosis (DISH). Note posterior displacement of the proximal cervical spine and loss of three-column fixation at C6–C7. Neurologic injury was complete. Extension injuries to the elderly spine most frequently occur at C6–C7. Extension injuries in the rheumatoid spondylitic or severe degenerative arthritic cervical spine may occur higher. (B) Lateral cervical spine radiograph of a 63-year-old man with rheumatoid spondylitis, demonstrating gross spine displacement at C5–C6. (C) AP tomogram of the same patient showing horizontal (transverse) fracture through osseous elements C4–C5. *(Figure continues.)*

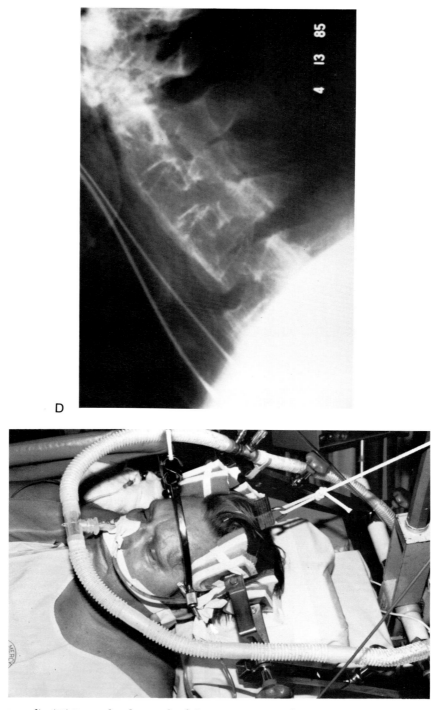

Fig. 15-21 *(Continued).* **(D)** Lateral radiograph of the same patient after recreation of prefracture cervical kyphosis. Note distraction instability. **(E)** Anterolateral photograph of the same patient. Note he required nasotracheal intubation for ventilatory support. Also note the use of two Gardner-Wells cervical tongs to restore cervical spine alignment (and cervical kyphosis). *(Figure continues.)*

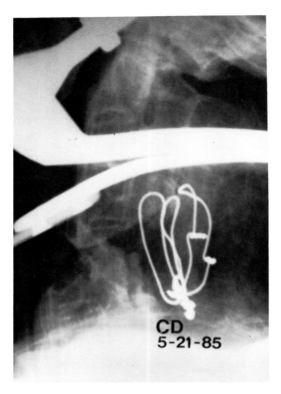

F

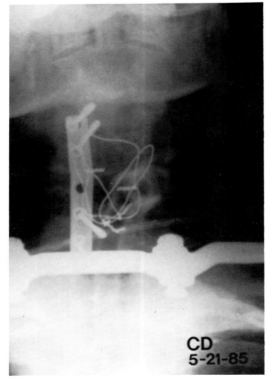

G

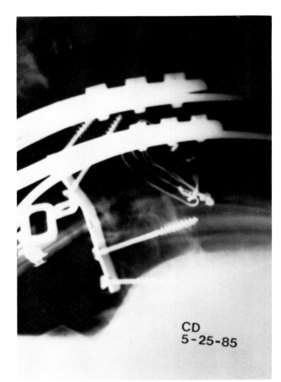

H

Fig. 15-21 *(Continued).* **(F)** Postoperative lateral radiograph of the patient maintained in halo vest fixation. Note distraction and posterior malalignment of upper cervical column. **(G,H)** Anterior and lateral radiographs of the cervical spine after insertion of anterior plate and screws. Postoperative immobilization was maintained by a halo vest orthosis.

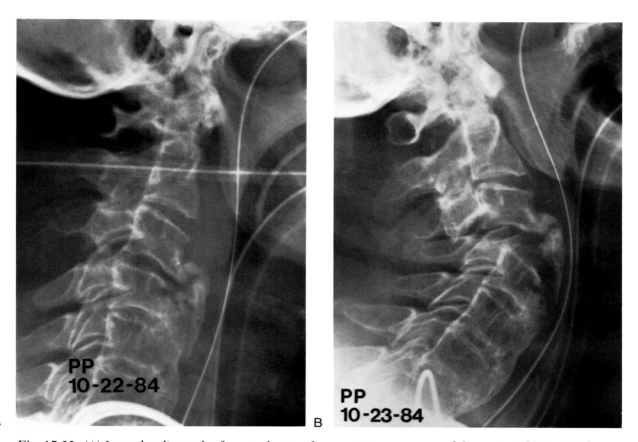

Fig. 15-22. (**A**) Lateral radiograph of cervical spine demonstrating presence of disseminated interstitial spinal hyperostosis. Patient sustained an extension injury resulting in complete neurologic injury at C3–C4. Note diastasis between spinous processes of C3 and C4. (**B**) Another lateral radiograph shows gross three-column instability, revealing diastasis anteriorly at C3–C4 and retrograde position of the upper cervical column above C4.

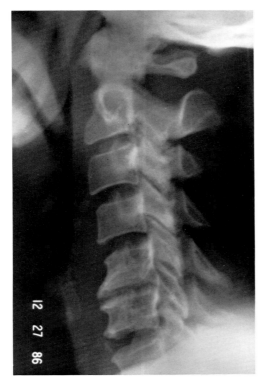

A

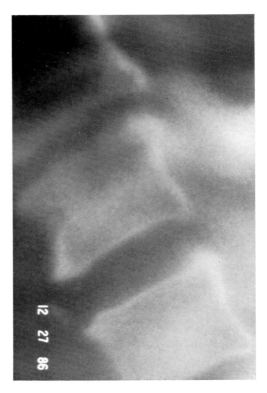

B

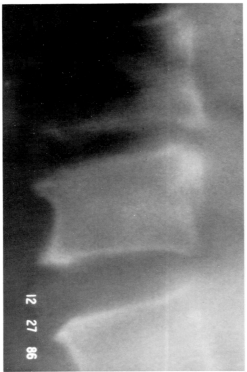

C

Fig. 15-23. (**A**) 45-year-old man with degenerative changes involving the cervical spine at C5–C6. Note fusion of C5 and C6, revealed by ossification of the posterior longitudinal ligament and obliteration of the disc space. Patient sustained hyperextension injury of the cervical spine by falling down the stairs. He had an incomplete central cord neurologic injury at C7. Note anterior widening of disc space C6–C7. (**B**) Lateral flexion tomogram of C6–C7 interspace. (**C**) Lateral extension tomogram. Note widening of C6–C7 interspace.

These spinal injuries require aggressive operative management. Some researchers have suggested conservative management as the alternative. In our experience, the resulting fracture exhibited such instability and extensive displacement, while maintained in traction, that the spine required early stabilization. For the spine fracture to be reduced, the initial spinal deformity required reconstituting. To gain this position, the patient's head and neck deformity was found to be more easily controlled by the insertion of two pairs of Gardner-Wells skeletal tongs. Without first reconstituting the pretrauma position of the cervical spine, appropriate alignment and internal fixation could not be accomplished. Likewise, the early reconstitution of the pre-existing (preinjury) neck deformity provides an opportunity for neurologic recovery, by bringing about an early reduction. This is vitally important in the patient with a neurologically incomplete injury.

In the older patient in whom the spine is restricted owing to disseminated interstitial osseous changes, but less restricted than in the rheumatoid spondylitic, the occurrence of a forceful extension force to the head (and neck) frequently results in an extension injury. We note that this usually occurs at the C6–C7 interspace, with rupture of the anterior logitudinal ligament (Fig. 15-23). If neurologic injury accompanies the spinal injury, it is more likely to be of the incomplete "central cord syndrome" type. While Denis's[13] and Holdsworth's[1] classifications of stable versus unstable injury of the spine were primarily descriptive of injuries involving the thoracolumbar spine, the "column theory" also applies to the cervical spine. Instability exists when any two of the three columns is disrupted.[1,13] Anterior surgery is the approach of choice, though in some cases it may not be possible owing to pre-existing spinal deformity. In these situations, posterior spinal fusion may be required, along with external halo vest stabilization.

The three surgical procedures most frequently utilized for extension injuries to the anterior cervical spine are (1) a one- or two-level anterior AO cervical plate and screw procedure, combined with an interbody tricortical bone graft, after disc excision;[14,15] (2) when fractured and retropulsed, a corporectomy of the involved vertebral body (with inlay bone graft) and anterior plate-screw fixation;

and (3) when a posterior fusion procedure is required, the interspinous process-strut graft (Meyer) technique, with either iliac or tibia donor bone as the graft.

UNILATERAL LAMINAR FRACTURE

Unilateral laminar fracture is the result of an axial load extension injury and is a stable injury. It is usually identified in a patient who has sustained a rollover motor vehicular injury or who has fallen on the apex of the head. While it is recognized that solitary or single-side fractures through a ring are virtually impossible without a fracture through another point, occasionally such appear. Management from the outset is identical to that of other cervical spine injuries: cervical tong traction. When the diagnosis is confirmed and no evidence of neurologic injury or spinal instability (arising from traction or flexion-extension radiographs) is identified, the injury can be managed with a SOMI orthosis, worn continuously for 10 weeks. At the completion of that time period, repeat flexion-extension films are obtained. If no abnormal motion exists, the patient may go unsupported. Follow-up radiographs are obtained at 6 months.

UNUSUAL NEUROLOGIC SYNDROMES ACCOMPANYING INJURY TO THE UPPER CERVICAL SPINE

Much mystique accompanies injuries to the occipitoatlantoaxial area of the cervical vertebral column. In large part this occurs because of the known vulnerability of this area of the spinal column to injury and the potentially devastating consequences that may follow.

Because the spinal cord, as it exits the foramen magnum, is but a downward extension of the cerebral cortex (brain stem), there are injuries to the upper cervical spinal cord that may simultaneously affect and influence brain function. Thus, there are some obscure neurologic syndromes that may arise with injury to the upper cervical spinal cord. While several are discussed in detail in Chapter 7, six are discussed here. Several are directly related to trauma, two are vascular in origin, and one is the involvement of a brain stem "nucleus" with extension into the upper cervical cord, resulting in a central nervous system neurologic finding.

The *sleep apnea* syndrome, known as "Ondine's curse," is the result of high cervical spinal cord-medullary injury. It results in the patient failing to maintain respiration should consciousness be lost, as with sleeping. A conscious effort must be made to breath, otherwise respiration ceases.

Another syndrome that follows injury to the occipitoatlantal area is *coma vigil*. With injury to the proximal spinal cord and reticular activating system, unconsciousness or "light coma" results.

An unusual syndrome occasionally associated with injury to the upper cervical spinal cord is the *locked-in syndrome*. Here, with severe trauma to the brain stem and midbrain (upper pontine), the patient's neurologic injury results in loss of all motor and sensory up to the level of the 3rd cranial nerve. The patient is cortically alert, but able to communicate only by blinking the eyes.

The *Dejerine effect* is produced by the involvement of the trigeminal sensory nucleus, as it extends down through the brain stem to the level of C4. With involvement, there is noted a slow-progressive loss of sensation over the trigeminal (5th) nerve distribution of the face. As involvement, or loss of function, progresses, careful sensory examination will reveal an "onion ring" or laminated loss of sensation in the 5th cranial nerve distribution, going from the periphery toward the center of the face.

The *man-in-the-barrel* syndrome results from a watershed loss of blood supply to the most superior aspect of the motor cortex during a period of hypotension. With hypotension and the loss of blood supply to the area of the motor strip representative of the *shoulder*, the patient will reveal loss of upper extremity (shoulder) muscular function, while the lower extremities continue to function. This disability was found to be present in 32 percent of individuals having severe enough hypotension to cause coma. Most patients die, but some do recover.[16,17]

The last syndrome of importance and relevance to injury to the upper cervical spine is a neurologic injury that follows a slow, progressive onset. Usually a patient with a cervical spine injury demonstrates findings similar to a stroke. Neurologically, the findings may be either unilateral or bilateral. The disability follows occlusion of the vertebral arteries, secondary to changes in head position, severe degenerative arthritis, or rheumatoid arthritic changes at the C1–C2 level[18] or occlusion of the vertebral arteries secondary to dislocation of the cervical spine at some level. The case in point: A patient, 55 years of age, after a dive into shallow water, sustained a bilateral facet dislocation at C3–C4. Because of the appearance of an unusual "hemiplegic" neurologic picture and facial involvement, an angiography was performed. It revealed occlusion of the vertebral arteries at C3–C4 (Fig. 15-24). The dislocation was reduced and stabilized posteriorly. From the vascular standpoint, the patient was managed conservatively.

OCCIPITOATLANTOAXIAL PATHOLOGY

Occipitoatlantal Injuries and Abnormalities

Fractures of the occipitoatlantal junction are very rare.[19] Until 1981, only eight cases had been reported in the world literature. The likely explanation is the rare survival of the patient after such an occurrence. Most patients with similar injuries succumb immediately or within days (Fig. 15-25). Initial management includes very light skeletal traction (2 to 3 lbs), just enough to maintain alignment. While trauma is the primary cause of injury, inflammatory diseases including rheumatoid arthritis, ankylosing spondylitis, and acute tonsillitis have been described as also producing injuries at this level.[20] In the patient with evidence of injury to the area of the occiput, diagnosis is best confirmed by tomography or CAT. Fracture in this area is often associated with unconsciousness and loss of voluntary respiratory function, and often is associated with fractures through the base of the skull, as well as the upper cervical spine (ring of C1 and the odontoid process.[21] Axial load forces that

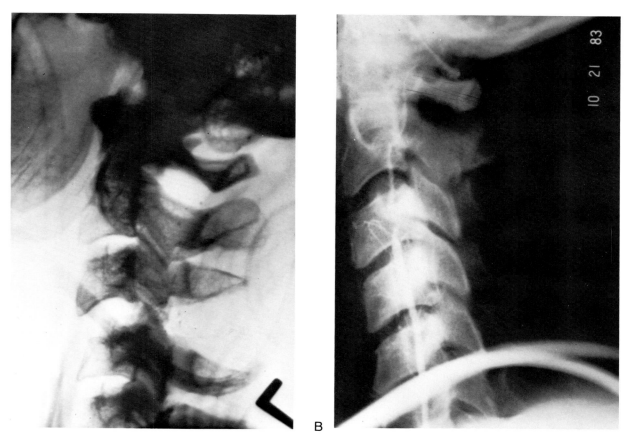

A   B

Fig. 15-24. (A) Lateral subtraction radiograph of cervical spine demonstrating unilateral facet dislocation at C3–C4. Note anterior displacement of the vertebral body of C3 on C4 by 20% and diastasis of interspinous space C3–C4. (B) The patient showed mild hemiplegic symptoms upon admission. Immediate postreduction vascular study demonstrates vertebral artery injury adjacent to the C3–C4 unilateral facet dislocation.

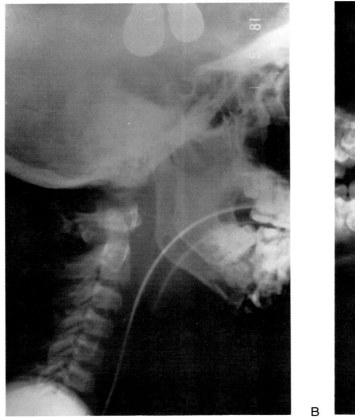

A

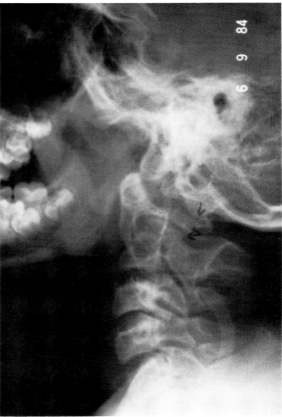

B

Fig. 15-25. (A) Lateral cervical spine radiograph of an 11-year-old child struck by a motor vehicle while crossing a street. The child was rendered immediately quadriplegic and apneic with altered consciousness (brain stem-spinal cord junction injury). Mouth-to-mouth resuscitation at the scene of accident saved the patient's life. Lateral radiograph on admission to the emergency department revealed occiput-C1 dislocation. Radiograph also demonstrates a fractured mandible. Note marked diastasis of the occiput-C1 interspace. The child died 24 hours after injury. (B) Lateral cervical spine radiograph in another child struck by a motor vehicle. The patient sustained extension injury to the head and neck, resulting in fracture of the posterior elements of C1 and C2 (hangman's fracture). Neurological examination revealed normal motor and sensory function.

result in injury at the occipitoatlantal junction produce compression fractures of the condyle. Although the diagnosis may be difficult to identify on standard radiographs, the presence of a localized extradural and suboccipital hematoma should alert the examiner to the presence of the injury. In a reported case, injury to the hypoglossal (12th cranial) nerve resulted from a fracture through the base of the skull that also involved the occipitoatlantal joint. Recovery in three of our eight cases occurred, using only conservative management.[10]

Ring Fractures of C1: The "Jefferson Fracture"

Burst fractures of the ring of C1 result from axial loading of the head, followed by a downward thrust of the calvaria, by way of the occipital condyles, to the lateral masses of the atlas. The result is a spreading of the lateral masses of C1, with fracture through either the arch anteriorly or the ring posteriorly. The extent of the lateral displacement of the lateral masses of C1 is variable (Fig. 15-26). A

Fig. 15-26. (A–C) Three CAT scans showing variations in axial load injuries to the cervical spine resulting in varied fractures to the C1 ring (Jefferson fracture). Figs. A and B show unilateral double ring fractures with associated disruption of the transverse ligament. Fig. C shows anterior ring fracture resulting from hyperextension injury. (*Figure continues.*)

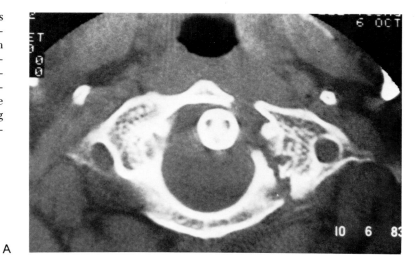

A

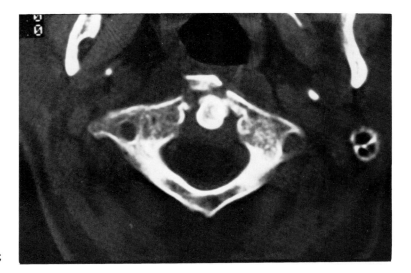

B

C

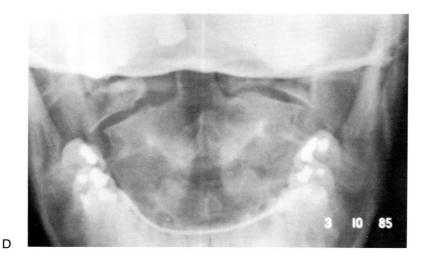

Fig. 15-26 *(Continued)*. **(D)** AP cervical spine radiograph revealing unilateral widening of the C1 (lateral mass) odontoid space and lateral displacement of the lateral mass of C1 on C2. The increased width of the C1 left lateral mass generally indicates malrotation at the C1–C2 interspace.

spread or lateral displacement of one of the lateral masses of C1 as much as 7 mm indicates rupture of the transverse ligament. The presence of this pathology contributes to further instability between the atlas and the axis (dens), allowing for anterior translation of the atlas on the axis (C1 on C2).[22] Management of fractures of C1 is normally conservative, traction followed by a halo vest.

A review of our cervical spine series revealed that Jefferson fractures were found in 15 patients (1 percent) of the 1,484 patients with cervical spine fractures. Neurologic injury occurred in four patients, two with complete neurologic injuries (13 percent) and two with incomplete injuries. Eleven were intact (73 percent) (Table 15-1).

The most effective means of providing immobilization is with the halo vest, though a lesser device may be used on occasions. When instability is identifiable, posterior arthrodesis between the occiput and C1 or C2 may be indicated[3,4] (see p. 484).

Complications Resulting from Atlas (C1) Fractures

Although rare, cranial nerve palsies have also been reported as complicating fractures of the ring of C1 (the Jefferson fracture). They included the 6th (abducens nerve), the 11th (spinal accessory nerve), the 9th (glossopharyngeal nerve), the 10th (vagus nerve), and the 12th (hypoglossal nerve) cranial nerves. The 9th, 10th, and 12th cranial nerves can simultaneously be injured in the following manner. Although the nerves do not exit the calvaria together, they pass over the lateral transverse process of the atlas together, lying medial to the styloid process of the occiput. With a downward or axial load on the head, and bursting of the ring of the atlas (C1), lateral displacement of a C1 lateral mass may result in entrapment or pinching of the three nerves.[22]

A not infrequent anomaly found to occur at the proximal end of the cervical vertebral column is failure of segmentation between the occiput and C1. The result is the presence of a congenital fusion between these structures. Disability is usually minimal. Gunther reported the occurrence of a fusion or failure in segmentation between the occiput, the atlas, and the dens of C2.[25] No other bony or soft tissue defect accompanied this finding. The resulting pathology included a decrease in the available range of rotary motion, neck pain, and abnormal motion between C1, the fused odontoid, and the body of C2. Radiographs of the deformity revealed what appeared to be a lack of continuity between the odontoid and the body of C2 (a congenital nonunion), through which some motion occurred.

Table 15-1.   Cervical Fractures: Fracture Type by Extent (Northwestern University Acute Spine Injury Center, 1972 to 1986)

Fracture Type	Total No.	Intact No.	Intact Percent	Incomplete No.	Incomplete Percent	Complete No.	Complete Percent	Unknown[a] No.	Unknown[a] Percent
Body	359	41	11.4	149	41.5	166	46.2	3	0.8
Axis body compression-burst fracture	185	32	17.3	79	42.7	73	39.5	1	0.5
Subluxation	97	29	29.9	49	50.5	17	17.5	2	2.1
Body compression	87	11	12.6	46	52.9	28	32.2	2	2.3
Bilateral facet lock and dislocation	77	6	7.8	35	45.4	36	46.8	0	0.0
Facet fixation	77	22	28.6	42	54.5	13	16.9	0	0.0
Unilateral facet lock	69	18	26.1	27	39.1	21	30.4	3	4.3
Type II odontoid	56	39	69.6	11	19.6	5	8.9	1	1.8
Bullet fragments	54	3	5.6	14	25.9	37	68.5	0	0.0
Hangman's fracture	41	33	80.5	5	12.2	2	4.9	1	2.4
Avulsed chip	39	15	38.5	15	38.5	8	20.5	1	2.6
Spinous process	34	17	50.0	12	35.3	5	14.7	0	0.0
Lamina	34	10	29.4	18	52.9	6	17.6	0	0.0
Pedicle	19	5	26.3	13	68.4	1	5.3	0	0.0
Posterior ligament disruption	19	6	31.6	5	26.3	8	42.1	0	0.0
Jefferson	15	11	73.3	2	13.3	2	13.3	0	0.0
Type III odontoid	15	11	73.3	3	20.0	1	6.7	0	0.0
Type I odontoid	10	7	70.0	2	20.0	1	10.0	0	0.0
Spondylolisthesis	8	1	12.5	7	87.5	0	0.0	0	0.0
Bilateral lamina	7	3	42.9	3	42.9	1	14.3	0	0.0
Anterior ligament disruption	5	1	20.0	3	60.0	1	20.0	0	0.0
Atlantoaxial subluxation	2	0	0.0	0	0.0	1	50.0	1	50.0
Transverse process	2	2	100.0	0	0.0	0	0.0	0	0.0
Bilateral pedicle	1	0	0.0	0	0.0	1	100.0	0	0.0
Other	62	23	37.1	31	50.0	6	9.7	2	3.2
None	110	3	2.7	66	60.0	38	34.5	3	2.7
Total	1484	349	23.5	637	42.9	478	32.2	20	1.3

[a] Extent is unavailable.

An unusual injury reported as having followed head trauma was a fracture of the posterior ring of the atlas, with intrapment of a segment of the posterior ring within the foramen magnum.[26] Neurologic symptoms (dysarthria and a left hemiplegia) were thought to have resulted from the head injury and were unchanged by the evacuation of a subdural hematoma. The resulting spinal deformity included the onset of upper cervical spinal lordosis, a cervicothoracic spinal kyphosis, a 20-degree fixed rotation to the right, and limitation in rotation to either side. Day et al. have also reported an untreated Jefferson fracture with associated neurologic symptoms resulting from basilar impression secondary to unilateral displacement of one C1 lateral articular mass.[27]

Transverse Ligament Injuries Involving the Atlas (C1)

The etiology of instability at the atlantoaxial (C1–C2) level, as found in the rheumatoid arthritis victim, results from (1) dissolution of the odontoid process by the highly vascularized pannus (or synovial granulation tissue) commonly found between the articulation of the dens and the anterior arch of C1 (Figs. 15-27, 15-28) and (2) the elasticizing effect of granulation tissue when in close proximity to the cruciate and transverse ligaments responsible for the stability between the odontoid process and the arch of C1. (3) Instability between the occiput and C1, and between C2 and C3, before the advent of antibiotic therapy or in the absence

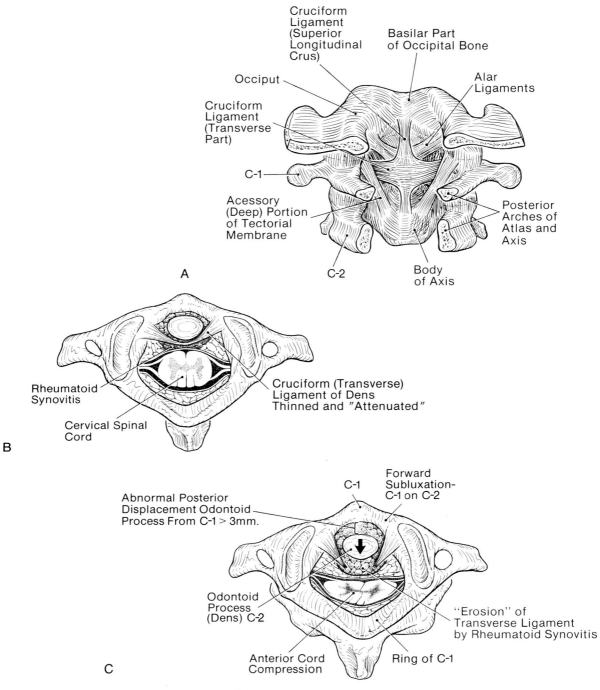

Fig. 15-27. (**A**) Ligamentous anatomy of the occiput C1–C2 articulation. (**B,C**) Mechanism of anterior cord compression as a result of rheumatoid synovitis and anterior subluxation of C1 on C2.

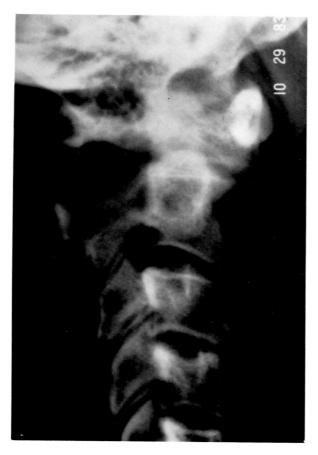

Fig. 15-28. Lateral radiograph of cervical spine demonstrating 5 mm displacement between odontoid process and ring of C1. This pattern indicates disruption of the transverse ligament and atlantoaxial instability.

Displacement of 5 mm or greater is definite evidence of disruption of the transverse ligament and indicates atlantoaxial instability. Fielding noted that often patients reveal significant injury at the C1 – C2 level, not by pain, but by neurologic symptoms. He also found that this same group of patients had greater instability (7.5 mm average) than those having no neurologic symptoms, and only pain (average, 6.5 mm of motion). *All patients having more than 5 mm of motion between the odontoid and the arch of C1 require surgical fusion.* Fusion of C1 to C2 has been found to result in 50 percent loss of rotation in the elderly and 20 percent loss of rotation in the younger patient. Other motions of the cervical spine were unaffected.

Rotary Fixation Injuries: Atlantoaxial Joint

A problem known to follow rotary trauma to the upper cervical spine is that of unilateral subluxation or dislocation of a lateral mass of C1 from its articulation with the lateral mass of C2. In a series of 17 patients, as reported by Fielding, the injury frequently had gone unrecognized, resulting in the disability being fixed or unreducible.[31] The resultant was a permanent torticollis involving the head-neck relationship, a flattening of one side of the face (in younger patients), and pain with any attempt at neck motion.

While the diagnosis is suggestive on plain radiographs, distortion in the bony anatomy can be confirmed on tomography (Fig. 15-29). Also of benefit, when asymmetry exists between the odontoid process and the lateral articular masses of the atlas, are 15-degree right and left "open mouth" views. Likewise, because of the tilt of the atlas on the anteroposterior view, owing to the absence of proper articulation of the articular masses (of C1 with C2), the two halves of the posterior arch will not be superimposed on each other. Although Fielding has effectively utilized cineradiography to study the pathology of this injury, this study has been essentially replaced by the use of CAT. Care must be taken not to confuse the CAT scan appearance of a type II odontoid fracture with that of a rotary subluxation at the atlantoaxial joint (Fig. 15-30).

Management can usually be conservative if the

thereof, frequently resulted from inflammatory involvement of the localized tissues after mastoiditis or acute retropharyngeal infections associated with tonsilitis.[28,29] All three processes result in bursal and facet joint (capsular) instability.

Injury to the primary restraining ligament, the transverse ligament, which extends between the lateral masses of the atlas (C1) and the posterior surface of the odontoid process, has always been a matter of concern. The question that exists is, what constitutes normal motion (in millimeters) between the anterior border of the odontoid process and the posterior surface of the arch of C1, with flexion and extension of the head and neck? Fielding et al. report this to be between 3 and 5 mm.[30]

patient is seen within days of the initial injury. The clinical picture will be a child with a vague history of trauma, a persistent torticollis of the head and neck, and a complaint of pain at the base of the skull. The patient should be placed in Gardner-Wells skeletal tong traction, on a Stryker wedge frame. The amount of weight normally required is 10 to 15 lbs initially, followed by maintenance in 5 lbs of traction once a reduction is obtained. The patient may require a sedative medication to facilitate the beneficial effects of traction. Because of the smallness of the child's frame, it is helpful to elevate the head of the frame, so that the child's body weight counteracts the traction weights. Reduction is normally gained within the initial 24 hours. The patient will often report that a reduction has occurred, by noting an audible or palpable pop, followed by the disappearance of all cervical spine pain. The reduction is confirmed by repeat CAT scan or tomograms. If a reduction has occurred, we suggest conservative management, with the child maintained in continued cervical traction for 1 to 2 weeks, followed by halo vest stabilization for 8 to 10 weeks. Should redislocation occur during therapy, a reduction should again be attempted utilizing traction, followed by a C1–C2 fusion. The techniques utilized by us include the Meyer posterior C1-C2 procedure (Fig. 15-30), and the Gallie procedure[31,32] (see p. 484).

If the patient on initial presentation is found to have evidence of a long-standing atlantoaxial subluxation or dislocation (months), surgical stabilization is recommended. The patient should be placed in cervical tong traction, and an attempt should be made to gain a reduction. Should this fail, the presence of linear traction before and during the performance of the procedure provides added spine stability during patient transfer on the operative frame. We strongly suggest that a Stryker wedge frame be utilized whenever a patient requires prone turning for a posterior spine procedure.

Fractures of the Odontoid Process of the Axis (C2)

Probably the most written about fractures of the spine, and certainly of the cervical spine, are frac-

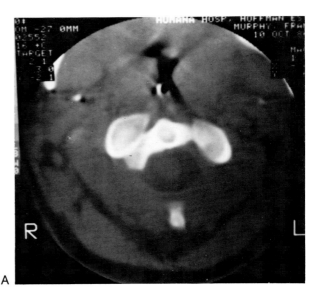

Fig. 15-29. (A) Tomogram of cervical spine demonstrating rotary subluxation-fixation involving the C1–C2 interspace. Radiograph reveals no evidence of fracture. This patient sustained multiple trauma requiring operative intervention for removal of brake pedal impaled through left thigh. Cervical spine reduction was achieved by Gardner-Wells traction. Cervical traction was maintained 4 weeks, followed by a SOMI orthosis 6 weeks. *(Figure continues.)*

tures of the odontoid process of the axis. The reasons are numerous: the perceived (and with some justification) vulnerability of the cervical spine to injury, the upper cervical spine's flexibility, and, the most obvious, the close proximity of the spinal cord to the bony elements. Many questions concerning the likelihood of nonunion and its etiology exist. Is it caused by motion at the fracture site or is it vascular in origin? The latter possibility can be put to rest, for an excellent arc of vessels encircles the odontoid process at its most proximal end. Nonunion, on the other hand, can be a problem (see Classification and Mechanism of Injury — Odontoid Process: C2, below). The ultimate questions that exist in the minds of most treating physicians are, what is the most appropriate management scheme, and when is surgery indicated?

For rheumatoid arthritis or unstable, nonunited fractures of the odontoid process (normally type II, occasionally type III), a variable occurrence of as-

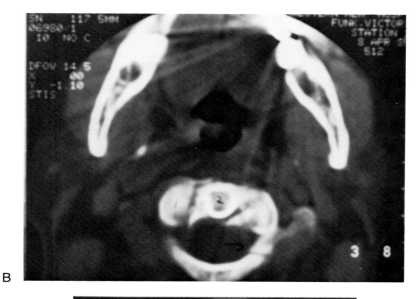

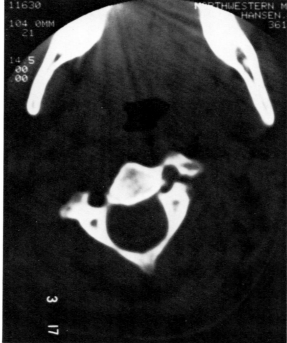

Fig. 15-29 *(Continued).* **(B)** CAT scan of a type III fracture of the odontoid involving vertebral body C2. Note suggestion of fracture through posterior ring C1. Patient was managed conservatively in Gardner-Wells traction followed by halo vest immobilization for 3 months. **(C)** CAT scan of bipedicle fracture involving the posterior elements of C2 (hangman's fracture). Fracture was reduced by Gardner-Wells skeletal traction for 4 weeks and SOMI orthosis for 8 weeks.

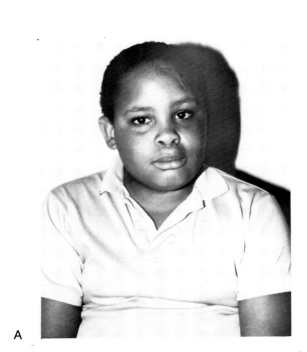

A

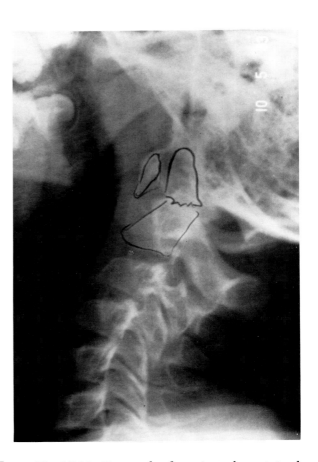

B

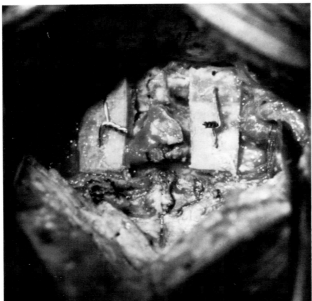

C

Fig. 15-30. Case study of a patient who sustained a fracture through the base of the odontoid and C2 (type II). The patient was transferred to the Spine Center six weeks after injury with a diagnosis of rotary subluxation of C1 on C2. **(A)** Clinical photograph of patient showing malrotation of the head. The patient's chin is displaced to the left and the head is angled to the right. Both suggest rotary subluxation (or unilateral facet dislocation). Note healed laceration over forehead. **(B)** Lateral radiograph demonstrating type II fracture through the base of the odontoid. **(C)** Operative view showing sublaminar wiring (Garber-Meyer fusion) of C1–C2 using posterior iliac bone graft. Occiput is toward top. *(Figure continues.)*

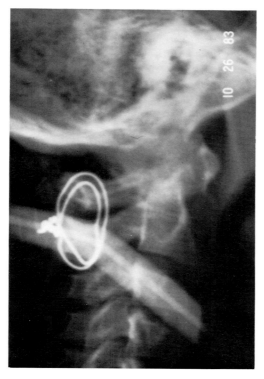

D

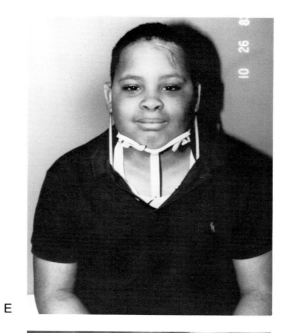

E

Fig. 15-30 *(Continued).* (**D**) Postoperative lateral radiograph showing improved alignment of odontoid process within body of C2. Note sublaminar wire-bone graft fixation of C1 and C2. The patient was managed postoperatively in a SOMI orthosis. (**E**) Postoperative photograph showing improved alignment of the head and neck. (**F**) Lateral radiograph 3 years after posterior fusion. Note intact wires on C1–C2, healing of odontoid process, and fusion of the posterior processes C1 and C2.

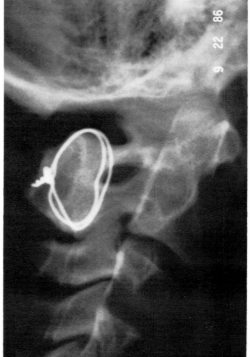

F

sociated neurologic involvement may arise. Fielding and Griffin noted an occurrence of neurologic involvement in approximately 33 percent with os odontoideum identified radiographically.[33] Anderson and D'Alonzo in 1974 noted a neurologic occurrence rate of 25 percent with type II and III fractures.[34] Osgood and Lund reported a death occurrence rate of 18.18 percent of patients sustaining fractures of the odontoid process.[35]

The fracture classification proposed by Anderson and D'Alonzo in 1974 for the evaluation and management of fractures of the dens process of C2[34] is still the most accepted and is utilized as the basis for management recommendations proposed by Bohler,[36] Brooks and Jenkins,[37] Fielding,[38] Ryan and Taylor,[39] Roy-Camille et al.,[40] and others.[41-43]

Classification and Mechanism of Injury — Odontoid Process: C2

Injury (type I, II, III) to the odontoid process of the axis (or dens) results from forces arriving at the head-neck interface from varying directions (Fig.

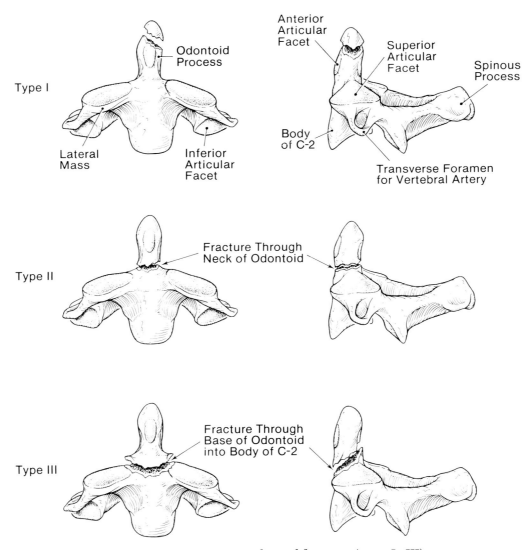

Fig. 15-31. Variations in odontoid fractures (types I–III).

15-31). Mouradian et al. proposed that fractures occurring through the base (type III) of the odontoid (and extending into the body, and probably representing a body fracture) are probably the result of flexion injuries and that fractures through the waist of the odontoid (type II) are the result of lateral forces applied to the head.[44] The latter injury results in loading of the odontoid against the lateral mass of C1, shearing off the body of the axis. The etiology of the infrequent fracture to the tip of the odontoid (type I) is thought to be the result of ligamentous avulsion.[34] When present, type I fractures are considered stable because the superior "apical" ligament and the two oblique "alar" ligaments, which attach to the tip of the odontoid, hold the fragments in place (see Fig. 15-27). A diagnostic observation that allows differentiation between ligamentous instability and trauma, seen on lateral radiographs (a fracture of the odontoid), is widening of the cervicolaryngeal space between the posterior wall of the larynx and the upper corner of the third cervical vertebra.[23,24] This space should not exceed 5 mm in the normal neck.

The incidence of odontoid fractures as reported by Ryan and Taylor[39] is between 7 and 14 percent. In our series of 1,484 cervical spine fractures, 81 (6 percent) odontoid fractures were diagnosed. Ten (12 percent) were type I, 56 (69 percent) were type II, and 15 (19 percent) were type III. Surgical stabilization was undertaken in 40 percent (4 patients) with type I fractures, 36 percent (20 patients) with type II fractures, and 27 percent (4 patients) with type III fractures. The combined incidence of surgical fixation in this series of odontoid fractures was 38 percent or 28 of 81 patients (Tables 15-1 and 15-2; Fig. 15-32).

Nonunion is the principal concern with fractures of the odontoid process. There are varying opinions as to the importance of blood supply to the proximal fragment. Schatzker and colleagues believe that it has no effect, rather that it is more likely related to the anatomic finding that fractures across the waist of the odontoid process are held distracted and away from the body of C2 by the apical and alar ligaments superiorly and, across the waist, by the thickened and posteriorly located transverse ligament (attached laterally on both sides to the medial aspect of the lateral mass of the atlas.[45] Anteriorly, two other ligaments, the accessory ligaments, are attached at the waist. These also attach laterally to the lateral mass of the atlas (C1). Consequently, when a fracture of the odontoid process occurs at the base, each of the above ligaments suspends the process, maintaining a fixed "unit" between the calvaria, the atlas, and the odontoid process. With articular motion through the facet joints of C1 and C2, a twisting motion is continually transmitted to the odontoid process, resulting in a rotary displacement and nonunion.[39]

Anderson and D'Alonzo reported no failures in union in type I fractures, a 63.7 percent primary healing rate in type II fractures, and a 92.3 percent healing rate in type III fractures.[34] Roberts and Wickstrom in 1972 reported a nonunion rate of 20 percent,[46] and Schatzker et al. (1975) reported a nonunion rate of 62 percent.[45] Ryan and Taylor in 1982 reported no nonunions in type I fractures, 77.8 percent unions in type II fractures, and no nonunions in type III fractures.[39] Similarly, Ackerson et al. in 1982 reported a union rate of 70 percent.[42] In 1983, Bell and Meyer reported the conservative management of 31 consecutive type II

Table 15-2.   Upper Cervical Surgery Sites: Fracture Type by Surgery Site (Northwestern University Acute Spine Injury Center, 1972 to 1986)

Fracture Type	Surgery Site						Total
	C1–C2	C1–C3	C1–C4	C1–C5	C2–C3	C3–C7	
Type I odontoid	4	0	0	0	0	0	4
Type II odontoid	17	2	1	0	0	0	20
Type III odontoid	2	0	0	1	0	1	4
Hangman's	0	3	1	0	1	0	5
Total	23	5	2	1	1	1	33

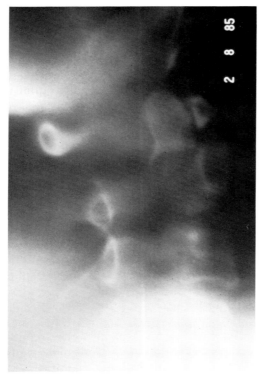

A

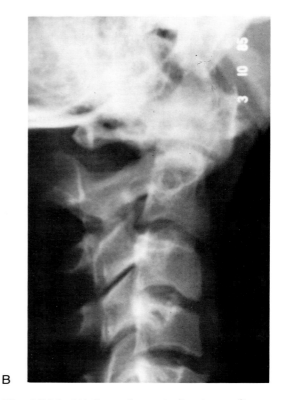

B

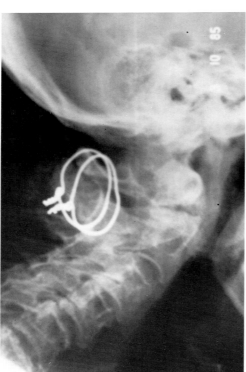

C

Fig. 15-32. (A) Lateral cervical spine radiograph showing a type II extension fracture of the odontoid with posterior displacement into the upper cervical canal at C2. Note the posterior oblique fracture fragment extending distally from the odontoid process. The location of this fragment indicates a fracture through the posterior superior aspect of the C2 vertebral body (in extension). (B) Lateral radiograph of a different patient showing reduction of a type III odontoid fracture in Gardner-Wells cervical traction. (C) Because of instability, signalled by frequent loss of position, the odontoid fractures seen in Figs. A and B, although they may be maintained in alignment by cervical traction, usually require posterior cervical fusion. (C) Posterior stabilization of the case shown in Fig. B shows maintenance of fracture reduction along the posterior border of C2, with extension of the fracture anteriorly resulting from the lordosis produced by posterior stabilization.

and type III odontoid fractures.[47] One death occurred (from pulmonary complications in an elderly patient on a ventilator while in traction) (3 percent); one nonunion occurred (in an elderly patient who died 7 months after trauma while on a ventilator) (3 percent); and 29 (94 percent) healed with Gardner-Wells skeletal traction for 4 to 6 weeks, followed by SOMI orthosis immobilization for 3 months.

Management of these fractures is, in most instances, conservative (halo vest). In most series, type II fractures most often required surgical stabilization. Fixation can normally be achieved by a C1–C2 fusion. The occiput may require inclusion when there is a fracture of the posterior element or a congenital deficiency in the ring of the atlas (C1).[14] Usually, inclusion of the spinous process of C3 is not necessary, unless there is a fracture involving the posterior process of the second cervical vertebra[34] (Table 15-2).

Deformities Involving the Odontoid Process of the Axis—Aplasia, Hypoplasia, Os Odontoideum: C2

Opinions differ as to whether the occasional deformity involving the upper two-thirds of the odontoid process is developmental or acquired. Fielding and Griffin make a qualified point that were the os odontoideum to be a congenital or developmental deformity, one would anticipate finding abnormalities in the development of the body of the axis as well.[33] The rationale for this is that the odontoid process of the axis arises from a union of the mesenchymal cells derived from the fourth cranial sclerotome and the first cervical sclerotome, and through the intricacies of segmentation at this level (see Ch. 3), the fourth cranial and the first cervical sclerotomes unite, migrate, and separate from the ring of C1 and unite with the body of C2. Thus, were the missing midportion segment of the odontoid process congenital, the body of C2 should also appear abnormal.

Aplasia. Aplasia is very rare, almost nonexistent, though congenital variations in the occipital-C1–C2 region of the cervical spine have been reported.[25] For such to be present, when involving

the odontoid process, it should also include that portion of the odontoid process that contributes to the upper part of the body of C2. Abnormalities in this region are usually confused with hypoplasia.

Hypoplasia. Hypoplasia of the odontoid process can be suspected when the radiographic finding of a partially developed odontoid exists. The "stump" of the odontoid will be very short and peglike. Variations exist from stump size to an almost normal size odontoid.

Nonunion of a fracture through the odontoid process: os odontoideum. There is no clear or differential picture between an os odontoideum and a traumatically induced fracture with nonunion. In the presence of a nonunion, however, there is usually a narrow fracture line separating the upper and lower segments, and the line is found at the base of the odontoid. Also, in the more clear-cut post-traumatic odontoid process fracture, the normal shape of the process is preserved.

An os odontoideum is a rounded ossicle, having a uniform cortex, and usually widely separated from the base of the odontoid. The ossicle appears in the same position that the tip of the odontoid process would and, during flexion and extension, moves with the arch of C1. This implies an attachment to the posterior arch of the atlas. Indeed, the alar ligament, as dissected by Fielding,[33] was found to attach to the occipital condyles. With the occurrence of this anatomic variant, that is, the os odontoideum, it is noted that the base of the odontoid is hypoplastic and extends upward only to the level of the superior facet of C2; the posterior ring of C1 is small; and the canal is narrow. Thus, the chances of a patient with this disability sustaining neurologic injury are greater than when the posterior ring of C1 is normal. Likewise, the amount of subluxation between C1 and C2, sometimes as much as 1 cm, is indicative of instability and is likely to result in neurologic injury were abnormal forces to be applied across the C1–C2 junction.

Because the canal is likely to be narrow, concern for the passage of wires into the sublaminar space must be taken into consideration (Fig. 15-33) (see Sublaminar Wire Stabilization, below). The techniques that we have used for fusion of the atlantoaxial junction include the Gallie technique,[32] the Garber-Meyer technique,[23] the Brooks procedure,[37] and the modified Brooks procedure.[48]

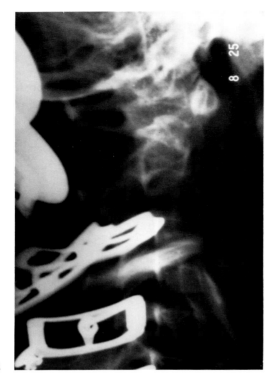

A

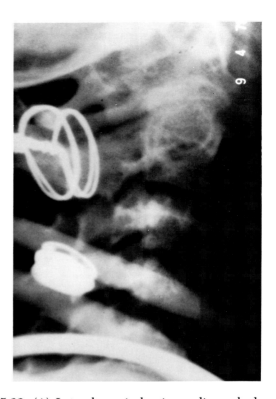

B

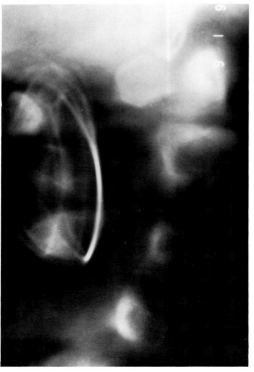

C

Fig. 15-33. (A) Lateral cervical spine radiograph demonstrating a defect through the waist of the odontoid process (either an os odontoideum or nonunion of a previous fracture). (B) Because of instability at C1–C2, a posterior sublaminar spine fusion of C1–C2 was undertaken. The width of the neural canal (posterior border of vertebral body to anterior cortex posterior element) must be taken into consideration before inserting sublaminar wires. When the preoperative canal is anatomically narrow, alternative methods of immobilization and stabilization must be considered. (C) Lateral radiograph showing an os odontoideum. The adequacy of the neural canal at the level of C1 may be seen. Note that the placement of the sublaminar wires (posteriorly and laterally) appears to compromise the neural canal space. Note also the sublaminar wires spanning C1–C3. Intraoperative radiographs must be obtained to ensure that the spinal canal (and spinal cord) are not compromised. SSEP is also highly recommended during placement of sublaminar wires.

NEURAL ARCH FRACTURES OF THE AXIS: HANGMAN'S FRACTURE

First described by Wood-Jones in 1913[49] and later named (and described by Schneider et al.) in 1965,[50] the "hangman's fracture" describes a group of fractures that involve the posterior architecture of C2 and occur as a result of an extension injury to the cervical spine. The mechanism of injury is thought to be the result of a sudden extension of the head and neck, which in turn results in the calvaria forcefully abutting against the poste-rior element of C1 and in turn C2. Because of the close approximation of the posterior elements of C2 and C3, a leverage effect fracture involving the C2 posterior element occurs. It is also presupposed that in many instances, a component of axial load contributes to the fracturing of the posterior elements. Because, in some instances, marked anterior displacement of the C2 vertebral body occurs (type III hangman's fracture), some investigators have postulated that a flexion-axial load mechanical component is implicated.[51] Francis and co-workers suggest that the etiology of the anterior body displacement is hyperextension.[52] Interest-

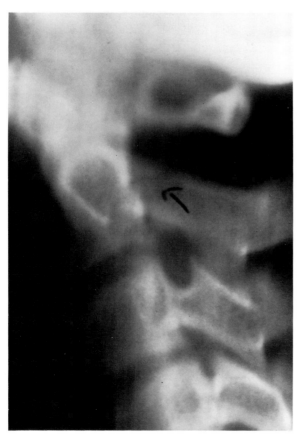

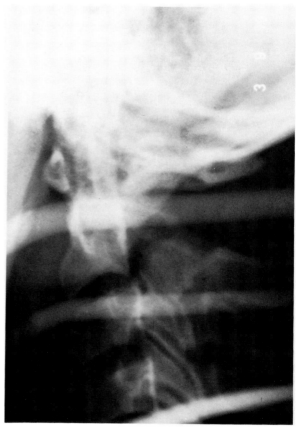

A   B

Fig. 15-34. (A) Lateral cervical spine radiograph demonstrating a nondisplaced fracture through the pedicle, posterior lamina, and posterior vertebral body of C2. The fracture was stable, and was managed conservatively by cervical traction and a SOMI orthosis. (B) Lateral cervical spine radiograph demonstrating a fracture through the pedicle and posterior lamina of C2 (hangman's fracture). Note that patient is managed in a cervical SOMI orthosis. The fracture is considered stable on the basis of follow-up radiographs. *(Figure continues.)*

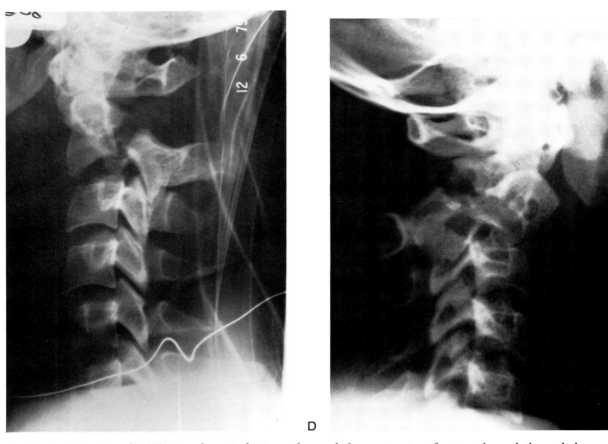

C   D

Fig. 15-34 *(Continued).* (C) Lateral cervical spine radiograph demonstrating a fracture through the pedicle, lamina, and posterior vertebral body of C2 (hangman's fracture) with a comminuted fracture of the posterior body of C2 and evidence of disruption of the posterior longitudinal ligament at C2–C3. Note intact facet joints. The fracture was considered stable, and neurologic status was normal. The patient was managed in Gardner-Wells traction for 4 weeks followed by a halo vest. (D) Lateral cervical spine radiograph demonstrating a fracture through the pedicle and posterior element of C2 (hangman's fracture) with acute angulation of the C2 vertebral body on C3. The latter defect indicates disruption of the posterior longitudinal ligament. The facet joints are intact, and neurologic status was normal. The patient was managed conservatively.

ingly, many variations of injury to the posterior elements of C2 occur (Fig. 15-34). In our series of 1,484 cervical spine injuries (1972 to 1986), 41 (type I to III) hangman's fractures (12 percent) occurred. Two patients with fractures (type III) revealed complete neurologic injury (4.9 percent), 5 patients had incomplete injury (12.2 percent), and 33 patients were intact neurologically (81 percent) (Table 15-1).

C2 posterior element fractures vary greatly. Some injuries involve only the lamina posteriorly,

whereas others involve various areas, including the anterior and middle segments.[1,13] The classification as described by Levine and Edwards[51] follows.

Grade I is a bilateral pedicle fracture, in which the fracture line lies anterior to the facet joints and results in a separation between the anteriorly located vertebral body of C2 and the posterior neural arch complex, including the facet-lamina and posterior spinous process segments. Although this injury appears ominous, it is not. The separation between the two components often measures 1 to 3 mm, but when flexion and extension radiographs are obtained, little if any abnormal motion at the fracture site occurs. Management of this fracture type, by most clinicians, is conservative: SOMI or a halo vest fixation is all that is required. An optional method favored by us of managing this fracture, particularly in the elderly patient, is the maintenance of the patient in skeletal (tong) traction for 4 to 6 weeks, followed by immobilization in a SOMI orthosis for a total of 3 months.[47,51,52]

Grade II hangman's fracture, as described by Effendi et al.,[53] occurs when both angulation and displacement are present. Though the anterior logitudinal ligament remains intact, because the displacement often exceeds the criteria established by White and Panjabi[54] (3-mm anterior body displacement, or 11 degrees of angulation), this injury type is thought to be unstable. Disruption of the posterior longitudinal ligament between C2 and C3 frequently is present and, on occasion, is associated with an avulsion fracture of the posteroinferior vertebral body of C2 (avulsed by the posterior longitudinal ligament) (Fig. 15-35). Reduction of the displaced components is usually accomplished by cervical traction alone (10 to 20 lbs). In some instances, posterior stabilization between C1 and C3 may be required. Most often, the injury can be managed by orthosis alone for a minimum of 3 months.[51-53]

Grade III hangman's fractures are grossly unstable injuries. The fracture line through the posterior segment of the vertebra varies. More often in this case, the fracture lies posterior to the facet rather than anterior (as in the grade I fracture) and will be accompanied by disruption of both the anterior and posterior longitudinal ligaments at the C2–C3 level, occurring as a result of either facet dislocation or C2 vertebral body dislocation. For the latter to occur, disruption of the anulus fibrosus and the disc must also have occurred. Thus, this C2 injury has three components: fracture of the pedicles or lamina, subluxation or dislocation of the facets, and disruption of the anterior and posterior longitudinal ligaments resulting in significant C2 vertebral body subluxation or dislocation (Fig. 15-36). Surgical management of the grade III hangman's fracture, when required, is to reduce the free segment containing the unreducible facet joints.

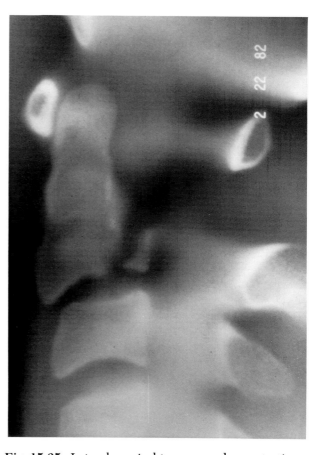

Fig. 15-35. Lateral cervical tomogram demonstrating a hangman's fracture involving the posterior element of C2 (poorly identified on this film). This film demonstrates the primary mechanism of injury to be flexion, resulting in avulsion fracture of the posteroinferior C2 vertebral body. The posterior longitudinal ligament is intact between fracture fragment C2 and C3.

The surgical procedure most often utilized is the straight posterior approach, with reduction of the facets under direct vision, followed by a stabilization procedure extending from C1 to C3. As noted, of the 41 hangman's fractures in our series, 5 (12 percent) required fusion: three between C1 and C3, one C2–C3, and one incorporating a lower level for an associated cervical spine fracture. The type of procedure most often utilized was the sublaminar wire-strut graft (Meyer) technique. Fardon and Fielding[55] and Francis et al.[52] have discussed

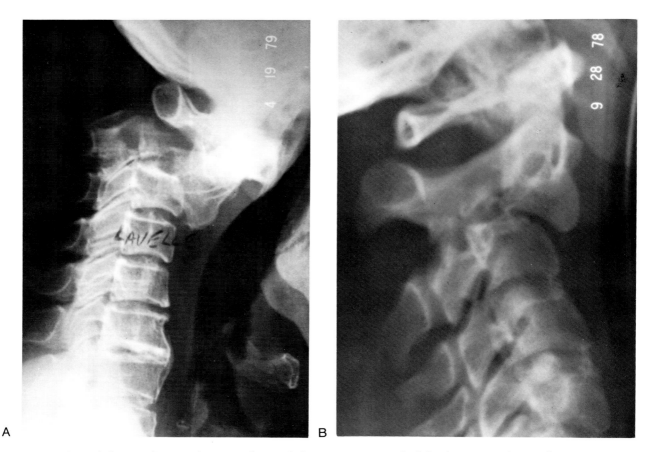

A   B

Fig. 15-36. (A) Lateral cervical spine radiograph demonstrating marked displacement of C1 and C2 vertebral bodies resulting from a fracture through the pedicle and posterior elements at C2 (hangman's fracture). The mechanism of injury was flexion. The patient had temporary loss of voluntary ventilation and neurologic function. Normal neurologic function and ventilation returned upon reduction of fracture. **(B)** Lateral radiograph of cervical spine demonstrating a type III flexion-induced fracture dislocation of C2–C3. Note dislocation of facet joints and fracture fragments along with 50% displacement of C2 and C3. While this radiograph does not demonstrate a hangman's fracture, it shows an acute displacement of the C2 vertebral body on C3, as seen in Figure 15-36A.

the use of an anterior approach at the C2–C3 interspace to maintain rotary motion at the C1–C2 level. Other posterior techniques are available and discussed below (see Posterior Surgical Fusion Techniques: Occiput, C1, and C2, below).

When traction reduction of a dislocation between C2 and C3 (hangman's dislocation) is successful, orthotic management, usually a halo vest, is recommended for 3 months.

FACTORS INFLUENCING MANAGEMENT OF CERVICAL SPINE INJURIES

Seven percent of cervical spine-injured patients sustained a neurologic injury (34 percent complete; 63 percent incomplete) in the absence of a recognized fracture. This finding indicates or suggests the presence of a pure soft tissue (interspinous ligament) disruption-type injury or a crushing pinch injury to the spinal cord between posterior vertebral elements (osteophytes, lamina) resulting in spinal cord hemorrhage, avascularity, or discontinuity (either anatomic or physiologic).

In our cervical spine injury patient population, multiple trauma was found to have occurred in 49 percent (Table 15-3) of patients with cervical spine fractures. Thirty-eight percent of all spine fractures required some method of stabilization and fusion. The most frequent operative stabilization procedures utilized in our cervical spine series were the interspinous process wiring procedure (27 percent), sublaminar wiring of fractures of the

Table 15-3. Cervical Fractures: Multiple Trauma (Northwestern University Acute Spine Injury Center, 1972 to 1986)

No. of systems involved	No.	Percent
None	761	51.3
One	566	38.1
Two	120	8.1
Three	32	2.2
Four	5	0.3
Total	1,484	100.00

odontoid process, C1–C2 (28 percent), wire fixation of hangman's fractures, C1–C3 (12 percent), and C3 to C7 posterior fusion (45 percent) (see Fig. 15-59). When a bilateral posterior fracture of the ring of C1 was accompanied by a fracture of the odontoid, posterior fusion could not be accomplished and therefore the fracture was managed conservatively (halo vest). One patient underwent an anterior screw fixation of an odontoid fracture (a patient with rheumatoid spondylitis and a previous healed fracture of the cervical spine). When fracture of the ring of C1 was not found posterior, but lay laterally (Fig. 15-25), we found that posterior wiring could be successfully accomplished without concern for loss of fixation or C1 ring displacement.

ANTERIOR COMPRESSION FRACTURES: CERVICAL VERTEBRAL COLUMN

Uncomplicated compression fractures of the vertebral column between C3 and C7 are often isolated injuries, not associated with either middle or posterior column injury. They are therefore considered "stable injuries" by definition, but as later discussed, the extent of vertebral body compression must be taken into account. When the vertebral body is fractured vertically, the etiology is axial loading. When the vertebral body reveals horizontal compression seen in the sagittal plane, this denotes flexion loading (Fig. 15-37).

Flexion-induced injuries often appear innocuous, although statistics in our series reveal the incidence of neurologic injury to be high: 32 percent complete, 53 percent incomplete, and only 13 percent intact. The likely rationale for this high incidence of neurologic injury is that the initial deformity at the time of injury is not that which is apparent on admission (owing to cervical spine alignment by the paramedic management team). These injuries therefore require careful attention, cervical traction for initial immobilization and restoration of alignment, and a careful evaluation for the presence of signs of instability (requiring surgery), or long-term (3 months) conservative care in either a halo vest or SOMI orthosis.

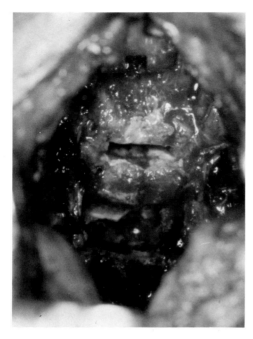

Fig. 15-37. Photograph taken of anterior vertebral column following excision of retropulsed disc at C4–C5 and C5–C6 following axial load injury to the cervical spine. Note vertical fracture involving C5 and anterior compression fracture of the C6 vertebral body. The cervical spine was stabilized by anterior A-O plate-screw fixation at C4 to C7. A cancellous bone graft was inserted in the disc space C4–5, C5–6.

Although many investigators attempt to grade the extent of vertebral compression on the basis of standard and tomographic radiographs, there is no accurate method of assessing cervical spine stability initially, other than by its visual appearance. We have noted that when there is evidence of vertebral compression of greater than 25 percent, along with widening of the interspinous ligament above or below the involved vertebral element and a measurable cervical kyphosis (greater than 11 degrees) (Fig. 15-38), a posterior stabilization (and fusion) is required. Attempts to maintain alignment in an orthosis will fail, the affected vertebral body will undergo further compression, and the cervical spine will develop greater kyphosis.

While there are contraindications to performing all operative procedures, the one that relates to the cervical spine is the presence of fracture involving multiple-level cervical vertebrae. When a posterior cervical spine fusion is attempted in such cases, considerable rigidity of the cervical spine results. Therefore, the recommended management for multiple-level fractures is immobilization of the cervical spine in an orthosis such as the halo vest for 3 months. The mere fact that fractures appear at multiple levels usually results in rapid healing of all fractures. We have also noted that when fractures occur at multiple levels, resulting in a "traumatic laminectomy," the patient is normally intact neurologically.

Flexion-Axial Load

With the application of an axial load to a cervical spine in an acutely flexed position, several types of vertebral element injuries can be anticipated: (1) a burst fracture of the vertebral body (with a vertical split fracture of a vertebral body, seen on a anteroposterior radiograph), (2) an anterointerior "teardrop" flexion-induced fracture of the involved vertebral body, (3) the occurrence of a unilateral (but normally bilateral) bipedicle fracture involving the posterior lamina of the vertebral body undergoing fracture, and (4) the *sine qua non* of a very unstable cervical spine fracture, the presence of posterior displacement of the fractured (upper) vertebral body posteriorly on the next inferior vertebral body. Such displacement is indicative of at least two-column instability and disruption of the inferior intervertebral disc. Although it is possible, the posterior elements do not usually undergo displacement because of the loss of continuity between the posterior and the anterior and middle columns. The above constellation of injuries results in gross spinal instability, acute angulation, and, almost uniformly, a complete neurologic injury (see Fig. 15-45). This type of cervical spine injury frequently follows a diving accident.

The opposite of this injury is the axial load extension injury. In this situation, multiple-level bilaminar (or pedicle) fractures may occur, but the effect is often a multilevel traumatic laminectomy type of spine injury, resulting in no or a minor neurologic injury.

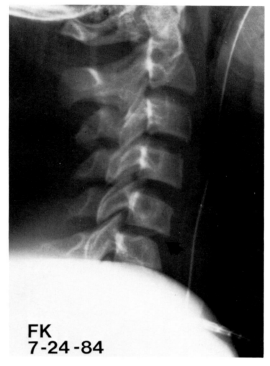

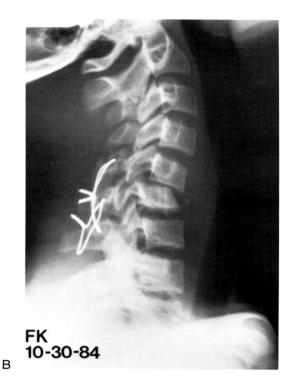

A
FK
7-24-84

B
FK
10-30-84

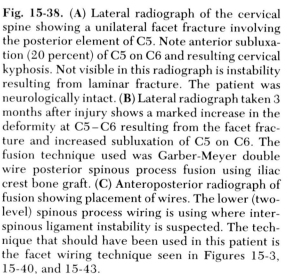

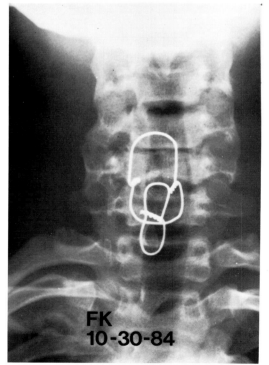

C

FK
10-30-84

Fig. 15-38. (A) Lateral radiograph of the cervical spine showing a unilateral facet fracture involving the posterior element of C5. Note anterior subluxation (20 percent) of C5 on C6 and resulting cervical kyphosis. Not visible in this radiograph is instability resulting from laminar fracture. The patient was neurologically intact. (B) Lateral radiograph taken 3 months after injury shows a marked increase in the deformity at C5–C6 resulting from the facet fracture and increased subluxation of C5 on C6. The fusion technique used was Garber-Meyer double wire posterior spinous process fusion using iliac crest bone graft. (C) Anteroposterior radiograph of fusion showing placement of wires. The lower (two-level) spinous process wiring is using where interspinous ligament instability is suspected. The technique that should have been used in this patient is the facet wiring technique seen in Figures 15-3, 15-40, and 15-43.

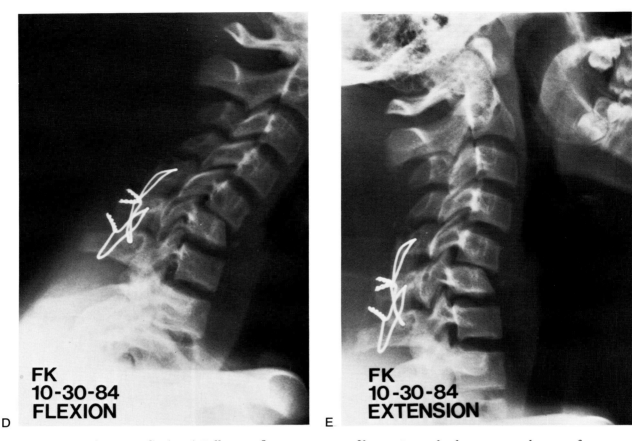

Fig. 15-38 *(Continued).* **(D,E)** Follow-up flexion-extension films at 3 months demonstrate absence of motion at C5–C6.

Management of the Axial Load Flexion-Induced Vertebral Body-Bipedicle Fracture

As noted above, the axial load flexion-induced vertebral body-bipedicle fracture is a grossly unstable injury and, in our experience, is more appropriately stabilized by an anterior surgical approach. Because the posterior laminar elements are "disconnected" from the retro-displaced anterior vertebral element, attempts at a posterior fusion have been found not to improve stability or to bring about a reduction of the anterior element. Thus, an anterior two- or three-level plate-screw (fusion) stabilization procedure is indicated. When the fracture pattern of the involved anterior vertebral body element permits rigid screw fixation, the use of an anterior cervical plate-screw apparatus (with intervertebral bone graft) and a postoperative

SOMI orthosis are usually sufficient for stability. When osteopenia or comminution of the affected vertebral body is present, the anterior plate-screw fixation may require augmentation with a posterior spine fusion or a halo vest orthosis for 3 months. If they are indicated, we prefer to perform both procedures at once, with the anterior procedure preceding the psoterior procedure.

UNILATERAL FACET JOINT DISLOCATIONS

Some researchers consider the presence of a unilateral facet dislocation a stable injury, particularly when unassociated with a fracture. This injury is interpreted as stable because this is a rotation and, to a lesser extent, flexion injury. Thus, there is less anteroposterior ligamentous disruption accompanying this injury than there is with the force-induced pure flexion injury, in which a bilateral facet joint dislocation occurs. With the latter, extensive ligamentous injuries result in gross spinal instability.

In the presence of a unilateral facet dislocation, the extent of vertebral element displacement upon the adjacent vertebra is usually one-third anterior vertebral body displacement of the superior vertebra on the inferior vertebra, as compared with one-half body displacement of one vertebral body on another with a bilateral facet joint dislocation (Fig. 15-39). Likewise, the neurologic injury with a unilateral facet dislocation is less (complete [31 percent] and incomplete [39 percent] = 70 percent), while the extent of the neurologic injury with the bilateral facet dislocation is greater (complete [47 percent] and incomplete [45 percent] = 91 percent) (Table 15-1). The neurologic injury associated with a unilateral facet joint dislocation is more often either a single "nerve root syndrome" or a "Brown-Séquard syndrome." Both have an excellent prognosis for improvement after reduction of the malalignment.

Although a unilateral facet dislocation may be stable,[56] when a neurologic injury occurs and a closed reduction (skeletal traction) is unsuccessful, particularly in the first 2 to 3 weeks after injury, an open reduction and stabilization procedure should be performed (Fig. 15-40). When a closed reduction is attained, a myelogram should be obtained in the early postreduction period to ensure that a herniated disc or fracture fragment in the neural canal is not overlooked. Should a change in neurologic function occur after reduction, a bolus of Decadron (dexamethasone) (50 mg) should be administered IV, a myelogram performed, and the patient surgically approached from anterior or posterior, depending on the radiographic findings.

On careful evaluation of the radiographs of a patient suspected of having a unilateral facet dislocation, several helpful findings will contribute to making the diagnosis. On the anteroposterior view, the spinous process of the affected vertebra will be found rotated from the midline toward the side of the subluxation or dislocation. This is not always an easily recognizable radiographic finding. Another helpful finding seen in the lateral radiograph is the oblique appearance of the facet joints above the level of injury. When a unilateral facet joint subluxation (or dislocation) exists, the involved vertebra and its facets and all of the facet joints above the level of injury will be more difficult to identify individually owing to "rotational overlapping" secondary to obliquity produced by the dislocation. Below the level of injury, the facet joints will be easily recognizable (Fig. 15-41).

Other considerations to be taken into account when managing a unilateral facet dislocation are the following. Is there an associated facet fracture? Is the dislocated facet reducible? How long has the dislocation existed, that is, is the injury old and "fixed"? Are there other associated injuries involving the cervical spine? We have found that when a unilateral facet dislocation is unreducible, this usually indicates a facet joint fracture. This can best be confirmed by tomography.

As noted above, it is not uncommon for a unilateral facet joint dislocation to occur without an associated neurologic injury. Of the 1,484 cervical spine injuries in our series, 69 (5 percent) were unilateral facet joint dislocations. In this group of patients, 26 percent were intact on admission, 39 percent had incomplete injury, and 30 percent revealed a complete neurologic injury.

When a unilateral facet joint dislocation is immediately unreducible, the rule is to discontinue further attempts at traction reduction. If the dislocation is an acute injury and is unaccompanied by any neurologic compromise, an elective surgical reduction and fusion is recommended. When Gardner-Wells skeletal traction is used and a reduction is easily attained, the ease of the reduction is often indicative of the state of stability. Should redislocation or an associated angular deformity exist or occur (the result of posterior ligamentous instability or an associated vertebral body compression fracture), elective surgical stabilization is indicated. Finally, because there is always a concern for producing injury to the nervous system while attempting reduction (as with a dislocated facet), should there be any suggestion of an alteration in neurologic function during the reduction attempt, the procedure should be discontinued and the dislocation surgically reduced.

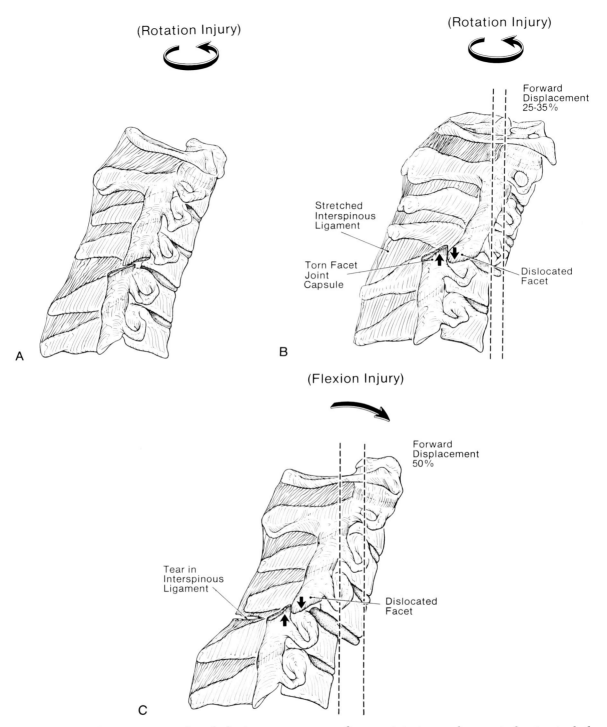

Fig. 15-39. The anatomic and pathologic consequences of rotary injuries to the cervical spine include degrees of facet joint dislocation. **(A)** Unilateral facet subluxation or incomplete displacement of facet joint surfaces. **(B)** Unilateral facet joint dislocation. The presence of this injury is identified by forward displacement of the affected vertebral element by 25 to 35 percent on the next lower element. **(C)** Bilateral facet joint dislocation results in forward displacement of vertebral elements by more than 50 percent. Unilateral facet dislocations result in complete neurologic injury in 30 percent of cases, bilateral facet dislocations result in complete neurologic injury in 47 percent of cases.

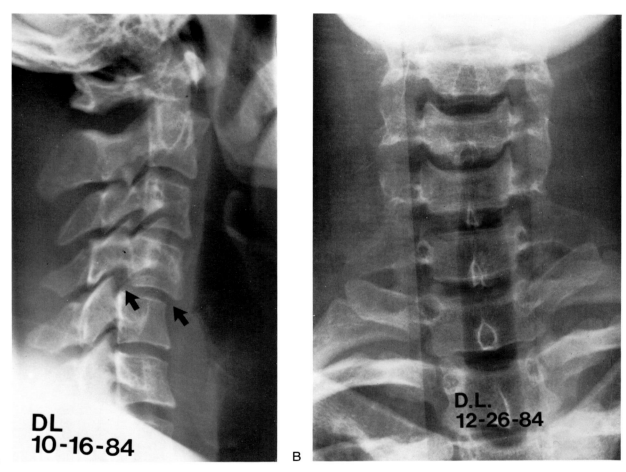

Fig. 15-40. (A) Lateral cervical spine radiograph demonstrating forward subluxation of C4 on C5 by one-third the width of the vertebral body. This finding is indicative of a unilateral facet dislocation. Note the lateral appearance of facet joints below C5 and the oblique view of the facet joints above C5. (B) A/P view. Note widening of joints of Luschka and C4–C5 disc space, right. While not apparent in this postreduction radiograph, injuries of this type result in displacement of the posterior spinous process to the same side as the facet dislocation. *(Figure continues.)*

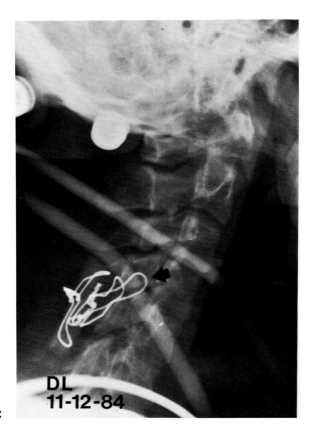

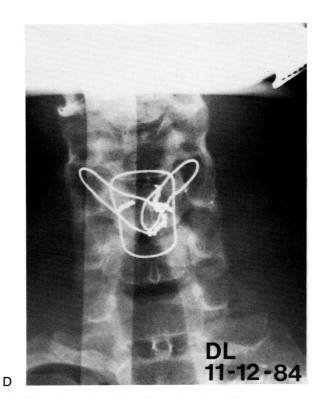

C

D

Fig. 15-40 *(Continued)*. **(C,D)** Postoperative lateral and AP radiographs following reduction. Facet-to-spinous-process wiring and posterior bone grafting were used for stabilization. Realignment of anterior cervical vertebra border is indicative of facet joint reduction. Also note restoration of parallelism of upper facet joints.

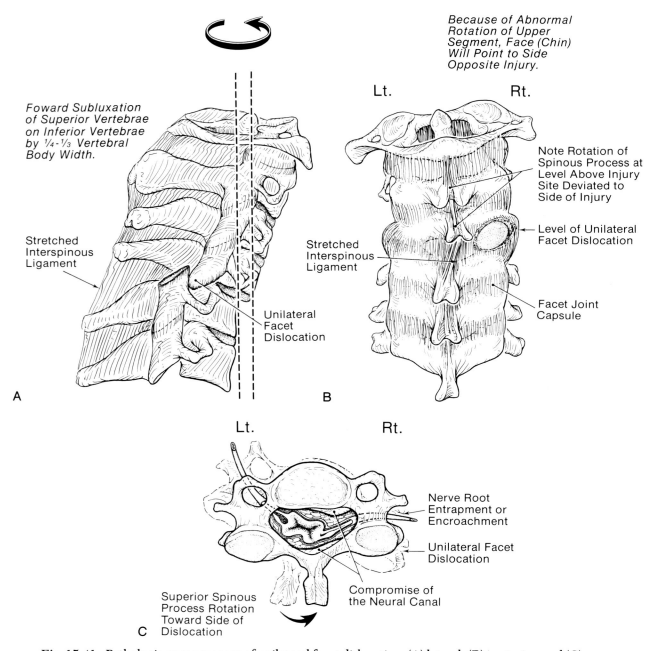

Forward Subluxation of Superior Vertebrae on Inferior Vertebrae by ¼-⅓ Vertebral Body Width.

Because of Abnormal Rotation of Upper Segment, Face (Chin) Will Point to Side Opposite Injury.

Lt.   Rt.

Note Rotation of Spinous Process at Level Above Injury Site Deviated to Side of Injury

Stretched Interspinous Ligament

Stretched Interspinous Ligament

Level of Unilateral Facet Dislocation

Facet Joint Capsule

Unilateral Facet Dislocation

A   B

Lt.   Rt.

Nerve Root Entrapment or Encroachment

Unilateral Facet Dislocation

Superior Spinous Process Rotation Toward Side of Dislocation

Compromise of the Neural Canal

C

Fig. 15-41. Pathologic consequences of unilateral facet dislocation. **(A)** lateral, **(B)** posterior, and **(C)** overhead transverse views.

Reduction Technique

The technique utilized for the reduction of a unilateral or bilateral facet dislocation is the following. All dislocations are reduced immediately, in the emergency room. All patients are evaluated physically, neurologically, and radiographically in the emergency room. Depending on the finding (on anteroposterior and lateral "scout" films), Gardner-Wells skeletal tongs are inserted as soon as possible. The patient is placed on a Stryker wedge frame and placed in weighted traction, using the level of the injury as the guide to the amount of weight to be applied (5 lbs per level of injury). Weight is increased in increments of 5 lbs, followed by new radiographs with each weight addition. Valium and an analgesic (meperidine or morphine sulfate) are used to relax the patient (when no contraindications such as allergy or a history of unconsciousness exist), to facilitate the reduction. Occasionally, assistive manipulation can be used to facilitate the reduction. Reduction can uniformly be obtained with weighted traction alone, whereas assistive manipulation is utilized when there is no evidence of an associated neurologic injury, no evidence of facet fracture, and reduction of the facet displacement has been reduced to the perched position (Fig. 15-42). When reduction is attained, the patient is maintained in cervical tong traction with the weights reduced to a maintenance level of 10 to 15 lbs. Should there exist a question of instability, flexion-extension films, under the supervision of a physician, are helpful.

Wagner, in an attempt to analyze the indications for operative intervention in cervical spine injuries, found that statistically, injuries resulting in compromise of the neural canal by more than 30 percent were severely dangerous.[57] This becomes a factor to be seriously considered for injuries occurring between the vertebral levels of C3 and C7. The anteroposterior diameter of the spinal canal in this region is at best narrow (a mean of 17 mm).

The surgical procedure recommended is wire stabilization of the adjacent posterior spinous processes when the facet joints are reduced and unaccompanied by fracture. When the facet joints are likely to undergo redislocation, spinous process wiring should be combined with bilateral inferior facet (the dislocated facet) to spinous process wiring.[56,58]

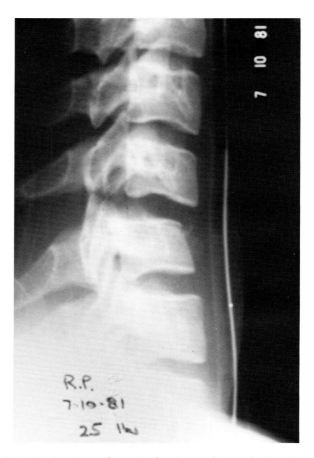

Fig. 15-42. Lateral cervical spine radiograph showing "perched" facets at C5–C6. Note anterior translation of C5 vertebral body on C6 by less than 25% and evidence of instability due to disruption of posterior interspinous and longitudinal ligaments and widening of posterior interspinous space C5–C6.

BILATERAL FACET JOINT DISLOCATIONS

Bilateral dislocation of the cervical facet joints usually results from the application of a violent flexion moment to the head and neck. The result is disruption in the posterior interspinous ligaments, the facet joint capsule, and the posterior and anterior longitudinal ligaments and the total disruption of the intervertebral disc. Because of the severity of the injury and the resulting vertebral element displacement, the incidence of neurologic injury is very high. In our series of 1,484 cervical spine injuries, 77 (5 percent) bilateral facet joint dislocations occurred. Forty-seven percent resulted in a complete neurologic injury, 45 percent in an incomplete injury, and only 8 percent were intact (without neurologic injury) a compared with 26 percent intact with unilateral facet dislocation.

Bilateral facet joint dislocations most frequently occur in the midportion of the cervical spine (C5 – C6), the area of maximum flexion motion. As reported above, Wagner et al. found that the mean sagittal diameter of the neural canal, in the midportion, was 17 mm.[57] Other measurements are reported to average 1.55 cm (15.5 mm), while the spinal cord proper measures approximately 0.90 to 0.85 mm.[59-61] (see Fig. 1-3). Thus, the high incidence of neurologic injury after bilateral facet joint

dislocation is the result of neural canal compromise secondary to facet dislocation, plus the displacement that likely occurred at the time of injury.

All bilateral facet joint dislocations are unstable,[56] and all require surgical stabilization. The surgical approach recommended is the posterior approach. Although it would be unusual to stabilize this injury by an anterior plate and screw procedure, the only time an anterior approach would be indicated would be for neural canal decompression. Reduction and stabilization can only be attained posteriorly by wire stabilization of each inferior facet (of the affected element) to the next inferior spinous process[56,58] (Fig. 15-43). Other posterior surgical procedures have been utilized[2-64] (see Posterior Surgical Fusion Technique: Occiput, C1, and C2, below).

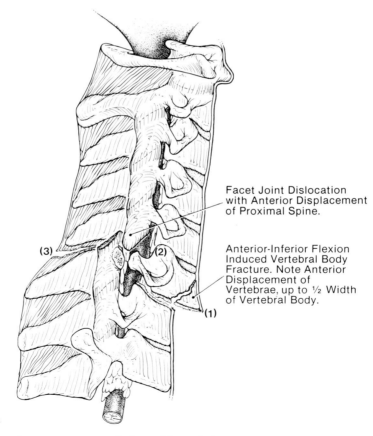

Facet Joint Dislocation with Anterior Displacement of Proximal Spine.

Anterior-Inferior Flexion Induced Vertebral Body Fracture. Note Anterior Displacement of Vertebrae, up to ½ Width of Vertebral Body.

(3)   (2)   (1)

A

Fig. 15-43. (A) Anatomic consequences of bilateral facet dislocation. Bilateral facet dislocations are secondary to flexion-distraction injuries, and result in three-column instability: disruption of the anterior (1) and posterior (2) longitudinal ligaments, and tear or fracture through posterior structures (3). *(Figure continues.)*

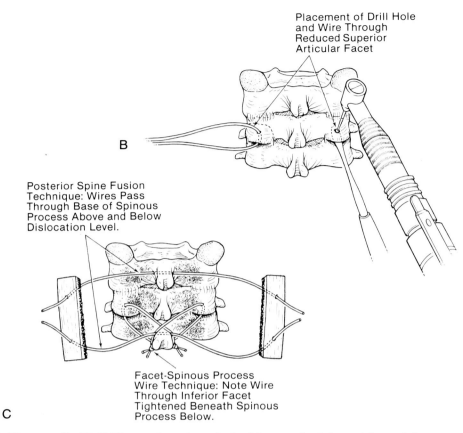

Placement of Drill Hole
and Wire Through
Reduced Superior
Articular Facet

B

Posterior Spine Fusion
Technique: Wires Pass
Through Base of Spinous
Process Above and Below
Dislocation Level.

Facet-Spinous Process
Wire Technique: Note Wire
Through Inferior Facet
Tightened Beneath Spinous
Process Below.

C

Fig. 15-43 *(Continued).* **(B,C)** The preferred method of fixation for bilateral facet dislocations: facet-to-spinous process wiring plus standard posterior Meyer fusion technique.

SURGICAL APPROACHES AND FIXATION PROCEDURES

Anterior Procedures

Anterior Surgical Incision Considerations: Right Versus Left

Although investigators[2,37] differ as to whether the right or left anterior approach is better, reference to *Morris' Human Anatomy*[65] shows that the recurrent laryngeal nerves, both right and left, are branches of the vagus (10th cranial) nerve, as is the left superior laryngeal nerve, which exits from the lower part of the ganglion nodosum. This latter nerve passes inferiorly and behind both the internal and external carotid arteries toward the larynx.

It enters this structure after having bifurcated into an internal branch to the upper border of the thyroid cartilage (accompanying the superior laryngeal artery) and an external branch to the lower border of the thyroid cartilage to end primarily in the cricothyroid muscle. Both supply the mucous membrane lining the larynx.

The right recurrent nerve, which arises from the vagus nerve at the root of the neck in front of the right subclavian artery, hooks posteriorly around the artery below and passes posteriorly behind the vessel, then ascending upward obliquely behind the common carotid artery (Fig. 15-44). As the nerve approaches the side of the trachea, it lies between the trachea and esophagus and accompanies branches of the inferior thyroid artery to supply the trachea, esophagus, and pharynx. Extend-

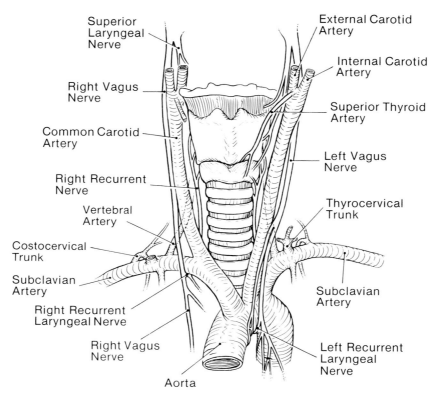

Fig. 15-44. Neurovascular relations of vagus (right and left recurrent laryngeal) nerves to the carotid artery.

ing proximally as a continuation of the right recurrent nerve is the inferior laryngeal nerve. This nerve continues to lie in a groove between the trachea and esophagus to enter the larynx, innervating the muscles (vocalis, cricoarytenoideus, thyroarytenoideus, etc.).

On the left side, the recurrent nerve arises in front of the aortic arch and winds around and under the vessel lateral to the ligamentum arteriosum. It crosses obliquely behind the root of the left common carotid artery to the interval between the esophagus and trachea and corresponds with the nerve of the right side.

The difference in opinion as to the appropriateness of an anterolateral right or left neck approach is thought to be that the left recurrent laryngeal nerve has a longer course (taking off lower on the left than the right), therefore being more prone to injury by retraction. Similarly, on the left side, the superior laryngeal nerve lies posterior to the exter-

nal carotid artery and is more exposed to trauma. Our preferred approach is the right anterolateral approach, either through a right anterolateral transverse incision at the level to be explored, or through the longer anterior oblique incision, anterior to the sternocleidomastoid muscle belly, to protect the laryngeal nerve innervation to the larynx.[2,65]

Surgical Concerns: In-place Tracheostomy
As previously noted (see Ch. 9), the safest method of protecting the airway and intubating the cervical spine-injured patient, when there is, or is not, a pre-existing neurologic injury, is by nasotracheal intubation. Endotracheal (transoral) intubation requires slight flexion of the cervical spine to facilitate the insertion of the endotracheal tube. Being carefully performed by an experienced anesthesiologist, this should not be a problem, as long as linear traction is maintained. The other choice of

maintaining the airway is by a tracheostomy. Here the proximity of the tracheostomy skin incision (and contamination therefrom) to the surgical skin incision is a consideration that must be taken into account. Usually, when a tracheostomy is in place, it has been in place for some time (and is more highly contaminated), in a patient with a high spinal cord injury requiring long-term ventilator support, or a patient who has sustained associated chest trauma.

The potential concern, as noted, is contamination of the surgical wound by the existing tracheostomy site. This hazard must be discussed with the patient or family (if appropriate) along with other hazards of surgery and anesthesia. Appropriate broad-spectrum antibiotics should be administered intravenously preoperatively, intraoperatively, and postoperatively for 72 hours. In place of the standard transcutaneous rigid tracheostomy tube, a flexible endotracheal tube can be inserted via the cutaneous tracheostomy into the trachea and shielded from the operative site by Betadine (povidone-iodine) Vyadrape.

Indications for Anterior Stabilization

Most injuries to the cervical spine result from either a flexion injury or an axial load injury (with or without rotation). When flexion, axial load, and rotation in combination have occurred, gross vertebral column instability and neural canal compromise with complete loss of neurologic function occur. The injury type that is least likely to occur is an extension, except in the elderly. Generally, it is the result of a fall.

Although extension injuries are not usually localized to any one area of the cervical spine, they do occur more frequently in the younger patient, in the posterior segments of C2 (the hangman's fracture), and in the elderly patient, at the C6–C7 level, where disruption of the anterior longitudinal ligament occurs.

As a general rule, flexion injuries require posterior surgical stabilization, whereas an anterior injury requires anterior stabilization. Although this concept is still adhered to, some flexion injuries to the spine (flexion-induced vertebral body retropulsion with narrowing of the neural canal or dural decompression) are now considered more amen-able to anterior stabilization than to posterior stabilization.

Anterior surgical stabilization is indicated under the following conditions: the need for excision of retropulsed vertebral body bone from the neural canal; excision of intervertebral disc at one or two levels, requiring intervertebral body spinal fusion; prominent posterior spondylosis requiring anterior decompression; disruption of the anterior longitudinal ligament with associated anterior interbody diastasis.

After the excision of an intervertebral disc, an anterior interbody fusion is usually performed. The anterior approach most often utilized is a right transverse anterolateral skin approach (Fig. 15-45). After the subcutaneous tissue is entered, the vertical striations of the platysma muscle are spread by blunt dissection. This brings one to the superficial investing fascia that envelopes all of the structures of the neck and surrounds the sternocleidomastoid. By following the interval just anterior to the sternocleidomastoid muscle, the thyroid, trachea, and esophagus (within the pretracheal fascia) can be retracted medially along with the recurrent laryngeal nerve (posterior to the trachea) (Fig. 15-45D). Laterally, the jugular vein, vagus nerve, and common carotid artery (all within the carotid sheath) are retracted (Fig. 15-45E). This brings into view the anterior aspect of the cervical vertebral column with its overlying anterior longus colli muscles and, in the midline, the anterior longitudinal ligament (Fig. 15-45G). When inserting retractors, bear in mind that the sharp points of a retractor may perforate a vital structure (such as the esophagus) even when care is taken. When such occurs, an esophageal cutaneous fistula results and may lead to a cervical vertebral osteomyelitis. The dissection is often easier if a nasogastric tube is placed into the esophagus after intubation. This greatly aids in palpation of the esophagus.

There are two ways to identify one's location. One is by palpating the very prominent transverse process of C6 (the carotid process). The other is by radiography. This is accomplished by placing a spinal needle into a disc space and obtaining a lateral radiograph. Two precautions: do not insert the needle too deeply into the disc space (Fig. 15-46), and be sure to include C1 or C2 in the lateral film,

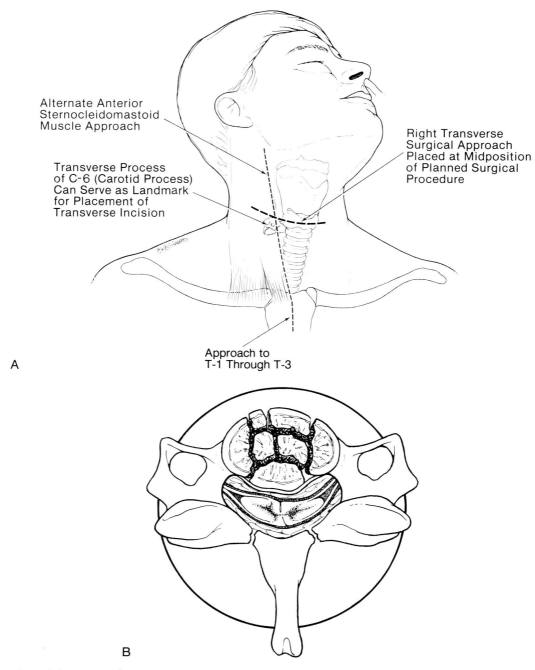

A

B

Fig. 15-45. (A) Suggested anterior approaches to the cervical spine. (B) Superior view of vertebral process showing comminuted vertebral body fracture with resulting narrowing of the neural canal and spinal cord compression. *(Figure continues.)*

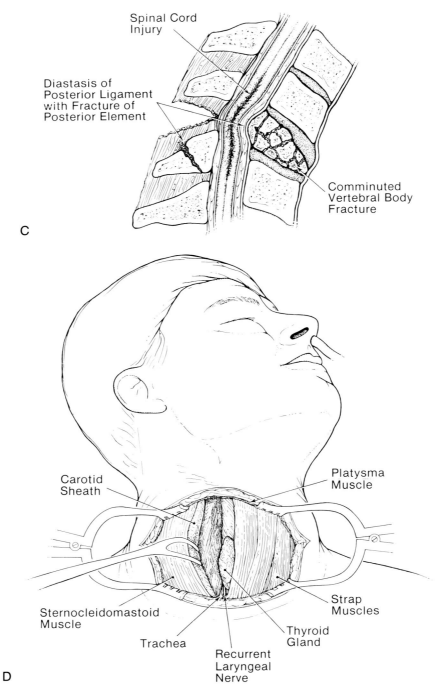

Spinal Cord Injury

Diastasis of
Posterior Ligament
with Fracture of
Posterior Element

Comminuted
Vertebral Body
Fracture

C

Carotid
Sheath

Platysma
Muscle

Sternocleidomastoid
Muscle

Strap
Muscles

Trachea

Thyroid
Gland

Recurrent
Laryngeal
Nerve

D

Fig. 15-45 *(Continued).* (**C**) Lateral view of cervical spinal column demonstrating spinal cord compression secondary to comminuted vertebral body fracture. (**D**) Anterior approach to the cervical spine through transverse incision. Major structures include the strap muscles, trachea, esophagus, thyroid cartilage, and recurrent laryngeal nerve medially, and the sternocleidomastoid and carotid sheath laterally.

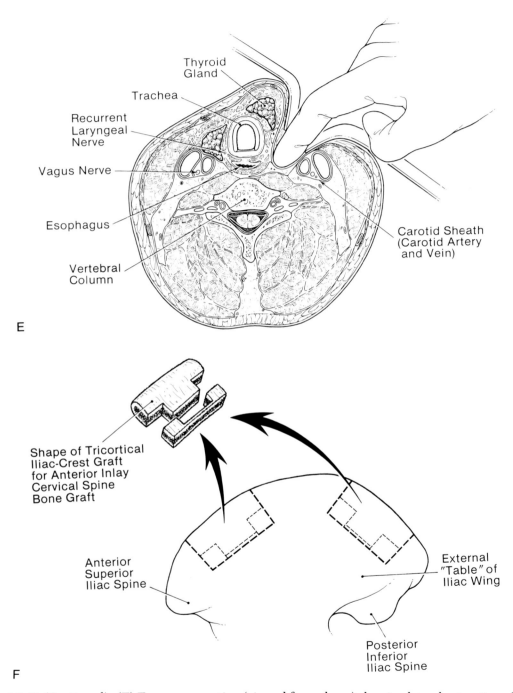

E

F

Fig. 15-45 *(Continued)*. **(E)** Transverse section (viewed from above) showing lateral retraction of carotid sheath and medial retraction of trachea and esophagus in approach to cervical spine. Finger palpates the anterior vertebral column. **(F)** Source of bone graft from anterior or posterior iliac crest. *(Figure continues.)*

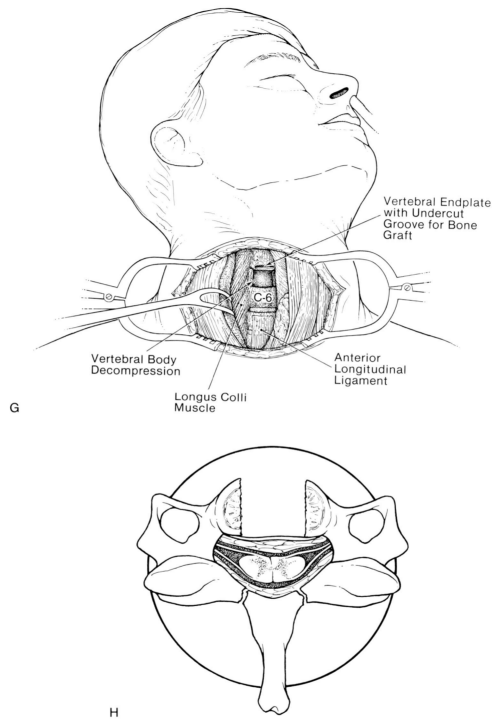

Vertebral Endplate
with Undercut
Groove for Bone
Graft

C-6

Vertebral Body
Decompression

Longus Colli
Muscle

Anterior
Longitudinal
Ligament

G

H

Fig. 15-45 *(Continued).* **(G)** Picture shows excision of the C5 vertebral body (corporectomy) and insertion of grooves on the undersurface of the C4 vertebral body and the superior surface of C6 for bone graft to be inserted as described in Figure 15-49. **(H)** Superior view showing removal of the central aspect of the affected vertebral body, allowing for decompression of the neural canal without complete excision of the vertebral body. (See Figure 15-45B.)

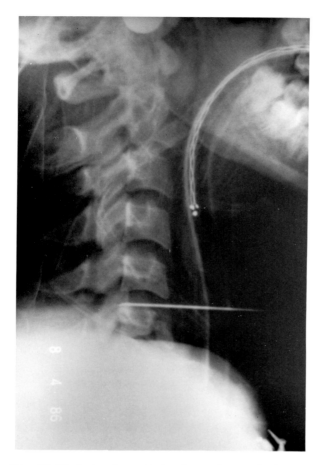

Fig. 15-46. Lateral cervical spine radiograph demonstrating the use of a needle marker for identification of the surgical level. Obtaining a marker film is a prerequisite before carrying out other procedures. Note anterior vertical fracture of C6 vertebral body (just below needle). Care must be taken not to insert the needle marker too far.

to accurately count down to the level of the needle. A helpful hint of use during surgery, particularly when operating at the C6–C7 and T1 level, is to place a bandage wrap or loop around each of the patient's wrists, with the tails of each brought to the foot of the operating table or frame. If during the operative procedure radiograph is required, these tails will allow an assistant to pull down on the arms (and shoulders), getting this area of the anatomy out of the way, to provide a better chance of visualizing the lower cervical vertebral column.

Bohler: Anterior Approaches to C1 – C2

We have limited experience with the anterior surgical stabilization procedure described by Bohler[36] and Whitesides and Kelley[66] for problems at the C1, C2, and C3 levels. The surgical approach is very similar to that utilized for approaches to the anterior cervical spine at lower levels. Although the transoral-retropharyngeal approach to the C1–C2 vertebrae serves as an additional approach, the hazard that this approach carries with it is infection. This approach was utilized by us on one occasion for the performance of an osteotomy through the base of the odontoid process, for a malunion of the dens. No infection occurred (Fig. 15-47).

Bohler[36] advises, in the presence of a nonunion of the odontoid process, that a posterior C1–C2 fusion be undertaken first. When there is a persistent nonunion of the odontoid process, Bohler advises that an anterior C1–C2 fusion also be undertaken. Should the fracture of the odontoid process reveal more than 3 mm of anterior displacement and be unreducible, or should there also be a concomitant fracture of the posterior arch of C1, then an anterior reduction, bone graft, and stabilization should be conducted first, followed by a posterior fusion. Bohler notes that the literature reveals that a posterior C1–C2 fusion procedure results in an odontoid nonunion rate of between 20 and 80 percent, with his nonunion rate being in the vicinity of 40 percent. We have found that the nonunion rate of odontoid fractures is not that high (12 percent) and that they are usually asymptomatic and seldom in need of further surgery. A combined anteroposterior procedure at the atlantoaxial joint is seldom necessary. Likewise, we have noted that the mere presence of a fracture involving the posterior ring of C1 does not automatically serve as a contraindication to the performance of a posterior procedure. It depends on where the fracture of the ring is located. The use of a CAT scan view of C1 is helpful in deciding this (Fig. 15-26).

The skin incision to the C1–C2 level is a transverse half-collar anteromedial aspect of the anterior aspect of the neck, usually on the right side, at the level of the cricoid cartilage. After retraction of the carotid sheath laterally, the anterior prominence of C1 can be palpated and the anterior body of C2 exposed. The prerequisite to the successful

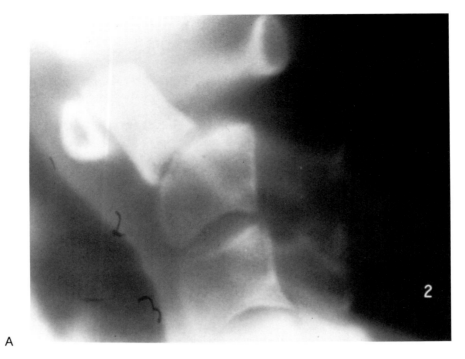

A

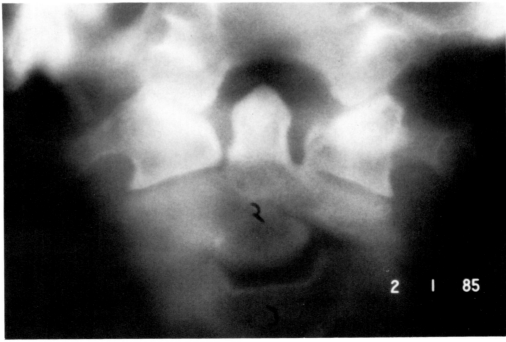

B

Fig. 15-47. **(A)** lateral and **(B)** AP cervical spine radiographs 8 weeks after trauma demonstrating an acutely flexed type III odontoid fracture healing in malposition. Note the obscure residual fracture line and the involvement of the anterosuperior C2 body. Note also the narrowness of the neural canal between the ring of C1 and the posterior aspect of the body of C2. At the time of this radiograph, the patient was neurologically normal. Flexion-extension films revealed no motion at the fracture site. The patient was managed in a SOMI orthosis for an additional 6 weeks. *(Figure continues.)*

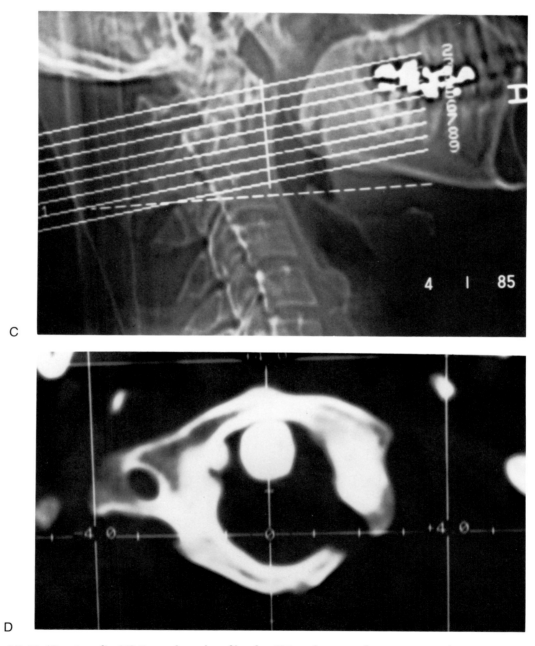

Fig. 15-47 *(Continued).* (**C**) Lateral marker film for CT evaluation of upper cervical spine. Note acute angular deformity of odontoid process in relation to the cervical spine. (**D**) Transverse CT scan (slice 3 in Fig. C) revealing larger than normal neural canal between posterior odontoid process and anterior border of posterior ring of C1. *(Figure continues.)*

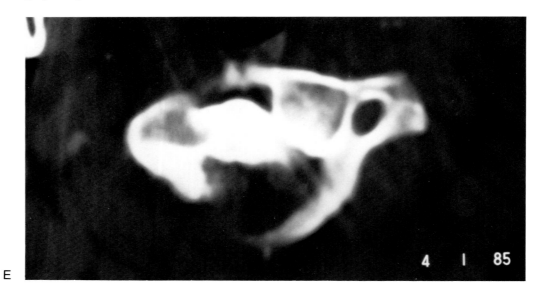

E

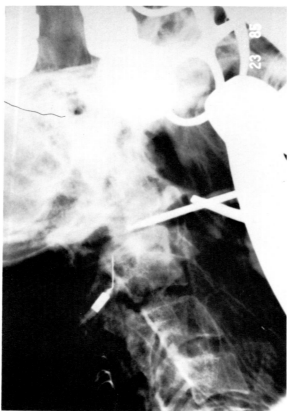

F

Fig. 15-47 *(Continued).* **(E)** CT scan (slice 4 in Fig. C). This view demonstrates narrowness of neural canal and alterations in anterior bony anatomy secondary to fracture through the base of the odontoid involving vertebral body C2. **(F)** Because of evidence of pyramidal tract spasticity secondary to malunion of the type III odontoid fracture, a transoral approach to the odontoid was undertaken and an osteotomy of the base of the odontoid was accomplished using a high speed burr. *(Figure continues.)*

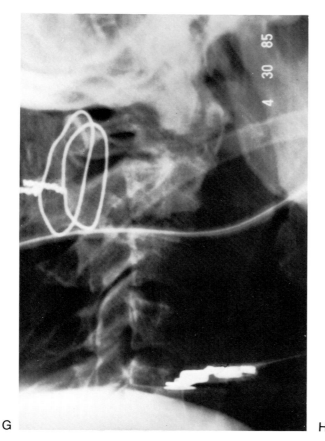
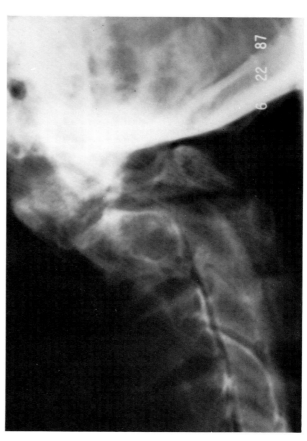

G   H

Fig. 15-47 *(Continued).* **(G)** Post-operative film following posterior C1–C2 modified Brooks-type posterior spine fusion. Note increased space of neural canal between anterior border of the C1 ring and the posterior aspect of the C2 vertebral body. **(H)** Because of continued pyramidal tract involvement and residual narrowing of the neural canal at C1–C2, the posterior internal fixation was removed. This lateral tomogram reveals maintenance of odontoid nonunion and increasing narrowness between ring of C1 and the posterior aspect of the vertebral body C2. *(Figure continues.)*

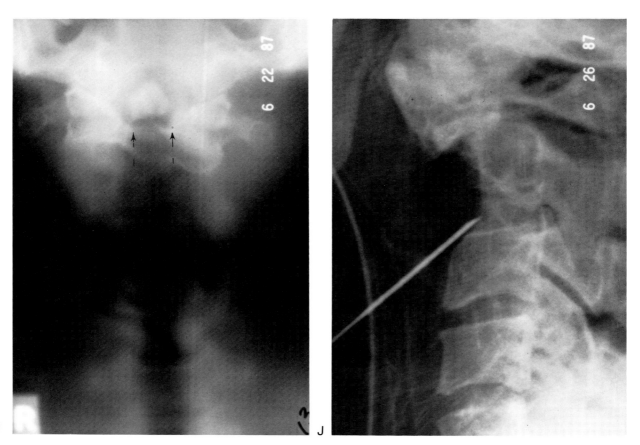

Fig. 15-47 *(Continued).* **(I)** Myelogram taken 2.5 years after original odontoid fracture confirms compression of upper cervical neural canal at C1–C2. **(J)** AP tomogram of upper cervical spine reveals continued presence of odontoid nonunion. Arrows outline proposed site of central C2 corporectomy for decompression of neural canal. **(K)** Lateral radiograph with needle marker in the C2–C3 interspace. Note that the anterior aspect of C2 is excised. A central corporectomy of C2 extending from the anterior to the posterior longitudinal ligament allows for anterior decompression of the dural column. Posterior fusion of C1–C2 is intact. Postoperatively, the patient demonstrated evidence of cervical subcutaneous emphysema. Barium swallow demonstrated a tracheal-esophageal fistula, thought to have been caused by retractor pressure during surgery. Patient required incision and drainage and tracheostomy. All wounds healed, tracheostomy was removed, and the patient was neurologically normal at 5 months postoperatively.

use of this approach and technique is the availability and use of an image intensifier, in both the anteroposterior and lateral planes. Though he did not personally utilize it, Bohler[36] describes a technique for the visualization and reduction of the displaced odontoid process (using a Hoffman retractor for leverage) through the fracture site. When managing an acute type II fracture, it is suggested that two drill holes be placed through the anteroinferior body of C2, using a power burr across the fracture site into the proximal tip of the odontoid process. Image intensification is mandatory. For a nonunion of the odontoid, corticocancellous bone graft dowls can be inserted via a trough in the body of C2 into the substance of the dens. For the unstable acute fracture involving the odontoid process (type II or III), usually seen in the head-injured or elderly patient, lag screw fixation is useful and indicated (Fig. 15-48). For a nonunion, bone dowels are placed across the fracture site to stabilize the fracture and prevent fragment rotation.

Postoperative immobilization suggested by Bohler was the use of a simple plastic collar for 6 to 8 weeks, or a cast.[36] We recommend either a halo vest (for a nonunion with bone grafts) or a SOMI orthosis when two screws are used.

Bohler reported one neurologic complication utilizing this surgical approach. This disappeared completely within 4 months. No failure of union occurred in his series of 27 procedures (15 having only the anterior compression screw fusion technique owing to the presence of accompanying posterior arch fracture involving C1).

Anterior Cervical AO Plate-Screws: Three-Level Fusion

In the situation, in which the surgeon plans an anterior cervical discectomy and fusion using plate-screw stabilization, the anterior surgical exposure of the spine is the same as that described in prior sections.

Once the anterior subperiosteal exposure of the vertebral bodies is completed, and the retractors are placed, the presence of a pulse in the superficial temporal artery is verified. A spinal needle is inserted into a disc space at the suspected level (superficially), and a lateral radiograph is obtained (including C1). After the level of the pathology is identified, the intervertebral discs above and

below the affected vertebra are excised. The anulus fibrosus is sharply incised, and the disc excision is completed with gentle currettage and with the use of pituitary rongeurs. Every attempt should be made to preserve the integrity of the posterior longitudinal ligament if it has not been interrupted by the trauma. The surgeon must be aware that with incision of the anterior longitudinal ligament (and a possible injury to the posterior longitudinal ligament), the possibility exists for overdistraction of the cervical spine by the Gardner-Wells traction. Generally this is not a problem.

Once the intervertebral discs have been excised above and below the injured vertebral body, the cartilaginous vertebral end plates can be removed, using a currette or high-speed burr with a small diamond tip. Exposure can be improved by inserting a small lamina spreader into the disc space. This must be done one level at a time, and the surgeon must avoid pressure by the lamina spreader on any unstable fragment of the injured vertebral body. If the vertebral body is comminuted, it can be excised and either a tricortical or tibial bone graft can be inserted.

At this point, anterior osteophytes overlying the three vertebral levels to be fused should be debrided with a high-speed diamond-tipped burr. This will allow the plate to lie flat along the anterior vertebral bodies. The anteroposterior dimensions of the end plates of the intact vertebrae are measured with a depth gauge. A 2.0 Kirschner wire is inserted into a Jacobs chuck, and using the drill guide placed over the k-wire and flush on the chuck, the length of the k-wire is then adjusted to match the measured anteroposterior dimension of the vertebral body. Either cancellous chips of bone graft are placed into the debrided intervertebral space or a tricortical graft can be appropriately shaped for each. It is imperative that the bone graft *not be packed* forcefully into the space owing to the risk of producing anterior epidural compression by extrusion of bone graft posteriorly (especially if the posterior longitudinal ligament was disrupted with the initial trauma). Traction is released, and an anterior cervical plate of appropriate size is selected and screwed in place along the three adjacent vertebral bodies.

Intraoperative lateral cervical spine radiographs are obtained, and the adequacy of reduction, hard-

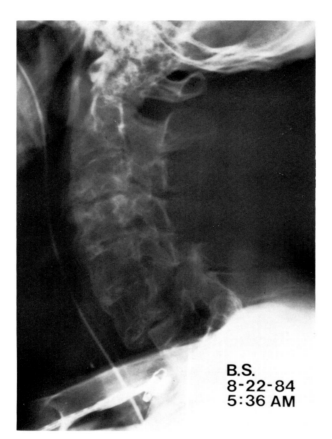

A

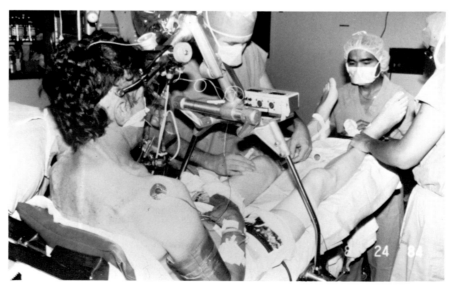

B

Fig. 15-48. (A) Lateral cervical spine radiograph in 56-year-old man with rheumatoid spondylitis involving the cervical/thoracic spine. Note displaced fracture at the C6–C7 interval. The patient sustained an incomplete central cord neurologic injury. (B) A posterior cervical spine fusion was undertaken with the patient in a sitting position in order to re-establish and maintain cervical spine alignment during the procedure. A tibial bone graft was obtained from the left anterior proximal tibia for posterior fusion. Note evoked potential monitoring needles in place. (*Figure continues.*)

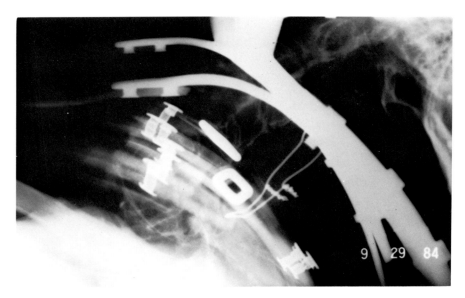

C

Fig. 15-48 *(Continued).* **(C)** Postoperative lateral radiograph demonstrating position of cervical spine and posterior wire fixation with patient in halo vest. **(D)** Lateral radiograph obtained 14 months postoperatively, demonstrating reduction and healed cervical spine fracture. The recommended surgical management of this fracture at the time of writing is anterior stabilization and halo fixation, not posterior wiring. *(Figure continues.)*

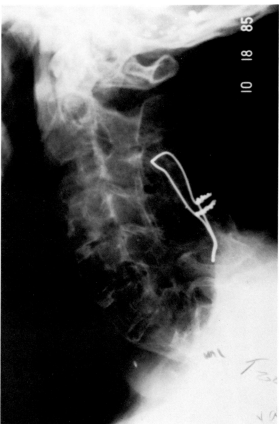

D

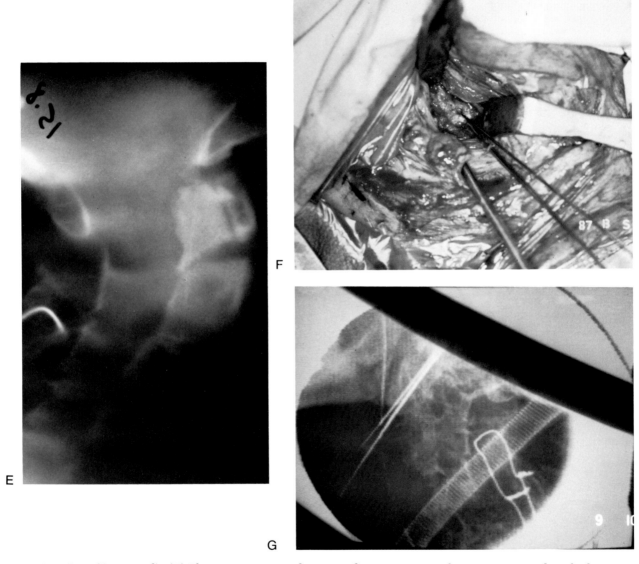

Fig. 15-48 *(Continued)*. **(E)** The patient returned 3 years after operation with an extension-induced odontoid fracture. Due to the rigid cervical/thoracic spine secondary to rheumatoid spondylitis, nonunion of the odontoid fracture was anticipated. **(F)** Insertion of Kirschner wire marker and stabilizing wires through the base of C2 across and into odontoid process. **(G)** Intraoperative x-ray monitoring of guidewire insertion. *(Figure continues.)*

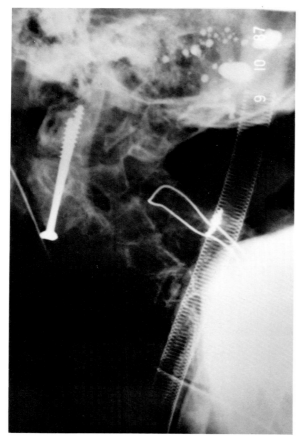

H

Fig. 15-48 *(Continued).* **(H)** Post-operative lateral radiograph showing two 40 mm 4.0 AO lag screws across the odontoid fracture at C2. Because of a rigid cervical spine secondary to rheumatoid spondylitis, anterior distraction at fracture site required acceptance. The threaded portion of the screws should not cross the fracture site.

ware placement, and bone graft placement is verified. If the fusion is considered stable, the Gardner-Wells tongs can be removed and the patient can be placed in a SOMI orthosis.

Anterior Cervical Vertebral Body Corporectomy and Three-Level Fusion

In those situations in which an acute flexion injury to the cervical spine results in a burst compression fracture of the vertebral body (Fig. 15-45B), or

metastatic carcinoma involves the vertebral body with extrusion of bone into the neural canal and neurologic compromise, an anterior approach with vertebral body corporectomy is indicated. This approach facilitates the complete excision of the vertebral body and two adjacent intervertebral discs (Fig. 15-49A) and allows for the insertion of a tibial bone graft obtained from the proximal medial aspect of the tibia (see Fig. 15-69A,B) or the iliac crest (Fig. 15-45F).

The right anterolateral surgical approach to the cervical spine is made with the patient supine on a Stryker wedge frame or operating table, with the patient in continuous Gardner-Wells tong traction. The patient is anesthetized, preferably by nasotracheal intubation. The intubation is done with the patient awake, with the assistance of local anesthesia in both the nasal and the retropharyngeal passages, along with the transcutaneous instillation of a local anesthetic agent directly into the trachea. A radial artery pressure transducer should be in place enabling monitoring of the mean arterial pressure (near 80 to 85 mm Hg) throughout surgery. Should the transoral endotracheal route be the only approach feasible, careful mild extension or flexion of the chin and head can be carried out without any ill effects. The safeguard is the in-place cervical traction, and the patient being awake. If the spinal lesion lies at C2, the spine should not be moved. Once the patient is intubated and stabilized under the general anesthetic, a nasogastric tube should be inserted. This is very helpful in identifying the esophagus by palpation during the dissection.

Although it is neither indicated nor contraindicated, the head, chin, and neck may be slightly turned toward the left to facilitate the right anterolateral approach to the neck. Palpation of the very prominent transverse process of C6 (the carotid process) serves as a landmark for placement of the transverse skin incision (Fig. 15-45A). The incision extends from just anterior to the belly of the sternocleidomastoid muscle, to just past the midline of the neck. After the subcutaneous tissue is entered, the vertical fibers of the platysma muscle are encountered and spread in line with the fibers by blunt dissection. This brings the surgeon to the superficial encapsulating fascia, which literally encompasses all of the strap muscles and superficial muscles of the neck. Beneath the sternocleidomas-

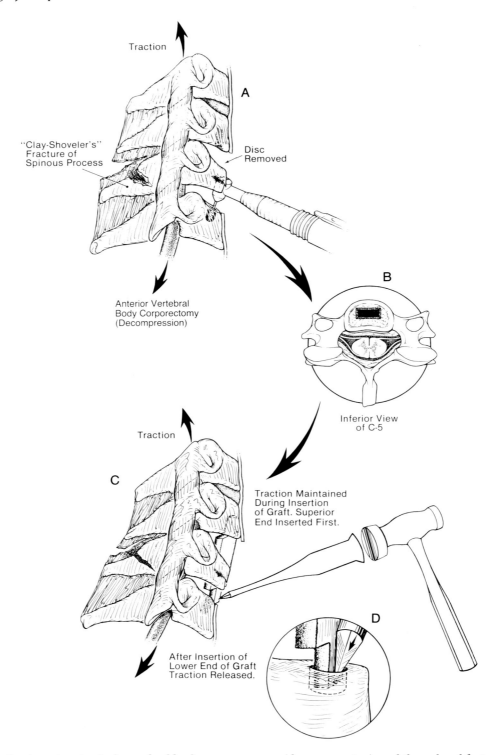

Fig. 15-49. Anterior cervical vertebral body corporectomy (decompression), and three-level fusion incorporating bone graft. (see Fig. 15-50C.) *(Figure continues.)*

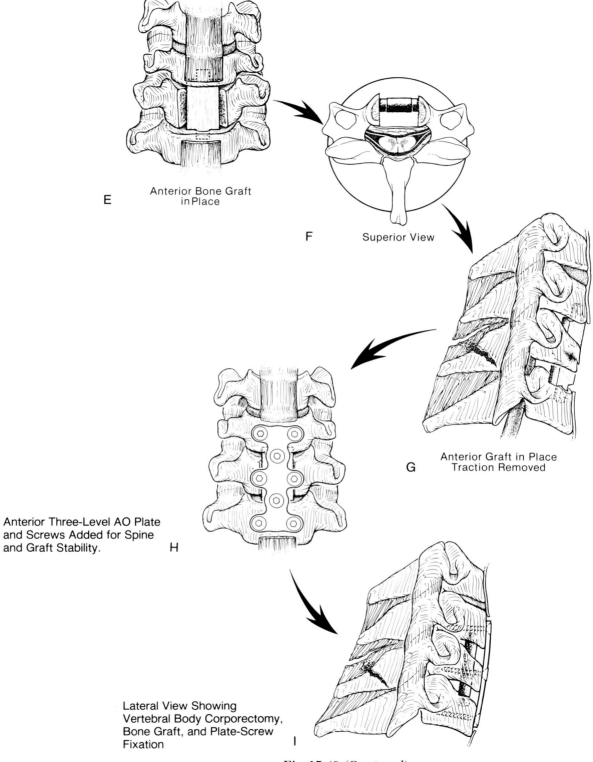

E   Anterior Bone Graft
in Place

F   Superior View

G   Anterior Graft in Place
Traction Removed

Anterior Three-Level AO Plate
and Screws Added for Spine
and Graft Stability.   H

Lateral View Showing
Vertebral Body Corporectomy,
Bone Graft, and Plate-Screw
Fixation   I

Fig. 15-49 *(Continued)*.

toid muscle, which is retracted laterally, the carotid sheath and pulse can be palpated. This bundle, which contains the jugular veins, the common carotid artery, and the vagus nerve, is retracted laterally (Fig. 15-45B). The surgeon's index finger can be inserted at approximately a 60-degree angle into the wound and easily pass deep and slightly medial to palpate the anterior cervical spinal column. Thus, everything medial to the finger (the trachea, thyroid, esophagus, and, between the trachea and esophagus, the right recurrent laryngeal nerve) can be retracted not only toward, but over the midline. This brings into view, with careful retraction, the anterior vertebral column, with its longus colli muscles on either side and the anterior longitudinal ligament along the midline. Particular care is taken for the sharp edges on retractor blades, for fear they may directly injure local vital structures. One should always have the anesthesiologist check for diminution of pulsation in the superficial temporal artery on the right, after placement or any adjustment of retractors, to ensure there is no carotid artery compression.

Using either sharp or electrocautery dissection, a longitudinal incision is made down the middle of the anterior longitudinal ligament, down to the vertebrae and discs. By subperiosteal dissections, the front of each vertebra is cleaned of soft tissue. The most difficult attachment to clear is the attachment of the anterior longitudinal ligament to the anulus fibrosus at each disc level. The two methods of identifying the correct operative level are: (1) by placing a sharp instrument (Keith needle) into the sought for disc level and obtaining a lateral radiograph identifying the fractured vertebra, or (2) to palpate the prominent transverse process (the carotid tubercle) of C6. This is a less certain method.

Having identified the correct disc spaces to be excised, it then becomes easy to visualize the comminuted vertebral body to be excised. Carefully, the intervertebral discs above and below are incised parallel to the vertebral end plates and excised either by sharp dissection or with the use of pituitary rongeurs. The vertebral body can then be removed by using a bone-biting Leckcell rongeur, a pituitary rongeur, or a diamond-tipped high-speed burr. With careful attention, both bone and disc fragments that have penetrated the posterior longitudinal ligament, or lie posterior to the vertebral body, are removed. At this point, one must be aware that the patient is in skeletal tong traction. Since the anterior longitudinal ligament has been surgically incised, and the posterior longitudinal ligament may have been traumatically injured, excessive traction may occur.

Using a Hall right-angle drill (Fig. 15-50A), with a variable size burr attached, a perpendicular burr hole is placed into the underside of the lower end of the vertebral body above, and the upper end of the vertebral body below (Fig. 15-50A,B). Great care is taken not to fracture the anterior border of either vertebral body. The holes are made approximately 0.7 to 0.9 mm deep, and extend across the end of the vertebral body in the coronal plane from side to side, approximately 2 to 3 mm posterior to the anterior cortex of the superior and inferior vertebral bodies.

A tibial bone graft is obtained from the most proximal portion of either tibia (see Fig. 15-69). Obtaining and carefully excising the graft from an area opposite and just inferior to the tibial tubercle greatly prevents excessive weakening of the proximal tibia and prevents the production of stress rises, which tend to weaken the tibia and allow the development of nondisplaced tibial fractures. In our experience of 355 such donor graft sites, only 15 (4 percent) fractures occurred. Their management consisted of a short-leg walking and weight-bearing cast for 6 to 7 weeks. One tibial fracture occurred 7 months postsurgery when the patient fell while working in a lumber mill.

After the graft is shaped (see Fig. 15-69E), the upper end of the graft is inserted first into the prepared hole in the end of the upper vertebra. Upon request, the anesthesiologist is asked to apply additional traction by hand. This increases the distraction across the corporectomy site and allows the appropriately shaped tibial graft to be tapped into place. The upper end of the graft is first inserted into the superior vertebra, followed by the lower end (Fig. 15-49C), using a Moe impactor. The lower end of the graft is driven or impacted posteriorly until its lower border enters the groove in the upper end of the inferior vertebra. Immediately, all traction and weights are removed. With the use of an awl, the graft is further tapped in place into the lower vertebral body. Attention is always directed toward preventing any compression on the posterior longitudinal ligament. With this in mind, one may carefully add available cancellous bone, but this is generally not necessary. A lateral radiograph of the cervical spine is obtained to check cervical spine alignment and bone graft position. When the retractors are carefully removed, the strap muscles will fall back into their anatomic position with no sutures required. The platysma muscle is closed by several superficially applied approximating sutures, and the subcutaneous tissue and skin are closed by either a 2–0 Dexon or a 2–0 Prolene subcuticular closure. Surgery completed, the Gardner-Wells tongs are removed and a SOMI orthosisis is applied. Somatosensory evoked potential monitoring throughout surgery is recommended.

Posterior Procedures

Although this chapter allots considerable space to the effects of trauma on the cervical spine, trauma is but one of the pathologic processes capable of altering in neurologic function. Others include cervical spondylosis secondary to degenerative arthritis; ankylosing spondylitis complicated by trauma; tumorous (usually metastatic) involvement of the spine with spinal cord compression and spine instability; and congenital (developmental) abnormalities resulting in neurological alterations. This latter group includes spinal stenosis, more frequently found in the midcervical spine and often associated with degenerative arthritic changes, and congenital processes, including the congenitally short and angular Klippel-Feil syndrome neck; cervical spine deformities resulting from the presence

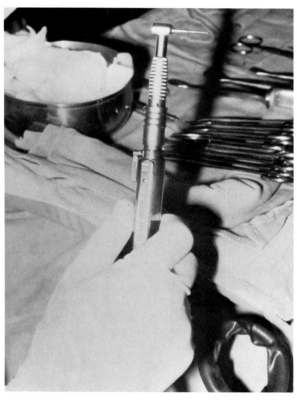

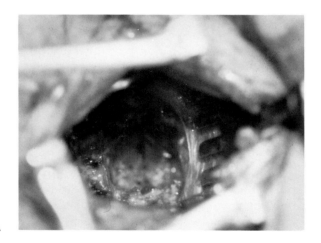

A

B

Fig. 15-50. (**A**) Intraoperative photograph of cervical vertebral body corporectomy. Left is cephalad. In the depth of the photograph is seen the posterior longitudinal ligament. (**B**) Right-angle high speed Hall burr is used for making grooves for acceptance of inlay bone graft in upper and lower ends of adjacent vertebral bodies. (See Fig. 15-49A.) *(Figure continues.)*

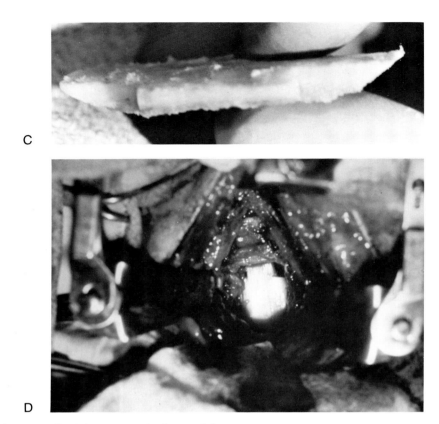

Fig. 15-50 *(Continued)*. **(C)** Bone graft obtained from anterior proximal tibia or iliac crest is shaped as shown in Figures 15-45F and 15-69. **(D)** Proximal end of bone graft inserted into undersurface of the proximal vertebra first; additional cervical traction is applied as the inferior end of the graft is inserted into the inferior vertebral body.

of congenital hemivertebra; and alterations in the architecture of the occipitoatlantal articulation with flattening of the occipital region of the skull (platybasia with basilar impression, resulting in compression of the brain stem by bony prominence of the surrounding foramen magnum and flattening of the base of the occipital bone). There may also be present an abnormal articulation between C1 and C2, with forward translation of the posterior ring of C1 (particularly when the anterior ring of C1 has been removed), resulting in further brain stem compression and further upward migration of the cervical spine, with intrusion of the odontoid process into the foramen magnum (Figure 15-51). The neurologic implications include brainstem com-promise with involvement of motor (pyramidal tract) function, and other alterations in brainstem functions such as respiration ("Ondine's curse").

Posterior Surgical Fusion Technique: Occiput, C1, and C2

While the purpose of this chapter is not to discuss the surgical solution to each potential problem affecting the cervical spine, one of the more compli-cated problems occuring in this anatomic region is the upward migration into the foramen magnum of the ring of C1 and/or the tip of the odontoid process. When either or both of these situations exists,

Fig. 15-51. (A) Lateral cervical spine radiograph in 23-year-old man with multiple cervical spine congenital abnormalities. Neurologic examination revealed upper and lower extremity spasticity. Radiograph shows that the odontoid process lies within the foramen magnum (basilar impression); the ring of C1 lies anterior to the posterior ring of the foramen magnum; and there is failure of segmentation of C5–C6. *(Figure continues.)*

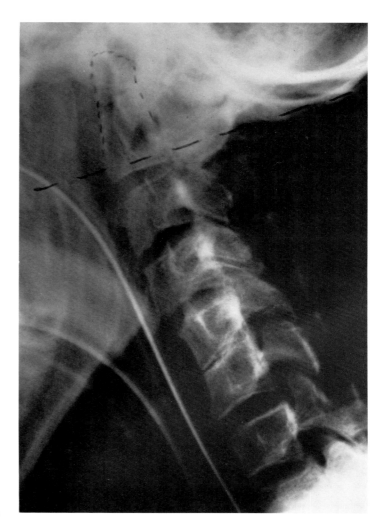

A

one or several surgical procedures may be indicated:

1. Resection of the anterior ring of C1
2. Amputation of the odontoid process
3. Excision of the clivus or the posteroinferior bony surface of the posterior cranial fossa, (the portion sloping upward from the foramen magnum to the dorsum sella
4. Excision of the posterior ring of C1
5. Posterior cervical spine fusion, extending from the posterior occiput to the posterior element of C2 or C3.

The first three procedures employ an anterior approach (Fig. 15-52)–either the retropharyngeal or the trans-oral approach.[66,69-71]

A comment concerning the performance of procedures 1 through 4. When procedures 1 and 2 are performed, resection of both the anterior rings of C2, excision of the odontoid, and resection of the clivas, may allow further penetration of the upper cervical spine into the already compromised foramen magnum. The further result of excising the anterior ring of C1 (along with the odontoid process) is anterior migration of the remaining segment of the posterior ring of C1, producing further

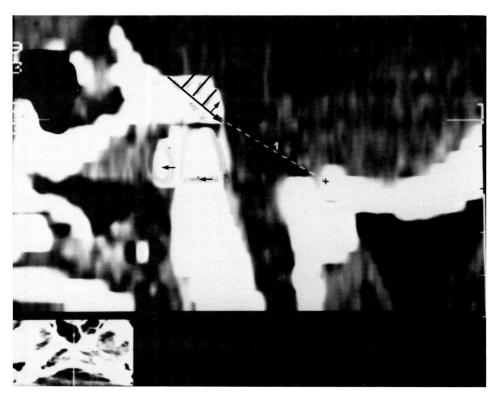

B

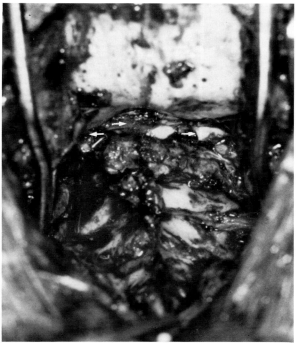

C

Fig. 15-51 *(Continued).* **(B)** Sagittal reformatted CT scan of the occipitoatlantal junction revealing prominence of the clivis portion of the base of the skull (hatch-marked area) and entrapment of the odontoid process within the foramen magnum resulting in compression of the brain stem. Before the planned posterior stabilization, the anterior ring of C1, odontoid process (see arrows), and clivis were removed through a transoral approach (by the neurosurgeon). The patient was maintained in cervical traction until the posterior cervical spine fusion was undertaken. For the fusion operation, the patient was placed in halo tong traction and evoked potential monitoring sensors attached to vertex region of scalp. Following initiation of anesthesia and prone placement on a Stryker frame, alternating pressure cuffs are applied to the lower extremities and are used throughout the operation to prevent deep venous thrombosis. **(C)** Operative view of posterior occipital cervical spine approach. Occiput revealing platybasia can be seen at top. Arrows show region from which posterior ring of C1 was removed, revealing the underlying dura. *(Figure continues.)*

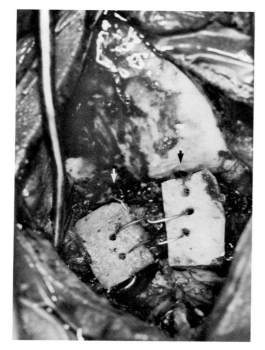

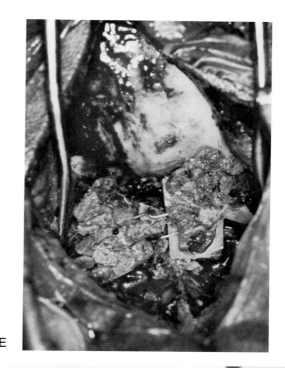

D

E

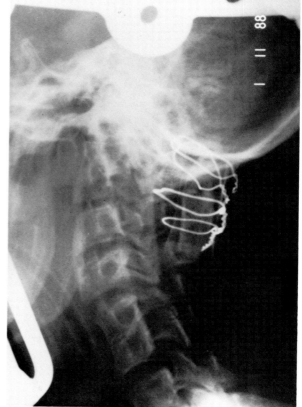

Fig. 15-51 *(Continued).* **(D)** Posterior cervical spine fusion using iliac crest bone graft. Wires for stabilizing the bone graft are placed through holes on either side of the occiput ¼ inch from the foramen magnum, but lateral to the midline so as not to enter the centrally located venous sinus. The bone graft is held to posterior elements C2 and C3 by wires placed through the base of the spinous process of each. **(E)** Cancellous bone graft is applied to the surface of the occiput and the iliac crest bone graft after roughening of the external surface. Care is taken not to allow bone graft to fall against the dura at C1. At the end of the operation, an antero-posterior halo shell was applied and the patient was removed from traction. **(F)** Intraoperative lateral radiograph of patient in halo vest showing cervical spine alignment and bone graft fixation and placement.

F

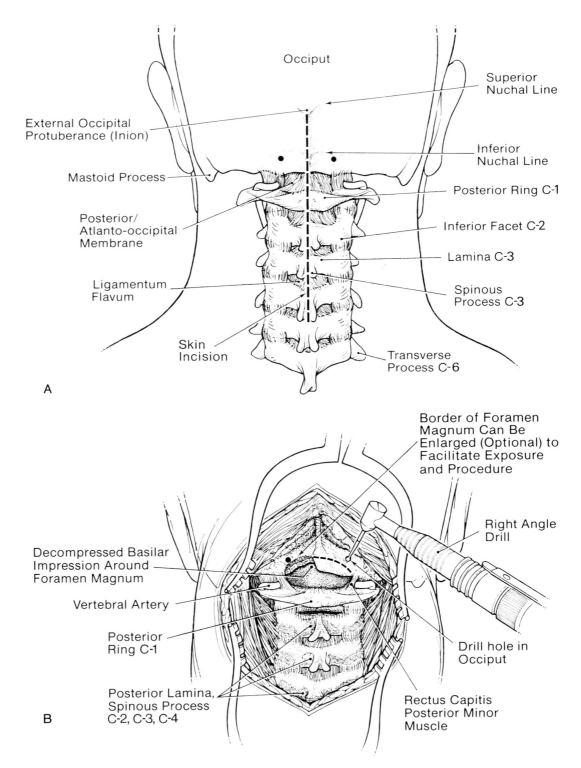

Fig. 15-52. Posterior surgical fusion technique: occiput–C1–C2. *(Figure continues.)*

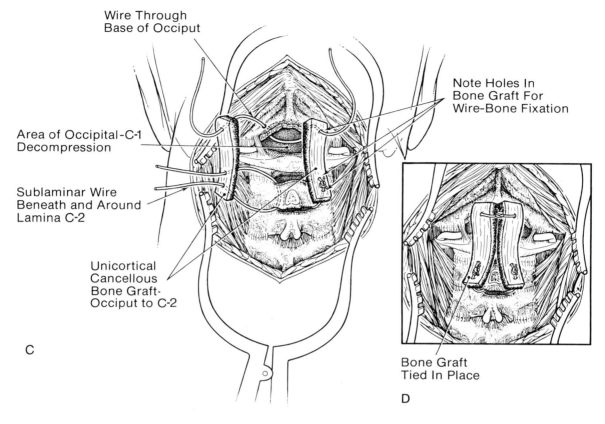

Wire Through
Base of Occiput

Note Holes In
Bone Graft For
Wire-Bone Fixation

Area of Occipital-C-1
Decompression

Sublaminar Wire
Beneath and Around
Lamina C-2

Unicortical
Cancellous
Bone Graft-
Occiput to C-2

C

D

Bone Graft
Tied In Place

Fig. 15-52 *(Continued)*.

compression on the brain stem or upper spinal cord. When possible, the posterior ring of C1 should not be excised. Its presence will facilitate obtaining a posterior fusion (along with the postoperative immobilization of the patient in a halo vest).

The surgical inclusion of the occiput into a posterior C1–C2–C3 fusion is essential when there is gross occipitoatlantal joint instability (as with rheumatoid arthritis), or a defect in the posterior ring of C1. Adding this procedure to the more standardized C1–C2 fusion adds significantly to the hazards. These include hemorrhage, epidural hematoma, and high spinal cord neurologic injury. Fusion from the occiput to C1–C2 is difficult and cumbersome to perform, even in the absence of any unusual anatomic variations (Fig. 15-52B). When congenital deformities exist, often there will be a shortening of the cervical spine, making the

occiput–C1–C2–C3 fusion difficult, dangerous, and sometimes almost impossible to visualize adequately. Even with an awareness of the region, complications may arise.[23,67]

The surgical approach to the posterior cervical spine, which includes the occipital region of the calvaria, is via the straight posterior midline approach (Fig. 15-52A). The incision extends from the inion of the calvaria distally to the level of the third or fourth cervical spinous process. The incision is carried down through the subcutaneous tissue to the occipital region of the calvaria and along the midline ligamentum nuchae to the underlying spinous processes. The muscle and fascial attachments to the spinous processes are dissected by sharp and electrocautery dissection. This technique significantly reduces interfascial-periosteal bleeding. The posterior aspect of the occiput and the posterior rings of C1, C2, and C3 (for exposure purposes) are denuded of their muscular and ligamentous attachments by dissecting scissor, electrocautery, and subperiosteal-periosteal elevator dissection. Care is necessary, as upper cervical spine instability may exist if C1 and the odontoid process have been removed.

The occiput–C1 membrane and the ligamentum flavum between C1 and C2 are carefully incised, allowing for the passage of sutures or wires as described below for the Meyer and Gallie techniques. The holes placed in the occiptial region, approximately 3/4 to 1 cm from the posterior border of the foramen magnum, are placed in the posterior occiput, one or two on either side of the midline, where fixation of the bone graft to the calvaria is required. Wertheim describes the placement of a transverse drill hole across the "keel" region of the occiput below the inion, in the midline overlying the cerebellum, into which a wire is placed for fixation of the bone graft to the calvaria.[71] This is an excellent technique if this bony prominence exists. If it does not, holes close to the border of the foramen are appropriate. (Fig. 15-52B). A wire suture (18 gauge) is passed through the holes in the occiput, and brought out through the foramen magnum (Fig. 15-51). Other wires for stabilization of the bone graft are placed through the base of the spinous process of C2 and C3, and tightened over the bone graft in the routine fashion (see Fig. 15-60), or beneath the lamina as shown in Figure 15-52. If the posterior ring of C1 is present, and is not displaced anteriorly, a sublaminar wire can be placed around C1 as shown in Figure 15-51, and the two strands used to tighten down the bone graft at this level. The most appropriate bone graft for this fusion procedure is that obtained from the external surface of the ilium (Fig. 15-12). With care, the bicortical bone graft can be removed from the ilium with breaking it across its midplane. The benefit of using a graft from this area is that the curve of the graft (due to the shape of the iliac wing) allows the graft to better match the area to be spanned.

Before inserting the bone graft, the external surface of the occiput and the lamina overlying the area to be incorporated in the fusion are roughened or partically decorticated with a Hall high-speed burr. Matching holes are drilled in the graft for the insertion of the pre-positioned wires, and the graft is tightened in place (Fig. 15-52D). Postopera-

tively, the patient can either be managed in Gardner-Wells tong traction for a variable period of time (if there is concern over the presence of a neurologic injury), or, where stability is a question, placed in a halo vest after surgery. In certain situations the use of a less stable orthosis may be indicated, but it is appropriate to wait several weeks before using a SOMI (sternal occipital mandibular immobilizer) type orthosis on a occiput-upper cervical spine fusion. The minimum duration of postoperative immobilization in an orthosis is 3 months.

Additional Concerns: Occiput-Cervical Spine Fusion

During the performance of a occipital-cervical spine fusion, because of the close proximity of the brain stem and the upper cervical spinal cord, that the anesthesiologist allow the patient to breathe by spontaneously throughout surgery. This allows both the anesthesiologist and the surgeon to constantly monitor the patients neurologic status. Similarly, the use of somatosensory evoked potential monitoring is indicated throughout surgery for the same reasons.

It is that patients with known cervical spine injury be transferred carefully to the operating table to prevent further injury. Whenever possible, the patient should be transferred awake, and in the supine position only. When the patient must be transferred from a frame or bed to the operating table, at least five or six individuals should be available to assist with the transfer. One person is always responsible for the head and neck alone. Patients requiring prone positioning for a posterior cervical spine procedure should always be placed preoperatively on a Stryker wedge frame in skeletal traction, whether the procedure is elective or for trauma. Patients that have been managed on a Roto-Rest bed in skeletal traction should be transferred to a Stryker frame preoperatively. This reduces the likelihood of causing or extending neurologic injury during transfer or prone positioning of the patient on the table.

While alterations in a patient's voluntary respiratory pattern usually indicate the presence of some form of neurologic embarrassment to the upper cervical spinal cord, the absence of such an alteration should not lull the surgeon into believing that all is well. Spine malalignment can and does occur during prone positioning of a patient on an operating table. For that reason it is recommended that the patient enter the operating room on a Stryker Wedge frame in skeletal traction, be anesthetized in a supine position, and then be turned to the prone position on the same Stryker frame. If any question exists, a lateral radiograph of the spine should then be obtained.

An alternative method of ensuring head-neck stability during the transfer-prone turning process is to place patients with gross instability into a halo vest preoperatively. If the patient is neurologically sound, it allows the patient to be pre-operative mobile, insures a stable spine relationship during turning, and provides for rigid post-operative immobilization. The halo vest is my preferred technique for managing patients who demonstrate pre-operative upper cervical spine instability, for example the cervical spine patient with dissolution of the odontoid process secondary to rheumatoid arthritis. The major disadvantage of having a patient in a halo vest during surgery is the occasional need to change the head-neck relationship during surgery. This is particularly a problem when the

surgeon is working in the occiput–C1 area. Even so, preoperative planning will allow a halo vest to be used, and when required, changes to be made.

Sublaminar Wire Stabilization

Using sublaminar wires to stabilize the cervical spine after a flexion injury is the most stable technique available, but it may not be the most safe. Care must be taken using this technique, even when the patient's neurologic level is complete. Because neurologic complications have followed the insertion of sublaminar wires between C3 and C7 in patients with an incomplete neurologic injury, *this procedure is not recommended in the patient with incomplete neurologic injuries. This rule holds true for all injuries below C3.*

Because the neural canal is wide at levels of the occiput–C1 (2.1 cm) and C2 (2.0 cm) (see Fig. 1-3), sublaminar wires can be used safely at these levels, with considerably less danger of producing neurologic injury. Nonetheless, patients should be carefully monitored by SSEP.

The insertion of sublaminar wires—that is, under the posterior elements between C3 and C7

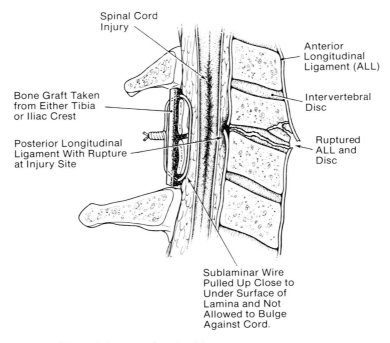

Fig. 15-53. Two-level sublaminar wire technique.

—necessitates considerable caution, as noted. When sublaminar wires are used across two levels only (Fig. 15-53), it has been noted that, when tightened, the wires tend to flatten out along the undersurface of the adjacent lamina. This reduces the risk of compromising the neural canal. On the other hand, when a sublaminar wire is passed beneath three laminae, there is a tendency for the wire to "bow" anteriorly, compromising the neural canal and encroaching on the dura and spinal cord (Figs. 15-54, 15-55). This occurred twice (0.06 percent), with severe neurologic sequea. The use of the technique was then discontinued in any patient who either had incomplete injury or was intact below C3.

In both patients in whom neurologic complications appeared, the patients reported their changing neurologic picture and both required immediate postoperative myelography. One myelogram

revealed encroachment on the dura without complete obstruction. It was thought that the wires did not require removal. The neurologic deterioration noted did not recover, despite immediate attempts to artifically increase the blood pressure by the IVs administration of sympathomimetic drugs (isoproterenol hydrochloride and dopamine hydrochloride). The second patient underwent a portable myelogram in the recovery room area. He was noted to have a complete obstruction (Fig. 15-56). The patient was immediately returned to the operating room where the operative site was explored and the sublaminar wires were found to be in an anterior bowed position, sufficient to produce positive compression (and compromise) of the dura and cervical spinal cord. The wires were removed and a partial laminotomy was performed. The bone graft inserted at the time for fusion was replaced without fixation. Postoperatively, the patient remained in cervical traction for 6 weeks. The neurologic loss that developed during surgery was incompletely recovered. Both of the complications occurred before the availability of SSEP monitoring at surgery. Both solidified the indications for its availability and use.

Thus, except at the C1–C2–C3 level, sublaminar wires should not be used in any patient with no or an incomplete neurologic injury and should be cautiously used even in the patient with a complete neurologic injury for fear of producing an upward extension of the already present neurologic injury. The technique now recommended for intact and incomplete neurologically injured patients with flexion-induced unstable cervical spine injuries is a Meyer modification of the Garber posterior cervical spine fusion technique (C3 to C7). (see Fig. 15-60).

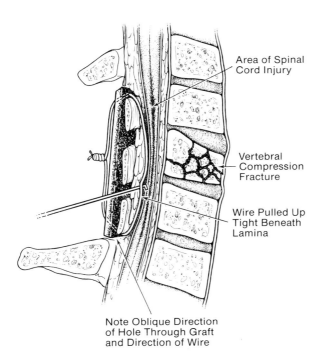

Area of Spinal Cord Injury

Vertebral Compression Fracture

Wire Pulled Up Tight Beneath Lamina

Note Oblique Direction of Hole Through Graft and Direction of Wire

Fig. 15-54. Three-level sublaminar wiring procedure to correct unstable compression fracture of vertebra resulting in kyphosis. Note the depiction of the major hazard of using sublaminar wires—anterior bowing. A hook is shown being used to reduce this hazard.

Passage of Sublaminar Wires: C1 to C3, C3 to C7

After the ligamentum flavum is incised between the occiput and the posterior arch of C1, with Gardner-Wells tongs in place and the head in slight flexion, and between the laminae of C1 and C2, and C2 and C3 if necessary, the epidural fat and the dura should be visible at each level. Using a vascular surgery instrument (the right- or left-turned aneurysm needle), the needle with a no. 2 Taudec suture is passed from inferior the respective lamina

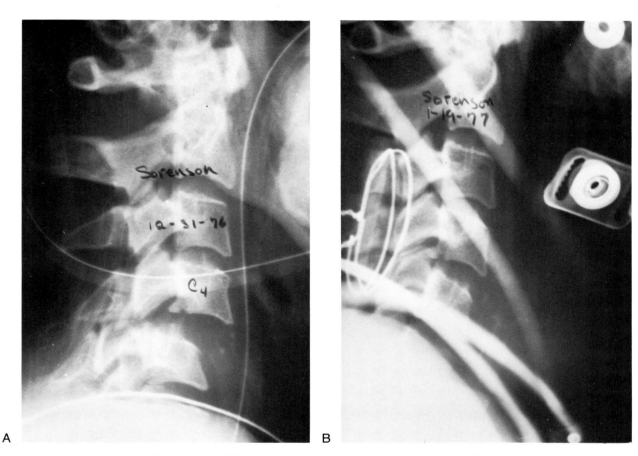

Fig. 15-55. **(A)** Bilateral facet joint dislocation at C4 – C5. Note avulsion fracture of the posteroinferior C4 vertebral body resulting from avulsion of the posterior longitudinal ligament. **(B)** Post-operative lateral radiograph. Note three-level sublaminar wire fixation. The hazard of three-level mid-cervical spine sublaminar wire fixation is anterior bowing of the internal fixation wires. While the procedure produces stable spine fixation, neural canal and neural tissue compromise may occur. Therefore, sublaminar wires should not be used between C3 and C4 when the patient is neurologically intact or has an incomplete neurologic injury.

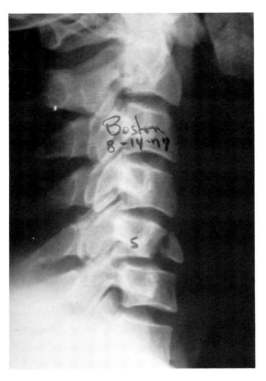

A

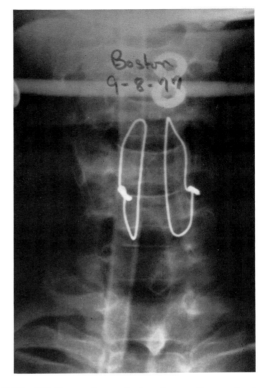

B

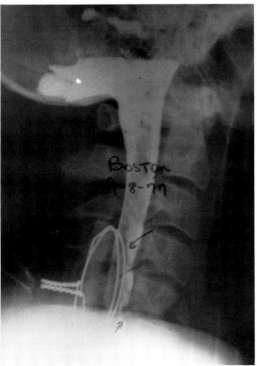

C

Fig. 15-56. (**A**) Lateral cervical spine radiograph showing retropulsion of C5 on C6 and anterior teardrop fracture involving the C5 vertebral body. Retropulsion of the upper vertebra is now known to indicate bilateral posterior element fracture. (**B**) Fracture stabilized by three-level sublaminar Garber-Meyer posterior fusion technique. Note position of sublaminar wires. (**C**) Lateral myelogram obtained in the recovery room after the patient reported progressive loss of motor and sensory function. Myelogram demonstrates anterior bowing of the sublaminar wires producing encroachment on neural canal and obstructing the flow of contrast medium past the fracture site. The internal fixation was immediately removed; the patient had incomplete return of motor and sensory function.

to superior at each level, in turn. Passage of the suture proximally is recommended because of the anatomic attachment of the ligamentum flavum (which passes from the superior border of each lamina to the undersurface of the lamina above). When the aneurysm needle and suture are passed from inferior to superior, beneath the ring of C1, the tip will exit between C1 and the occiput. The Taudec suture in the eye of the aneurysm needle (approximately 14 to 16 inches in length) is passed beneath each successive level (C1, C2, then C3) with the needle rethreaded each time at each lower level. The suture, when in place, should lie beneath the C1, C2, or C3 lamina, if all three levels are to be incorporated in the fusion (Fig. 15-57). This technique is either done again on the opposite side (one suture on either side of the midline), or a longer suture can be used initially, pulling the looped end inferiorly, upon which the loop can be cut inferiorly, and each suture in turn attached to a 10-inch straight length of 18-gauge wire. The wire is carefully bent into a small loop at one end, and the Taudec suture is tied to the loop with a "fisherman knot" (Fig. 15-51D). The loop should be flattened with needlenose pliers. Care must be taken during the passage of the wire that the wire at the loop does not injure the dura (anterior to the wire) as it passes proximally. Such injuries can occur, but have not ever produced an injury of consequence. When the wire is pulled beneath the lamina, the suture is held taut at both ends and is pulled in a proximal direction with tension maintained inferi-

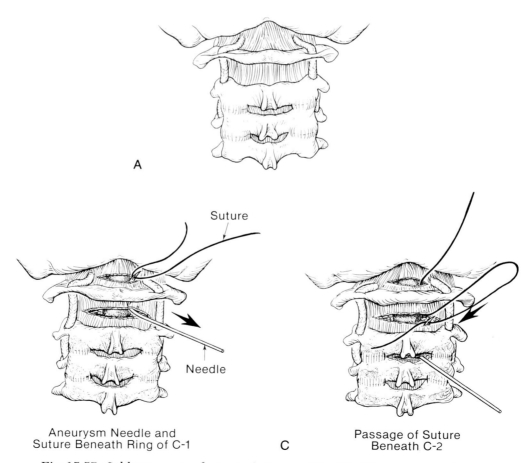

A

Suture

Needle

B   Aneurysm Needle and
Suture Beneath Ring of C-1

C   Passage of Suture
Beneath C-2

Fig. 15-57. Sublaminar wire fusion technique at C1–C2. *(Figure continues.)*

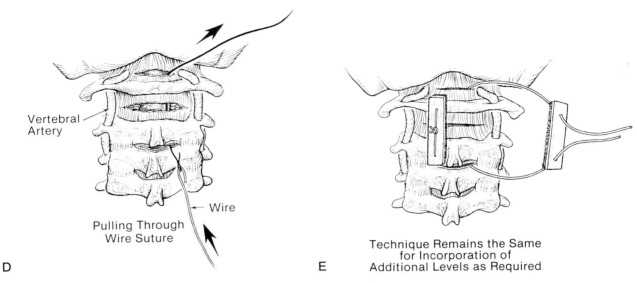

Fig. 15-57 *(Continued).*

orly on the wire, preventing any anterior bowing of the wire in the direction of the neural elements. When the wire is in place, a hook instrument is passed between each lamina into the interspace, and any anterior bowing of the wire is removed by lifting dorsally on the wire.

If the Gallie wire technique is used, a single Tau-dec suture is passed (as described above) and tied at the center of a loop of 18-gauge wire (measuring approximately 16 inches long). The center of the wire loop (or Luque wire) is then pulled proximally, beneath the appropriate laminae (of C1 and C2), leaving the two free ends inferiorly. For a two-level fusion, such as C1 – C2, this technique is adequate. For more than two levels, the passage of a single, doubled wire becomes more difficult. A sublaminar wire should not be utilized below the level of C3, in any patient with an intact neurologic level (see pp. 491 and 498) (Figs. 15-53, 15-58).

Meyer Modification of the Garber Posterior Cervical Spine Fusion Technique: C1 to C3, C3 to C7

The technique described here, while initially thought of as original, is not. Similar bone graft fixation techniques have been proposed by others and originality often expressed. The initial descrip-tion, although not identical to ours, is very similar. The procedure is credited to Neil J. Garber of Indi-anapolis, IN, in 1961.[23,24] The present procedure is so titled to denote those aspects of the present technique thought unique.

This procedure follows the placement bilaterally of sublaminar wires, which span the two or three lamina to be incorporated in the fusion mass (in the patient rendered neurologically complete). As noted in Figure 15-18, because of the use of a pos-terior approach and the use of interspinous process wire, fixation of the unstable bilaminar fracture usually failed. For this reason, this particular frac-ture is now stabilized via the anterior approach. For the cervical spine that is stable and requiring a posterior fusion, the technique utilized is as fol-lows: one wire is placed through the base of the spinous process at the upper end and a second wire is placed through the base of the spinous process at the lower extent of the area to be fused (Fig. 15-60A,B). One 18-gauge wire is used proximally, and one is used distally. This allows the bone graft to be placed down upon the laminae being incorpo-rated in the fusion, with the proximal wire through the proximal end of the graft and the distal wire through the distal end of the graft. This is done bilaterally. Before the application of the bone graft (cancellous side down) against the posterior sur-

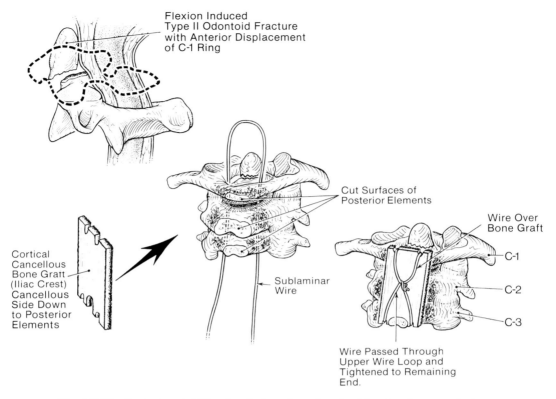

Flexion Induced
Type II Odontoid Fracture
with Anterior Displacement
of C-1 Ring

Cut Surfaces of
Posterior Elements

Wire Over
Bone Graft

C-1

C-2

C-3

Cortical
Cancellous
Bone Graft
(Iliac Crest)
Cancellous
Side Down
to Posterior
Elements

Sublaminar
Wire

Wire Passed Through
Upper Wire Loop and
Tightened to Remaining
End.

Fig. 15-58. Posterior stabilization fusion three-level sublaminar bone technique.

face of the lamina, the surface of each lamina is superficially denuded of all soft tissue and the cortex is roughened on the outer surface (Fig. 15-60C,D). After this procedure, the wires are simultaneously tightened at the midpoint. During the act of tightening, vertical (dorsal) tension is maintained on the twisting wires. The wires are cut appropriately short, and the tip of each spinous process throughout the extent of the fusion is rongeured (permitting exposure of bleeding bone to the cancellous bone graft). Additional cancellous bone is then applied along each gutter and over both cortical strips (Fig. 15-60E).

If cervical traction is in place during the operative procedure, all weight should be removed while the wires are being tightened. Traction may be discontinued if the spine is considered stable. If the patient is to be turned supine and an anterior spine procedure performed, the head and neck should be maintained in modest traction for support.

If an exposed area of the dura mater lies between the posterior elements in the area of the fusion, a small shaped Gelfoam pad can be applied to prevent accidental encroachment of the dura by cancellous bone graft. The wound is carefully closed in layers, with figure-of-eight 2–0 Dexon sutures in the muscle and fascia, 3–0 Dexon in the subcutaneous tissue, and a 2–0 Prolene subcuticular skin closure.

Use of CO_2 Laser for Supine Dissection

A more recent surgical technique used in the performance of the posterior approach to the cervical spine is the use of a CO_2 laser for making the skin incision, the subperiosteal muscle dissection down to the posterior lamina, and the transverse hole through the base of the spinous process.

Using the laser to make the skin incision does cause some delay in skin healing (owing to radiated heat). This necessitates the use of either staples or interrupted sutures in the skin for a slightly longer

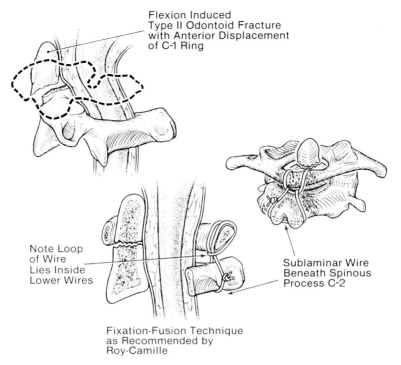

Flexion Induced
Type II Odontoid Fracture
with Anterior Displacement
of C-1 Ring

Note Loop
of Wire
Lies Inside
Lower Wires

Sublaminar Wire
Beneath Spinous
Process C-2

Fixation-Fusion Technique
as Recommended by
Roy-Camille

Fig. 15-59. Roy-Camille posterior fusion technique for flexion fracture of odontoid process of C2.

period (3 weeks) than with a subcuticular closure. The resulting scar is slightly wider when made by a laser incision than that resulting from sharp dissection. The use of the laser does, however, reduce the time required for the operative procedure, significantly reduces the amount of blood loss, and allows for the continuous monitoring of spinal cord function by the evoked potential unit, without the electrical interference noted when using the standard electrocautery instrument.

The Gallie Posterior (C1–C2) Fusion

When no fracture or no unstable fracture of the posterior arch of C1 exists, and reduction of the odontoid process has been accomplished by skeletal traction (using 5 to 10 lbs), the posterior approach with the sublaminar placement of wires and the application of a bone graft described by Gallie is indicated.[32] With the patient anesthetized and in the prone position, a posterior midline incision is made extending from the inion process of the occiput to the level of the posterior spinous process of C3 (Fig. 15-52). The only real difficulty of this approach is the close proximity between the inferior occiput and the posterior arch of C1. This can usually be adjusted by placing the head and neck into a slightly flexed position. To facilitate this, a transverse roll across the upper aspect of the patient's chest, at the level of the shoulders, or tilting the head by means of tong traction will open up the occipitoatlantal interspace. Additional traction may also be carefully added. Cortical SSEP monitoring of spinal cord function should be conducted throughout the surgical procedure, particularly in the presence of an intact or incomplete neurologic system.

The Gallie procedure[32] requires the passing of an 18-gauge wire beneath the laminae of the posterior elements of C1 and C2 or (in some cases when there exists an associated posterior element hangman's fracture through the pedicle of C2) beneath the posterior element of C3. While the technique of passing a sublaminar wire requires some experience and manipulative dexterity, with care it can be accomplished without problem. Caution must be taken, however, inasmuch as there is only a

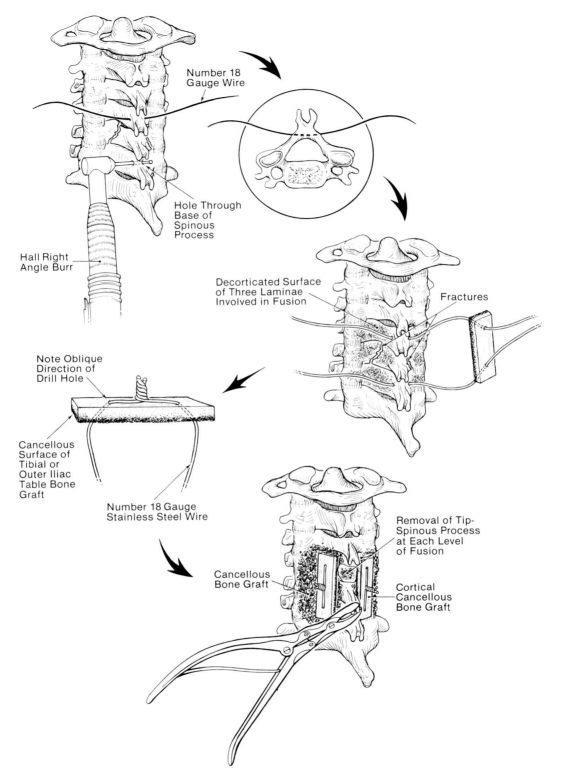

Fig. 15-60. Posterior spinous process wiring technique using cortical-cancellous bone graft (Garber-Meyer) technique.

2-mm space between the interior border of the lamina and the most posterior portion of the dura. Another caution taken during exposing of the posterior ring of C1 is to remain in the midline, carefully stripping subperiosteally only 1 cm in either direction laterally. This will prevent potential injury to the vertebral artery as it loops over the posterior ring of C1 to enter the cranium through the foramen magnum (Fig. 15-57).

After sublaminar placement of a loop of 18-gauge stainless-steel wire beneath the laminae of C2 and C1, an H-shaped bone graft obtained from the external surface of the posterior iliac crest is tightened in place by the passage of one free end of the wire inferiorly, through the loop of wire superiorly, and then tightened to the remaining free end of the wire on the other side inferiorly. This, in effect, tightens the sublaminarly placed wire on the external surface of the H-shaped graft and compresses this graft against the posterior laminae of C1 and C2 (Fig. 15-61). Before the application of the H-shaped graft, the external surfaces of the laminae at C1 and C2 are denuded of all soft tissue and external cortex with a high-speed burr.

Cervical traction can be discontinued, and the patient can be managed postoperatively in a **SOMI** orthosis or Philadelphia collar.

Brooks Fusion Technique

The Brooks posterior C1–C2 fusion technique[37] differs only slightly from the standard C1–C2 sublaminar technique described by Meyer (Fig. 15-62). The Brooks technique includes the introduction of a bone graft between the inferior ring of C1 and the superior surface of the spinous process and lamina of C2. The technique calls for the use of

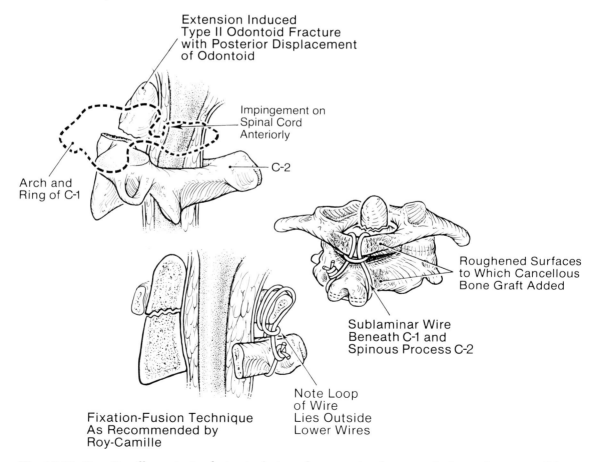

Extension Induced
Type II Odontoid Fracture
with Posterior Displacement
of Odontoid

Impingement on
Spinal Cord
Anteriorly

C-2

Arch and
Ring of C-1

Roughened Surfaces
to Which Cancellous
Bone Graft Added

Sublaminar Wire
Beneath C-1 and
Spinous Process C-2

Note Loop
of Wire
Lies Outside
Lower Wires

Fixation-Fusion Technique
As Recommended by
Roy-Camille

Fig. 15-61. Roy-Camille posterior fusion technique for extension fracture of odontoid process of C2.

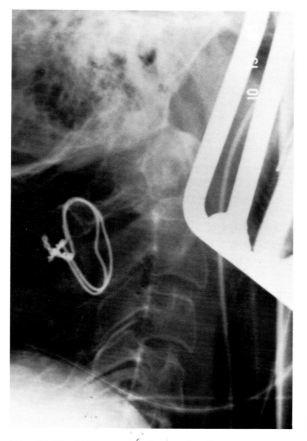
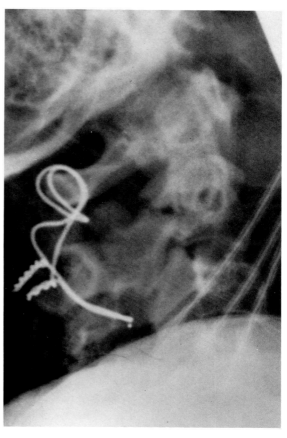

A   B

Fig. 15-62. (A) Lateral radiograph of a posterior cervical spine fusion of C1–C2 using the sublaminar wire fixation technique for type III odontoid fracture. Note approximation of posterior elements of C1 and C2. (B) Lateral radiograph of a cervical spine fusion of C1–C3 for an unstable C2 posterior element (hangman's) fracture. The fusion is a combination of the Roy-Camille and Brooks fusion techniques. Note the wire loop on the posterior ring of C1 and the inclusion of bone graft between posterior elements C1 and C2.

a single wire on the right and left sides, to prevent displacement of the bone graft anteriorly between C1 and C2 and to provide compression of the ring of C1 against the bone graft and the lamina of C2 (Fig. 15-63).

Callahan Modification of the Brooks C1–C2 Fusion

The Callahan modification is identical to the Brooks procedure described above, except for the position of the wires at the level of C1. When the neural canal is severely compromised at the C1 level, contraindicating placement of sublaminar wires beneath the posterior ring of C1, Callahan et al. recommend the placement of a perpendicular

hole through the ring of C1 bilaterally, permitting the sublaminar wire at C2 to be passed proximally through the ring of C1 and then tightened in the standard Brooks technique dorsally, over bone grafts inserted bilaterally between the C1 and C2 posterior spinous processes.[48]

Roy-Camille Posterior Fusion Technique For Flexion-Extension Fractures of Odontoid Process (C2)

Roy-Camille and colleagues recommend C1 sublaminar-C2 spinous process wire fixation for fractures involving the odontoid process of C2.[40] Their technique varies only in the position of placement of the wire loop around the posterior ring of C1 (Figs. 15-59, 15-61). The two alternatives are as follows. For flexion injuries of the odontoid process, when the odontoid lies anterior to the body of C2, to pull the ring of C1 posteriorly, the loop of the wire lies inside the ring of C1 (Fig. 15-59). For extension fractures of the odontoid, when the odontoid is posteriorly displaced, the wire loop lies outside the posterior ring of C1 (Fig. 15-61). Whether these variations truly alter the position of the C1-odontoid (C2) complex is difficult to say for certain. With either variation, however, the two free ends of the wire are not sublaminar to C2; rather, they are external to the C2 posterior element and beneath the inferior border of the spinous process of C2. A complication of this pro-

cedure is an inadvertent angulation or translatory displacement of the odontoid process in relation to the body of C2, as the posterior ring of C1 is approximated with the posterior process of C2. Neurologic alterations with this complication have been reported, prompting Brooks and Jenkins in 1978 to describe their variation of the Roy-Camille fusion technique.[37] Their suggestion was that a bicortical segment of iliac crest be removed (as for a Robinson-Southwick anterior interbody fusion[14]; Fig. 15-63) and placed between the posterior ring of C1 and the spinous process of C2. Such a bone graft will allow the sublaminar spinous process wires to be tightened without the likelihood of overcompression of the C1 and C2 posterior element and the potential displacement of the frac-

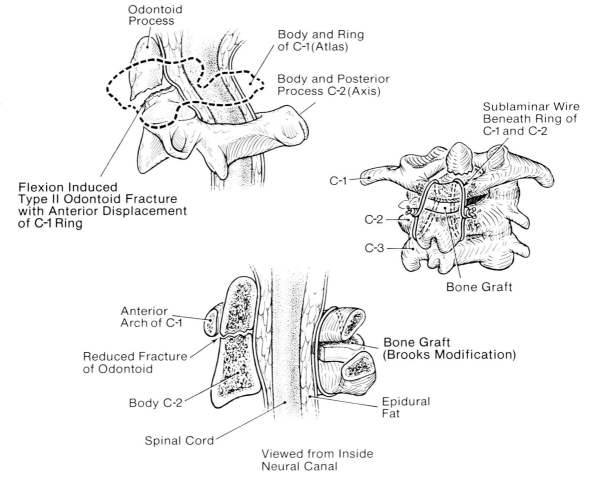

Fig. 15-63. Posterior fusion technique combining the use of sublaminar C1–C2 wire fixation with the addition of bone graft between spinous processes C1 and C2 (Brooks modification).

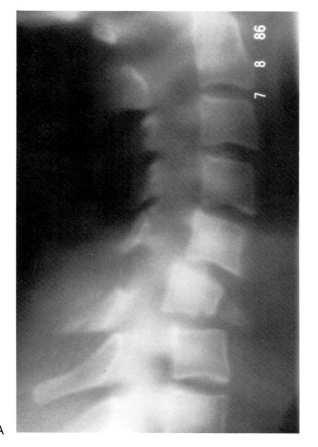
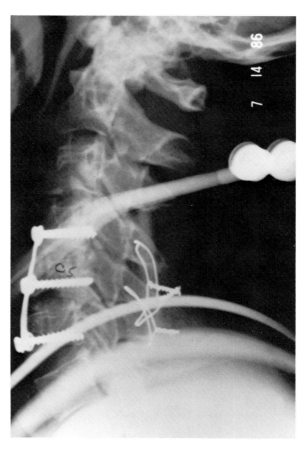

A   B

Fig. 15-64. (A) Lateral cervical spine radiograph showing unstable axial load flexion injury of the cervical spine resulting in a wedge compression fracture of C6, posterior displacement of the C6 vertebral body on C7 (indicating posterior bilaminar fracture), and diastasis of the posterior elements of C5 and C6. (B) Lateral radiograph after posterior and anterior spine fusion. A double-wire posterior fusion technique was used. Because of postoperative evidence of instability after the initial posterior fusion, a three-level anterior AO plate-screw procedure was used for C4–C6. Bone graft was inserted anteriorly before application of plate within disc spaces C4–5, C5–6. This fracture pattern is now recognized as grossly unstable and best-managed by anterior plate and screw fixation.

tured segment of the odontoid process (Fig. 15-64).

Roy-Camille Plate-Screw Fusion Technique

Roy-Camille and co-workers designed a plate and screw combination to stabilize the unstable occiput-C1 junction by stabilizing the posterior calvaria to the posterior elements of C1 and C2 (Fig. 15-65).[40] This technique has not been utilized by us, but is included for completeness. In a recent conversation (1987), Professor Roy-Camille noted that the procedure continues to be utilized in France without complications.

The use of the Roy-Camille posterior cervical spine plate and screw fixation technique is popular in Europe. It addresses the posterior structure injuries directly. In the United States and Switzerland, the anterior plate and screw technique would probably be more appropriate, allowing for intervertebral disc removal at the level of injury.

Use of Methyl Methacrylate: Bone Graft Technique

The use of methyl methacrylate in gaining rigid spine stability has been suggested by numerous re-

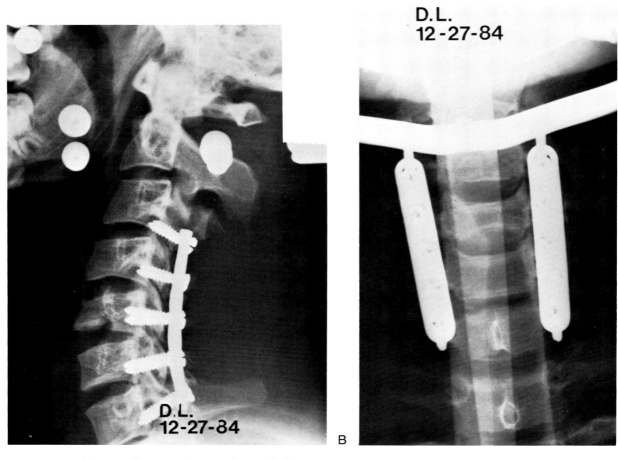

Fig. 15-65. (A) Lateral cervical spine radiograph showing Roy-Camille plate and screws used for an unstable fracture of the posterior elements of the C5 vertebral body. Note resection of spinous processes C4–C6. (B) AP view showing screw placement lateral to pedicles, overlying the facet joints and facing laterally approximately by 20 degrees.

searchers.[62,68] The principal indication has been its use in patients with tumorous involvement of the spine resulting in gross vertebral element instability.

Methyl methacrylate is sometimes used to enhance fixation. It is applied over the external surface of the bone graft fixed to the posterior elements of the cervical spine by wire fixation. The technique devised by Davey et al. specifically for spinal instability incorporated the use of transverse Steinmann pins through bone grafts placed in approximation with the base of the spinous processes above and below the area of pathology.[63] Methyl methacrylate has been used in conjunction with the wire bone graft technique by other surgeons (Fig. 15-66).

A major concern with the use of methyl methacrylate is whether or not there is a higher incidence of infection or nonunion when this substance is used. The literature reveals neither. Concern for the amount of methyl methacrylate used and good standard wound closure are both important in attaining primary uncomplicated wound healing.

Combined Anteroposterior Spine Fusion
Occasionally, the surgical procedure utilized as the stabilizing procedure for a spinal injury fails. Under these circumstances, an additional opera-

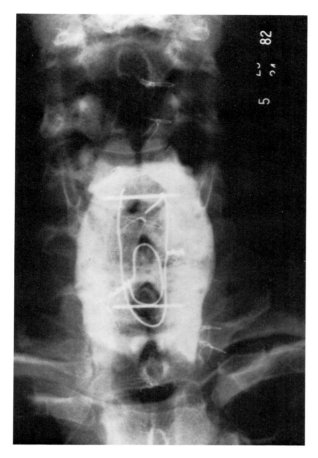

Fig. 15-66. AP radiograph showing transverse Stein-mann pin and circular wire fixation used beneath and within methylmethacrylate. This method of fracture fixation is unorthodox and not recommended.

tive procedure becomes necessary to ensure stability.

As noted in Figure 15-64, a compression fracture of the vertebral body of C6 with diastasis of the posterior interlaminar space at C5 – C6 appears to demonstrate that the area of maximum instability lies posteriorly. For this reason, a posterior double wire fusion procedure was performed, utilizing one wire across the area of distasis between the spinous processes of C5 – C6 and an overall fusion from C4 – C6 with an iliac or, as in this case, a tibial bone graft (Meyer technique).

Upon completion of this operative procedure, it was apparent that further posterior displacement of the C5 vertebral body on C6 was occurring. This

problem has been previously identified and discussed (see Unstable Flexion-Axial Load-Induced Bilaminar Vertebral Body Injuries, above). To correct the existing cervical instability, an anterior AO plate and screws were used with interbody fusion performed on C4 to C6. Postoperatively, the patient was immobilized for 3 months in a SOMI orthosis.

Other situations in which a combined anteroposterior approach performed either simultaneously or separately may be indicated are for patients having posterior procedures that have failed to maintain stability, or when the patient demonstrates postoperative signs of increasing neurologic disability (anterior herniated nucleopropulsus that follows a previous posterior stabilizing procedure) (Fig. 15-67C).

Bone Graft (Donor) Procedures

Selection of Bone Graft Site
The source of a bone graft is dictated by the type of graft required, whether two surgical teams (neurosurgery and orthopaedics) are operating simultaneously, and the surgeon's choice. When a large amount of bone is required for the surface area being fused, or in the presence of a large bony defect, the outer table of the posterior iliac wing is probably the best source, outside the use of femoral head allografts. An additional advantage to the use of the iliac wing is access to a copious amount of both cortical and cancellous bone.

When an anterior cervical spine fusion (either single or multiple levels) is proposed, without the need for a vertebral body corporectomy, the vertebral cortical end plates should be maintained and a tricortical iliac bone graft from the anterior iliac crest utilized (Fig. 15-45F). When an anterior vetebral body inlay graft is required, either a tricortical iliac crest bone graft or a corticocancellous bone graft from the proximal anteromedial tibia can be used. This latter site is selected when the operative procedure is performed simultaneously by both the orthopaedic and neurosurgery services (taking a tibial bone graft allows both teams to proceed at opposite ends of the table simultaneously and unencumbered); a strong, stable bone graft is required; or when copious cancellous bone graft is also required. Such graft material can be simulta-

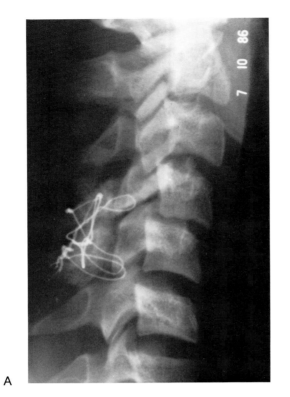

A

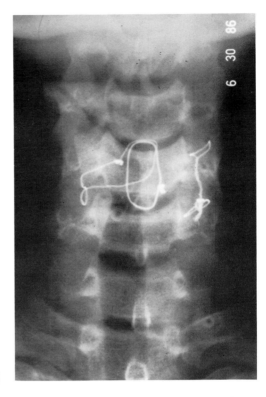

B

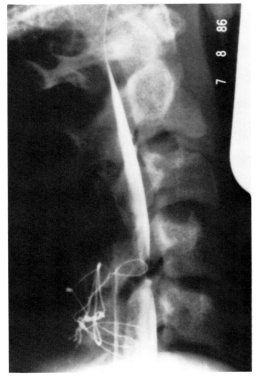

C

Fig. 15-67. (A,B) Lateral and AP cervical spine radiographs of a patient referred to the Spine Center after an unorthodox two-level posterior fusion. Note forward subluxation of the C4 vertebral body on C5. The patient had a neurologic deficit (C5) commensurate with subluxation of C4 on C5. (C) Myelogram confirming the presence of an extruded disc. *(Figure continues.)*

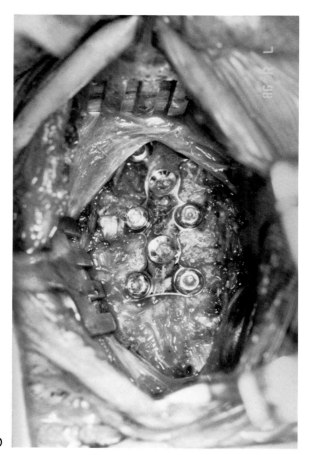

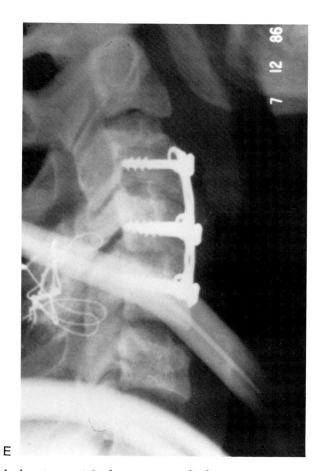

Fig. 15-67 *(Continued).* **(D)** Intraoperative photograph showing an AO plate-screw applied across vertebral bodies C3–C5. **(E)** Lateral radiograph after anterior disc removal and intervertebral body fusion of C3–C4, C4–C5, and plate-screw fixation of C3–C5. The patient was supported in a SOMI orthosis for 3 months.

neously obtained from the proximal tibia metaphyseal region. A tibial bone graft can be obtained with the patient in either the supine or prone position, during either an anterior or posterior procedure (see Fig. 15-69A).

Anterior Tricortical Iliac Bone Graft. Like a posterior iliac crest bone graft, an anterior graft can be obtained from the anterior aspect of the iliac crest (Fig. 15-68). The only anatomic consideration involved in making the incision is the lateral femoral cutaneous nerve that exits inferior to the antero superior iliac spine, directly posterior, anterior, or through the sartorius tendon, which inserts on the anterior superior iliac crest.

Once the iliac wing has been cleansed of its muscle and soft tissue attachment by subperiosteal dissection, both the internal and external surfaces of the iliac crest are cleansed. Using either a straight (1 to 1½ inch) osteotome or an oscillating Stryker saw, a section of iliac crest (Fig. 15-7) is removed, measuring approximately 1½ to 2 inches in length, and approximately 1 inch in depth. Both the inner and outer tables are removed intact along with the crest. This makes up the tricortices. Such a graft can be cut into multiple sections, preserving the three cortices. After disc excision, the grafts are inserted as anteriorinterbody grafts, between the two cervical vertebrae being fused. Care must be

taken to insert the bone graft sufficiently deep so that it lies inside and under the anterior ledge of adjacent vertebrae. Wound closure is similar to that of other graft sites, with the muscle-fascial attachments, removed from either the anterior or posterior iliac crest at the time of the approach, reattached with 0 or 2–0 Dexon suture, after the placement of a Hemovac drain in the wound, if thought required.

Posterior Iliac Bone Graft: Technique. Not a primary concern, but one taken into consideration, is the presence of neurologic function in the lower extremities. When motor function exists and it can be anticipated that the patient will return to an active ambulatory status within a reasonable period of time after surgery, it is appropriate to obtain a needed bone graft from the posterior iliac spine rather than the proximal tibia.

An incision is made over the posterior iliac crest (see Fig. 18-17, 18-42), along the posterior brim of the crest to the level of the sacroiliac joint. The incision is carried down to the crest, where the muscles and lumbodorsal ligaments and fascia are excised off the crest by sharp dissection. The outer table of the ilium is subperiosteally stripped of its soft tissue attachments, and with a curved osteotome, both the external cortical bone and the intervening cancellous bone are removed, leaving the

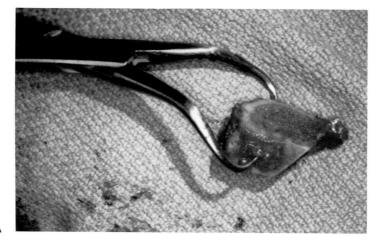
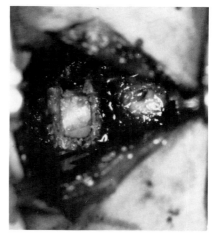

A   B

Fig. 15-68. (A) Tricortical graft obtained from the anterior iliac crest using a Stryker oscillating saw. (B) Interbody fusion after insertion of the tricortical graft. The posterior depth of the bone graft is critical. Care must be taken to insert the graft deeply enough to lie inside and under the anterior ledge of the adjacent vertebra. An intraoperative lateral radiograph should be obtained to confirm that the bone graft is deep enough yet does not encroach on the neural canal. (see Fig. 15-15C)

inner table intact. Care must be taken when removing cancellous bone from the inner cortex, for in some areas, the inner table is very thin. It is possible for the osteotome to penetrate the inner table and pass into the iliacus muscle inside the pelvis. Although this rarely causes problems, it is possible to produce intrapelvic bleeding in this manner.

The outer table bone graft is carefully removed to maintain its integrity. The size of the graft should depend on the length of the area to be fused. The graft can be cut into two cortical strips later, measuring approximately 3 inches in length and $\frac{3}{8}$ to $\frac{1}{2}$ inch in width, of sufficient strength to stabilize the posterior cervical spine when wired in place. This means that the overall size of the graft is approximately 3 to $3\frac{1}{2}$ inches long and 2 inches wide.

After removal of the cortical and cancellous bone from the outer aspect of the posterior iliac wing, the interstices of the cancellous bone are occluded with medical-grade bone wax. The latter is used to prevent bone "oozing" and hematoma formation. Care must be taken not to leave behind fragments of wax in the soft tissues. The wax will serve as a foreign body and may result in wound infection. The wound is otherwise closed in a routine fashion (in layers) over Hemovac drains.

Tibial Bone Graft Technique. Although an iliac bone graft will often suffice, the thinness of the outer table varies considerably, making this type of bone graft unreliable in strength. When strength is an important consideration, the proximal anteromedial tibia serves as an excellent source for a rigid corticocancellous graft. The procedure used for obtaining this graft from the proximal tibia is the following. A tourniquet is applied to the upper thigh. The leg is appropriately prepped and draped from the midthigh to the tip of the toes. The leg is exsanguinated, and the tourniquet is inflated to 300 mm Hg. The graft is obtained through an anteromedial proximal tibial longitudinal incision (Fig. 15-69A), extending from just above and medial to the attachment of the patellar tendon to the tibial tuberosity, to a point approximately 6 inches distal. In a child less than 17 years old, in whom the epiphysis remains, care must be taken not to injure the epiphysis. The incision is carried down to and through the periosteum. The periosteum is opened

on either end in an H fashion (Fig. 15-69C), with care taken during subperiosteal stripping not to disrupt the periosteal sleeve to ensure its accurate closure. Proximally, the attachment of the pes anserinus tendons will be encountered (Fig. 15-69B). A small area is subperiosteally dissected along with the periosteum, to expose the anterior and medial tibial borders. A Chandler retractor or flat-blade instrument is passed along the anteromedial and posteromedial tibial borders, allowing for exposure of the medial "face" of the proximal tibia. Careful attention is paid to the upper level from which the graft is obtained. Ideally, the upper end of the graft lies opposite the tibial tubercle (protecting the insertion of the patellar tendon). If the graft is removed lower on the tibia, where the tibia becomes more narrow, the tibia can be sufficiently weakened to allow a "stress fracture." When a stress fracture occurs (with ambulation, less than 4 percent), it occurs at the lower end of the graft site. Rarely does this occur in the quadriplegic patient; rather, it occurs in the patient with a more normal neurologic level as postoperative activities are increased.

The length of the bone graft to be removed is determined by the length of the area to be fused. The width of the graft is constant. An effort is made to stay away from the anteromedial (crest) and posterio borders of the tibia, leaving at least a $\frac{1}{4}$- to $\frac{3}{8}$-inch border on either side of the long axis of the graft (Fig. 15-67C). The width of the graft usually measures approximately $\frac{3}{4}$ inch.

The outer border of the graft is marked on the tibia by drill holes placed at the four corners of the proposed graft and along the boundary of the graft as desired (Fig. 15-69B). With a power saw, the anteromedial cortex of the tibia is cut through to the interior of the tibia. The anterior border is cut at an oblique angle so as not to cut into the thickened "anterior column" of the tibia (Fig. 15-69C,D). The graft is cut longitudinally along the posterior border and perpendicularly at both ends. Before its removal, the graft is sawed in the midline longitudinally, allowing the graft to be removed as two grafts measuring approximately 3 inches long and each $\frac{3}{8}$ inch wide. With a flat osteotome at each corner, the two grafts can be easily pried out. After removal of the two cortical strips, copious cancellous bone can be obtained from the

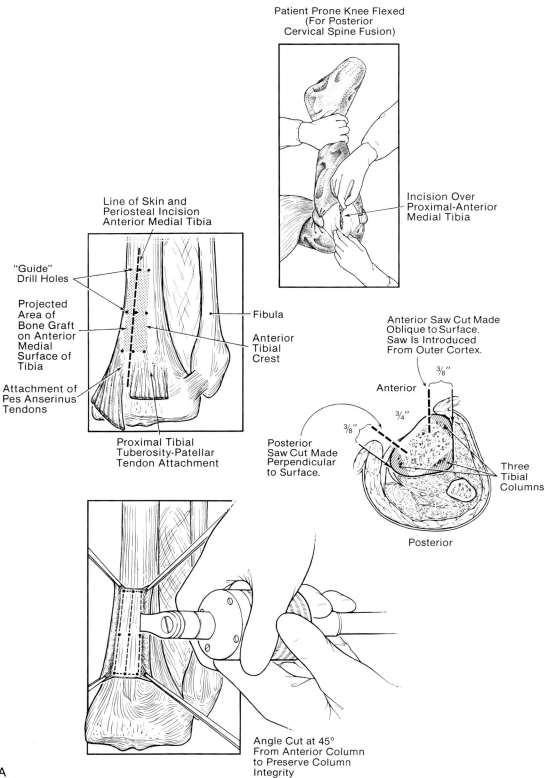

Patient Prone Knee Flexed
(For Posterior
Cervical Spine Fusion)

Incision Over
Proximal-Anterior
Medial Tibia

Line of Skin and
Periosteal Incision
Anterior Medial Tibia

"Guide"
Drill Holes

Projected
Area of
Bone Graft
on Anterior
Medial
Surface of
Tibia

Attachment of
Pes Anserinus
Tendons

Fibula

Anterior
Tibial
Crest

Proximal Tibial
Tuberosity-Patellar
Tendon Attachment

Anterior Saw Cut Made
Oblique to Surface.
Saw Is Introduced
From Outer Cortex.

Anterior

3/8"

3/4"

3/8"

Posterior
Saw Cut Made
Perpendicular
to Surface.

Three
Tibial
Columns

Posterior

Angle Cut at 45°
From Anterior Column
to Preserve Column
Integrity

A

Fig. 15-69. Method of obtaining tibial bone graft. *(Figure continues.)*

Bone Graft Not Cut in Two.

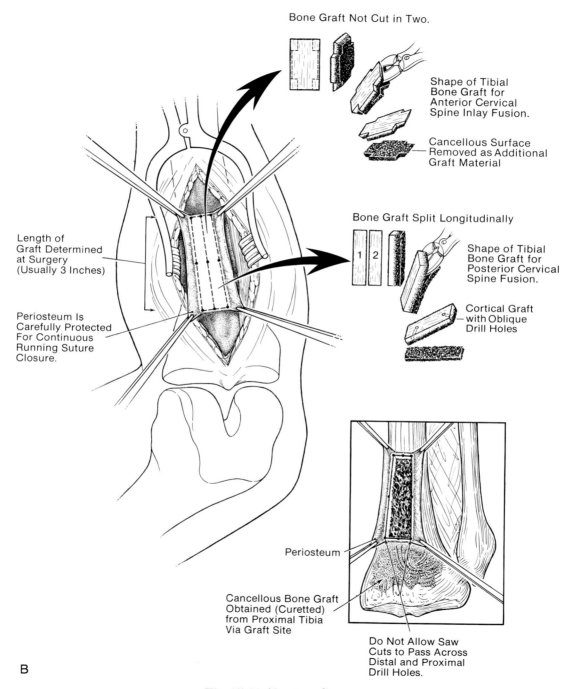

Shape of Tibial
Bone Graft for
Anterior Cervical
Spine Inlay Fusion.

Cancellous Surface
Removed as Additional
Graft Material

Bone Graft Split Longitudinally

Shape of Tibial
Bone Graft for
Posterior Cervical
Spine Fusion.

Cortical Graft
with Oblique
Drill Holes

Length of
Graft Determined
at Surgery
(Usually 3 Inches)

Periosteum Is
Carefully Protected
For Continuous
Running Suture
Closure.

Periosteum

Cancellous Bone Graft
Obtained (Curetted)
from Proximal Tibia
Via Graft Site

Do Not Allow Saw
Cuts to Pass Across
Distal and Proximal
Drill Holes.

B

Fig. 15-69 *(Continued).*

proximal tibial metaphysis (Fig. 15-69F). After removal of the bone graft, the periosteum is carefully sutured with interrupted figure-of-eight 0 chromic or 2–0 Dexon sutures. The subcutaneous tissue is closed with 3–0 Dexon, and the skin is closed with either a subcuticular 2–0 Prolene suture or the suture of choice. A sterile dressing is applied over the wound, along with a pressure dressing and Ace bandage from the toes to the level of the knee, and the tourniquet is released. Care should be taken to determine that the tourniquet has deflated, if the procedure has not ended.

"Direct" Bone Graft Application Technique. A method of attempting to gain a fusion, as in the area of the occipitocervical angle of the upper spine (where visualization is difficult and the anatomy either abnormal or difficult to visualize clearly or dissect safely), is to apply cancellous bone graft directly onto or into the area of the proposed fusion, without extensive dissection (Fig. 15-70). This procedure has been utilized in the elderly patient and the rheumatoid arthritic, in whom erosion of the odontoid has occurred, resulting in subluxation between the odontoid and the ring of C1, and in whom the bone substance required for wire fixation is insufficient to withstand wire fixation because of the disease process.

The patient is first placed into a halo vest, followed by the required surgical exposure (the occiput, the posterior ring of C1, and C2). Cancellous iliac crest bone graft is carefully packed into the area of attempted fusion. The patient is maintained in the halo vest for 3 months, or for as long as possible. Six weeks is striven for. Should some other orthotic device be required for a short period, the orthosis of choice would be the SOMI orthosis. Fusion from the occiput to C2 is seldom attempted, although should it occur, it has not been found to be a handicap. The usual area of fusion is C1 to C2. In the case of occipital-C1 instability, fusion from the occiput to C2 or C3 is appropriate.

Postoperative Immobilization

Postoperative orthoses are recommended for the support of all patients requiring spinal stabilization. This is particularly the case in two groups of patients: those rendered severely neurologically compromised (quadriplegic), and those in whom the surgical stabilization alone, unsupported, is insufficient for the time required for bony stability (or fusion) to occur.

For the neurologically intact patient requiring a stabilization procedure, minimal external support for the 2 to 3 months required for fusion is required. The orthosis usually recommended is the SOMI orthosis. An alternative would be the Philadelphia collar. A "soft" collar is never recommended (Fig. 15-71) (see Ch. 12).

For the patient sustaining either a complete or incomplete neurologic injury in association with a spine injury requiring surgical stabilization, the orthosis recommended is either the SOMI orthosis or some modification of the same.

The indication for the preoperative or postoperative use of a halo are clear. They include those patients with vertebral column injuries requiring the most rigid immobilization that can be attained with an orthosis, without surgery, or those fractures considered unstable even though operated on.

In the first category fall fractures of the ring of C1, odontoid fractures of types II and III, and in most cases, fractures of the posterior element of C2 (the hangman's fracture). Also included is the group of patients who have sustained fractures over multiple levels, or who otherwise are without surgical indications.

In the second category fall the patients who require both surgical stabilization and rigid postoperative immobilization (3 months), that is, rheumatoid arthritics and elderly patients with fractures involving the C1–C3 complex, and Marie-Strümpell rheumatoid spondylitis patients, whose fractures are known for their gross instability (even after internal fixation), owing to the presence of extensive osteopenia.[9–11]

An alternative or optional management technique available for either the operated or the nonoperated patient with a cervical spine injury is immobilization of the fracture by skeletal traction (Gardner-Well tongs) for a period sufficient to allow the traumatized spine to gain some stability, before placing the patient in an orthosis. This technique is often utilized in the elderly or fragile patient in whom skeletal traction is used for the initial 4 to 6 weeks, followed by placement in an orthosis

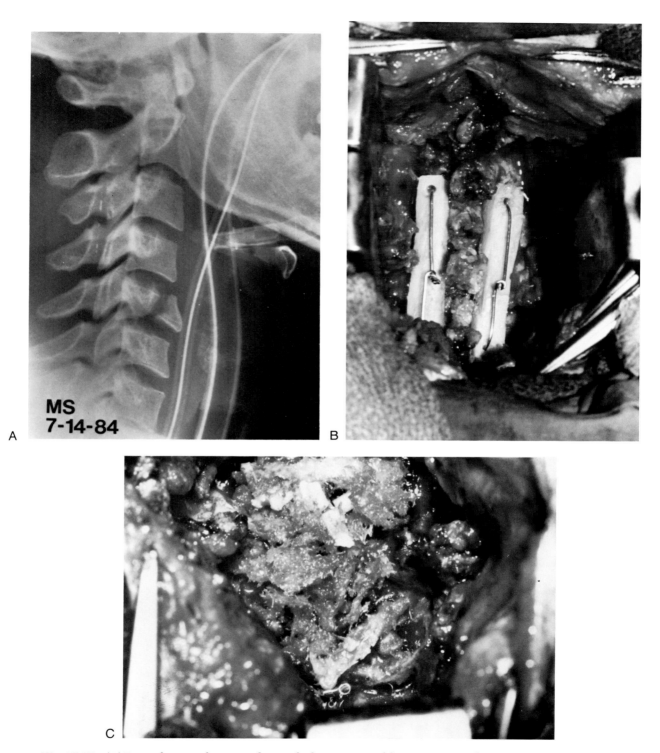

Fig. 15-70. (A) Lateral cervical spine radiograph showing unstable compression fracture with retropulsion of the C5 vertebral body. (B) Intraoperative photograph showing bilateral tibial strut-spinous process wiring technique. (C) Intraoperative view showing application of additional cancellous bone. *(Figure continues.)*

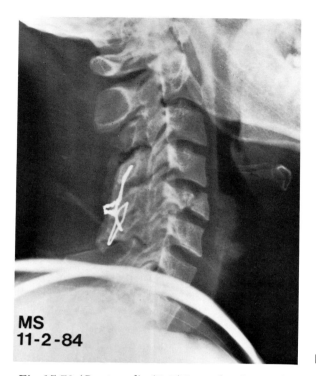

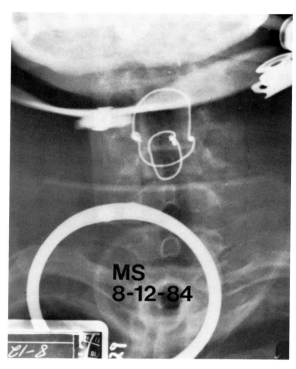

D   E

Fig. 15-70 *(Continued).* **(D,E)** Lateral and AP radiographs taken 4 months after operation, showing double wiring posterior fusion with incorporation of posterior elements of C4–C6. The lower wire stabilizes the posterior spinous process of C5–C6. The larger wire incorporates the spinous process of C4–C6 with posterior tibial strut grafts.

for the remainder of the 3 months. This allows the spine injury to undergo sufficient stability that the patient can be placed into a less restrictive device (SOMI orthosis) rather than a halo vest. This routine is often used for odontoid fractures, hangman's fractures, multiple-level fractures, and those patients in whom evidence exists that neurologic recovery is occurring and continued maintenance in traction is thought protective. This technique is also utilized to shorten the period of time a patient will require immobilization in a halo vest (see Ch. 12).

which surgery might have been inadequate, stable postoperative immobilization may be a positive influence on the patient's eventual outcome. This was exemplified by two rheumatoid patients who underwent occiput-C2 fusions followed by placement in a halo vest for 10 to 12 weeks. Because osteopenia was so severe, only cancellous bone was laid on a decorticated surface of the occiput and the laminae of C1 and C2. Fusion occurred in both. It is generally agreed that when an attempt is made to incorporate the occiput in the fusion mass, the most appropriate immobilization is the halo vest.

POSTOPERATIVE NONUNION RATE

Of all series reviewed, nonunion after surgery was noted in only the most unusual case and generally was the result of difficulty in immobilization during the postoperative period. In situations in

NEUROLOGIC COMPLICATIONS WITH SURGERY

Neurologic complications can and do occasionally follow spine surgery. Bohler[36] and others, including us, have recorded such occurrences. For-

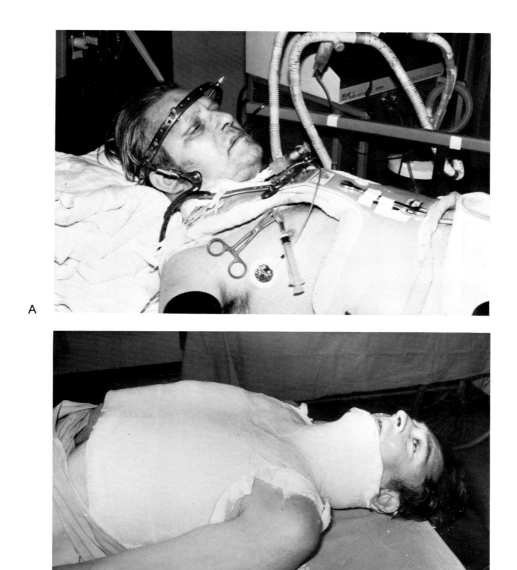

Fig. 15-71. **(A)** A patient with Marie-Strümpell rheumatoid spondylitis (see Figs. 15-13, 15-21) managed postoperatively in a halo vest. **(B)** A patient in a plaster of paris minerva jacket. This type of immobilization is used for patients whose medical condition is stable but whose ability to cooperate with postoperative management is doubtful. *(Figure continues.)*

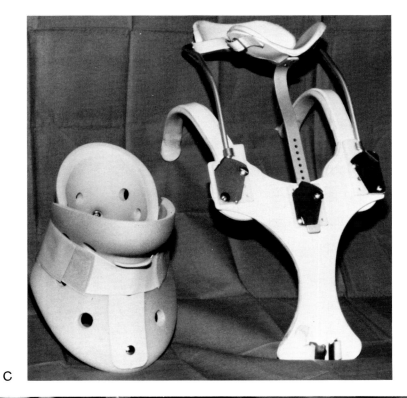

C

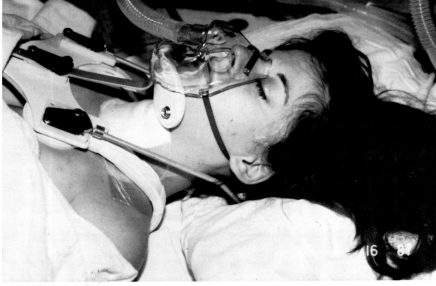

D

Fig. 15-71 *(Continued).* **(C)** Commonly used cervical orthoses: Philadelphia collar (left) and SOMI (sternal-occipital-mandibular immobilizer) orthosis (right). Both orthotic devices require a stable spine. **(D)** Patient immediately after posterior cervical spine fusion placed in a SOMI orthosis. Note patient's anterior neck reveals recent removal of tracheostomy. When a tracheostomy tube remains in place, the chin upright requires addition of a circle insert (see Fig. 15-70E).

tunately, the incidence is low, with serious neurologic complications occurring in less than 1 percent of the spinal surgical procedures; minor, transient changes requiring no treatment occurring in 15 to 20 percent; and moderate, incomplete neurologic complication, which follows a second operative procedure to eliminate or rule out a cause, occurring at a rate of 7 to 10 percent (Table 15-4). There are instances, for which we were consulted, in which a patient postoperatively revealed significant neurologic injury of an unknown etiology. Usually the etiology, with sudden onset, is vascular.

Displacement of the odontoid process, with the patient in a prone position, can produce a neurologic deficit. Occasionally, without either spine displacement or surgery, an unexplained quadriparesis or quadriplegia may occur, after trauma. Direct encroachment on the cord is always a concern. It is important to recall that the space available for the spinal cord is greatest at the foramen magnum and C1–C2–C3 levels, thus neurologic injury at this level is either rare or lethal owing to injury to the brain stem (see Fig. 1-3). At C1, the spinal cord measures 1 cm and the neural canal measures 2.1 cm. At the C2 level, the spinal cord measures 0.95 cm and the neural canal measures 1.98 cm. At the C3 level, the spinal cord measures 0.85 cm, and the neural canal measures 1.85 cm.

Below the C3–C4 level, the spinal canal becomes most narrow and neurologic injury is likely to result when it is compromised. Should a fluctuation in the level of neurologic performance occur, the following pathologic processes must be consid-

ered: direct spinal cord compression by a herniated disc (Fig. 15-72); the loss of bony position or reduction resulting in neural tissue compromise; vascular embarrassment of the spinal cord; hemorrhage and hematoma; direct spinal cord manipulation at surgery; and spinal cord compromise after the passage of internal fixation (i.e., sublaminar wires) (Figs. 15-53, 15-54).

EXTENSIVE CERVICAL SPONDYLOSIS

With the radiographic finding of extensive cervical spine degenerative arthritis, one can anticipate the presence of a very immobile and almost rigid vertebral column. The motion that is most affected is flexion-extension and lateral bending, with rotation least affected (65 to 70 percent of which occurs at the C1–C2 atlantoaxial articulation). Thus, falls, primarily occurring in the elderly, result in the occurrence of an extension injury at C6–C7. When there is limited motion available, trauma results in the abnormal displacement of vertebral elements resulting from disruption of calcified or inelastic ligamentum flavum, and the resultant injuries are occasionally an overt fracture or bone injury; an associated cervical spinal cord-central cord syndrome, resulting from pinching of the spinal cord between posterior vertebral body osteophytes and inelastic ligamentum flavum posteriorly (Fig. 15-73); and a compression of the anterior spinal cord against posterior vertebral body osteophytes. Because of the already less than optimal blood supply to the cervical spinal cord, in the face of localized pinching injuries of the spinal cord, central gray matter hemorrhage with trauma, and anterior spinal artery thrombosis, etc., poor and unexpected recovery or improvement is anticipated after even relatively minor trauma.

Such injuries, like all others to the cervical spine, must be initially managed by some form of cervical splinting (cervical tong traction) for 3 to 6 weeks. After tomograms and a myelograph are obtained, particularly when there is no direct correlation between radiologic and neurologic findings, if the problem is vascular and the patient is reliable, the

Table 15-4. Cervical Fractures: Change in Neurologic Status[a] (Northwestern University Acute Spine Injury Center, 1972 to 1986)

Type of Change	No.	Percent
Improvement	112	7.5
No change	1,234	83.2
Degradation	9	0.6
Missing[b]	129	8.7
Total	1,484	100.00

[a] Change criterion is one or more Frankel grades, higher or lower.
[b] Change in neurologic status is unavailable.

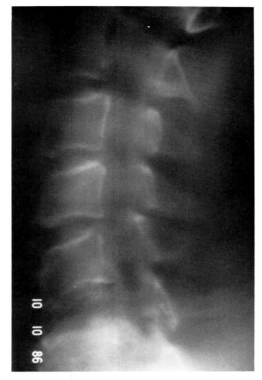

A

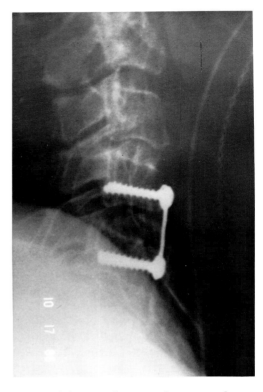

B

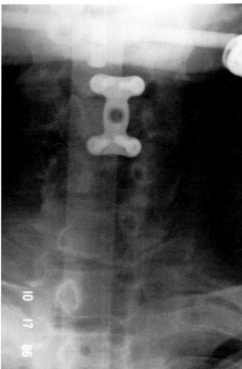

C

Fig. 15-72. (A) Lateral cervical spine radiograph demonstrating cervical spondylitis of C5–C6. Flexion-extension radiograph failed to demonstrate cervical spine instability. Myelogram demonstrated spinal cord encroachment by a herniated C5–C6 disc. (**B,C**) Lateral and AP radiographs after excision of the herniated disc and insertion of a bone graft at C5–C6, followed by anterior stabilization using AO plate-screws. Note widening of interspace and depth of bone graft.

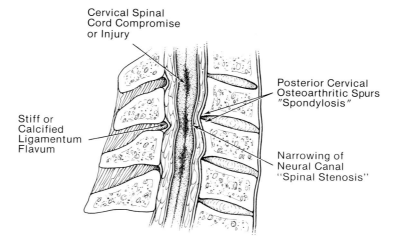

Fig. 15-73. Cervical central cord syndrome resulting from pinching of the spinal cord between posterior vertebral body osteophytes and the inelastic ligamentum flavum.

injury can be managed in a light orthosis of the SOMI type for 6 to 9 weeks. When the patient is unreliable, cervical traction must be maintained for up to 4 weeks, followed by a light orthosis. Surgery is rarely required. If vascular encroachment secondary to osteophytes is thought to be the etiology, anterior decompression is appropriate.

EXCEPTIONS TO RETURNING TO IMPACT SPORTS

When an individual has either sustained an injury that has resulted in ligamentous injury without bone fracture or incurred a bone or ligamentous injury that has required a spinal fusion procedure, a return to contact (impact) sports is not deemed wise.

In either situation, when ligamentous injury has occurred and healed by scar formation, followed by no obvious pathologic motion across the injury site, this spine injury will require a period of observation for at least a year. Without question, ligamentous injuries do not heal with the same strength as a fracture. The only reprieve here might be when spontaneous bony union occurs between the two adjacent vertebrae. In the presence of an essentially well-defined ligamentous injury, resulting

from a flexion-stretch injury to the posterior interspinous ligaments and facet joint capsule, it is unwise to allow an athlete to return to competitive impact sports in anything less than 1 year, and only then after a very careful reappraisal (including stress flexion-extension films). Any significant signs of degenerative spondylosis, above or below the previous level of injury, should rule out further participation organized sports.

For injuries to the cervical spine that have resulted in either bone or ligamentous injury, with evidence of cervical spinal instability that requires a one- or two-level fusion, a return to competitive sports is contraindicated. The rationale for this is that the normal flow of bending, rotational, etc., motion of the cervical spine at each level is lost. Although 60 to 70 percent of all rotation of the cervical spine occurs at the C1–C2 articulation, the same is true for flexion and extension between C3 and C7. With fusion of one, two, or more joints or levels, a proportionate amount of motion is lost. To compensate for this loss, increased motion through alternate joints above and below the level of fusion must occur. For the individual involved in competitive sports, required to take abnormal stresses, those stresses or forces would be concentrated at and would be of greater magnitude across those joints immediately above and below the level of fusion. With a repeat injury, injury at an alternate level will occur. This has been identified in two situations those persons with a previously unknown multiple-level congenital fusion (dislocating at a level just below the congenital fusion), or the patient who has undergone a fusion for a fracture, falls again, and sustains a second dislocation at the level just above or below the previous fusion (Fig. 15-74).

Any patient who has undergone a surgical or congenital fusion at one or more segments of the cervical spine should be discouraged from participating in contact or impact sports. We are aware that some authorities believe that individuals with congenital fusions (which commonly occur at C2–C3) should not be disqualified from impact sport activity. In this situation, the decision can be made by the extent of "abnormal" translatory motion that exists between C3 and C4. If, with flexion-extension radiographs, such motion is greater than 3 mm, or if degenerative arthritic changes are identified, no contact sports should be allowed.

PREVENTION OF POSTOPERATIVE DEEP VENOUS THROMBOSIS

A general rule for all patients from whom a tibia bone graft has been obtained, and particularly for those patients without protective lower extremity sensation, is the need for the removal of any protective dressing on the extremity within 24 hours. Only the dressing immediately over the incision is left in place. TED support hose, alternating Jobst air compression stockings, or some appropriate compression device is used on both calves for the first 2 to 3 postoperative days for those patients with active motor power in the lower extremities, or for longer periods for the quadriplegic or paraplegic patient. The development of deep venous thrombosis is an inherent complication in the patient placed at forced recumbency for prolonged periods of time, and is more likely to occur in the patient rendered paralyzed. It is recommended

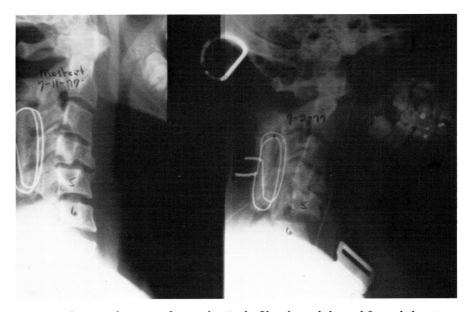

Fig. 15-74. (A) Lateral cervical spine radiographs. Right film shows bilateral facet dislocation at C5–C6 4 years after previous fracture dislocation and compression fracture at C4–C5. The initial injury produced complete C5 quadriplegia. Left film shows reduction of the C5–C6 dislocation. Patient's fusion was extended one level, and stabilized in a cervical orthosis.

that heparine sodium be used both preoperatively and postoperatively for the prevention of deep venous thrombosis. Various drugs and techniques have been utilized to prevent the occurrence of deep venous thrombosis. These include ASA, Dextran, alternating pressure stockings, elevation, TED hose, etc. The most effective method of prevention has been found to be the use of "adjusted dose heparin" (which requires repeated evaluation of blood-clotting factors) in which the clotting time is kept at approximately one and one-half to two times normal. A more simplified method of utilizing heparin is the administration of subcutaneous heparin (5,000 units b.i.d.). This routine can be maintained for either 6 weeks or until the patient is placed on longer-term therapy. For long-term prophylaxis against the occurrence of deep venous thrombosis, or its complication of pulmonary embolism, Coumadin (sodium warfarin; 2.5 to 5 mg) is administered each day. Levels of this drug are adjusted by monitoring the prothrombin time, which is kept at one and one-half to two times normal for a 3- to 6-month period, or until the threat of venous thrombosis is gone. This usually occurs when the patient returns to a preinjury level of activity.

REFERENCES

1. Holdsworth FW: Review article: fracture, fracture-dislocations of the spine. J Bone Joint Surg 52A:1534, 1970
2. Bulger RF, Rejowski JE, Beatty RA: Vocal cord paralysis associated with anterior cervical fusion: considerations for prevention and treatment. J. Neurosurg 62:657, 1985
3. Micheli LJ: Sports following spinal surgery in the young athlete. Clin Orthop 198:152, 1985
4. Gassman J, Seligson D: The anterior cervical plate. Spine 8:700, 1983
5. Calenoff L, Chessare J, Rogers LF et al.: Multiple levels, spine injuries: importance of early recognition. AJR 130:665, 1979
6. Kewalramani LS, Taylor RG: Multiple non-contiguous injuries to the spine. Acta Orthop Scand 47:52, 1976
7. Scher AT: Hyperextension trauma in the elderly: an easily overlooked spinal injury. J Trauma 23:1066, 1983
8. Hunter T et al.: Spinal fractures complicating ankylosing spondylitis. A long-term followup study. Arthritis Rheum 26:751, 1983
9. Fardon DF: Odontoid fracture complicating ankylosing hyperostosis of the spine. Spine 3:108, 1978
10. Grisolia A, Bell RL, Peltier LF: Fractures and dislocations of the spine complicating ankylosing spondylitis. J Bone Joint Surg 49A:339, 1967
11. Kewalramani MB, Taylor RG, Albrand OW: Cervical spine injury in patients with ankylosing spondylitis. J Trauma 15:931, 1975
12. Meeks LW, Renshaw TS: Vertebral osteophytosis and dysphagia. J Bone Joint Surg 55A:197, 1973
13. Denis F: The three column spine and its significance in the classification of acute thoracolumbar spine injuries. Spine 8:817, 1983
14. Robinson RA, Southwick WO: Surgical approaches to the cervical spine. AAOS Instructional Course Lectures 17:299, 1960
15. Cloward R: Surgical treatment of dislocations and compression fractures of the cervical spine by the anterior approach. p. 26. Proceedings of the 17th Veterans Administration Spinal Cord Injury Conference, New York, 1969. Veterans Administration, Washington, DC, 1969
16. Sage JI, Van Uitert RL: "Man-in-the-barrel" syndrome. Neurology 26:1102, 1986
17. Delavelle J, Lalanne B, Megret M: "Man-in-the-barrel." Neurology 29:501, 1987
18. Robinson BP, Seeger JF, Zak SM: Rheumatoid arthritis and position vertebrobasilar insufficiency. J Neurol 65:111, 1986
19. Harding-Smith J, MacIntosh PK, Sherbon KJ: Fractures of the occipital condyle. J Bone Joint Surg 63A:1170, 1981
20. Evarts CM: Traumatic occipito-atlantal dislocation. Report of a case with survival. J Bone Joint Surg 52A:1653, 1970
21. Eismont FJ, Bohlman HH: Posterior atlanto-occipital dislocation with fractures of the atlas and odontoid process. J Bone Joint Surg 60A:3, 1978
22. Zielinski CJ, Gunther SF, Deeb Z: Cranial-nerve palsies complicating Jefferson fracture. A case report. J Bone Joint Surg 64A:1382, 1982
23. Garber JN: Surgery in cervical spine injuries. AAOS Instructional Course Lectures, 26:67, 1961
24. Garber JN: Abnormalities of the atlas and axis vertebrae. J Bone Joint Surg 46A:1782, 1964
25. Gunther SF: Congenital anomaly of the cervical spine: fusion of the occiput, atlas, odontoid process. J Bone Joint Surg 62A:1377, 1980
26. Kahanavotiz N, Mehringer MC, Johanson PH: Intracranial entrapment of the atlas complicating an un-

treated fracture of the posterior arch of the atlas. A case report. J Bone Joint Surg 63A:831, 1981

27. Day GL, Jacoby CG, Dolan KD: Basilar invagination resulting from untreated Jefferson's fracture. AJR 133:529, 1979

28. Cattell HS, Clark GL, Jr.: Cervical kyphosis and instability following multiple laminectomies in children. J Bone Joint Surg 49A:713, 1967

29. Bailey DK: The normal cervical spine in infants and children. Radiology 59:712, 1952

30. Fielding JW, Cochran G, Lawsing JF, III, Hohl M: Tears of the transverse ligament of the atlas. J Bone Joint Surg 56A:1683, 1974

31. Fielding JW, Hawkins RJ: Atlanto-axial rotatory fixation. J Bone Joint Surg 59A:37, 1977

32. Gallie WE: Fractures and dislocations of the cervical spine. Am J Surg 46:495, 1939

33. Fielding W, Jr., Griffin PP: Os odontoideum: an acquired lesion. J Bone Joint Surg 56A:187, 1974

34. Anderson LD, D'Alonzo RT: Fractures of the odontoid process of the axis. J Bone Joint Surg 56A:1663, 1974

35. Osgood RB, Lund CC: Fractures of the odontoid process. N Engl J Med 198:61, 1928

36. Bohler J: Anterior stabilization for acute fractures and non-union of the dens. J Bone Joint Surg 64A:18, 1982

37. Brooks AL, Jenkins EB: Atlanto-axial arthrodesis by the wedge compression method. J Bone Joint Surg 60A:279, 1978

38. Fielding JW: Cervical spine surgery. Past, present and future potential. Clin Orthop 200:284, 1985

39. Ryan MD, Taylor TKF: Odontoid fractures, a rational approach to treatment. J Bone Joint Surg 64:416, 1982

40. Roy-Camille R, Saillant G, Berteaux D, Marie-Anne S: Early management of spinal injuries. p. 57. In McKibbin B (ed): Recent Advances in Orthopaedics. Vol 3. Churchill Livingstone, Edinburgh, 1979

41. Clark CR, White AA III: Fractures of the dens. A multicenter study. J Bone Joint Surg 67:1340, 1985

42. Ackerson TT, Patzakis MJ, Moore TM et al.: Fractures of the odontoid: a ten-year retrospective study. Contemp Orthop 4:54, 1982

43. Pepin JW, Bourne RB, Hawkins RJ: Odontoid fractures, with special reference to the elderly patient. Clin Orthop 193:178, 1985

44. Mouradian WH, Fietti VG, Cochran G et al.: Fractures of the odontoid: a laboratory and clinical study of mechanisms. Orthop Clin North Am 9:985, 1978

45. Schatzker J, Rorabeck CH, Waddell JP: Non-union

of the odontoid process: an experimental investigation. Clin Orthop 108:127, 1975

46. Roberts A, Wickstrom J: Prognosis of odontoid fractures. J Bone Joint Surg 54A:1353, 1972

47. Bell W, Meyer P: Non-halo/non-surgical management of C1–C2 fractures. Orthopaedic transactions. J Bone Joint Surg 7:481, 1983

48. Callahan RA, Lockwood R, Green B: Modified Brooks fusion for an os odontoideum associated with an incomplete posterior arch of the atlas. A case report. Spine 8:107, 1983

49. Wood-Jones F: The ideal lesion produced by judicial hanging. Lancet 1:53, 1913

50. Schneider RC, Livingston KE, Cave AJE, Hamilton G: Hangman's fracture of the cervical spine. J Neurosurg 22:141, 1965

51. Levine AM, Edwards CC: The management of traumatic spondylolisthesis of the axis. J Bone Joint Surg 67:217, 1985

52. Francis WR, Fielding JW, Hawkins RJ et al.: Traumatic spondylolisthesis of the axis. J Bone Joint Surg 63B:313, 1981

53. Effendi B, Roy D, Cornish B et al.: Fractures of the ring and axis. A classification based on the analysis of 131 cases. J Bone Joint Surg 63B:319, 1981

54. White AA, Panjabi MM: Functional spinal unit and mathematical models. In Clinical Biomechanics of the Spine. JB Lippincott, Philadelphia, 1978

55. Fardon DF, Fielding JW: Defects of the pedicle and spondylolisthesis of the second cervical vertebra. J Bone Joint Surg [Br] 63B:526, 1981

56. Ducker TB, Bellegarrigue R, Saleman M: Timing of operative care in cervical spinal cord injury. Spine 9:525, 1984

57. Wagner FC, Chehrazi B: Surgical results in the treatment of cervical spinal cord injury. Spine 9:523, 1984

58. White, AA, III, Panjabi MM, Tech D: The role of stabilization in the treatment of cervical spine injuries. Spine 9:512, 1984

59. Lusted LB, Keats TE: Atlas of Roentgenographic Measurements. p. 97. 4th Ed. Year Book Medical Publishers, Chicago, 1978

60. Wolf BS, Khilnani M, Malis L: Measurement of the sagittal diameter of the cervical spinal cord in adults. J Mt Sinai Hosp NY 23:283, 1956

61. Lowman RM, Finkelstein A: Radiology 39:700, 1942

62. Clark CR, Keggi KJ, Panjabi MM: Methyl methacrylate stabilization of the cervical spine. J Bone Joint Surg 66:40, 1984

63. Davey JR, Rorabeck CH, Bailey SI et al.: A tech-

nique of posterior cervical fusion for instability of the cervical spine. Spine 10:722, 1985

64. Whitehill R, Schmidt R: The posterior interspinous fusion in the treatment of quadriplegia. Spine 8:733, 1983

65. Schaeffer JP: Morris' Human Anatomy: A Complete Systematic Treatise. 11th Ed. Blakiston, New York, 1953

66. Whitesides TE, Jr., Kelly RP: Lateral approach to the upper cervical spine for anterior fusion. South Med J 59:879, 1966

67. Bohlman HH: Complications of treatment of fractures and dislocations of the cervical spine. p. 681. In Epps CH (ed): Complications in Orthopaedic Surgery. 2nd Ed. Vol. 2. JB Lippincott, Philadel-phia, 1985

68. Bryan WJ, Inglis AE, Sculco TP, Ranawat CS: Methyl methacrylate stabilization for enhancement of posterior cervical arthodesis in rheumatoid arthritis. J Bone Joint Surg 64:1045, 1982

69. Whitesides TE, Jr., Kelly RP: Lateral approach to the upper cervical spine for anterior fusion. South Med J 59:879, 1966

70. McAffee PC, Bohlman HH, Riley LH, et al: The anterior retropharyngeal approach to the upper part of the cervical spine. J Bone Joint Surg 69A:1371, 1987

71. Wertheim SB, Bohlman HH: Occipitocervical fusion. Indications, technique, and long term results in 13 patients. J Bone Joint Surg 69A:833, 1987

16

Fractures of the Thoracic Spine: T1 to T10

Paul R. Meyer, Jr.

This chapter begins by emphasizing the distinction between the cervical and the thoracic spine that underlies the discussion of fractures of the thoracic spine. Anatomically and fundamentally, the cervical spine is a clearly defined area of the vertebral column. There is little tendency for fractures of the cervical spine to be associated directly with adjacent injuries of the thoracic spine, that is, fractures and dislocations across the cervicothoracic junction are rare. Likewise, it is rare for internal fixation to cross the cervicothoracic junction. At our spinal trauma center, of 688 patients undergoing surgical procedures involving the cervical and thoracic spine, only 48 (7.0 percent) had internal fixation that crossed the junction.

In contrast, the thoracic spine is not such a clearly defined area. When looked at in the traditional manner, the thoracic spine is defined as T1 to T12, the thoracolumbar junction is the area between T12 and L1, the lumbar spine is defined as L1 to L5, and the sacrum is defined as S1 to S5 (Table 16-1). Our spine center's data reveal that the most frequent area of spine injury (excluding the cervical spine) is the region between the thoracic and lumbar spine (T12–L1). However, the lower spine's "junctional" area cannot always be restricted to the fixed anatomic locale of these two adjacent levels (T12 and L1) and, as such, may require redefinition to comprehend the concept of the "thoracolumbar junction." There are two primary statistics to substantiate this redefinition: the high frequency of injuries in this area (T12–L1),

and the high incidence of cross-junctional internal fixations, attributable to the practice of achieving stabilization by going two levels above and two levels below the injury site. For example, of the 426 thoracic spine fractures (T1 to T12) and lumbar spine fractures that required surgery, 298 (70 percent) had internal fixation that crossed the T12–L1 junction. Moreover, most of these internal fixation procedures spanned the region from T11 to L2. Thus, I suggest that the "thoracolumbar junction" ought logically to refer to an area that extends beyond the adjacent T12–L1 levels and includes the entire range of levels from T11 to L2. Consequently, in this text, all future references to the "thoracolumbar junction" will in fact be describing the area from T11 to L2 (Fig. 16-1; Table 16-2).

This chapter focuses attention on the mechanisms and patterns of vertebral injury within the thoracic spine (T1 to T10). Other aspects relative to injury in this region are also considered: the types of neurologic injuries that were identified, the association of spine injury and neurologic injury to multiple trauma, unusual injuries that infrequently appear (avulsion vascular injuries to the thyrocervical trunk and brachial artery with proximal thoracic spinal fractures), the use of skeletal traction for the reduction of proximal thoracic spine fractures, and the postoperative and conservative orthotic management of spine fractures (see Chap. 12). Chapter 17 will review the surgical management of thoracic spine fractures.

Table 16-1.   Modified Level of Injury (Northwestern University Acute Spine Injury Center, 1972 to 1986)

Injury Level	No.	Percent
None	294	10.8
Cervical	1,484	54.8
Thoracic (T1–T10)	376	13.9
Thoracolumbar (T11–L2)	470	17.3
Lumbar (L3–L5)	73	2.7
Sacral	13	0.5
Total	2,710	100.0

Table 16-2.   Highest Level of Multi-Level Vertebral Fracture (Northwestern University Acute Spine Injury Center, 1972 to 1986)

Highest Level of Fracture	No.	Percent
T01	23	3.5
T02	11	1.7
T03	29	4.4
T04	57	8.7
T05	27	4.1
T06	36	5.5
T07	22	3.3
T08	28	4.3
T09	21	3.2
T10	54	8.2
T11	35	5.3
T12	110	16.7
L01	74	11.3
L02	41	6.2
L03	35	5.3
L04	28	4.3
L05	16	2.4
S01	6	0.9
S03	4	0.6
Total	657	100.0

ACUTE SPINE INJURY DATA: THORACIC SPINE FRACTURES

Between 1972 and 1986, 2,710 patients with acute vertebral column injuries were admitted to the acute spine injury service of the Midwest Regional Spinal Cord Injury Care System (MRSCICS), Northwestern Memorial Hospital, Chicago, IL. Within this group, 1484 were fractures of the cervical spine and 294 (11 percent) sustained traumatic neurologic injuries without fracture and were thus ineligible for inclusion (Table 16-1). Of the remaining 932 fractures involving the thoracic, lumbar, and sacral spine, 376 (14 percent) were fractures of the thoracic spine between T1 and T10, and 470 (17 percent) were fractures of the lower thoracic and upper lumbar spine, T11 through L2 (the area defined as the thoracolumbar junction), and only 86 (3 percent) of the fractures occurred from L3 through S5.

The redefined classification of thoracic (T1 to T10) and thoracolumbar junction (T11-L2) fractures correlates well with the torsional stiffness findings of White and Panjabi[1] and Markolf.[2] These investigators call attention to the fact that torsional stiffness increases from T7–T8 to L3–L4, with the peak at T12–L1. They also noted a direct correlation with the change in the anatomic facing of the facets in these areas. A nearly unhindered rotation of one vertebral articular process on another (low torsional stiffness) occurs at T5–T6; few rotational injuries occur in this area but there is a high incidence of axial load injuries. As one approaches

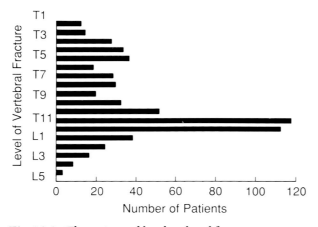

Fig. 16-1.   Thoracic- and lumbar-level fractures presenting at Northwestern University Acute Spine Injury Center from 1972 to 1986.

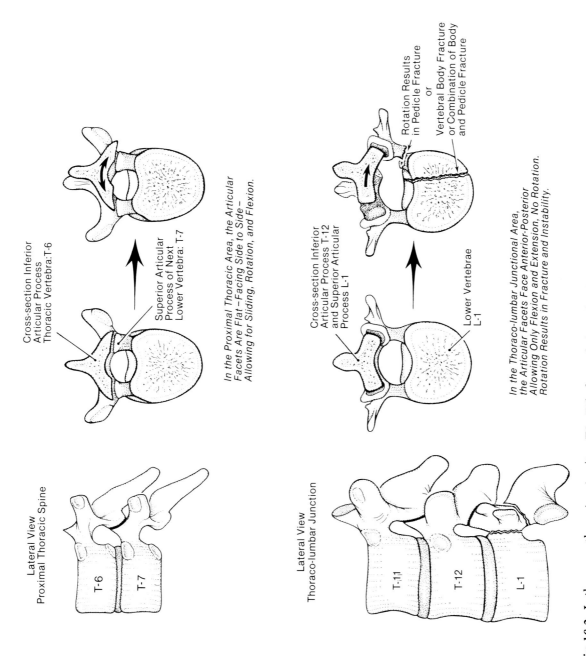

Lateral View
Proximal Thoracic Spine

T-6

T-7

Cross-section Inferior
Articular Process
Thoracic Vertebra: T-6

Superior Articular
Process of Next
Lower Vertebra: T-7

In the Proximal Thoracic Area, the Articular Facets Are Flat—Facing Side to Side—Allowing for Sliding, Rotation, and Flexion.

Lateral View
Thoraco-lumbar Junction

T-11

T-12

L-1

Cross-section Inferior
Articular Process T-12
and Superior Articular
Process L-1

Lower Vertebrae
L-1

Rotation Results
in Pedicle Fracture
or
Vertebral Body Fracture
or Combination of Body
and Pedicle Fracture

In the Thoraco-lumbar Junctional Area, the Articular Facets Face Anterior-Posterior Allowing Only Flexion and Extension. No Rotation. Rotation Results in Fracture and Instability.

Fig. 16-2. In the upper thoracic spine (*top*, T6–T7), the mediolateral and oblique vertical alignment of the facet joints allows freedom of motion in flexion, extension, and rotation. In the thoraco-lumbar spine (*bottom*, T12–L1), note that the inferior facet T12 is "locked" in by the cupped, lateral constraint produced by the superior facet at L1. Rotary injuries at this level result in fractures of the pedicle, the vertebral body, or both due to the lack of freedom of motion.

T12–L1, the facet joint construction is such that axial torsion is essentially blocked (Fig. 16-2). This abrupt change in stiffness between a flexible upper spine segment and an inflexible lower segment creates an area of high stress concentration, leading to rotational mechanical failure at T9 through L1.[1,2] Comminuted posterior element fractures (Fig. 16-3) may thus occur at any level between T9 and L1. These mechanical findings of White[1] and Markolf[2] explain the apparent bimodal occurrence of injuries to the thoracic spine (T4 to T6) and the thoracolumbar junction (T11 to L2) in our series (Fig. 16-1). This bimodal occurrence was reported earlier.[3]

The relevance of the area of stress concentration is apparent in our series. Most injuries, 470 (50 percent), occurred within the thoracolumbar junctional area of peak stiffness (T11 to L2). Between T1 and T10, 376 (40 percent) of the fractures occurred, and 73 (8 percent) of the fractures occurred between L3 and L5. Thirteen (1 percent) fractures were identified in the sacrum (S1 to S5) (Table 16-3).

Primary and Secondary Fracture Patterns

Given the predilection for fractures of the spine to occur most frequently at the T11 to L2 level, one must anticipate the occurrence of spine injuries over multiple, widely separated levels in cases of sudden positive deceleration (the application of sudden, high mechanical loads over a short period, with a focal surface area and little time for energy absorption or dissipation). It is necessary to evalu-

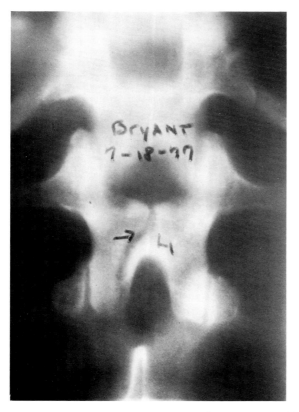

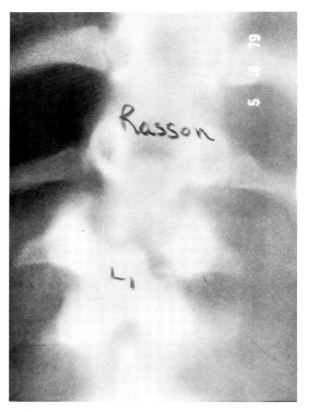

A   B

Fig. 16-3. Anteroposterior views of two patients, illustrating fractures of the posterior elements. **(A)** Axial load "split" of posterior element of L1. This injury is usually associated with a sagittal split of the vertebral body. **(B)** Typical presentation of torsional injury between T9 and L2, involving entrapment of the inferior facets of the vertebra above with rotation fracture of one of the superior articular facets of the next lower posterior vertebral elements.

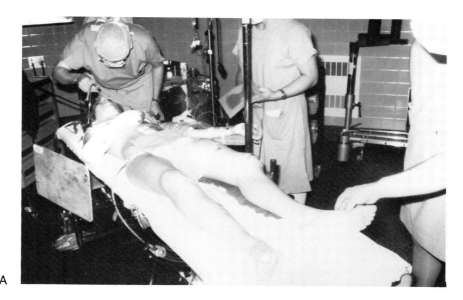

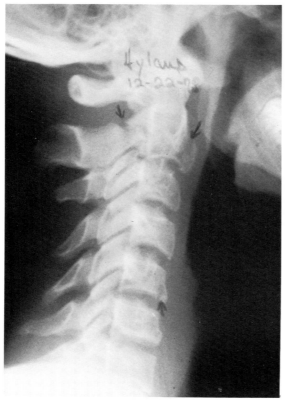

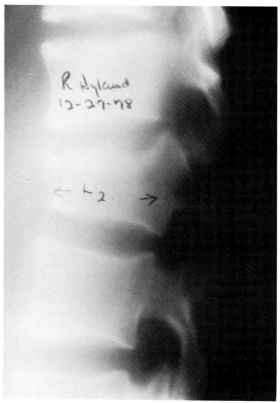

Fig. 16-4. (A) 22-year-old woman who sustained multiple skeletal injuries in a motor vehicle accident. (B) Lateral radiograph showing hangman's fracture through the posterior elements of C2, avulsion fracture of the anteroinferior lip of C2, and nondisplaced fracture of the anteroinferior area of the C5 vertebral body. (C) Flexion axial load comminuted fracture of the L2 vertebral body. The patient was neurologically normal.

Table 16-3.   Gross Level of Lower Spine Fractures (Northwestern University Acute Spine Injury Center, 1972 to 1986)

Gross Level of Fracture	No.	Percent
Thoracic	376	40.3
Thoracolumbar (T11–L2)	470	50.4
Lumbar	73	7.9
Sacral	13	1.4
Total	932	100.0

ate the entire spine radiographically after trauma. Calenoff and co-workers substantiated this need by demonstrating the frequent occurrence of three clearly defined patterns of acute primary and secondary fractures within the vertebral column[4,5] (see Fig. 10-8). In their review, in the 710 patients with fractures admitted to the Acute Spine Injury Program, Northwestern University, three fracture patterns were revealed:

Pattern A: Fractures occurring primarily in the cervical spine between C4 and C7 are frequently accompanied by a secondary fracture in the lower thoracic and lumbar spine between T11 and L5 (Fig. 16-4).

Pattern B: Fractures that occur primarily in the area of the upper thoracic spine between T1 and T4 are frequently accompanied by a secondary fracture within the cervical spine between C1 and C7.

Pattern C: Fractures involving primarily the lower thoracic and upper lumbar spine, T12 to L2, frequently have a secondary fracture of the lumbar spine between L4 and L5 (Fig. 16-5).

The incidence of multiple (widely spaced) vertebral column fractures in their series was 4.5 percent. This is compatible with the incidence other researchers cited (3 percent to 5 percent). Calenoff found the incidence of neurologic injury to be as high as 80 percent in those patients who sustained multiple contiguous vertebral element fractures and postulated that the high rate of neurologic injury was likely due to the violence required to produce vertebral injury over adjacent levels.[5]

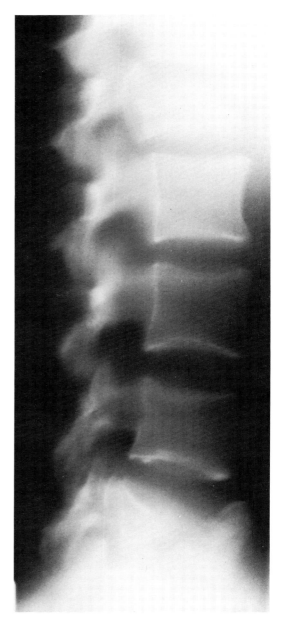

Fig. 16-5. Lateral spinal radiograph of a 27-year-old patient who jumped from the third storey while evading an intruder. The patient sustained an axial load burst injuries of L1 and L5, with incomplete neurologic injury at S1 and S2.

Table 16-4. Etiology of Thoracic Spine Injury (Northwestern University Acute Spine Injury Center, 1972 to 1986)

Etiology	No.	Percent
Gunshot wound	106	28.2
Auto	90	23.9
Fall	81	21.5
Other trauma[a]	38	10.1
Motorcycle	34	9.0
Other medical	23	6.1
Other sports	4	1.1
Total[b]	376	100.0

[a] Total represents those patients with complete admission data.
[b] Other trauma includes those with multiple etiologies.

Table 16-5. Biomechanical Fracture Type (Thoracic Spine) (Northwestern University Acute Spine Injury Center, 1972 to 1986)

Biomechanical Type	No.	Percent
Axial	120	31.9
Flexion	114	30.3
Rotation	8	2.1
Direct	2	0.5
Extension	1	0.3
Other	81	21.6
None[a]	50	13.3
Total	376	100.0

[a] Force undefined.

Etiology of Injury of the Thoracic Spine

Somewhat surprisingly, of the 376 thoracic spine fractures, the primary etiology in the Northwestern University thoracic spine series (1972 to 1986) was gunshot wounds: 106 (28 percent). In the overall spinal cord injury population, gunshot wounds were the fourth most common cause at 10.2 percent. The anticipated primary cause, motor vehicle accidents, was actually second (90 patients, 24 percent), and falls from heights were the third most common cause (81 patients, 22 percent). The remaining causes of injury, in descending order, were: motorcycle (9 percent), other trauma (10 percent), medical (tumor) (6 percent), and sports (1 percent) (Table 16-4). As noted below, because of the anatomic construction of the chest, injury to the thoracic vertebral column usually followed the occurrence of unrestrained violent trauma.

Fracture Patterns: T1 to T10

Because of the "cage" construction of the thorax (ribs, sternum, and vertebral column complex) and the encapsulation of the thoracic spine within this protective shell, the thoracic vertebral column has

an inherent stability and rigidity.[6] Despite this mechanical protection against perpendicular forces, the thoracic spine is vulnerable to axial (compression) loads, followed by flexion loads, particularly within the most proximal segment of the thoracic spine (T1 to T6). This is verified by data contained in Tables 16-5 and 16-6. The most common injury is the axial load, flexion (wedge burst) fracture of

Table 16-6. Fracture Type (Northwestern University Acute Spine Injury Center, 1972 to 1986)

Fracture Type	No.	Percent
Axial body compression	118	31.4
Miscellaneous body fracture	92	24.5
Bullet fragments	73	19.4
Wedge compression fractures	11	2.9
Facet fracture	4	1.1
Chance fracture	4	1.1
Spinous process	3	0.8
Unilateral facet lock	2	0.5
Bilateral facet lock	2	0.5
Transverse process	2	0.5
Subluxation	2	0.5
Other	13	3.5
None	50	13.3
Total	376	100.0

the vertebral body, in association with a resulting anterior (kyphotic) angulation (Fig. 16-6). Between T1 and T10, forward subluxation of one vertebra on another may occur, in the presence of significant burst comminution of the inferior vertebra, but significant anteroposterior translation can and does occur with bilateral facet lock or bilateral facet fracture, resulting in mechanical anterior translation of the superior vertebra.

The principal mechanical forces that contribute to the thoracic vertebral element fractures listed in Table 16-6 were identified by radiologic findings to be the following.

Axial compression fractures were the most frequently observed injury, (118, 31 percent). This agrees with the biomechanical fact that the thoracic spine is well protected by the ribcage from perpendicular forces, but is highly susceptible to compressive loads. With high compressive loads, the intervertebral disc is driven into the adjacent vertebral body end plate, producing either the typical codfish indentation on the superior and inferior surfaces of the vertebral body, or a burst, as a result of excessive axial loading.

Nonspecific body fractures were recorded as the primary fracture in 92 patients (25 percent). The injury is usually a form of a wedge compression fracture to the vertebral body without translation, and of a lesser nature.

Seventy-three penetrating injuries to the spine (19 percent) occurred. As noted, gunshot wounds are the primary cause for injury to the thoracic spine. The presence of a foreign body projectile (retained partially or completely within a vertebral element or neural canal) is implied. As described later in this chapter, the presence of a migrating foreign object (bullet) in the canal, in a patient with a neurologically incomplete lesion, is usually the single accepted indication for removal of the (bullet) foreign body, unless there is evidence of infection. Under such circumstances, the projectile should be removed. (It is routine on the acute spine injury service at Northwestern University not to remove a bullet foreign body just because it is present.) Infection usually follows passage of the projectile through a major, highly contaminated, hollow viscus such as the large bowel, the trachea, or the esophagus. All patients with gunshot wounds have the wound of entrance debrided and are

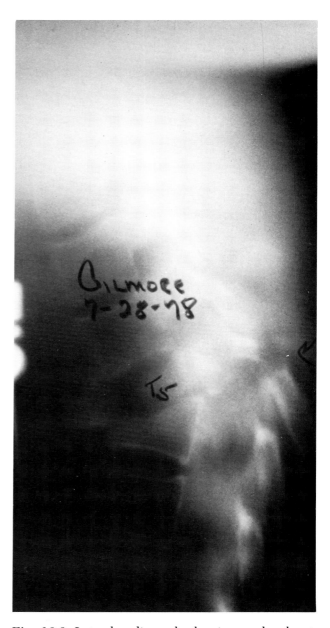

Fig. 16-6. Lateral radiograph showing wedge burst compression fracture of T5 and T6 vertebral bodies. Note fracture of the posterior elements and angular deformity (traumatic kyphosis) at the fracture site. Note also bone in the neural canal.

placed on antibiotics. The rule is to not attempt removal of the foreign body.

Explanation for the very low occurrence of facet dislocation (2 [0.5 percent]) lies with the fact that while the proximal facets (T1 through T7) more freely allow torsional motion, below this level, facet torsion stiffness is the rule because of the anteroposterior facing of the facets. This anatomic variance produces restrictive rotation. Bones with restrictive motion, when stressed, fracture (Fig. 16-7). Facet dislocation within the upper or middle thoracic spine (T1 and T10) seldom occurs. Such injuries are not uncommon in the lower thoracic and upper lumbar spine. The etiology is a distraction and flexion force, as occurs over a seat belt.[7]

To demonstrate that a relationship exists between the anatomic structure of the thorax and tho-racic spine and the mechanical origin of the spine fractures that occur in the region, an attempt has been made to analyze the biomechanical forces involved (Table 16-5) and translate this information into a most probable force moment (or mechanism of injury). A second potential benefit, while not absolute, derived from the biomechanical analysis of fracture patterns is the matching of the mechanism of injury with the resulting fracture and resulting neurologic injury.

The thoracic fractures were classified as having originated from one of the following mechanisms: axial (32 percent), flexion (30 percent), rotation (2 percent), or direct force (0.5 percent) (Table 16-5). Penetrating (gunshot) wounds resulted in a consistently high incidence of neurologic injury; 80 percent of patients suffered complete and 20

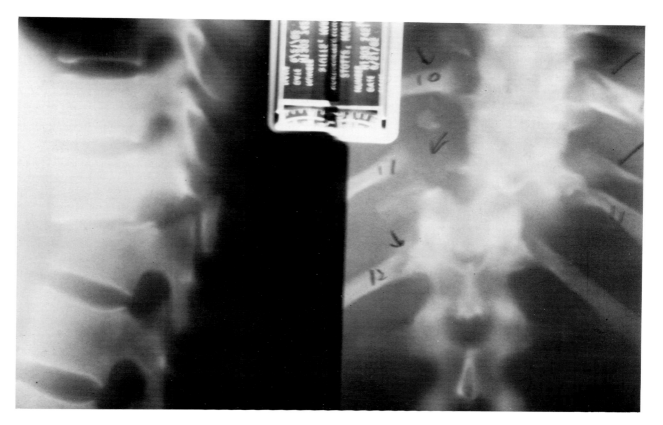

Fig. 16-7. AP and lateral radiographs of multisegmental fractures involving the thoracolumbar junction area. The injury involved axial load, flexion, and rotational components, and resulted in a comminuted fracture of the T12 vertebral body, comminuted fracture of the posterior elements of T11 and T12, and multiple rib fractures of T10 through T12.

Table 16-7. Biomechanical Type by Extent (Northwestern University Acute Spine Injury Center, 1972 to 1986)

Fracture Type	Total	Intact		Incomplete		Complete	
		No.	Percent	No.	Percent	No.	Percent
Axial	120[a]	21	17.5	31	25.8	65	54.2
Flexion	114	12	10.5	31	27.2	71	62.3
Rotation	8	0	0.0	3	37.5	5	62.5
Direct	2	1	50.0	1	50.0	0	0.0
Other	82	3	3.7	16	19.5	63	76.8
None	50	0	0.0	19	38.0	31	62.0
Total	376	37	9.8	101	26.9	235	62.5

[a]Extent is unavailable for three subjects.

percent incomplete neurologic injuries. Axial load and flexion injuries produced similar neurologic injury patterns, with flexion injuries more often severe (62 percent complete and 11 percent intact). With axial load injuries, 54% of patients suffered complete neurologic loss, and 18% were neurologically intact (Table 16-7). One might conclude from these data that axial load injuries less frequently result in "space compromising" injuries, whereas flexion forces more often obstruct the neural canal with either disc or bone, or momentarily occlude the canal by a sudden angular deformity. Either may result in crushing of the spinal cord or in injury to the anterior spinal artery with resulting vascular occlusion.

MECHANISM OF INJURY: THORACIC SPINE

Determining the single mechanical force that when applied to the thoracic spine will result in vertebral element fracture is not possible. Frequently, the radiographic appearance will indicate the likely direction of the offending force. The mechanism of injury is usually arrived at indirectly through history, physical examination (abrasion [Fig. 16-8A], malalignment [Fig. 16-8B], the presence of a gibbus [Fig. 16-8C], etc.), and an analysis of the initial postinjury radiographs [Fig. 16-8D].

The actual directional force (flexion, axial [or vertical] load, rotation, extension, or translation), that produces the vertebral element fracture or malalignment with resulting neurologic injury is seldom appreciated. What has been appreciated is the relationship between neurologic injury and the combination of forces: flexion, axial loading, and rotation. Bedbrook is of the opinion that it is rotation and crushing of the spinal cord that ultimately results in neurologic injury.[8]

Axial (Compression) Load Fractures

In this series of 376 fractures of the thoracic vertebral column (T1 to T10), the mechanical load most often implicated as the cause of injury was found to be axial load. The fracture follows direct vertical loading of the spine, either from above, as from a falling object, with injury to either the cervical or upper thoracic spine, or falling directly on the proximal thoracic spine (T1 to T5) (Fig. 16-9). The fracture may also be induced from below, as with a fall from a height, landing on the feet or buttocks. With a fall, a burst compression-type fracture more frequently occurs, either in the lower or midthoracic spine (T10) or at the thoracolumbar junction.

Fall injuries usually result in both axial and flexion load fractures at or above the normal thoracic kyphosis (T3 to T7). The result is a compression

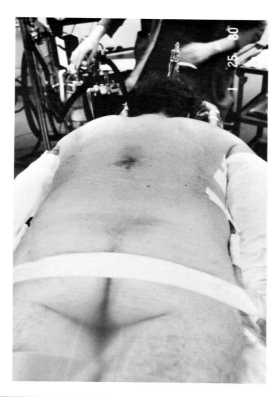

A

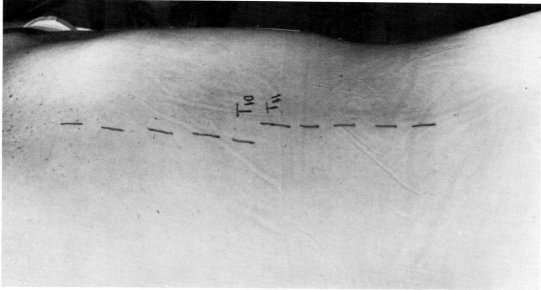

B

Fig. 16-8. (A) Area of abrasion over posterior thoracic spine showing the level of the direct trauma. **(B)** Malalignment of posterior spinous processes as a result of fracture and displacement of the posterior elements of T10 and T11. *(Figure continues.)*

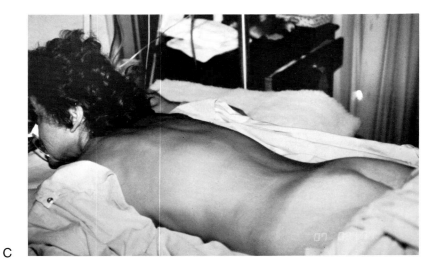

C

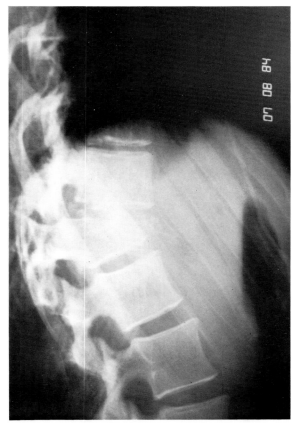

D

Fig. 16-8 *(Continued)*. **(C)** Gibbus overlying lower thoracic spine indicates the level of vertebral element displacement. **(D)** Lateral radiograph of the T11–T12 fracture subluxation injury of the patient shown in Fig. C.

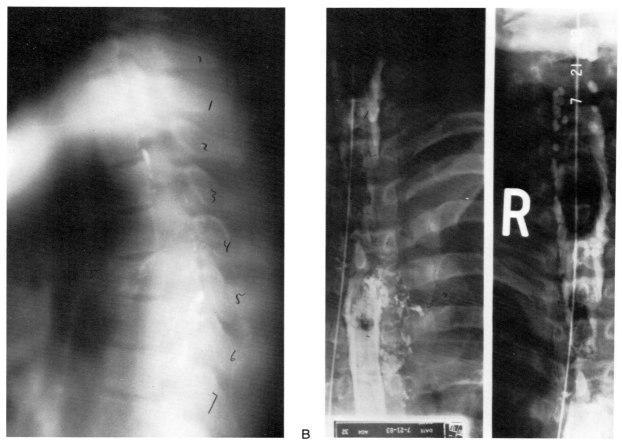

A   B

Fig. 16-9. (A) Radiograph showing axial load injury to thoracic vertebral elements posteriorly at T4 and T5 and axial load compression injury of T5 vertebral body. Because the patient had bilateral incomplete paraparesis (motor and sensory) below T5, a myelogram was performed. The patient also had associated hemopneumothorax. **(B)** Myelogram on the left shows incomplete obstruction at T4–T5, dural tear with extravasation of contrast, and associated rib-transverse process injury. The AP myelogram on the right reveals secondary spinal cord edema at C5–C7. The patient had no neurologic involvement of the upper extremities.

fracture. Holdsworth labeled this fracture, in the absence of any translation, as "stable."[9,10] As a rule, a pure vertical load injury to the spinal column will not be associated with either anterior or lateral translation of the superior vertebral body on the adjacent lower vertebral body, unless there is an associated combination of vertical load, flexion, and rotation and some component of translational forces applied in a horizontal direction. This combination, when present, dictates the presence of instability and an "unstable fracture."[9,10] Pure ver-

tical loading results in either compression or bursting of the vertebral body. Retropulsion of bone from the posterior vertebral body wall into the neural canal (Fig. 16-10) not infrequently occurs, producing a neural canal space compromise of greater than 50 percent. In the thoracic spine, this amount of neural canal and neural tissue compression is poorly tolerated and will result in neurologic sequelae. Bedbrook is of the opinion that compression of the neural canal up to 50 percent can be tolerated without harm.[8] His statement in no way

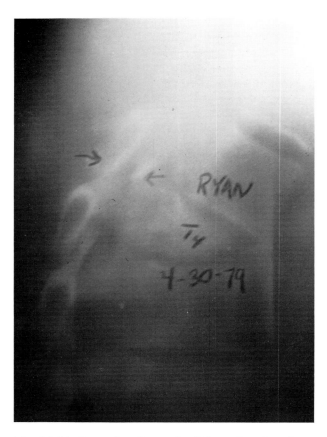

Fig. 16-10. Lateral radiograph of thoracic spine shows retropulsion of bone at the posterior aspect of the T4 vertebral body. The patient sustained complete T4 neurologic injury.

Flexion Injuries

The mechanical force most often suspected of producing injury to the thoracic spine is flexion, yet evidence reveals that it was second in mechanical occurrence (see Table 16-5). In large part, this occurs because of the already present proximal thoracic spine kyphosis, which varies in magnitude from individual to individual. After gunshot wounds, motor vehicle accidents are the most frequent cause for this mechanical injury to the thoracic spine, followed by falls or falling objects (see Table 16-4). Because the vascularity of the thoracic spinal cord is poor at best in its proximal and midportions (see Chap. 4) and is accompanied by an anatomic narrowing of the neural canal[3] (1.2 by 1.2 cm) (Table 16-8), the frequency of associated spinal cord injury is high. In my series of 114 T1 to T10 flexion fractures, 62 percent were complete, 27 percent were incomplete, and only 11 percent were intact (Table 16-7).

In my opinion, there are three factors that contribute to the 62 percent frequency of complete neurologic injury after the occurrence of a flexion mechanical load (and fracture) to the thoracic spine: a high-magnitude force; an acute angular deformity occurring at the time of injury; and the traumatic interruption of the blood supply to the anterior spinal cord. This thesis is supported by the history of a flexion injury to the spine, the find-

indicates either the magnitude or the direction of force that produced that compromise. It is my opinion that the compromise of the canal more likely was at or near 100 percent at the moment of injury. The presence of the rib cage serves as a vital support for the vertebral column. As long as the ribs remain attached to the sternum and the vertebral column, much of the axial load forces falling on the spine will be dissipated into the surrounding skeletal structure and reduced. Thus, when fracture of a vertebral body does occur, its force has, in all likelihood, been dissipated by the surrounding and adjacent structures. Again, the extent of the injury is based on the force and direction of the original injury.

Table 16-8.   Measurement of Thoracic Spinal Cord in the Sagittal Plane

	Diameter of Spinal Cord (mm)		
Spinal Cord Level	Minimum	Average	Maximum
T3		6.0	
T4	5.6	6.2	7.3
T5	3.7	6.1	7.2
T6	3.7	6.1	7.8
T7	5.3	6.3	7.9
T8	3.4	6.3	7.8
T9	3.7	6.2	8.0
T10	6.0	6.5	7.0
T11	4.5	6.9	10.5
T12	3.8	7.4	9.3

ing of a wedge compression fracture (usually greater than 50 percent) or compression-burst fracture in the midthoracic (T4 to T6) region, and a neurologic injury at or near the same neuroanatomic level. Vascular injury, as the most suspect factor causing neurologic dysfunction, is supported by the gradual appearance or ascent over a 24 to 36 hour period of a neurologic injury, when time is the only variable. This phenomenon is not uncommon with vertebral-vascular injuries in the area of the lower thoracic spinal cord (T10-T11 level).

Flexion injuries of the thoracic spine may be minor and inconsequential (with a less than 25 percent compression of the superior and anterior vertebral body) and have little or no threat of injury to the nervous system or may be more serious (more than 35 to 50 percent compression of the height of the vertebral body). If not initially injurious to the nervous system, this latter group has a potential for producing neurologic injury later. To do so, this fracture would be considered unstable by virtue of being a fracture of the vertebral body height of 25 to 35 percent or greater, with other associated vertebral element injuries; having diastasis of the posterior interspinous and interlaminar ligaments; having diastasis of the facet joint capsule; having rupture of the posterior longitudinal ligament; having a fracture of the posterior bony elements; angular deformity (kyphosis) of the spine, resulting in a shifting of the center of gravity through the vertebral body center of gravity such that the weight-bearing line through the upper thoracic spine lies sufficiently anterior to cause further flexion angular deformity (from either vertebral body collapse secondary to altered biomechanics or bone resorption as a process of fracture healing). The presence of this degree of angular deformity (greater than 35 percent, with evidence of progressive collapse) will require internal stabilization.[7,9–14] (Fig. 16-11A,B).

While the progressive deformity fracture requires stabilization, there are many with an initial lesser degree of angular deformity that require only close observation, bed care, or orthotic support for 6 weeks to 10 weeks. Some of these fractures, however, despite their initial benign appearance, may collapse, resulting in not so much a neurologic injury as the development of a prominent gibbus or kyphosis. These fractures initially appear with a loss in anterior vertebral body weight of less than 25 percent. In time, there is further alteration in vertebral body architecture, and within 2 to 3 weeks of injury, probably as a result of unrecognized comminution, the vertebral body undergoes resorption and compression. Once kyphosis reaches 35 percent of the vertebral body's height, this alone indicates instability and a possible need for stabilization. It is this occurrence that prompts obtaining tomograms on each spine fracture as a method of fracture evaluation, regardless of the fracture's initial benign appearance.

Rotation (Torsion) Fractures

The most frequent mechanical force that appears in combination with other more direct forces that alone produce vertebral column injuries is rotation. Bedbrook and colleagues, reviewing the posttraumatic pathology (autopsy specimen) of neurologic injury victims, noted that compression of the spinal cord was not the most common mechanism of irreversible injury.[8,15] Rather, crushing, stretching, and rotational shearing stresses were the three forces that most often caused permanent spinal cord injury.

Bedbrook and his co-worker made other important pathologic observations.[15] Examination of the spinal cord at autopsy revealed that neural damage frequently extended over a distance of 1 cm to 5 cm opposite the site of spinal injury. This followed fracture of the posterosuperior border of the vertebral body below, with the intervertebral disc debris serving as a fulcrum over which the spinal cord was stretched, producing secondary cord impression. The pathologic changes that occurred subsequent to trauma were noted to be a continuous process. Initially, the cord appeared normal between 1 hour and 24 hours after injury. Thereafter, there was increasing evidence of gliosis and fibrosis associated with necrosis and liquifaction and death of the central gray matter. These changes may have been the result of direct trauma, followed by edema and ischemia. In some instances, these changes were noted with infection. These pathologic findings within the spinal cord, secondary to spinal trauma, are not amenable to improvement by surgical decompression, except in

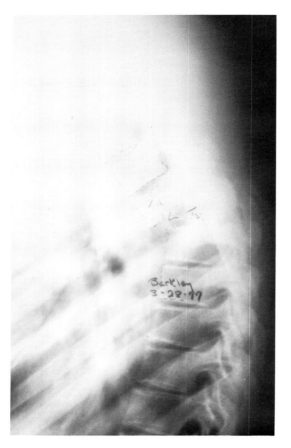
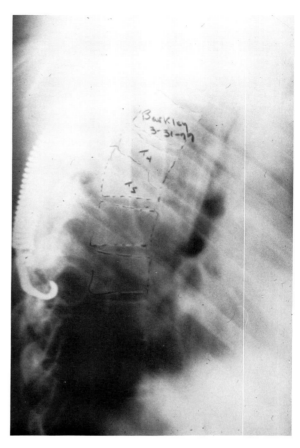

A

B

Fig. 16-11. (A) Lateral radiograph of thoracic spine showing flexion wedge compression fracture of the T5 vertebral body with anterior subluxation of T4 on T5. The patient had complete paraplegia at T5. (B) Postoperative lateral radiograph showing improved spinal alignment. Compression (Weiss) springs were used for internal fixation, and a Knight-Taylor orthosis with pectoral horns and cervical extension to the posterior occiput was used for external immobilization for 3 months.

specific incidences of well-localized spinal cord hematomyelia or spinal cord compromise secondary to cord compression, and even then, the correct surgical approach is from the direction of the compression, not categorically by means of laminectomy.

After thoracolumbar and lumbar spinal trauma in which nerve root injury results in a completely flaccid motor response and sensory loss of function, the nerve root has likely been torn in a ragged fashion, with disruption of both axonal fibers and nerve sheath (neurotomesis). Bedbrook has noted that only those rootlets having intact sheaths surrounding the axonal fasciae are capable of recovery.[16]

Should the sheath be intact and the axon disrupted (axonotomesis), axonal regeneration will occur as long as the cell body is intact.

Rotation injuries appear at all levels of the vertebral column. They are usually associated with a neurologic deficit. With the focus and concentration of a rotary force to a localized area, the resultant injury will likely be a comminuted fracture involving the posterior elements at one level, with either instability or dislocation; involvement of multiple adjacent vertebra with comminution; bone displacement into the neural canal; translation of one vertebra on another; or a combination of all the above.

In the midthoracic spine, the type of fracture most frequently seen is the one noted in Figure 16-12A,B. An oblique fracture extends through one vertebral body (to include the posterior element, the pedicle, and the facet joint on one side), and the fracture is carried downward across the adjacent inferior disc space to involve the next inferior vertebral body. This body will frequently demonstrate a fracture across its superior plate.

Because of the magnitude of the force of the compression and rotation, there will usually be an associated element of lateral translation of the upper vertebral body segment on the lower and comminution involving one or both of the two vertebrae. As noted, the appearance and extent of lateral displacement of the superior on the inferior vertebra will depend on the extent of rotation and the various degrees of horizontal or translatory forces present. Regardless of the resultant appearance, a complete neurologic injury will be present.

Extension and Bending Fractures

Although isolated extension and bending forces may induce injury in the thoracic spine, they are rare because of the construction of the rib cage, sternum, and the multiple rib attachments to the

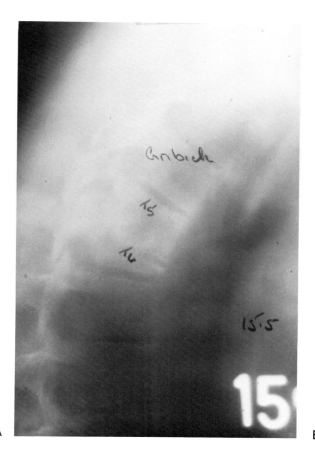

A

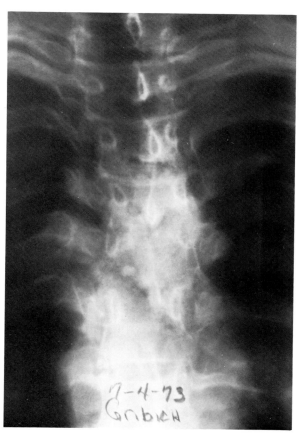

B

Fig. 16-12. (A) Lateral radiograph of thoracic spine showing axial load flexion-rotation injury involving vertebral bodies T5 and T6. This fracture is usually associated with comminution of both involved anterior and posterior vertebral elements. (B) Radiograph showing rotational component resulting in oblique fracture through posterior and anterior elements of T5–T6 and lateral translation of the upper segment. The fracture was managed conservatively with bed rest and an orthosis.

spine. The ribcage also provides resistance to lateral bending and absorbs perpendicular forces striking the chest from the anteriorly and laterally.

No extension injury occurred in our series of 376 T1 to T10 fractures. This rarity is not isolated to the thoracic spine alone. Only three such injuries have been observed in our series 470 thoracolumbar and 86 lumbosacral injuries. One extension injury occurred in the lumbar spine (see Fig. 16-14B), and two at the lumbosacral junction. In the area of the lower thoracic and upper lumbar spine, lateral bend fractures do occur, but hyperextension fractures are rare. Bedbrook reported only 3 of 180 injuries to the lumbar spine in his own series.[16] Although the dorsal aspect of the thoracic spine is certainly vulnerable to extension forces and injuries, at present this type of injury has not been identified.

The mechanism of extension injury is usually a sharp, severe translation force across the posterior spine resulting in sudden trunk or torso hyperextension (as being struck from behind by a swing beam). To occur, the force must be of short duration, focused or highly localized, and produced by a moderately heavy and wide object. The injury must be across an area of the spine and body where there exists above the level of the injury sufficient body mass (trunk) to acutely lever the torso posteriorly, above and over the anteriorly displaced lower segment. Such an injury may result from a blow across the frontal region of the chest, producing a fractured sternum (Fig. 16-13). A rheumatoid spondylitis victim involved in a motor vehicle ''rear-end'' accident sustained two hyperextension fractures: one in the cervical spine, the other in the lumbar spine (Fig. 16-14A,B).

The type of vertebral injuries one is likely to see with an extension moment to the spine are anterior disruption of the anterior longitudinal ligament and anterior diastasis through the anulus fibrosus in the normal spine. In the hyperextended osteoporotic spine, one would expect to find anterior distraction of the vertebral bodies, with avulsion of the anterior longitudinal ligament from the vertebral body either inferiorly or superiorly. In the rheumatoid spondylitic patient as illustrated in Fig. 16-14B, a hyperextension fracture through the midportion of the involved vertebral body is characteristic.

Although no extension fractures occurred in this

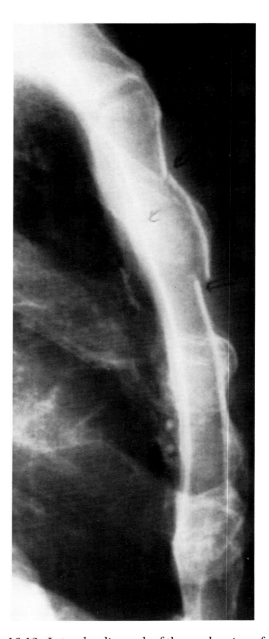

Fig. 16-13. Lateral radiograph of thorax showing a fracture of the sternum. This type of fracture is often accompanied by intrathoracic trauma such as pericardial tamponade, hemopneumothorax, multiple fractured ribs, and great vessel injury.

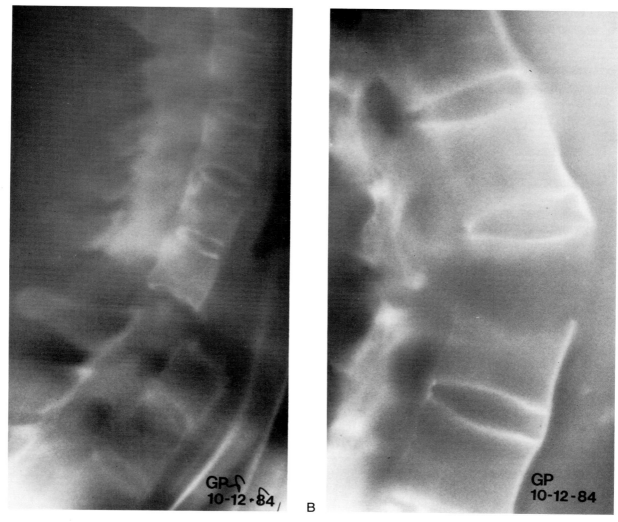

A   B

Fig. 16-14. (A) Lateral cervical spine radiograph of a 53-year-old man with Marie-Strümpell rheumatoid spondylosis involving the entire spine. The victim's automobile was struck from the rear, causing sudden extension injuries. The radiograph shows devastating fracture dislocation with retroluxation of the upper segment and immediate onset of quadriplegia at C7. (B) Lateral radiograph of lumbar spine showing an extension injury through the substance of the superior aspect of the L3 vertebral body. Both fractures were grossly unstable, and both required internal fixation to achieve alignment and stability. The lesson to be learned from this case is that a previously deformed spine should be placed in its previous angular deformity at the time of internal fixation. No attempt should be made to achieve improved vertebral column alignment through "traumatic osteotomy" of the spine.

series of patients and there are no statistics to relate the likelihood of complete to incomplete or intact neurologic injury after such injury, it is worthwhile to draw on the experience of neurologic injury after extension injuries in the cervical spine. As noted in Chapters 14 and 15, extension injuries do occur in the cervical spine. Extension injuries rarely produce significant neurologic injury (only 5.8 percent of cervical extension injuries produced complete neurologic injury; see Chap. 14).

ASCENDING NEUROLOGIC LOSS AFTER SPINAL CORD INJURY

Of 109 thoracic and lumbar injuries with associated complete neurologic injury, three patients were found on admission to have the injury levels at T11 to L1, with a neurologic level that ascended to the level of the T6 to T8 interval. Two of the three patients demonstrated ascending neurologic deficits (decreased sensation) within the first few hours after admission. The etiology of these events could not be accounted for by any other means than vascular, with an absence of a more proximal bony injury or an injury that could have reduced spontaneously, while demonstrating an obvious injury with fracture dislocation at T11–T12 or T12–L1. The logical cause was a progressive, ascending spinal cord ischemia. One patient demonstrated on myelogram a medullary obstruction to contrast medium seven vertebral levels above the site of injury (Fig. 16-15). This obstruction resolved spontaneously on repeat myelogram at 3 weeks.

Frankel, discussing the problems of ascending cord lesions in the early stages of acute spinal cord injury, noted the onset of neurologic changes within the first days to weeks after injury.[6] He reported seven patients who sustained injuries to the thoracic and thoracolumbar junction that resulted in ascending lesions between 2 days and 18 days after injury. Five fractures were at the T12 level, one was at T11, and one was at T4. Although the incidence was only 7 in 808 reported cases (0.8 percent), Frankel was of the opinion that closer review of lesions involving the lower thoracic spine would reveal an incidence between 1.5 percent and 2 percent. (The incidence in our 1978 series of 109 patients was 2.8 percent[17].)

The most common cause of an ascending neurologic level is some form of vascular embarrassment to the spinal cord, or an ascending lesion secondary to spinal cord edema or hematomyelia, or, as suspected in six of Frankel's cases, the presence of an inflammatory necrotizing lesion. The lesions in these patients were accompanied by hyperpyrexia above 102°F (38.9°C).

Frankel and others describe varied approaches to the management of these ascending lesions.

Guttmann discussed the possibility of surgery, particularly when an ascending lesion was due to an epidural hematoma, or in the more rare presence of a subdural or medullary hematoma with associated cord edema.[18] Each of these could result in vascular compromise of the spinal cord as a consequence of

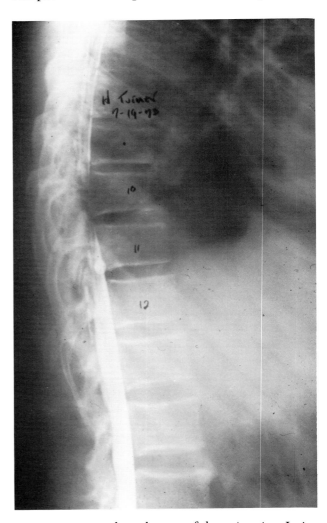

Fig. 16-15. Lateral myelogram of thoracic spine. Insignificant vertebral displacement is visible at T10–T11, but the patient had complete T10 paraplegia. The myelogram reveals cord swelling opposite the level of the neurologic injury. The diagnosis was spinal cord ischemia secondary to loss of primary vasculature (the vessel of Adamkiewicz or arteria radicularis magna). Other local pathologic causes of vascular obstruction include subdural or medullary hematoma (hematomyelia), cord edema, and epidural hematoma.

either intrinsic (hematomyelia) or extrinsic pressure on the anterior spinal artery, resulting in arterial thrombosis. Hardy[3] was of the opinion that when an ascending lesion occurred, it was more likely the result of one, rather than more than one, radicular vessel supplying the cord. In seven similar cases, he reported that heparin treatment was not successful.

Thus, the sequence of events that leads to an upward progression of the neurologic injury is the following. A fracture occurs at a lower level, accompanied by a neurologic injury (complete or incomplete) at the same neurologic level. Within hours to a day or two, there is an ascension of the neurologic level to as high as T6. The ascent of the neurologic level most likely follows the onset of vascular ischemia to the spinal cord secondary to direct injury to the anterior spinal artery or secondary to spinal cord edema or other potential causes, such as the angular (fracture) deformity or direct bony compression. Vascular injury may be confirmed only by vascular angiography (which carries the hazard of vascular thrombosis or infarction of the spinal cord by "stealing" of its arterial vascular support by the contrast material during the performance of the study).[19] A good indication that vascular compromise is the logical etiology is an absence of radiographic evidence of vertebral fracture and a negative myelogram. Further confirmation is the pattern of onset of the neurologic deterioration. If it is sudden, vascular thrombosis is suspected. If it is gradual, it is most likely secondary to spinal cord edema. The key to neurologic prognosis under such conditions is the evidence that the change in neurologic deterioration was gradual and incomplete. When neurologic deterioration is sudden, this is a poor prognostic sign and indicates infarction of the spinal cord and very little likelihood of neurologic recovery. On the other hand, when the loss is gradual, function will frequently (and gradually) return.

ASSOCIATED MULTIPLE TRAUMA

It has long been recognized that fractures of the scapula (see Fig. 2-2A), a flat bone, will frequently be associated with severe chest injury and multiple rib fractures (approximately 75 percent of the cases). The reason is both anatomic and biomechanical. The scapula lies protected against the posterior chest, beneath and between several thick muscles (the trapezius and the supraspinous and infraspinous muscles dorsally and the subcapularis and serratus muscles anteriorly). It lies on a flattened posterior rib cage. For a fracture to occur, a significant and well-focused force must be directed to the scapula. Thus, with the delivery of a concentrated force to the upper back, it is possible to produce a stellate (star-shaped) fracture of the scapula. This force, when transmitted through to the chest, may result in multiple underlying rib fractures. In the present series of 376 fractures of the thoracic spine, 41 percent of the victims had trauma to the chest. Frequently associated with multiple rib fractures are hemopneumothorax (see Fig. 1-2B), vascular injury (either thyrocervical trunk, subclavian artery, or aorta), and fractured clavicles (see Fig. 2-2A). Injuries to the chest require careful monitoring for evidence of respiratory stridor (difficulty), hemorrhage, tachypnea (increased respiratory rate), or decreased pulmonary compliance with alterations in arterial blood gases, etc. (see Chap. 9). Injuries that can and do accompany fractures of the thoracic spine (T1 to T10) include:

Fractures of the scapula (2 percent) (see Fig. 2-2A)
Fractures of the clavicle (5 percent) (see Fig. 2-2A)
Fractures of multiple ribs (carefully observe for ribs 1 and 2) (10 percent) (Fig. 16-16)
Hemothorax and pneumothorax (13 percent and 10 percent, respectively) (see Fig. 2-9A)
Rupture of a mainstem bronchus with tension pneumothorax
Injury to the great vessels (subclavian) (see Fig. 2-2A)
Avulsion of the brachial plexus (see Fig. 1-2E)
Pneumopericardium, pneumomediastinum
Cardiac tamponade (see Fig. 2-4C)
Tracheal fractures (see Fig. 2-3D)
Injuries to the arch of the aorta (see Fig. 2-2C)
Rupture of the diaphragm (Fig. 16-17)
Ruptured viscus or spleen (see Fig. 2-6B)
Extremity fractures (11 percent) (Fig. 16-18)
Head injuries (42 percent) (Fig. 16-19)
Hematemesis (3 percent)?

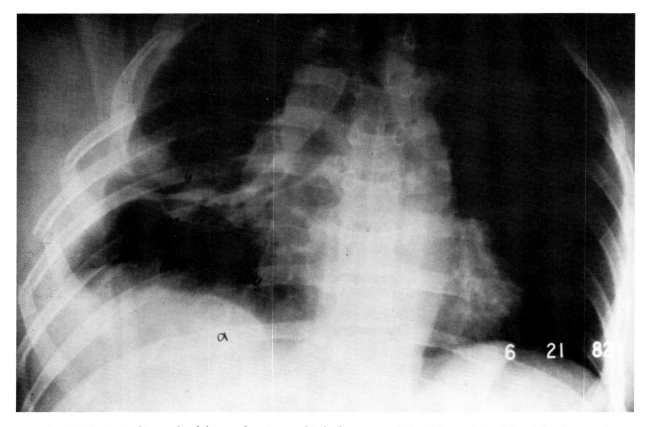

Fig. 16-16. AP radiograph of thorax showing multiple fractures of ribs 2 through 9 of the right chest with associated hemopneumothorax. The patient was the victim of a motor vehicle accident, and also suffered a cervical spine fracture at C5–C6.

VASCULAR INJURIES TO THE THORACIC SPINAL CORD

The intent of this brief overview of the spinal cord's vascular supply is to emphasize once again the vulnerability of the thoracic spinal cord to vascular injury with trauma. An in-depth review of the vascular supply of the entire spinal cord blood supply is found in Chapter 4.

Although it is relatively easy to affix the cause for loss of neurologic function in the presence of gross vertebral column fracture, occasionally no evidence of vertebral fracture exists, yet there will be neurologic injury. As noted in Table 16-1, this oc-

curred in 294 of 2,710 fractures of the spine (11 percent). The etiology is most often thought to be vascular interruption of the anterior spinal artery. Because the blood supply to the thoracic spinal cord between T4 and T11 is precarious and marginal even under normal conditions, there is little wonder that vascular changes follow known injury, particularly when associated with fractures demonstrating displacement.

The answer lies in the insufficient blood supply[20-23] and the anatomic narrowness of the thoracic neural canal (see Fig. 2-18).[24] An appreciation of both the spinal cord's blood supply and the anatomic construction of the thoracic neurol canal is important. In the patient with a neurologically

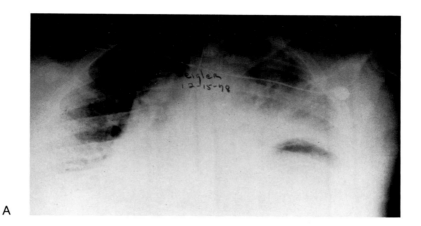

A

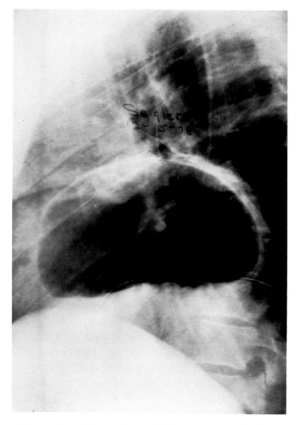

B

Fig. 16-17. Sequential AP chest films of a patient with multiple trauma including spinal cord injury. **(A)** Film showing occlusion of both right and left lung fields secondary to hemothorax and pneumothorax. The air shadow in the left chest is ominous. **(B)** Lateral thoracic radiograph reveals a large air shadow in the lower chest. Note the air shadow above the level of the liver shadow. Diagnosis: ruptured diaphragm with stomach in chest. *(Figure continues.)*

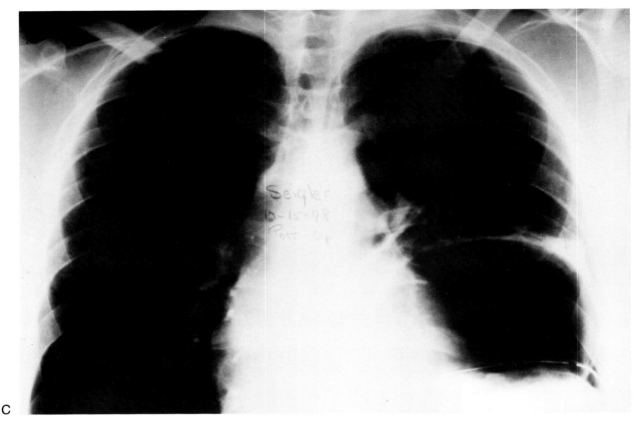

C

Fig. 16-17 *(Continued)*. (C) Postoperative AP radiograph after repair of diaphragm. Note thoracostomy tube in left lung field.

incomplete lesion, the patency of the canal must be determined. This can be ascertained by computed tomography (CT) scan; myelogram; tomogram; or magnetic resonance imaging (MRI). When the canal is compromised and the neurologic evaluation reveals the injury to be incomplete, this is one of the few indications for surgical decompression based on evidence of surgically relievable compromise. The structures most often compromised are the anterior spinal artery and, to a lesser extent, the two posterior spinal arteries. The persistence of this compromise may with time result in neural (spinal cord) tissue ischemia and permanent neurologic loss.[23] *Surgery may have no effect on the outcome, and in some instances, may even contribute to the already present defect by extending the neurologic deficit.*

Allen, in 1908 and 1911, described the histopathologic changes that appeared in the spinal cord after laboratory experimental trauma.[23] The experiments consisted of dropping a known weight a known distance onto the exposed dorsal surface of an anesthetized animal's thoracic spinal cord. The sequential changes that appeared in the traumatized spinal cord after death of the animal were recorded. Allen's animal studies have been revived by other researchers.[24-26] The following sequence of tissue changes has been identified.

Immediately (within the first hour) after the injury, Allen found edema and hemorrhage to the superficial area overlying the dorsal column. There was associated hemorrhage in the pia mater and bluish purple discoloration overlying the dorsal columns.

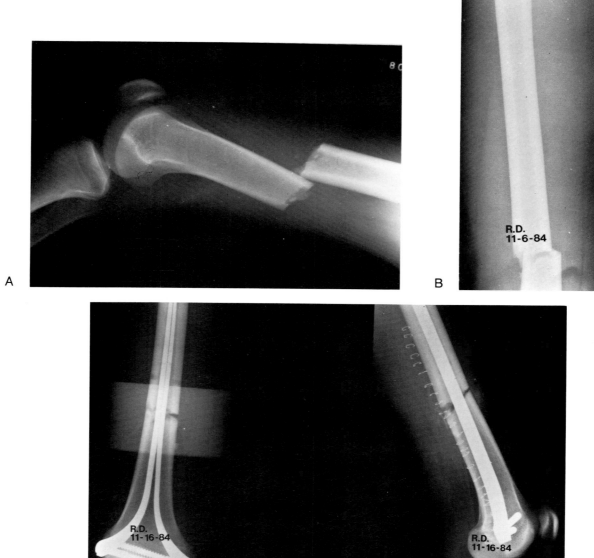

Fig. 16-18. (A,B) Lateral and AP radiographs of distal femur showing closed transverse fracture. (C) Internal fixation of femur with Zickel supracondylar nails. The patient suffered multiple trauma including L1 fracture dislocation. The femur was internally fixed before the spine injury was stabilized because of the supine position of the patient on the fracture bed and an unalterable neurologic injury.

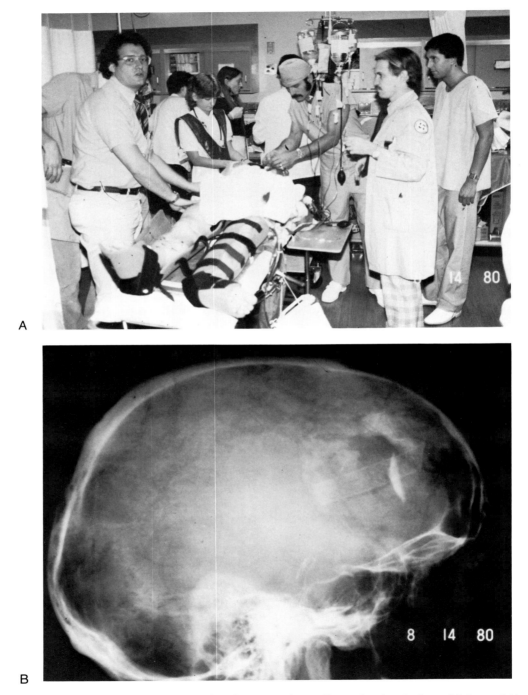

Fig. 16-19. (A) Emergency room scene of multitrauma (aircraft accident) spinal cord injury victim. **(B)** Depressed skull fracture requiring immediate operative intervention. *(Figure continues.)*

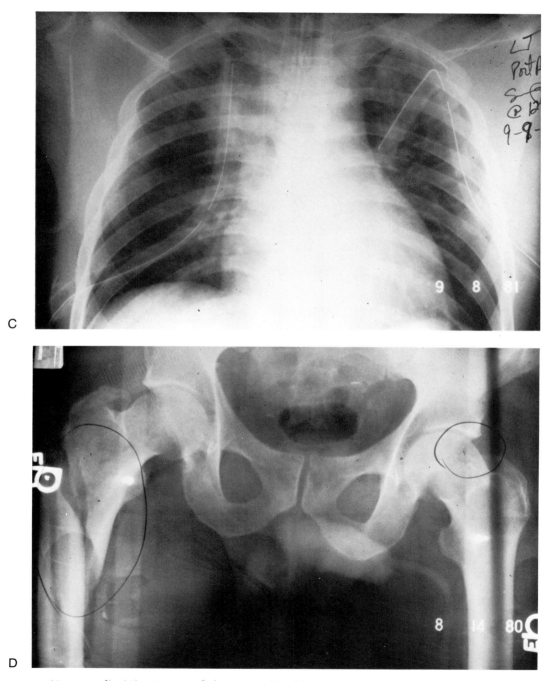

Fig. 16-19 *(Continued).* **(C)** AP view of chest revealing bilateral thoracostomy tubes for bilateral hemo-pneumothoraces. **(D)** AP view of pelvis and upper femurs revealing comminuted (open) fracture, proximal right femur. Immediate debridement was required. *(Figure continues.)*

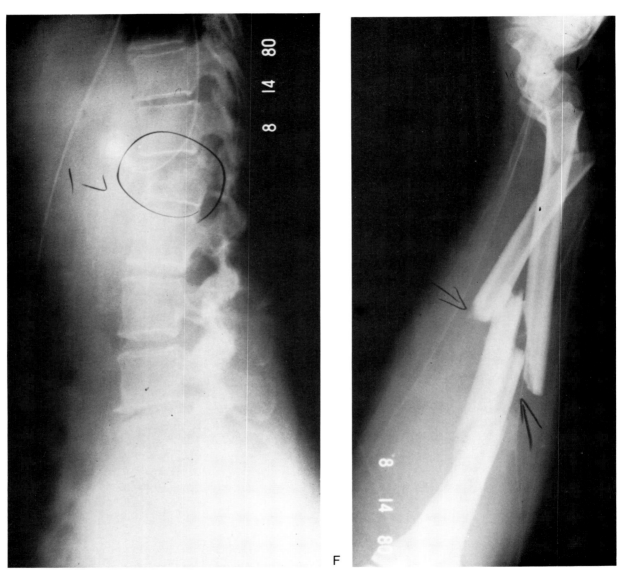

E

F

Fig. 16-19 *(Continued).* **(E)** Lateral radiograph of lumbar spine revealing compression fracture of vertebral body of L1 with subluxation of T12 on L1. The patient was unconscious and the neurologic level unobtainable. (Upon awakening from head trauma, the patient was found to have spastic quadriparesis from head injury and loss of L5 through S2.) **(F)** Open bone fractures of the right forearm requiring immediate debridement and secondary internal stabilization.

At 2 hours, hemorrhage was noted in the central gray matter. Most of the gray matter was invaded by red blood cells. Portions of the white matter were similarly involved. The most central portion of the central gray matter of the spinal cord took on the appearance of hyaline degeneration. Edema of the white matter was extreme.

At 4 hours, additional changes were noted. Numerous swollen axis cylinders were identified within the white matter, particularly in the lateral and posterior columns. Whether this was the result of injury from impact or biochemical changes from outpouring of serum or blood could not be ascertained.

At 5 to 6 hours, there was only an exaggeration of the findings described above.

At 6 hours, obvious evidence of spinal cord destruction was noted.

The anterior spinal artery in the thoracic region of the spinal cord is the principal provider of blood supply to the central gray matter. It receives tributaries from three sources (see Chap. 4):

The first intercostal artery, a rather large vessel, arising from the first thoracic segmental artery off of the aorta

The vessel of Adamkiewicz (or the arteria radicularis magna) via its upward watershed blood supply, ascending through the anterior sulcus of the spinal cord, from below (this vessel is a direct segmental branch off of the thoracic aorta [usually at the level of T10–T11])

Multiple less important segmental intercostals, which contribute to the overall arterial flow within the anterior spinal artery (or the anterior medial spinal artery below the level of the fourth thoracic cord segment). The contribution from these sources is small, variable and unreliable.

Because the central gray matter requires a relatively rich blood supply, it cannot escape periods of avascularity without injury. Because of its comparatively rich vascularity, the central gray matter is more susceptible to hemorrhage and its effects (autodestruction of the central gray matter secondary to the byproducts of neural tissue trauma).

The two posterior or dorsal arteries, which derive their blood supply from adjacent intercostal arteries, contribute little to the overall vascular support of the thoracic spinal cord. Their primary support is to the dorsal and peripheral areas of the white matter, which are principally composed of myelinated fibers and are relatively avascular. This explains the decreased vascular demand to the exterior areas of the spinal cord and serves as the rationale for survival of peripheral long tracts of the spinal cord (i.e., the spinothalamic tract [pain, temperature, and light touch] and the corticospinal [motor] tract) under conditions of relative spinal cord ischemia. The posterior vessels contribute little to the anterior spinal artery, although there are connections between the two, the arteriae coronae. Likewise, anatomic dissection of the anterior spinal artery reveals a very sparce number of penetrating (or perforating) vessels (the anterior sulcus arteries) entering into the interior of the central gray matter and little evidence that these vessels contribute to the surrounding peripheral white matter (see Fig. 4-7).

Clinical Support of Compromised Spinal Cord Vascularity

From the standpoint of clinical management, direct vascular support of or to the spinal cord is not possible. Any support for the spinal cord vascular network is indirect and is primarily influenced by enhanced support of the cardiovascular system centrally. When shock is the principal clinical picture or when the patient's cardiovascular system is unstable, certainly under those conditions of trauma to the nervous system (brain or spinal cord), there is concern for ischemic injury to neural tissue with systemic shock. Should cardiogenic shock be the primary cause, this must be addressed immediately, along with the prevention of systemic metabolic acidosis. Other causes of shock (such as hidden blood loss) after known trauma must also be kept in mind. Several empirical management techniques are suggested:

1. Fluids, crystalloids, lactated Ringer's solution; 0.1 N normal saline; 5% dextrose and water
2. The use of blood (preferred over other plasma expanders) because of its oxygen-carrying capacity
3. A cardiopressor such as dopamine hydrochloride (a myocardial inotropic drug that increases

cardiac output and renal and mesenteric vascular flow while having little or no effect on the peripheral vasculature)

4. Isoproterenol hydrochloride (Isuprel). This is another (and similar) inotropic drug that when titrated, increases cardiac output and decreases peripheral resistance.

With the objective being to enhance spinal cord capillary flow, the following may be used:

Mannitol (500 ml of 20% solution) is infused over 1 hour. It is employed as an osmotic diuretic and as such helps reduce tissue edema after trauma to central nervous system tissue. It also pulls extracellular fluid into the intravascular space. This treatment produces a relative hemodilution and improves capillary flow.

Dextran 40 (Reomacrodex; 500 ml) is utilized as a plasma expander and a platelet deaggregator, and to reduce intravascular sludging.

While positive evidence does not exist that dexamethazone (50 mg) is selectively effective on traumatized neural tissue,[27] I have found the drug beneficial in the patient with an incomplete neurologic injury. In the presence of vascular compromise, the drug is recommended. It is administered initially as a bolus and is followed over the next 5 to 6 days with a tapering of the dosage.

NEUROLOGIC INJURIES ASSOCIATED WITH THORACIC SPINE INJURIES

Of 376 fractures of the thoracic spine (T1 to T10), 235 (63 percent) resulted in complete neurologic injuries to the spinal cord. This predominence of complete neurologic injuries is anticipated because of the reduced size of the neural canal, the smallness of thoracic spinal cord[28] (Table 16-8), and the already discussed anatomic sparseness of the arterial vascular supply to the thoracic spinal cord. The width of the cervical and thoracic spinal cord has been accurately determined by air myelography. The diameter of the thoracic spinal cord

is small at this level (6.0 mm at T3, 6.5 mm at T10, and 7.4 mm at T12). The size of the neural canal at the level of T6 is the circumference of the tip of an index finger (see Fig. 2-18).[24] The thoracic spinal cord has only a small number of neurons within the central gray matter and is principally composed of peripheral white matter (long tracts). It is slenderer than the cervical spinal cord (the central gray matter area of the cervical cord is much larger than that of the thoracic cord, and it has an enlarged peripheral white matter as well — 10 mm at C1 – C2, 9.5 mm at C3, 8.5 mm at C6, etc.).[28]

Thus, the tolerance of the thoracic spinal cord for vertebral displacement with trauma to the thoracic spinal column is small. Interestingly, the literature states that while spinal stenosis is a problem to be contended with in the cervical and lumbar spine area, it apparently is rare in the thoracic spine.[30]

As noted, complete neurologic injuries (63 percent dominate the type of injuries that occurs in the thoracic vertebral column. Incomplete injuries represented only 27 percent of the injuries (101 of 376), and only 37 were intact injuries (10 percent) (Table 16-7). The relationship of neurologic injury to the occurrence of various types of spine fracture is a correlation attempted by other investigators.[31,32] No consistent correlation appears, although research continues.

Reviewing a fractured vertebral process radiographically, along with its relationship to adjoining vertebral processes, may suggest the anticipated neurologic injury, but not accurately. The answer lies in the specific nature of the vertebral processes fractured: anterior vertebral body, pedicle and facets, lamina or spinous process.[9-11] The neurologic injury depends on the type, extent, and combination of fractures and the instability resulting (Fig. 16-20).

With axial loading of the spine, wedge compression anteriorly, or bursting of the posterior aspect of the vertebral body, or fracture of the posterior elements may occur. The key to the neurologic level lies in the presence or absence of extrusion of the bone from the posterior vertebral wall into the neural canal, with fracture of the middle column (posterior vertebral body plus the pedicles and facets); the presence of subluxation or dislocation (translation) of one vertebral process on another;

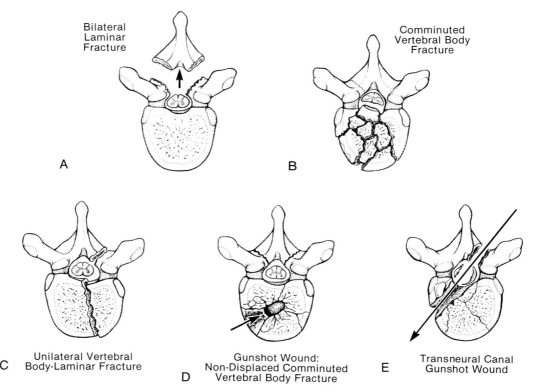

Fig. 16-20. Injuries to the vertebral column vary in origin and complexity, and may or may not result in neurological injury. **(A)** Axial load-extension injuries resulting in posterior bilaminar fractures without vertebral element displacement are stable injuries and often escape neurological injury. Essentially, these are "traumatic laminectomies." **(B)** Axial load-flexion injuries with vertebral body comminution are unstable and require internal stabilization. The spinal cord may be injured by bone extrusion into the neural canal. **(C)** Axial load-lateral bending injuries resulting in unilateral anterior and posterior column fractures are unstable. The severity of neurologic injury varies with the extent of initial displacement. **(D)** "Civilian" (low velocity) gunshot wounds of the vertebral column do not result in spine instability. Neurologic injury may result from impact or missile-induced tissue cavitation. **(E)** High-velocity missile injuries of the vertebral column, traversing both the anterior and posterior columns, do not result in spine instability. When the projectile traverses the neural canal, complete neurologic injury results.

or the presence of crushing or stretching of the cord. Occasionally, with vertical loading, fractures at multiple posterior element (pedicle, facet, and lamina) levels will occur with no neurologic injury at all. There are two reasons: the injury had an extension component (which produces fewer neurologic injuries), or the posterior canal was made wider by a "traumatic laminectomy." This injury has been identified in the cervical and lumbar

spine, but not in the thoracic spine (Fig. 16-21). The importance of these radiographic findings are that each element of spinal fracture plays a role in the cause or effect of neurologic injury, but cannot always be expected to correlate directly. This lack of correlation becomes important in my series of 2,710 patients, in which 294 (11 percent) had traumatic neurologic injuries without fracture. Similar experiences have been identified by others.[33]

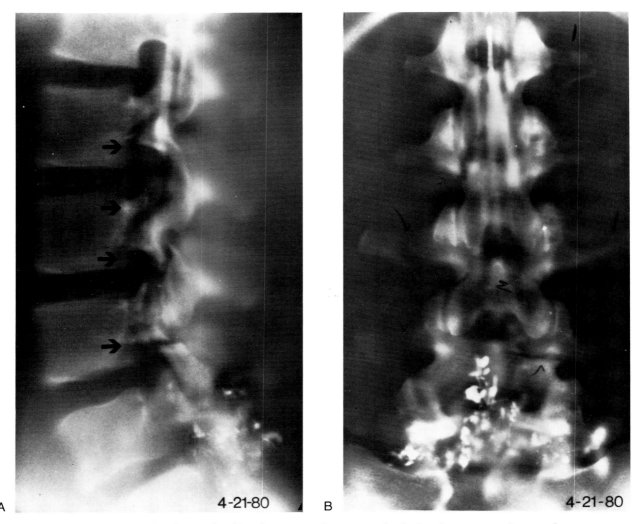

A   4-21-80   B   4-21-80

Fig. 16-21. (**A**) Lateral radiograph of lumbar spine showing multiple-level posterior element fractures secondary to acute sudden axial load extension injury. The patient was riding a motorcycle and fell through a hole in the street at a construction site, landing sharply on his buttocks and falling backward off of the motorcycle. The patient's neurologic injury was bilateral L5 axonotomesis. (**B**) AP radiograph of the lumbar spine showing extravasation of contrast as a result of multiple pedicle fracture and dural lacerations. Whenever bilateral pedicle fractures are identified, dural laceration should be suspected.

Aside from the predictability of specific neurologic injuries occurring with specific vertebral column fractures, certain associations of fractures occur (Table 16-9). Surprisingly, the axial compression (or burst) fracture in this series produced the fourth highest rate of complete neurologic injuries (54 percent). In a more generalized category

of vertebral fractures, identified as miscellaneous body fractures, which include compression fractures of the anterior, posterior, unilateral, or bilateral vertebral body and coronal and sagittal fractures, etc., 67 percent resulted in complete neurologic injury of the two patients with bilateral fracture dislocation, one had complete and the

Table 16-9. Fracture Type by Extent (T1 through T10) (Northwestern University Acute Spine Injury Center, 1972 to 1986)

Fracture Type	Total	Intact		Incomplete		Complete	
		No.	Percent	No.	Percent	No.	Percent
Axial body compression	118[a]	20	16.9	31	26.3	64	54.2
Miscellaneous body fracture	92	5	5.4	25	27.2	62	67.4
Bullet fragments	73	0	0.0	12	16.4	61	83.6
Wedge compression fracture	11	5	45.5	2	18.2	4	36.4
Facet fracture	4	0	0.0	2	50.0	2	50.0
Chance fracture	4	2	50.0	2	50.0	0	0.0
Spinous process	3	0	0.0	1	33.3	2	66.7
Unilateral facet lock	2	0	0.0	0	0.0	2	100.0
Bilateral facet lock	2	0	0.0	1	50.0	1	50.0
Transverse process	2	1	50.0	1	50.0	0	0.0
Subluxation	2	0	0.0	1	50.0	1	50.0
Other	13	4	30.8	4	30.8	5	38.5
None	50	0	0.0	19	38.0	31	62.0
Total	376	37	9.8	101	26.9	235	62.5

[a]Extent is unavailable for 3 subjects.

other incomplete neurologic injury. Interestingly, neurologic levels caused by facet dislocations in the thoracic spine area were either complete or incomplete. Gunshot wounds had the highest rate of neurologic injury in a category, with more than 10 observations (80 percent). One distraction-flexion injury of the thoracic spine occurred (without fracture). It resulted in a complete neurologic injury. This was probably due to cord stretching and vascular injury.[30]

MUSCULAR ANATOMY: THORAX AND THORACIC VERTEBRAL COLUMN

From the standpoint of orthopaedics, the thoracic vertebral column is a formidable structure to deal with. The posterior musculature consists of the superficial layer (trapezius, rhomboids, and levator scapulae), the intermediate layer (serratus superior and inferior, lumbodorsal fascia); and the deep muscles (erector spinae, spinalis, multifidus, semispinalis, rotators).[24]

Some of these muscles extend over several levels (in a rostral-to-caudal direction), and some over as few as one level (rotators brevis). Posteriorly and medially, between the lower (12th) rib and the superior rim of the posterior iliac crest, lies the quadratus lumborum. This muscle is responsible for stabilizing the 12th rib and has major responsibilities with stabilizing the spine and rib cage with lateral bending.

On the anterolateral and inferior borders of the thoracic cage, the muscles that affect the thoracic vertebral column lie in two distinct planes, one intercavitary along the vertebral column (the paraspinal muscles), and the other externally along the anterolateral chest wall. Both influence the behavior and function of the thoracic vertebral column.

Muscles of the Anterior Lateral Chest

Overlying the anterior and lateral chest are the pectoralis major and minor and the serratus anterior muscles. Inferiorly and anteriorly are the rectus abdominis and its rectus sheath, which stretches from the anterior surfaces of the fifth, sixth, and seventh costal cartilages and from the xiphoid process of the sternum to the pubic crest. From the 7th through the 12th rib anteriorly and laterally, inferior to the crest of ilium and to the pubic crest, pass the obliquus internus and externus and the transversus abdominis, and in between each rib are found the intercostal muscles.

Intercavitary Paraspinous Vertebral Muscles

Along the anterior aspect of the thoracic vertebral column (within the chest cavity) there are no muscular structures present other than the intercostal muscles. Inferiorly, still within the chest and abdomen, along the lateral sides of the vertebral column, lie the origin of the psoas major muscle (it originates at T12 and L1 to L5). Inferiorly and posteriorly along the thoracic vertebral column, extending from T12 inferiorly (to include the upper two or three lumbar vertebrae) is the origin of the diaphragm. This very strong and important structure inserts anteriorly along the costochondral border of the lower six ribs (Fig. 16-22).

From the standpoint of orthopaedic surgery, unless there are specific orthopaedic problems involving the thorax or thoracic spine (e.g., scoliosis), the musculature of the area is seldom addressed. In the average orthopaedic office practice, the only anterior chest maladies requiring attention include the sternoclavicular joint or a costochondritis of the second or third rib at its attachment to the sternun (Tietze's syndrome). Posteriorly, the problem most frequently addressed (over the posterosuperior thorax) is pain in the area of the insertion of the levator scapular muscle to the superomedial border of the scapula or pain in the area of the rhomboid muscles. The thoracic spine is not an area of frequent complaint, whereas the cervical and lumbar spine are. Therefore, from a biomechanical standpoint, the thoracic vertebral column is less well understood. It is possible, therefore, under conditions of trauma to the thoracic spine, that structural failure, muscle weakness, and imbalance, including the early onset of secondary paralytic scoliosis, may go undetected. When paralytic diseases such as anterior poliomyelitis were prevalent, early changes in vertebral column alignment were observed. Often, in the case of paralytic changes resulting from trauma, there is less of an

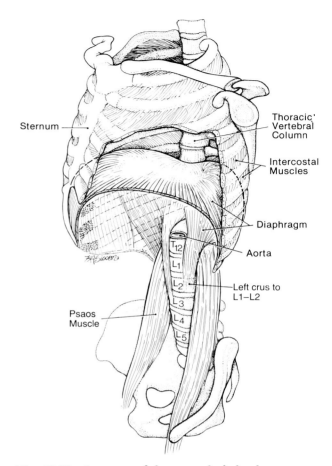

Fig. 16-22. Anatomy of the musculoskeletal structures at the thoracolumbar junction. The diaphragm attaches to the 10th rib anteriorly and to the 12th rib posteriorly, and to the vertebral column from T12 to L2. Note the relationship of the crux of the diaphragm to the aorta, and the attachment of the iliopsoas muscle to the vertebral column from L1 to L4.

early tendency to observe these changes because the victim is wheelchair bound, bedridden, inactive, etc., therefore not as prone to reveal a disability (scoliosis). As with other scoliosis curves, hereditary curves are S-shaped, and paralytic curves are C-shaped.

Scoliosis is a definite complication of spinal column trauma, particularly when there is neurologic involvement, and particularly in the child younger than 16 years[8,16,33-35] (Fig. 16-23). Traumatic scoliosis has also been identified in adult patients (such as a 43-year-old man with a complete neurologic

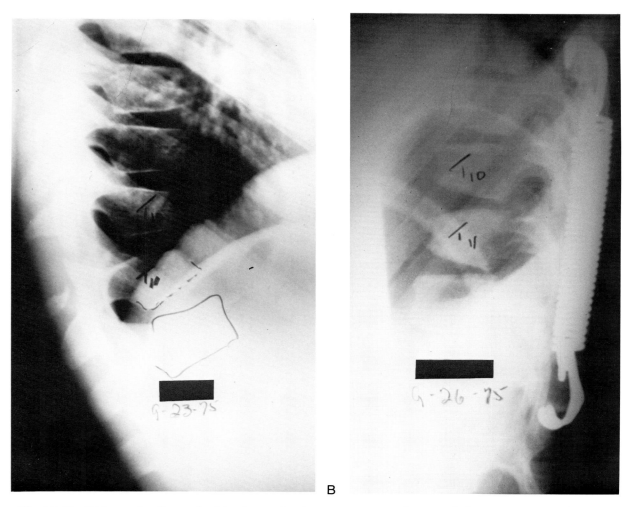

A
B

Fig. 16-23. (A) Lateral radiograph of the thoracolumbar spine reveaing fracture dislocation at T10–T11 in an 11-year-old girl. Note fracture of posterior element to include facet joints and anterior wedge compression of T11. Patient was rendered complete T11 paraplegic. (B) Lateral radiograph showing reduction of T10–T11 fracture dislocation and correction of traumatic kyphosis. Internal fixation device is Weiss spring. *(Figure continues.)*

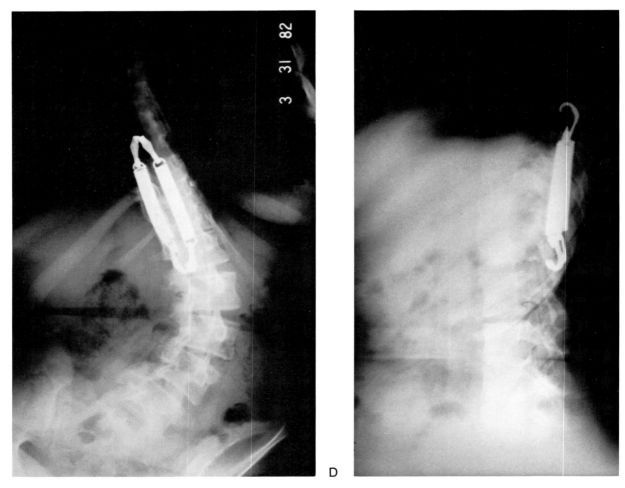

C

D

Fig. 16-23 *(Continued)*. (C) AP radiograph 7 years later. Note marked lumbar scoliosis and maintenance of alignment at the thoracolumbar junction. (D) Lateral radiograph showing maintenance of thoracolumbar alignment in the lateral plane despite the anteroposterior scoliosis. A spine fusion using Luque rod instrumentation from T7 to the sacrum was performed. *(Figure continues.)*

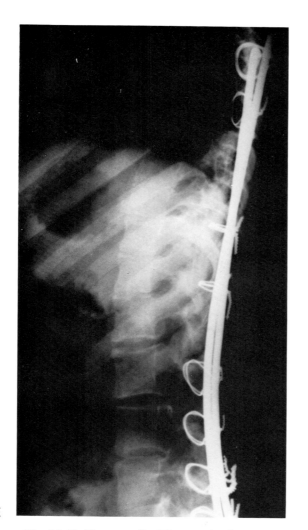

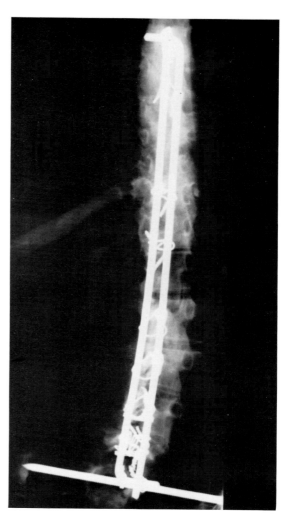

E   F

Fig. 16-23 *(Continued)*. **(E)** Lateral radiograph 15 months after spine fusion. **(F)** AP radiograph 5 years after spine fusion.

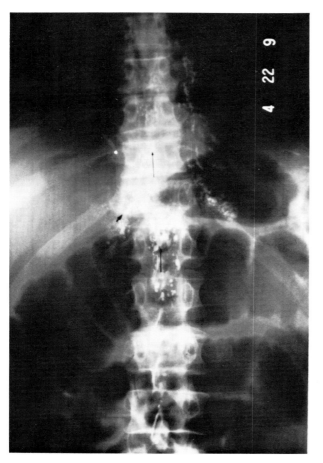
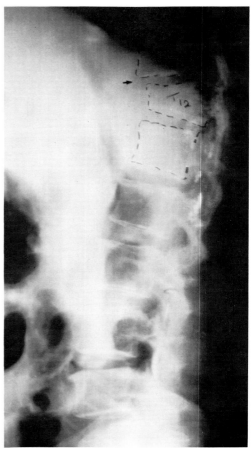

A   B

Fig. 16-24. A 43-year-old man who sustained fracture dislocation of T12–L1 from a truck accident. (A) AP radiograph of the thoracic spine showing the translatory fracture dislocation of T12–L1. Patient had a complete T12 neurologic injury. Note extravasation of myelographic contrast material. (B) Lateral view of the thoracolumbar spine showing a wedge compression fracture of T12 and forward subluxation of T11 on T12. *(Figure continues.)*

injury below T12, Fig. 16-24). The fact that it occurs at all is not unreasonable. The closer we observe the patient for its onset, the greater will be the frequency of its appearance.

OSTEOLOGY: THORACIC VERTEBRAL COLUMN

The thoracic vertebral column consists of 12 vertebrae and supports the ribs directly and the sternum indirectly. The combination of the thoracic spinal column and the paired ribs forms the root of the chest cavity, serving as a protective envelope around the major organs: the heart, the esophagus, the trachea, the lungs, the great vessels, the diaphragm, and the thoracic spinal cord. The vertical stance and stability of the thoracic vertebral column provide a foundation for the carriage of the trunk and torso, directly enable upright skeletal mobility, and serve as a mechanical fulcrum, allowing such things as raising the arms and shoulders, bending, twisting, etc. White and Panjabi[1] note that the stiffness of the spine is enhanced 2.5 times by the presence of the rib cage over the "ligamentous spine alone."

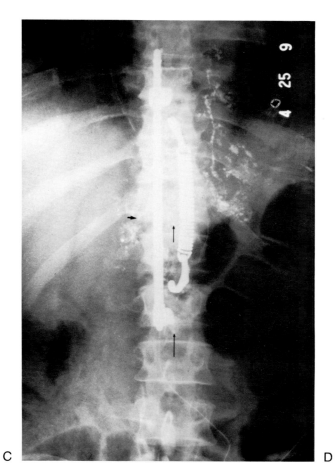
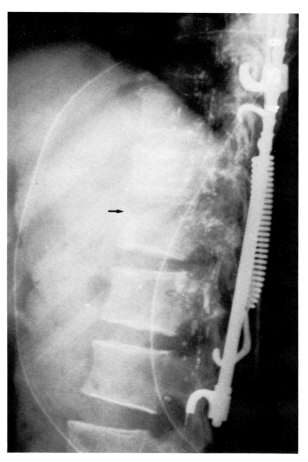

C   D

Fig. 16-24 *(Continued)*. **(C)** AP view of the thoracolumbar spine after open reduction internal fixation using Harrington distraction rods on one side of the vertebral compression fracture and Weiss springs on the opposite side to apply compression across the fracture-dislocation site. Note improvement in lateral translatory displacement of T12. **(D)** Lateral view showing improved alignment of T11 and T12 and correction of the traumatic kyphosis seen in Fig. B. Note improvement in wedge compression of the T12 vertebral body anteriorly. *(Figure continues.)*

Viewed in the anteroposterior projection, the thoracic spine is normally straight. In the lateral projection, the thoracic spine displays an accommodating posterior convexity (or kyphosis) in its upper and midportions, extending from approximately the second to the ninth vertebra. The thoracic vertebrae are consistent in size and shape (Fig. 16-25). Each vertebra is composed of several major identifiable parts: the vertebral body proper; a superior and inferior costal pit on each side of the vertebral body for the attachment of the ribs (except the 1st, 10th, 11th, and 12th verte-

brae); the posterior (laminar) arch, serving as a roof over the dura and its contents (the spinal cord); the intervertebral neuroforamen (for the exit of the spinal nerves and the entrance of a segmental blood vessels); and the vertebral canal, which is round at the midpoint and becomes more triangular as it approaches both the cervical and the lumbar ends of the thoracic vertebral column.

The thoracic neural canal is smaller than it is in either the cervical or lumbar spine. This is because of the smallness of the thoracic spinal cord. Unlike the cervical and lumbar regions of the spinal cord,

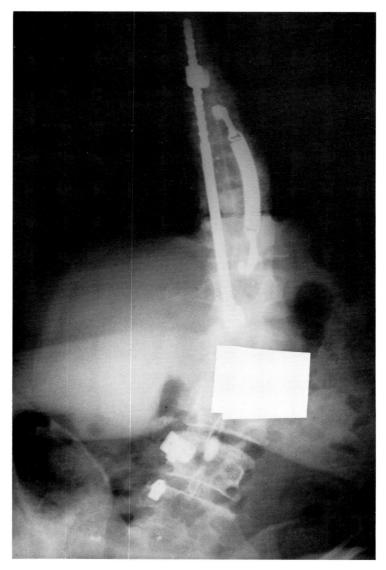

E

Fig. 16-24 *(Continued)*. **(E)** AP view 7 months later shows development of significant paralytic scoliosis and close proximity of right 12th rib to right iliac crest. Note maintenance of **AP** alignment of the thoracolumbar junction. Traumatic scoliosis is a complication that affects both children and adults following upper middle thoracic spine neurologic injuries.

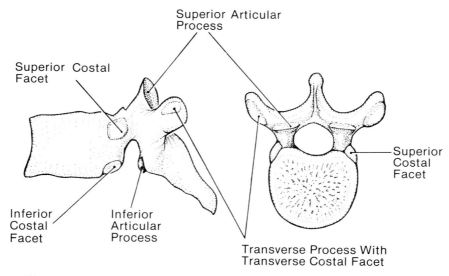

Fig. 16-25. Prominent anatomic landmarks of a typical thoracic vertebra.

where there are enlargements resulting from the large number of nerves entering and exiting the cord which pass to the extremities, in the thoracic region there are only those nerves to the cutaneous regions and the intercostal nerves and branches to the anterolateral and posterior musculature exiting the cord at each level. This single anatomic finding takes on major significance when it is appreciated that the incidence of significant neurologic injury after trauma to the thoracic vertebral column is higher than with injury to other areas of the vertebral column. As noted above, 63 percent of spine injuries in the area of the thoracic spinal column are complete, 27 percent are incomplete, and 10 percent are intact. Because of the smallness of the thoracic spinal cord, there is a natural reduction in the extent of the vascular supply to the thoracic cord (see Chap. 4). Along with a sparcity in the blood supply, there is an associated smallness to the neural canal. Together, these indicate the seriousness of any injury to the thoracic spinal cord.

Each vertebral body has seven processes: two superior and two inferior articular facets, two transverse processes, and one spinous process (see Fig. 16-25). The superior articular processes face dorsally, cranially, and laterally (viewed from above), while the inferior articular processes face in a ventral, caudal, and medial direction. As noted

above, the fit between the facet joints at T5-T6 is minimal (facing horizontally at each other), while at T12–L1 there is literally locking of the facets (owing to the anatomic facing of the facets medially and laterally) (Fig. 16-2).

Between the superior and the inferior articular processes laterally lies a vertebral neuroforamen (see Fig. 4-6). Through it passes a nerve root and a blood vessel (see Chap. 4). Like the articular processes, the laminae in the upper thoracic region are imbricated, slope caudally, and result in the cranial laminar processes overlapping the caudal laminar processes.[29]

Generally, thoracic vertebral bodies appear similar throughout. The first thoracic vertebra is a transitional vertebra and has general configurations very similar to those of the seventh cervical vertebra. Both have concave cranial surfaces, and both are more wide transversely than in the anteroposterior direction. The most distinguishing characteristic of the first thoracic vertebra, differentiating it from the seventh cervical vertebra, is the presence of the first thoracic rib. This rib makes its articulation with the first thoracic vertebra along its superolateral border at the so-called costal pit. As stated earlier, each vertebral body has two (a superior and an inferior) costal pits. This normal anatomic finding varies in the 1st, 10th, 11th, and

12th thoracic vertebra where only one pit appears. Another area where costal pits are found is along the anterolateral border of each of the transverse processes, except the 11th and 12th thoracic transverse processes.

Radiographically, C7 and T1 appear quite different. Besides the presence of the first thoracic rib, the lateral mass-transverse processes of the seventh cervical vertebra and the first thoracic vertebra face in different directions. The lateral mass-transverse process of C7 slopes in a caudal direction, while the transverse process of the first thoracic vertebra slopes in a cranial direction. Radiographically, a visible difference is seen in the appearance of the posterior spinous process, in the lateral projection. Throughout the thoracic spine, the spinous processes are large and strong in appearance. The first thoracic vertebra spinous process generally lies in a horizontal position, whereas the seventh cervical vertebra spinous process slants in a more caudal direction. Consequently, the spinous process of T1 is frequently more prominent than that of C7. *This fact should be remembered at surgery.* The remainder of the spinous processes of the thoracic vertebra below T1 slope caudally, down to the level of T9-T10, where they become horizontal again.

CONSERVATIVE MANAGEMENT PHILOSOPHY

As a rule, fractures of the thoracic spine between T1 and T10 without neurologic compromise should be managed conservatively. This is particularily true for those fractures in which the neurologic level is completely normal. The rationale is as follows. You cannot improve on the neurologic level, but it is possible to make it worse. The thoracic spine is inherently stable because of the rib cage, making conservative care the first choice. The anatomy of the thoracic spinal (neural) canal is such that one must constantly be aware of the hazard of inducing neurological injury with surgical intervention. With the normal anatomic presence of a thoracic kyphosis, the use of any internal fixation device presently available requires that the

device be bent into a conforming shape; that (if distraction is used) the fixation will be posterior to the vertebral body center of motion, producing distraction anteriorly and straightening of the thoracic spine; that any internal fixation device inserted can, by virtue of its sublaminar position (hooks, wire), potentially serve as a mechanism of injury and compromise the narrowness of the neural canal. This statement does not rule out such instrumentation. Rather, it only serves as a reminder of the hazards during insertion. Careful monitoring of the somatosensory evoked potential during this period of the operative procedure is suggested (see Ch. 6).

Northwestern University Series, 1972 to 1986

Of the 932 fractures of the thoracic, lumbar, and sacral spine admitted to the acute spinal cord center at Northwestern University between 1972 and 1986, 376 (40 percent) of the fractures involved the thoracic spine between T1 and T10, and of those, 64 percent were managed conservatively (Table 16-10). The type of biomechanical force inducing injury to the thoracic vertebral column is summarized in Table 16-5. The radiologic fracture classification is given in Table 16-6.

As noted in Table 16-5, the most frequent mechanical cause for injury to the thoracic spine was

Table 16-10. Treatment by Change in Status[a] (Northwestern University Acute Spine Injury Center, 1972 to 1986)

Change in Status	Total	Conservative Treatment		Surgical Treatment	
		No.	Percent	No.	Percent
Improve	26	14	5.8	12	9.0
No change	325	211	87.2	114	85.1
Degradation	4	1	0.4	3	2.2
Unknown[b]	21	16	6.6	5	3.7
Total	376	242	64.4	134	35.6

[a]Change in status is change in Frankel score.
[b]Extent is unavailable.

axial loading (32 percent) from either the cranial or the caudal direction. Where the axial load is high, "bursting" of the vertebral body occurs, and neurologic injury is common (80 percent). The effect of this loading is vertebral body compression. Where an angular or flexion mechanical moment is also present, causing wedging of the vertebral body, the occurrence of neurologic injury increases to 90 percent (complete and incomplete) (Table 16-7). The latter occurs where the loss of anterior vertebral body height is greater than 35 percent.

Flexion injuries follow axial load injuries in frequency (30 percent), with 62 percent resulting in complete neurologic injury. Fractures of the vertebral column that occur secondary to an angular (flexion) injury also result in disruption of the posterior interspinous and interlaminar ligaments, rupture of the posterior longitudinal ligament, and are sometimes accompanied by either facet fractures or facet dislocations. Neither of these latter injuries is common in the thoracic spine, because of the restrictions on translatory motion provided by the rib cage. Our series of 376 thoracic fractures included only 4 facet fractures and 4 facet dislocations (unilateral or bilateral) (Table 16-9). All of these involved neurologic injury.

The next most common biomechanical force producing vertebral (and neurologic injury — 100 percent) was rotation (Table 16-7). It is stretching, crushing, and rotation of the spinal cord that most frequently results in neurologic injury. Rotation rarely occur as an isolated biomechanical force in spine injuries. It is usually associated with two other components — axial and flexion loads. The combination of the three is devastating.

Gunshot wounds to the thoracic spine were actually the primary cause of injury to the thoracic vertebral column, accounting for 106 of 376 thoracic injuries (28 percent). Eighty percent of the gunshot wounds resulted in a complete neurologic injury, and 20 percent in an incomplete neurologic injury. As a rule, gunshot wounds do not produce spine instability unless they become secondarily infected. Infection usually occurs only when the projectile passes through a highly contaminated hollow viscus, such as the trachea, esophagus, or colon. Infection rarely follows gunshot wounds to the small bowel, due to the absence of highly contaminated bacterial flora.

Fractures: T1 to T10

As stated above, there are numerous advantages to attempting conservative management initially. They include the following.

Most fractures occurring in the thoracic spine produce serious (complete) neurologic injury, accompanied by paraplegia (63 percent). Assuming that spinal column realignment has been accomplished before surgery or that the initial injury producing neurologic injury was not one with gross spine malalignment, surgical realignment and rigid fixation do not contribute to neurologic recovery. In the remaining 38 percent of patients with residual neurologic function (27 percent incomplete and 10 percent intact), it is reasonable to assume that surgical stabilization in this group may have contributed to the preservation of the residual neurologic function (Table 16-7).

The thoracic vertebral column has various degrees of anatomical kyphosis, making the insertion of internal fixation (Harrington, Wisconsin, Jacobs rods and hooks) difficult. To do so requires bending the internal fixation device to match the anatomic curve.

Bending any type of internal fixation device reduces the mechanical and structural strength and increases the chances for implant material (fatigue) failure (Harrington rod). Exceptions would be AO, C-D, and Luque rods.

The shallowness of the neural canal must be considered. Insertion of anything sublaminar within the epidural space (Harrington, Wisconsin, or Edwards hooks, Luque sublaminar wires, etc.), particularly in the incomplete neurologically injured patient, serves as a potential hazard to the thoracic spinal cord. Contributing factors are the narrow canal, spinal cord edema, and anatomic variants. Surgery should be utilized when the needs for and the benefits derived by its use outweigh the modest gains anticipated by applying only conservative management.

Fractures of vertebral segments at multiple (two or three) adjacent levels in the absence of major surgical indications (vertebral element dislocation, gross instability at one level, etc.) are best managed by recumbency until stable (usually 6 weeks to 8 weeks), followed by rigid orthotic support for an additional 6 to 8 weeks. Loss of skin sensation is not a deterrent to the wearing of an orthosis. Postoperative spine stabilization also requires orthotic management for periods of up to 3 months.

If multiple-level fractures require surgical stabilization, stability may be more rapidly attained, but the area of required stabilization may be more extensive than desired and result in unnecessary or excessive spine rigidity.

Because there are fractures that meet the criteria for internal fixation and stabilization, regardless of potential hazards, Chapter 17 contains this discussion and the options available. Basically, the indications for surgical management include gross spine instability, with the likelihood of being progressive; gross spine deformity with instability; need for patient mobility (skin, enhancement of pulmonary toilet, etc.); widely separated fractures (anatomically), one fracture above the level of neurologic injury, the other below, etc. (see Fig. 16-14AB); widely separated fractures, both mechanically unstable (see Fig. 16-14AB).

Thoracic Spine Fractures of T1 to T5: Adjunctive Management

A fracture that is not infrequent, yet when confronted is potentially difficult to manage, is the severe (greater than 50 percent) compression fracture of an upper thoracic vertebra (between T1 and T5 or T6). The fracture follows a direct fall onto, or a blow by an object to, the upper thoracic spine, resulting in a wedge compression fracture to an upper thoracic vertebra. The injury is almost always associated with a complete neurologic injury. There is usually present on radiographic evaluation an acute kyphotic angulation at the level of injury, accompanied by posterior displacement of fracture fragments into the canal. It is envisioned that this fracture occurs with the victim landing inverted on the ground in such a manner that all of the body weight (or weight of the object) is concentrated at a single level, producing an extremely high mechanical load on a small concentrated area.

A patient with the type of fracture described above was scheduled for surgical reduction and internal fixation of a severe compression fracture of T3. During the preoperative evaluation, an electrocardiogram revealed evidence of myocardium contusion secondary to the associated chest trauma. Surgery was not advised. The patient was therefore placed in cervical Gardner-Wells skull tong traction to maintain a straightaway head-neck-thorax relationship and to allow the patient to be managed on a Stryker wedge fracture frame. The amount of skeletal traction was 5 lb per level of injury (C1 to T3 = 10 segments × 5 lb = 50 lb). Within 2 hours the fracture was reduced (Fig. 16-26A). That patient was managed conservatively throughout his entire course, and at 6 weeks was placed in a Knight-Taylor orthosis with cervical extension (cervicothoracolumbosacral orthosis, CTLSO), stabilizing the head and neck as well as the thoracic spine (see Fig. 12-19). Since this first patient, seven others with similar fractures have been so managed, and at our suggestion, other centers have found this technique to be equally effective in bringing about a reduction of a similar fracture. It must be noted that fracture realignment in these situations has no influence on neurologic recovery. Neurologic injury in this area of the thoracic spinal canal is almost always all or none. The reasons are obvious: high concentration of forces over a small area; narrow neural canal with little spinal cord clearance; poor blood supply to the spinal cord (see Chap. 4). At the junction of T3-T4, the very abundant blood supply of the cervical spinal cord meets the very sparce watershed blood supply of the upper thoracic spinal cord (from below). Therefore, injury to the area either totally destroys the spinal cord mechanically or interrupts the spinal cord's blood supply, despite the first intercostal artery being a major segmental feeder to the anterior spinal artery at about this same level.

Effects of Management on Neurologic Function

As noted, of the 376 fractures of the thoracic spine, 242 (64 percent) were managed conservatively, while 134 (36 percent) were managed surgically (Table 16-10). Of the fractures managed conservatively, 14 patients (6 percent) demonstrated neurologic improvement and 1 patient (0.4 percent) demonstrated neurologic deterioration. Of the 134 patients managed surgically, 12 patients (8.9 percent) demonstrated neurologic improvement and 3 (2.2 percent) demonstrated neu-

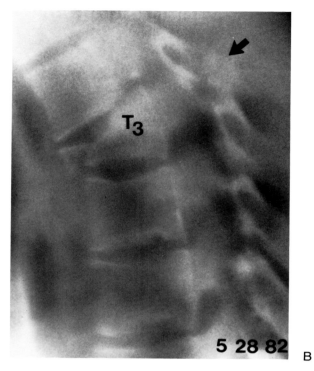 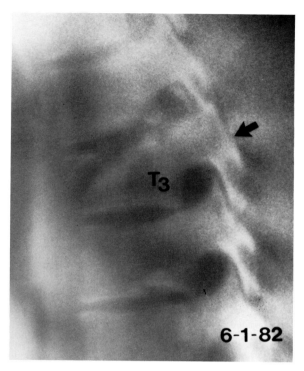

Fig. 16-26. (A) Lateral radiograph of the thoracic spine showing a flexion angulation anterior subluxation of T2 on T3, with complete T2 paraplegia. The patient also sustained a cardiac contusion, preventing surgical stabilizaton of the spine fracture. (B) Because surgical stabilization could not be carried out, the patient was placed in Gardner-Wells cervical tongs (5 lb per level of injury). Note that the alignment of the thoracic spine fracture is improved. The patient was maintained in skeletal traction, bed rest, and a Knight-Taylor orthosis with cervical extension and pectoral horns. The thoracic spine was held in good alignment with this conservative care.

rologic deterioration. Although surgical management resulted in a higher number of neurologic improvements, so also did surgical intervention result in a greater number of patients demonstrating evidence of neurologic deterioration. The beneficial effects of surgery is therefore statistically insignificant at a level of $P < .05$.

Orthotic Management

As noted earlier, when fracture of the upper thoracic spine has occurred at or above T6, the standard orthotic device, supporting the vertebral column at the sacrum and upper thoracic spine, cannot be utilized without the addition of a cervical

extension. The addition is required because without it, the anterior and proximal portion of the orthosis will not have sufficient body surface contact to prevent further forward kyphotic deformity. This orthosis is known as a **CTLSO** (see Chap. 12).

Below T6, there are several types of orthotic devices that may be utilized: the standard Knight-Taylor (or Arnold) orthosis (see Fig. 12-18), the Jewett hyperextension orthosis (Fig. 16-22), the modified cruciate Jewett orthosis (see Fig. 12-15), and the plastic laminated orthosis (see Fig. 12-20). Each of these orthoses should be worn at all times, including those patients required to spend short periods in bed. The orthosis is utilized to protect the spine from torsional forces while turning in bed or coming to a sitting position. For the patient with minimal vertebral injury without neurologic injury, the orthosis may be removed during recumbency. Patients with a thoracic spine injury between T1 and T10, when not using an orthosis, should maintain a flat position while in bed, without the use of a pillow. This should be adhered to for a period of 6 weeks, or until stability at the injury site has been verified.

The primary precaution for all patients having sustained a spine injury with neurologic injury is the hazard for skin breakdown beneath the orthosis. It is suggested that each patient wearing an orthosis wear a T-shirt beneath the orthosis at all times to protect the skin from shear forces. The skin should be carefully observed frequently for any signs of skin breakdown. This implies all areas of skin contact: orthosis, clothes, bed, or chair.

REFERENCES

1. White AA, Panjabi MM (eds): Functional spinal unit and mathematical models. In Clinical Biomechanics of the Spine. JB Lippincott, Philadelphia, 1978
2. Markolf KL: Deformation of the thoracolumbar intervertebral joint in response to external loads: a biomechanical study using autopsy material. J Bone Joint Surg 54A:511, 1972
3. Hardy AG: The treatment of paraplegia due to fracture-dislocations of the dorsolumbar spine. Paraplegia 3:112, 1965
4. Calenoff L, Chessare J, Rogers LF, et al.: Multiple levels, spine injuries: importance of early recognition. AJR 130:665, 1979.
5. Calenoff L (ed): Radiology in Spinal Cord Injury. CV Mosby, St. Louis, 1981
6. Frankel HL: Ascending cord lesion in the early stages following spinal injury. Paraplegia 7:111, 1969.
7. Kaufer H, Hayes JT: Lumbar fracture-dislocation. A study of twenty-one cases. J Bone Joint Surg 48A:712, 1966
8. Bedbrook GM: Some pertinent observations on the pathology of traumatic spinal paralysis. Paraplegia 1:215, 1963
9. Holdsworth FW: Review article. Fracture-dislocation and fracture-dislocations of the spine. J Bone Joint Surg 52A:1534, 1970
10. Holdsworth FW, Hardy, AG: Early treatment of

paraplegics from fracture of the thoracolumbar spine. J Bone Joint Surg 35B:540, 1953
11. Denis F: The three column spine and its significance in the classification of acute thoracolumbar spine injuries. Spine 8:817, 1983
12. Harrington PR, Dickson JH: An eleven year clinical investigation of Harrington instrumentation. Clin Orthop 112:113, 1973
13. Jacobs RR, Asher MA, Snider RK: Thoracolumbar spine fractures, a comparative study of recumbent and operative treatment in 100 patients. Spine 5:463, 1980
14. Soreff J, Axdorph G, et al.: Treatment of patients with unstable fractures of the thoracic and lumbar spine. A follow-up study of surgical and conservative treatment. Acta Orthop Scand 53:369, 1982
15. Kakulus BA, Bedbrook GM: Pathology of injuries of the vertebral column. p. 27. In, Vinken PJ, Bruym GW, (eds): Handbook of Clinical Neurology. Vol. 25. North Holland, Amsterdam, 1976
16. Bedbrook GM: Treatment of thoracolumbar dislocation and fractures with paraplegia. Clin Orthop 112:27, 1975
17. Meyer PR: Complications of treatment of fractures of the dorsolumbar spine. p. 643. In Complications in Orthopaedic Surgery. 2nd Ed. Vol. 2. JB Lippincott, Philadelphia, 1978
18. Guttmann LJ: Surgical aspects of the treatment of traumatic paraplegia. J Bone Joint Surg 31B:389, 1949
19. Djindjian R, Houdart R, Hurth M: Angiography of the Spinal Cord. p. 52. University Park Press, Baltimore, 1970
20. Lazorthes G, et al.: Arterial vascularization of the spinal cord. J Neurosurg 35:253, 1971
21. Dommisse CF: The blood supply of the spinal cord. J Bone Joint Surg 56B:225, 1974
22. Dommisse GF: The Arteries and Veins of the Human Spinal Cord from Birth. Churchill Livingstone, New York, 1975
23. Allen, AR: Surgery of experimental lesions of spinal cord equivalent to crush injury of fracture dislocation of spinal column. JAMA 57:878, 1911
24. Ducker TB, Hamit HF: Experimental treatment of acute spinal cord injury. J Neurosurg 30:693, 1969
25. Osterholm J, Matthews GJ: Altered norepinephrine metabolism following experimental spinal cord injury. Part I. Relationship to hemorrhagic necrosis and post-wounding neurological deficits. J Neurosurg 36:384, 1972
26. Osterholm J, Matthews GJ: Altered norepinephrine metabolism following experimental spinal cord injury. Part II. Protection against traumatic spinal

cord hemorrhagic necrosis by norepinephrine synthesis blockade with alpha methyl tyrosine. J Neurosurg 36:395, 1972

27. Brachken MB, Collins WF, Freeman DF, et al.: Efficacy of methylprednisolone in acute spinal cord injury. JAMA 251:45, 1984

28. Lusted LB, Keats TE: Atlas of Roentgenographic Measurement. 4th Ed. p. 123. Year Book Medical Publishers, Chicago, 1978

29. Anderson JE: Grant's Atlas of Anatomy. 7th Ed. Williams & Wilkins, Baltimore, 1978

30. Hinck VC, Hopkins CE, Savara BS: Sagittal diameter of the cervical spinal canal in children. Radiology 79:97, 1962

31. Bedbrook GM: Spine injuries with tetraplegia and paraplegia. J Bone Joint Surg 61B:267, 1979

32. Riggins RS: The risk of neurological damage with fractures of the vertebra. J Trauma 17:126, 1977

33. Cheshire DJE: The pediatric syndrome of traumatic myelopathy without demonstrable vertebral injury. Paraplegia 15:74, 1977

34. Brown HP, Bonnett CC: Spinal deformity subsequent to spinal cord injury. J Bone Joint Surg 55A:441, 1973

35. Kilfoyle RM, Foley JJ, Norton PL: Spine and pelvic deformities in childhood and adolescent paraplegia. J Bone Joint Surg 47A:659, 1965

17

Surgery of the Thoracic Spine

Paul R. Meyer, Jr.

The thoracic portion of the spinal cord between the neurologic segments of T3 and T12 (vertebral elements T2 to T10) is delicate and more susceptible to injury than the cervical spinal cord. The smallness of the neural canal within this area of the thoracic vertebral column (at T3 the sagittal measurement of the neural canal is approximately 6.0 mm)[1] leaves only a small margin for error with respect to anterior or posterior translatory motion. Similarly, the thoracic spinal cord vascular supply is sparse. Thus, the thoracic spinal cord is very vulnerable to injury.

The rigidity that exists in the thoracic spinal column (owing to the sternum-rib-spine complex) puts positive limits on the degrees of freedom in flexion, extension, rotation, or translation before abnormal motion produces severe neurologic injury. Sixty-three percent of patients sustaining thoracic spine injury sustained a complete neurologic injury (Table 17-1). Therefore, it is imperative that patients with a history of injury be carefully observed for evidence of neurologic deterioration. Often subtle, the changes may be sudden and irreversible.

Depending on the presence or absence of neurologic or vertebral column injury, the problem-management response varies. The important variable is the type of bony-ligamentous injury. When neurologic injury is identified without vertebral fracture (13.5 percent) (Table 17-2), and other studies (flexion-extension radiographs) for instability are negative, only conservative care is indicated.

Absolute measurements of the sagittal diameter of the thoracic spinal canal are difficult to obtain because of overlapping bony elements and intervening structures. Nonetheless, between T1 and T12 (principally at T6), the thoracic neural canal is narrower than the cervical neural canal. In the cervical spine, the sagittal diameter of the canal (20 mm) is 100 percent larger than the cord at C1 and C2 (10 mm) and 75 percent larger than the spinal cord between C3 and C7. At T3, the sagittal measurement of the thoracic spinal canal is 6.0 mm[1] and offers very little leeway for translatory motion between the vertebrae and the spinal cord. What might be only a minor degree of displacement in other areas of the spinal column often results in neurologic deficit in the thoracic spine. As noted earlier, there is a high incidence of complete neurologic injuries (63 percent) associated with injury to most levels of the thoracic spinal column (Table 17-1). Reasons why less serious neurologic injuries are noted in the lumbar region are a significantly wider neural canal (as compared with the thoracic canal) and the presence of cauda equina nerve roots rather than spinal cord tissue, except for the conus medullaris (which consists of spinal cord segments L5 to S5 and lies posterior to the T12-L1 vertebrae).

Table 17-1.   **Thoracic Fractures: Level by Extent (Northwestern University Acute Spine Injury Center, 1972 to 1986)**

Fracture Level	No.	Intact		Incomplete		Complete	
		No.	%	No.	%	No.	%
T01	19	1	5.3	5	26.3	13	68.4
T02	20	3	15.0	4	20.0	13	65.0
T03	32	1	3.1	9	28.1	22	68.6
T04	49[a]	5	10.2	13	26.5	30	61.2
T05	47[a]	4	8.5	8	17.0	34	72.3
T06	22	5	22.7	6	27.3	11	50.0
T07	32	4	12.5	4	12.5	24	75.0
T08	34	7	20.6	5	14.7	22	64.7
T09	32[a]	6	18.8	10	31.3	15	46.9
T10	38	1	2.6	18	47.4	19	50.0
Other[b]	51						
Total	376	37	9.8	82	21.8	203	54.0

[a]One subject's extent is unavailable.
[b]Either no fracture or level is unavailable.

THORACIC SPINAL INSTABILITY

The thoracic spine is the most stable area of the entire vertebral column. It possesses this inherent stability because of the anatomic relationship between the spine, the rib cage, and the sternum. White and Panjabi noted that the presence of the rib cage stiffens the thoracic spine and provides resistance to vertebral element displacement, from either trauma or destructive disease. Moreover, the ribs provide a manifold increase in the mechanical transverse dimensions to the thoracic spine, increasing its strength and energy absorption capa-

Table 17-2.   **Thoracic: Treatment by Fracture (Northwestern University Acute Spine Injury Center, 1972 to 1986)**

Treatment	No.	Fracture		No Fracture	
		No.	%	No.	%
Conservative	242	195	80.6	47	19.4
Surgical	134	131	97.8	3	2.2
Total	376	326	86.7	50	13.3

bilities. This is particularly valuable in counteracting the forces of trauma.[2] Other structural components contributing to the strength and stability of the thoracic vertebral column (primarily realized in extension) are the anatomic overlapping of the posterior elements and the strong interlaminar (ligamentum flavum) and interspinous process ligaments. These ligaments increase the spine's stiffness 2.5 times.

There is a relatively "unrestrictive" amount of lateral intersegmental rotation in the upper thoracic spine between T1 and T9, owing to the presence of horizontally facing facet joints. The direction in which these facets face varies significantly from that which exists at or near the thoracolumbar (T10 to L2) junction. Here, rotation and lateral translatory motion is greatly restricted by the "closed facing" of the facets, which allows only flexion and extension[2] (see Ch. l6, Fig. 16-2). With torsional forces (often produced through a combination of axial loading, flexion, and rotation), thoracic pedicle-facet and/or vertebral body fractures result. With the concentration of significant mechanical forces (and energy) across a relatively small area (pedicle-facet joint), neurologic injury is practically unavoidable (62.5 percent of rotational

Table 17-3. **Thoracic Fractures: Biomechanical Type by Extent (Northwestern University Acute Spine Injury Center, 1972 to 1986)**

Fracture Type	Total	Intact		Incomplete		Complete	
		No.	%	No.	%	No.	%
Axial	120[a]	21	17.5	31	25.8	65	54.2
Flexion	114	12	10.5	31	27.2	71	62.3
Rotation	8	0	0.0	3	37.5	5	62.5
Direct	2	1	50.0	1	50.0	0	0.0
Other	82	3	3.7	16	19.5	63	76.8
None	50	0	0.0	19	38.0	31	62.0
Total	376	37	9.8	101	26.9	235	62.5

[a]Extent is unavailable for three subjects.

injuries were associated with neurologically complete injuries) (Table 17-3). The stability of the thoracic vertebral column is provided by the rib cage and the sternum. Its resistance to certain trauma-induced injuries contributes to the buildup of torque and rotational forces that, when released or exceeded at one area, result in vertebral column fracture and, frequently, an associated neurologic injury.

THORACIC VERTEBRAL FRACTURES

Neurologic Injury without Fracture

The incidence of neurologic injury is highest (73 percent) when accompanied by a compression fracture of the vertebral body; however, neurologic injury is also prevalent in a group of spinal injuries in which no evidence of fracture was found to exist (13 percent). In this series of nonfracture neurologic injuries, 62 percent resulted in complete neurologic injury (Table 17-3). This results primarily from the fragility of the thoracic spinal cord's blood supply and that blood supply's alteration by any or all of the following: spinal cord stretching associated with rupture of the posterior interspinous, interlaminar, and facet joint ligaments (Fig. 17-1); compression of the anterior spinal cord (and artery) (Fig. 17-2) over a kyphotic spine deformity; extruded intervertebral disc material; pressure resulting from hematoma; or cen-

tral spinal cord hemorrhage secondary to direct spinal cord compression type trauma (Fig. 17-3A,B).

Anterior Wedge Compression Fractures

Anterior wedge thoracic vertebral compression fractures of 35 to 50 percent tend to result in a progressive increase in thoracic kyphosis, thus requiring stabilization, even in the presence of preserved neurologic function (55 percent of wedge fractures were managed surgically) (see Fig. 17-7D) (Table 17-4). When vertebral fractures of this magnitude occur, the mechanical effect is a shift of the thoracic axial weight-bearing line anteriorly. This results in increased compressive forces (axial and angular) across the fracture site, terminating in increased thoracic kyphosis.[2] With bone resorption at the fracture site (during fracture healing), further loss of vertebral body height and bone substance occurs. In the presence of high anterior compressive loads and a maintenance of posterior vertebral body wall height, kyphosis occurs. This leads to gibbus formation, altered facet joint mechanics, and degenerative changes. When neurologic function is normal, potential compromise of the neural canal may result in either early or delayed alterations in neurologic function. Thus, an appropriate indication for stabilization is the prevention of angular deformity of the spine. Fractures resulting in little structural damage and no

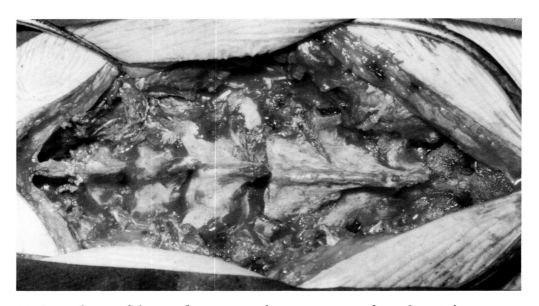

Fig. 17-1. Surgical view of thoracic flexion injury demonstrating significant diastasis between posterior elements T4–T5–T6. Injuries to the spine as represented in this view are generally associated with significant compression involving anterior elements and complete neurologic injuries.

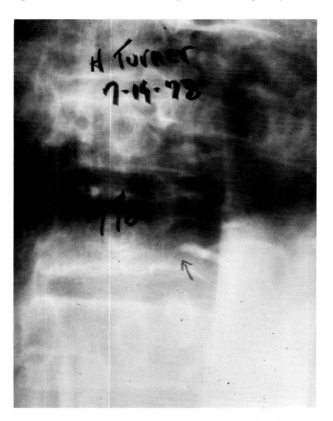

Fig. 17-2. Selective thoracic aorta angiography demonstrating vessel of Adamkiewicz entering spinal cord at T10–T11 on the left. Patient had complete neurologic injury.

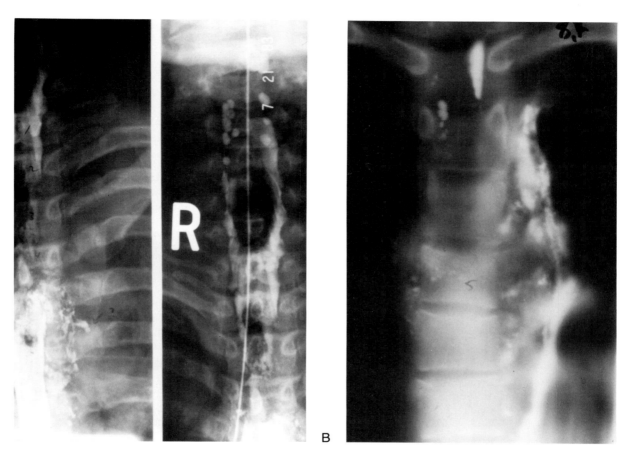

A

B

Fig. 17-3. (A) Anteroposterior (AP) view of myelogram demonstrating spinal cord swelling at the C6–C7 level and evidence of dural injury at T5–T6. (B) Tomogram of same patient revealing no evidence of fracture of the thoracic vertebrae but evidence of paraspinal hematoma and extravasation of contrast material into the adjacent paraspinal area. Note in A suggestion of injury at exit of T5 nerve root. This may be the source of the dural tear. Patient demonstrated incomplete paraplegia. During period of hospitalization, neurologic improvement occurred. Patient was also managed for left hemopneumothorax.

Table 17-4.   **Thoracic: Fracture Type by Treatment**
(Northwestern University Acute Spine Injury Center,
1972 to 1986)

Fracture Type	No.	Conservative No.	Conservative %	Surgical No.	Surgical %
Axial body compression	118	52	44.1	66	55.9
Body fracture	92	45	48.9	47	51.1
Bullet fragments	73	70	95.9	3	4.1
Anterior body compression	11	5	45.5	6	54.5
Facet fracture	4	4	100.0	0	0.0
Chance fracture	4	3	75.0	1	25.0
Spinous process	3	3	100.0	0	0.0
Facet lock	2	1	50.0	1	50.0
Bilateral facet lock	2	1	50.0	1	50.0
Transverse process	2	2	100.0	0	0.0
Subluxation	2	1	50.0	1	50.0
Other	13	8	61.5	5	38.5
None	50	47	94.0	3	6.0
Total	376	242	64.4	134	35.6

instability justify conservative management and careful observation. This is particularly indicated for the patient who sustains multiple trauma and other injuries, the management of which preempts spine surgery (see Fig. 17-8). On the other hand, when neurologic deterioration occurs during conservative care, surgical management of the spine becomes the highest priority.

Burst Fractures

Burst fractures (see Fig. 17-19) of the thoracic vertebral bodies are rare. Compression fractures (see Fig. 17-7A) are not. When present, burst fractures are usually associated with other signs of vertical (axial) loading, including multiple rib fractures and hemopneumothorax (Fig. 17-4A). Occasionally there may be some degree of associated translatory displacement of one vertebral body on another. According to Holdsworth, burst fractures can be thought of as having some residual "intactness" in the anterior or posterior longitudinal ligaments and can be classified as stable.[3] Whether or not the respective anulus fibrosus and

nucleus pulposus remain intact is a matter of conjecture. My data reveal that burst fractures are frequently associated with neurologic injury (59 percent complete neurologic injuries) (Table 17-5), particularly when they occurred in the thoracic spine and upper lumbar spine areas. In these two locales, burst fractures cause fragments from the posterior vertebral body to extrude into the canal (revealed radiographically) and are thus thought to be the cause of neurologic injury. Both the thoracic and upper lumbar spine are prone to neurologic trauma because of an anatomically narrow bony neural canal in relation to the size of the spinal cord and conus medullaris and the known anatomic disparity in the thoracic spinal cord blood supply.

When a burst-compression fracture occurs, the most appropriate means of obtaining spinal realignment and stabilization is by the application of a posterior distraction force across the fracture site. This management philosophy is correct, whether neurologic injury is present or not. The methods of fixation most frequently considered are the Harrington rod,[4] AO (Jacobs) rod,[5] and Edwards rod.[6] Each method is capable of accomplishing the task of restoring vertebral body height, reducing bone

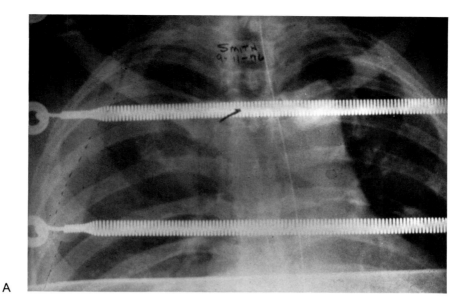

A

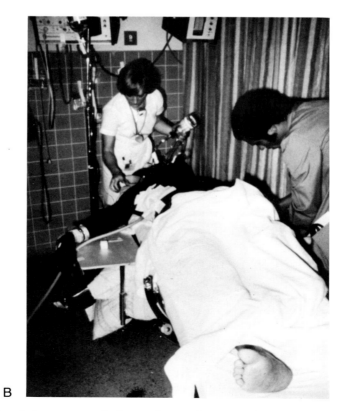

B

Fig. 17-4. Patient admitted after motor vehicle accident with T3 neurologic injury. **(A)** Note hemothorax in right chest and widened mediastinum. Question of injury to great vessels or esophagus. **(B)** Chest tube being inserted in emergency room. Patient is supine on Stryker frame. *(Figure continues.)*

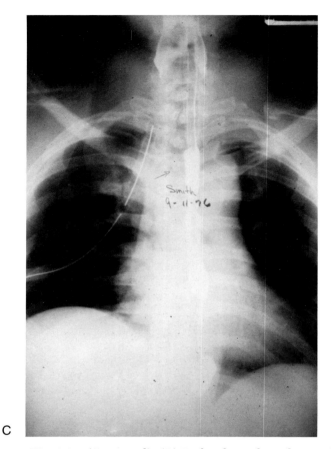
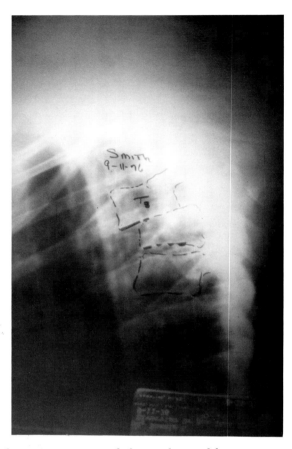

C

D

Fig. 17-4 *(Continued)*. **(C)** Right chest cleared immediately upon insertion of chest tube, and barium swallow performed in emergency room reveals continuity of the esophagus. Vascular studies showed no injury to the thoracic aorta. **(D)** Lateral radiograph of thoracic spine shows fracture subluxation of T3 on T4 with fracture of posterior elements and complete neurologic injury.

compromise of the neural canal, providing stabilization, and improving alignment.

Restoration of vertebral body height by distraction (when continuity remains between the posterior longitudinal ligament and the posterior fragments) may result in retraction of posterior bony fragments from within the neural canal. This does not necessarily apply to the extraction of soft tissue (intervertebral disc) from within the canal. Also, the application of a distractive force across a burst fracture can, because of fracture fragment distraction, result in a fracture healing delay (see Complications with Internal Fixation Devices, below).

Given the methods of fracture fixation and stabilization available, distraction is more favorable

than compression (and particularly in the presence or incomplete neurologic injury of neurologic intactness). The risks of compromising the spinal canal or inducing vertebral body translation with compression are hazards to be considered. When the neurologic examination reveals a complete neurological injury, other methods of internal fixation techniques can be utilized (see Compression: Fracture Management, below).

Anterior Longitudinal Ligament

A frequent concern in vertebral column trauma is the role of the anterior longitudinal ligament, and whether its continuity affects fracture reduction or

Table 17-5.   Thoracic Fractures: Fracture Type by Extent (Northwestern
University Acute Spine Injury Center, 1972 to 1986)

Fracture Type	Total	Intact		Incomplete		Complete	
		No.	%	No.	%	No.	%
Axial body compression	118[a]	20	16.9	31	26.3	64	54.2
Body fracture	92	5	5.4	25	27.2	62	67.4
Bullet fragments	73	0	0.0	12	16.4	61	83.6
Anterior body compression	11	5	45.5	2	18.2	4	36.4
Facet fracture	4	0	0.0	2	50.0	2	50.0
Chance fracture	4	2	50.0	2	50.0	0	0.0
Spinous process	3	0	0.0	1	33.3	2	66.7
Facet lock	2	0	0.0	0	0.0	2	100.0
Bilateral facet lock	2	0	0.0	1	50.0	1	50.0
Transverse process	2	1	50.0	1	50.0	0	0.0
Subluxation	2	0	0.0	1	50.0	1	50.0
Other	13	4	30.8	4	30.8	5	38.5
None	50	0	0.0	19	38.0	31	62.0
Total	376	37	9.8	101	26.9	235	62.5

[a]Extent is unavailable for three subjects.

stabilization. This a major concern in the thoracolumbar and lumbar regions of the spine. Jacobs et al.[7,8] and Bradford,[9] in a review of this subject, reported that the anterior longitudinal ligament plays a dominant role when Harrington distraction rods are utilized and contributes to the restoration of anterior vertebral column (body) height, alignment, and stability. Its presence (or continuity) allows the Harrington rod-hook complex to reach an end point by encountering resistance during the application of a distraction force. In its absence, distraction can be too easily accomplished and can become a cause of instability. Ultimately, overdistraction of the vertebral column will result in failure of internal fixation.

A method of mechanically testing the integrity of the anterior longitudinal ligament at surgery is as follows. A Kirschner wire is inserted perpendicularly into two adjacent spinous processes, opposite the site of spinal injury, either slightly divergent or parallel to each other (Fig. 17-5A). With the insertion of bilateral Harrington distraction rods, as the distraction force is applied across the fracture site, one of the following will occur:

The tips of the Kirschner wires will further diverge, indicating continuity of the anterior longitudinal ligament and an instability in the posterior structures (spreading of the posterior structures by the Harrington rods) (Fig. 17-5B);

The Kirschner wires will remain parallel, indicating that the vertebral bodies are distracting anteriorly (with the application of the distraction force) and that there is discontinuity within the anterior longitudinal ligament (Fig. 17-5C).

Unilateral Vertebral Body, Pedicle, and Facet Fractures

A unilateral compression or vertical oblique shear fracture through one side of a vertebral body, as seen in the coronal or frontal projection, results from the application of an excessive and unbalanced axial load (with associated lateral bending) to the spine. When this force is in excess of normal load dynamics, localized segmental bending (or scoliosis) occurs, resulting in unilateral vertebral body, pedicle, and/or facet fracture (Fig. 17-6).

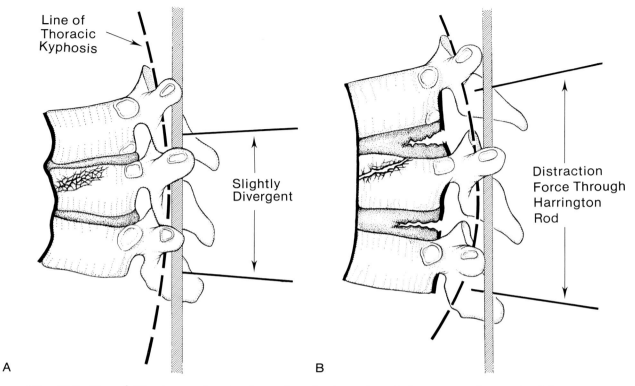

Fig. 17-5. Use of Kirschner wires to determine the integrity of the anterior longitudinal ligament. (A) Kirschner wires are inserted perpendicularly into two adjacent spinous processes. They will be slightly divergent or parallel to each other. Bilateral Harrington distraction rods are inserted, and a distraction force applied across the fracture site. One of the following two events will occur. (B) Application of force leads to distraction kyphosis secondary to opening of structures posteriorly. There is no opening anteriorly, indicating that the anterior longitudinal ligament is intact. The posterior opening will be indicated by further divergence of the Kirschner wires. *(Figure continues.)*

The resultant deformity is a concavity toward the side of the depressed fragment. This particular fracture type is most commonly identified at or near the junction of the thoracic and lumbar spine. When fractures of the ipsilateral vertebral body, pedicle, and facet are demonstrated, acute lateral angular deformity may result. The most appropriate method of internal stabilization in such a case is bilateral distraction rods. Although Luque rods could be utilized, with axial loading, lateral translation of the fracture can occur.

When the vertebral fracture results from a combination of lateral bending and forward flexion, kyphosis occurs and will be prominent at the fracture site. Correction of the resulting anterior angulation correctly suggests the application of a posterior compressive force (i.e., Harrington compression rods or Wisconsin compression system), but correction with this method of internal fixation is difficult to achieve. Therefore, again, owing to the unbalanced nature of the fracture, should compression be applied across the fracture, iatrogenic scoliosis is likely to occur (Fig. 17-6C). The most appropriate method of internal fixation is with bilateral Harrington distraction rods (Fig. 17-6E,F). The posterior force applied through the rods must be sufficient to correct the traumatic kyphosis without resulting in fracture fragment distraction.

Axial-angular loads to the vertebral column result in unilateral fractures of the pedicle and facet on the same side as compression of the vertebral body. If little or no evidence of neural canal com-

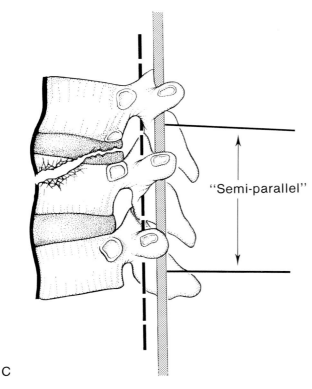

"Semi-parallel"

C

Fig. 17-5 (Continued).

promise occurs, neurologic injury is uncommon. Should it occur, it is more likely to be associated with fractures of the body than the facet or pedicles (Table 17-5).

As noted, neurologic injury can occur with unilateral vertebral body fractures, but this injury as described above usually occurs in the area of maximum mobility (the junction of the thoracic and lumbar spine) and coincides with that portion of the neural canal having the greatest diameter. When neurologic injury occurs, it is either a single nerve root injury (if in the area of the cauda equina) or an incomplete spinal cord injury (if in the area of the spinal cord or conus medullaris). When anterior or lateral vertebral body shear occurs, complete neurologic injury is likely to result (See Fig. 17-18A).

Other management considerations include the insertion of AO internal fixator with threaded rods and Shanz pins, or Luque rods (see Fig. 17-15). If vertebral column angulation (kyphosis or scoliosis)

does not exist, these fractures will heal with conservative orthotic management in a manner similar to that of traumatic spondylolisthesis.

Fractures over Multiple Adjacent Levels

When multiple posterior element fractures occur, the mechanism of injury is axial load, a combination of axial load plus a hyperextension moment, or the result of avulsion ("clay shoveler's") fractures of the posterior spinous processes. White and Panjabi noted that the thoracic spine is rigid in hyperextension because of the overlapping of the posterior elements and the stability provided by the rib cage.[2] It is not unreasonable to anticipate, therefore, that with an axial load and a hyperextension force, a more severe injury to the vertebral column will occur (Fig. 17-7). When neurologic injury accompanies this fracture, it is likely to be the result of direct injury to the spinal cord from fracture fragments, rupture of ligamentum flavum, disc protrusion, or a combination of any of the above (Fig. 17-8). Because thoracic neural canal space is limited (see Ch. 16, Table 16-8), even small alignment deformities can result in significant neurologic injury. When neurologic injury occurs in the presence of normal radiographs, myelogram, computed axial tomography (CAT) scan, or magnetic resonance imaging (MRI), the likely cause is vascular injury (see Ch. 4).

Axial load or extension injuries to the spine over multiple levels are usually best managed by conservative means. This includes immobilization of the spine in a body cast or similar orthosis, followed by early mobilization. This regimen is dependent on the presence of spinal stability in two of the three anatomic columns (Table 17-6). Injuries to the thoracic spine above T6 are managed by an orthosis having a cervical extension to incorporate the head and neck (See Ch. 12) (see Fig. 17-13).

When neurologic injury is present and there is evidence of anterior-posterior translation of the vertebral segments in the sagittal plane, it is appropriate to assume that spinal instability exists. This can be determined by flexion-extension radiographs, tomograms, or CAT scan. If instability is identified, the spine will require operative stabili-

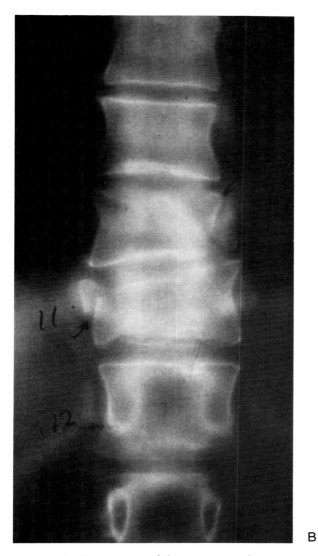

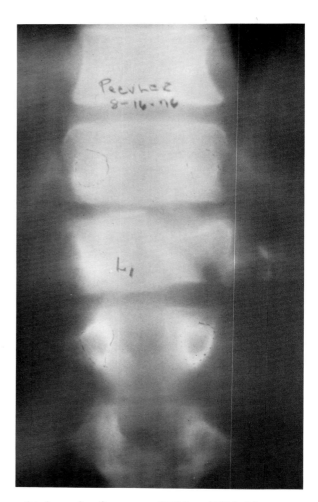

A   B

Fig. 17-6. **(A)** AP view of thoracic spine demonstrating multiple wedge fractures of T10 and T11. Note unilateral decompression of vertebral body with associated widening of pedicle. **(B)** AP view demonstrating classic lateral bend-type fracture resulting in unilateral vertebral body-pedicle-facet fracture (L1). *(Figure continues.)*

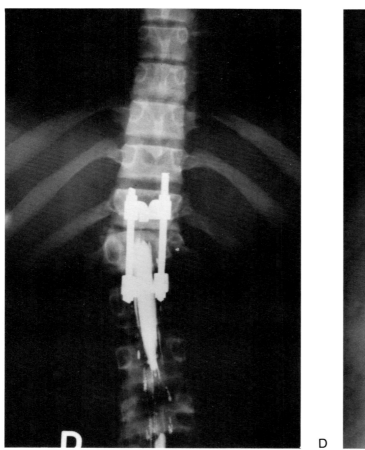
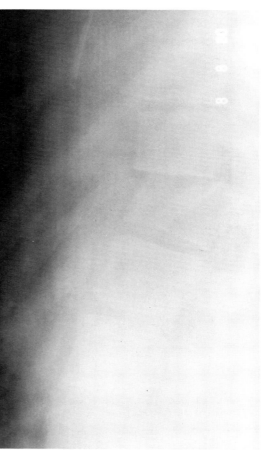

C   D

Fig. 17-6 *(Continued).* **(C)** AP radiograph showing compression fixation at fracture site L1. Note resulting scoliosis convexity on the side of the displaced pedicle and facet. This type of fracture is a contraindication for compression fixation. **(D)** Unilateral vertebral body fracture of T12 seen in lateral view. Note associated subluxation of T11 on T12. *(Figure continues.)*

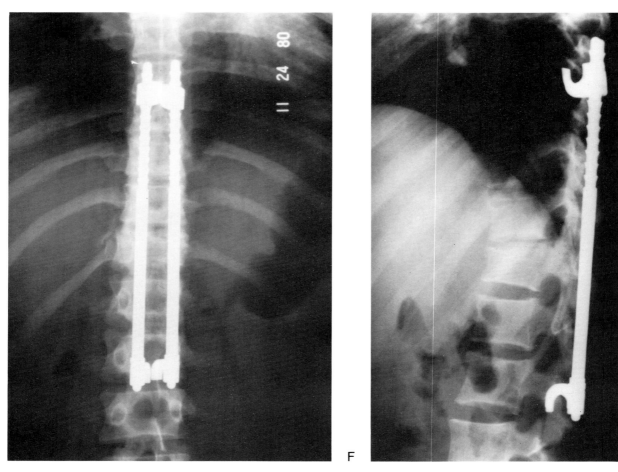

E   F

Fig. 17-6 *(Continued).* **(E,F)** AP and lateral radiographs demonstrating reduction of displaced T11 on T12 and appropriate vertical alignment maintained by the use of Harrington distraction rods. This is the appropriate method of internal fixation for unilateral compression fractures.

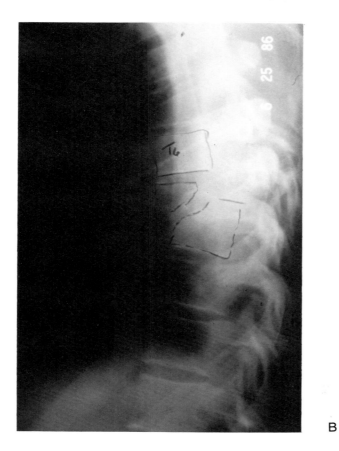 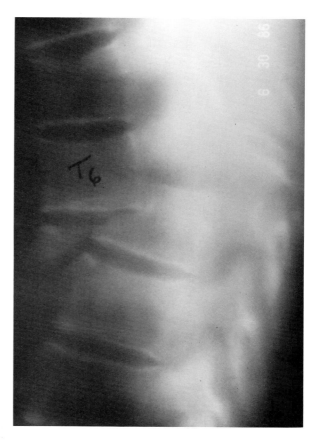

A   B

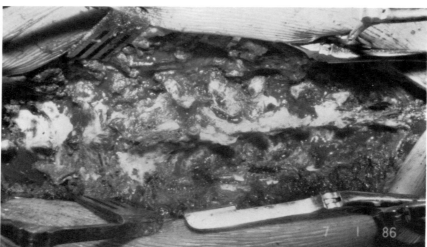

C

Fig. 17-7. (A) Lateral radiograph of thoracic spine demonstrating anterior shear or compression fracture of vertebral body of T7. Patient's neurologic level was T6 complete. (B) Lateral tomogram of thoracic spine demonstrating further displacement of T6 on T7 on date of admission (5 days after injury). Note multiple posterior element fractures. Despite dislocation in the sagittal plane, alignment was good. (C) Intraoperative view of thoracic spine revealing multiple posterior element fractures of T5 – T6 – T7. *(Figure continues.)*

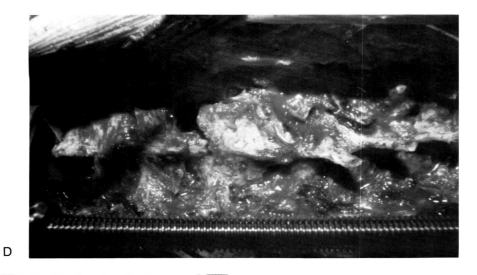

D

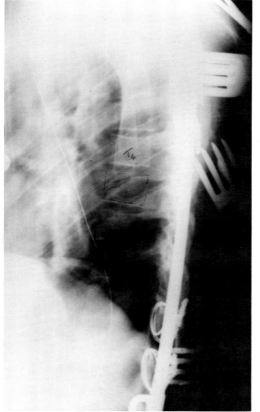

E

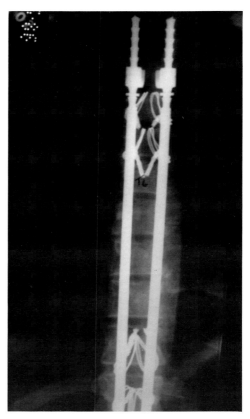

F

Fig. 17-7 *(Continued).* (**D**) Harrington distraction apparatus used to reduce the dislocation at T6 – T7. Note intact dura in center of picture. (**E,F**) Postoperative view of reduction and internal fixation fracture dislocation of T6 and T7, utilizing Harrington rods and supplemental sublaminar Luque wires. Note straightening of thoracic curvature. Note also placement of shank-notch junction at distance from level of injury. Harrington rods are not prebent. Upper ends of rods are shortened before closure.

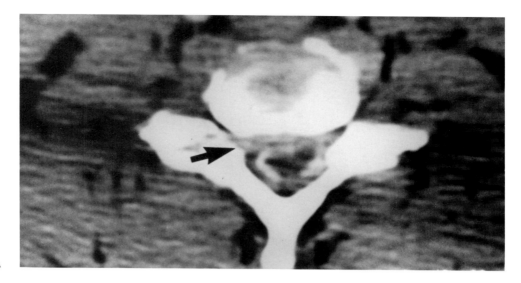

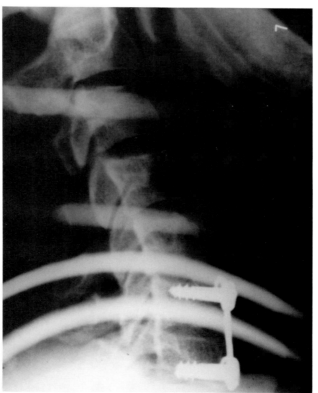

Fig. 17-8. 21-year-old male multiple trauma victim. Patient's neurological injury on admission was a C6 incomplete (mixed) motor-sensory injury. This patient also sustained multiple extremity and secondary skeletal trauma. (A) CAT scan view at C6–C7, revealing posterior extrusion of the cervical disc at this level. (B) Following disc excision, an anterior cervical spine fusion using a tricortical interbody graft and AO plate-screw fixation was performed at C6–C7. The cervical spine was managed postoperatively in a SOMI orthosis. *(Figure continues.)*

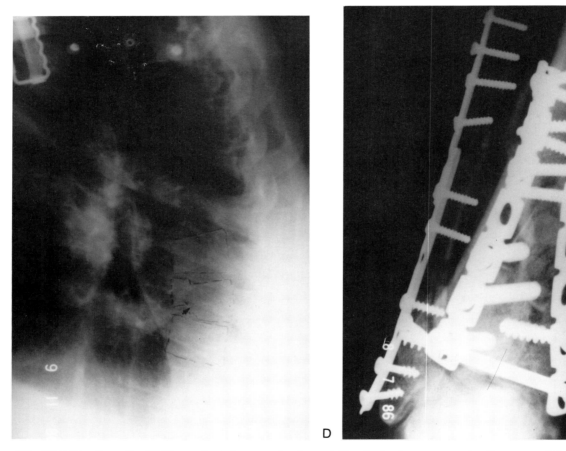

C   D

Fig. 17-8 *(Continued).* **(C)** The patient also sustained an axial load–flexion compression fracture at T6. Due to multiple extremity and abdominal trauma, the thoracic spine was managed conservatively in a Knight-Taylor orthosis with pectoral pads. **(D)** Comminuted distal tibia-fibula fracture involving the tibial plafond, stabilized with malleable Synthes plate and screws. *(Figure continues.)*

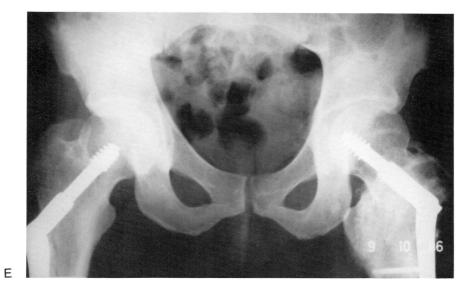

E

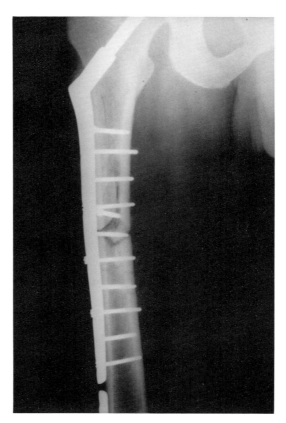

F

Fig. 17-8 *(Continued)*. The patient also sustained a basilar neck–intertrochanteric fracture of the left hip (**E**), and a comminuted transverse fracture of the proximal middle third of the right femur (**F**). The fracture was stabilized with a Richards sliding nail–long side plate. Note AO right angle plate at lower end of right femur, used as internal fixation of a distal femur fracture. *(Figure continues.)*

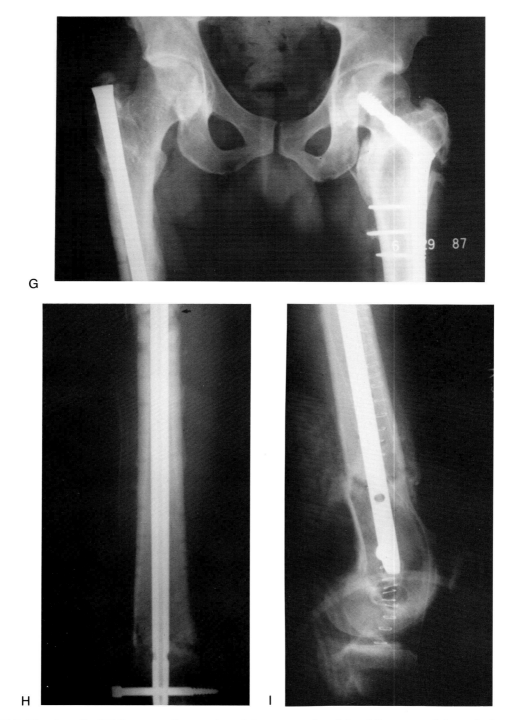

Fig. 17-8 *(Continued).* **(G)** Because of nonunion of the proximal and distal fractures of the right femur and bending of the internal fixation, the patient required removal of previous internal fixation devices, and replacement with Gross-Kempf nail and trans-fixation screw, plus bone graft. **(H)** Proximal and distal femoral fractures aligned and stabilized by Gross-Kempf nail and distal trans-fixation screw. **(I)** Lateral view, distal femoral fracture. All fractures healed following this procedure.

Table 17-6. Column Theory of Spine Construction and Stability

Two-Column Theory (Holdsworth)	Three-Column Theory (Denis)
Posterior bone-ligament complex Posterior laminar arch Supraspinous ligament Interspinous ligament Posterior lateral capsule Ligamentum flavum	Same[a]
	Middle column[a] Posterior longitudinal ligament Posterior anulus fibrosus Posterior vertebral body wall
Anterior column Anterior vertebral body Anterior longitudinal ligament Anterior anulus fibrosus	Same

[a]Disruption of any two indicates instability.

zation by Harrington distraction rods, (see Fig. 17-7D–F) AO (Synthes) rods,[5] or Luque rods (see Fig. 17-18).

FRACTURE SURGERY VERSUS SCOLIOSIS SURGERY

During the preceding 30 years, orthopaedic training programs have continually readjusted their disease-oriented management scheme based on advances and improvements in surgical skills, new technology, and findings from accumulated medical data. In the area of the spine, these changes have been most profound, particularly in regard to scoliosis management. Because of a drastic change in the etiology of the scoliosis (from paralytic [anterior poliomyelitis] to familial [or idiopathic] scoliosis as the principal cause), there has been a constant change in the method of management. Numerous internal fixation devices have appeared in the orthopaedic surgeon's armamentarium. They include Harrington compression and distraction rods[4] (Fig. 17-6E,F), Weiss compression springs[10] (Fig. 17-9D), combination use of distraction and compression (Fig. 17-11), Murig Wil-

liams plates[11] (Fig. 17-9A–C), Roy-Camille plate and screws,[12] Dwyer anterior cable, Luque segmental spinal rod instrumentation[13] (see Fig. 17-18), and the recent addition of the AO (Jacobs-Synthes) locking hook-rod system (see Fig. 18-39), and the even more recent AO internal fixator (see Fig. 18-40).

In a time when technical growth is continuously expanding, more and more opportunities are found to utilize the new technology. An excellent example of this has been the attempt to translate "problem-solving management" in the area of scoliosis management to spine trauma management; that is, using scoliosis surgical techniques to solve spinal fracture surgical management problems. While this "technology transfer" in many instances has been appropriate, in other situations it has not. Certainly, an example of the latter situation is the attempt to provide spine stability (with Harrington distraction rods) in most situations of spinal trauma, without taking into account the adverse effects of trauma on spinal stability. It thus becomes imperative for the surgeon to appreciate that specific biomechanically oriented surgical techniques developed with one disease entity in mind, may not, under differing situations, be compatible with another entity. An example of this is found in the use of Harrington rods for scoliosis management, in which failure results from:

The utilization of distraction scoliosis instrumentation out of a "blind obedience."

The difference between tissue instability caused by abnormal spinal alignment in scoliosis, and tissue instability caused by fractures. The result is the misapplication of internal fixation across unstable segments, or across an inappropriate number of segments.

The use of distraction (often overdistraction) rather than compression.

The use of distraction rods across dislocated thoracic or lumbar facet joints, with failure to gain either reduction or stability.

The use of compression devices across fractured vertebral segments where the body, pedicle, or facet fracture is unilateral. This results in surgically induced lateral spine column angulation (scoliosis).

The use of inappropriate internal fixation devices (i.e., plate-bolt fixation of the spinous process)

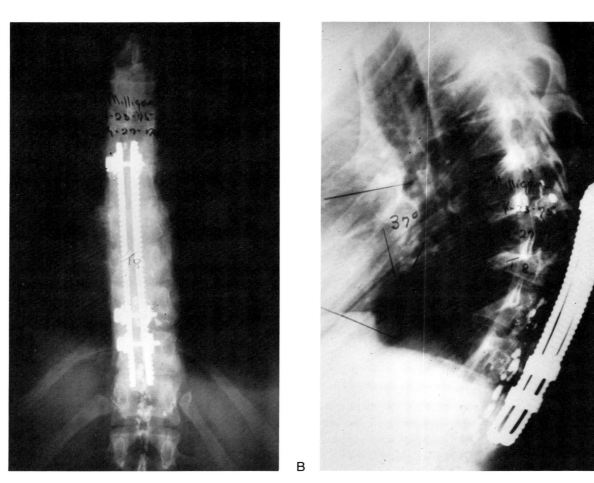

Fig. 17-9. (A,B) AP and lateral radiographs of thoracic spine in patient who sustained compression fracture of T8 and was internally stabilized with Murig-Williams plate and bolts. Note displacement of proximal thoracic spine from internal fixation. Radiograph was taken 6 months after injury. *(Figure continues.)*

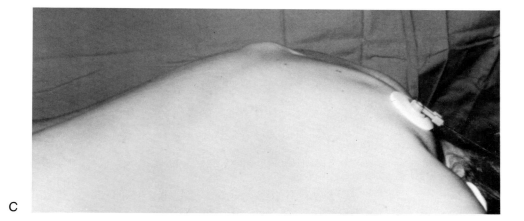

C

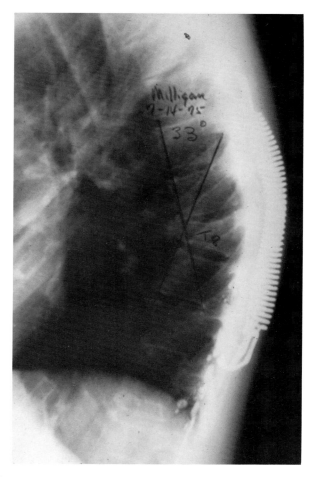

D

Fig. 17-9 *(Continued).* **(C)** Patient prone on operating table. Note acute prominence of Murig-Williams plate beneath skin. **(D)** Lateral radiograph of thoracic spine after insertion of Weiss springs. Patient was managed postoperatively in a Knight-Taylor orthosis with pectoral horns.

for unstable flexion-distraction injuries of the spine.

Individually, the above examples do not represent significant errors in technique. What they do represent is overspecialization in a narrow area of orthopaedic surgery, a hazard that is compounded by the impulse to transport problem-solving surgical techniques from one specific orthopaedic surgical area (scoliosis) to related problems in another (spinal fractures). Occasionally this can be accomplished in a generalized sense, but more often, the results will be less than optimal, and the eventual outcome will be hampered by frustration and failure.

With respect to the Luque rods, the same problems exist; that is, directly utilizing scoliosis correction and stabilization techniques for the management of spinal fractures. In scoliosis, when the procedure is performed where the neural canal is wide (in the lumbar region) and the neural contents are highly resilient to trauma (the cauda equina), the passage of sublaminar rod fixation wires is less likely to produce neural tissue injury. However, the same is not necessarily true when managing spinal trauma, particularly in the thoracic or thoracolumbar area where there has likely been associated trauma to the neural contents. With traumatically induced neural tissue edema and a compromised vascular supply, the inherently highly sensitive neural tissue of the spinal cord or conus medullaris is quite vulnerable to further injury as a result of the passage of wires through the sublaminar or epidural space. It is for this reason that great care must be taken when performing instrumentation requiring sublaminar wires in the thoracic or thoracolumbar spine areas (particularly when neurologic function remains intact or incomplete). This procedure, like all others of its kind, must include the use of somatosensory evoked potentials (SSEP) or the "wake-up test" for intraoperative monitoring of neurologic function.[14]

ANATOMIC CONSIDERATIONS: THORACIC SPINE SURGERY

From the standpoint of a surgical approach, the thoracic spine is very similar to the cervical spine in that vital organs lie anteriorly. These include the esophagus, the trachea, the ascending vessels arising from the arch and descending from the aorta, the vena cava, and the right and left lungs. Regarding the posterior thoracic approach, there are many similarities to the approach to the posterior cervical spine, with the addition of the following: the prominence of the first thoracic spinous process; the oblique cephalad slant of the first thoracic vertebral transverse process (differing from the same process of the seventh cervical vertebra which angles obliquely caudal) (see Ch. 16); the laminae of the upper thoracic spine lie in a shingled or overlapping position (in relation to each other). There are palpable ribs that articulate with the transverse processes laterally; radiographically, they lie opposite the upper third of the vertebral body in the anteroposterior plane, and on the lateral plane, are in line with their respective pedicles. From T2 through T10, the spinous processes are angled slightly inferiorly, and like the lamina, overlap the next lower posterior element process. The T11 and T12 posterior spinous process elements, like those in the lumbar spine, lie in a more horizontal position.

Therefore, in radiographic views of the thoracic vertebral column in the anteroposterior direction, the spinous process of one vertebral element overlies the next lower vertebral body. Because of this anatomic relationship, when approaching a posterior thoracic interlaminar space it may be necessary to remove the more superior spinous process to uncover the ligamentum flavum lying within the interlaminar space. It may also be necessary to remove a small portion of the overlapping lamina from above (a "partial hemilaminotomy") to enter the interlaminar space (Fig. 17-10). This is a routine procedure in the performance of a surgical excision of a herniated intervertebral disc in the lower lumbar spine and is frequently required for the insertion of the sublaminar-positioned Harrington hooks during the Harrington rod procedure (Fig. 17-7) (see Harrington Distraction Rods Procedure, below).

Variations in the posterior elements between the thoracic and the lumbar spine are to some extent obvious, yet can be confusing. When the anatomic appearances are similar at the transitional junction, or in the presence of congenital variations (such as a transitional rib at L1), radiographs are the most accurate means of identifying the level. Those ana-

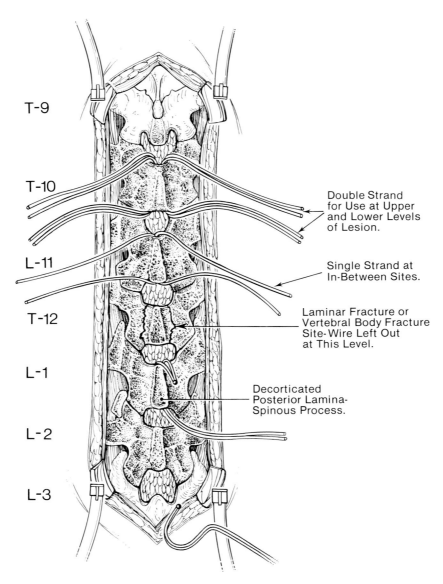

T-9

T-10

L-11

T-12

L-1

L-2

L-3

Double Strand
for Use at Upper
and Lower Levels
of Lesion.

Single Strand at
In-Between Sites.

Laminar Fracture or
Vertebral Body Fracture
Site-Wire Left Out
at This Level.

Decorticated
Posterior Lamina-
Spinous Process.

Fig. 17-10. Technique for inserting sublaminar wires. The Luque wire is first bent, then passed superiorly from one interlaminar space to the next. A double wire is used at the proximal and distal ends of the operative field. Sublaminar wires are not used on vertebrae with a fractured lamina (T12 in this case).

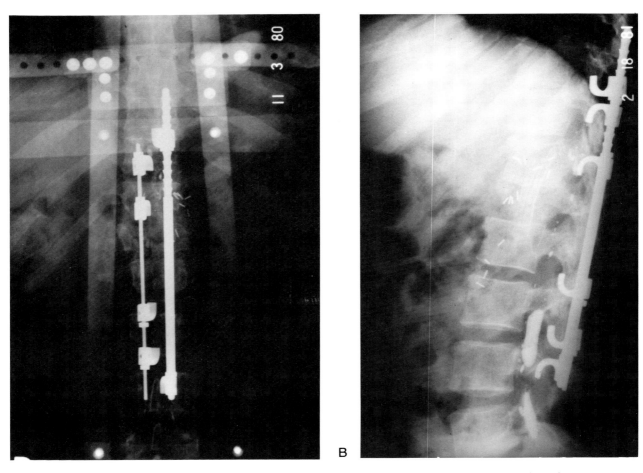

A   B

Fig. 17-11. (A,B) Views showing use of combined distraction-compression Harrington rods for a fracture occurring at the level of T12-L1. Note position of Harrington hooks in sublaminar space. *(Figure continues.)*

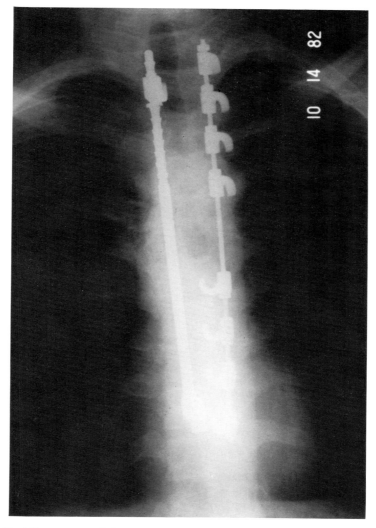

C

Fig. 17-11 *(Continued).* **(C)** AP view of thoracic spine fracture at T6. Note that Harrington compression hooks proximally are attached to lateral transverse processes, and inferior hooks are in sublaminar position.

tomic features that can aid level identification are the 12th thoracic rib, a "float" rib (confusing if a 1st lumbar "rib" is present); the presence of an enlarged and more posteriorly directed spinous process at L1; the anteroposterior direction of the T12-L1 facet joints; the presence of visible and palpable mammary bodies lateral to the facet joints at L1 (Fig. 17-12).

The noticeably short and mobile last thoracic rib is occasionally confused with the transverse pro-

cess of L1; therefore, care must be taken to identify the absence of mobility of the L1 transverse process. Similarly, it is important to identify preoperatively (on an anteroposterior radiograph), the presence or absence of a short "nubbin" of a rib, lateral to what appears to be the transverse process of L1. Usually, this level is T12 and is an important anatomic reference to the surgeon who must determine the appropriate injury level and the appropriate internal fixation level. Another useful anatomic

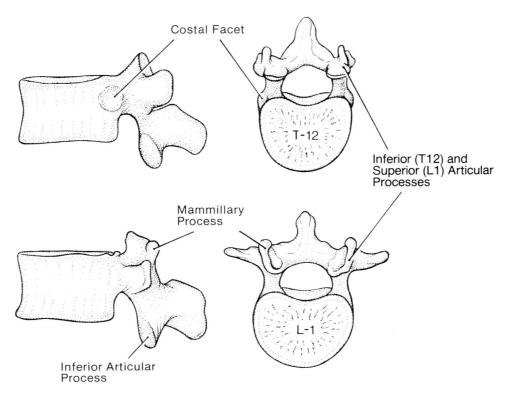

Fig. 17-12. Anatomic landmarks of the thoracolumbar junction.

precept to consider is the appearance of a transitional thoracolumbar junctional vertebra, which often will be accompanied by a sacralization and enlargement of the transverse process of L5 with S1, or some other lower lumbar anatomic variation. Occasionally, the last lumbar vertebra may appear as a 6th lumbar vertebra, while in fact it is a failure of fusion of the first sacral segments.

ANTERIOR SURGICAL APPROACH: THORACIC SPINE

Customarily, the anterior approach for the scoliosis surgeon[15] is through an anterior right chest approach. This is due to the presence of a high right thoracic convex (congenital) curve. In the case of traumatic injuries to the spine, when a choice exists, the preferred approach is through the left side. This allows for the "falling away," retraction, or displacement of the aorta, the vena cava, and the lungs, as well as causing a depression of the diaphragm on the side of the smaller lobe of the liver (left). Moderate displacement of these organs to the right, away from the vertebral column, allows for their protection. Although this places the aorta closer to the operative field, in the event of intraoperative complication, repair of the aorta is more easily accomplished than repair of the vena cava because the aorta has a well-defined muscular layer.

In view of these vascular and anatomic considerations, as a rule, the chest approach is made by the chest service or with a member of the chest service assisting the orthopaedic service. Once the approach has been accomplished, the procedure is complete by the orthopaedic surgeon. Although less complicated than the approach, closure of the chest is usually performed by the chest service (instances do exist, however, when this rule is waived).

Rationale: Anterior Spine Approach

The decision to approach the thoracic spine via a left anterolateral transthoracic approach is based on either a chance of preserving residual neurologic function that is being compromised by anterior encroachment on the spinal cord,[16,17] or the need to stabilize or reduce gross vertebral column malalignment or dislocation (for more than 2 to 3 weeks). The alternative to the latter is to accept the deformity and allow the spine to stabilize by conservative means (bed rest) and orthotic immobilization for a period adequate for healing to occur (3 to 5 months) (see Fig. 16-26).

The choice of surgical or conservative management in the presence of gross spinal malalignment is difficult at best. Two questions that invariably arise are: Why bother to achieve an anatomic reduction of a fracture-dislocation knowing that a complete neurologic injury exists at and below the level of spine injury? and, Can such an injury, if conservatively managed, be allowed to stabilize over time without the development of further deformity? These questions are difficult to answer, and an "always" answer does not exist; however, the concerns in such an instance are clear:

Appearance: can the patient tolerate an unsightly spinal deformity?
Pain: can the patient tolerate the pain experienced as a result of the deformity?
Skin breakdown: can the skin withstand the possibility of breakdown over the area of the deformity?
Sit-balance: can the patient tolerate the loss of sit-balance caused by the deformity?

A "no" response to any of these questions is almost enough to indicate surgical management, provided the patient is fully aware of the hazards of such management. It is the physician's responsibility to explain to the patient these potential hazards (e.g., lacerated aorta or vena cava), as well as the potential benefits (enhanced neurologic recovery, the prevention of neurologic deterioration, the regaining of spinal stability lost secondary to fracture) of such an operative procedure so that the patient (and family) may carefully consider the two alternatives and decide accordingly. I have observed 86 (33 percent) fracture-dislocations and pure dislocations of the thoracic spine over a 13-year period, and my experience has shown that the majority did require reduction and stabilization because of gross spinal instability or the presence of an unacceptable spinous process prominence (gibbus) (Fig. 17-13A,B) or malalignment that, if left unattended, would ultimately cause skin breakdown over the area of prominence.

After identification of the type of vertebral fracture and the extent of displacement of the vertebral column, certain considerations arise, such as: Can stability be achieved in the presence of a complete dislocation of one vertebral segment from its adjacent member? and, Can stability be achieved when an extensive anterior or lateral wedge compression fracture is associated with fracture of an articular processes, fractures of a posterior element, or gross ligamentous disruption? The "Denis theory"[18] of vertebral column instability (instability is indicated by the loss of stability in two of the three vertebral columns) can be beneficial (Table 17-6). Once a particular injury is determined to be either unstable or stable, the question of the necessity of internal stabilization is immediately resolved. However, the following questions should be discussed with the patient before implementing either the surgical or conservative managerial alternatives:

What characteristics are indicative of instability?
What is the most appropriate method of internal stabilization?
Is it possible to anticipate which thoracic spine fracture will demonstrate instability and late malalignment if not initially stabilized?
Is the fracture likely to become stable with bed immobilization alone?
Will the unoperated spine remain stable with increased patient activity and mobilization?
How much deformity is "acceptable"?
How much time is required for stability to occur, and is the same time period adequate for all deformities?
What might be the consequences of prolonged immobilization, bed care, and inactivity?
What are the consequences of previous "laminectomy" without stabilization (as a result of the loss of "chain link" stability attained via the lamina-ligamentum flava-interspinous ligament-spinous process linkage)?

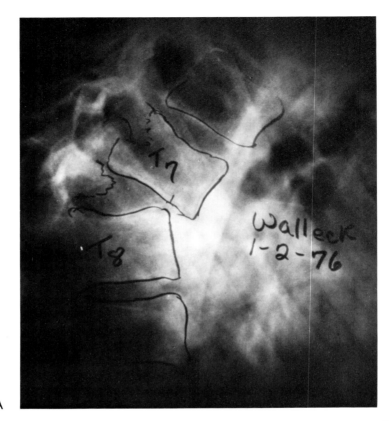

A

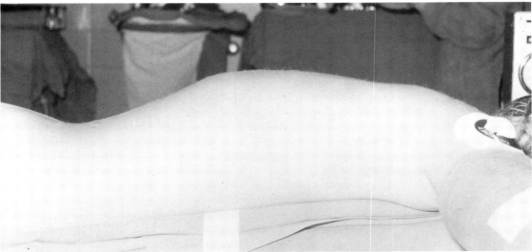

B

Fig. 17-13. (**A**) Lateral radiograph of thoracic spine showing fracture subluxation of T7 on T8, with fracture through pedicle easily identified. (**B**) Lateral view of patient prone on operating table, showing proximal thoracic kyphosis secondary to fracture seen in **A**. *(Figure continues.)*

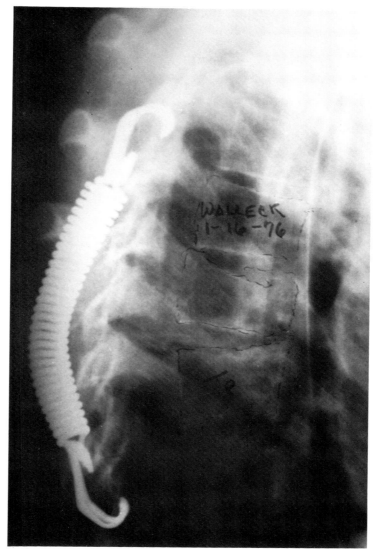

C

Fig. 17-13 *(Continued).* (C) Lateral radiograph of thoracic spine after open reduction and internal fixation and stabilization with Weiss springs.

COMPLICATIONS WITH INTERNAL FIXATION DEVICES

Neurologic Dysfunction with Internal Fixation

A well-known and serious complication that can occur with internal stabilization of thoracic vertebral column fractures is the loss of neurologic func-tion during or after the procedure. Such a complication is always possible with surgery anywhere in the spine. The more common causes for its occurrence are interference with an already precarious blood supply to the thoracic spinal cord (described in Ch. 4, Vascular Supply of the Spinal Cord) caused by direct pressure on the spinal cord by bone fragments, soft tissue (disc), hematoma, or direct pressure during surgical intervention);

stretching of the spinal cord at the time of the fracture (flexion-distraction-type injuries); or post-traumatic spinal cord myelopathy secondary to direct bruising or trauma to the spinal cord, resulting in edema or central spinal cord hematomyelia with secondary vascular interruption.

Diastasis with Distraction Fixation

A hazard of distraction-type internal fixation of vertebral column (compression) fractures is the occurrence of diastasis between fracture vertebral body fragments or intersegmentally. Although infrequently encountered (or recognized), and more likely to occur in the lumbar spine region (see Ch. 19, Fig. 19-15), diastasis after instrumentation can and does occur in the presence of a fracture through the posterior wall of a vertebral body (likely indicating a discontinuity within the posterior longitudinal ligament) (Table 17-6); an anterior wall compression fracture of greater than 50 percent (also indicating a likely involvement of the anterior longitudinal ligament); "posterior column" facet joint-interlaminar segmental separation; or the presence of a prominent (or traumatically induced) kyphosis.

In the situation described above, a single and always preferred method of internal fixation is not available. Distraction with the Harrington rod system[4] or the Jacob's distraction rod systems[5] appears to be the more appropriate method of internal stabilization because these systems are capable of producing restoration of vertebral body height, correction of the kyphosis, and stability.

Loss of Reduction with Compression and Alignment Devices

A question that arises is, What are the indications for use of Luque (or Harrington compression) rod systems? In the presence of preserved neurologic function, compression is not indicated, but with great care and monitoring the Luque system is perhaps indicated. The hazard is encroachment on the canal, either by compression or by the fixator itself. Likewise, postoperative axial loading may result in further fracture compression and neural canal nar-

rowing (see Luque Segmental Spinal Instrumentation, below). As the thoracic neural canal is already anatomically small, increased canal compromise is always to be avoided.

As noted above, not all compression fractures require surgical management. This is particularly true of some fractures with no evidence of instability, malalignment, or associated neurologic injury. Thus, simple compression fractures (less than 25 to 35 percent of the vertebral body height lost) can usually be managed by 4 weeks of recumbent bed rest followed by orthotic immobilization for 2 to 3 more months (see Ch. 12).

SURGICAL APPROACHES AND INTRAOPERATIVE TECHNIQUES

Standard Posterior Approach

The posterior approach to the vertebral column usually requires that the patient be placed on the standard operating table or the Stryker frame in the prone position. Although this is the utility approach for the performance of all of the posterior instrumentation procedures (Harrington rod, Luque rod, Jacobs [AO] rod, Weiss spring, etc.), each of the aforementioned procedures can be also performed with the patient in the lateral decubitus position. Placing the patient in the lateral decubitus position implies the performance of a simultaneous approach (transpleural, transperitoneal, or retroperitoneal)[4,10,12,19] to the anterolateral vertebral column (Fig. 17-14). Before the procedure is initiated, certain prerequisites must be met:

The patient must always be intubated before turning

The patient must have a radial artery pressure-monitoring transducer in place (with the transducer at the level of the spinal cord, not the level of the heart)

The patient must have an indwelling urinary catheter in place

When there is intact neurologic function, SSEP electrodes should be in place and tested

An additional monitoring device, such as a temperature transducer in the rectum, is often utilized

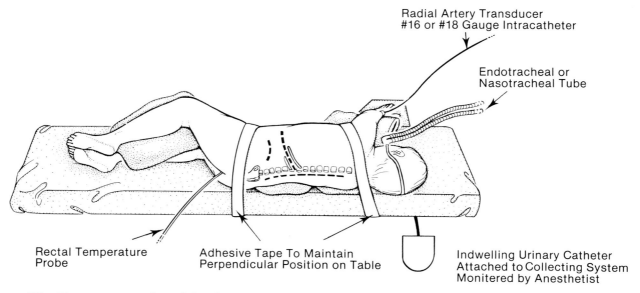

Radial Artery Transducer
#16 or #18 Gauge Intracatheter

Endotracheal or
Nasotracheal Tube

Rectal Temperature
Probe

Adhesive Tape To Maintain
Perpendicular Position on Table

Indwelling Urinary Catheter
Attached to Collecting System
Monitered by Anesthetist

Fig. 17-14. Patient in lateral decubitus position, with back close to the outer edge of the operating table. This position allows simultaneous anterior transthoracic and posterior approaches to the spine by two surgical teams.

Prone Positioning on the Operating Table

With the patient in the prone position on the operating table, care must be taken to position longitudinal rolls along each side of the chest and abdomen, from the level of the shoulders to the iliac crests. These rolls semi-suspend the patient and allow for a more complete chest expansion along with freedom of motion of the diaphragm during surgical anesthesia. The rolls also protect the pelvic rim's bony prominences from pressure sore problems. Special attention must also be taken to place the roll around and alongside the anterior superior iliac spine, not directly over it. If the patient lies directly on these bony areas for lengthy periods, skin pressure problems may arise secondary to a lack of adequate subcutaneous tissue over these areas. When it is desirable to maintain the patient in a hyperextended position while prone, one pillow or log roll can be placed transversely across the upper chest at or slightly below the level of the sternal notch, and a second transverse roll can be placed across the lower pelvis, just inferior to the anterior superior iliac spine.

Surgical Incision

If the fracture under management is at T6, with the patient in the prone position, a mild to moderate gibbus or accentuated thoracic kyphosis produced by angular deformity of the thoracic spine secondary to fracture and by the prominence of the thoracic spinous processes will be visually identifiable and likely palpable (along with the spinous process of T6-T7). This site will be the center point of a straight midline posterior incision, which extends from the third posterior lamina above the injury site to the third lamina below the injury site. Once the incision is made by sharp dissection, it can be carried down through the subcutaneous tissue to the fascia overlying the posterior spinous processes by electrocautery dissection. I prefer this technique to sharp dissection because of the vascular nature of the posterior musculature (the latissimus dorsi inferiorly, the trapezius superiorly, along with the underlying erector spinae, multifidi, and rotator muscles). Also present are the small vessels that lie opposite each spinous process and lateral to each posterior element. Use of the electocautery, which at first may seem slower than the standard technique, will significantly conserve blood loss.

Preparation of the Posterior Elements

The interlaminar and interspinous ligaments are excised either by sharp dissection or by a Kerrison rongeur. The electrocautery blade is used in a continuous running fashion along, around, and through the posterior fascia and interspinous ligaments, exposing the tip of each spinous process along the planned length of the approach. Once each of the appropriate spinous processes have been exposed, a Cobb or Key periosteal elevator is used to free the perispinous muscles from the lateral sides of each of the spinous processes. Careful attention is taken to dissect all soft tissue from the posterior bony structures. To enhance this procedure, I have found that by "scarifying" the tissue over each of the posterior elements (and facet joint capsules) with the electrocautery, the removal of the periosteal layer of soft tissue is greatly facilitated. A Stryker "Hall" burr is used to debride the external surface of the lamina and posterior spinous processes. No attempt is made to decorticate the external surface of the lamina; only to clean it. This is carried out to the lateral border of each of the thoracic (or lumbar) posterior elements (lamina and facets). Occasionally it is necessary to dissect out to the base of the transverse process, in the thoracic spine, to enhance the exposure and facilitate the performance of the procedure. With respect to facet joints, in scoliosis, great care is taken to decorticate the articular surfaces. In spinal trauma, I have found the high-speed burr an effective means of denuding the articular surfaces of the facet. I have also noted that in trauma, the need to perform extensive facet debridement (as required with scoliosis) is not necessary. Possibly the tissue pathology (at the root of the etiology of scoliosis) influences the healing and fusion process. Regardless, with trauma, the spine appears to require less tissue manipulation to accomplish a solid fusion.

Management of Operative Blood Loss

Every attempt should be made to prevent and control all bleeding during the procedure. When substantial intraoperative bleeding is anticipated,

arrangements should be made preoperatively for the use during surgery of a Haemonetic Cell Saver. The use of this device (Mark 4 model, capable of processing 300 ml of blood per minute) for blood collection and readministration is very effective. Blood bank packed cell or whole blood is only necessary when supplemental blood is required, or when it is thought that fresh blood (containing clotting factors washed out during the collection of the Cell Saver blood) is inadequate. The Northwestern University (1981 to 1985) experience has revealed that the estimated blood loss during a standard posterior instrumentation procedure is approximately 1,567 ml. For the ever present small segmental blood vessels that lie in close proximity to the lateral border of the lamina, the availability of a "bipolar" coagulator is essential. When using the electrocautery for dissection, I recommend only coagulation dissection. Use of the instrument in the coagulation rather than cutting mode facilitates small vessel coagulation. To achieve effective coagulation with the electrocautery, it may be necessary to turn the coagulation segment of the instrument up to 5, rather than using a normal coagulation setting of 3 to 4.

Intraoperative Antibiotic Usage

Before the incision is made, an appropriate intravenous antibiotic should be administered. In the absence of a penicillin allergy history, I utilize one of the cephalosporin antibiotics (cephalothin sodium [Keflin]). One gram is administered preoperatively or with the administration of the anesthetic and is repeated every 3 to 4 hours during the procedure. Antibiotic coverage is continued at the same dosage level every 6 hours over the next 48 hours. Throughout the operative procedure, the wound is frequently irrigated with an antibiotic irrigating solution (mixed by the pharmacy: bacitracin [250,000 U] and neomycin [2.0 g] in 1,000 ml of normal saline.)

Intraoperative Fracture Reduction

When a fracture-dislocation of the thoracic spine exists, the deformity may be the result of a flexion-distraction injury with facet dislocation, a translatory fracture-dislocation with fracture of the facets, or an axial load compression-burst-type vertebral fracture with translation. Frequently, this fracture will require intraoperative reduction. To accomplish this, a distraction force is required (using the Harrington distraction device) for fracture reduction or spine realignment and reduction. It is necessary to expose the posterior elements from the third level above to the third level below the fracture site, as this third level will be used as the fixation points for the superior (1253) and inferior (1254) distraction hooks. Preparation of the lamina includes (1) excision of the ligamentum flavum, by sharp dissection, from the interspaces between the respective adjacent lamina into which the hooks will be inserted (i.e., the second and third laminae above and below the fracture level), and (2) notching of the lamina *(inferomedial surface of the upper lamina and the superomedial aspect of the lower lamina)* with a right-angle Kerrison rongeur so it can accept the appropriate hooks. If sublaminar (Luque) wires are required for enhanced internal fixation device stability, the ligament is excised at each intervening level (Fig. 19-10). This is followed by the insertion of hooks and the distraction device. Care is required to ensure the stable placement of the hooks against the appropriate laminar surface. If not, the lamina may fracture. It may also be helpful to notch the adjacent (opposite) laminar surface to facilitate the insertion of the hooks. When the distraction force has been applied, the extent of the reduction can be determined by an intraoperative cross-table lateral radiograph (Fig. 17-7E,F). In general, it is important to be aware that Weiss compression hooks used in the lumbar spine area are larger than those used in the thoracic area and that Harrington distraction hooks vary in size depending on the type used (the size of the Harrington compression hooks is uniform).

Intraoperative Myelogram

If the question arises whether neural canal compromise has resulted from the reduction of a dislocation or the insertion of the internal fixation device (identified by a change in the intraoperative SSEP), a metrizamide myelogram can be obtained with the patient in the prone position, during the operative procedure. The head of the operating table can be lowered and elevated, permitting the contrast material to flow through the spinal canal across the level in question.

Loss of Intraoperative Somatosensory Evoked Response

Should significant loss or alteration in the observed SSEP occur during an operative procedure, and particularly during the insertion of the posterior instrumentation, the device should be removed and sufficient time allowed for the evoked response to return, before reinsertion. If the potential does not return to the same level and a myelogram does not reveal encroachment, the change in the SSEP may be secondary to distraction on the dura, the anesthetic agent being used (see Ch. 6), hypotension, change in environmental temperature, or loss of an electrode (check all). It is advisable not to reinsert the fixation device until the source of the change in the SSEP has been found. It may be necessary not to reinsert the planned internal fixation device at this time, and rather return to do so at a later date, or to perform the fixation anteriorly as a staged procedure. If, on the other hand, the potential demonstrates continued improvement, reinstrumentation can be attempted. Usually during the "wait" period between depression of the evoked response, removal of the fixation device, and the return of the SSEP, Decadron (dexamethasone) (50 mg) should be administered intravenously and the area of spine trauma bathed in cool to cold saline.

Posterior Spinal Fusion

After insertion of the internal fixation device, a posterior spinal fusion should be performed. The length of the fusion may be commensurate with the length of the internal fixation, or across only the fractured vertebra(e) and the level above and below the injury site. Bone graft material is obtained by a second incision over one of the posterior iliac crests in the routine manner if the procedure involves the upper end of the thoracic spine.

If the instrumentation and fusion are at the lower end of the lumbar spine, the bone graft may be obtained by the same midline incision, with dissection between the subcutaneous tissue and the paraspinous muscles, down to the appropriate posterior iliac crest (Fig. 17-15). Before the application of the cancellous bone graft obtained from the iliac crest, the spinous processes should be rongeured down to their base, and the external surface of the lamina further denuded of its external cortex, if it is believed that further decortication is required.

Wound Closure

Before the closure of the posterior spine wound and iliac crest donor site wound, both should be thoroughly irrigated with antibiotic irrigation solution and saline. A medium or large (depending on the surgeon's choice) Hemovac is inserted into each wound. Wound closure is usually preceded by debridement of the paraspinous muscles along the wound edges, followed by a muscle-fascial closure using figure-of-eight 0 Dexon interrupted sutures. Once this layer is tightly closed, the subcutaneous

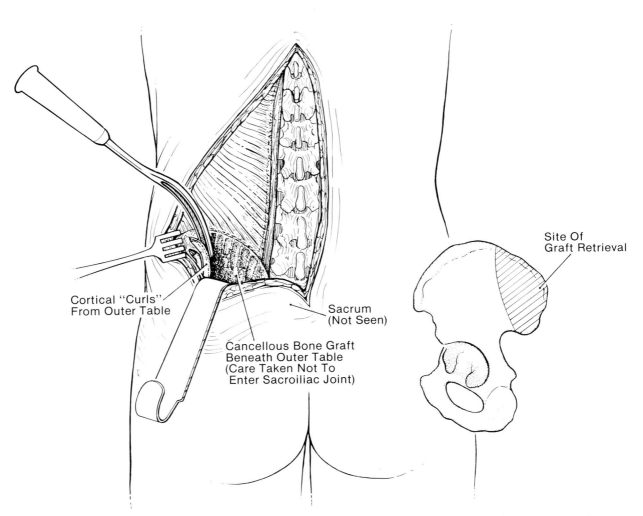

Cortical "Curls" From Outer Table

Sacrum (Not Seen)

Cancellous Bone Graft Beneath Outer Table (Care Taken Not To Enter Sacroiliac Joint)

Site Of Graft Retrieval

Fig. 17-15. Posterior superior iliac crest graft taken through same incision used for lumbar spine procedure.

tissue is approximated with 0 Dexon interrupted sutures, and the skin is closed with either skin staples or a 2-0 subcuticular Prolene suture. A standard external dressing is applied.

Postoperative Orthotic Device Usage

The spine should be supported by an external orthosis for at least 3 months postoperatively. The choice of orthosis depends on the type of fracture, the mechanism of internal fixation, prescribed conservative care, the surgeon, and the orthotist. The kind of orthosis most frequently utilized at Northwestern University for fractures below the level of T6 is the Knight-Taylor orthosis with pectoral horns (see Ch. 12), followed by the plastic laminated body jacket. For fractures above the level of T6, the type of orthosis recommended is the Knight-Taylor orthosis with both pectoral horns and a cervical extension (Fig. 17-16).

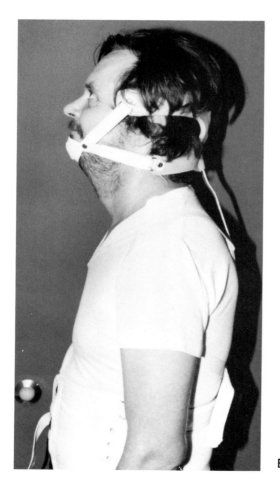
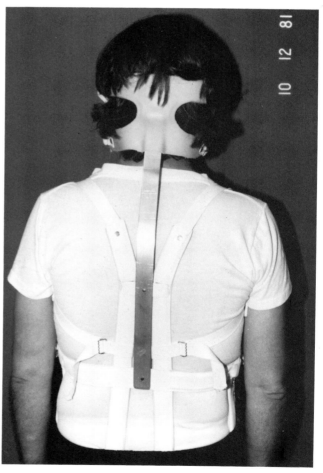

A   B

Fig. 17-16. (A) Lateral and (B) posterior views demonstrate use of Knight-Taylor orthosis with cervical extension. This device is utilized for fractures of the thoracic spine above the level of T6. This orthosis is frequently modified to include pectoral pads if other fractures of the thoracic spine exist and an upper thoracic extension moment is required.

SURGICAL INSTRUMENTATION
TECHNIQUES

Luque Segmental Spinal Instrumentation

The introduction of the Luque segmental fixation ("L" or "rectangular") rods and the use of sublaminar wire for fixation of the rods to the posterior elements has provided a significant advancement in the armamentarium of spinal instrumentation. First introduced by Eduardo Luque of Mexico in the late 1970s and early 1980s, and reported in a series of 14 patients in 1982,[13] the procedure now

serves as the major alternative to Harrington rod[4] spinal fixation. The Luque rod technique of spinal stabilization provides immediate spinal stability by direct fixation of the implant to uninjured posterior spinal elements (lamina) above and below the fracture site at multiple levels. With the use of the original L-shaped rods, a paralytic curve could be positively corrected by the application of transverse wires between the two upright rods, appropriately placed along the curve (Fig. 17-17A,B). With fracture management, the same improved alignment opportunity exists (Fig. 17-18A,B,C,D,E). With the use of the rectangular Luque rods, correction of the spine in the lateral

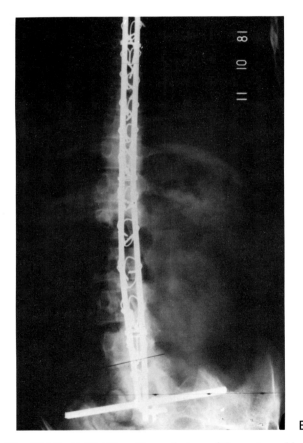 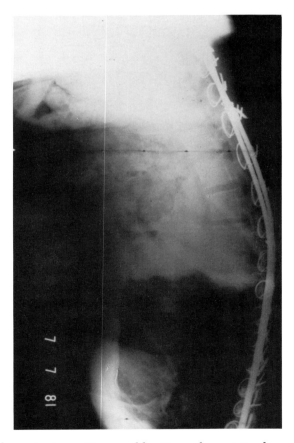

A   B

Fig. 17-17. (A,B) AP and lateral view of thoracic and lumbar spine in an 18-year-old patient who sustained cervical spine fracture dislocation of C3 on C4 in 1973 at age 11. Follow-up revealed onset of severe thoracolumbar paralytic scoliosis. Patient required spine stabilization procedure from T4 to the sacrum for maintenance of sit-balance and to overcome increased spinal deformity associated with spasticity. Note transverse wires on AP view at T7, T12, and L3-L4. Tightening of these wires assists in correcting scoliotic curve and prevention of lateral displacement of individual L rods.

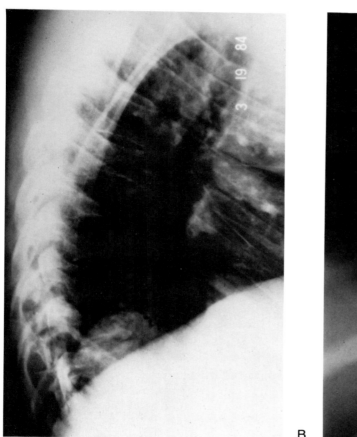
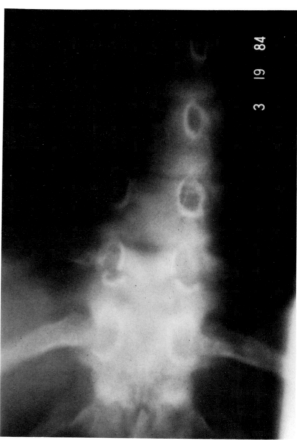

A

B

Fig. 17-18. **(A,B)** AP and lateral radiographs of thoracic spine demonstrating Chance fracture through T10. On AP view a horizontal fracture through the pedicles bilaterally is easily identified. This fracture results from flexion distraction forces. *(Figure continues.)*

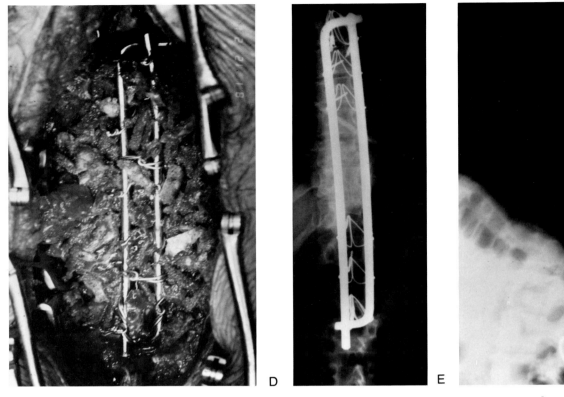

C   D   E

Fig. 17-18 *(Continued).* **(C)** Operative view of L-shaped Luque segmental instrumentation and transverse wires to assist in maintaining vertical alignment. Note extent of spine fusion. **(D,E)** AP and lateral radiographs of thoracic spine demonstrate improved alignment with L-shaped Luque segmental rods.

projection can be accurately obtained (Fig. 17-19); however, the same corrective advantage does not exist in the anteroposterior plane. Therefore, indications for the use of the L-shaped or rectangular Luque system should be considered. Prebending the rods in the sagittal plane allows for both the accommodation of the normal thoracic and thoracolumbar kyphosis or lumbar lordosis, or for the correction of a fracture deformity. Therefore, with the use of the Luque rod spine stabilization system, scoliosis or acute (trauma-induced) lateral angular deformities can be corrected; sagittal deformities (kyphosis or lordosis) can be maintained, corrected, or eliminated; in the presence of spinal fracture instability, stability can be immediately restored.

Luque rod instrumentation is an excellent stabilizing procedure for fractures of the lumbar spine, particularly when neurologic function remains intact and where the neural canal is wide. It is very well suited for fractures of the anterior vertebral column (wedge compression fractures). This is not the case with fractures of the thoracic vertebral column. Here the neural canal is quite narrow, and because the blood supply to the spinal cord is already precarious, great care must be exercised when passing Luque wires beneath the lamina of the thoracic spine (T2 to T10) (Fig. 17-20). Similar to the use of Harrington rods, fixation of the Luque system to the spine requires fixation two levels above and below the level of injury. The technique can be effectively utilized by going only one level above or below (with the careful use of a postoperative orthosis for 3 months) when no other alternative exists.

After making the appropriate incision and thoroughly exposing the appropriate vertebral elements (see Standard Posterior Approach, above), a right-angle Luque rod (¼-inch short rod) is cut to the appropriate length. If the rectangular rod system is used, the appropriate length rectangular rod is selected. This system is much less cumbersome than the use of two L rods.

When using two L rods (one rod has the L shape at the top, the opposite rod has the L at the bottom (Fig. 17-18D,E), each rod is bent in the sagittal plane to provide, maintain, or restore the normal (prefracture) vertebral column curve. With the rods lying in place, the upper L should lie transversely between the second and third spinous process above the fractured vertebral element, and extend distally to the second and third interspinous space below the fracture site. What may force the surgeon to extend the fixation more distally would be the presence of posterior element fractures over multiple levels (Fig. 17-7B,D).

Prepared Luque wire loops (18 gauge) are used for fixation of the rods to the lamina. The wires are

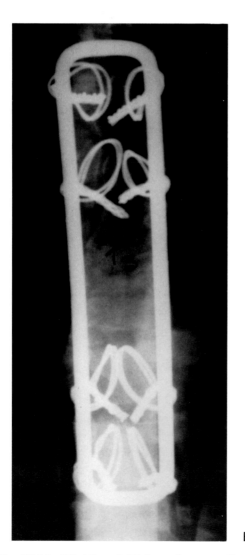
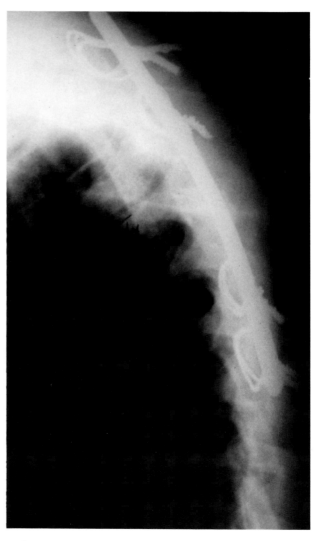

Fig. 17-19. (A) AP and (B) lateral views of rectangular Luque rods and postoperative alignment of the thoracic spine in a patient with axial load-flexion fracture dislocation of T3 on T4.

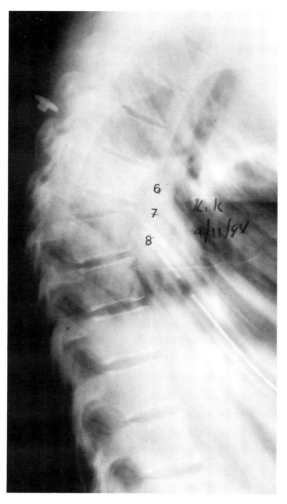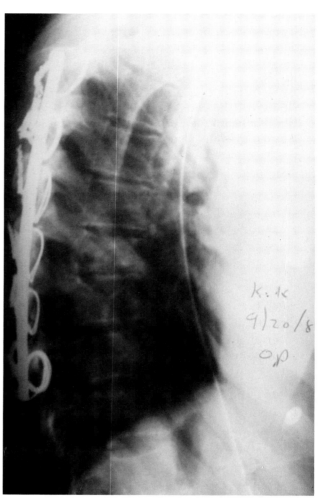

A   B

Fig. 17-20. (A) Lateral radiograph of thoracic spine showing a severe wedge compression fracture at T7. (B) Postoperative lateral radiograph after insertion of Luque rods and sublaminar wires shows significant improvement in the height of the T7 vertebral body and relief of the acute traumatic thoracic spine kyphosis.

appropriately bent to pass easily beneath and between each lamina, after a small "window" has been made in the ligamentum flavum at each level. The wire is passed into each intralaminar sublaminar space from an inferior to a superior direction. As the wire exits the intralaminar space above, it is pulled through to approximately one-half the length of the wire. The wire is left doubled at the upper and lower four corners. At each intervening level, the wire loop is cut with a wire cutter, and one side of the wire is taken to the right, the other

side to the left. This means there will be a double wire on the right and the left sides of the lamina at T4 and T8, and a single wire on the right and left sides of the lamina of T5, T6 (if stable and not comminuted, otherwise omit), and T7.

The Luque rods are now inserted, weaving them in and out of each successive wire from top to bottom. The rule "down and out" is used to consistently place the Luque wires around the rods. The double wires at each of the four corners are tightened first to fix two Luque rods (or rectangular rod) in place. Special wire tighteners are available, but standard vise grip wire tighteners will suffice. As the wires are tightened they are pulled taut, perpendicular to the surface of each lamina. When the four outer corners are tight, each of the other wires is sequentially tightened. To further enhance the stability of the rods, a double transverse wire is placed beneath the Luque rods (when the two-rod system is used) at a level above and below the fracture level (Fig. 17-18C). Tightening these wires (usually double strands) pulls the two Luque rods toward the midline, straightening out any existing curve and significantly increasing the stability of the system.

Before the Luque rod system is inserted, the external surface of each lamina is decorticated on its external surface by a high-speed burr. When the rods and wires are in place and tightened, the spinous processes are rongeured down to the level of the Luque rods, but not below. This bone, along with an axillary bone graft obtained from one of the posterior iliac wings, is inserted along the fusion site. It is the surgeon's choice whether the fusion is carried out along the entire internal fixation, or only in the middle, to include one level above and one level below the injury site.

Distraction: Fracture Management

Because of the recognized success of Harrington distraction rods (Figs. 17-6E,F, 17-7E) in the surgical correction of scoliosis, many believed the device to be equally effective in restoring and maintaining spinal alignment after trauma.[7,8,20] The instrumentation does provide stabilization, but may not be indicated (as with distraction-dislocation injuries) in every instance of spinal trauma. It is necessary, therefore, to establish "indication criteria" for distraction instrumentation in spinal trauma. Thus, the following traumatic injuries to the spine are thought to be the more obvious indications for the use of distraction-fixation, particularly in the presence of intact or incomplete neurologic function:

Anterior compression fractures of the vertebral body (Fig. 17-7A)
Burst fractures of the vertebral body (Fig. 17-21)

Unilateral vertebral body, pedicle, facet fractures (Fig. 17-6B)
Fractures over multiple levels (Fig. 17-7B)

Harrington Distraction Rod Procedure

After making the appropriate incision and thoroughly exposing the appropriate vertebral elements, an appropriate length Harrington distraction rod is selected. *Care is taken not to use a rod that places the junction between the ratchet portion of the rod and the smooth shank portion of the rod directly over the fracture site.* This junction is biomechanically the weakest area of the rod. When applied directly over the level of the fracture, should there be any repetitive (or oscillating) bending moments applied to this area of the rod, "stress risers" will result in rod "fatigue failure." Therefore, select a longer rod (with a longer smooth shank) and cut notches in the end of the rod to an appropriate length (leaving three notched levels above the upper hook). This will also facilitate the removal of the system at an appropriate time, if deemed necessary.

With the inferior surface of the upper lamina notched (three above the fracture site or sometimes higher if fractures of the posterior elements exist just above the level of the fracture), and the superior surface of the inferior lamina similarly notched, using a Kerrison rongeur, a 1253 hook is inserted superiorly. This hook is impacted in place with the hook impactor. The ratchet portion of the rod is inserted into the proximal hook sufficiently far to allow the inferior portion of the rod to fit into the inferior (1254) hook (which has been inserted into the superior surface of the lower lamina) at the third lamina below the involved or fractured lamina. Occasionally, because of the kyphosis associated with the presence of a thoracic or thoracolumbar fracture, it may be necessary to use the high-speed burr on the posterior cortical surface of the lamina, just above the lower hook lamina, making a vertical groove for the rod to lie in. This will allow the rod to be depressed down against the posterior lamina, thus allowing the lower end of the Harrington distraction rod to fit into the lower hook. This accomplished, the ratchet-hook spreader is inserted superiorly, and distraction between the upper hook (bilaterally) is applied to the rods. Care must be taken not to overdistract the

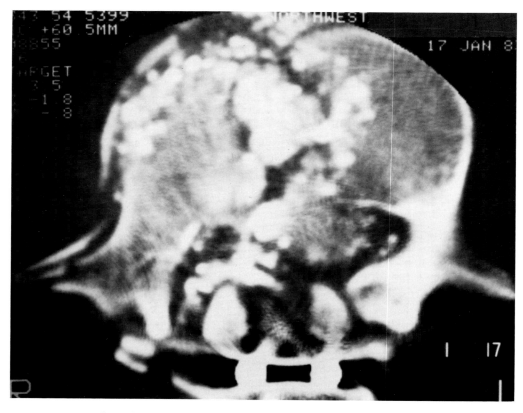

Fig. 17-21. CAT scan of T12 burst fracture with posterior Harrington distraction rods in place. The patient had an incomplete neurologic injury. The patient underwent staged anterior resection of comminuted fragments in canal.

spine. This is a particularly sensitive problem when there has been associated vertebral diplacement or significant vertebral body comminution (though Holdsworth believed these fractures to be stable[3]). A consideration to be taken into account is the presence or absence of stability within the anterior longitudinal ligament. A method of determining this is described in Figure 19-5. Remember, distraction of vertebral elements contributes to internal fixation instability and delay in fracture fragment healing.

If, because of anticipated instability, the surgeon elects to insert Luque wires under each of the intervening laminae, these wires should be inserted (as described in Luque Segmental Spinal Instrumentation, above) before the posterior Harrington distraction apparatus is inserted. Care must be taken during the passage of the sublaminar wires

not to further injure the already traumatized dura and contained neural elements.

Once the rods are in place and appropriate distraction is applied, the wires may be tightened around the Harrington rods (using an appropriate wire tightener). To prevent lateral displacement of the Harrington rods, a wire may be placed (and tightened) transversely between the two Harrington rods, one superior and inferior to the level of the fracture.

Posterior "Locking Hook-Spinal Rod System" (AO Synthes-Jacobs)

The AO Synthes-Jacobs locking hook-spinal rod system[5,7,8] is mentioned here, under thoracic spine injuries, to complete the section on thoracic instrumentation. Although there may be occasion to utilize this method of internal fixation for fractures occurring between T1 and T10, the device is more often indicated for injuries in the region of the thoracolumbar junction (T11 through L2) or the lumbar spine. See Chapter 18 for a more thorough discussion.

Compression: Fracture Management

The Harrington compression rod system was found to be the most stable of the internal fixation instrumentation procedures when tested in the laboratory.[21,22] However, the major problem with Harrington compression rods is the cumbersome nature of inserting the component parts bilaterally: rods, washers, multiple hooks, and numerous nuts. In fact, the insertion of all these components is a significant disincentive to its usage. A second reason for the Harrington compression system not being more frequently utilized is that most fractures of the thoracic spine have a flexion component as a mechanism of injury, producing compression of one (usually the more inferior) vertebra. Thus, this injury was frequently associated with either a comminuted compression fracture or a posteroinferior vertebral body fracture, which, if placed under compression, could be extruded into the neural canal and potentially cause (or further exaggerate) neural compromise. With this potential hazard in mind, the criteria for application of compression across a vertebral column fracture are that there be no fracture of the posterior wall of the affected vertebral body; that there be no evidence of gross instability (anteroposterior vertebral body translation) diagnosed on the original radiograph, or vertebral element distraction (meaning loss of disc, or loss of major ligamentous continuity anteriorly or posteriorly; and that there not be an unbalanced fracture of the vertebral elements under consideration — that is, the vertebral body must not be fractured in the coronal plane in such a manner that one side of the vertebral body-pedicle-facet complex is intact and the opposite side is depressed, or displaced laterally. (When this exists, the application of compressive forces bilaterally will produce an iatrogenic scoliosis toward the concavity on the side of the depressed, displaced elements). Upon satisfying any of the above criteria, stabilization via a compression device is indicated.

The devices of choice are Harrington compression rods, the Wisconsin compression rod system, or Weiss compression springs.

Harrington Compression Rods

After the appropriate incision is made and the appropriate vertebral elements are thoroughly exposed, Harrington compression (threaded) rods of appropriate length are selected. The number of segments to be crossed will determine the number of compression hooks required bilaterally. Usually, only two above and two below (bilaterally) are required. Because of the necessity of having the hooks aligned along the Harrington compression rod before and during insertion of the rods (the hooks facing inferiorly above the level of injury and superiorly below the level of injury), the application of this device is somewhat difficult, cumbersome, and time consuming.

Each hook is loosely applied over the rod with its tightening nuts present proximally for the more proximal hooks and inferiorly for the lower hooks. As each hook is placed beneath its adjacent laminar border, it is lightly tightened in place. It is necessary to remember that because compression is being applied, the hooks must be tightened closest to the fracture first, and then alternately between the superior and inferior hook so that the rod-hook complex remains in place. Once the entire apparatus is inserted bilaterally, further compression above and below the level of injury can be applied, until the desired amount of compression or correction has been achieved. This can be determined radiographically during surgery.

Wisconsin Compression Rod System

After the appropriate incision is made and the appropriate vertebral elements are thoroughly exposed, (threaded) Wisconsin compression rods[23] of appropriate length are selected. They may be further cut with a rod cutter to an appropriate length before insertion. The number of segments to be crossed depends on the number of compression hooks required bilaterally. The advantage of the Wisconsin rod-hook system is that each hook can be inserted under its respective lamina, independent of the compression rod. This greatly simplifies the procedure and allows each hook to be inserted singularly into the appropriate laminar interspace, and the lamina to be rongeured for fit if need be.

When each hook-laminar complex has been prepared, the Wisconsin compression (threaded) rod can literally be laid into the groove of each of the 1204 hooks. Along the rod, appropriately placed on the side opposite the hook, a "Keene" bushing is slid over the rod, one for each of the four hooks (two above and two below the fracture) on each side. Also applied is a "hex nut" at each location. The Keene bushing prevents displacement of the rod from the hook once applied. The hex nut is for the application of compression on each nut-bushing-hook complex as they are set into place. Counterforce is required from the opposite direction to maintain the position of the device and apply compression across the fracture site. This procedure is carried out alternately at each level bilaterally until the device is appropriately tightened in place. Intraoperative radiographs can be used to check for the desired surgical correction.

Weiss Compression Springs System
Historically, the use of the Weiss compression springs system of spinal trauma instrumentation (producing dynamic compression) became a surgical alternative in the mid-1970s. The procedure was popularized by Marion Weiss of Warsaw, Poland, following its initial introduction into the spinal instrumentation armamentarium in the late 1950s and early 1960s as a means of correcting scoliosis secondary to poliomyelitis. The instrumentation was less successful with scoliosis than with trauma, although in the management of the latter, its level of success was modest and its stability both surgically and in the laboratory was less than required. The primary deficit in stabilization was in rotation. Through personal experience with the use of Weiss springs, this device has revealed itself to be indicated almost solely for those injuries to the spine in which only ligamentous disruption has occurred (with dislocation of facets without fracture), and it is not indicated when significant fracture of either the anterior or posterior elements has occurred.

Using fresh cadaver specimens, Pinzer et al. observed four-point loading-stability characteristics of Harrington distraction and Harrington compression rods and compression (Weiss) springs.[21] The elastic modulus of each device was compared with the preinjured state. Fixation with Harrington compression rods was found to have the highest elastic modulus (i.e., the most stiff), yet failed with the least amount of displacement. Similar findings were reported by Stauffer and Neil.[22] Weiss compression springs were found to have the least elastic modulus, yet maintained internal fixation continuity with pure flexion displacement. Failure occurred when the combination of flexion and rotation was present.[10,24] Again, similar findings were identified by Stauffer and Neil.[22] Thus, from laboratory analysis, it was determined that Weiss springs were more favorably indicated for anterior lumbar vertebral body fractures of minor degree or for ligamentous disruption of the posterior column, with the middle columns remaining intact and without evidence of sagittal or coronal translation. The device in this case, is indicated because of already inherent stability of the spine remaining, ease of insertion, fixation at only two points (proximally and distally, rather than at four points as with the Harrington compression or Wisconsin compression devices), fewer segments are crossed (than with the Harrington compression rod), and because the system is dynamic and tends to produce posterior compression with mild anterior distraction when the anterior longitudinal ligament is intact, resulting in correction of the traumatically induced kyphosis (Figs. 17-13C, 17-22A,B, 17-23A,B).

After the appropriate incision is made and the appropriate vertebral elements are thoroughly exposed (see Standard Posterior Approach, above), the appropriate length spring is selected. The length used (5 to 12 cm) is commensurate with the distance between the upper and lower lamina, minus approximately 1.5 to 2 cm (the length to which the spring will stretch if it is 9 cm long). The shorter the spring, the less stretch is available, and thus there is the need for the spring to be almost the length of the area being spanned. As a rule, a distraction force across a stretched spring system (between the upper hook and lower hook) is approximately 30 to 40 lbs. It is this "dynamic" compression load that is capable of providing minor correction of a traumatic kyphotic deformity.

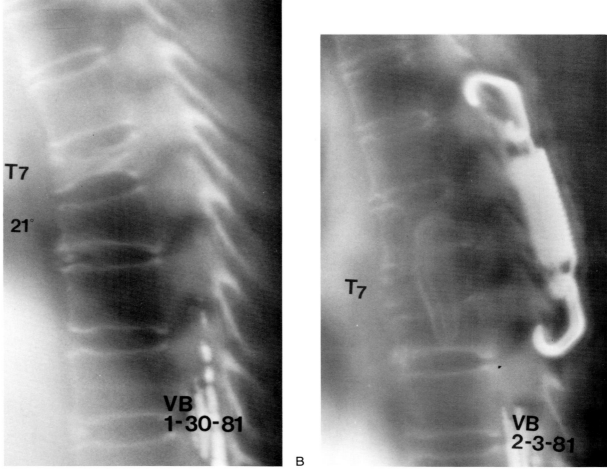

A   B

Fig. 17-22. (A) Lateral radiograph of severely osteoporotic thoracic spine with compression fractures at T7 and T8. Patient had incomplete neurologic injury with obstruction to flow of contrast material. (B) Lateral radiograph of thoracic spine showing postoperative result after simultaneous AP approach and internal fixation with posterior compression spring system. Note anterior bone graft at T6 – T7 – T8. Patient's incomplete neurologic injury improved after operation (Frankel grade B to Frankel grade D).

Posterior Spinous Process Wiring

After the reduction of spinal column malalignment or facet dislocation, particularly when produced by a flexion or distraction force, it is suggested that the two adjacent posterior spinous processes at the level of injury (if not fractured) be stabilized by means of an 18-gauge compression wire across the base of the two respective processes. Some surgeons prefer placing this wire without any special preparation of the spinous pro-

cess. With a concern for wire displacement, however, the following technique has been utilized at Northwestern University. A transverse hole is made through the base of the proximal spinous process and an 18-gauge stainless-steel wire is passed through their bases. The hole is carefully placed anteriorly in the superior spinous process and slightly more posteriorly in the inferior process. This ensures good fixation of the wire within the spinous process and prevention of fracture of the spinous process with tightening of the wire. If a

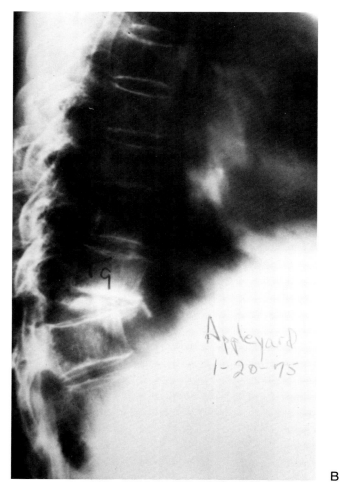

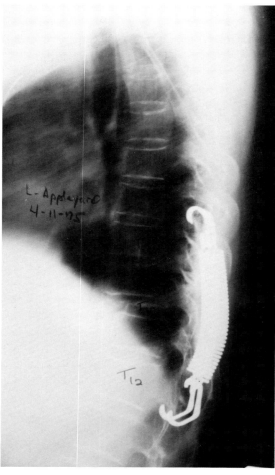

A   B

Fig. 17-23. (A) Lateral radiograph of thoracic spine showing tumorous distraction of T10 (metastatic carcinoma of the breast). (B) Lateral radiograph of thoracic spine after compression spring instrumentation. Note that the mild forward displacement of T9 on T10 seen in the preoperative view did not change, but the flexion deformity at the site of pathology is decreased.

double-loop 18-gauge wire is used, a small notch is made at the anterior base of the proximal spinous process, providing a fixation point for the wire when it is tightened into place. At the base of the inferior spinous process, a small notch can be made, either with a rongeur or a burr, but because of compression with tightening, it is less important. The two ends of the strand wire are brought together and tightened with a wire twister (or vise grip pliers). The wire should be tightened sufficiently to bring the adjacent spinous processes toward each other and allow maintenance of the

reduction of the facets. Reduction is frequently confirmed by intraoperative radiographs (Fig. 17-24).

Combination Use of Posterior Fixation Devices

Fractures of the spine frequently combine axial load, producing burst-type injuries; flexion, producing compression fractures; and lateral bend or rotation, producing translatory injuries with uni-

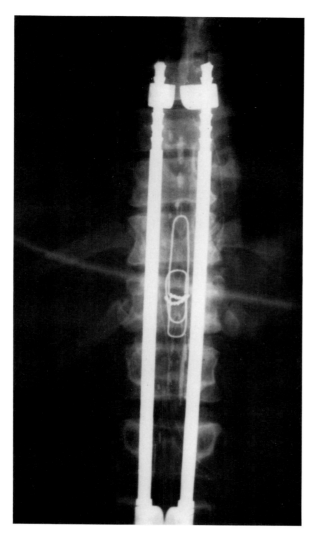

Fig. 17-24. AP radiograph of thoracic and thoracolumbar flexion dislocation. Open reduction of dislocated facets was followed by wire fixation through spinous processes T11–L1 and T12–L1. This was followed by insertion of a Harrington distraction apparatus.

The two most frequently utilized devices have been the Harrington distraction rod on one side of the vertebral column and the Harrington compression device on the opposite side. On several occasions, the Weiss compression spring has been utilized opposite the distraction rod. The rationale for the use of compression on one side and distraction on the other is the presence of a traumatic scoliosis. When present, the fracture findings include compression of one side of the vertebral body, with depression or widening of the pedicle and facet on that same side. This serves as the indication for distraction on this side. On the opposite side, one is likely to find a lateral shift of the upper vertebra to the side of compression, and a traumatically induced flexion (kyphotic) deformity of the spine at the fracture site. This serves as the indication for compression. As noted, the usual combination is the use of both Harrington compression and distraction rods. Note in Figure 17-11C the placement of the hooks at one level (inferiorly) into the sublaminar area and superiorly across the thoracic transverse processes. This latter method is very ineffective and unreliable.

Three factors must be taken into account. First, the results are often less than desired. Second, in several adults paralytic scoliosis has occurred secondary to muscle imbalance. The combination probably has no influence on the occurrence, but it has been noted. Although more infrequent in the adult, paralytic scoliosis secondary to traumatically induced quadriplegia or high paraplegia is not unusual. Finally, the state of the neurologic injury must always be taken into account. When neurologic function is intact, or the vertebral body is comminuted, one should be cautious about applying compression across the fracture site.

lateral (body-pedicle-facet) fracture on one side of the vertebral body and maintenance of anteroposterior element integrity on the opposite side. Because of the "compound" nature of these mechanically induced fractures, simultaneous distraction-compression fixation is occasionally used as the method of achieving spinal stability (Fig. 17-11).

ORTHOTIC MANAGEMENT

As noted above when a thoracic fracture occurs above the level of T6, it is necessary to extend the orthosis upward to the occiput. This prevents the inherent tendency (weight) of the head and shoulders to produce a kyphotic deformity across the fracture site. Thus, the cervical extension and anterior pectoral pads (or horns) of the orthosis, for injuries above T6, tend to prevent this complication from occurring (Fig. 17-16). This orthosis is known as a CTLSO or cervicothoracolumbosacral orthosis. Below T6, a standard thoracolumbosacral (TLSO) orthosis can be used.

Below T6, there are several types of orthotic devices which may be utilized: The standard Knight-Taylor (or Arnold) orthosis, the Jewett hyperextension orthosis, the modified cruciate Jewett orthosis, or a plastic laminated orthosis (see Ch. 12). Each is recommended to be worn at all times when sitting or standing, and for many patients (depending on spine stability), use of the orthosis is required during periods of recumbency to increase spinal stability and to reduce torsional forces on the spine when turning in bed or coming to a sitting position. For those patients without neurologic injury, the orthosis may be removed during periods of recumbency. All patients when in bed without an orthosis should be instructed to lie flat, without a head pillow, particularly when the fracture is in the upper two-thirds of the spine. This continues until approximately 6 weeks postinjury.

The primary precaution for all patients having sustained spinal trauma with associated neurologic injury is the potential hazard for skin breakdown over areas of insensitive skin beneath the orthosis. It is therefore suggested that the patient wear a T-shirt beneath the orthosis at all times and that the skin be carefully and frequently observed for indications of skin irritation or pressure sore development.

THORACIC SPINE SURGICAL OUTCOME DATA

Surgical versus Conservative Management

Of the 376 thoracic spine fractures managed (1972 to 1986), 242 were managed conservatively (64 percent) and 134 surgically (36 percent) (Table 17-7).

Of those managed conservatively, 14 (6 percent) demonstrated neurologic improvement, a slightly lower rate of improvement than those surgically

Table 17-7. Thoracic Fractures: Type of Management (Northwestern University Acute Spine Injury Center, 1972 to 1986)

Management Type	No.	%
Conservative	242	64.4
Surgical	134	35.6
Total	376	100.0

managed (9 percent). No patient managed conservatively demonstrated neurologic deterioration.

Of the patients undergoing surgical stabilization, 12 (9 percent) demonstrated neurologic improvement, and 3 (2 percent) demonstrated neurologic deterioration (Table 17-8).

Neurologic improvement was slightly higher in those patients managed surgically, whereas the risk of neurologic deterioration (2 percent) with surgical intervention is a recognized hazard.

Instrumentation

Of the 134 thoracic spine fractures managed between 1972 and 1986 (Table 17-9), Harrington distraction rods were used in 20 (15 percent) patients with 1 deterioration (5 percent) and 3 (15 percent) neurologic improvements. This was the highest rate of improvement of any of the three major instrument types utilized. Harrington com-

Table 17-8. Thoracic Fractures: Treatment by Change in Status[a] (Northwestern University Acute Spine Injury Center, 1972 to 1986)

Change in Status	Total	Conservative No.	%	Surgical No.	%
Improve	26	14	5.8	12	9.0
No change	325	211	87.2	114	85.1
Degradation	4	1	0.4	3	2.2
Unknown[b]	21	16	6.6	5	3.7
Total	376	242	64.4	134	35.6

[a]Change in status is change in Frankel score.
[b]Extent is unavailable.

Table 17-9. **Thoracic: Surgical Instrumentation by Change in Status (Northwestern University Acute Spine Injury Center, 1972 to 1986)**

Instrumentation	No.	Improve No.	%	No Change No.	%	Degrade No.	%	Missing No.	%
Single facet-spinous process	6	0	0.0	5	83.3	0	0.0	1	16.7
Double facet-spinous process	2	0	0.0	1	50.0	1	50.0	0	0.0
Luque rods	43	5	11.6	35	81.4	0	0.0	3	7.0
HRI[a] compression	1	0	0.0	1	100.0	0	0.0	0	0.0
HRI[a] distraction	20	3	15.0	16	80.0	1	5.0	0	0.0
Weiss compression	52	3	5.8	49	94.2	0	0.0	0	0.0
Other	1	0	0.0	1	100.0	0	0.0	0	0.0
Missing	9	1	11.1	6	66.7	1	11.1	1	11.1
Total	134	12	9.0	114	85.1	3	2.2	5	3.7

[a]HRI, Harrington rod.

pression rods were utilized in one patient. Fifty-two compression spring procedures (39 percent) were performed during a national evaluation of this device. Three improved (6 percent) and none deteriorated neurologically in this patient group. Forty-three (32 percent) patients were stabilized with Luque instrumentations, with five improvements and no deteriorations. Four (4 percent) patients had primary wiring of the spinous process (one with neurologic deterioration), and four patients had spinous process wiring combined with other posterior procedures (Table 17-9).

The data seem to indicate that compression is less of an overall hazard than distraction (though only slightly), but is likely biased owing to the high frequencies of certain types of fractures that necessitated compression management.

Surgical Approach

Of the thoracic spine patients undergoing surgical stabilization, 112 (84 percent) underwent posterior stabilization only. Within this group, nine

Table 17-10. **Thoracic: Surgical Approach by Change in Neurologic Status (Northwestern University Acute Spine Injury Center, 1972 to 1986)**

Approach	No.	Improve No.	%	No Change No.	%	Degrade No.	%	Missing** No.	%
Anterior	3	0	0.0	2	66.7	0	0.0	1	33.0
Posterior	112	9	8.0	99	88.4	2	1.8	2	1.8
Combined	8	1	12.5	6	75.0	0	0.0	1	12.5
Anterior then posterior	2	1	50.0	1	50.0	0	0.0	0	0.0
Posterior then anterior	1	0	0.0	1	100.0	0	0.0	0	0.0
Missing[a]	8	1	12.5	5	62.5	1	12.5	0	0.0
Total	134	12	9.0	114	85.1	3	2.2	4	3.0

[a]Approach is unavailable.
[b]Neurologic change is unavailable.

patients (8 percent) improved and two (2 percent) deteriorated neurologically. Of the three patients who underwent primary anterior decompression (2 percent), and the eight who had the combined anteroposterior decompression-stabilization procedure (6 percent), none deteriorated neurologically (Table 17-10). Of the three patients who underwent a staged anteroposterior stabilization procedure (2 percent), two revealed no neurologic change, and one improved neurologically.

No patient undergoing anterior approach decompression and fusion demonstrated neurologic deterioration. Nonetheless, the overall risk (vascular and neurologic) is still greater with this approach.

REFERENCES

1. Lusted LB, Keats TE: Atlas of Roentgenographic Measurement. 4th Ed. p. 123. Year Book Medical Publishers, Chicago, 1978
2. White AA, Panjabi MM: Functional spinal unit and mathematical models. Clinical Biomechanics of the Spine. JB Lippincott, Philadelphia, 1978
3. Holdsworth FW: Review article-fracture-dislocation and fracture-dislocations of the spine. J Bone Joint Surg 52A:534, 1970
4. Harrington PR, Dickson JH: An eleven year clinical investigation of Harrington instrumentation. Clin Orthop 112:113, 1973
5. Jacobs RR, Schlapfer F, Jacobs RR, et al.: A locking hook spinal rod system for stabilization of fracture-dislocations and correction of deformities of the dorsolumbar spine. Clin Orthop 189:168, 1984
6. Edwards CC: The spinal rod sleeve: its rationale and use in thoracic and lumbar injuries. J Bone Joint Surg Orthop Trans 6:11, 1982
7. Jacobs RR, Asher MA, Snider RK: Thoracolumbar spine fractures, a comparative study of recumbent and operative treatment in 100 patients. Spine 5:463, 1980
8. Jacobs RR, Casey MP: Surgical management of thoracic-lumbar spinal injuries: general principles and controversial considerations. Clin Orthop 189:22, 1984
9. Bradford DS: Treatment of severe spondylolisthesis. A combined approach for reduction and stabilization. Spine 4:423, 1979
10. Weiss M: Dynamic spine alloplasty (spring loading correction device) after fracture and spinal cord injury. Clin Orthop 112:150, 1975
11. Holdsworth FW, Hardy AG: Early treatment of paraplegics from fracture of the thoracolumbar spine. J Bone Joint Surg 35B:540, 1953
12. Roy-Camille R, Saillant G, Berteaux D, Marie-Anne S: Early management of spinal injuries. p. 57. In McKibbin B (ed): Recent Advances In Orthopaedics. Vol. 3. Churchill Livingstone, Edinburgh, 1979
13. Luque ER, Cassis N, Ramirez-Wiella G: Segmental spine instrumentation in the treatment of fractures of the thoracolumbar spine. Spine 7:312, 1982
14. Waldman J, Kaufer H, Heuringer RH, Callaghan ML: Wake-up technique during Harrington rod procedure; a case report. Anesth Analg 56:733, 1977
15. DeWald R, Faut MM: Anterior and posterior spine fusion for paralytic scoliosis. Spine 4:401, 1979
16. Spencer DL: Simultaneous anterior and posterior surgical approach to the thoracic and lumbar spine. Spine 4:29, 1979
17. Meyer PR: Complications of treatment of fractures of the dorsolumbar spine. p. 643. In Epps CH (ed): Complications in Orthopaedic Surgery. 2nd Ed. Vol. 2. JB Lippincott, Philadelphia, 1978
18. Denis F: The three column spine and its significance in the classification of acute thoracolumbar spine injuries. Spine 8:817, 1983
19. Dickson JH, Harrington PR, Erwin WD: Results of reduction and stabilization of the severely fractured thoracic and lumbar spine. J Bone Joint Surg 60:799, 1978
20. Soreff J, Axdorph G et al.: Treatment of patients with unstable fractures of the thoracic and lumbar spine. A follow-up study of surgical and conservative treatment. Acta Orthop Scand 53:369, 1982
21. Pinzer MS, Meyer PR, Lautenschlager EP et al.: Measurement of internal fixation device support in experimentally produced fractures of the dorsolumbar spine. Orthopaedics 4:28, June, 1979
22. Stauffer ES, Neil JL: Biomechanical analysis of structural stability of internal fixation in fractures of the thoracolumbar spine. Clin Orthop 112:159, 1975
23. Keene JS, Drummond DS: Wisconsin Compression System Surgical Technique. Zimmer, 1981
24. Meyer PR: Weiss spring spinal internal fixation. p. 22. Surgical Technique. Zimmer,

18

Indications: Anteroposterior Surgical Approach to the Thoracolumbar Spine

Paul R. Meyer, Jr.

The thoracolumbar junction is the second most frequently injured area of the spine. Review of injury data for 1972 to 1986 from the Midwest Regional Spinal Cord Injury Care System (MRSCICS) reveals that, of 932 injuries to the thoracic, lumbar, and sacral spine, in patients admitted to the acute spinal injury service, 376 were thoracic (T1–T10), 73 were lumbar (L3–L5), and 13 were sacral (S1–S5) (Table 18-1). Of these 932 injuries, 470 involved the thoracolumbar junction (T11–L2). Because most lower spine injuries occur between T11 and L2, for the purposes of this chapter this junctional area is recognized as a distinct region of the spine. This chapter examines specific injuries encountered and treatments indicated for fractures occurring in the thoracolumbar junctional area.

Vertebral injuries vary greatly in location, type, number, and severity. Three major variants that influence these fractures are the direction of the applied force, the severity (or magnitude) of the force, and, unmeasurable for the most part (except in the laboratory), the length of time or duration a force is applied. Between T11 and L2, the most frequent site of injury was L1 (36 percent). This was followed closely by T12 (29 percent), T11 (14 percent), and L2 (13 percent).

Injury to the T11–L2 area frequently produces a variety of neurologic injuries, some of which totally handicap the victim, and some of which almost go unrecognized. Because of the anatomic makeup of the area of the nervous system that lies posterior to the vertebral column at the T11 through L2 levels, neurologic injuries (when averaged) are usually incomplete, with sufficient residual neurologic function remaining in the lower extremities to allow ambulation.

ASSOCIATED INJURIES

Fractures occurring between T11 and L2 correlate well with the primary mechanisms of injury, falls or falling objects, motor vehicle accidents, and gunshot wounds. The first and second of these expend large amounts of energy over a short time period, often resulting in "burst"-type injuries to the vertebral bodies. As noted by other authors, when injury to the spine follows a fall or jump-type injury with the victim landing feet first, large amounts of energy will be absorbed. This frequently results in less of a neurologic injury than

626 Surgery of Spine Trauma

Table 18-1. Thoracolumbar Fractures: Gross Level of Lower Spine Fractures (Northwestern University Acute Spine Injury Center, 1972 to 1986)

Gross Level of Fracture	No.	Percent
Thoracic	376	40.3
Thoracolumbar (T11–L2)	470	50.4
Lumbar	73	7.9
Sacral	13	1.4
Total	932	100.0

Table 18-3. Thoracolumbar: Associated Injury (Northwestern University Acute Spine Injury Center, 1972 to 1986)

	Associated Injury[a]	No.	Percent
External	Scalp laceration	14	3.0
	Face laceration	13	2.7
	Other laceration	13	2.7
	Miscellaneous abrasion	6	1.3
Fracture	Skull	11	2.3
	Face	2	0.4
	Mandible	4	0.9
	Clavicle	6	1.3
	Scapula	5	1.1
	Radius-ulna	5	1.1
	Wrist	11	2.3
	Hand	5	1.1
	Metatarsal	8	1.7
	Rib(s)	54	11.5
	Pelvis	21	4.5
	Femur	12	2.6
	Tibia-fibula	16	3.4
	Ankle	17	3.6
	Foot	3	0.6
	Other	67	14.3
Internal	Loss of consciousness	91	19.4
	Cranial nerve defect	5	1.1
	Other head trauma	53	11.3
	Pulmonary contusion	13	2.8
	Pneumothorax	42	8.9
	Hemothorax	36	7.7
	Other thoracic	88	18.7
	Other abdominal trauma	85	18.1
	Other internal trauma	25	5.3

[a]Listed categorically and anatomically, head to foot.

one would anticipate. The relationship between multiple trauma (to extremities) and injuries to the thoracolumbar spine is high (14.9 percent in the thoracolumbosacral spine group and 16.2 percent in the thoracolumbar junction group) (Table 18-2). The incidence of associated head injury is 34.4 percent in the former group and 29.8 percent in the latter group, and abdominal injuries occur to 14.5 and 18.1 percent, respectively. Specific skeletal system injuries associated with thoracolumbar fractures are: tibia (3.4 percent), femur (2.6 percent), and ankle-os calcis (3.6 percent) (Table 18-3). Of the 470 patients with junctional injuries, 42.8 percent had only injury to the vertebral column, 33.4 percent had one other system injured (i.e., head, chest, abdomen, long bone injury, etc.), and 16.6 percent had two other systems injured (Table 18-4).

Most patients admitted with these injuries are males (72 percent). Patients fall into two major age

Table 18-2. Thoracolumbar (TL) versus Lower Anatomic Systems Traumatized (Northwestern University Acute Spine Injury Center, 1972 to 1986)

Traumatized System	TL No.	Percent	Lower Spine No.	Percent
Head	140	29.8	321	34.4
Chest	118	25.1	281	30.2
Abdomen	85	18.1	135	14.5
Extremity	76	16.2	139	14.9

Table 18-4. Thoracolumbar (TL) versus Lower Spine: Multiple Trauma (Northwestern University Acute Spine Injury Center, 1972 to 1986)

No. of Involved Systems	TL No.	Percent	Lower Spine No.	Percent
None	201	42.8	375	40.2
One	157	33.4	316	33.9
Two	78	16.6	170	18.2
Three	30	6.4	64	6.9
Four	4	0.9	7	0.8
Total	470	100.0	932	100.0

categories: 44 percent are 25 years or younger, and 43 percent are between 26 and 50 years of age. A question frequently asked is whether alcohol is associated with the occurrence of spine injuries. In this series of 490 thoracolumbar injuries, alcohol was implicated in 11.5 percent.

ETIOLOGY OF INJURIES

The principal causes of injury to the thoracolumbar junctional area of the spine are falls from heights (34.5 percent) (e.g., ladders, windows, porches, scaffolding, employment-related job activities, etc.), motor vehicle accidents (25.5 percent), and gunshot wounds (12.8 percent) (Table 18-5).

Injuries to the spine do occur despite the use of seatbelts; however, fractures and dislocations are less likely to occur when a chest-lap belt combination is used. Should fracture occur in a patient involved in an automobile accident who is wearing a chest-lap belt, via sudden positive deceleration (flexion-distraction) or rollover (axial load) injuries, neurologic injury is rare.

Table 18-5. Thoracolumbar: Etiology of Spine Injury (Northwestern University Acute Spine Injury Center, 1972 to 1986)

Etiology	No.	Percent
Fall	161	34.5
Auto	119	25.5
Other traumatic[a]	70	14.9
Gunshot wound	60	12.8
Motorcycle	30	6.4
Other sports	17	3.6
Other medical	7	1.5
Diving	3	0.6
Unknown	3	0.6
Total	470	100.0

[a]"Other traumatic" includes those with multiple etiologies.

THORACOLUMBAR VERTEBRAL FRACTURES

Extent of Vertebral Column Injury

Injury to the thoracolumbar region of the vertebral column after major trauma is frequently accompanied by severe neurologic injury to the conus medullaris and/or the cauda equina (Fig. 18-1). The biomechanical rationale for the high incidence of injury at the T11–L2 interval is the sharp transition between an area of thoracic spine rigidity (fixed by the rib cage-spine-sternum complex) and the more highly mobile lumbar spine, uninhibited by any anatomic structures. In fact, the facet joints in the upper lumbar region actually promote flexion, extension, and lateral bend with rotation, by virtue of their flat coronal facing (see Ch. 17) and, as such, are in stark contrast to the lowermost thoracic facet joints, the anteroposterior facing of which greatly restricts the allowable degrees of flexion, extension, and rotational motion. (Fig. 18-2). In the lower lumbar region, these facet joints again take on a more sagittal anteroposterior orientation, thus limiting rotation and allowing only flexion and extension.

Findings

A review of vertebral element fractures within the junctional area T11 through L2 revealed that fractures or dislocations were either associated with an overall larger group of injuries, that is, dislocations and fracture-dislocations, or fell into a specific morphologic group, that is, the lamina, pedicle, spinous process, etc. (Table 18-6). The five major biomechanical types of injuries noted were: (1) axial, (2) flexion; (3) other (including gunshot wounds); (4) rotation; and (5) direct (Table 18-7).

Classification of Spinal Fractures

Sir Frank Holdsworth classified fractures of the vertebral column by the mechanism or "direction" of injury into five categories: flexion, extension, axial (or compression) load, shear, rotation, and a

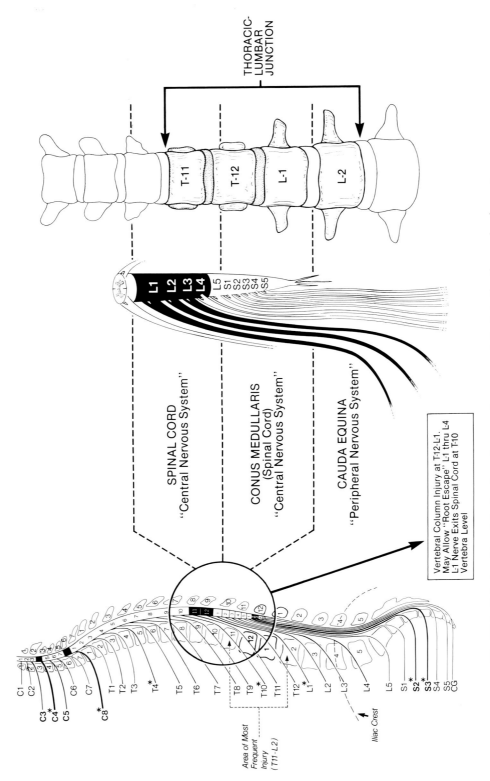

Fig. 18-1. Relationship of the lumbar plexus and conus medullaris to the thoracolumbar spine.

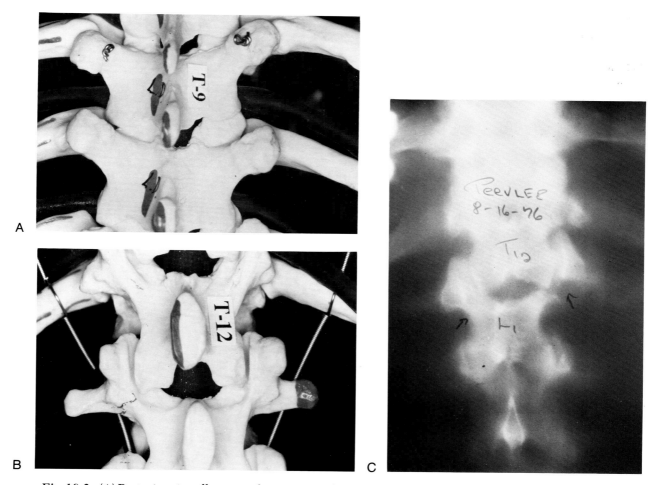

Fig. 18-2. (A) Posterior view illustrates the posterior elements of T9 overriding the superior articular facets of the next lower process. Note the flat facing of facets in a superoinferior direction. Such joints allow unrestricted flexion-extension and rotation. (B) Posterior view the articular facet joint of T12 with L1. Note the lateral wall of the superior facet joint of L1. This anatomic construction allows flexion-extension only. Rotation results in fracture of the pedicle. (C) Radiograph showing rotational injury to the thoracolumbar junction with fracture through the L1 pedicle.

Table 18-6. Thoracolumbar: Neurologic Extent by Fracture Type (Northwestern University Acute Spine Injury Center, 1972 to 1986)

Fracture Type	Total Cases	Intact		Incomplete		Complete	
		No.	Percent	No.	Percent	No.	Percent
Axial compression	221[a]	80	36.2	103	46.6	37	16.7
Body	105	21	20.0	37	35.2	47	44.8
Bullet fragments	46	2	4.3	16	34.8	28	60.9
No fracture	40	0	0.0	25	62.5	15	37.5
Anterior compression wedge	19	8	42.1	10	52.6	1	5.3
Chance	11	4	36.4	6	54.5	1	9.1
Avulsed chip	6	4	66.7	1	16.7	1	16.7
Bilateral facet lock	5	1	20.0	1	20.0	3	60.0
Transverse process	2	1	50.0	1	50.0	0	0.0
Pedicle	2	1	50.0	1	50.0	0	0.0
Facet	2	0	0.0	1	50.0	1	50.0
Subluxation	2	0	0.0	1	50.0	1	50.0
Other	9	4	44.4	2	22.2	3	33.3
Total	470	126	26.8	205	43.6	138	29.4

[a]One subject's extent is unavailable.

combination of two or more.[1] Interesting was his inadvertant omission of "distraction" or tension fractures as a mechanism of injury. I have taken the liberty of inserting this mechanism into his classification.

Holdsworth also categorized fractures into two groups that, when evaluated, revealed either disruption ("unstable") or preservation ("stable") of the "posterior complex." Combining the mechanism of injury and fracture type categories provides a framework for fracture management (Table 18-8). The scheme as developed, however, omitted several processes that, affecting the spine, would result in instability and would likely require a need for surgical stabilization. Examples are the typical "flexion-distraction" seatbelt injury to the

Table 18-7. Thoracolumbar: Neurologic Extent by Biomechanical Type of Injury (Northwestern University Acute Spine Injury Center, 1972 to 1986)

Biomechanical Type of Injury	Total Cases	Intact		Incomplete		Complete	
		Number	Percent	Number	Percent	Number	Percent
Axial	221[a]	80	36.2	103	46.6	37	16.7
Flexion	139	33	23.7	54	38.8	52	37.4
Rotation	7	1	14.3	2	28.6	4	57.1
Extension	4	2	50.0	2	50.0	0	0.0
Direct	3	1	33.3	2	66.7	0	0.0
Other	56	9	16.1	17	30.4	30	53.6
None	40	0	0.0	25	62.5	15	37.5
Total	470	126	29.4	205	42.0	138	28.7

[a]One subject's extent is unavailable.

Table 18-8. Fractures of the Thoracolumbar Junction

Mechanism of Injury	Stable-Unstable	Management
1. Pure flexion (wedge)	Stable	Conservative
2. Flexion-rotation	Unstable	Surgical
3. Extension (cervical)	Stable (in flexion)	Conservative[a]
4. Compression	Stable	Conservative[a]
5. Shear	Unstable	Surgical
6. Flexion-distraction (lumbar)[b]	Stable (in extension)[b]	Surgical

[a]Depends on disease process (example 3, rheumatoid spondylolisthesis; 4, extent of injury (surgical if >25 to 35 percent) or tumor).
[b]Not in Holdsworth classification.[1]
(From Holdsworth,[1] with permission.)

thoracolumbar and lumbar spine, and an extension injury to the rigid Marie-Strümpel rheumatoid spondylitic "bamboo" spine. Injuries to the spine in these patients are grossly unstable, and with pre-existing spinal deformity, are difficult and sometimes impossible to reduce or maintain without surgical intervention.

Interpretation of Stability by Altered Spinal Anatomy

Numerous researchers have described the occurrence of interesting, unusual, or previously unidentified fractures of the spine. Others have categorized neurologic injury with fracture type, while some have demonstrated a relationship between fracture type and spinal stability. Each consideration is of importance and must be taken into account when interpreting and prescribing the most appropriate management course to follow.

Two investigators stand out in this area: Sir Frank Holdsworth[1,12] and Francis Denis (1983[2]). For simplicity and a need for conformity, the classification and definition of spinal fractures and stability has been narrowed to these two researchers, because of their similarity and the fact that most fractures occurring within the spine fall within their classifications (Table 18-9).

Holdsworth described what he believed to be the pattern of injuries occurring to the thoracolumbar spine and what represented stability and instability. He noted that the common denomina-

tor of instability was the interruption of what he described as the posterior complex. The structures that fell within this grouping were the posterior bone processes (the spinous process and the lamina), the supraspinous and interspinous ligaments,

Table 18-9. Column Theory: Spinal Stability

Two-Column Theory (Holdsworth)[1,12]	Three-Column Theory (Denis)[2]
Posterior bone-ligament complex	Posterior bone-ligament complex as in two-column theory[a]
Posterior laminar arch	
Supraspinous ligament	
Interspinous ligament	
Posterior lateral capsule	
Ligamentum flavum	
	Middle column[a]
	Posterior longitudinal ligament
	Posterior anulus fibrosus
	Posterior vertebral body wall
Anterior column	Anterior column as in two-column theory
Anterior vertebral body	
Anterior longitudinal ligament	
Anterior anulus fibrosus	

[a]Disruption of any two indicates instability.

the posterolateral (facet) capsular ligaments, and the ligamentum flavum connecting any two adjacent laminae. Holdsworth also noted that those spines demonstrating gross instability also demonstrated interruption of the anterior column, with tearing through the anulus fibrosus and the anterior longitudinal ligament. Although he did not emphasize this latter (anterior) column as the second "column" and a cause for instability when also injured, he did mention its simultaneous presence.

Denis[2] in 1983 classified injuries to the spine into "three-column" injuries. Drawing on Holdsworth's overall concepts, he respectfully disagreed. Denis was of the opinion that the posterior complex was not solely responsible for vertebral column stability. Were this the case, Denis notes, with all the spines operated on by surgeons attempting to improve spinal malalignment (scoliosis), which required the taking down of the posterior complex to insert corrective internal fixation

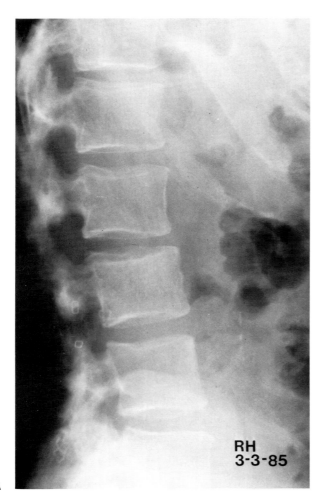

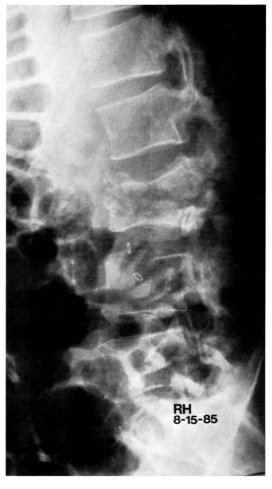

A   B

Fig. 18-3. **(A)** Lateral radiograph of the thoracolumbar spine showing normal architecture of the vertebral bodies as seen in the sagittal plane. **(B)** Lateral radiograph taken 5 months later shows collapse and total destruction of the L3 vertebral body secondary to radiation necrosis. Note lumbar kyphosis secondary to vertebral collapse (see Figure 18-15).

and to perform a fusion, there would have been evidence of gross spinal instability in many of these spines. Since this apparently was not the case, it was his contention that the instability lies with disruption of two columns, and that a third column, the "middle column," which included the posterior longitudinal ligament, the posterior anulus fibrosus, and the posterior aspect of the vertebral body wall, existed and was instrumental in providing spinal stability.

Examples of Spinal Instability

Fractures of the thoracolumbar spine demonstrating both subtle and gross evidence of instability all have one thing in common, as described by both Denis and Holdsworth: disruption of two columns, and in some instances three. A situation noted on several occasions is progressive spinal (gibbus) deformity, where no apparent disruption of any column appeared originally. This occurrence raises the question of instability. It is contended that when progressive spinal deformity results from progressive vertebral compression fracture collapse, when the initial film fails to reveal anterior body wall compression greater than 50 percent, surgical instrumentation may be required for stability or the prevention of deformity, whether stable or unstable (Fig. 18-3). This applies to vertebral body compression fractures with as little as 25 to 35 percent compression when there is evidence of progressive deformity. This concept adheres to Holdsworth's interpretation that separation of the posterior ligamentous structures serves as an indicator of instability.

Other processes affecting the spine and requiring stabilization include tumors involving the vertebral body (Fig. 18-4), gross spinal malalignment in either the anterior or lateral plane (Fig. 18-5), or burst fractures (although Holdsworth did not consider this an unstable fracture because of continued continuity within the anterior and posterior longitudinal ligaments; see Fig. 18-40). The rationale for surgical stabilization is that if the patient is managed conservatively, there is need for prolonged horizontal bed care. Even with such, change in position of the fracture may occur, either

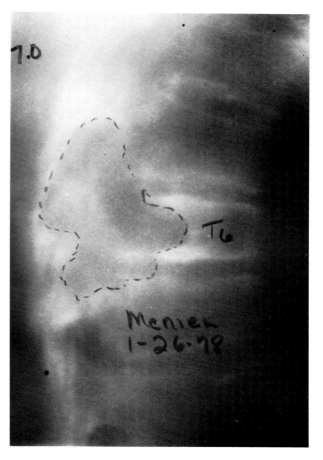

Fig. 18-4. Lateral film of thoracic spine revealing evidence of metastatic tumor involvement of T5–T7. This spine required radiation therapy and instrumentation for stability.

with bed care or axial loading. This becomes of primary importance in those patients in whom the neurologic level remains incompletely intact. Other considerations are the occurrence of complications such as deep venous thrombosis (8.9 percent incidence rate) (Table 18-10). Finally, another injury to the spine that requires consideration for surgical intervention is the spine that reveals displacement without the presence of fracture. This is the typical "dislocation" injury. Experience has demonstrated that such injuries will not develop sufficient ligamentous healing to induce spinal stability.

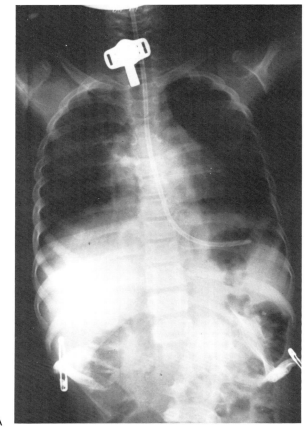
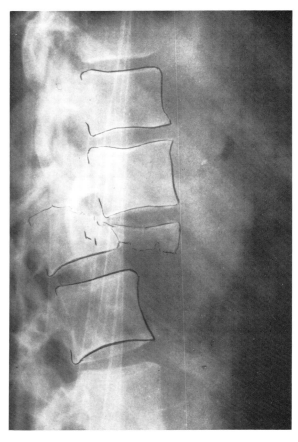

A   B

Fig. 18-5. (A) AP radiograph revealing total dislocation at L2–L3 in the coronal plane. (B) Sagittal view of lumbar spine in another patient showing "slice" fracture through L1 with total dislocation of T12 on L1.

VERTEBRAL INJURY CLASSIFICATION

Dislocations

Dislocations of the vertebral column imply violent trauma resulting in gross ligamentous rupture and vertebral instability, usually involving two or more of the three spinal columns. These include disruption of the interspinous ligaments, posterior longitudinal ligaments, or anterior longitudinal ligaments. Dislocations may occur within the superior portion of the column displaced anteriorly on the inferior column (Fig. 18-5B) or the superior column displaced posteriorly on the anterior column (see Fig. 18-40B). The direction of the dislocation is the resultant effect of forces applied to either the proximal or the distal segment of the vertebral column.

The extent of dislocation can vary from subluxation (incomplete displacement of one vertebral element on another, in which the facets are not dislocated) to total facet dislocation of the adjacent vertebral element. With total dislocation, the extent of displacement of one segment from the other may vary from one-half of the width of the vertebral body to total dislocation of one body on another (Fig. 18-5B).

As a rule (and also noted in the cervical spine), extension injuries are less often associated with severe neurologic injury for two reasons: expansion or enlargement of the neural canal with extension between segments, and a lack of anatomically available extension range of motion. With extension,

Table 18-10. Thoracolumbar: Medical
Complications (Northwestern University Acute
Spine Injury Center, 1972 to 1986)

Medical Complication	No.	Percent
Arrythmia	6	1.3
Bradycardia	4	0.9
DT	4	0.9
Deep venous thrombosis	42	8.9
Gastrointestinal bleed	4	0.9
Hypotensive	18	3.8
Hyperthermic	19	4.0
Paralytic ileus	4	0.9
Pleural effusion	5	1.1
Pneumo-hemothorax	2	0.4
Pneumonia	20	4.3
Pulmonary embolism	9	1.9
Pressure sore	26	5.5
Renal failure	3	0.6
Respiratory failure	8	1.7
Sepsis	3	0.6
Urinary tract infection	157	33.4
Other	47	10.0

the anterior abdominal musculature restricts hyperextension, and because of the anatomic shape of the posterior elements, fracture is less likely to occur or the elements to be placed in such an anatomic position as to result in neurologic injury.

Dislocations may result from either a flexion injury (greater than 90 percent) or from an extension forces. As already noted, the latter is rare.

Flexion-Dislocations

Flexion-dislocations usually follow sudden, positive deceleration of the fixed pelvis resulting in the thoracolumbar portion of the spine simultaneously elongating (through distraction) and flexing over a fixed point (as around a lap belt). The effect is tearing or rupture of interlaminar ligamentous structures posteriorly, allowing the facets to distract to an extent that they can dislocate and flex into facet overriding without resulting in fracture to either of the superior or inferior facet elements. For the latter to occur, a straight anterior translatory force vector must be an accompanying component of this injury. Generally speaking, when axial loading is not a mechanical component of the injury, major fractures of the vertebral bodies do not occur,

though minor, ill-defined avulsion fractures from ligamentous structures may result. Such fractures do not influence management.

Neurological Injury. Flexion injuries to the spine resulting in spinal dislocation do frequently result in neurologic injuries (38.8 percent incomplete; 37.4 percent complete) (Tables 18-7, 18-8). Neural elements within the neural canal are either held captive within the canal or they are "dragged" forward by the upper segments displacement resulting "pinching or tearing" of the dura and its contents between the posterior surface of the inferior vertebral element and the anteriorly displaced posterior element of the superior vertebral segment. Although the extent of the initial dislocation will not be apparent on initial radiographs, it should be appreciated that the amount of displacement likely to have occurred at the time of the initial injury was extensive. The type of neurologic injury to occur will depend on the level of injury and the type of neurologic tissue (spinal cord, conus medullaris, cauda equina) involved (see p. 655).

Treatment (Conservative). Initial management of distraction-flexion dislocations of the thoracolumbar junction should be very conservative (Table 18-8), particularly when neurologic function remains intact. The presence of a dislocation does require early surgical intervention to restore anatomic realignment of the vertebral column, decompression of the neural canal, and restoration of vertebral column stability. If neurologic tissue encroachment is a complication (identified by greater than 50 percent narrowing of the neural canal on either tomography or computed axial tomography [CAT] scan, along with evidence of continued neural function distal to the level of injury), surgical open reduction of the dislocation becomes more immediate. The patient's condition after admission determines how the patient should be managed before surgery. Either way, the patient must be managed in a strictly horizontal plane, preferably with some component of hyperextension (extension on either a standard bed or a Stryker frame). When the patient is managed supine, transverse pillows are placed at the level of the spinal gibbus. When the patient is prone (as on the Stryker frame), a pillow is placed transversely across the lower pelvis and the upper chest (Fig. 18-6). This "pillow positioning" allows for the

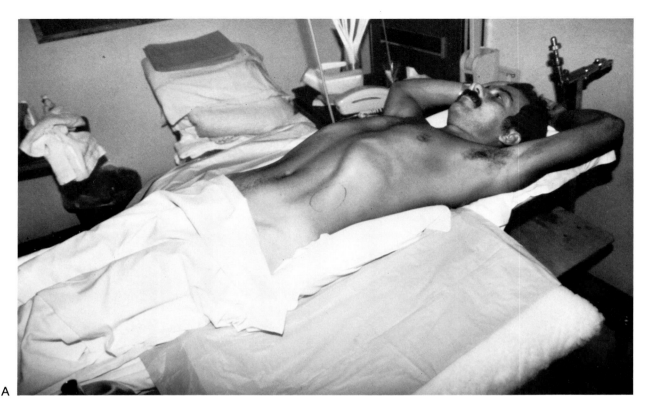

A

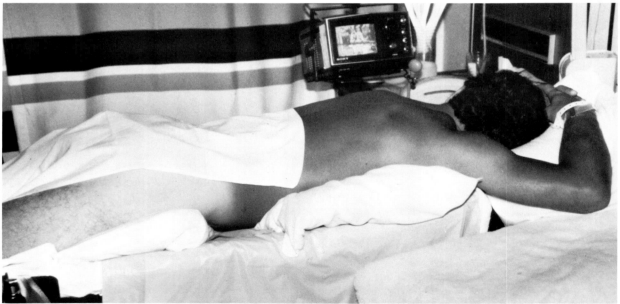

B

Fig. 18-6. (A) Patient with fracture involving the thoracolumbar junction. To assist in achieving closed reduction and/or maintaining sagittal alignment, the patient's thoracolumbar junction is maintained in hyperextension. (B) Patient in prone position on a Stryker frame. The transverse pillow across the upper chest and lower pelvis maintains the spine in hyperextended position.

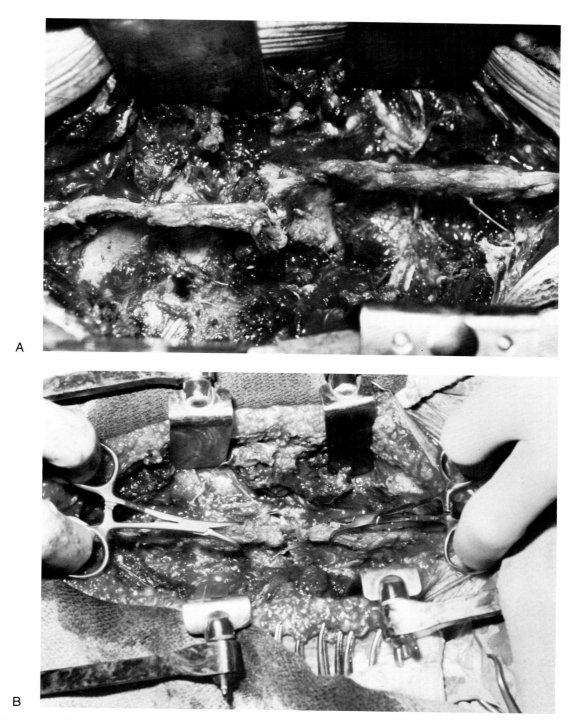

Fig. 18-7. (A) Operative view of fracture dislocation at T11–T12. Note significant lateral malalignment between posterior and distal segments. Patient's neurologic deficit was: T12 complete. (B) Towel clips placed in the spinous process are used for operative manipulation of fracture segments. *(Figure continues.)*

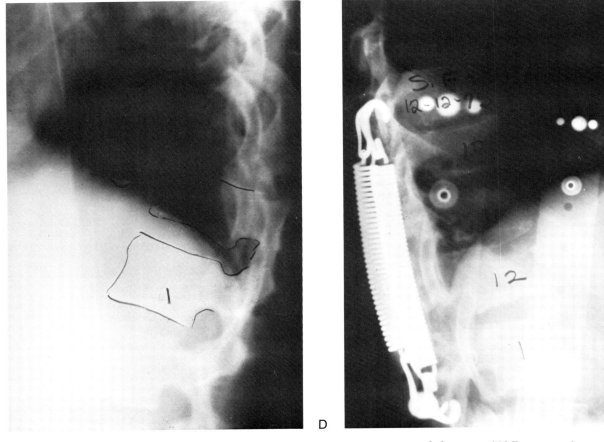

C

D

Fig. 18-7 *(Continued)*. **(C)** Lateral radiograph showing complete T11–T12 dislocation. **(D)** Postoperative lateral radiograph showing reduction of fracture and use of compression springs for internal fixation. This procedure was performed in 1973.

maintenance of a semi-extension moment on the spine, which, if not producing a reduction, prevents further flexion displacement.

Surgical management.   At surgery, with the use of a Harrington distraction apparatus, dislocated elements can be distracted, the adjacent vertebral elements can be gently manipulated, distraction can be reduced, and with the use of towel clips in the adjacent displaced posterior spinous process, reduction of the dislocated facets can be accomplished. (Fig. 18-7). The appropriate surgical internal fixation device, in the presence of intact facets, is one producing compression (Wisconsin device, Harrington compression rods, Weiss compression springs), or is the Luque instrumentation system or the more recently introduced AO Internal Fixator. Each method has its advantages and disadvantages (see p. 675).

Extension-Dislocations

Extension injuries to any area of the spine are infrequent. In the cervical spine, they usually occur at the C6–C7 level (see Ch. 15). In the thoracolumbar region, they occur at the L1–L2 level (Fig. 18-8), and in the lumbar spine, they occur at or near the L3 level (see Ch. 19). The injury usually occurs just below an area of relative greater "mass" (head, chest, etc.) superiorly.

With the application of a direct and forceful ex-

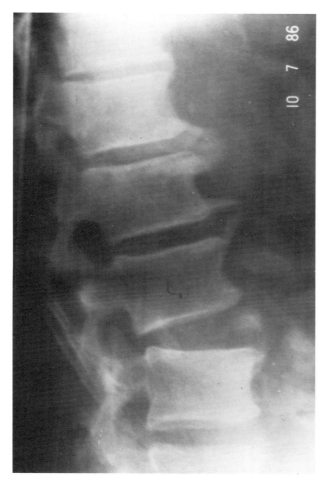
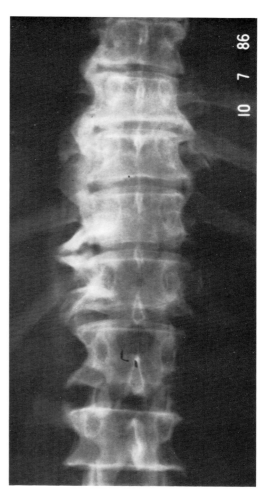

A   B

Fig. 18-8. (A) Lateral radiograph of lumbar spine showing a hyperextension injury at L1–L2. In the intervening disc space an avulsion fragment from the anteroinferior L1 osteophyte is visible. (B) AP radiograph showing straightaway alignment. Note significant evidence of DISH (disseminating interstitial spinal hyperostosis) syndrome. *(Figure continues.)*

tension moment across the upper anterior chest (proximal thoracic spine), in the presence of relative fixation of the lower spinal segment, hyperextension occurs at a site or level of maximum mobility. One segment of the spine is suddenly forced into flexion while the other moves into extension. The result is disruption of the anterior longitudinal ligament at the transition point (Fig. 18-8A). Minor avulsion fractures of the vertebral bodies may occur as a result of the disruption of the anterior longitudinal ligament, but independently they have little relevance. Fractures of the facets, al-

though infrequent, may occur. The extent of dislocation of the upper spinal segment on the lower segment (in extension injuries) demonstrates less variation than that seen with flexion injuries. The extent of displacement (retrolisthesis) of the superior vertebra on the inferior vertebra, although not known at the moment of injury, has been noted on the initial radiographs to be less than half the lateral width of the superior vertebra on the lower adjacent (inferior) vertebral body.

A representative case of the above mechanism of injury is demonstrated in Fig. 18-8. There is noted

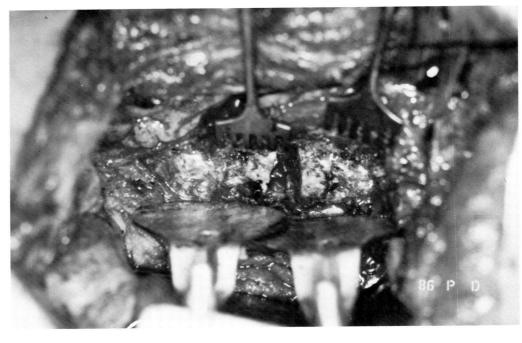

C

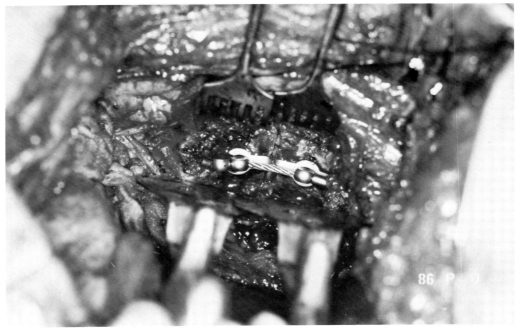

D

Fig. 18-8 *(Continued).* **(C)** Operative view showing the hyperextension defect between L1 and L2. **(D)** Operative view of lumbar spine with staple-screw-Dwyer cable compression apparatus in place on L1–L2. *(Figure continues.)*

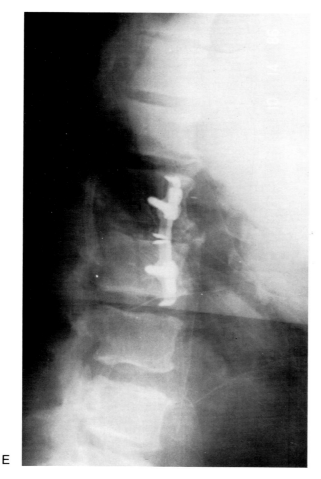
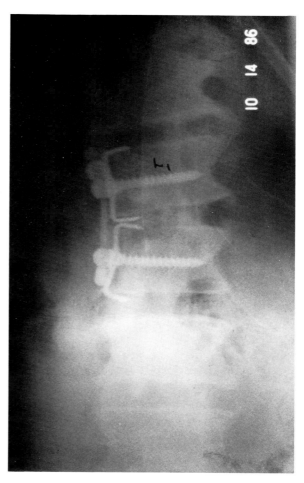

E   F

Fig. 18-8 *(Continued)*. (E) Postoperative lateral radiograph showing reduction of hyperextension deformity by the Dwyer apparatus. A bone graft was inserted between L1 and L2 before compression was applied. (F) Postoperative AP radiograph. Note opening of the interspace opposite the Dwyer apparatus due to unilateral application of compression forces.

disruption of the anterior longitudinal ligament at the level of L1–L2, with resulting hyperextension between L1 and L2 (Fig. 18-8A–C). The deformity was corrected and the spine was stabilized by the application of a compressive force between L1 and L2, using the Dwyer apparatus, as seen in Fig. 18-8D,F.

Neurologic Injury. With extension-dislocation type injuries, neurologic examination is likely to reveal residual neurologic intactness (Tables 18-7, 18-8). This is accompanied by a greater likelihood of some neurologic recovery than one might anticipate with a flexion-dislocation injury. As noted ear-

lier, the extent of vertebral column displacement with extension is less than with the flexion injuries. Thus, vascular injury is less likely to result with distraction (and stretching) than with a flexion injury (in which direct neural tissue vascular contusion occurs).

Conservative Management. The patient is best managed on a standard bed without pillows when in the supine position, or preferably, on a Stryker frame (Table 18-8). Stryker frame management allows total skin care anteriorly and posteriorly without concern for spine displacement during "logrolling." When the patient is in the prone po-

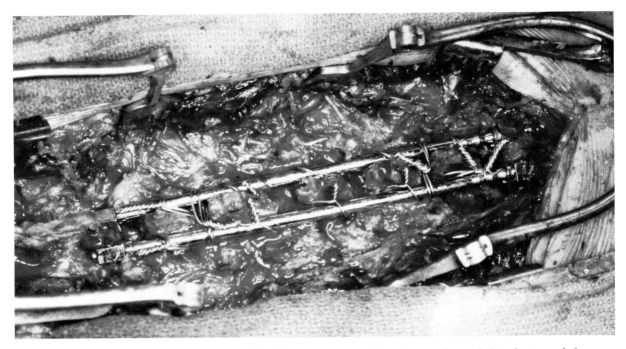

Fig. 18-9. Surgical view of Harrington rod-sublaminar wire combination used to stabilize fracture dislocations of the thoracolumbar spine.

sition on a Stryker frame, transverse pillows can be used across the abdomen to maintain a semi-flexed position of the spine and prevent hyperextension from occurring.

Surgical Management. The same urgency for surgical intervention does not exist with extension-dislocation as with flexion-dislocation injuries because of the expansion of the neural canal with hyperextension and the less often associated encroachment of the canal by disc or bony elements. The ideal and most frequently indicated surgical instrumentation for reduction and stabilization of this vertebral column injury is Harrington distraction rods with sublaminar wires proximal and distal to the level of injury (Fig. 18-9). Care must be taken during distraction to ensure that overdistraction (of the already dislocated facets) does not occur. A variation in the use of Harrington rods with sublaminar wire stabilization would be the concomitant use of the "Edwards sleeves" (Fig. 18-10, see Fig. 18-33J,K). Luque instrumentation

can also be used for stabilization of this injury (Fig. 18-11).

Fracture-Dislocations

Fracture-dislocation suggests that some segment of the vertebral column has undergone both displacement and fracture. The types of fractures normally anticipated are avulsion fractures of the posterior elements (i.e., spinous processes, laminae) and, with anterior translatory fracture-dislocation, fracture of the superior or inferior facets of the respective vertebral elements. If flexion and axial loading are major components, fracture of the anterior vertebral body element (wedge compression) (see Fig. 18-11) or burst fracture (see Fig. 19-27) with or without ligamentous avulsion fractures of the anterior superior or inferior lips of the adjacent vertebral bodies may result. The extent of the associated vertebral body compression injury is highly variable and may be associated with fracture fragments displaced posteriorly into the neural canal. Al-

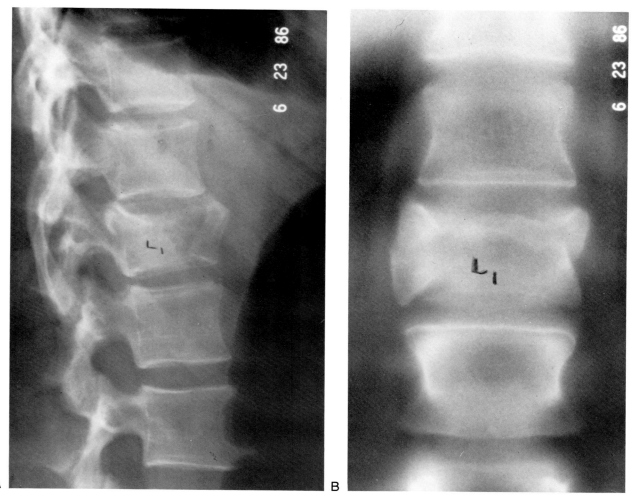

Fig. 18-10. (A,B) Lateral and AP views of an axial load burst fracture of L1. *(Figure continues.)*

though extension-fracture dislocation is possible, in the absence of an axial load component, it is not likely.

Neurologic Injury. Serious neurologic injuries normally accompany fracture-dislocations of the thoracolumbar junction (Table 18-11). Injury follows pinching or entrapment of the neural elements between anterior and posterior bony elements or encroachment by fracture fragments, or extruded intervertebral disc material, into the neural canal from the posterior vertebral body wall.

Conservative Management. When posterior facet-laminar elements are no longer intact, fracture-dislocations are grossly unstable. Without attention to bed or frame positioning, these fractures may undergo significant unrecognized displacement even with strict recumbent (logrolling) care. Careful radiographic follow-up is required. Recommended methods of immobilization are straight-away standard bed management or positioning on a Stryker frame (Table 18-12). A transverse pillow at the level of fracture-dislocation, with the patient in the supine position, and transverse pillows across

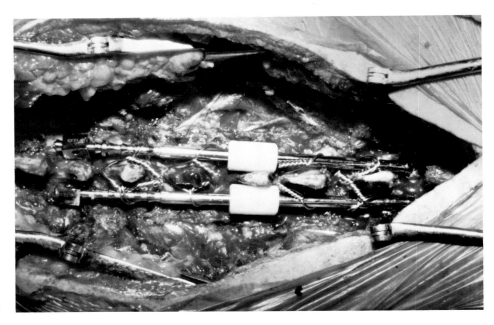

C

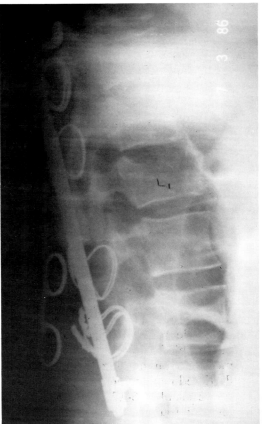

D

Fig. 18-10 *(Continued)*. **(C)** Operative view showing internal fixation using Harrington distraction apparatus, sublaminar wires, and Edwards sleeves at the level of fracture to produce hyperextension. A bone graft was applied over this instrumentation. **(D)** Postoperative radiograph shows alignment achieved using Harrington rods, Edwards sleeves, and sublaminar wires.

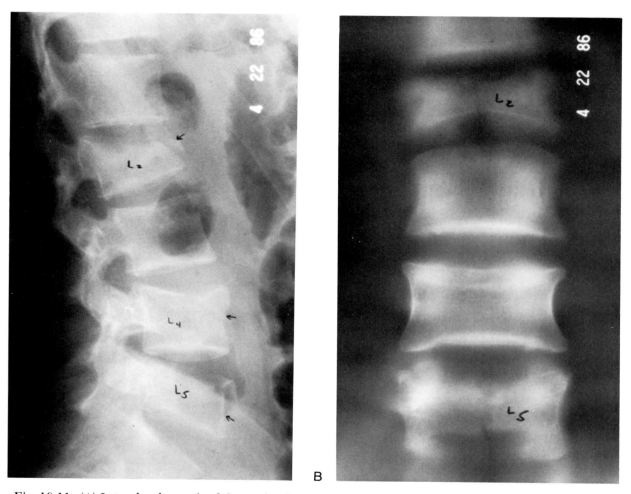

Fig. 18-11. (A) Lateral radiograph of thoracolumbar spine showing numerous compression fractures involving L2–L4–L5. **(B)** AP tomogram shows fractures of L2 and L5. *(Figure continues.)*

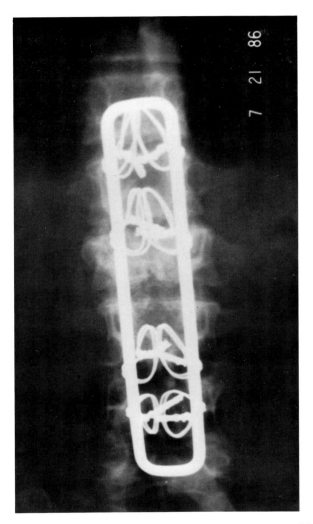 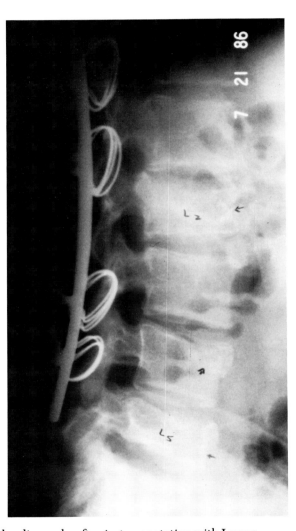

C   D

Fig. 18-11 *(Continued)*. **(C,D)** Postoperative AP and lateral radiographs after instrumentation with Luque rectangular rod system. Sublaminar wires could not be used at L5 due to unrecognized posterior element fractures. The option was to use instrumentation across the lumbosacral joint. The patient was neurologically normal and was managed in a thoracolumbar orthosis with external hip joint and thigh lacer to the knee on the right side.

Table 18-11. Thoracolumbar (TL) versus Entire Thoracic, Lumbar, and Sacral Spine: Extent of Neurologic Injury (Northwestern University Acute Spine Injury Center, 1972 to 1986)

Extent	TL		Lower Spine	
	No.	Percent	No.	Percent
Intact	126	26.8	191	20.5
Incomplete	205	43.6	362	38.8
Complete	138	29.4	375	40.2
Missing[a]	1	0.2	4	0.4
Total	470	100.0	932	100.0

[a]Extent is unavailable.

the upper chest and lower pelvis, when the patient is prone, reduce spinal displacement during bed care and turning.

Surgical Management. The method of surgical stabilization of fracture-dislocations of the vertebral column is subject to the presence or absence of residual neurologic function. In those situations in which no residual neurologic function exists below the level of injury, Luque instrumentation with sublaminar wires is likely to be the most effective method of spinal stabilization.[3] In those situations in which neurologic function persists, care must be taken when considering the use of sublaminar wires, because of the potential for further injury to the already traumatized dura and its contents. Luque rod instrumentation can be utilized if somatosensory evoked potential (SSEP) monitoring is utilized during the operative procedure. Depending on the extent of spinal instability, Harrington distraction rods,[4] in conjunction with the Edwards sleeve,[5] can be utilized to maintain mild hyperextension across the fracture site, using sublaminar wires superiorly and inferiorly to increase instrumentation fixation and stability. Available for several years and now more frequently used for spinal stabilization are the Roy-Camille plate and screws[6] (Fig. 18-12). I have not used this device, but I have observed it in use by its developer. When complete anatomic reduction has been obtained, this device provides excellent internal spinal stabilization. Technically, it is demanding because of the need for appropriate pedicle-screw placement in the vertebral elements. A similar criticism applies to

Table 18-12. Thoracolumbar: Type of Management by Fracture Type (Northwestern University Acute Spine Injury Center, 1972 to 1986)

Fracture Type	Total Cases	Conservative		Surgical	
		No.	Percent	No.	Percent
Axial compression	221	43	19.5	178	80.5
Body	105	34	32.4	71	67.6
Bullet fragments	46	44	95.7	2	4.3
No fracture	40	36	90.0	4	10.0
Anterior compression wedge	19	7	36.8	12	63.2
Chance	11	2	18.2	9	81.8
Avulsed chip	6	2	33.3	4	66.7
Bilateral facet lock	5	1	20.0	4	80.0
Transverse process	2	1	50.0	1	50.0
Pedicle	2	1	50.0	1	50.0
Facet	2	1	50.0	1	50.0
Subluxation	2	1	50.0	1	50.0
Other	9	3	33.3	6	66.7
Total	470	176	37.4	294	62.6

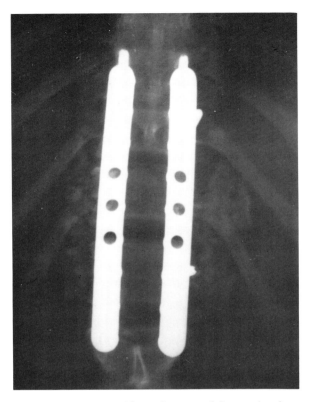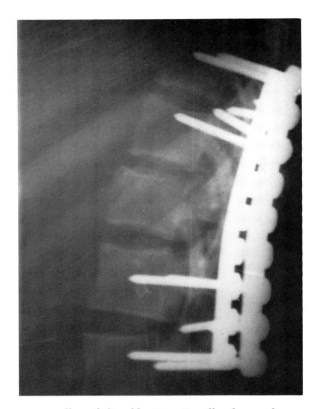

Fig. 18-12. AP and lateral views of thoracolumbar junction internally stabilized by Roy-Camille plate and screws.

the recently introduced (and still considered experimental) AO Internal Fixator[7] (see Fig. 18-40). This device allows for internal stabilization across fewer segments of the vertebral column while providing very stable internal fixation.

Vertebral Body Fractures

Avulsion Fractures

Avulsion-type fractures result from "tearing" away of ligaments from bone. They are more commonly found in the area of the posteroinferior quadrant of the superior vertebra, from the avulsion of bone by the posterior longitudinal ligament when vertebral element dislocation occurs. Other areas of bony avulsion are the anteroinferior border of the superior vertebral element (secondary to avulsion through the anterior longitudinal ligament) with extension injuries. This latter fracture is stable, requiring only vertebral column alignment. The fracture heals with stability.

Wedge Compression Fractures

Wedge compression fractures result from anteriorly placed axial compression load forces across a vertebral element. The extent of this load determines the amount of compression. Compression may result in no more than 10 to 15 percent of the vertebral body height as seen on lateral radiographs, and requires no management other than prolonged bed care and an orthosis or the application of a hyperextension orthosis. However, when the wedge is 35 to 50 percent or greater, surgical stabilization is required. Under these circumstances, this fracture will frequently be associated with extensive vertebral body comminution, resulting in loss of vertebral body height and a thoracolumbar gibbus deformity with vertical or axial loading (Fig. 18-13). Although the deformity may not be painful, it may result in intolerance to pressure over the posterior elements or skin breakdown with wheelchair sitting or lying. Neurologic injury with this fracture is often less serious than with burst fractures. The appropriate methods of internal stabilization include: Harrington distraction rods[4] (with or without Edwards sleeves),[5] Luque rods, and the AO (Synthes) locking hook-rod system.[8,9]

Burst Fracture

Burst fracture is the most severe of the vertebral element fractures and implies a very high degree of axial load forces applied at the time of injury (Fig. 18-10). This fracture frequently results in extrusion of bone from the posterior wall of the vertebral body into the neural canal, resulting in dural (and neurologic tissue) compression with neurologic injury. Although the extent of the vertebral body injury is extensive, it was considered by Holdsworth that continuity of the posterior longitudinal ligament was maintained in the presence of a burst fracture. This interpretation is most likely correct. This being the case, distraction across the fracture site should allow for the closed reduction of these

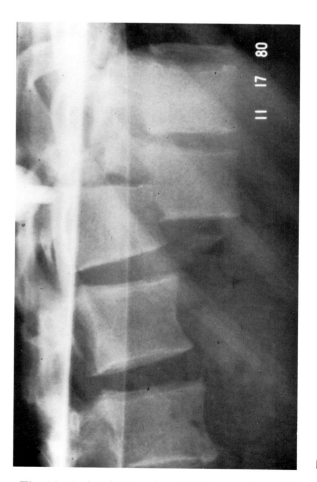
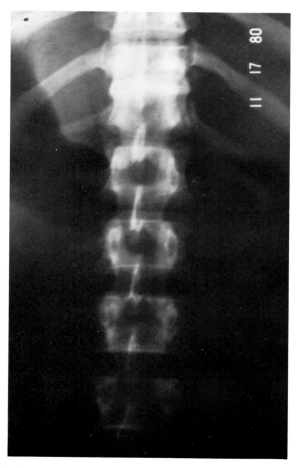

A   B

Fig. 18-13. (A,B) Lateral and AP views of total fracture dislocation at T11–T12. Note on AP view the absence of an interspace at T11–T12. The patient had complete T11 neurologic injury. *(Figure continues.)*

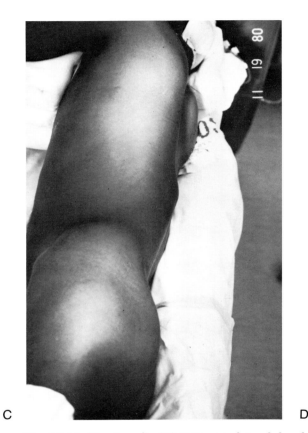

C

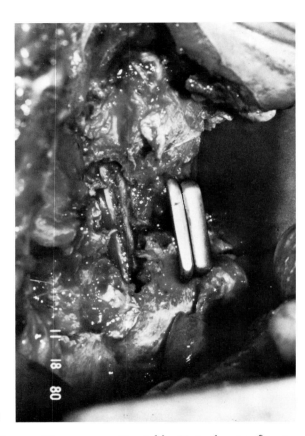

D

Fig. 18-13 *(Continued)*. **(C)** Patient in lateral decubitus position on operating table. Note the significant "gibbus" involving thoracolumbar junction at the midportion of the back. The gibbus coincides with the level of dislocation. The patient underwent a simultaneous anteroposterior spine stabilization procedure. **(D)** Operative view of thoracic spine via thoracotomy approach. T11 has been brought into continuity with T12, and is held with staples and inlay bone graft. *(Figure continues.)*

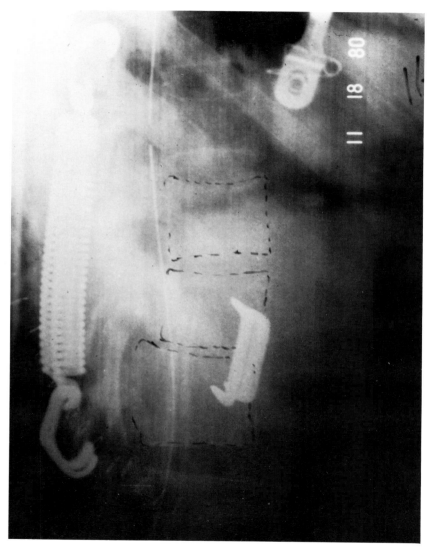

E

Fig. 18-13 *(Continued).* **(E)** Postoperative view. Compression apparatus (Weiss springs) was applied after anterior reduction of dislocation, bone grafting, and stapling.

fracture fragments into the neural canal from the posterior vertebral body with the application of distraction forces. This is not always the case, and depending on the extent of neurologic injury, it may not be the approach or solution to attempt decompression of a nervous system injured by bone fragmentation. The decision then becomes one of approach to this burst fracture anteriorly (for decompression purposes) or posteriorly, with distraction when neurologic function is less of a consideration. The appropriate methods of internal stabilization at this time are Harrington distraction rods (with or without Edwards sleeves) and sublaminar wires for greater internal fixation and device stabilization, the AO Synthes (Jacobs) locking hook-rod system,[8,9] and the Luque rod system. This latter technique can be utilized, though it is less indicated because of the absence of distraction opportunity and the loss of anterior vertebral element stability, the result being extensive vertebral body compression with axial loading (see Fig. 19-1E).

Posterior Element Fractures

Fractures of the posterior elements are most likely to result from the application of direct forces to the posterior vertebral column. Fracture of the posterior spinous process at one or several levels is the most frequent injury to occur. Often an associated fracture of a lamina may occur. This fracture does not require anything per se other than short-term conservative care. If, however, fracture of the posterior elements is associated with significant diastasis of the interspinous and interlaminar spaces, one must be very careful to determine the presence or absence of associated anterior posterior column ligamentous injury, indicating vertebral column instability. Depending on the presence or absence of neurologic injury, and the extent of neurologic injury, it is often helpful to obtain "moderate" flexion-extension radiographs to determine the extent of instability. If the spine is unstable, management often becomes surgical rather than conservative.

Gunshot Wounds

Gunshot wounds of the spinal column, regardless of the caliber or projectile velocity, normally result in stable injuries of the vertebral column because of the lack of total bone stock or ligamentous disruption (Fig. 18-14). It is appropriate to appreciate that the higher the velocity, the greater the tissue destruction and contamination. Data at Northwestern University (Table 18-12) reveal that very few gunshot wounds required surgical excision of the projectile (4.3 percent). This approach has been taken for the following reasons: severe gunshot wounds are produced by low-velocity hand guns; surgical decompression or debridement in no way influences neurologic recovery after a gunshot wound. As a matter of fact, it has been noted that gunshot wounds demonstrate the lowest rate of neurologic improvement after injury of any mechanism of neurologic injury (Table 18-13). At present, the only indications for surgical management of gunshot wounds are high-velocity wounds (rifle or Magnum pistols with muzzle velocities greater than 1,300 to 1,500 feet/sec); gunshot wounds of the neck where associated structure injury is a frequent occurrence (carotid arteries, esophagus, trachea); or when some neurologic intactness remains, the projectile lies in the neural canal, and there is evidence of deteriorating neurologic function. When there is evidence of projectile fragmentation, even with a major fragment in the neural canal, generally speaking, neurologic function will not remain and therefore the need for fragment removal is not likely or indicated.

Other

Other injuries include such isolated fractures as unusual vertebral body fractures, isolated pedicle fractures, transverse process fractures, etc. Alone, these fractures do not contribute to vertebral column instability. Most require only conservative management and very short periods of recumbency.

Multiple-Level Fractures

Fractures of vertebral elements within the thoracolumbar junction area, T11 to L2, were found to involve one level in 59 percent of the cases, two levels in 27 percent, three levels in 5 percent, and four levels in 1 percent of the injuries. In those

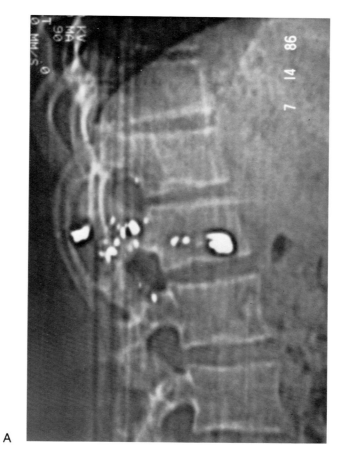

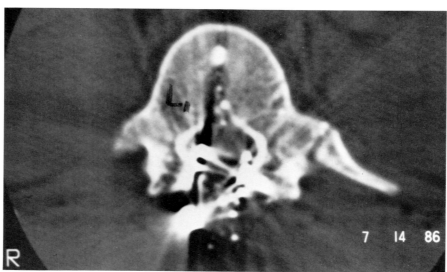

Fig. 18-14. (**A**) Lateral CT scan of a gunshot wound to the thoracic spine (L1). Note fragments of the bullet from the point of impact over the posterior structures to the anterior aspect of the vertebral body. (**B**) Transverse CT scan at same level. Note bone destruction involving posterior elements and vertebral body, and fragments in canal.

Table 18-13.   Thoracolumbar: Neurologic Status by Fracture Type[a] (Northwestern University Acute Spine Injury Center, 1972 to 1986)

Fracture Type	Total Cases	Improvement		No Change		Deterioration		Missing[b]	
		No.	Percent	No.	Percent	No.	Percent	No.	Percent
Axial compression	221	31	14.0	168	76.0	9	4.1	13	5.9
Body	105	11	10.5	87	82.9	0	0.0	7	6.7
Bullet fragments	46	2	4.3	42	91.3	0	0.0	2	4.3
No fracture	40	4	10.0	26	65.0	0	0.0	10	25.0
Anterior compression wedge	19	3	15.8	16	84.2	0	0.0	0	0.0
Chance	11	1	9.1	10	90.9	0	0.0	0	0.0
Avulsed chip	6	0	0.0	6	100.0	0	0.0	0	0.0
Bilateral facet lock	5	0	0.0	5	100.0	0	0.0	0	0.0
Transverse process	2	0	0.0	2	100.0	0	0.0	0	0.0
Pedicle	2	1	50.0	1	50.0	0	0.0	0	0.0
Facet	2	0	0.0	2	100.0	0	0.0	0	0.0
Subluxation	2	0	0.0	2	100.0	0	0.0	0	0.0
Other	9	0	0.0	7	77.8	1	11.1	1	11.1
Total	470	53	11.3	374	79.6	10	2.1	33	7.0

[a]Change criterion is one or more Frankel grades, higher or lower.
[b]Neurologic change is unavailable.

instances in which multiple fractures occurred (defined as fractures involving adjacent or distant vertebral elements within the thoracolumbar junctional area), conservative management was the primary method of management, particularly for those injuries involving three or more levels. The rationale for this approach has been as follows. In my experience, fractures occurring at multiple levels with widespread bony injury have been found to produce excellent fracture callus and evidence of early fracture stability within 3 to 5 weeks, when the patient was treated in a recumbent position followed by an orthosis for a total of three months. Attempts at surgical stabilization of the spine with extensive fractures at multiple levels often result in more extensive spine stabilization than necessary (extending two levels above and below the fracture site closest to the fixation device, to gain internal fixation stability). An extensive instrumentation fusion results in loss of spine mobility over a wider area than necessary or desired. I have not found that fractures over multiple levels are any less likely to heal than any other area or fracture type. Rather, the converse has been found.

NEUROLOGIC INJURY

Injury to the thoracolumbar region of the vertebral column results in a variety of neurologic lesions. The type of injury that occurs depends on the anatomic level of vertebral injury and the corresponding neuroanatomy at that level. An analysis of vertebral column fractures between T1 and L5 (932 fractures) revealed a 79 percent incidence of neurologic injury (Table 18-11). Of the 470 injuries occurring in the thoracolumbar (T11–L2) region, 29.4 percent were neurologically complete, 43.6 percent were incomplete, and 26.8 percent were intact (Table 18-11).

The decreased incidence of complete injuries in the thoracolumbar area (29.4 percent), compared with the incidence of complete injuries in the entire lower spine (40.2 percent), occurs because of the "mixed" neuroanatomy found within the T11–L2 region of the vertebral column (spinal cord, conus medullaris, cauda equina) (Fig. 18-1); the width of the neural canal between T11 and L2; and the inherent resistance to injury demonstrated by the cauda equina (peripheral nerve rootlets).

The area above the level of T10 is just the opposite. Here the spinal cord is extremely susceptible to even the slightest injury; the neural canal is narrow (see Ch. 16, Fig. 16-8); and the blood supply to the thoracic spinal cord is the poorest of all areas of the spinal cord (see Ch. 4, p. 97).

T11 – L2 Neuroanatomy

Traumatic injuries to the thoracolumbar (T11 – L2) junctional area of the vertebral column are capable of producing one or more of three potential types of neurologic injuries (Fig. 18-1). These include the following.

Spinal cord. The spinal cord proper, that is, the central gray and peripheral white matter area of the spinal cord, terminates with the S5 segment of the conus medullaris at the approximate level of the lower border of vertebral body L1. The structure is looked on as "spinal cord" because of its normal, "central gray, peripheral white matter" architecture.

Conus medullaris. The conus medullaris is that segment of the spinal cord that contains the cell bodies and dendrites (axons) exiting to "peripheral nerves" of the sacral plexus between L5 and S5. This neuroanatomic area lies between the superior border of T12 and the inferior border of L1.

Cauda equina. The caudi equina is neuroanatomically representative of the peripheral nervous system (i.e., nerve roots). It is composed of axon cylinders surrounded by tough, fibrous sheaths that are fortunately resistant to injury. The cauda equina begins its take off at the bony vertebral level T10, where the nerve root L1 exits the spinal cord (Fig. 18-1). The L1, L2, and L3 nerve roots exit the spinal cord opposite the T10 and T11 vertebra and descend through the neural canal, traversing the thoracolumbar junction posterior to the vertebral bodies of T12 and L1 along with the conus medullaris. An injury at T12 – L1 can, therefore, produce a "combination" injury to the conus medullaris and the cauda equina. It is also possible to sustain an injury at this level without injuring the cauda equinal nerve roots, L1, L2, or L3, which exit the spinal cord opposite the T10, T11, and T12 vertebral bodies (Fig. 18-1). Thus, with persistent function in the L1, L2, and L3 nerve roots and destruc-

tion of the conus medullaris (L5 – S5), producing motor or sensory loss or both in the sacral plexus, such an injury would be described as "root escape." By itself, this observation has no other special neurologic prognostic significance other than to indicate the presence of residual peripheral nerve function in the segments L1 through L3. Thus, these nerve roots escape injury with vertebral column trauma at the T12 – L1 level.

Neurologic Assessment

Because an injury to the vertebral column between the levels of T11 and L2 neurologic can result in a mixed central and peripheral nervous system injury, between the segments of L2 to S5, sensation will be lost from the level of the inguinal ligament (L1) to the perianal region (S5)[10,11] (Fig. 18-1). Simultaneously, motor function will be lost from the neurologic level of L2 (the nerve root exiting the spinal cord opposite the T11 vertebral body to innervate the iliopsoas muscle, producing hip flexion), to the level of the perianal muscles, which arise from S2 to S5. Two frequent questions asked are: is it possible to differentiate between a central nervous system (spinal cord) injury and a peripheral (nerve) nervous system injury on rectal examination, and does the information derived from the rectal examination serve any prognostic value? The answer comes in three parts.

1. If a spinal cord injury occurs above the level of T11 and produces a complete motor and sensory injury, the resultant complete neurologic injury will likely result in priapism of the penis (resulting from noncortical control of autonomic nervous system outflow), the presence of a bulbocarvernosus reflex (contraction of the perianal muscles with pin prick, and perianal muscle contraction with squeezing of the glands penis, or pulling on an inflated catheter balloon in the male or female bladder). The combination of these findings indicates little chance of neurologic return.

2. With injury at the level of the conus medullaris (T12 – L1), the central gray matter neuronal cells are frequently destroyed (both motor and sensory). This results in flaccid paralysis in the

perineum and loss of all bladder and perianal muscle control. The irreversible nature of this injury to the sacral segments would reveal itself by the absence of a bulbocavernosus reflex, and no perianal "wink." Given this situation, motor function in the lower extremities between L1 and L4 may (with root escape) or may not exist.

3. In the presence of a complete cauda equina injury, all peripheral nerves to the bowel, bladder, perianal, and lower extremities would be lost. This would result in a flaccid paralysis to the bowel, bladder, and lower extremities, and an absence of the bulbocavernosus reflex, absence of an anal wink, and absence of all reflex activity in the lower extremities. This indicates an absence of any function in the cauda equina, but because the cauda equina is in reality the peripheral nervous system, there does exist an opportunity for some function to return if the nerve rootlets have not been completely transected or destroyed as a result of the injury. This type of injury frequently reveals itself to be neurologically incomplete (Table 18-14).

Of the 470 thoracolumbar junction injuries, 29.4 percent resulted in complete neurologic injuries and 43.6 percent resulted in incomplete neurologic injuries. Of the 470, 16 percent were cauda equina (peripheral nervous system) injuries, 3.2 percent were anterior cord injuries (involving the motor portion of the conus medullaris [central nervous system], 1.5 percent were mixed motor-sensory injuries, and 1 percent were Brown-Séquard injuries.

Injury to the thoracolumbar junction of the vertebral column therefore has the potential of producing five various types of neurologic injuries. They include:

1. Complete motor sensory spinal cord lesion. No neurologic function below the highest level of neurologic injury.
2. Incomplete motor-sensory spinal cord-peripheral nerve lesion. Some function exists below the level of injury.
3. Loss of conus medullaris function (L2–S5). No bowel, bladder, perianal, or lower extremity function below L4.
4. Central cord–conus medullaris injury. A small segment of the conus medullaris is lost, result-

Table 18-14. Fractures of the Thoracolumbar Junction: Neurologic Assessment and Interpretation

Assessment	Interpretation
Immediate complete absence of motor and sensory function, with absent reflexes below the injury level	(Suspected) complete
Complete absence of motor and sensory function without any return in the first 24 hours	Complete
Immediate complete absence of motor and sensory function with questionable peripheral reflex (i.e., patellar)	(Suspected) incomplete
Immediate complete absence of motor function with preservation of perianal sensation	Incomplete
Return of peripheral reflex activity below the level of spinal cord injury with absent motor and sensory function	Complete
Isolated nerve root injury	Incomplete
Bilateral nerve root (central cord) injury	Incomplete

ing in absent bladder and perianal motor function, in the presence of perianal (saddle) sensation.

5. Cauda equina lesion. Absence of bowel, bladder, perianal, and lower extremity motor and sensory function from L1 to S5. There will frequently be some degree of (late) neurologic return with this injury.

Spinal Shock

What is and when is "spinal shock"? There seems to be an expectation that with time, and return of "reflex" activity, there may be the return of something that may provide evidence of return of neurologic function. In my experience, this has not been so.

The principal neurologic finding indicating the presence of spinal shock is total absence of all motor, sensory, and reflex activity during the post-traumatic period. Frequently associated with this shock period is the absence (or presence) of the bulbocavernosus reflex, thought by some to indicate completeness or incompleteness of neurologic function. In actuality it is neither, only a reflex that returns (or never ceases) in the early minutes after injury.

Reflex activity involuntary muscle function, artificially activated, below the level of the injury. Whether its presence serves as a predictor of neurologic incompleteness is doubtful, and whether it serves in any way as an indicator of neurologic incompleteness or as a prognosticator of recovery remains doubtful. Appended to the question of the importance of spinal shock is the concern over the presence or absence of penile priapism (produced by loss of cortical control over peripheral autonomic nervous system function). The presence and significance of the bulbocavernosus reflex and penile priapism as prognosticators of neurologic function were raised by Holdsworth,[1,12,13] though the finding and first statement concerning "the presence of priapism in the absence of bowel or bladder control" was found in the Edwin Smith surgical papyrus written between 2500 and 3000 BC.[14] There the presence of priapism was indicative of a complete neurologic injury.

To place the subject in proper perspective and offer some grade of importance to various aspects of the perineal neurologic exam, the following interpretation is a compilation of 15 years of experience of neurologic examinations.

When perianal "voluntary" motor function is present, this is absolute evidence of incompleteness and serves as the best indicator of future neurologic activity. This finding also serves as a major neurologic monitoring function and, like a loss of neurologic function in other areas, can serve as an important early warning of neurologic deterioration.

Intact perianal senation unquestionably indicates the presence of posterior column function within the spinal cord. If present immediately after injury, it serves as a major indicator of incomplete-

ness and bears continued observation for any evidence in neurologic deterioration.

Absent voluntary perianal motor function and absent perianal (pain) sensation, with the presence or absence of priapism of the penis, is an indication of a complete neurologic injury, with little likelihood of neurologic recovery.

Absence of perianal sensation and no voluntary perianal motor function, in the presence of intra-anal proprioception, is a weak but definite indicator of neurologic incompleteness. It is determined by the presence of intra-anal recognition (by the patient) of the position of the examining finger during rectal examination. It indicates some remaining electrical continuity within the posterior columns of the spinal cord.

Presence of a peripheral reflex (patellar or Achilles tendon), with a total absence in motor or sensory function below the level of injury, within the first 48 to 72 hours after trauma may be a weak indicator of some residual (and questionable) spinal cord long tract continuity below the level of the spinal cord injury. In the presence of a residual anterior and posterior column function reflex (arc), function may persist during the otherwise silent period of spinal shock in a patient who otherwise appears to have a complete motor-sensory injury.

None of the above five findings have any special meaning with respect to spinal shock. Some investigators are of the opinion that the total absence of motor and sensory function, in the absence of reflex activity, indicates spinal shock. This may be correct but has no predictor values. Some researchers are of the opinion that the presence of a complete neurologic injury in which reflex activity has returned (usually within 3 to 6 weeks postinjury) serves as an indication that the period of spinal shock has passed. It may, but again has no predictive value. The presence of any incomplete injury sign is very important, and the bulbocavernosus reflex, an involuntary reflex, normally present in all, is the first reflex to return in the presence of a complete neurologic injury, and generally is noted to be present within 45 minutes after injury. This finding is almost always found during the period when the remainder of the neurologic examination demonstrates spinal shock. Absence of the bulbocavernosus reflex indicates direct injury to the conus medullaris, with destruction of the central gray matter cells and axon dendrites that are required for reflex activity (S1–S2), or vascular injury to the spinal cord (conus medullaris) resulting in flaccid paralysis below the level of the spinal cord injury.

SURGICAL APPROACHES AND PROCEDURES

Among surgeons providing care of the spine-injured patient, some controversy seems to exist as to the most opportune time to surgically approach a patient having evidence of a fracture (subluxation, dislocation, burst, etc.) with an associated incomplete neurologic injury. It is appreciated that there is a growing body of knowledge to indicate that the earlier a patient with multiple trauma is mobilized, and the shorter the recumbency period, the greater the reduction in the hazards of secondary complications (vascular, pulmonary, and urologic).[15] The question that exists in reference to the spinal column and the presence of a spinal cord injury is whether immediate surgery on the vertebral column of a neurologically traumatized or potentially neurologically traumatized patient warrants the early introduction of the hazards of surgical manipulation. The option would be, in the absence of neurologic deterioration, to allow the injury to stabilize for a variable period before instituting surgical stabilization. The philosophy on the acute spinal cord injury service at Northwestern University, developed after observing patients deteriorate neurologically after immediate or early post-trauma surgery, has been to delay surgery until such time as neural tissue edema and hematoma development have subsided. While some researchers advocate early surgery, believing that such might enhance neurological function,[4,16,17] Willen[16-18] found no difference after a prolonged follow-up in a controlled study of 24 patients managed conservatively and 26 patients managed by early operative stabilization.[18] Willen did note that postoperative reduction was better in those patients undergoing surgery within 3 days of injury.

When multiple trauma to other areas of the body has occurred, spine surgery is often delayed 1 to 2 weeks. Northwestern University data reveal the average preoperative wait period between injury and surgery to be 10 days. The prerequisite for spinal stabilization after stabilization of other fractures is that there not be any evidence of further neurologic deterioration as a result of spinal instability.

In the presence of persistent vertebral column displacement, the performance of early surgery depends on the extent of the displacement and the presence of an incomplete neurologic injury. Under most circumstances, early reduction of the dislocation is indicated. When the neurologic injury is complete, however, or as long as the neurologic injury is not deteriorating and the spinal malalignment is neither increasing nor demonstrating gross evidence of instability, surgery may be delayed until a more opportune time. The deciding factor is whether there is any evidence of neurologic deterioration. If none, waiting allows other trauma sites (chest, head, etc.) to stabilize, the patient's cardiovascular status to equilibriate, and the neurologic and vertebral column evaluation to proceed to completion (somatosensory evoked responses, CAT scan, myelogram [if the neurologic injury is incomplete], and tomograms). If displacement of vertebral elements exist, even in the presence of a complete neurologic injury, and surgical reduction is indicated, it should be performed within the first 3 weeks. If not, reduction of the vertebral column displacement will often be incomplete, difficult, or both.

During the intervening time between admission and proposed surgery, the patient is managed on a Stryker frame, turned every 2 hours (supine to prone), and placed on either an indwelling or intermittent urinary catheter care program, and a decision is made concerning the most appropriate surgical stabilization procedure to use. During this decision-making process, all hazards of the proposed surgery are reviewed with the patient and, when required or beneficial, with the family. Our belief is, the patient and the family should be aware of and share in the decision-making process.

Surgical Approaches

Of 470 patients sustaining injury to the thoracolumbar area of the spine, 294 (62.6 percent) were managed surgically and 176 (37.4 percent) were managed conservatively. Within the surgical group, 218 (74 percent) were operated on through the posterior approach, for both spinal stabilization and spinal fusion. The posterolateral approach (grouped with the posterior approach) was seldom utilized for decompression of the neural canal (five times), and when used, was done so specifically for neurologic symptoms in the form of "nerve root encroachment" and a vertebral deformity that was unilateral radiographically.

The second most frequent approach was the combined anteroposterior approach (simultaneous in 16 percent and staged in 2 percent). This approach was almost exclusively utilized for the anterior decompression of neural tissue compromise, secondary to bone or soft tissue, in a patient with an incomplete neurologic injury.

The anterior approach alone is not used for stabilization, rather it is reserved for failure of a previous attempt at posterior stabilization, which requires an anterior supplementary stabilization and fusion, or when, after previous posterior surgery, there is evidence of anterior neurologic compromise requiring decompression. There are other situations that might require anterior stabilization. An example is seen in Figure 18-15, in which radiation necrosis of L1–L2 followed excision of a posterior spine tumor. This was performed in nine patients (3 percent).

Anterior (Transthoracic-Transabdominal) Approach

As noted above, the decision to approach the spine via the anterior approach indicates that the injury is an incomplete neurologic injury, accompanied by an unacceptable degree of gross vertebral column malalignment, and that there is spinal cord compromise, either by bone or soft tissue, identified by preoperative myelogram, CAT scan, tomograms, and somatosensory evoked potential studies. From each of these evaluative procedures, a determination can be made as to whether decompression of the area of compromise is appropriate or whether anterior surgery offers any potential of enhancing neurologic recovery.

Conditions that require consideration before undertaking the anterior or the combined anteroposterior surgical approach are:

The presence of other systemic injuries that may serve as a contraindication to surgery (an infection not under control). In reference to infections, it is not uncommon for a patient with an indwelling catheter to run a protracted febrile course. The policy on the acute spine injury service is: if the patient has been on antibiotic therapy for 24 hours before surgery, surgery can usually be carried out, knowing that the involved system is most likely the urinary tract.

Pulmonary trauma (hemopneumothorax) or pulmonary infection. This is not an uncommon complication with thoracic spine fractures. Data reveal that the incidence of pulmonary infection was 14 percent in the thoracolumbosacral spine group and 4.6 percent in the thoracolumbar junction group (see Table 18-14). The rationale here is that acute chest trauma more often follows upper thoracic spine fracture than lower spine injuries.

Skin loss or abasions over the proposed operative site. It is occasionally necessary to manage such abrasions with topical antibiotics for several days, followed by open (to dry) management. Surgery through an area incompletely healed has not proved to be a problem, though it produces some concerns. All patients are administered broad-spectrum antibiotics at the institution of the operative procedure (Kefzol [cefazolin sodium], 2 intravenously [IV]; Cefadyl [cephapirin sodium], 1 or 2 g IV, etc.) and repeated every 3 to 4 hours during the procedure and every 6 hours IV for 3 days postoperatively.

Preoperative anemia. This problem is usually noted in a patient having sustained multiple trauma or long bone fractures. It may also be more apparent than real, with rehydration after fluid management in the immediate post-trauma period. Therefore, several days are allowed to pass for the patient to equilibriate and the etiology and defect to be managed.

Selection of the Surgical Approach

Normally, the incision site is based on two things: the level (or location) of the fracture, or the condition of the local skin. Occasionally after trauma, abrasions, superficial lacerations, or infection may require altered positioning of the incision. If this is

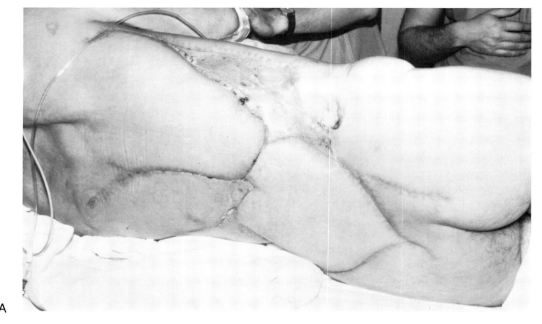

A

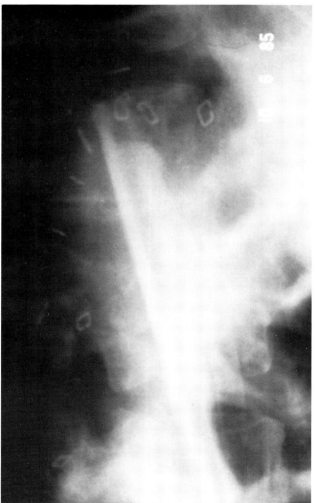

B

Fig. 18-15. (A) Posterior view of referred patient following multiple skin and pedicle grafts for radiation necrosis of the L1 vertebral body and the skin over the lumbar spine. Radiation therapy was used for malignant lymphoma. (B) Lateral radiograph showing radiation necrosis of multiple vertebral bodies. Note previous operative procedure with inlay of fibular bone graft across T12–L1–L2. *(Figure continues.)*

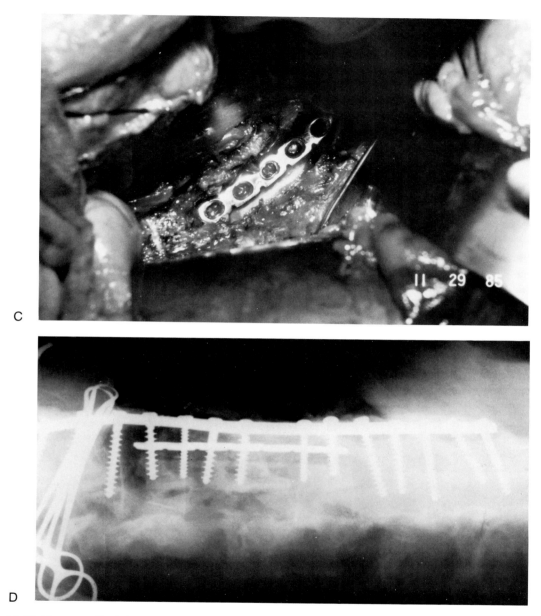

C

D

Fig. 18-15 *(Continued).* **(C)** AO compression plate inserted into the trough overlying the inlay fibular bone graft, engaging the proximal and distal vertebrae. After application of the long AO compression plate over the external surface of the thoracolumbar spine, methylmethacrylate (in fluid form) was injected into the interstices and drill holes prior to screw insertion. **(D)** Postoperative lateral radiograph showing external and internal AO compression plates and previous fibular inlay graft. The screw fixation of the external plate passes through the internal plate. The patient was neurologically normal. At 7 months after the procedure, the patient was neurologically normal and the nonunion was healed.

not a consideration, the incision is centered at the level of the fractured vertebral process, or elements, composing the center of the area to be stabilized by internal fixation. This applies primarily to the placement of the posterior spinal incision, or the incision for obtaining a bone graft from the posterior iliac crest (Fig. 17-15). Other considerations must be taken into account in the selection of the anterior thoracotomy approach (Fig. 18-16).

Selection of Chest Incision Site

As a general rule, the selection of the site or location of the incision is based on the vertebral body to be excised; however, although the rib serves as an excellent anatomic guide to the location of the ver-

tebral body in question, it does not necessarily happen that the same rib incision and excision are used for the vertebral body that is to undergo corporectomy. The customary surgical positioning is with the patient lying right side down (lateral decubitus position), with the back perpendicular to the table top. The back and buttock should be as close to one side of the table as possible, facilitating the posterior approach. This position allows performance of a posterior approach simultaneously with the anterolateral transthoracic or retroperitoneal (abdominal) approach (Fig. 18-17).

In my experience, the most utilitarian approach to the chest has been the left 11th rib approach. This rib and this site have been selected for several reasons.

The 11th rib is sufficiently long (if removed al-

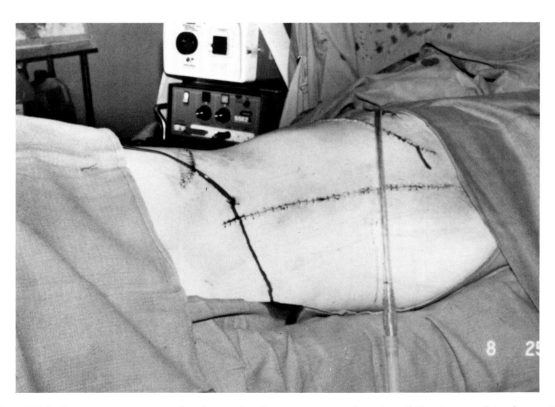

Fig. 18-16. Postoperative view of a thoracolumbar spine-injured patient following combined anterior decompression of the thoracic spine and posterior stabilization of the thoracolumbar spine. The thoracotomy approach was via the 11th rib. Bone graft was obtained from the posterior left iliac crest. The posterior incision allowed stabilization three levels above and three levels below the fracture site.

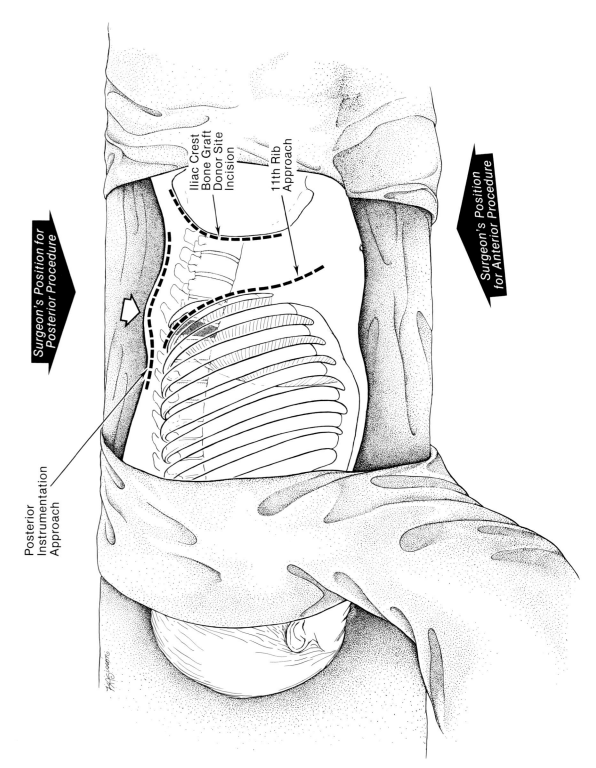

Surgeon's Position for Posterior Procedure

Iliac Crest
Bone Graft
Donor Site
Incision

11th Rib
Approach

Surgeon's Position
for Anterior Procedure

Posterior
Instrumentation
Approach

Fig. 18-17. Anterior and posterior approaches to the thoracolumbar vertebral column.

most entirely) for making "matchstick" grafts to span the area of vertebral body excision and to be inlaid into the vertebral body above and below the corporectomy site (for example, T11 above and L1 below).

The curve of the 11th rib actually places the T12–L1 interspace in the center of the operative field.

Because the diaphragm and the upper reaches of the iliopsoas muscles attach at or just below the level of T12–L1, it is often necessary to incise the diaphragm and to split the psoas muscle, in line with its fibers, at or near its origin (L1 and L2 vertebral body). Use of the T11 approach allows for sufficient mobilization of the tissues and a wide exposure.

The "stump" of the excised 11th rib serves as an anatomic guide to the vertebral body to which it is attached and provides positive identification of the subsequent vertebral bodies above and below. If a question continues to exist, it is suggested that an anteroposterior radiograph of the spine (with the patient in the lateral position on the table) be obtained. If a combined anteroposterior approach is being performed, the radiograph should await exposure of the posterior elements. In this manner, the correct anatomic level, both anteriorly and posteriorly, can be visualized simultaneously.

Anterior Surgical Approach: Considerations

With the rib incision site selected (transpleural 11th rib resection), the incision is usually made by the thoracic surgery service (accompanied by orthopaedic surgery) from a point 3 inches lateral of the posterior midline over the 11th rib. The incision is carried anteriorly and inferiorly in line with the 11th rib, to a point about an inch distal to the tip

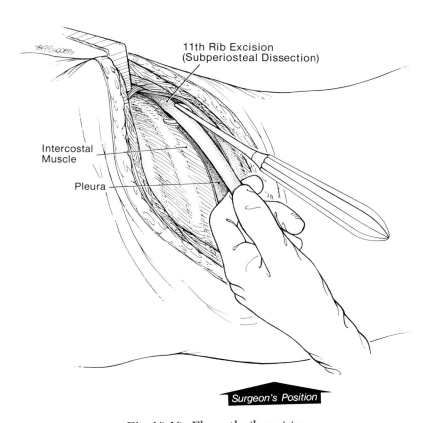

11th Rib Excision (Subperiosteal Dissection)

Intercostal Muscle

Pleura

Surgeon's Position

Fig. 18-18. Eleventh rib excision.

of the cartilaginous tip of the rib. The incision is carried down through the skin and subcutaneous tissue to the periosteum overlying the rib. By sharp subperiosteal dissection, the periosteum is stripped from the 11th rib posteriorly as far as the transverse process of the 11th vertebra, or just slightly lateral to this point (Fig. 18-18). The rib is resected with a guillotine rib cutter, leaving a stump of the posterior rib 1½ to 2 inches long (Fig. 18-19). The rib is placed in moist sponges for safekeeping until it is cut into matchstick grafts and ready for insertion (Fig. 18-20). With the rib removed, an incision is made by sharp scissor dissection through the pleura, in line with the periosteal cuff of the 11th rib (Fig. 18-21). The anesthesiologist should be notified when the chest is entered. Care must be taken not to injure the lung parenchyma (Fig. 18-22). The lower lobe of the left lung is packed upward into the left chest cavity with a moist lap sponge, and a self-retaining chest retractor inserted. Inferiorly, the diaphragm is incised

transverse to its fibers (Fig. 18-23). Superiorly lies the lower lobe of the left lung; anteriorly, the aorta and the peritoneum (beneath the diaphragm); and directly posteriorly, the vertebral column. The vertebral bodies are vaguely visible beneath the reflected pleura, the anterior longitudinal ligament, and the periosteum laterally (Figs. 18-24, 18-25). The attachment of the periosteum and the anterior longitudinal ligament to the anulus fibrosus at each disc level is great. I have found that the easiest method of facilitating the surgical exposure of the vertebral column is by electrocautery dissection of the periosteum, followed by the use of a periosteal elevator to dissect the periosteum off of the lateral walls of the vertebral bodies (done rather easily). When an interval has been established anteriorly between the periosteum and the vertebra, a Chandler or Bennett retractor is inserted beneath the periosteal sleeve (to protect the aorta lying just anterior to the vertebral column) (Fig. 18-26). The electrocautery has been found to

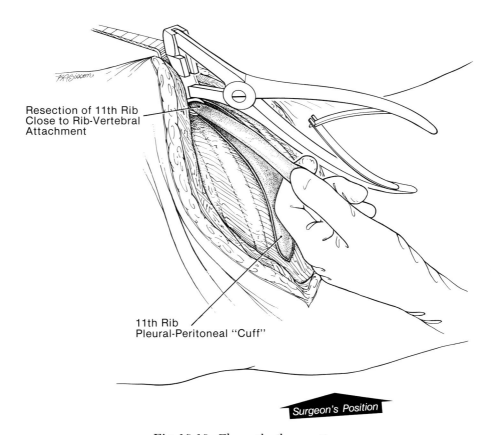

Resection of 11th Rib
Close to Rib-Vertebral
Attachment

11th Rib
Pleural-Peritoneal "Cuff"

Surgeon's Position

Fig. 18-19. Eleventh rib resection.

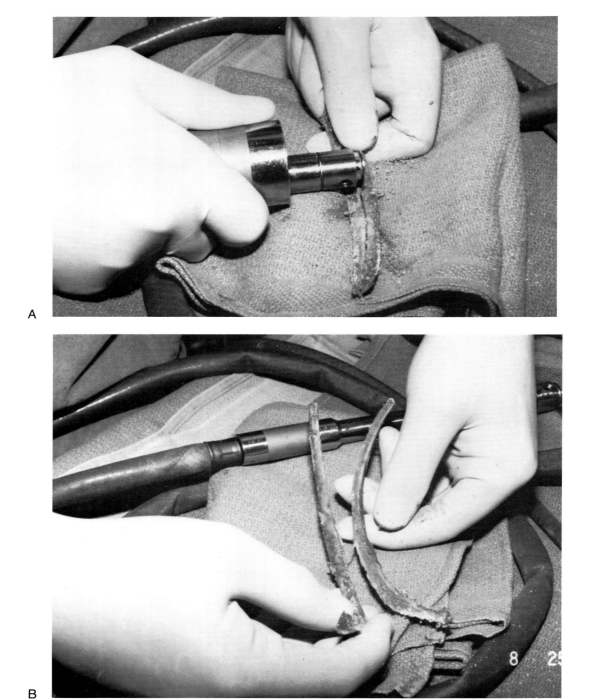

A

B

Fig. 18-20. **(A)** 11th rib removed during a thoracotomy approach to the anterior thoracic spine being cut longitudinally with an oscillating saw. **(B)** After longitudinal incision of the rib, transverse cuts are made at appropriate lengths, from which "matchstick grafts" are made, to be inserted anteriorly.

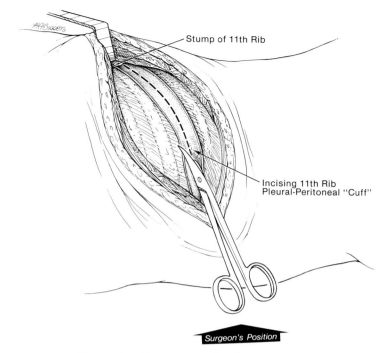

Fig. 18-21. Entrance to the pleura.

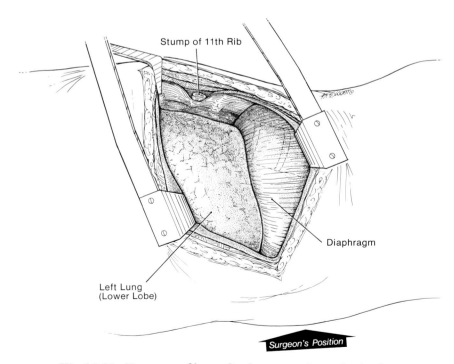

Fig. 18-22. Exposure of lung, diaphragm, and vertebral column.

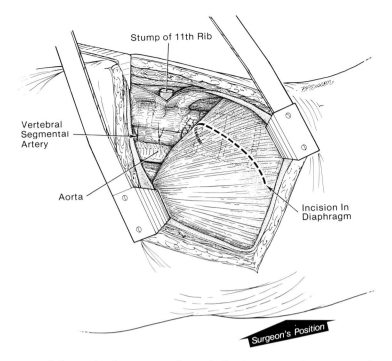

Fig. 18-23. Resection of eleventh rib, incision through diaphragm, and exposure of vertebral column and vessels.

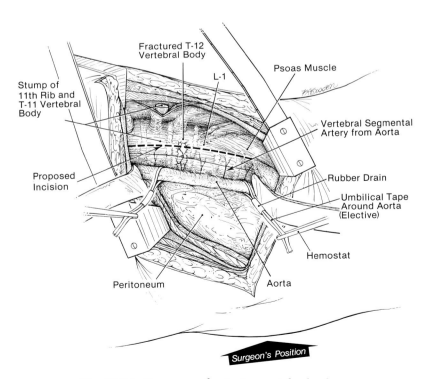

Fig. 18-24. Exposure of anterior vertebral column.

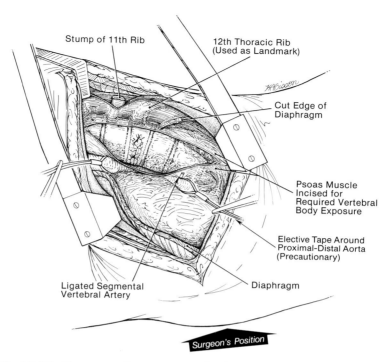

Fig. 18-25. Exposure of anterior vertebral column and fracture site.

be an effective method of detaching the very closely adherent anterior longitudinal ligament from the anulus fibrosus. A long electrocautery tip is used during the chest approach to facilitate working in the depths of the wound (Fig. 18-27).

The only vital structures encountered during the approach to the vertebral column, beside the aorta, are the segmental arteries running transversely from the aorta (anteriorly and laterally), in the direction of the neuroforamen (posteriorly) (see Chapter 4). Transecting these vessels anterolaterally can be performed without fear of producing vascular embarrassment to the spinal cord. This is not the case with coagulating a segmental vessel in the area of the neuroforamen. Here, coagulation is likely to injure the small branches exiting the segmental vessel, serving as medullary feeders known as the "anterior radicular arteries." Injury to these latter vessels can produce neurologic injury, including paraplegia. The routine method of occluding the segmental vessels in my hands is by electrocautery. Some surgeons prefer small vascular clips, or surgical ligatures. The latter technique is more

time consuming and has not been found to be more effective.

With the vertebral injury site identified, the anterior longitudinal ligament and periosteum are dissected free from the anterior vertebral column extending from one level above the injury to one level below the injury. The soft tissues and the aorta are protected by the insertion of either Bennett or large Chandler retractors in the space between the vertebral bodies and the anterior longitudinal ligament-periosteum cuff developed opposite the fractured vertebra(e). This accomplished, removal of the offending vertebra is begun (Figs. 18-26, 18-28, 18-29). This is done very carefully, protecting the aorta and the peritoneal structures. Other anatomic structures requiring identification and protection are the anterior rami of the nerve roots L1 and L2, as they exit the spine via the neuroforamen and pass into the substance of the psoas muscle, coursing anteriorly and inferiorly as components of the ilioinguinal (L1), iliogenital (L1–L2), and femoral nerves (L2, L3) (Fig. 18-28). The major and highest branch easily identified is

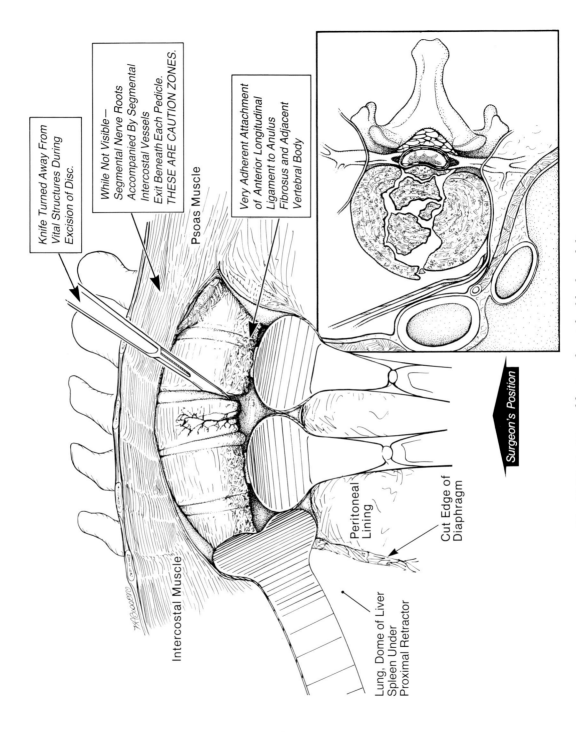

Knife Turned Away From Vital Structures During Excision of Disc.

While Not Visible— Segmental Nerve Roots Accompanied By Segmental Intercostal Vessels Exit Beneath Each Pedicle. THESE ARE CAUTION ZONES.

Psoas Muscle

Very Adherent Attachment of Anterior Longitudinal Ligament to Anulus Fibrosus and Adjacent Vertebral Body

Surgeon's Position

Intercostal Muscle

Peritoneal Lining

Cut Edge of Diaphragm

Lung, Dome of Liver Spleen Under Proximal Retractor

Fig. 18-26. Excision of fractured vertebral body and disc.

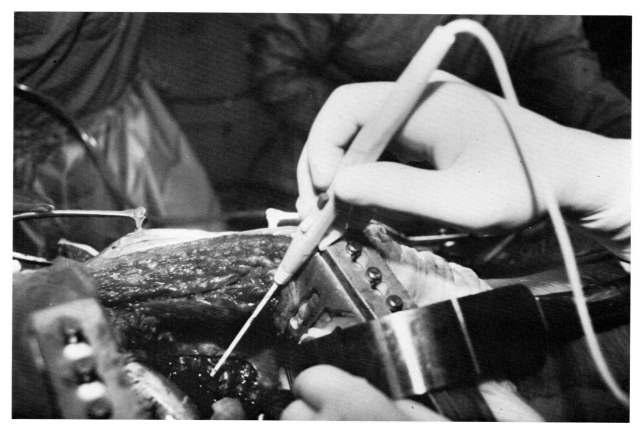

Fig. 18-27. Use of electrocautery (with a long tip) during dissection of anterior vertebral column via thoracotomy approach. Electrocautery dissection is particularly helpful in dissecting the attachment of the anterior longitudinal ligament from the anulus fibrosis at each disc level.

L2. Care must be taken when stripping the psoas muscle from the L2 vertebral body anterolaterally to identify it and protect it. The L2 nerve root would only be encountered if working at the L2 level (T12 to L2).

By sharp dissection, the intervertebral discs above and below the vertebra are excised. The instruments found most effective for this portion of the procedure are a sharp number 10 knife blade on a long handle (always incising in a posterior direction, away from the vital structures anteriorly, if possible) (Fig. 18-26), a Lecksel rongeur, a high-speed burr, and a curette. I have found the use of a pituitary forceps very unrewarding during the removal of the anulus fibrosus and the central disc, though it logically would be the appropriate in-

strument to use in this area. Using a bone-biting rougeur, a large pituitary rougeur, an angled curette, and a diamond-tipped burr, the fractured vertebral body impinging on the neural canal can be excised (Fig. 18-28). Usually, the area of vertebral body excised is that portion anterior, left lateral, and posterior, with the right side of the vertebral body left in place unless there is a need for its removal. Otherwise it serves as protection for the vena cava anteriorly on the right side of the vertebral body.

Approaching the posterior portion of the vertebral body, a high-speed burr, a curette, and a small pituitary forceps are utilized for decompression of the dura. At Northwestern University, this portion of the procedure is performed either by the neuro-

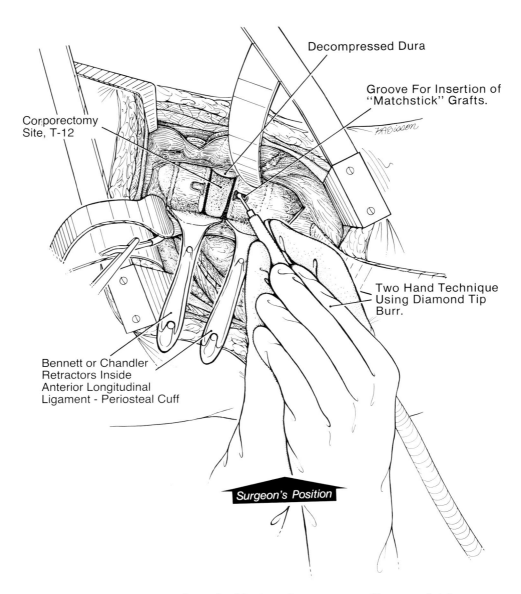

Decompressed Dura

Groove For Insertion of "Matchstick" Grafts.

Corporectomy Site, T-12

Two Hand Technique Using Diamond Tip Burr.

Bennett or Chandler Retractors Inside Anterior Longitudinal Ligament - Periosteal Cuff

Surgeon's Position

Fig. 18-28. Excision of vertebral body and preparation of bone graft inlay.

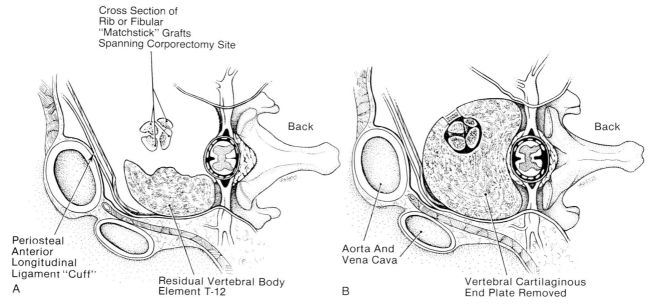

Fig. 18-29. Cross-sectional views of the relationship between bone graft and vertebral bodies. (**A**) View proximally from superior surface of L1. (**B**) View from inferior surface of T11.

surgical consultant (following protocol) or the orthopaedic surgeon. The surgeon should instruct the technician performing the evoked potential to carefully observe the responses for changes. After removal of the vertebral body (for example, T12), the dura should be clearly visible from the area posterior to T11 to the superior border of L1. When the surgeon is satisfied that an adequate debridement of the dura has been accomplished, the end plates of the vertebral bodies above and below are curetted or burred free of their cartilaginous surfaces. The high-speed burr is very useful for this task. This completed, grooves are then placed in the lower half of the upper vertebra (in this instance, T11) and in the upper half of the lower vertebra (L1) along their anterior lateral borders (Fig. 18-28). Into these grooves will be placed inlay rib matchstick or fibular grafts (Fig. 18-30). To accomplish this task, a Stryker saw is used to cut the rib longitudinally into two equal parts. The length of the space between the two vertebral grooves and the corporectomy site is measured after the insertion of the posterior internal fixation (Harrington[4] or Luque[3] rods). This is done after the posterior instrumentation because distraction of the internal fixation or vertebral column lengthens the space

prepared for the bone graft. If the grafts are cut early, they will be too short when the internal fixation is applied. The grafts are cut into appropriate lengths and inserted into the planned grooves. This accomplished, care is taken to insert cancellous bone grafts only anterior to or between the matchstick grafts and the anterior longitudinal ligament periosteal cuff, not allowing the graft to come in contact with the dura posteriorly (Fig. 18-30).

The reflected pleural sheath posteriorly is closed with a running, locking 0 chromic or Vicryl suture. This accomplished, a number 28 or 32 chest catheter is inserted into the eighth interspace, in the anterior axillary line, making sure that the tip of the catheter is placed up to and alongside the apex of the left upper lobe. The remainder of the chest procedure is performed by the thoracic surgery service in a routine manner. The diaphragm is approximated with interrupted 2-0 silk sutures. This is followed by the approximation of the 10th to the 12th rib by a rib clamp, and approximation of the intercostal muscles with interrupted 2-0 silk or Vicryl sutures. The subcutaneous tissue is closed with 2-0 Dexon sutures, and the skin is closed with staples, interrupted mattress, or a running subcuticular skin closure, using a 2-0 Dermalon suture.

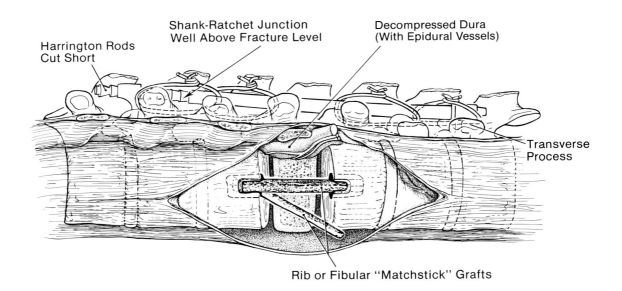

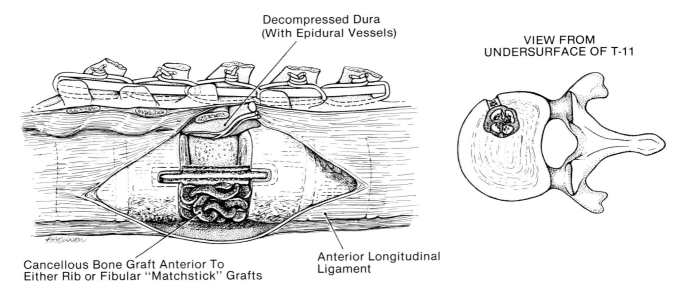

Fig. 18-30. Inlay of vertebral body bone graft across corporectomy site.

Standard Posterior Approach

The posterior approach is the standard midline exposure of the posterior vertebral elements, extending from the third level above to the third level below the area of the spine to be stabilized. The vertebral process that will serve as the center of the posterior incision can usually be identified by the presence of a gibbus or prominence of that posterior element as a result of the kyphotic angulation of the thoracolumbar spine, secondary to anterior compression of the involved vertebral element.

As noted elsewhere, if the anterior and posterior approaches are performed simultaneously, the correct identification of the appropriate vertebral process posteriorly becomes important for the correct localization of the surgical incision. Because of the curve of the ribs from superior to inferior, posteriorly to anteriorly, the chest incision overall will extend more proximal than the vertebral body being approached. This frequently leads to confusion and the making of the posterior approach at an incorrect level (Fig. 18-17). This can be prevented by recognizing that the error is easy to make, and if difficult to determine accurately, obtain a radiograph to correctly identify the proper posterior element. The posterior incision can then be centered on this process.

The posterior approach, whether performed singularly or in combination with an anterior approach, is the most appropriate approach for obtaining posterior vertebral element reduction, stabilization, and multilevel spine fusion. If performed during the early weeks after trauma, and if no overriding reasons exist for making the anterior approach (i.e., decompressing an incomplete neurologic injury, or the taking down of a longstanding vertebral column malalignment), it is the most appropriate approach for gaining or improving spinal alignment. The posterior approach is also the only means of obtaining reliable spinal stability over multiple levels.

Posterior Stabilization: Techniques

The selection of the appropriate posterior internal stabilizing device is dependent on several important variables. They include the following:

The extent of the gross spine malalignment, and how long it has been present

Whether the neurologic injury is complete or incomplete (distraction when incomplete)

Whether there is evidence of posterior vertebral body wall fracture

Whether there has been dislocation of intact facets (a result of flexion-distraction forces) or fracture through facets resulting from a horizontal shear injury with anterior translation of the upper segment on the lower segment

Whether the vertebral body fracture is unilateral, bilateral, anteriorly compressed, comminuted, or burst

How many levels of the spine require stabilization

Whether kyphosis or lordosis deformity is present, and to what extent

Whether the lumbosacral joint is involved (making every effort not to include it if normal)

Review of 218 thoracolumbar (T11–L2) junction posterior stabilization procedures reveals the most frequently utilized internal fixation device to be Harrington distraction rods (50.7 percent), followed by the (previously used but now substituted by other device) compression springs device (30.3 percent), and Luque rods (11.2 percent) (Table 18-15). Other procedures were occasionally utilized. Experience with the compression springs device (Weiss springs)[19] was gained during a time

Table 18-15. Thoracolumbar: Type of Surgical Stabilization (Northwestern University Acute Spine Injury Center, 1972 to 1986)

Type of Stabilization	No.	Percent
Harrington distraction	149	50.7
Weiss compression springs	89	30.3
Luque rods	33	11.2
Cottrel-Debousett	1	0.3
Other	9	3.1
Missing[a]	13	4.4
Total surgery	294	100.0
No surgery	176	
Total	470	

[a] Stabilization is unavailable.

when this device was being evaluated in a multi-center collaborative research program.[20]

With the rapid change in internal fixation philosophy and numerous new internal fixation techniques, a review of the procedures performed between 1985 and July 1986 revealed the following. There has been a real increase in the number of fractures of the thoracolumbar region stabilized with Luque rod instrumentation. There has been, as a result of the influence of the Luque system of internal fixation, a significant increase in the use of sublaminar wires in the fixation of Harrington rods. This latter fact has occurred despite the concerns over the passage of sublaminar wires in the presence of known spinal cord (conus medullaris–cauda equina) injury. The successful use of this technique has probably been made possible with increased dependency and reliance on the information obtained from the use of SSEP. There has been a trend toward the use of new procedures such as the "Dunn,"[21] the "AD Internal Fixator," the "Jacobs" AO Synthes rods, etc. Since the Dunn procedures were performed, this device has been removed from the market owing to the report of late abdominal great vessel complications. Also of note is the almost total cessation of the compression Weiss spring procedure. The latter was not discontinued because of failures (though, as with other procedures, these have occurred and have been reported). Rather, the Weiss springs were much less stable, and the Luque system was the appropriate technique to replace the springs, that is, it produced compression (or allowed the same, as with Luque rods) or provided linear alignment.

Inappropriate Use of Harrington Rods

Most spine surgeons agree that there is no more utilitarian orthopaedic instrument than the Harrington rod. This device has been the most utilized spine intrumentation since its development in 1957. Clinically introduced as a new and effective means of gaining both correction and stability for such spinal disabilities as paralytic and developmental scoliosis and meningomyelocele, in time it was being used for fractures, tumors, etc. Despite the instrument's utility and ease of insertion, there are indications and situations when it may not be the most appropriate device for use. These include the presence of a developmental and prominent thoracic kyphosis; the presence of an uncorrectable compression thoracic fracture gibbus, with marked thoracic kyphosis; use in the area of the lumbar spine, complicated by the presence of a prominent thoracolumbar kyphosis, where it may be difficult to insert the lower lumbar hooks, without requiring the inappropriate use of a longer (sacral alae) hook; the Harrington rod to be prebent to be inserted (producing "stress risers" in the metal rod at the shank-notch interval, making the rod more likely to undergo fatigue failure with loading; less of a problem with the new Synthes locking hook-spinal rod system, owing to improved rod construction[9]); or the placement of a groove in the posterior lamina at the level immediately above the lamina into which the lower Harrington hook are to be inserted. Of the three techniques above, this latter technique has been found to be the most appropriate solution.

Two other occasions when Harrington rods may be less appropriate (than Luque rods) are across the cervicothoracic junction (for tumor stabilization), and across the lumbosacral junction (Fig. 18-31). The primary rationale for their not being used across these two major joint areas is the extent of motion that occurs at each. In the cervical spine, rotary and flexion-extion motion is essentially unrestricted, except for that which results from the construction of the joints. Below this, in the thorax, motion is restricted by the ribs. Likewise, in the lumbar spine, while rotation at the L5 interval is limited, flexion, and to a lesser degree, extension are not. On the other hand, no motion occurs below the L5–S1 junction. It is this contrast that results in failure of internal fixation when it is used across these two intervals. However, Harrington rods, or for that matter, other means of internal fixation, may be required out of necessity (as with fractures of L5 or S1 requiring distraction for fracture reduction and maintenance, scoliosis, or fusions).

When used, Harrington rods (or Luque rods) are usually fixed to the pelvis or, by the use of a transverse sacroiliac transfixation pin, into the sacral ala (see Fig. 18-42), where Harrington rods are less effective. When motion persists, loss of fixation of the lower hooks from the lamina occurs (Fig. 18-31), or the lower end of the Harrington rod dislocates from the lower hooks (Fig. 18-31). Furthermore, the insertion of Harrington rods across the lumbosacral joint is capable of producing a loss

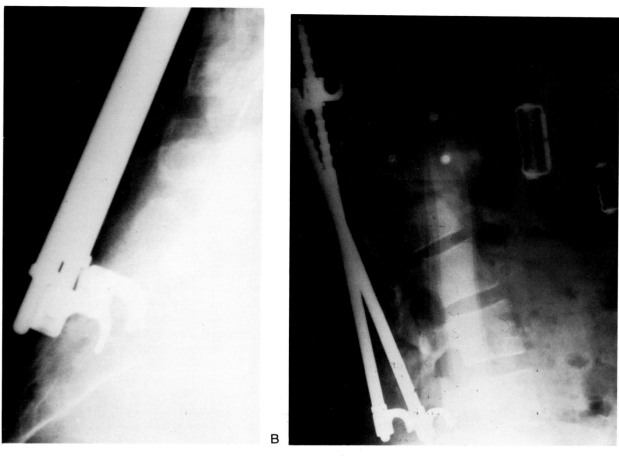

Fig. 18-31. (A) Radiograph showing insertion of Harrington hooks into the second sacral foramen, and the displacement of the rods from the hooks bilaterally. (B) Displacement of Harrington rod internal fixation both proximally and distally. Note that one rod has displaced superiorly, the other inferiorly. The fracture site is T12–L1.

in the normal lumbosacral angle. In my experience, the result is the production of an abnormal patient "stance posture" owing to the presence of an abnormal anterior pelvic tilt. This results in an abnormal gait.

Anterior Corporectomy with Posterior Instrumentation

For the purposes of this section, it is assumed that the involved fractured vertebra is T12. The posterior skin incision extends posteriorly from T9 above to L3 inferiorly (particularly if the plan is to insert Harrington distraction rods). This procedure requires that the superior hooks and the inferior hooks be applied to the third lamina above and below the injury site. This is done to have at least two intact posterior elements above and below, to prevent the tendency for the spine to fall into kyphosis. This occurs secondary to further collapse of the fractured vertebra and as a result of further stress relaxation of the intervertebral ligaments secondary to the forces of distraction brought about by the distraction rods.

Some surgeons have suggested that the combined anterior-posterior management technique is "too extensive." Review of 47 procedures reveals that the average blood loss for the combined procedure is 5,827 ml (Table 18-16) and that the mor-

Table 18-16. Thoracolumbar Fractures: Estimated Blood Loss for Approach Types (Northwestern University Acute Spine Injury Center, 1972 to 1986)

Surgical Approach	Mean Blood Loss (ml)	No. of Cases
Anterior	4,257	7
Posterior	1,894	199
Combined	5,827	47
Anterior then posterior	4,600	2
Posterior then anterior	2,600	4
Missing[a]		211
Total	2,704	470

[a] Estimated blood loss is unavailable.

bidity from the procedure is reasonably low. Operative time required for the combined procedures averages 7 to 8 hours (the posterior procedure takes just under 3 hours and the anterior procedure takes approximately 7 hours). The incidence of complication with the combined anterior-posterior procedure is less than 2 percent. Of 49 anterior spine procedures, one surgical death resulted (2 percent) (in a patient 1.5 years after sustaining a war wound, with original spine, abdominal, and chest injuries). Because of an incomplete neurologic injury and an accompanying gross spinal angulation, with pseudarthrosis at the thoracolumbar junction, an attempt to resect the involved vertebra and perform a spinal fusion resulted in injury to the aorta, from which the patient died postoperatively.

It is appropriate, therefore, to attempt correction of spinal fracture deformity early, to circumvent spinal deformity requiring late bone resection, the application of unusually high correction forces, the need to overcome tissue contracture secondary to shortening, the need to perform extensive internal fixation to gain a fusion, and prolonged immobilization, particularly when accompanied by neurologic injury. Holdsworth stated in 1970,[1] "attempts at correcting longstanding (or late) spine malalignment, is fraught with hazards and complications." In my experience, gross spinal malalignment can only be accurately reduced surgically if done in the first 2 to 3 weeks post-trauma.

After this, soft tissue contractures and fracture callus prevent anatomic correction. To attain correction when performed "late" (2 to 3 weeks), extensive dissection will be required.

SPINAL INSTRUMENTATION PROCEDURES

Harrington Distraction Rod Procedure with Modification

After the appropriate incision is made, thoroughly exposing the appropriate vertebral elements, an appropriate length Harrington distraction rod[4] (Fig. 18-32E,F) is selected. Care is taken not to use a rod that places the smooth shank-ratchet portion of the rod at the level of the fracture site. This junctional area of the rod is biomechanically weak. When applied across the level of the fracture, with repetitive (or oscillating) bending moments to this area, stress risers result, and rod fatigue failure occurs (Fig. 18-33). Select a longer rod (with a longer smooth shank) and with a rod cutter, shorten the ratchet end of the rod to an appropriate length (leaving three or four notched levels above the upper hook) (Fig. 18-32). This will also facilitate the removal of the system at an appropriate time, if deemed necessary.

The inferior surface of the upper lamina is notched, usually three levels above the level of the fracture site (and sometimes higher when fractures of the posterior elements exist at several levels above or below the level of the fracture), and the superior surface of the inferior lamina, three levels below the fracture, is similarly notched, using a "Kerrison" rongeur. A 1253 hook is inserted superiorly, and a 1254 hook is placed inferiorly. The hooks are impacted in place with the hook impactor. The superior ratchet portion of the rod is inserted into the proximal hook sufficiently far to permit the inferior aspect of the rod to fit into the inferior (1254) hook. Occasionally, when kyphosis, associated with the fracture, is prominent and must be contended with, it may be necessary to use the power burr on the posterior cortical surface of the lamina, at the level just above the lower hook, to provide a vertical groove for the rod to lie in (Fig.

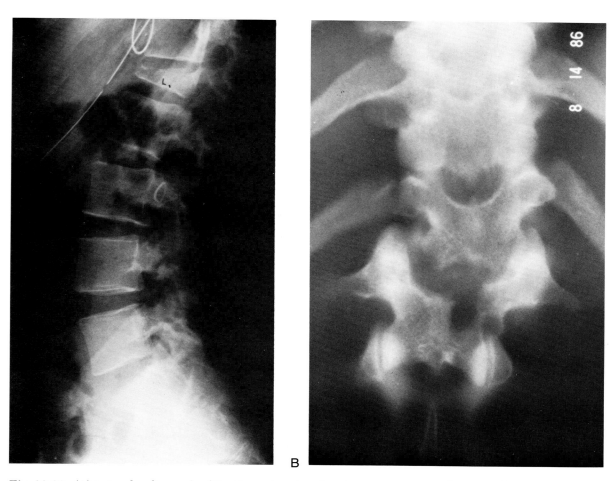

A   B

Fig. 18-32. **(A)** Lateral radiograph of the thoracic spine showing a compression fracture of L1 by greater than 60% of its height. The patient was neurologically intact. **(B)** AP tomogram showing a typical rotation-induced fracture through the pedicle of L1. (see Fig. 18-2) *(Figure continues.)*

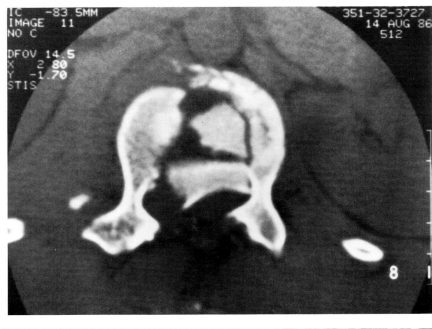

C

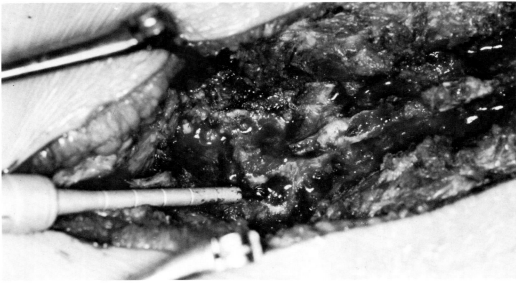

D

Fig. 18-32 *(Continued)*. **(C)** Transverse CT scan shows comminuted burst fracture of L1 with extrusion of bone fragments posteriorly. **(D)** Operative view showing posterior surface of lamina one level above the lamina into which the Harrington rod hook is inserted. A longitudinal groove is being cut in the lamina, lateral to the spinous process, to facilitate insertion of the Harrington rod. *(Figure continues.)*

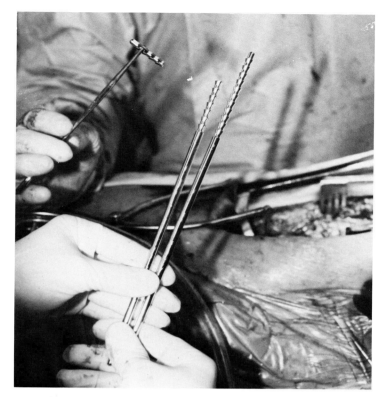

E

F

Fig. 18-32 *(Continued)*. **(E)** To prevent mechanical failure of Harrington rods, the shank-ratchet area of the rod should not lie opposite the fracture site. Selecting a longer shank rod requires removing part of the ratchet area. Enough of the ratchet portion is removed to allow for adequate distraction across the fracture site. To facilitate removing the rods, excess length proximal to the hooks must be removed. **(F)** Harrington rods, cut to the correct length, in place following insertion of sublaminar wires and appropriate distraction. High-density polyethylene Edwards sleeves are placed posterior to the lamina at the level of the vertebral body fracture. The Harrington rod is not bent; rather, the Edwards sleeves produce the hyperextension moment. Note also the transverse wires maintaining midline approximation of the Harrington rods. Sublaminar wire was not passed at the level of the fracture site. *(Figure continues.)*

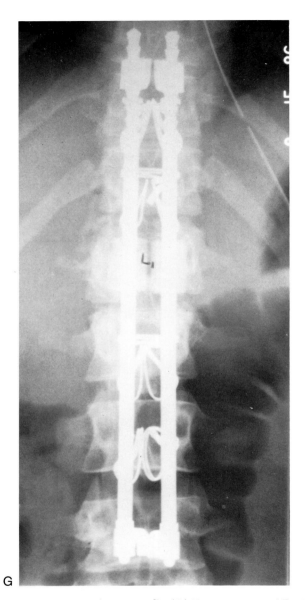

G

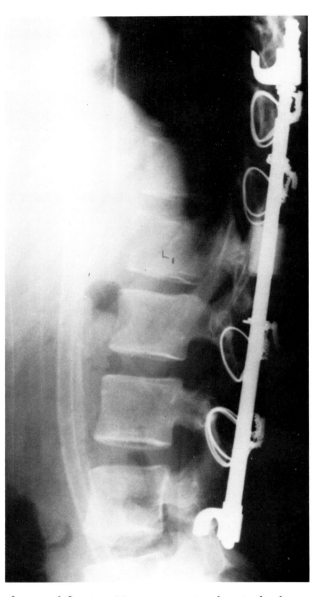

H

Fig. 18-32 *(Continued)*. **(G)** Postoperative AP view of internal fixation. Note appropriate longitudinal alignment vertebral column. **(H)** Lateral view. Note complete reconstitution of vertebral body height and reduction of traumatic kyphosis. Edwards sleeve is approximated to posterior element L1. *(Figure continues.)*

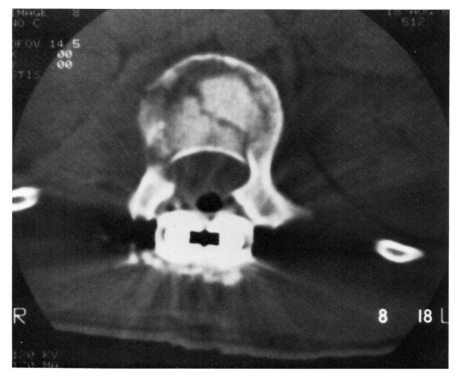

Fig. 18-32 *(Continued).* **(I)** Postoperative CT scan showing reconstitution of vertebral body alignment and retraction of bone from posterior canal. Note Harrington rods posteriorly.

18-32). This groove allows the rod to be depressed down against the posterior lamina, and allows the lower end of the Harrington distraction rod to fit into the 1254 hook. When the lower rod-hook attachment is secured, the ratchet-hook spreader is inserted superiorly, and distraction between the Harrington rod and the upper hook is applied. Care must be taken not to overdistract the spinal segments (Fig. 18-34). This is a particularly sensitive problem when there has been associated vertebral element displacement or significant vertebral body comminution (though Holdsworth believed these fractures to be stable[12]) and the likelihood of loss of continuity. A consideration to be taken into account is the relative stability of the anterior longitudinal ligament. A method of determining this is described in Chapter 17 (see Fig. 17-5A,B,C). When intact, along with the posterior longitudinal ligament, distraction across the fracture may result

in significant reduction of the fracture, including fragments extruded into the neural canal (Fig. 18-32).

Distraction at the fracture site has two adverse affects: it contributes to internal fixation instability, and it delays fracture fragment healing (Fig. 18-35).

In the presence of anticipated instability or excessive kyphosis, and the likely loss of internal fixation as a result, it may be appropriate to ensure rod-vertebral element stability by inserting Luque wires under one or two of the intervening lamina above and below the fracture (see Luque Segmental Spinal Instrumentation, below) before the insertion of the posterior Harrington distraction apparatus (see Fig. 18-42). Great care must be taken during the passage of the sublaminar wires not to further injure the already traumatized dura and contained neural elements.

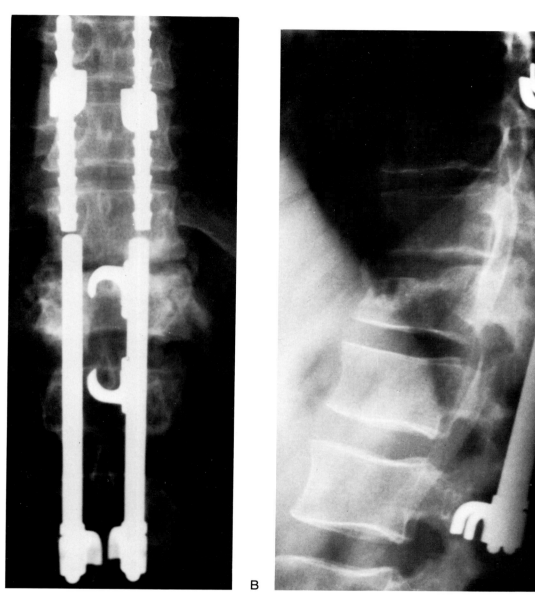

A   B

Fig. 18-33. (A) AP thoracolumbar radiograph showing healed fracture of T12. Note fracture of Harrington rods at ratchet-shank junction, which approximates the previous T12 fracture level. The patient was referred for hardware removal. (B) Lateral view shows the level of fracture and the shank-ratchet portion of the Harrington rod. Note also the combined usage of Harrington compression rod on posterior spinous processes of T11–T12.

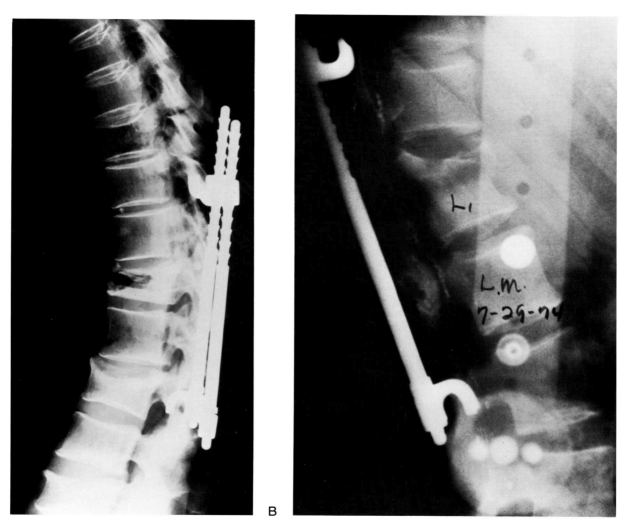

A   B

Fig. 18-34. (A) Lateral radiograph of autopsy specimen. Note distraction through the fracture site when a distraction force applied to the Harrington rods. (B) Lateral radiograph of thoracolumbar spine showing distraction through the fracture site in a patient with a compression fracture of L1.

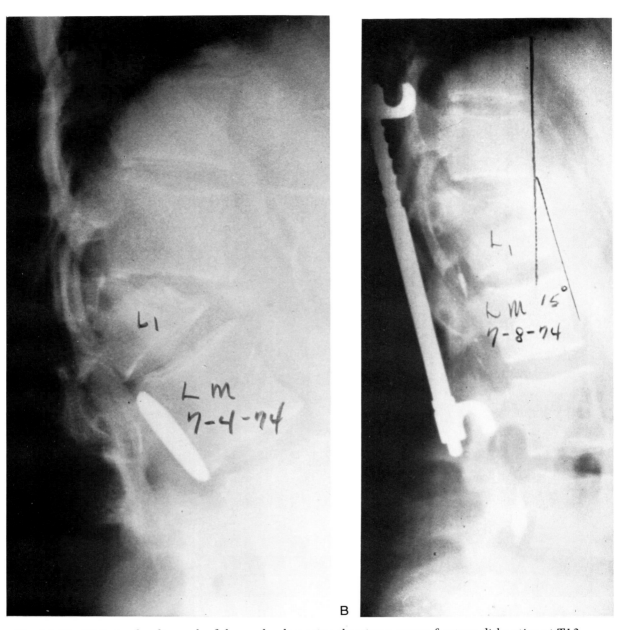

A

B

Fig. 18-35. (A) Lateral radiograph of thoracolumbar spine showing a severe fracture dislocation at T12–L1. Patient had L2 complete neurologic injury. (B) Lateral radiograph showing compression fracture of the L1 vertebral body. Note that Harrington rod apparatus is inserted only one level above and one level below the fracture site. The vertebral body height has been reconstituted by distraction forces applied through the Harrington rod system. *(Figure continues.)*

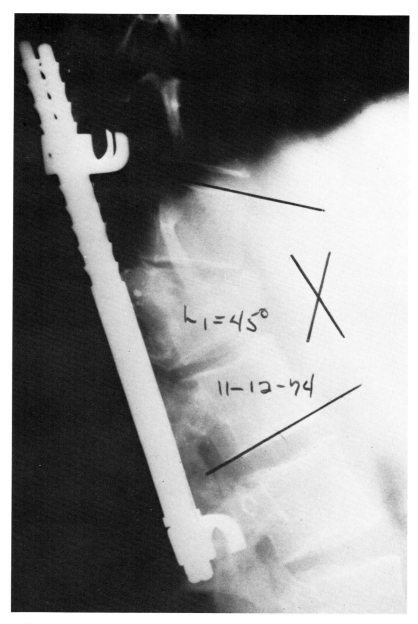

C

Fig. 18-35 *(Continued)*. **(C)** Lateral radiograph showing increased angulation across the fracture site due to insufficient length of Harrington rod proximal and distal to fracture site. Apparatus of proper length should allow two intact laminae above and below the fracture site.

Once the rods (and wires) are in place and appropriate distraction has been applied, the wires are tightened around the Harrington rods (Fig. 18-33). To prevent lateral displacement of the Harrington rods, wires may be inserted transversely between the two Harrington rods, one superior and one inferior to the level of the fracture. Once in place, they are tightened. These latter wires contribute to linear stability.

Wisconsin Compression Rod System

After the appropriately placed posterior incision is made, exposing the posterior vertebral elements, threaded Wisconsin compression rods[22] of appropriate length are selected. They may be further cut (with a rod cutter) to appropriate length before insertion. The number of compression hooks required bilaterally depends on the number of segments to be crossed. The advantage of the Wisconsin rod-hook system is that each hook can be inserted under its respective lamina, independent of the compression rod. This greatly simplifies the procedure, and allows each hook to be singularly inserted into the appropriate laminar interspace, and the lamina to be rongeured for fit if need be.

When each hook-laminar complex has been prepared, the Wisconsin compression (threaded) rod is laid into the groove of each of the in place 1204 hooks. Along the rod, appropriately positioned on the side facing opposite the hook, a "Keene" bushing is slid over the rod, one for each of the four hooks (two above and two below the fracture) on each side. Also applied is a hex nut at each location. The Keene bushing prevents displacement of the rod from the hook once applied. The hex nut is for the application of compression on each nut-bushing-hook complex as they are set into place. Counterforce is required from the hook facing the opposite direction, to maintain the position of the device and apply compression across the fracture site. This procedure is carried out alternately at each level, bilaterally, until both rods are tightened in place. Intraoperative radiographs can be used to check for the desired surgical correction.

Luque Segmental Spinal Instrumentation

The introduction of the Luque segmental fixation ("L" or "rectangular") rods, and the use of sublaminar wire for fixation of the rods to the posterior elements, has provided a significant advancement in the armamentarium of spinal instrumentation. First introduced by Eduardo Luque of Mexico in the late 1970s and early 1980s, and first reported as a series of 14 patients in the journal *Spine* in 1982,[3] the procedure now serves as a major alternative to Harrington rod[10] spinal fixation.[4] The Luque rod technique of spinal stabilization provides immediate spinal stability by direct fixation of the implant to uninjured posterior spinal elements (lamina) above and below the fracture site, at multiple bilateral levels. With the use of the original L shaped rods, a paralytic curve could be positively corrected by the application of the Luque rods above and below the curve apex and the placement of transverse wires between the two upright rods, appropriately placed along the curve (Fig. 18-36). With early spinal fracture management, the same improved alignment opportunity exists (Fig. 18-36). With the use of the rectangular Luque rods, correction of the spine in the sagittal projection can be accurately obtained; however, the same corrective advantage does not exist in the coronal plane. Therefore, the rationale for the use of the L or rectangular-shaped Luque system should be considered. Prebending the rods in the sagittal plane allows the accommodation of both the normal thoracic and thoracolumbar kyphosis or lumbar lordosis, or for the correction of a fracture deformity (Fig. 18-36). The use of the Luque rod spinal stabilization system allows scoliosis or acute (trauma-induced) angular deformities to be corrected; sagittal deformities (kyphosis or lordosis), either naturally occurring or traumatically induced, to be maintained, corrected, or eliminated; in the presence of spinal fracture instability, stability can be immediately restored.

Luque rod instrumentation is an excellent stabilizing procedure for fractures of the lumbar spine, particularly when neurologic function remains intact and where the neural canal is wide. It is very well suited for fractures of the anterior vertebral column (wedge compression fractures) in the thor-

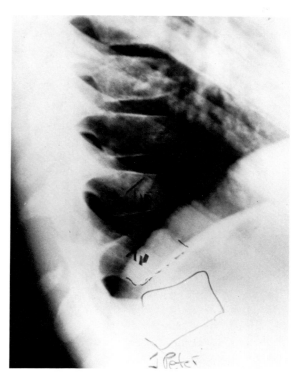
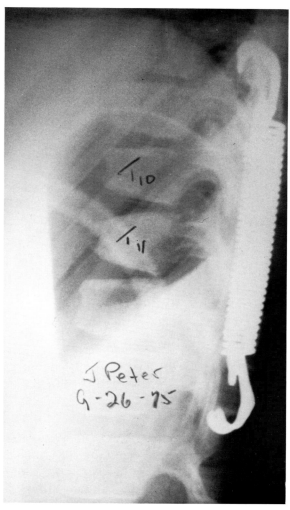

A   B

Fig. 18-36. (A) Lateral radiograph of lower thoracic spine showing a fracture dislocation of T10 on T11 in a 9-year-old girl. Note the extent of kyphosis secondary to the fracture. (B) Postoperative lateral radiograph showing correction of the traumatic kyphosis and reduction of the dislocated T10-T11 facets. Internal fixation is by compression (Weiss) springs (no longer utilized). The internal fixation device crosses two intact laminae above and below fracture site. *(Figure continues.)*

acolumbar and lumbar areas of the spine. This is not the case in the thoracic vertebral column, where the neural canal is narrow and the blood supply to the spinal cord is precarious. Great care must be exercised when passing Luque wires beneath the lamina. Similar to the use of Harrington rods, fixation of the Luque system to the spine requires fixation two levels above and below the level

of injury. The technique can be utilized only one level above or below a fracture (when no other alternative exists), as long as careful use of a postoperative orthosis for 3 months is part of the management regimen.

After the appropriate incision is made, thoroughly exposing the appropriate vertebral elements (see Standard Posterior Approach, above), a

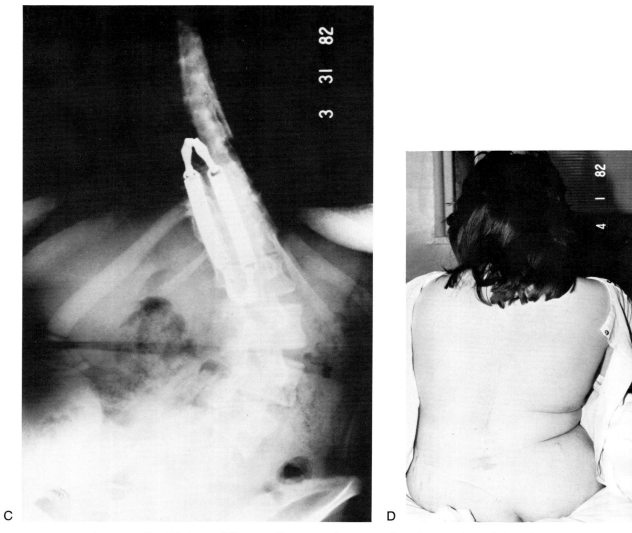

C

D

Fig. 18-36 *(Continued)*. **(C)** 7-year follow-up film. Note the onset of paralytic scoliosis below the level of the fixation device. The patient's neurologic level was T11 complete. **(D)** Posterior view of the patient showing the paralytic scoliosis. The patient was reoperated, and sublaminar (Luque) wires and a transverse Harrington sacral bar were inserted. *(Figure continues.)*

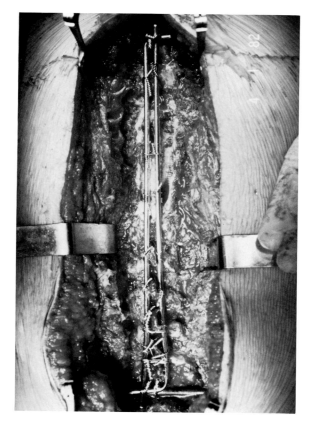

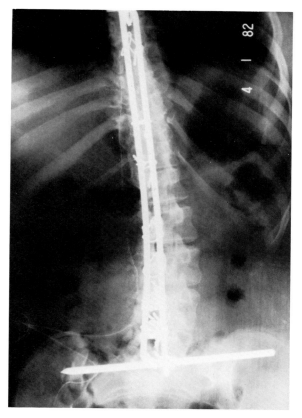

E

F

Fig. 18-36 *(Continued)*. **(E)** Surgical view of Luque rods in place. Note fixation inferiorly to transverse sacral bar, and transverse wires maintaining central alignment of the Luque rods. **(F)** Post-operative radiograph demonstrating significant improvement in the scoliosis.

right-angle Luque rod (¼-inch short rod) is cut to the appropriate length. If the rectangular rod system is used, the appropriate length rectangular rod is selected. This system is much less cumbersome than the use of two L rods. The disadvantage is the lack of tailor-made lengths available in some instances.

When using two L rods (one rod has the L shape at the top, the opposite rod has the L at the bottom) (Fig. 18-36), each rod is bent in the sagittal plane to provide, maintain, or restore the normal (prefracture) vertebral column alignment. With the rods in place, the upper L should lie transversely between the second and third spinous process above the fractured vertebral element, and extend distally to the second and third interspinous space below the fracture site. The presence of posterior element

fractures over multiple levels may force the surgeon to extend the fixation more proximal or distally than normal.

Prepared Luque wire (18-gauge) loops are used for fixation of the rods to the lamina. The wires are appropriately bent to pass easily beneath and between each lamina, after a small "window" laminotomy has been made in the ligamentum flavum and lamina at each level (Fig. 18-37B). The wires are passed into each intralaminar and sublaminar space from an inferior to a superior direction. As the wire exits the intralaminar space above, it is pulled through to approximately one-half the length of the wire. The wire is left doubled at the upper and lower four corners. At each intervening level, the wire loop is cut with a wire cutter and one side of the wire is taken to the right, the other side to the left. This means there will be a double wire on the right and the left sides of the lamina at the upper and lower four corners, and a single wire on the right and left sides of each of the intervening laminae (if stable and not comminuted, otherwise omit).

The Luque rods (both L and rectangular rods) are inserted by the weaving of the sublaminar wires (at each level one wire internal to the rod and one external) at each successive level. The rule "down and out" is used to uniformly place the Luque wires around the rods. The double wires at each of the four corners are tightened first to fix the Luque rod systems in place. Special wire tighteners are available, but standard vise grip wire tighteners will suffice. As the wires are tightened they are pulled taut, perpendicular to the surface of each lamina. When the four outer corners are tight, each of the other wires is sequentially tightened. To further enhance the stability of the rods, a double transverse wire is placed beneath the Luque rods (when the two-rod system is used) at a level above and below the fracture level (Fig. 18-36). Tightening these wires (usually double strands) pulls the two Luque rods toward the midline and tends to straighten out any existing curve, while also increasing the stability of the system.

Before the Luque rod system is inserted, the external surface of each lamina is decorticated with a high speed burr. When the rods and wires are in place and tightened, the spinous processes are rongeured down to the level of the Luque rods, but not below. This bone, along with an axillary bone graft obtained from one of the posterior iliac wings, is inserted along the fixation site. It is the surgeon's decision to extend the fusion along the entire length of the internal fixation, or only in the middle, to include one level above and one level below the injury site.

Posterior "Locking Hook-Spinal Rod System" (AO Synthes-Jacobs)

The posterior locking hook-spinal rod (AO-Jacobs rod) system of internal spinal stabilization, while not new, has recently (1985) achieved sufficient acceptance that clinical experience is now being gathered.[8,9,15] At present, its use is less than

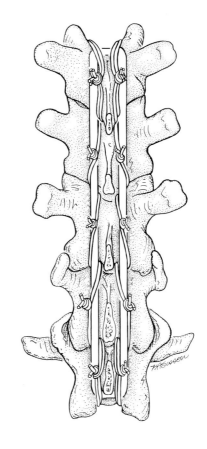

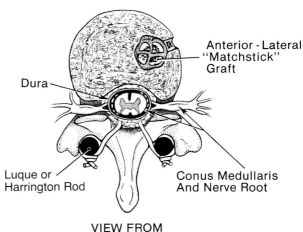

Dura

Anterior - Lateral "Matchstick" Graft

Luque or Harrington Rod

Conus Medullaris And Nerve Root

VIEW FROM UNDERSURFACE OF T-11

Fig. 18-37. Technique for the insertion of sublaminar wires. *(Figure continues.)*

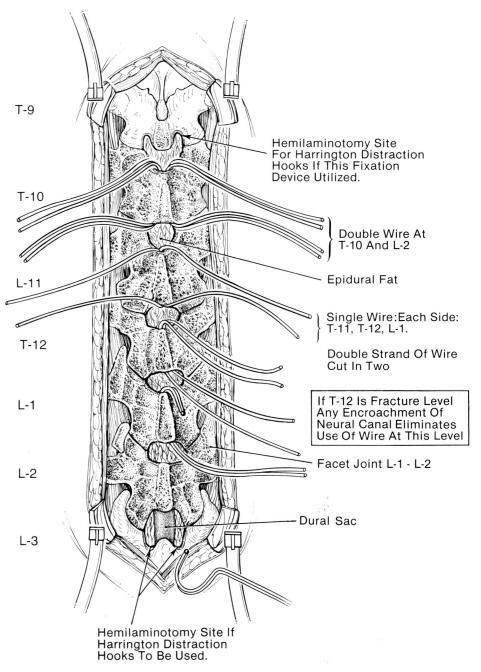

T-9

T-10

L-11

T-12

L-1

L-2

L-3

Hemilaminotomy Site
For Harrington Distraction
Hooks If This Fixation
Device Utilized.

Double Wire At
T-10 And L-2

Epidural Fat

Single Wire:Each Side:
T-11, T-12, L-1.

Double Strand Of Wire
Cut In Two

If T-12 Is Fracture Level
Any Encroachment Of
Neural Canal Eliminates
Use Of Wire At This Level

Facet Joint L-1 - L-2

Dural Sac

Hemilaminotomy Site If
Harrington Distraction
Hooks To Be Used.

Fig. 18-37 (*Continued*).

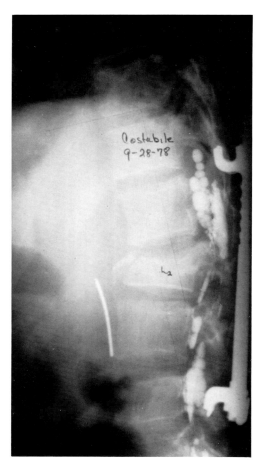

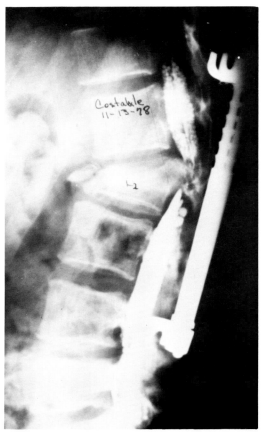

A   B

Fig. 18-38. (**A**) Lateral radiograph showing internal fixation of a compression fracture of the L2 vertebral body by Harrington distraction rods. Note the inappropriate length of the rod-hook complex. Two intact laminae should be spanned proximal and distal to fracture site, not including the hook fixation level. (**B**) Lateral radiograph 3 months later. Note displacement of the upper hooks and resulting increase in the thoracolumbar kyphosis at L1–L2. *(Figure continues.)*

initially anticipated. This is due to minor degrees of difficulty with insertion, a need for "exactness" with device fixation to the lamina, and the proven acceptance of the Harrington distraction procedure.

The AO Synthes rods have many of the characteristics of the Harrington distraction rod system and can thus be viewed as a modification of that device. There are nonetheless, two specific differences: the thickness of the AO rod (7 mm versus the 4-mm Zimmer rod) and the locking of the top hook into the upper lamina. Threaded at both ends, hooks are rotationally locked to meshed washers (with radial grooves) that are then tightened in

place by nuts, and "keyed" to the two flat sides of the rod. This portion of the apparatus is designed to prevent rod-hook rotation with respect to axial alignment, and upper lamina-hook displacement. Like any procedure, the anticipated results do not always measure up to the surgical result. Occasionally, the upper hook becomes displaced from the upper lamina because of loose fixation of the locking device, or tearing away of the hook from the lamina. This has been found to occur in the presence of an increasing kyphotic deformity (Fig. 18-38), due to either further collapse of the fracture or insufficient distraction applied initially.

After the appropriate incision is made, thor-

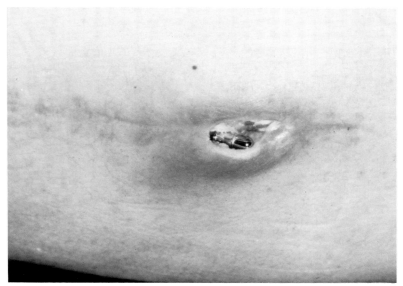

C

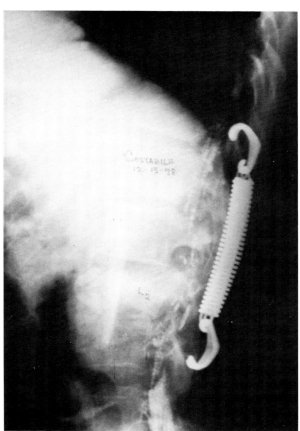

D

Fig. 18-38 *(Continued)*. (C) View of thoracolumbar junction showing the tip of the Harrington rod eroding through the skin secondary to the onset of acute kyphosis and pressure against the orthosis upright. (D) Lateral radiograph after removal of the Harrington rods and correction of the kyphosis by compression springs.

oughly exposing the appropriate vertebral elements, the AO rod is bent into either a lordotic or kyphotic shape in its midportion, to conform to or reestablish a thoracic kyphosis or lumbar lordosis, often lost with vertebral fracture. The solid (nonthreaded) portion of the rod, in its middle third, should lie opposite and adjacent the level of the fracture site. The lower unit, composed of a nut, a mesh washer, a lower hook, and the lowermost nut, is assembled onto the lower threaded rod. Only a very short portion of the threaded rod should be allowed to extend beneath the lower hook (Fig. 18-39). This portion of the device is then inserted as a unit beneath the lowermost lamina. Sometimes, because of the prominence of the defect (kyphosis), the lamina just above the one into which the lower hook attaches will be so prominent as to impede the insertion of the lower rod-hook assembly (similar to that discussed with Harrington rod insertion). If so, I have found it helpful to make a vertical groove, using a high-speed burr, in the next higher lamina (outer cortex only) just lateral to the spinous process (Fig. 18-32). This will allow the lower rod-hook complex to lie in closer approximation with the lamina just above the hook-lamina attachment level, and greatly facilitate rod insertion.

The insertion of the upper hook is more difficult and time consuming. It requires that the hook be inserted at an angle, pointing in the direction of the dura and superiorly. Pressure directed anteriorly on the rod-hook complex, against the vertebral column, is required to produce correction of the traumatic kyphosis (if present), and to start the superior hook beneath the upper lamina. Once beneath the lamina, the hook is tapped anteriorly and superiorly to obtain a solid seating. When the hook is in place, the upper border of the lamina under which the upper hook lies is notched, and a locking device is slid down over the top of the rod, turned in line with the upper hook, and tightened down over the superior lamina, producing a locking of the upper hooks to the lamina (Fig. 18-39). This then allows the application of a distraction force beneath the upper hook-lamina assembly by the lower hook-nut assembly, and should provide a solid fitting of the superior hook to the adjacent superior lamina. The nuts superiorly and inferiorly are crimped along their lateral sides, causing the nuts to con-

form with the lateral (flattened) sides of the rod superiorly and inferiorly. The system is thus locked, preventing rotation or shortening of the rod-hook complex. To help prevent dislodgement of the upper hooks, distraction between the upper and lower hooks must be applied from the inferior end. Should gross instability and loss of ligamentous stability be present both anteriorly and posteriorly (along with comminution of the anterior vertebral body), sublaminar wires might be used to supplement stability at selected levels, similar to their use with the Luque or the Harrington rod system (Fig. 18-39).

AO Internal Fixator System

The technique for the insertion of the AO posterior internal fixator (Fig. 18-40) is identical to the insertion of the Roy-Camille posterior plate and screws (Fig. 18-12). The posterior approach is utilized, followed by the appropriate identification of the pedicles with the assistance of a "C" arm image intensifier and a radiologic table top in the following manner.

Anatomically in the thoracic spine, the position of insertion of the threaded Schanz screws is at the lower edge of the joint and 2 mm lateral to the middle of the joint.

In the lumbar spine, the pedicle position lies directly lateral to the cranial articular process, at the level of the middle of the transverse process (Fig. 18-40).

To prevent injury to the nervous system during insertion of the Schanz screws, it is advised that the screws are directed 10 degrees anteromedial in the thoracic spine area and approximately 5 degrees anteromedial in the lumbar spine (Fig. 18-40).

Preceding the insertion of the Schanz screw, a 2.0-mm smooth k-wire should be inserted into the pedicles, to a depth of 30 mm, and its position checked by image intensification in the anteroposterior and lateral planes.

One Kirschner wire is removed at a time and replaced with a 3.5-mm Schanz screw. The depth of the screw's insertion in the thoracic region is approximately 40 to 45 mm, and in the lumbar and sacral regions, the depth is 40 mm. The ac-

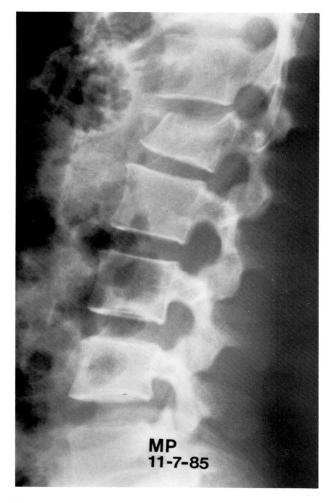

A

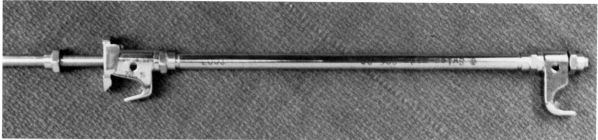

B

Fig. 18-39. (A) Lateral radiograph of thoracolumbar spine showing a compression fracture of L1. (B) AO Synthes (Jacobs) posterior locking hook spinal rod. This rod is threaded at each end. Lower end is thread-nut locked to prevent rod hook displacement. Distraction across the fracture site is gained through the threaded proximal rod end. Note shelf (laminar locking device) over proximal hook. Rod is 7 mm thick and is less likely to suffer fatigue fracture with bending prior to insertion. *(Figure continues.)*

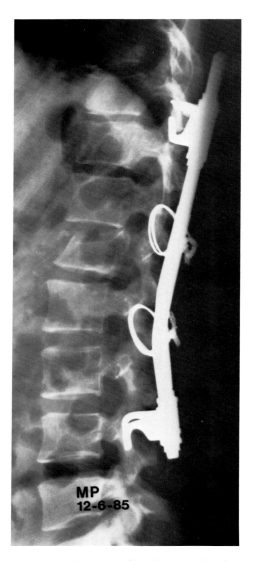

C

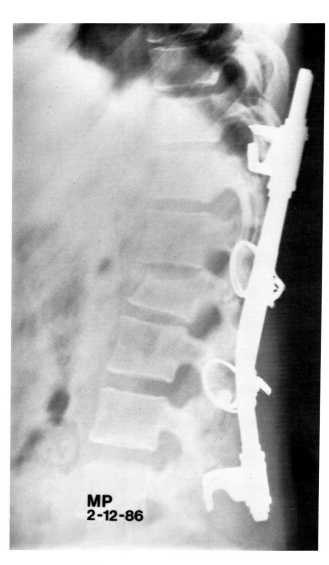

D

Fig. 18-39 *(Continued).* (**C**) Lateral radiograph showing improved thoracolumbar alignment and internal fixation by AO rods. (**D**) Lateral radiograph 6 days after operation show dislocation of the AO rod inferiorly, with resulting increase in the thoracolumbar kyphosis. The rods had to be replaced.

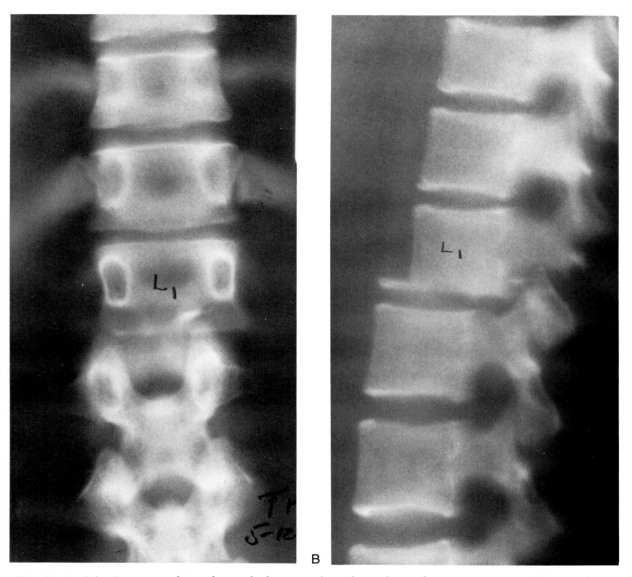

A   B

Fig. 18-40. (A) AP tomographic radiograph showing a lateral translation fracture at L1–L2. (B) Lateral tomogram showing retroluxation of L1 and L2 with associated slice fracture through inferior surface L1. Note fracture through posterior elements L1. On a myelogram, the flow of contrast was obstructed at L1–L2. *(Figure continues.)*

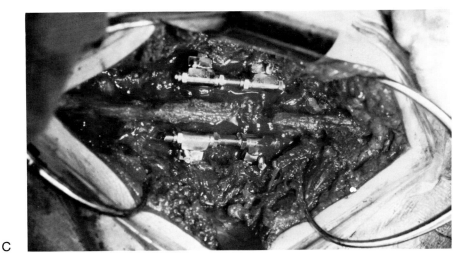

C

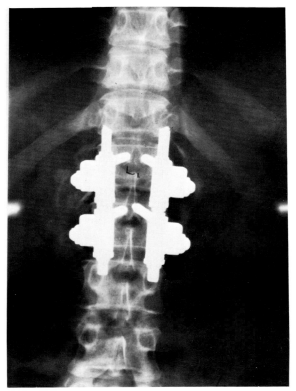

D

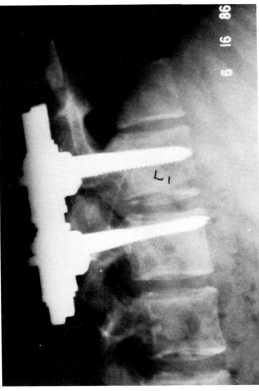

E

Fig. 18-40 *(Continued).* **(C)** Operative view showing final position of AO internal fixator. The construction of this device allows angular corrections as well as compression or distraction to improve fracture alignment. **(D)** Postoperative AP radiograph showing lateral-to-medial, inferior-to-superior placement of schanz pins into vertebral bodies L1 and L2. **(E)** Lateral radiograph showing total reduction of inferior slice fracture through L1 and improved alignment of the vertebral column.

tual depth is controlled by lateral imaging until the screws reach the anterior cortex of the vertebral body.

Image intensification guidance of the Schanz screw is advised for obtaining the correct level; passage through the pedicle; and passage through the vertebral body parallel to the superior vertebral end plate, directed toward the middle of the vertebral body anteriorly (Fig. 18-40). It is important to remember that the vertebral bodies are round anteriorly, so one must be careful that the Schanz screws do not pass out anteriorly too far before they are seen radiographically.

The internal fixator is applied over the Schanz screws. Before cutting, the screws are manipulated to correct the spinal deformity present. The correction is monitored by image intensification. When the spinal correction and alignment are acceptable, the fixator is tightened onto the Schanz screws.

By means of the nut on the internal fixator, distraction or compression of the fracture is possible. When the desired position is attained, the nuts are tightened and crimped in place, along the flat sides of the rod (Fig. 18-40).

Postoperative management should include the use of an external orthosis, particularly when the injury is accompanied by the presence of a neurologic deficit or in the presence of tumor. The device is worn for 8 to 12 weeks postoperatively. This should provide sufficient time for healing of the fractured vertebral elements. If the problem is tumor related, the spine may require external orthotic protection for a more indefinite period of time.

Weiss Compression Springs System

Historically, the Weiss compression spring procedure (Fig. 18-41) is included for completeness. While reserved for select occasions, the use of this method of spinal trauma instrumentation (producing dynamic compression) became a surgical alternative in the mid 1970s, having been popularized by Marian Weiss of Warsaw, Poland. The spring compression concept was initially introduced into the spinal instrumentation armamentarium in the

1950s and early 1960s as a means of correcting paralytic scoliosis. Because of the transverse process placement of the spring-hooks for fixation, failure of the fixation was a complication. For trauma, the compression springs demonstrate a modest level of success, though their stability surgically and in the laboratory was less than required. The primary deficit in stabilization was failure in rotation. Through personal experience, the device was found most indicated for injuries to the spine in which posterior ligamentous disruption occurred (in association with facet dislocation without fracture). It is not indicated when significant fracture of either the anterior or posterior elements has occurred.

Using fresh cadaver specimens, Pinzer et al.[23] observed four-point loading-stability characteristics of Harrington distraction rods, Harrington compression rods, and compression (Weiss) springs. The elastic modulus of each device was compared with that of the preinjured state. Fixation with Harrington compression rods was found to have the highest elastic modulus (i.e., was the most stiff), yet failed with the least amount of displacement. Similar findings were reported by Stauffer and Neil.[24] The compression springs were found to have the least elastic modulus, yet maintained internal fixation continuity with pure flexion displacement the longest. Failure occurred when the combination of flexion and rotation was present.[6,23] Again, similar findings were identified by Stauffer and Neil.[24] Thus, from laboratory analysis, it was determined that compression springs were more favorably indicated for anterior lumbar vertebral body fractures of minor degree and for ligamentous disruption of the posterior column, while the middle column remained intact and without evidence of sagittal or coronal translation. The device in this case was thought indicated because of the already inherent stability of the spine remaining, ease of insertion, fixation at only two points (proximally and distally, rather than at four points as with the Harrington compression or Wisconsin compression devices), fewer segments crossed (than with the Harrington compression rod), and because the system was dynamic and tended to produce posterior compression with mild anterior distraction (when the anterior longitudinal ligament was intact), resulting in correction of the traumatically induced kyphosis (Figs. 18-36,

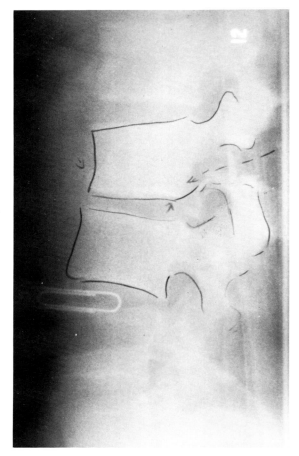

A

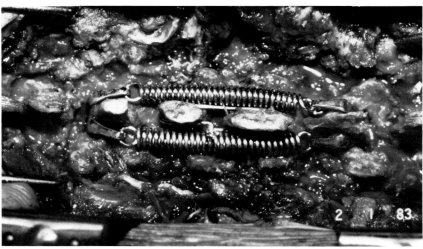

B

Fig. 18-41. (A) Lateral radiograph of thoracolumbar spine showing a Chance-type fracture of L2, extending through the posterior elements and posteroinferior aspect of the L2 vertebral body. (B) Surgical view showing posterior internal fixation with double stainless steel wires between adjacent spinous processes and compression springs across fracture site. Wiring between posterior spinous processes is used to maintain reduction of dislocated facets during insertion of internal fixation device. *(Figure continues.)*

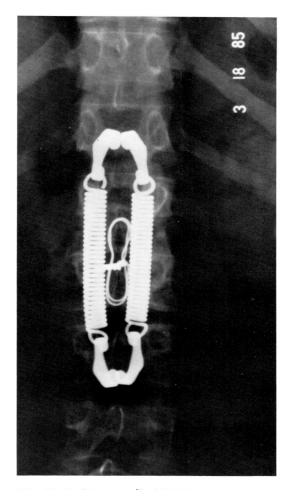

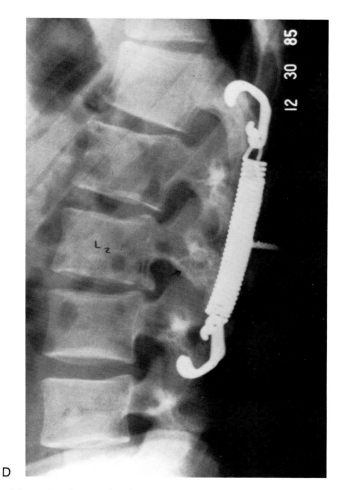

C   **D**

Fig. 18-41 *(Continued)*. (C,D) Postoperative AP and lateral radiographs showing improved alignment in sagittal plane secondary to healing of the fracture.

18-37, 18-41). As noted, the device was most attractive for maintaining compression fixation (with an external orthosis) in the presence of pure facet dislocation.

After the appropriate incision is made, thoroughly exposing the appropriate vertebral elements (see Standard Posterior Approach, above), the appropriate length spring is selected. The length used (5 to 12 cm) is commensurate with the distance between the upper and lower laminae, minus approximately 1.5 to 2 cm (the length to which the spring will stretch if it is 9 cm long). Shorter springs have less stretch available. As a rule, a distraction force across a stretched spring

system (between the upper hook and lower hook) is approximately 30 to 40 lbs. This dynamic compression load is capable of producing minor degrees of correction of a traumatic kyphotic deformity (Fig. 18-42).

Iliac Crest Bone Graft Approach

The position of the patient, that is, supine, prone, or in the lateral decubitus position, relates directly to the procedure to be performed. If only a straight posterior procedure is to be performed in the thoracolumbar junctional area of the spine, then bone

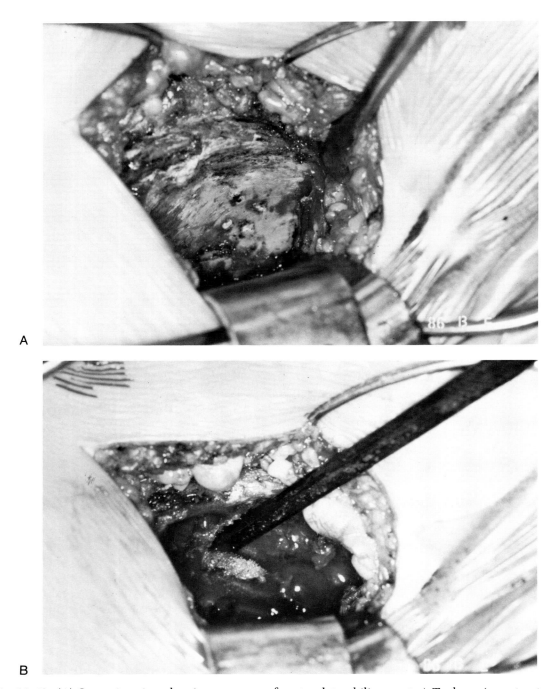

A

B

Fig. 18-42. (A) Operative view showing exposure of posterolateral iliac crest. A Taylor spine retractor is used inferiorly to displace the gluteus maximus muscle laterally. (B) Bone gouge used to remove a cancellous bone curl from the space between the inner and outer tables of the iliac crest. *(Figure continues.)*

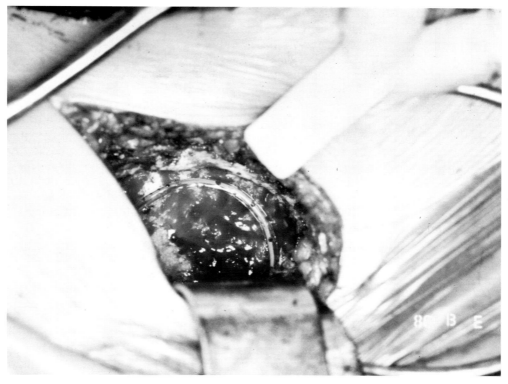

C

Fig. 18-42 *(Continued)*. (C) Bone graft donor site following harvesting of the bone graft. The interstices of the remaining cancellous bone are closed with sterile bone wax (seen in the photo in brick form), followed by insertion of a hemovac catheter prior to closure. Care must be taken to remove all excess bone wax. The wound is closed in the routine manner.

can be obtained from the posterior iliac crest through a separate posterior iliac crest incision (Fig. 18-42; and see Fig. 17-15). If the patient is to undergo a combined transthoracic and posterior spine procedure, a posterior iliac crest incision again is the method utilized for harvesting the posterior iliac crest graft. Rarely, either the anterior or middle area of the iliac crest has been used for bone graft. The problem is that the ilium is narrow, bicortical, and has less bone available for harvesting. Because the patient is normally placed in the right lateral decubitus position for the performance of the combined anterior-posterior procedure, the left iliac crest becomes the donor site. When the patient is prone, either crest is utilized.

The posterior crest is approached through a curved incision over the posterior crest, from the posterior sacroiliac joint to the lateral aspect of the posterior ilium. Without entering the sacroiliac joint, the incision is carefully carried down to the crest, first by sharp dissection and then by electocautery dissection. This latter technique is used to reduce bleeding (Fig. 18-42C). Care is taken not to incise the muscles inserting onto the iliac crest, rather to dissect them off of the iliac crest directly, by electrocautery dissection. Similarly, with subperiosteal dissection, the gluteus maximus muscle is stripped away from the external iliac table and held in a retracted position by a pair of Taylor spine retractors. This accomplished, curls of external cortical table and cancellous bone are then removed with a straight or curved gouge (Fig. 18-42). As much cancellous bone is removed from the space between the two cortical tables of the iliac crest as possible, taking care not to go through the inner table of the ilium owing to its thinness, into the substance of the iliacus muscle (on the inner side), and not to enter the sacroiliac joint while obtaining cancellous bone from the most posterior iliac crest.

Upon completion of the harvesting of the bone graft, bone wax is carefully and evenly compressed with the finger and a sponge (4×4) into the interstices of the remaining cancellous bone. This is done to prevent the formation of a postoperative wound hematoma. To further discourage the formation of a hematoma, a medium Hemovac is placed into the wound before closure. (Fig. 18-42). Great care must be taken to remove all loose pieces of bone and loose wax (capable of acting as foreign bodies) before wound closure. When this is accomplished, the wound is closed in a routine fashion.

SURGICAL COMPLICATIONS

It is a major consideration to undertake the anterior approach because of the potential hazards of the approach, the possibility of producing injury to major structures or vital organs, the hazard of extending the already present neurologic injury with surgical decompression of the anterior dura, or some other unsuspected problem. I have experienced these problems, making it worthwhile to briefly review each and the management process utilized in their resolution. Parenthetically, it is important that each of the problems herein described, be discussed in detail with the patient and his or her family before surgery. Their being preoperatively aware of the hazards, and sharing in the burden, enhances the surgeon-patient relationship, and smooths out the postoperative management. It also ensures that the patient has been duly informed.

Bleeding

Bleeding or hemorrhage during the anterior chest approach is always a potential hazard. Although generalized bleeding from a complication such as "consumption coagulopathy" is a possibility, usually its onset can be recognized early, and management procedures instituted, that is, ensuring the availability of fresh frozen plasma, platelets, fresh whole blood, etc.

Drugs or Medications
Bleeding may follow the preoperative use of heparin or coumadin (used in the prophylactic prevention of deep venous thrombosis). Although heparin is rapidly metabolized (4 hours), coumadin requires days unless reversed by vitamin A (3 to 6 hours). Aspirin, used preoperatively as a prophylactic platelet adhesive for the prevention of deep venous thrombosis, may result in diffuse, continuous bleeding and failure to coagulate. Treatment is the administration of platelets, fresh frozen plasma, and fresh blood.

Small Vessel Bleeding
Small vessel bleeding usually arises from one of two sources: a vertebral segmental vessel or an intercostal artery. The consequence of this slow bleeding (usually appearing late) is a second operative procedure to correct the problem. An intercostal artery should be expected if the blood from the chest tube is bright red. Finally, bleeding may result from injury to a major vessel such as the vena cava or aorta. Injury to either is immediately recognizable and requires the assistance of a vascular surgeon (Fig. 18-24).

Major Vessel Bleeding
As described under Anterior Surgical Approach: Considerations, great care must be taken to isolate and protect the aorta in the area of vertebral column injury, when one is performing a vertebral body corporectomy or removal of disc material. Because the wall of the aorta has a well-defined muscular layer, allowing for a stable surgical repair (whereas the vena cava is thinner and unaccompanied anatomically by prominent muscular layers), the preferred approach to the chest is the left anterolateral approach. This allows the surgeon to work in the proximity of the aorta (which lies anterior to the vertebral column; (Fig. 18-24) rather than in the vicinity of the vena cava. To prepare for the uncommon and unusual complication of injury to the aorta, an umbilical tape can be placed circumferentially around the aorta, above and below the levels where the surgeon may be working (Fig. 18-24). The tails of the tapes can be pulled through

a rubber catheter, and a hemostat applied to the ends of the tapes. Should injury to the aorta occur, the tapes and the rubber catheter can be immediately tightened down on the aorta. This is not a routine procedure, but is recommended when dissection around the aorta is difficult.

Pulmonary

Bleeding from the pulmonary parenchyma is infrequent and usually results from direct trauma to a vascular segment of the lung. What is more common is bleeding associated with the insertion of a chest catheter (with injury to an intercostal vessel). Bleeding will be brisk, moderate, and progressive. On only one occasion (in 70 patients with a diagnosed hemothorax) did this complication occur (1.4 percent), requiring surgical intervention. Under such circumstances, blood in the chest catheter and Pleur-evac will be bright red. If the amount lost in 1 hour exceeds 750 ml, surgical exploration is required. Blood from a hemothorax, on the other hand, will be thin, nonclotting, slightly pink, and combined with reactive fluid from the chest. After closure of the chest, at the completion of an anterior procedure, bleeding may be continuous, at the rate of 1 to 200 ml per hour for several hours, but will then begin to slacken. The source of such bleeding is usually from the interstices of the cancellous vertebral body which was removed, or from the vertebral bodies where inlay bone grafts have been inserted. The chest tube is usually removed within 3 to 5 days. After removal of the tube, the patient should be carefully observed for the reappearance of a hemothorax.

Bone Graft Site Hematoma

Hematoma of the bone graft site is fortunately uncommon. It usually results from the presence of an unrecognized bleeding vessel at the time of wound closure. Because the graft site is in close proximity to the back and chest wound sites (on the combined approach), infection in one area is a concern for the other areas. To reduce the chances of wound hematoma and sepsis, four things are done.

(1) The wound should not be closed until any troublesome bleeding points have been carefully identified. The superior gluteal artery is a vessel that can be injured (as it passes through the substance of the gluteus maximus muscle) with the taking of a posterior iliac bone graft. Other areas to be observant of are the thin portions of the iliac wing posterolaterally. With the removal of cancellous bone in this thin area of the pelvis, it is possible to penetrate the inner table and injure the iliac muscle or a vessel within the pelvis proper.

(2) Generally, most if not all bleeding from the area of cancellous bone can be stopped by the careful use of bone wax in the area from which a bone graft is removed. Care must be taken to remove any excessive wax. If it is left behind, it may serve as a nidus for a foreign body reaction and/or infection.

(3) The operative area must be thoroughly irrigated with saline and operative antibiotic irrigating solution (2 g of neomycin and 250,000 units of bacitracin in 500 ml of 0.9 normal saline, or, as now recommended by the pharmacy: 1 g of cefazolin sodium (Kefzol, Ancef) and 80 mg of gentamicin sulfate (Garamycin, Gentamicin), in 500 ml of 0.9 normal saline).

(4) Before a tight three-layered closure is made, a medium Hemovac catheter is inserted into the depth of the posterior spine wound, where, because of the large exposed surface areas of bone and soft tissue, as well as the amount of free bone graft placed in the wound, prevention of wound hematoma is absolutely required. Either a large or a medium Hemovac catheter is utilized, depending on the anticipated bleeding. The average postoperative loss of blood is 1,894 ml for the posterior procedure alone (Table 18-16).

A question frequently asked is whether there is a difference in the extent of bleeding associated with the different internal fixation techniques. Table 18-17 reveals that the estimated blood loss was highest with the Harrington distraction rod procedure and the Luque procedure. It stands to reason that the combined anterior (thoracotomy)-posterior procedure causes the greatest overall procedural blood loss.

Excessive bleeding during surgery has been found to follow the use of aspirin, as administered prophylactically for the prevention of deep venous thrombosis. This complication has been found to occur even when aspirin has been discontinued 3 to 4 days before the anticipated surgery. What seems to occur at surgery, in the absence of any abnormalities in the bleeding or clotting profile, is excessive bleeding and an absence of clot formation. This

Table 18-17. Thoracolumbar: Estimated Blood Loss by Type of Fixation (Northwestern University Acute Spine Injury Center, 1972 to 1986)

Fixation	No. of Cases	Estimated Blood loss (ml)	SD
Harrington distraction	141	2,964	3,030
Weiss springs	89	2,375	1,975
Luque rods	24	2,488	3,218
Cotrell-Debousett	1	1,500	
Other	7	1,367	671
Missing[a]	208		
Total	470	2,683	2,701

[a]Missing either estimated blood loss or instrumentation.

most likely results from an altered platelet aggregation produced by the aspirin. It is suggested that aspirin not be used preoperatively. When deep venous thrombosis prophylaxis is suggested or required, management should be with subcutaneous heparin (5,000 units bid) or adjusted dose heparin (3,000 to 7,000 units of heparin, bid). The attempt here is to maintain the activated partial thromboplastin time (APTT) at the upper limits of the respective hospital's normal range (Northwestern Memorial Hospital's range is 23 to 35 seconds). Because in b the patients treated with adjusted dose heparin the APTT is actually within the upper range of normal, should unscheduled surgery be required, a delay or "wait" period would not be required. If however, the patient is fully heparinized (the APTT being in the range of 2 to 2.5 times the normal range) and unplanned surgery is required, a wait of 4 to 6 hours (for heparin metabolism) would be required before surgery could proceed. As with aspirin and coumadin therapy, flexibility is lost.

Changes in Neurologic Function

A change in postoperative neurologic function, whether temporary or permanent, is a major concern and must be taken into consideration. Should it occur, more than likely it will be secondary to partial or complete loss in the vascularity of the nervous tissue in the area of the surgery. This complication has been identified after surgical correction of an abdominal aortic aneurysm, which the aorta was cross-clamped to facilitate the repair. After the release of the clamp and upon awakening, the patient reported and demonstrated paraplegia. The complication in this instance was the result of an abnormal lumbar take-off (off the lower abdominal aorta) of the vessel of Adamkiewicz (normally present at the T10 vertebral level). The determination of the permanency of this complication depends on the rapidity of its onset. Rapid or sudden onset of paralysis (upon awaking from a procedure) indicates a high probability of permanent injury. On the other hand, when the neurologic change (or deterioration) is slow and progressive in onset, the experience has been a slow, progressive return of function (weeks to months later). These findings are more likely to be observed in the area of the spinal cord than in the area of the cauda equina.

This vascular complication has been seen as an immediate complication of trauma to the T10–T11 area of the thoracolumbar junctional area of the spine. Fractures within the T11 area may result in "watershed" vascular injury to the spinal cord, hours to days after the fracture. The patient may suddenly demonstrate an ascending neurologic injury, unrelated to obstruction or compromise of the neural canal (proven by CAT scan or myelography). The rationale for the ascending neurologic injury is the occurrence of ischemia of the spinal cord, secondary to injury to the anterior spinal artery. When loss of neurologic function results from ischemia of the spinal cord, flaccid paralysis below the level of injury occurs. Flaccid paralysis is identified with transection of peripheral nerve roots, as with injuries to the cauda equina.

When trauma occurs directly to the spinal cord, resulting in "central cord" syndrome, flaccid paralysis occurs in the area of loss of the anterior horn cells. The area below the injury will, in time, demonstrate spasticity.

Infection

Wound sepsis after elective surgery is fortunately a complication with a low occurrence rate. Care is taken in its prevention in the following manner.

Antibiotics are administered at the institution of each major operative procedure. The protocol calls for the use of a broad-spectrum antibiotic, usually of the cephlosporin variety. The drug of choice has been Kefzol (1 or 2 g administered by IV push at the beginning of an elective operative procedure). This is followed with a repeat of the drug (1 g IV push) every 3 to 4 hours throughout the operative procedure. Antibiotics are continued by IV administration at the rate of 0.5 g every 6 hours for 48 hours, at which time they are discontinued, unless indicated.

As previously noted, all operative wounds (chest approach, posterior spine approach, and bone graft sites) are copiously irrigated with saline and antibiotic irrigation solutions throughout each procedure (see Bone Graft Site Hematoma, above).

Dislodgement of Anterior Bone Graft

Dislodgement of an anterior bone graft, while not unheard of, is not all that common. Inlay grafts may be compressed into the vertebra with axial load, or may be completely displaced. The latter has occurred on one occasion. A patient requiring a posterolateral decompression for neural canal compression secondary to degenerative changes after spine trauma had an interbody bone graft inserted between two unfused segments. The graft extruded itself upon ambulation without a protective orthosis. Re-exploration required removal of the graft, because of neurologic changes (nerve root symptoms), associated weakness, and sensory changes. Decompression of the nerve root was followed by neurologic recovery.

Because of this concern, care is taken to countersink each matchstick graft into the vertebral bodies when performing the anterior approach. Also, to ensure no loss of graft position, postoperative upright radiographs, with the patient in an orthosis, are routinely obtained. This ensures that the patient is stable, before active mobilization. Dislodgement of an anterior bone graft would not be anticipated in a patient stabilized by the combined anterior-posterior approach because of the rigidity gained by the simultaneous posterior stabilization procedure, although it is always a possibility. This complication is a concern in the patient requiring only the anterior approach, as with anterior instru-

mentation procedures, or anterior decompression for resection or decompression of a tumor.

Should dislodgement occur, the hazard is compression of the dura and its contents. Close observation of the postoperative neurologic status is important.

Loss of Internal Fixation

Loss of internal fixation can occur either anteriorly or posteriorly, but because of the frequency of procedures, was more frequently seen posteriorly. The reasons for loss of fixation include stress relaxation of tissues;[23-25] failure of bone at the implant fixation site; fatigue failure of the internal fixation device; inappropriate selection or indication for use of internal fixation device.

Anterior
The type of fixation utilized on the anterior aspect of the vertebral column is usually an inlay matchstick type of bone graft, using iliac crest, rib, or fibula graft. When excision of a primary or metastatic bone tumor is required, resulting in excision of the vertebral body and instability of the vertebral column, stabilization by the addition of some fixation device anteriorly is required. The AO plate and screws and methyl methacrylate procedure has been successfully utilized here (Fig. 18-15). The Dunn device,[21] when it was available, was also used successfully under similar circumstances. This latter device has since been removed from the market because of vascular complications.

Posterior
The two most frequently utilized internal fixation devices are the Harrington distraction rods (Figs. 18-33, 18-35), with and without sublaminar wires, and the Luque rods (Fig. 18-36). The latter require, in each instance, the use of sublaminar wires. Both provide rigid fixation, particularly when the Harrington rod procedure is combined with the use of sublaminar wires (Fig. 18-32F). Several possible reasons for posterior internal fixation failure are inadequate fixation of hooks onto the lamina and sublaminar spaces (Fig. 18-31); placement of the junction of the smooth portion of the Harrington rod at the level of the vertebral fracture (due to anticipated cycling of the implanted rods with

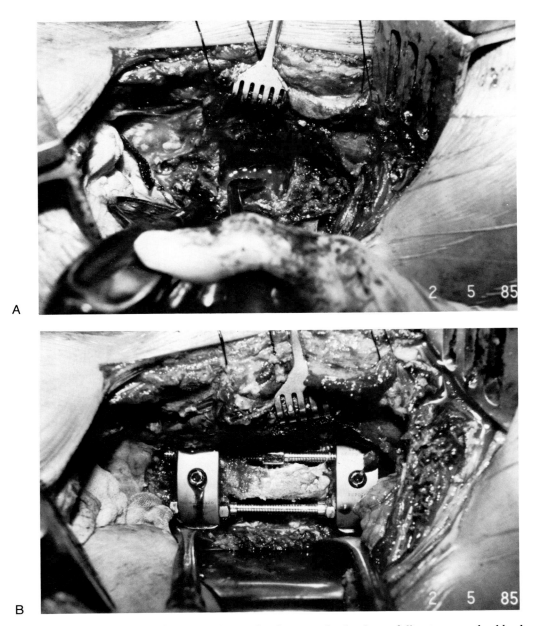

Fig. 18-43. **(A)** Operative view of anterior thoracolumbar vertebral column following vertebral body corporectomy and decompression of dura (seen posteriorly). **(B)** Dunn internal fixator in place producing stable fixation anteriorly (this device is no longer available). Note tricortical iliac crest graft inserted between T12 and L2. *(Figure continues.)*

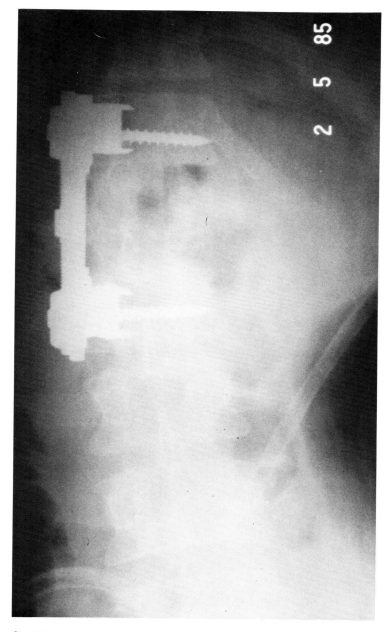

Fig. 18-43 *(Continued).* (C) AP radiograph of thoracolumbar junction following insertion of Dunn apparatus.

functional activity, fatigue failure of the implant of this junction occurs) (Fig. 18-33); disengagement of the lower portion of the Harrington rod from the hook (Fig. 18-31); stress relaxation of the vertebral column secondary to either the application of great amounts of distraction forces on a spine or unrecog-nized ligamentous instability; an inadequate length or inadequate fixation of the device above and below the site of injury. The result is the development of further spinal deformity (kyphosis) at the fracture site (Fig. 18-35).

When Harrington rods are utilized without sublaminar wires, the most frequent cause for failure is stress relaxation of the tissues (interspinous, interdiscal, anterior and posterior longitudinal ligaments) secondary to the application of distraction forces.[23,25] The result is vertebral column elongation—the Harrington rods become "too short for the spine" and the spine lengthens owing to stress (distraction) relaxation. This generally results in dislodgement of the lower hooks, particularly when a bending moment is applied across the lower segment of the spine. This may occur even after a fusion has been accomplished across the fracture site. With bending or flexion of the unfused segments of the spinal column, the column becomes "longer" than the rod, causing the Harrington rods to dislocate themselves from the lower hooks (Fig. 18-31).

One of the two complications identified with the use of the Luque rods is collapse or compression of vertebral elements with axial loading, after stabilization of a burst or comminuted fracture of the lumbar spine with the rectangular or L-shaped rods (see Ch. 17, Fig. 17-19A). The second major complication occurs with the passage of the sublaminar wires. During the process of passage it is possible to traumatize the dura and its contents, producing either a tear in the dura or a neurologic injury. This dural tear complication is frequently inconsequential, although the injury may produce a significant "leak" requiring repair.

Because of the hazard of neurologic injury during the insertion of the Luque wires, this portion of the procedure is closely monitored by SSEP. The method of management usually utilized is maintenance of strict bed rest and, in the presence of a persistent leak, neurosurgical consultation, the performance of a spinal tap, and short-term use of a subarachnoid catheter to maintain a lowered spinal fluid pressure. This will normally allow the rent in the dura to seal over within a week.

FINDINGS AND CONCERNS

It is both interesting and important to observe the neurologic changes that occur between admission and discharge, in the thoracolumbar junction patient group.

Looking at the admission neurologic injury of the thoracic, lumbar, and sacral injury group as a whole, 40.2 percent were complete, 20.5 percent were intact, and 38.8 percent were incomplete. In the thoracolumbar junction injury group, 44 percent were incomplete on admission, 27 percent were intact, and 29 percent were complete (Table 18-16).

On discharge evaluation, using the Frankel scale as the measuring system, an important improvement in the neurologic function appeared. In the T11–L2 junction group, 11.3 percent improved neurologically (one Frankel grade) from admission to discharge, compared with 10.1 percent in the thoracolumbosacral group (Table 18-18).

Table 18-18.   Thoracolumbar versus Lower Spine: Change in Neurologic Status[a]
(Northwestern University Acute Spine Injury Center, 1972 to 1986)

Type of Change	Thoracolumbar No.	Thoracolumbar Percent	Low Spine No.	Low Spine Percent
Improvement	53	11.3	94	10.1
No change	374	79.6	761	81.7
Degradation	10	2.1	15	1.6
Missing[b]	33	7.0	62	6.7
Total	470	100.0	932	100.0

[a]Change criterion is one or more Frankel grades, higher or lower.
[b]Neurologic change is unavailable.

RESULTS

Of the 470 patients with thoracolumbar spine fractures admitted to the acute spine injury service (with complete data) of Northwestern University between 1972 and 1986, the median admission time was 8 hours postinjury. The median time from injury to surgery was 12 days. The median length of hospitalization was 27 days (mode = 14). Seven patients died.

The procedure most frequently performed was the Harrington distraction rod procedure. Within this group, 6 patients (4 percent) demonstrated one Frankel grade of deterioration in their postoperative neurologic examination, while 24 (16 percent) demonstrated at least one Frankel grade of improvement (Table 18-19). A nearly identical degradation and improvement rate was seen with the compression spring device (3 percent degradation and 20 percent improvement). No patient with the Luque system (used in 33 cases) demonstrated loss of function.

The surgical approach most frequently performed was the posterior approach. Within this group, 5 patients (2 percent demonstrated one Frankel grade of deterioration in their postoperative neurologic examination, while 25 (12 percent) demonstrated at least one Frankel grade of improvement (Table 18-20). In the combined anterior-posterior approach (used in 47 cases), 1 pa-

tient (2 percent) demonstrated loss of function, and 12 (25.5 percent) demonstrated evidence of one Frankel grade of improvement.

Of the thoracolumbar fracture patients managed both surgically and conservatively, 79.6 percent remained the same neurologically after admission, while 2.1 percent revealed some evidence of neurologic deterioration, and 11.3 percent demonstrated evidence of neurologic recovery by at least one Frankel grade[26] (Table 18-21).

Although it is difficult to determine accurately whether surgery was indeed the major event resulting in the postoperative return of neurologic function, this finding did occur. As noted in Table 18-21, of the patients operated on, 15.0 percent demonstrated evidence of neurologic recovery, whereas only 5.1 percent of those managed conservatively demonstrated evidence of neurologic recovery. Similarly, in the surgical group, 3.1 percent (nine patients) revealed some neurologic deterioration. In the nonoperative group only one patient (0.06 percent was noted to demonstrate a decrease in neurologic function.

Finally, it appears that surgical stabilization and, when indicated, surgical decompression have a positive influence on neurologic recovery, particularly in the area of the thoracolumbar spine. From the above information, it appears that the risk versus benefits of surgery are significant ($P < 0.001$) and do contribute to neurologic recovery.

Table 18-19. Thoracolumbar: Neurologic Change by Type of Spine Stabilization[a] (Northwestern University Acute Spine Injury Center, 1972 to 1986)

Type of Stabilization	Total Cases	Improvement		No Change		Deterioration		Unknown[b]	
		No.	Percent	No.	Percent	No.	Percent	No.	Percent
Harrington rod distraction	149	24	16.1	110	73.8	6	4.0	9	6.0
Weiss springs	89	18	20.2	66	74.2	3	3.4	2	2.2
Luque rods	33	0	0.0	33	100.0	0	0.0	0	0.0
Cotrell-Debousett	1	0	0.0	1	100.0	0	0.0	0	0.0
Other	9	1	11.1	8	88.9	0	0.0	0	0.0
Missing[c]	189	10	5.3	156	82.5	1	0.5	22	11.6
Total	470	53	11.3	374	79.6	10	2.1	33	7.0

[a]Change criterion is one or more Frankel grades, higher or lower.
[b]Neurologic change is unavailable.
[c]Either no surgery, or instrumentation is unavailable.

Table 18-20.   Thoracolumbar: Surgical Approach by Neurologic Status[a] (Northwestern University Acute Spine Injury Center, 1972 to 1986)

Surgical Approach	Total Cases	Improvement		No Change		Degradation		Unknown[b]	
		No.	Percent	No.	Percent	No.	Percent	No.	Percent
Posterior	218	25	11.5	181	83.0	5	2.3	7	3.2
Anterior	9	2	22.2	4	44.4	1	11.1	2	22.2
Combined	47	12	25.5	32	68.1	1	2.1	2	4.3
Anterior then posterior	2	1	50.0	0	0.0	1	50.0	0	0.0
Posterior then anterior	4	2	50.0	2	50.0	0	0.0	0	0.0
Missing[c]	190	11	5.8	155	81.6	2	1.1	22	11.6
Total	470	53	11.3	374	79.6	10	2.1	33	7.0

[a] Change criterion is one or more Frankel grades, higher or lower.
[b] Neurologic change is unavailable.
[c] Either no surgery, or surgery approach is unavailable.

Table 18-21.   Thoracolumbar: Neurologic Status by Management[a] (Northwestern University Acute Spine Injury Center, 1972 to 1986)

Management	Total Cases	Improvement		No Change		Degradation		Unknown[b]	
		No.	Percent	No.	Percent	No.	Percent	No.	Percent
Conservative	176	9	5.1	144	81.8	1	0.6	22	12.5
Surgical	294	44	15.0	230	78.2	9	3.1	11	3.7
Total	470	53	11.3	374	79.6	10	2.1	33	7.0

[a] Change criterion is one or more Frankel grade, higher or lower.
[b] Neurologic change is unavailable.

REFERENCES

1. Holdsworth FW: Review article—fracture-dislocation and fracture-dislocations of the spine. J Bone Joint Surg 52A:534, 1970
2. Denis F: The three column spine and its significance in the classification of acute thoracolumbar spine injuries. Spine 8:817, 1983
3. Luque ER, Cassis N, Ramirez-Wiella G: Segmental spine instrumentation in the treatment of fractures of the thoracolumbar spine. Spine 7:312, 1982
4. Dickson JH, Harrington PR, Erwin WD: Results of reduction and stabilization of the severely fractured thoracic and lumbar spine. J Bone Joint Surg 60:799, 1978
5. Edwards CC: The spinal rod sleeve: its rationale and use in thoracic and lumbar injuries. J Bone Joint Surg Orthop Trans 6:11, 1982
6. Roy-Camille R, Saillant G, Berteaux D, Marie-Anne S: Early management of spinal injuries. p. 57. In McKibbin B. (ed): Recent Advances in Orthopaedics. Vol. 3. Churchill Livingstone, Edinburgh, 1979
7. Internal Fixator for the Spine. Synthes Bulletin. No. 70, November 1985
8. Jacobs RR, Casey MP: Surgical management of thoracic-lumbar spinal injuries: general principles and controversial considerations. Clin Orthop 189:22, 1984
9. Jacobs RR, Schlapfer F, Mathys R: A locking hook spinal rod system for stabilization of fracture-dislocations and correction of deformities of the dorsolumbar Spine. Clin Orthop 189:168, 1984
10. Last RJ: Innervation of the limbs. J Bone Joint Surg 31B:450, 1949
11. Chusid JG: Correlation Neuroanatomy and Functional Neurology. 17th Ed. p. 173. Appleton & Lange, East Norwalk, CT, 1979
12. Holdsworth FW: Symposium on Spinal Injury. p.

161. Edinburgh Royal College of Surgeons, Edinburgh 1963

13. Holdsworth FW, Hardy AG: Early treatment of paraplegics from fracture of the thoracolumbar spine. J Bone Joint Surg 35B:540, 1953

14. Elsberg CA: The Edwin Smith surgical papyrus, and the diagnosis and treatment of injuries to the skull and spine 5000 years ago. Am Med Hist 3:271, 1931

15. Seibel R, LaDuca J, Hassett JM et al.: Blunt trauma (ISS36), femur traction and the pulmonary failure-septic state. Ann Surg 202:283, 1985

16. Jacobs RR, Asher MA, Snider RK: Thoracolumbar spine fractures, a comparative study of recumbent and operative treatment in 100 patients. Spine 5:463, 1980

17. Soreff J, Axdorph G, Bylund P: Treatment of patients with unstable fractures of the thoracic and lumbar spine. A follow-up study of surgical and conservative treatment. Acta Orthop Scand 53:369, 1982

18. Willen J: Unstable Thoracolumbar Fractures — An Experimental and Clinical Study. p. 1. Department of Orthopaedic Surgery and Diagnostic Radiology, Sahlgren Hospital, University of Goteborg, Goteborg, Sweden, 1984

19. Weiss M: Dynamic spine alloplasty (spring loading correction device) after fracture and spinal cord injury. Clin Orthop 112:150, 1975

20. Meyer PR: Weiss Spring Spinal Internal Fixation Surgical Technique. p. 1. Zimmer USA, Warsaw, NY, 1975

21. Dunn HK, Danials AU, McBride GG: Comparative assessment of spine stability achieved with a new anterior spine fixation device. J Bone Joint Surg Orthop Trans 4:269, 1980

22. Keene JS, Drummond DS: Wisconsin Compression System Surgical Technique. Zimmer USA, Warsaw, NY, 1981

23. Pinzer MS, Meyer PR, Lautenschlager EP et al.: Measurement of internal fixation device support in experimentally produced fractures of the dorsolumbar spine. Orthopaedics 4(6):28, 1979

24. Stauffer ES, Neil JL: Biomechanical analysis of structural stability of internal fixation in fractures of the thoracolumbar spine. Clin Orthop 112:159, 1975

25. Nachemson A, Elfstrom G: Intravital wireless telemetry of axial forces in Harrington distraction rods in patients with idiopathic scoliosis. J Bone Joint Surg 53A:445, 1971

26. Frankel HL: Ascending cord lesions in the early stages following spinal injury. Paraplegia 7:111, 1969

19

Fractures of the Lumbar and Sacral Spine: Conservative and Surgical Management

Paul R. Meyer, Jr.

No other area of the vertebral column has elicited such an "explosion" of interest and surgical innovativeness, as has been directed toward the management of problems of the lumbar and lumbosacral spine.[1] Not since the advent of total joint arthroplasty, beginning with John Charnley in the 1960s, has so much happened in such a short period of time. It is as though the orthopaedic community awaited "the peer acceptance of surgical management philosophy" for maladies of the spine, for there to be a sudden rush of surgical procedure variety. International authorities, including Roy-Camille[2] and Louis[3] of Paris, Luque[4] of Mexico, Zielke[5,6] and Magerl[7,8] of Germany and Switzerland, Kostuik[9] of Canada, and Wiltse,[1] Steffee,[10] and Bradford[1] of the United States, along with countless others, have contributed. Pathologic problems spanning the spectrum from congenital and developmental deformities to degenerative arthritis and disc diseases are now being approached surgically. Similar surgical management enthusiasm for problems related to the lumbar spine was noted at the 45th AO-ASIF Spine Conference, Davos, Switzerland, in December 1986.

This chapter will not attempt to analyze or interpret all of the procedures now being proposed for the management of problems relating to the lower spine and pelvis. Rather, an attempt will be made to provide a foundation on which to make appropriate decisions as to surgical or conservative management. Some basic discussion of several of the procedures will be included when personal experience applies. No discussion of nontraumatic disorders will be included, for it is certain that an accurate corollary between the two pathologies (traumatic and nontraumatic), mechanically or pathologically, can be accurately drawn.

As noted in Chapters 16 and 18, for the purposes of this text, the area of the vertebral column defined as the lumbar spine is the area between L3 and L5. It is appreciated that the traditional area of the lumbar spine parallels the normal vertebral column anatomy, L1 through L5. Data from the Spine Injury Center of Northwestern University (1972 to 1986) revealed that "fracture-injury" patterns and the areas of their required instrumentation, throughout the spine, fell into defined groupings that lay outside the "normal" anatomic vertebral column distribution. An excellent example of this was the finding that the preponderance of the 928 fractures of the thoracic and lumbar segments of the vertebral column fell into specific areas of distribution: T1 to T10 (376 [40.3 percent]). Outside the cervical spine, the most frequently injured area of the vertebral column was the thoraciolumbar junction, T11 to L2 (470 [50.4 percent]). The third major injury area was that area of the spine between L3 and L5 (73 [7.8 percent]). The least number of injuries occurred between S1 and S5 (13 [1.4 percent]). Comparative "traditional" and "redefined" vertebral column fracture data appear in Table 19-1.

Of the 73 L3 to L5 lumbar spine fractures discussed below, 27.4 percent followed the occurrence of a motor vehicle accident, 30.1 percent were caused by a fall, 15.1 percent were secondary to gunshot wounds, and 27.5 percent resulted from some other traumatic mechanism (Table 19-2).

LUMBAR STATISTICS

Our series of lumbar fractures and dislocations number 73. As previously defined, fractures occurring in this area of the spine are those lying between L3 and L5 (Tables 19-1 and 19-4). Of 24 fractures occurring at L3, 12 (50 percent) were the result of axial loading. Of 25 fractures occurring at L4, 13 (52 percent) resulted from axial loading, while fractures occurring at L5 were the result of either direct trauma or gunshot wound (7 or 50 percent).

Table 19-1. Traditional versus Modified Breakdown of Lower Spine Vertebral Fractures (Northwestern University Acute Spine Injury Center, 1972 to 1986)

Modified			Traditional		
Levels of Injury	No.	Percent	Levels of Injury	No.	Percent
T1–T10	376	40.3	T1–T12	600	64.4
T11–L2	470	50.4			
L3–L5	73	7.8	L1–L5	319	34.2
S1–S5	13	1.4	S1–S5	13	1.4
Total	932	100.0	Total	932	100.0

Table 19-2. Lumbar versus Sacral Etiology (Northwestern University Acute Spine Injury Center, 1972 to 1986)

Etiology	Lumbar		Sacral	
	No.	Percent	No.	Percent
Fall	22	30.1	6	46.2
Motor vehicle accident	20	27.4	2	15.4
Other trauma[a]	14	19.2	3	23.1
Gunshot wound	11	15.1	1	7.7
Motorcycle	4	5.5	0	0.0
Other	2	2.8	1	7.7
Total	73	100.0	13	100.0

[a] Other trauma represents those patients with multiple etiologies.

As noted in Table 19-2, falls were the primary cause of injury to the lumbar spine (30 percent). This cause is followed closely by motor vehicle accidents and direct trauma.

The mechanical forces influencing the type of fractures occurring in the lumbar spine are quite consistent. Because of the high incidence of falls, axial load or compression injuries are most frequent (50 percent). This is followed by flexion injuries with associated compression loading (37 percent), and direct trauma resulting in lateral shear injuries (8 percent). Combinations of mechanical forces were most frequently seen at the L3–L4 level with a high occurrence of flexion-distraction (Chance) fractures, and direct "punch" trauma re-

Table 19-3. Lumbar versus Sacral Biomechanical Type of Injury (Northwestern University Acute Spine Injury Center, 1972 to 1986)

Biomechanical Injury	Lumbar		Sacral	
	No.	Percent	No.	Percent
Axial	28	38.4	2	15.4
Flexion	18	24.7	3	23.1
Other[a]	13	17.8	4	30.8
No fracture	8	11.0	4	30.8
Rotation	3	4.1	0	0.0
Extension	3	4.1	0	0.0
Total	73	100.0	13	100.0

[a] Other includes direct trauma and gunshot wounds.

Table 19-4. Lumbar: Biomechanical Type of Injury by Injury Level (Northwestern University Acute Spine Injury Center, 1972 to 1986)

Biomechanical Injury	Total	L3		L4		L5		Other[a]	
		No.	Percent	No.	Percent	No.	Percent	No.	Percent
Axial	28	12	50.0	13	52.0	3	21.4	0	0.0
Flexion	18	9	37.5	9	36.0	0	0.0	0	0.0
Rotation	3	1	4.2	1	4.0	1	7.1	0	0.0
Extension	3	0	0.0	0	0.0	3	21.4	0	0.0
Other	13	2	8.3	2	8.0	7	50.0	2	20.0
No fracture	8	0	0.0	0	0.0	0	0.0	8	80.0
Total	73	24	32.9	25	34.2	14	19.2	10	13.7

[a] Includes those with no fracture site.

sulting in fractures of transverse processes and lateral translatory dislocations as seen at the lumbosacral junction (Fig. 19-1). Fractures of the transverse and spinous processes at multiple levels also resulted from the effects of forceful paraspinous muscle contractions, resulting in avulsion fractures. Gunshot wounds of the spine were classified as direct injury.

As noted in Table 19-4, most frequent injuries occurring at L5 were at the L5–S1 junction and resulted from axial loading, translatory loading, and extension injuries. In the presence of high vertical loading secondary to construction falls or suicide attempts, multiple lower extremity fractures were not uncommon (Fig. 19-8).

There were 13 fractures and dislocations involving the sacrum. Each followed a somewhat different biomechanical mechanism of injury, but the end result was the same — direct trauma (Table 19-3).

NEUROLOGIC INJURY ACCOMPANYING LUMBOSACRAL FRACTURES

Of the 73 patients sustaining injury to the lumbar spine, 37 percent remained neurologically intact, 60.3 percent sustained some form of incomplete neurologic injury, while only 2.7 percent sustained complete neurologic injury. As discussed below, there is a good anatomic rationale for the low incidence of complete neurologic injury accompany-

ing fractures to the lumbar spine. In the sacral fracture group, one patient remained intact, and 12 had some form of sacral nerve root (incomplete) injury (Table 19-5).

Axial load trauma to the lumbar spine resulted in incomplete neurologic injury in 50 percent of cases. In the thoracolumbar junctional area, 46.6 percent of injuries were incomplete. The explanation is the type (or preponderance) of neurologic tissue found present at each level (Table 19-6).

Comparing flexion injuries at both the thoracolumbar junction and the lumbar regions, 50 percent were incomplete in the lumbar region and 38.8 percent were incomplete in the thoracolumbar region (Table 19-6).

Comparing all mechanical etiologies of injury in both regions, only 2.7 percent of lumbar fractures resulted in a complete neurologic injury, whereas 29.4 percent of the fractures at the thoracolumbar junction resulted in complete neurologic injury (Table 19-6). This obvious and significant differential in the incidence of neurologic injury at both levels resulted from three important factors: the size of the neural canal at each level; the vascular supply to the neurologic tissue within each region; and most importantly, at the thoracolumbar junctional region, the nervous system is best described as "mixed." Above T12 lies solely the spinal cord, and between T12 and L1 is found the conus medullaris portion of the spinal cord (neurologic segments L5 through S5). This neurologic area lies opposite or posterior to the vertebral bodies of T12 and L1. Beginning at T10 is the exit of the L1 (cauda equina) nerve root. The nerve roots L1 through L4 exit the spinal cord opposite the T10

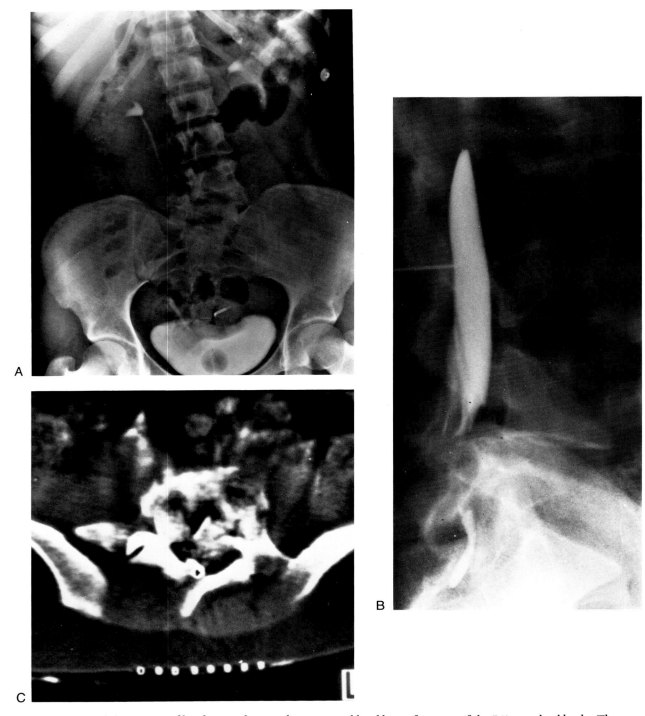

Fig. 19-1. **(A)** AP view of lumbosacral spine showing axial load burst fracture of the L5 vertebral body. The patient jumped from a bridge in a suicide attempt. **(B)** Lateral myelogram of the lumbar spine. Note total obstruction of the spinal canal at L5. The patient had complete neurologic loss of the S1–S2 segments. **(C)** CT scan of L5 showing the nature of the burst fracture. *(Figure continues.)*

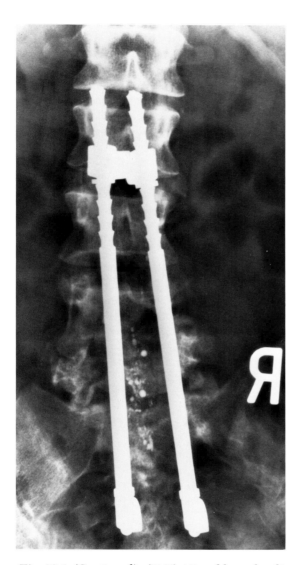

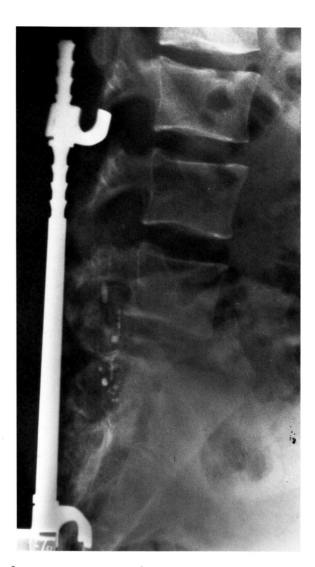

D

E

Fig. 19-1 *(Continued)*. **(D,E)** AP and lateral radiograph after instrumentation with Harrington rods. Note placement of inferior hook directly into the sacrum. Note also posterior luxation of L5 on S1 and loss of lumbosacral angle with distraction internal fixation.

Table 19-5. Lumbar versus Sacral Neurologic Extent of Injury (Northwestern University Acute Spine Injury Center, 1972 to 1986)

Extent of Injury	Lumbar		Sacral	
	No.	Percent	No.	Percent
Intact	27	37.0	1	7.7
Incomplete	44	60.3	12	92.3
Complete	2	2.7	0	0.0
Total	73	100.0	13	100.0

vertebral body down to a position opposite and posterior to the L1 vertebral body and below L1 lies "pure" cauda equina representing "peripheral nerves." This latter structure, the cauda equina, is significantly more resistant to trauma than is the spinal cord, which is the reason for the low incidence of complete neurologic injuries occurring in this region of the spine. It is difficult to predict the neurologic outcome in the region of the lumbar spine for the following four reasons.

1. The nerve root L1 has its cell bodies within the anterior horn cell mass of the spinal cord opposite T10. The nerve per se exists the spinal canal at L1-L2 (see Fig. 18-1). For the same reason, the cell bodies for the L3 nerve root lie opposite the T11–T12 vertebrae (well above any bony injury to L3, should that be the level of fracture) and exit at L3–L4. Here the nerve is a peripheral nerve.

2. The neuroanatomic construct of a peripheral nerve root is such that it is resistant to injury. The exiting axon cylinder is ensheathed within a lipoprotein myelin matrix (produced by Schwann cells), and these two structures lie within a fibrous connective tissue known as the epineurium.[11] This sheath provides strength and protection to the axon against trauma (impingement by herniated disc, fractured vertebral body elements, compression, stretching, angulation, laceration, etc.). Although infrequent, a peripheral nerve (root) can be so injured as to result in loss of axonal continuity (axonotomesis). If the nerve sheath remains intact, axon regrowth may occur, with variable amounts of neurologic recovery.

3. The same is not necessarily true with injury to the sensory portion of a peripheral nerve root. Though its axons may lie within the same nerve sheath, its cell bodies of origin lie with the dorsal root ganglion, outside of the spinal cord, in continuity with entrance sensory fibers, entering the dorsal column from the dorsal root ganglion. The same sensory cell sends off a peripheral axon, composing the second component of a peripheral nerve, the sensory portion. Destruction of the dorsal root ganglion inhibits recovery or regrowth of sensory axons.

4. The cauda equina (which in fact are peripheral nerves) is resistant to trauma. Half (50 percent) of the lumbar spine fractures result in incomplete neurologic injuries. Trauma may induce a temporary loss of nerve root function known as neurapraxia (in which neurologic function is lost but

Table 19-6. Thoracolumbar Area: Neurologic Extent by Biomechanical Type of Injury (Northwestern University Acute Spine Injury Center, 1972 to 1986)

Biomechanical Type of Injury	Total Cases	Intact		Incomplete		Complete		Missing[a]	
		No.	Percent	No.	Percent	No.	Percent	No.	Percent
Axial	221	80	36.2	103	46.6	37	16.7	1	0.5
Flexion	139	33	23.7	54	38.8	52	37.4	0	0.0
Rotation	7	1	14.3	2	28.6	4	57.1	0	0.0
Direct	3	1	33.3	2	66.7	0	0.0	0	0.0
Extension	4	2	50.0	2	50.0	0	0.0	0	0.0
Other	56	9	16.1	17	30.4	30	53.6	0	0.0
No fracture	40	0	0.0	25	62.5	15	37.5	0	0.0
Total	470	126	26.8	205	43.6	138	29.4	1	0.2

[a] Extent is unavailable.

Table 19-7. Lumbar versus Sacral: Change in Neurologic Status[a] (Northwestern University Acute Spine Injury Center, 1972 to 1986)

Type of Change	Lumbar		Sacral	
	No.	Percent	No.	Percent
Improvement	14	19.2	1	7.7
No change	55	75.3	7	53.8
Degradation	1	1.4	0	0.0
Missing	3	4.1	5	38.5
Total	73	100.0	13	100.0

[a] Change criterion is one or more Frankel grades, higher or lower.

nerve sheath and axon remain in continuity). In neurapraxia, nerve function can reappear anytime, from hours to months after injury. In fact, 14 (19.2 percent) of the 73 patients with lower lumbar injuries demonstrated neurologic improvement (one or more neurologic Frankel grades) (Table 19-7). Total severance of a nerve root (sheath and axon) is neurotmesis.

MULTIPLE TRAUMA

The incidence of multiple trauma noted in those patients sustaining fractures to the lumbar spine was high (Tables 19-8, 19-9). This is due in part to the fact that patients sustaining lower spine injury after falls most frequently strike the ground feet first (or lower extremity first). This results in the absorption of high-energy forces through the lower extremities, with an associated high compressive load from above (trunk and thorax — a large body mass [50 percent] centered above the level of L1) undergoing sudden deceleration (Table 19-8).

A high incidence of multiple trauma was not seen in the patient population sustaining sacral fractures. One was an open fracture (Fig. 19-2), three patients required no attempt at fracture reduction, and two required open reduction or debridement. Two patients with a fracture of the sacrum sustained a secondary fracture of the spine or extremity.

Other than injury to the lumbar spine, the most

Table 19-8. Lumbar versus Sacral: Associated Injury (Northwestern University Acute Spine Injury Center, 1972 to 1986)

	Associated Injury[a]	Lumbar		Sacral	
		No.	Percent	No.	Percent
External	Scalp laceration	4	5.5	0	0.0
	Facial laceration	4	5.5	0	0.0
Fracture	Skull	5	6.8	0	0.0
	Facial	5	6.8	0	0.0
	Radius-ulna	3	4.1	0	0.0
	Metatarsal	3	4.1	0	0.0
	Rib(s)	3	4.1	1	7.7
	Pelvis	5	6.8	1	7.7
	Femur	3	4.1	0	0.0
	Tibia-fibula	5	6.8	1	7.7
	Ankle	10	13.7	1	7.7
	Foot	4	5.5	0	0.0
	Other	15	20.5	2	15.4
Internal	Loss of consciousness	10	13.7	2	15.4
	Pulmonary contusion	2	2.7	0	0.0
	Pneumothorax	2	2.7	0	0.0
	Hemothorax	2	2.7	0	0.0
	Other thoracic	6	8.2	1	7.7
	Other abdominal	21	32.7	3	24.1
	Other	9	12.3	4	31.8

[a] Listed by gross type and then anatomically.

Table 19-9. Lumbar versus Sacral: Multiple Trauma (Northwestern University Acute Spine Injury Center, 1972 to 1986)

No. of Involved Systems	Lumbar		Sacral	
	No.	Percent	No.	Percent
None	35	47.9	7	53.8
One	17	23.3	3	23.1
Two	16	21.9	2	15.4
Three	4	5.5	1	7.7
Four	1	1.4	0	0.0
Total	73	100.0	13	100.0

frequently associated multiple trauma sites were the lower extremities (26 percent), the abdomen (26 percent), and the head (26 percent), followed by the chest (11 percent) (Table 19-10). In this series, two patients sustained a hemothorax and two sustained a pneumothorax. Two patients with lumbar or sacral fractures required exploratory laparotomy for a positive peritoneal lavage. One of these two patients was found to have sustained a traumatic injury to the colon, requiring a colostomy. Peritoneal lavage by the minilaparotomy approach is an evaluative procedure routinely performed in the emergency room (by the general surgery trauma team) on any patient with a suggested history or physical examination of abdominal injuries. A positive (mild yet requiring surgery) peritoneal tap in lumbar spine injuries is not uncommonly seen. It is usually the result of retroperitoneal hemorrhage associated with the lumbar spine fracture. Other areas of the anatomy considered vulnerable to injury are the head and the extremities (Tables 19-8, 19-10). During our 14-year experience, no deaths occurred in either the lumbar or sacral spine-injured patient populations.

ASSOCIATED AREAS OF SKELETAL TRAUMA

Injuries to the lower extremity are quite frequently associated with fractures involving the lumbar spine. This is particularly the case when spinal fractures result primarily from clearly de-fined axial loading. Orthopaedic educators frequently remind the student of the slightly more than subtle relationship between fractures of the os calcis and compression fractures of the lumbar spine (particularly L1). The fracture types more frequently associated with lower lumbar spine injuries were multiple trauma to the lower extremities (fractures of the tibial shaft [6.8 percent], fractures of the ankle [13.7 percent], fractures of the pelvis [6.8 percent], and the fractures of the femur [4.1 percent]) (Table 19-8).

INITIAL PATIENT AND RADIOLOGIC EVALUATION

In the presence of a lumbar (and less often sacral) vertebral fracture, with the presence of multiple trauma, a negative neurologic picture or a minor initial symptom may be overlooked. It may not be until motion such as rolling, twisting, or straight leg raising occurs that pain occurs. Postinjury, the patient will likely demonstrate two important physical findings: paravertebral muscle spasm and abdominal distention secondary to paralytic ileus, induced by the presence of a vertebral fracture. As it is possible to overlook injury to the lumbar or sacral spine, it is also possible to overlook other areas of trauma including the os calcis, the pelvis, the clavicle, the carpal navicular bone, and other areas of trauma within the vertebral column[12] (Fig. 19-1). It becomes imperative, therefore, during the evaluation process for the examiner to figuratively and literally "walk" down each of the extremities, the trunk, and the vertebral column from

Table 19-10. Lumbar versus Sacral: Anatomic Systems Traumatized (Northwestern University Acute Spine Injury Center, 1972 to 1986)

Traumatized System	Lumbar		Sacral	
	No.	Percent	No.	Percent
Head	19	26.0	3	23.1
Chest	8	11.0	2	15.4
Abdomen	19	26.0	3	23.1
Extremity	19	26.0	2	15.4

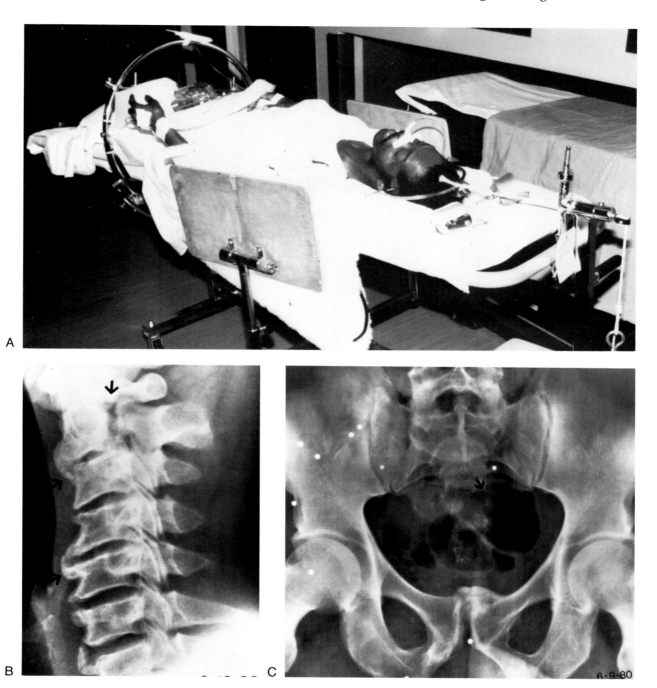

Fig. 19-2. (A) Patient with multiple spine fractures managed in Gardner-Wells tongs for fracture of the cervical spine and open fracture of the sacrum. (B) Lateral cervical spine radiograph showing the fracture through the pars articularis (hangman's fracture of C2) and avulsion fracture of osteophytes at C2 – C3, C4, C5. (C) Anterior pelvic radiograph showing comminuted fracture of the sacrum. Note the loss of symmetry of the sacral foramen. Loss of symmetry is indicative of fracture. *(Figure continues.)*

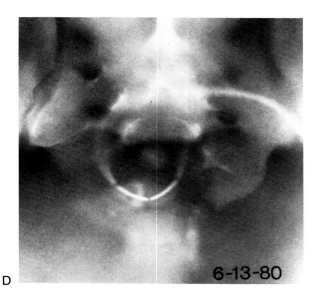

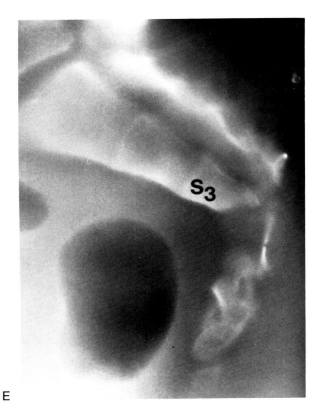

D   E

Fig. 19-2 *(Continued)*. **(D,E)** Postoperative **AP** and lateral radiographs of the sacral fracture.

end to end with the examining hand. Direct pressure over the spinous process of a fractured vertebral element will elicit pain at the site of injury. The examiner, with several assistants, carefully log rolls the patient into the lateral position to evaluate (and observe) the skin over the lumbar spine. What may be identified, and not anticipated, is either significant abrasion overlying a spinous process (opposite the level of injury) or the presence of a spinal deformity secondary to the prominence of one or more spinous processes, evidence of spinal column malalignment (a gibbus) (Fig. 19-3). Such displacement may be in either the anteroposterior (sagittal) or lateral (coronal) direction. Palpation (with pain) of a space between two spinous processes is a reliable indicator of injury to the vertebral column.

Because multiple sites of trauma are likely with lumbar spine fracture, which as noted earlier most frequently follows a fall (23 percent), at some point shortly after admission, the patient must be totally disrobed and all areas of the body examined. A careful initial (admission) neurologic assessment must be performed, recorded, and repeated every 30 minutes to 1 hour for the first 6 to 8 hours after admission. Included in the examination is a rectal exam, observing for the presence or absence of perianal sensation, perianal reflex activity (the bulbocavernosus reflex), intra-anal proprioception, and voluntary perianal muscle function and control. During the first 24 hours, the neurologic examination should be repeated every hour and recorded. A suggested format for maintaining such information is a neurologic form used by the nursing staff (Fig. 19-4).

All areas of questionable or potential injury (secondary areas of spine or skeletal system trauma) require early radiologic evaluation. Initially, spine films are obtained only in the anteroposterior and lateral views. Additional views can be obtained later as required. Oblique films of the spine are not

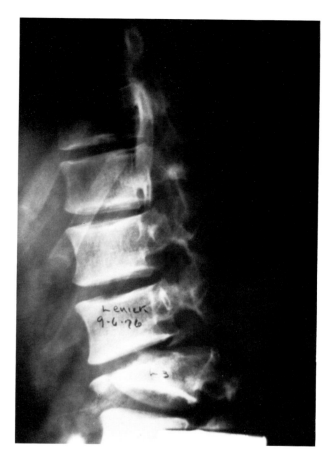

Fig. 19-3. Lateral radiograph showing three-column disruption resulting in fracture dislocation of L2 on L3.

stretcher to an emergency room cart, bed, or Stryker wedge frame, so as to allow the ambulance personnel to leave?" The answer is multifaceted, yet simple: Not until one knows what injuries one is dealing with. In the presence of adequate help (four or more persons), the patient can be safely moved if sufficient knowledge, evaluation, or radiologic data are available. In the presence of neurologic injury, radiographs must be available and reviewed before patient transfer. If they are not available, they must be obtained first. When the patient is ready for transfer, it must always be performed in the supine position. Once the patient is found to be stable in the supine position, prone radiographs can be obtained to establish alignment of the lumbar spine in this position. The addition of appropriately placed pillows has been found to contribute positively to improving spinal alignment. (see Pillow Fracture Reduction Technique, below).

TECHNICAL EVALUATIVE PROCEDURES

Various radiographic and nonradiographic evaluative techniques can be most helpful in the assessment of injuries to the lumbar spine.

Radiographic Procedures

Standard anteroposterior and lateral radiographs of the lumbar spine should include the thoracolumbar junction as well as the lumbosacral joint. Oblique radiographs are not as helpful in the evaluation of trauma as they are in the assessment of developmental, degenerative, or tumorous involvement of the spine (in light of other, more demonstrative techniques such as MRI, CAT, tomography). When specific defects in the pars interarticularis are sought, oblique views of the spine are most valuable.

Tomograms are made of the vertebral column under evaluation, in both the anteroposterior and lateral planes. It is important to appreciate that injuries to the vertebral column may occur at mul-

immediately required, and with computed tomography (CT), magnetic resonance imaging (MRI), or standard polytomography, not necessary. If the patient requires management on a Stryker frame, it is often advantageous to turn the patient prone to facilitate visualization of the vertebral column away from the bed or frame surface. Also, the spine can be visualized in extension, which tends to reduce a flexion-induced injury. When translatory malalignment between two vertebrae exists, in either the coronal or sagittal plane, a serious (and unstable) vertebral column injury exists. Most likely, the displacement seen was much greater at the time of initial trauma.

The question arises: "When is it safe to transfer a patient on a spine board from an ambulance

Northwestern Memorial Hospital
Form No. 501248 Rev. 7/83

SPINAL CORD
NEUROLOGICAL ASSESSMENT

LEVEL OF CONSCIOUSNESS:

A = Alert
C = Confused

PUPIL REACTION:

PERL, L > R or R > L

MUSCLE GRADING:

0 = Absent
1 = Trace
2 = Poor
3 = Fair
4 = Good
5 = Normal

DATE/TIME:							
SIGNATURE:							
LEVEL OF CONSCIOUSNESS							
PUPIL REACTION:							

KEY MUSCLE FUNCTIONS:		RT	LT	RT	LT	RT	LT	RT	LT	RT	LT	RT	LT	RT	LT
Shoulder Elevators	C-4														
Elbow Flexion	C-5														
Wrist Dorsiflexion	C-6														
Elbow Extension	C-7														
Finger Abducters, Adducters	C-8														
Hip Flexion	L-2														
Knee Extension	L-3														
Ankle Dorsiflexion	L-4														
Great Toe Extension	L-5														
Ankle Plantar Flexion	S-1														
Voluntary Rectal Tone	S-2,3														

SENSORY LEVELS:		RT		LT		RT		LT		RT		LT		RT		LT		RT		LT		RT		LT		RT		LT	
		Pain	D.T.	Pain	D.T.	Pain	D.T.	Pain	D.T.	Pain	D.T.	Pain	D.T.	Pain	D.T.	Pain	D.T.	Pain	D.T.	Pain	D.T.	Pain	D.T.	Pain	D.T.	Pain	D.T.	Pain	D.T.
CERVICAL	2																												
	3																												
	4																												
	5																												
	6																												
	7																												
	8																												
THORACIC	1																												
	2																												
	3																												
	4																												
	5																												
	6																												
	7																												
	8																												
	9																												
	10																												
	11																												
	12																												
LUMBAR	1																												
	2																												
	3																												
	4																												
	5																												
SACRAL	1																												
	2																												
	3																												
	4																												
	5																												
Complete (C): Incomplete (Inc.)																													

DEEP TOUCH:

+ = Present
- = Absent

PAIN SENSATION:

S = Sharp to Pinprick
D = Dull to Pinprick
A = Absent to Pinprick

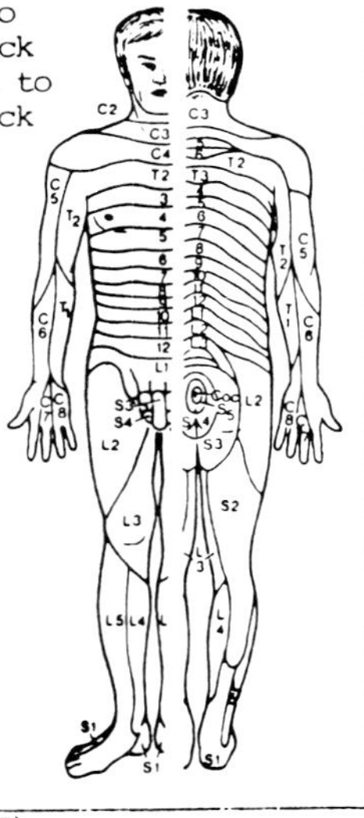

Fig. 19-4. Nursing spinal cord neurological assessment form. This form is maintained on every spine fracture patient pre-operatively. (Northwestern Memorial Hospital, Acute Spinal Cord Injury Center)

tiple levels; therefore, this study should include a reasonable area of the spine above and below the known area of injury (Fig. 19-5).

In those patients in whom no apparent fracture is identified, yet evidence of neurologic injury is present, carefully performed and monitored *flexion-extension radiographs* (either standard or tomographic) in the lateral projection may be very helpful in eliciting unrecognized instability.

Computed axial tomography for horizontal viewing of the neural canal, when encroachment of neural structures and canal by bone or soft tissue is sought, is most valuable when attempting to determine the efficacy of neural tissue decompression in the neurologically incompletely injured patient (Fig. 19-6).

Myelography is indicated when based on a prescribed criterion. It is most indicated when there is

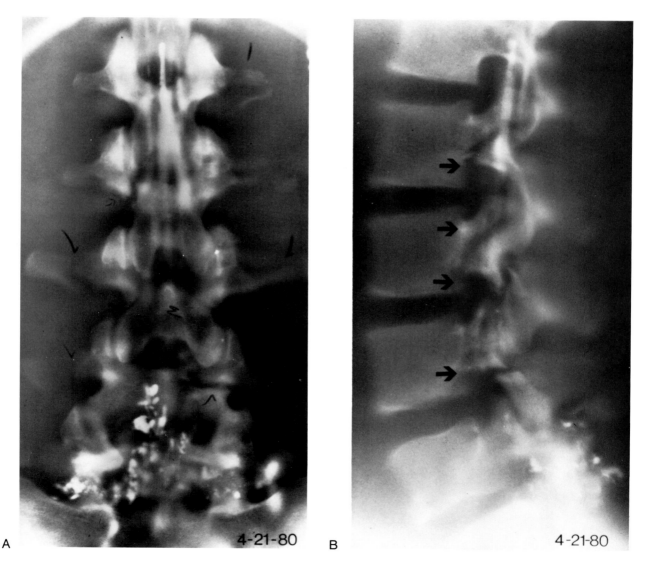

Fig. 19-5. AP (**A**) and lateral (**B**) radiographs showing multiple spine fractures of L2 through L5. Note fractures of pedicles at each level, of posterior elements, and of transverse processes, and dural tears evidenced by contrast material in the extradural space. Patient had loss of S1 and S2 neurologic segments.

evidence of neurologic compromise in the absence of trauma, or when there is a history of trauma that is inconsistent with neurologic findings (see Fig. 19-21).

Nonradiographic Procedures

Magnetic resonance imaging is becoming a valuable diagnostic trauma tool, as specific indications are developed. A deterrent to the use of this evaluative technique has been the success to date of using other evaluative procedures such as CAT scan and tomography. The major deterrent to the use of MRI has been the magnetic field required for the function of these units. Patients undergoing treatment on or with ferrous-containing splints, frames, vascular clips, or staples, etc., cannot be placed in the vicinity of this equipment. On the other hand, patients having undergone surgical procedures in which nonferrous hardware has been used can be evaluated with this device. This includes most orthopaedic internal fixation devices. Magnetic resonance imaging is a very effective means of ascertaining the patency of the neural canal and provides excellent detail of bone and soft tissue anatomic structures in the sagittal plane. It is likely that this procedure will eventually replace alternative procedures now being used (Fig. 19-7).

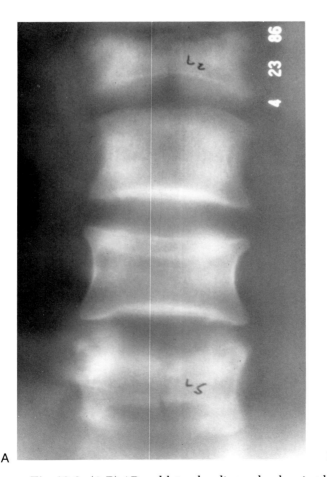

A

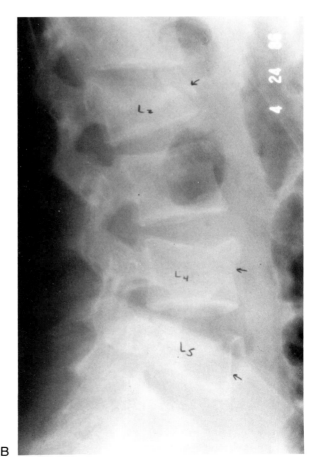

B

Fig. 19-6. (A,B) AP and lateral radiographs showing burst fractures of L2, L4, and L5. The patient was neurologically normal. *(Figure continues.)*

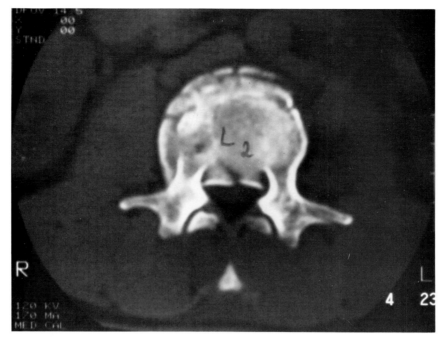

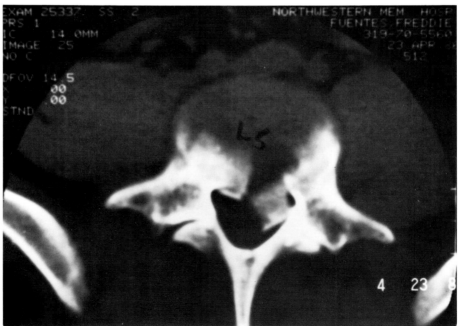

Fig. 19-6 *(Continued)*. **(C)** Transverse CT scan showing fracture pattern of L2. **(D)** CT scan showing different fracture pattern of the L5 vertebral body. This fracture pattern represents axial loading and flexion.

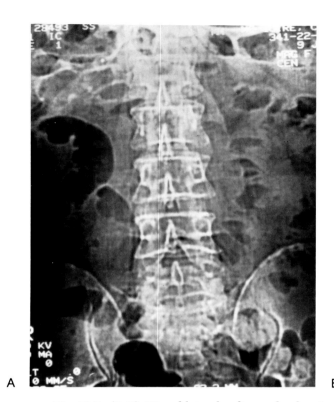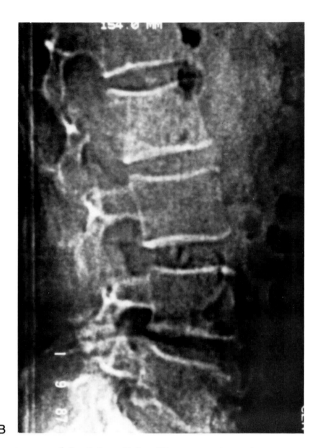

A   B

Fig. 19-7. (A,B) AP and lateral radiographs showing a tumor of the L2 pedicle. *(Figure continues.)*

Bone scanning with technetium 99m has become most useful in the evaluation of the spine in patients having undergone known trauma in whom standard radiographic techniques have failed to reveal the site of injury. When neurologic changes accompany trauma without radiographic correlation, bone scanning is not only helpful in identification of the site of trauma, but also assists in answering the question as to whether or not multiple sites of injury exist.

Somatosensory evoked potential (SSEP) is used to evaluate each patient sustaining spine trauma with neurologic injury, to assess the extent of neurologic injury, and to determine a baseline. The procedure is also utilized as a nervous system-monitoring device during surgery and for postoperative evaluation of patients in whom there is question of either neurologic improvement or deterioration.

Indications for Myelography

Indications for myelography in the spine-injured patient, in the past, were founded almost solely on a history or the presence of "spinal" trauma. Specific criteria for this evaluative procedure did not exist; rather they varied loosely from physician to physician. Between 1972 and now, specific guidelines and indications were jointly developed by the Northwestern University orthopaedic surgery and neurosurgical services.

1. *The presence of neurologic deterioration.* This indication is somewhat broad. Differences or variations in neurologic performance may occur after trauma, resulting in subtle neurologic changes secondary to neural tissue edema. Such changes are insidious in onset. Deterioration resulting from vascular compromise is more sud-

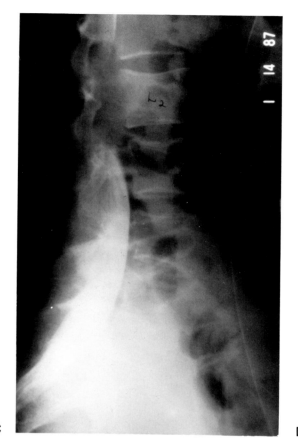

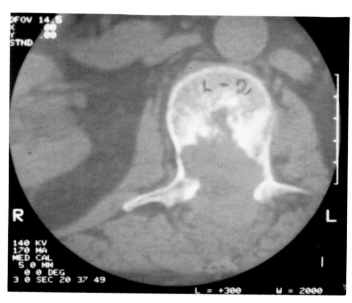

Fig. 19-7 *(Continued).* **(C)** Myelogram showing obstruction of contrast material at L2. A posterior laminectomy performed for biopsy showed the tumor to be a chordoma. **(D)** CT scan of the L2 vertebral body shows involvement of vertebral body and posterior laminectomy.

den in onset and may be associated with loss of spinal alignment or entrapment of neural tissue by fracture fragments, ruptured disc material, etc. Neurologic deterioration rapidly follows vascular obstruction. Although emergency myelography is rarely contraindicated (allergy to contrast media) when only subtle neurologic changes have occurred that are more than likely due only to neural tissue edema, nonetheless, it must be considered and the question asked, is the study indicated or required? Just moving the patient from frame or bed to myelographic table, placing the patient into a prone or Trendelenburg position (for the study), followed by return to the frame or bed, is also potentially

injurious to the patient, and must be considered along with the indications.

2. *A patient requiring operative intervention in the presence of an incomplete neurologic injury.* Appreciating the hazard of all surgery, and the fact that neurologic injury can occur during the performance of an operative procedure, it is appropriate to rule out known or potential contributing causes preoperatively. Example: If a patient with traumatic cervical spine instability requires a posterior stabilization procedure, either prone placement on the operating table or the planned surgical stabilization procedure will result in reconstitution of the lost cervical lordosis. Should there exist anteriorly a hereto-

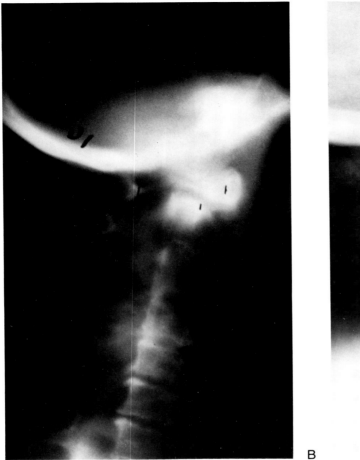
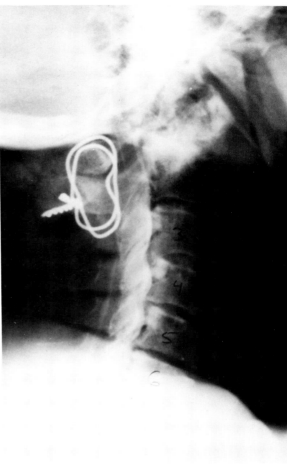

A   B

Fig. 19-8. (A) Lateral cervical spine radiograph in a patient who sustained a fracture of the odontoid process and forward subluxation of C1 and C2. (B) The patient underwent posterior spine fusion of C1–C2 without complications, but postoperatively demonstrated incomplete C5–C6 quadriparesis which extended to C6 quadriplegia over the next 7 days. This myelogram reveals previously unrecognized cervical spondylosis at C5–C6 resulting in quadriplegia. The explanation for the neurological injury was compression of the spinal cord by cervical spondylosis while the patient was in the prone position for the posterior fusion of C1–C2.

fore unrecognized, nonsymptomatic cervical disc, with the recreation of cervical spine hyperextension it is possible (and it has occurred) that the anterior spinal cord and anterior spinal artery will undergo compromise and that neurologic injury will be either accentuated or caused. It is also appropriate to note that identical causes for neurologic injury (prone positioning hyperextension) from marked cervical spondylosis (Fig. 19-8) are also possible.

3. *Presence of partial neurologic recovery after vertebral column trauma, with early neurologic pla-*

teauing. After spinal column injury, when an incomplete neurologic injury results, a patient may demonstrate early evidence of partial neurologic recovery, followed by sudden cessation of progress. Anticipating further improvement, it is necessary to rule out neurologic tissue or spinal canal compromise as the etiology.

4. *Inconsistent relationship between the extent of neurologic injury and radiologic evidence of vertebral column trauma.* In the presence of known trauma and neurologic injury identified on physical examination, one would anticipate a

correlation between the neurologic injury and the vertebral column trauma. When correlation does not exist, either not at all or at different levels, other causes must be ruled out, (i.e., spinal cord edema, extradural hematoma, herniated disc, unsuspected tumor, etc.).

5. *Inconsistency between findings on neurologic examination and SSEP examination.* The patient whose initial postinjury physical examination reveals so evidence of residual motor or sensory function, yet upon SSEP testing shows sparse evidence of neurologic function, suggests electrical neurologic "incompleteness." This becomes an indication for a myelogram, giving the patient the benefit of the doubt.

MECHANICAL (DISTRACTION) FORCES RESULTING IN COLUMN INJURY

The direction and magnitude of mechanical forces applied across the vertebral column alter its structure and result in either specific or combinations of ligamentous and vertebral element injuries. These in turn, depending on the extent of vertebral element injury and anatomic level of that injury, produce either a neurologic or non-neurologically related injury:

Flexion injuries cause disruption of posterior (interspinous) ligaments and are frequently associated with a compression fracture of a vertebral body.

Flexion-distraction forces cause disruption of the posterior interspinous ligaments, facet joint capsule, posterior longitudinal ligament, ligamentum flavum, and anulus fibrosus resulting in loss of stability in at least two of the three vertebral column stabilizers. The result is spinal instability.[13] The combination of flexion and distraction force vectors may result in facet dislocation without facet fracture, or facet dislocation with anterior column vertebral body fracture.

Shear or translatory forces cause partial displacement (subluxation) or complete horizontal displacement (dislocation) of one vertebra on another. For either to occur, either facet subluxation or facet fracture occurs, in combination with stretching or tearing of the interspinous and supra-spinous ligaments, the ligamentum flavum, the posterior and anterior longitudinal ligaments, and the posterior and anterior anulus fibrosus, in a posterior to anterior horizontal direction. These may occur with or without vertebral element fracture. The extent of injury depends on the magnitude of the force.

Axial load or compression injuries produce various forms of compression-type injuries. Primarily, they include wedge compression vertical vertebral body fractures or explosive "burst" (comminuted) fractures. Bursting occurs when the total body mass above the fracture level (head and neck, upper extremities, chest cavity, and abdomen) rapidly decelerates in line with the lower vertebral column.

Rotational (or torsion) injuries; as a result of complex forces that together terminate in the occurrence of gross vertebral element instability, are fracture-dislocations.[14–17] Vertebral fractures, when they occur, usually extend through the upper aspect of the lower vertebra, with the injury resulting inligamentous and bone instability from anterior to posterior.

Ferguson's and Allen's classification of "thoracolumbar" spine fractures[17] included two mechanisms of injury in addition to those listed above. They were *distraction-extension* injuries to the spine and pure *lateral flexion* injuries. While I accept the two additional mechanisms, my experience, like Ferguson's, was that distraction-extension injuries were rare. In our series, only two "hyperextension" injuries to the entire thoracolumbar spine occurred (Figs. 19-10, 19-11), and no pure lateral flexion injury occurred without an associated axial load or flexion component identified in the sagittal plane (Fig. 19-1). All revealed on tomography an element of anterior vertebral compression.

Anatomically, it is well recognized that two important variables exist in the area of the lumbar vertebral column not found in other regions: a large (or wider laterally than anteroposteriorly) canal, and a nervous system composed of the cauda equina, which, in essence, is an area containing only peripheral nerves. As a consequence, the nervous system is very often spared injury. Statistics reveal that only two (of 73) L3–L5 fractures resulted in a complete neurologic injury (Table 19-5).

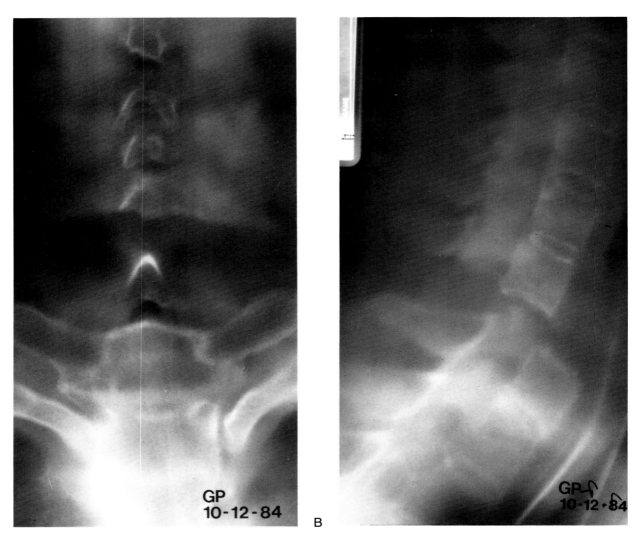

Fig. 19-9. (A,B) AP and lateral radiographs showing cervical spine fracture in a patient with Marie-Strüm-pell rheumatoid spondylitis. The patient was riding in a vehicle that was struck from the rear. The accident produced devastating hyperextension fracture-dislocation of C5–C6 with complete quadriplegia. *(Figure continues.)*

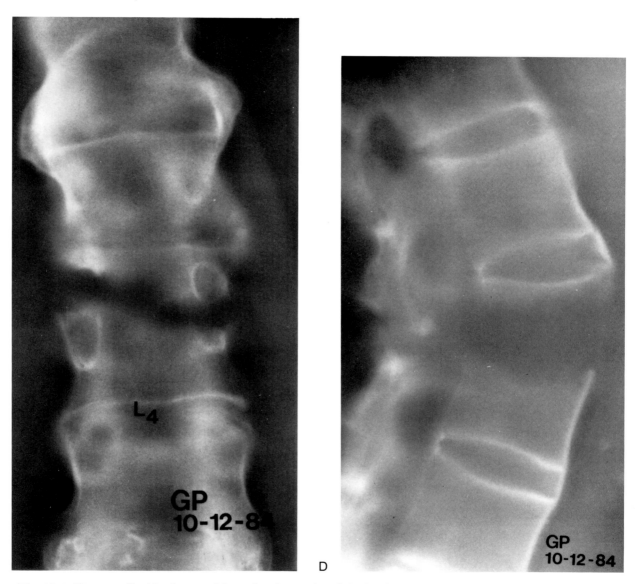

C

D

Fig. 19-9 *(Continued).* **(C,D)** AP and lateral radiographs of the lumbar spine showing extension fracture-dislocation through L3. *(Figure continues.)*

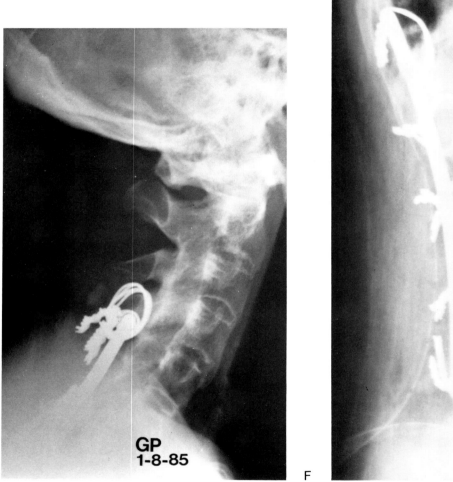

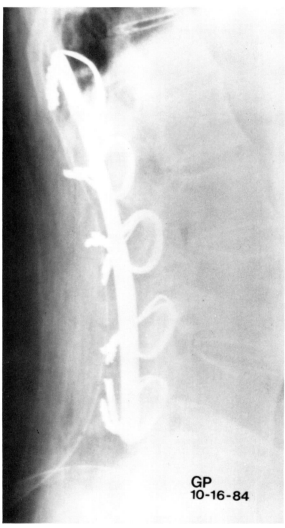

E   F

Fig. 19-9 *(Continued).* (E) Postoperative lateral cervical spine radiograph showing internal fixation and anatomic reduction using Luque instrumentation. (F) Lateral radiograph of the lumbar spine showing anatomic reduction and stabilization following Luque instrumentation. Anterior AO plate fixation of cervical spine fractures was not yet in use at the time of this repair; it would now be the treatment of choice. Similarly, the recently introduced transpedicular rod-screw fixation technique would be the treatment of choice for the lumbar injury.

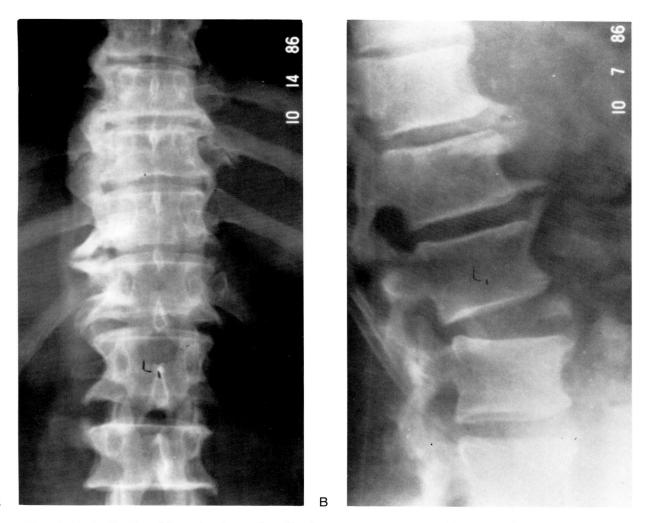

Fig. 19-10. (A,B) AP and lateral radiographs of lumbar spine in a 69-year-old patient who sustained an extension injury of L1–L2 following a fall. Note presence of extensive degenerative spondylosis. *(Figure continues.)*

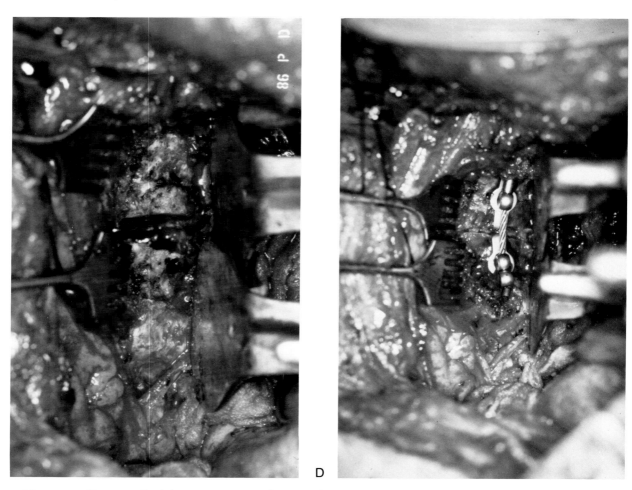

C

D

Fig. 19-10 *(Continued).* **(C)** Intraoperative photograph showing Bennett retractors protecting the aorta anteriorly, and the widened space between L1 and L2 representing the extension injury. The intervertebral disc has been excised. **(D)** Dwyer cable inserted and compression applied. Before compression was applied, a bone graft was inserted between L1 and L2. *(Figure continues.)*

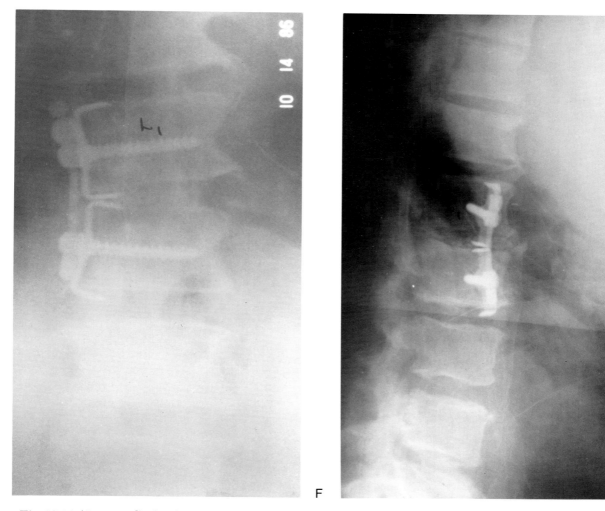

E   F

Fig. 19-10 *(Continued).* **(E,F)** AP and lateral radiographs showing Dwyer staples and cable between L1 and L2. Note closure of L2–L3 intervertebral disc space and presence of the bone graft. The patient was neurologically normal.

BIOMECHANICAL, ETIOLOGIC, AND FRACTURE PATTERNS OF INJURIES OF THE LUMBAR VERTEBRAL COLUMN

When varied mechanical forces are applied to the spine, they result in identifiable patterns of injury [13,17–19] (i.e., ligamentous injury without vertebral body fracture; compression injuries [including angular or wedge fractures or axial burst vertebral body fractures]; flexion distraction injuries; lateral translatory injuries, and those injuries that result from a combination of mechanical forces: flexion-axial load-rotation injuries).

In the lower lumbar region, particularly between L3 and L5, falls from heights (construction injuries or attempted suicides) most often resulted in vertical (axial) load (burst)-type injuries. As noted earlier, when mechanical forces are "uncontaminated" by complex or multiple force vectors, the absorption of high-energy loads usually resulted in a burst fracture (38.4 percent) (Table 19-3). Flexion injuries occurred in 24.7 percent of cases and occurred secondary to forces varying from pure flexion to flexion-distraction (as with lap or seatbelt injuries) to flexion-rotation injuries (including dislocations). Translatory or shear-type injuries followed direct injury to the torso or vertebral column.

Of the 73 fractures occurring between L3 and L5, 28 (38.4 percent) were burst fractures. This was the most frequently identified fracture. The

second most frequent fracture (10) was a vertical vertebral body fracture (in either the coronal or sagittal plane) in 19.2 percent (see Figs. 19-1, 19-21); 8 were gunshot wounds (11 percent) (Fig. 19-12); and 4 were Chance[20] fractures (5.5 percent) (Fig. 19-13). The remaining 11 vertebral injuries (15 percent) were of various types including spinous process, pedicle, facet fractures, two dislocations, and three traumatic spondylolistheses (Table 19-11).

Injuries to the sacral spine failed to demonstrate

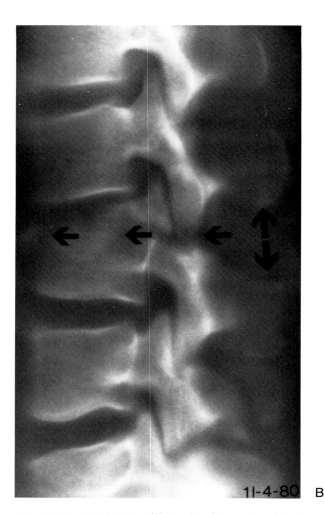
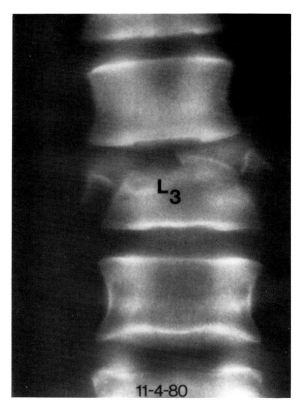

Fig. 19-11. (A,B) AP and lateral radiographs of lumbar spine showing Chance-type fracture through L3. Note distraction identified by increased space between the L2–L3 posterior spinous processes, and flexion axial load identified by the presence of a comminuted compression fracture of the superior plate of L3. The patient was neurologically intact.

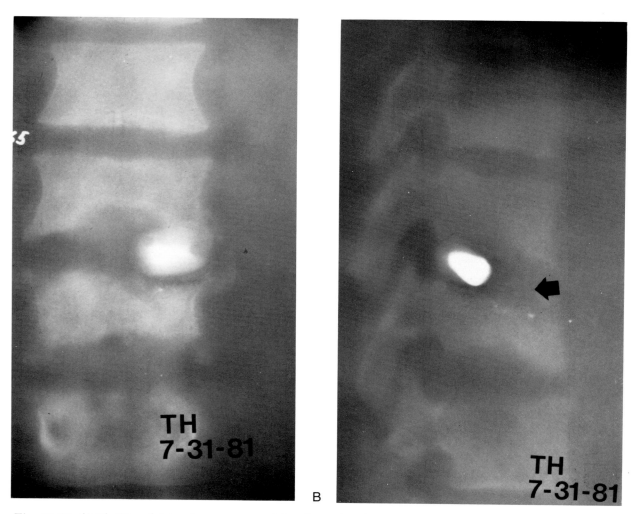

Fig. 19-12. **(A,B)** AP and lateral tomograms of the thoracolumbar spine revealing a bullet lying in the T12–L1 interspace. Note the presence of bone resorption in both views, evidence of disc space infection. *(Figure continues.)*

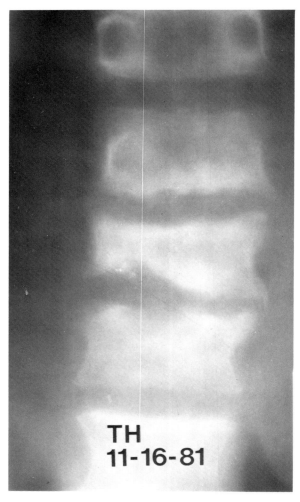

C

Fig. 19-12 *(Continued).* (C) AP view of T12–L1 disc space after removal of the bullet. Note healing of the disc space and maintenance of vertebral column alignment.

Table 19-11. Lumbar versus Sacral: Type of Spinal Fracture (Northwestern University Acute Spine Injury Center, 1972 to 1986)

Type of Spinal Fracture	Lumbar		Sacral	
	No.	Percent	No.	Percent
Axial body compression	28	38.4	2	15.4
Body	10	13.7	3	23.1
Bullet fragments	8	11.0	1	7.7
No fracture	8	11.0	4	30.8
Chance	4	5.5	0	0.0
Facet	3	4.1	0	0.0
Spondylolisthesis	3	4.1	0	0.0
Other	5	6.8	3	23.1
Total	73	100.0	13	100.0

LUMBAR FRACTURE CLASSIFICATION AND INTERPRETATION OF SPINAL STABILITY

Kaufer and Hayes, in 1966, reviewed a series of 21 lumbar spine injuries and noted that most fractures in this area of the vertebral column (the lumbar spine) result in "instability."[18] The definitions of instability by Holdsworth[14-16] and Denis,[13] although not identical, ultimately arrived at the same conclusion: the loss of two of the three structural columns results in instability of the vertebral column (Fig. 19-14). The structures composing each of the three columns from anterior to posterior are the anterior column (the anterior longitudinal ligament, the anterior two-thirds of the vertebral body, and the anterior portion of the anulus fibrosus); the middle column (the posterior one-third of the vertebral body including the pedicle, the posterior longitudinal ligament, and the posterior portion of the anulus fibrosus); and, the posterior column (the posterolateral (facet) capsular ligaments, the ligamentum flavum, the posterior laminar structures, and the supraspinous and interspinous ligaments).

As noted above, each spine fracture classification has been an attempt at combining structural loss of

any pattern. It was not possible to identify the specific mechanical force resulting in fracture. Fracture often followed direct (violent) force to the sacrum or the lumbosacropelvic region of the vertebral column. Of the 932 fractures of the lower spine treated at Northwestern University, only 13 injuries occurred in the area of the sacrum (1972 to 1986) (Table 19-1).

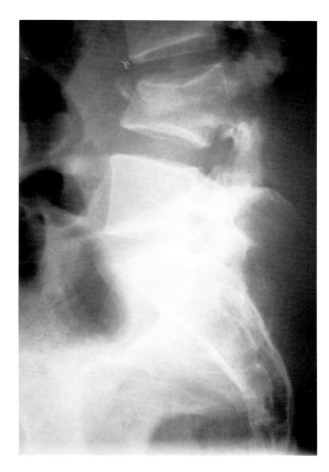

Fig. 19-13. Lateral radiograph of the lumbar spine showing distraction-flexion Chance fracture through the midportion of the anterior middle vertebral column. Note the presence of traumatic lumbar kyphosis and the widened space posteriorly between the posterior elements of L4 and L5.

Table 19-12.   Scheme to Estimate Vertebral Column Stability

Column Injury	Structural Injury	Severity
A. Anterior	Bone	Mild
B. Posterior	Ligament	Moderate
C. Combined	Combined	Severe

tous injuries are more likely to require surgical intervention because of their recognized failure to heal with stability by conservative means alone.

The extent of internal (or external) fixation was determined by the structures undergoing loss of integrity and the severity of that injury. The attempt made, with this new and more simplified classification, was to suggest a uniform, descriptive method of communicating the indications for and the type of necessary stabilization between colleagues, much as the Frankel classification provides a descriptive method of denoting neurologic injury recovery over time.[22] The surgeon must keep in mind, when using any of the presently available spine fracture classifications, that structural injury does not correlate with either the extent or the type of neurologic injury present or the potential for that neurologic injury to recovery. Therefore, management must be based solely on the structures undergoing injury and the interpretation of resulting loss of stability.

The fracture classification described by Kaufer and Hayes,[18] although simple, remains accurate and represents the lumbar spine injury variations most commonly identified in their series.

Type 1: Dislocation of facets and vertebral body without fracture (Fig. 19-15)

Type 2: Dislocation of facets with vertebral body fracture (Fig. 19-11)

Type 3: Dislocation of articular processes without dislocation of the vertebral body

Type 4: Dislocation of one pair of facets with the fracture line through the opposite pars interarticularis, pedicle, articular process, and into either the vertebral body or disc space

Type 5   Dislocation of the posterior processes without dislocation of the vertebral body (bilateral fracture through the pedicle or pars interarticularis)[23]. This latter injury

integrity with residual instability, indicating a need for surgical stabilization. The most recent (suggested) classification of spinal stability-instability was presented at the 1986 AO-ASIF Spine Course (Davos, Switzerland) by Fritz Magerl of St. Galen, Switzerland, and Jurgen Harms of Karlsbad, Federal Republic of Germany.[21] Their suggested method of determining vertebral column stability or lack thereof was based on the scheme in Table 19-12. Surgical stabilization was indicated by the presence of *any* two-column injury (row C), with a moderate or severe severity level. Pure ligamen-

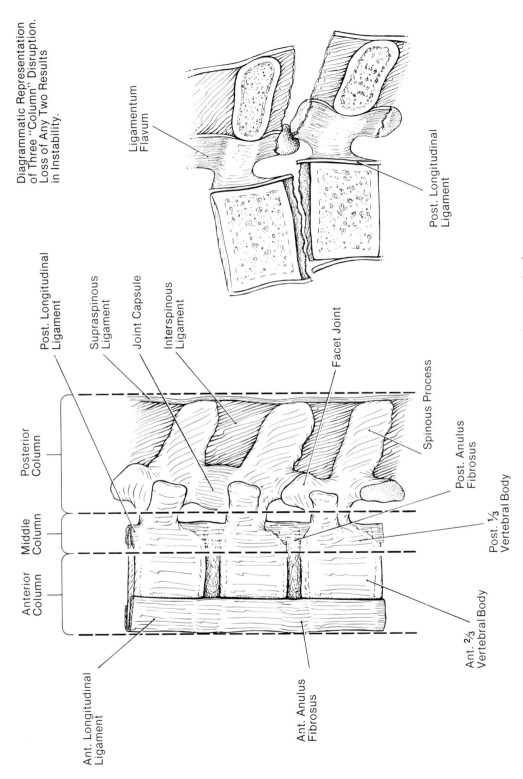

Diagrammatic Representation of Three "Column" Disruption. Loss of Any Two Results in Instability.

Ligamentum Flavum

Post. Longitudinal Ligament

Post. Longitudinal Ligament

Supraspinous Ligament

Joint Capsule

Interspinous Ligament

Facet Joint

Spinous Process

Post. Anulus Fibrosus

Posterior Column

Middle Column

Anterior Column

Post. ⅓ Vertebral Body

Ant. ⅔ Vertebral Body

Ant. Longitudinal Ligament

Ant. Anulus Fibrosus

Fig. 19-14. The "three-column" model of the spinal column.

is a variation seen rather than frequently identified.

Most researchers agree that sufficient structural integrity has been lost with the following injuries, as to require surgical stabilization:[13,14,18,21,23-26] Translatory (horizontal) displacement (greater than 3.5 mm) of one vertebral segment on another; torsion (or rotation) injuries of the vertebral segments, in which one pedicle and facet are fractured, with vertebral body displacement; comminuted (burst) vertebral body fractures; wedge compression fracture of the vertebral body of greater than 35 percent; or distraction injuries (seatbelt injury) with dislocation or subluxation.

In the series of 73 lumbar fractures presented here (L3 and L5), 52.1 percent or 38 fractures required surgical stabilization (Table 19-13). The majority of the fractures were burst fractures (75 percent) (Table 19-14) (see Figs. 19-1, 19-21).

As noted in Figures 19-6, 19-21, and 19-11, other variations and combinations of fractures frequently occurred. Although noteworthy and of low incidence, they still required surgical stabilization.

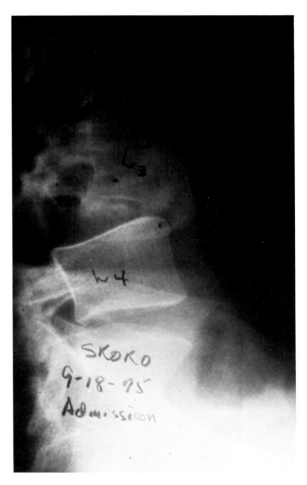

A

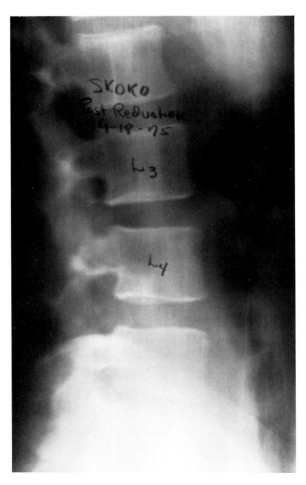

B

Fig. 19-15. (A) Lateral radiograph of the lumbar spine showing a flexion-distraction injury at the L3–L4 interspace. The radiograph reveals dislocation of the inferior facets of L3 without visible fractures of the facets. Note anterior translation of L3 on L4, demonstrating three-column instability. (B) Lateral radiograph following closed manipulation in the emergency room shortly after admission (see Figs. 19-3, 19-5). *(Figure continues.)*

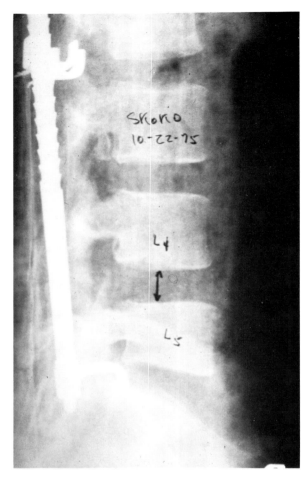

C

Fig. 19-15 *(Continued).* (C) Postoperative lateral radiograph following insertion of Harrington distraction apparatus from L2 to the sacrum. Note the widened intervertebral space at each level resulting from forceful distraction apparatus, with a bony defect noted in the area of the spinal canal at L3–L4. Note intact facets at the same level.

Table 19-13. Lumbar versus Sacral:
Management (Northwestern University Acute
Spine Injury Center, 1972 to 1986)

Management	Lumbar		Sacral	
	No.	*Percent*	*No.*	*Percent*
Conservative	35	47.9	11	84.6
Surgical	38	52.1	2	15.4
Total	73	100.0	13	100.0

As noted, the most frequent fracture patterns identified in the lumbar spine included burst fractures (see Figs. 19-1, 19-21); compression fractures of the superior plate of the inferior vertebral body associated with anterior displacement of the superior vertebral body on the inferior, with fracture of one or both facets (often associated with kyphosis); and fractures of the posterior elements with involvement of the upper third (middle and anterior columns) of the inferior vertebral body (as with the Chance fracture).[20] Numerous variations of this fracture exist (Figs. 19-11, 19-13).

The least frequently identified mechanism of injury in my series of 73 lumbar spine fractures was flexion-distraction (particularly at the L5-S1 junction) (Fig. 19-16) Although it was infrequent in our

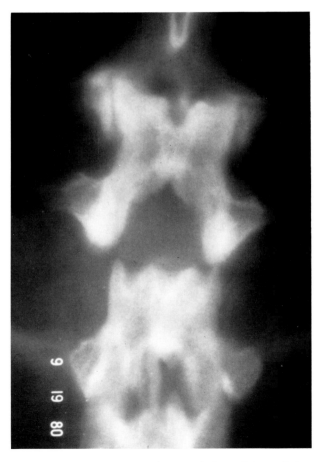

Fig. 19-16. AP tomogram showing bilateral facet dislocation resulting from a flexion-distraction type injury to the midlumbar spine.

Table 19-14. Lumbar: Type of Management by Fracture Type (Northwestern University Acute Spine Injury Center, 1972 to 1986)

Fracture Type	Total Cases	Conservative No.	Conservative Percent	Surgical No.	Surgical Percent
Axial compression	28	7	25.0	21	75.0
Body	10	4	40.0	6	60.0
Bullet fragments	8	7	87.5	1	12.5
No fracture	8	8	100.0	0	0.0
Anterior compression wedge	4	2	50.0	2	50.0
Chance	4	2	50.0	2	50.0
Facet	3	0	0.0	3	100.0
Spondylolisthesis	3	3	100.0	0	0.0
Other	5	2	40.0	3	60.0
Total	73	35	48.0	38	52.1

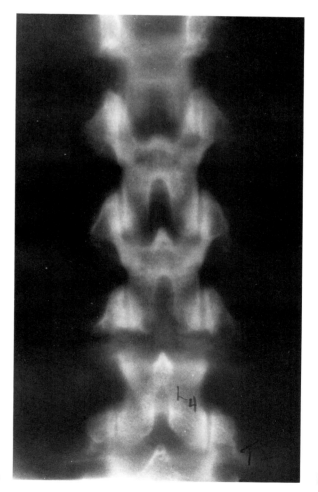

A

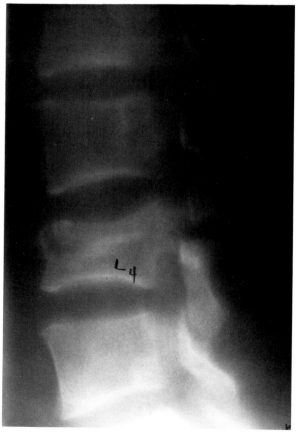

B

Fig. 19-17. (A,B) AP and lateral radiographs reveal Chance fracture involving the posterior elements and vertebral body of L4. Note horizontal fracture through posterior transverse processes and pedicles of L4. Patient required colostomy for closed injury to the colon resulting in perforation of the large bowel and contamination of the peritoneal cavity. Intraabdominal injuries not infrequently accompany injuries to the lumbar spine. The patient was neurologically intact. *(Figure continues.)*

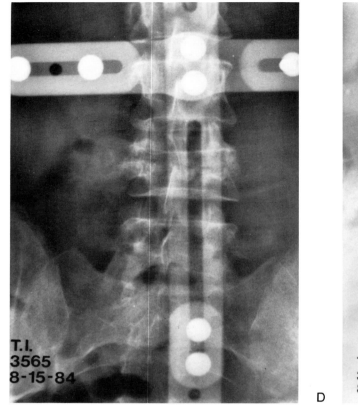
C

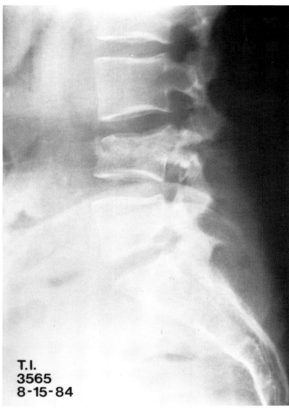
D

Fig. 19-17 *(Continued)*. **(C,D)** AP and lateral radiographs of the lumbar spine showing position of fixation in "CASH" cruciate hyperextension external orthosis.

series, Gumley et al. in 1982 reported on 20 flexion-distraction injuries occurring in the lumbar spine.[27] Similar to my findings, no injuries in their series occurred at either L4 or L5. Most appeared at L1 (9) and L3 (6). Four occurred at L2, and one occurred at T12. Because seatbelt usage is uniformly mandatory in Australia, most of the injuries followed motor vehicle accidents in which the seatbelt was implicated (65 percent). The remaining patients (35 percent) sustained injury after either a fall or unknown causes. Gumley, et al. also noted a high incidence of associated abdominal injuries in their series (40 percent)[27] (Fig. 19-17). The most serious intra-abdominal trauma was seen in those patients sustaining injury at L3 (cecal perforation).[27,28] The additional abdominal injuries were divided over adjacent levels.

The typical flexion-distraction injury or fracture to the lumbar spine is a Chance fracture.[20] As described by Chance[20] and correlated with "over the belt" or extension flexion-distraction injuries by others,[18,27,29–31] the resulting vertebral column injury may be in the form of a fracture, passing from posterior to anterior through all bone and ligamentous structures (Fig. 19-9), or in the form of a dislocation (in which the nonfractured facet dislocates, allowing forward displacement of the superior vertebra on the inferior vertebra (see Fig. 19-18)[32]; also, fractured facets allow anterior vetebral element displacement.

When the forces of distraction allow displacement of one vertebral element from another without fracture, there results an obvious loss of structural integrity that involves the posterior interspinous and supraspinous ligaments, the posterior anulus fibrosus, the facet joint capsules, the

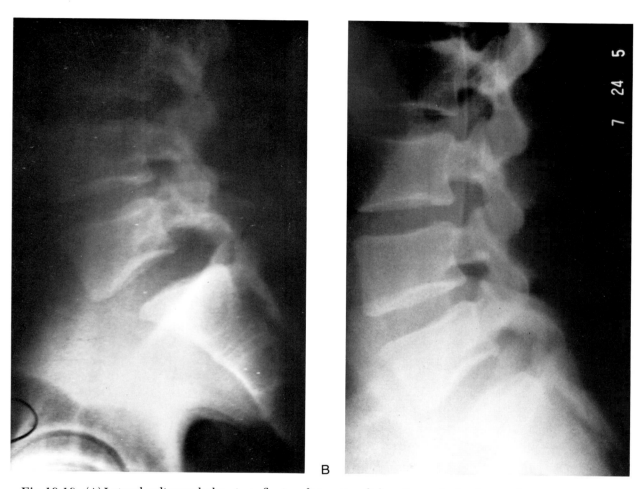

Fig. 19-18. (A) Lateral radiograph showing a flexion-distraction dislocation at the lumbosacral joint without fracture of the facets. The patient was neurologically normal. (B) Lateral radiograph of the lumbosacral spine showing closed reduction of dislocated facets L5–S1. *(Figure continues.)*

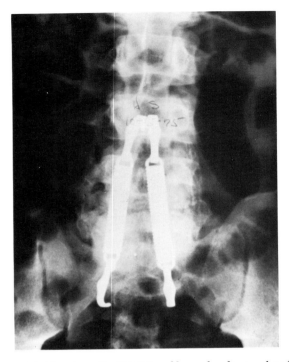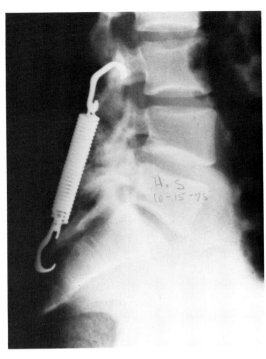

C

Fig. 19-18 *(Continued)*. **(C)** AP and lateral radiographs of the lumbosacral spine demonstrating reduction of facet dislocation and reconstitution of lumbosacral lordosis. Weiss compression springs were used for internal fixation; the inferior hooks were placed directly into the second sacral foramen and the upper hooks over the superior surface of the L3 lamina. Lateral spine fusion was also performed. This internal fixation device is no longer used; transpedicular three-level fixation is more appropriate.

ligamentum flavum, and the posterior longitudinal ligament (Fig. 19-15). Associated fracture of the anterior and middle column may or may not occur, though forward luxation of the superior vertebra on the inferior vertebra may result. These latter injuries were identified at the lumbosacral joint on two occasions (Figs. 19-18, 19-19). Both were managed by initial prone positioning of the patient on a Stryker frame. The patient with intact facets had a closed reduction. The patient with fractured facets underwent open reduction and surgical excision of a posterior herniated disc (Fig. 19-19). Initial neurologic examination of both patients revealed permanent loss of one or more unilateral lumbar or upper sacral segments, and one patient was revealed on myelography to have a gross contrast column defect owing to a large extruded intervertebral disc at the L5–S1 interval. Both required surgical procedures for either decompression or stabilization (Figs. 19-18, 19-19).

A third patient (an elderly pedestrian) sustained a lateral translatory fracture-dislocation at the L5–S1 level (Kaufer type 4 injury). The patient had a unilateral L5 nerve root defect. She was managed conservatively (4 weeks of bed care, followed by the wearing of an orthosis for 2 months) and the application of a below-knee ankle-foot orthosis.

It is worth noting that the three injuries just demonstrated each show five of the seven basic mechanisms of injury: flexion-extension; distraction; rotation; lateral translation; and a combination of forces (including compression, extension, and lateral flexion).

Extension injuries to the thoracic and lumbar vertebral column are considered uncommon. Only one lumbar hyperextension injury occurred in the 73 L3 to L5 lumbar fractures appearing in my series. (Of 319 traditional L1-L5 fractures, 4 were extension injuries [2.0 percent]. This latter incidence figure collaborates with that of Ferguson and Allen.[17]) This single injury occurred in a motor vehicle passenger (with Marie-Strümpel rheuma-

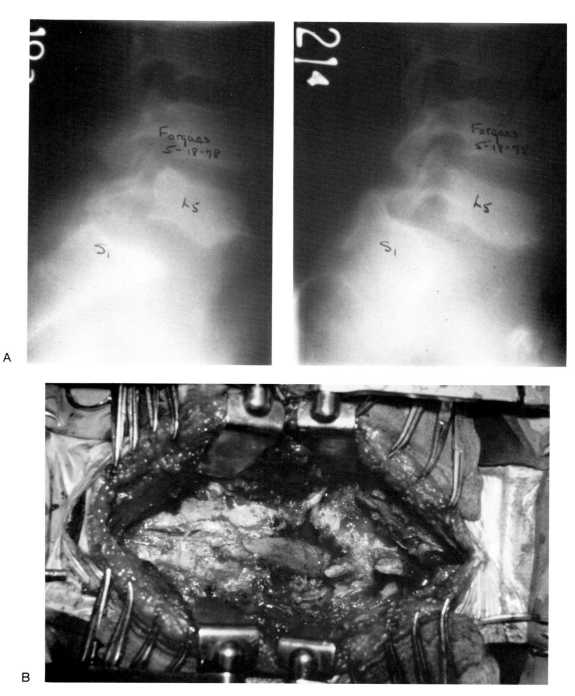

Fig. 19-19. (A) AP and lateral radiographs of the lumbosacral joint showing bilateral facet dislocation of the joints and anterior displacement of the L5 vertebral body on S1. (B) Intraoperative photograph of surgical pathology following removal of herniated L5–S1 intervertebral disc. Sacrum is toward the left. Note remaining continuity of dural sheath. *(Figure continues.)*

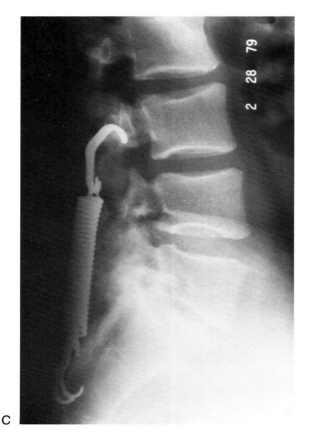

C

Fig. 19-19 *(Continued)*. **(C)** Postoperative lateral radiograph (9 months after operation) showing reduction of L5–S1 dislocation and fusion of L4 to the sacrum. Internal fixation is maintained with Weiss compression springs. Cotrel-Dubousset fixation now utilized for fixation at this level (Fig. 19-46).

toid spondylitis) whose car was struck from the rear. The patient sustained two simultaneous extension fracture-dislocation injuries to the spine: one at C5-C6, the other at L2-L3 (Fig. 19-9). Gross spinal instability[33–35] occurred at both sites, with the injury at C5 resulting in a C5 quadriplegia (complete). The patient underwent a posterior Luque rod spinal stabilization procedure at both levels of injury. Though it is suggested in the literature that there may be posterior hematoma formation contributing to the presence of the neurologic injury, the only evidence of etiology of the neurologic injury was the extent of the initial injury and the amount of spinal instability resulting from that injury.

MULTIPLE SPINAL LEVEL INJURY PATTERNS

Calenoff and Rogers[12,36] (Northwestern University, Department of Radiology) reviewed the pattern of vertebral column fractures in a patient population of greater than 700 acute spine injury patients between 1976 and 1981. Three repeatable injury patterns appeared (Fig. 19-20). Each is divided into two subgroups: a primary lesion (capable of producing neurologic injury or spinal instability or both), and a secondary lesion (not responsible for neurologic deficit or spinal instability). The patterns were as follows:

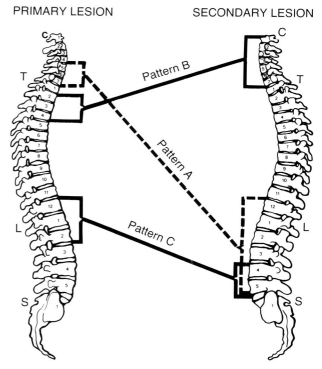

Fig. 19-20. The three most common multilevel fracture patterns involving the vertebral column. The *primary lesion* is the fracture for which the patient was admitted or from which neurologic symptoms arise. The *secondary lesion* accompanies the primary injury. Pattern C is the least common occurring pattern of spinal injuries.

Pattern A: Primary injury at C5 to C7 was a secondary injury occurring between T11 and L5. This was the most frequently appearing pattern of spinal column injury.

Pattern B: Primary injury occurs between T2 and T4 and the secondary injury occurs in the cervical spine between C1 and C7. As unusual as this grouping may appear, the injury is not rare, though infrequent.

Pattern C: Primary injury at T11 to L2 and secondary injury at L4–L5.

The value of recognizing pattern injuries occurs during patient evaluation. Two lumbar spine-injured patients are described below and represent the most frequently appearing pattern (A) and the least frequent pattern (C).

The patient sustaining a pattern A injury was a 62-year-old man with a stable but severe spinal deformity, secondary to Marie-Strümpel[37,38] rheumatoid spondylitis.[39,40] The patient's preinjury status, according to history, was that the patient was fully ambulatory, yet, because of severe spinal deformity, was unable to see the horizon without bending his knees and leaning backwards. On the date of admission to the acute spine injury service, the patient was reported to be a passenger in the rear seat of a motor vehicle stopped at a street light. The victim's vehicle was struck from the rear by a truck, causing the patient to be thrown acutely into extension. Paramedics arriving at the scene found the patient conscious but quadriplegic at the C5 level, with complaints of pain in the cervical spine (Fig. 19-20). Evaluation of the patient revealed total radiologic disruption of the anterior, middle, and posterior columns[13,20,33] and complete loss of motor and sensory function below the C5 neurologic level. Radiologic evaluation demonstrated the presence of an extension-disruption injury involving the anterior, middle, and posterior columns of the lumbar spine at L3 (Fig. 19-20). The patient was managed initially on a Stryker wedge frame. When it was determined that both fractures were grossly unstable and that reduction was lost after rotation of the patient into extension, the patient was managed on a Roto-Rest bed in a supine position. Some consideration was given to taking advantage of the fractures by placing the patient in slightly more hyperextension at both fracture sites,

so as to improve the patient's eventual upright (vertebral column) stance position. The cervical spine fracture, even with total recumbency, was grossly unstable. Therefore, the cervical spine was immobilized with a halo vest. Even this proved unsuccessful, requiring stabilization posteriorly with a Luque rod system. Failure to gain stability with a halo vest differs from the experience of Burgman and Stauffer,[39] yet was also noted by Bohler and Gaudernak.[41]

As noted, this same patient had a similar management problem (instability) in the area of the lumbar spine fracture. The literature describes difficulty in maintaining alignment.[38,39] Some investigators have suggested taking advantage of the opportunity to improve the preinjury position of the spinal deformity by managing the vertebral column in a straightaway (horizontal) position. Again, instability was a problem. I found that both the cervical and lumbar spine fracture areas were enhanced in their healing by placing the ankylosed spine in the pretrauma flexed or extended position, depending on the level of injury. It is appreciated that this may not always be attainable, particularly when operating on a patient in the prone position. The lumbar fracture was likewise stabilized with the Luque rod segmental instrumentation system. Neurologically, the patient had a C5 quadriplegia resulting from injury at the C5 level of the cervical spine (Fig. 19-9). It can be stated emphatically that the use of SSEP monitoring during surgery on the spine can and does give the surgeon a margin of safety not previously available, and for which the "wake-up" test was frequently required, particularly when operating on an intact patient or on one with an incomplete neurologic injury. It is appreciated that real concerns exist with various surgical procedures, including the passage of sublaminar wire; however, with qualified monitoring, these hazards can be reduced or eliminated.[42,43] When there is evidence of incomplete neurological injury, definite care must be taken with the passage of sublaminar wires, and/or alternate methods of stabilization should be undertaken.

An example of a C pattern patient, that is, fracture of the vertebral column at both the thoracolumbar and the lumbar spine, is that of a 22-year-old woman who sustained an injury to the lumbar spine after a three-story fall, jumping from a burning building. Although sustaining a relatively minor neurologic injury (an L5-S1 conus medullaris-type injury bilaterally), she sustained a compression (burst) fracture at both the L1 and the L5 levels of the lumbar spine and a suspected fracture of the odontoid (Fig. 19-21B). The cervical spine was managed in Gardner-Well tong traction for 3 weeks, followed by a SOMI orthosis. Management of the two noncontiguous level vertebral body injuries included lumbar myelography (Fig. 19-21C) and tomography (which revealed two-level neural canal compromise) (Fig. 19-21A). This necessitated a "staged" multilevel anterior decompression, with rib and fibular inlay bone graft used across the T12 to L2 interval and likewise across the L4 to S1 levels. Posteriorly, the patient's spine was stabilized from T11 to S2 with Harrington distraction rods (Fig. 19-21D,E). Postoperatively, the patient was placed in a plaster of paris pantaloon body cast-spica for 3 months. Her neurologic strength at 1 year revealed improvement from a Frankel C level[22] to a Frankel D level.

CONSERVATIVE MANAGEMENT OF FRACTURES OF THE LUMBAR SPINE

Advocates of conservative thoracic and lumbar spine fracture management were the same physicians who actually put spinal injury care into perspective, beginning in the 1940s up until the early 1970s.[23,44,45] To give credit where it is due, these physicians, surgeons and nonsurgeons, managed spinal injuries under entirely different circumstances. Although it appears that a significant contrast exists between then and today, actually what has changed is everything but the fracture, that is, greatly improved patient retrieval and initial care, anesthesia, metallurgy, antibiotics, spinal cord monitoring, operating conditions, recognition of complications from long-term recumbency and their prevention, costs, etc. While Guttmann suggested prolonged conservative bed care and for such developed the Guttmann Bed,[44] today a very close facsimile, the Roto-Rest bed, is used, as well as the standard method of managing acute spinal injuries, the Stryker wedge frame. There is general agreement that there are certain fractures that

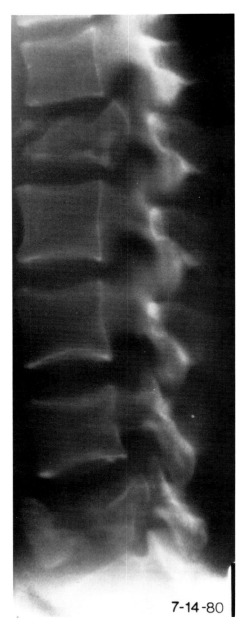

A   7-14-80

Fig. 19-21. (A) Lateral radiograph of the lumbar spine showing a severe burst compression fracture of vertebral bodies L1 and L5. Note posterior extrusion of vertebral body elements into the neural canal at L1 and L5. *(Figure continues.)*

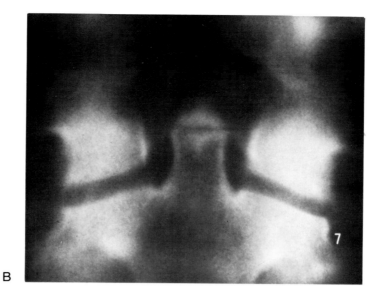

B

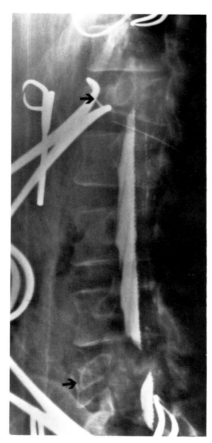

C

Fig. 19-21 *(Continued)*. **(B)** Anterior tomogram of C1–C2 demonstrating suspected fracture of the proximal tip of the odontoid process. The patient was managed in cervical tong traction and a Stryker frame during the initial phase of hospital care. **(C)** Lateral myelogram revealing obstruction at L1 and L5. *(Figure continues.)*

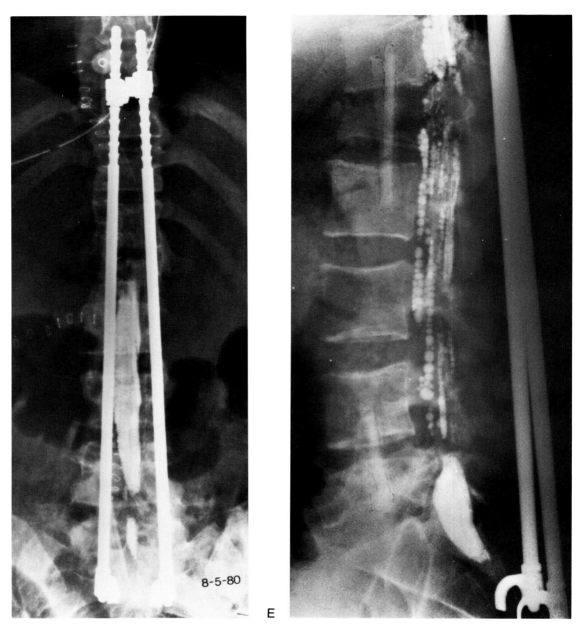

D   E

Fig. 19-21 *(Continued).* **(D,E)** AP and lateral radiographs showing postoperative internal fixation with Harrington rods and evidence of anterior decompression with inlay bone grafts at T12–L2 and L4–S1. *(Figure continues.)*

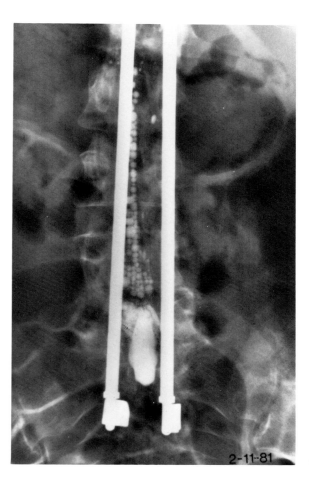
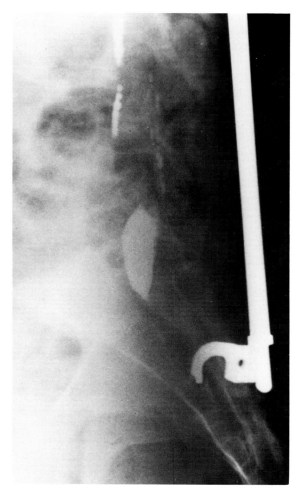

Fig. 19-21 *(Continued)*. **(F,G)** AP and lateral radiographs taken six months after operation, demonstrating bilateral loss of fixation of the Harrington rod hooks from the sacrum.

warrant conservative management (48 percent in the Northwestern University series). These include:

Compression fractures of the anterior vertebral body (less than 25 to 35 percent), with less than 3.5 mm of vertebral element displacement.

Multiple fractures of the vertebral column, which exist not only at adjacent levels, but at varying distances from one another. The presence or absence of neurologic injury really does not alter this basic concept. This rule (conservative management of multiple-level fractures) is closely adhered to. Surgical stabilization-fusion at-

tempts would require the inclusion of multiple levels, resulting in excessive spinal rigidity. One of the complications of attempting a long fusion, other than producing excessive vertebral column rigidity, is failure of fusion owing to the large numbers of segments being crossed.

Patients with injuries (and significant deformity) more than 3 weeks postonset. By the third week, there is usually evidence of early fracture healing. Attempts to gain improved spinal column realignment (even operatively) are extremely difficult and often are accompanied by the occurrence of multiple complications: further loss of neurologic function owing to the excessive dissection or distraction force required; loss of fixation secondary to the relative "osteoporosis" resulting from injury to the area and hypervascularity; medical complications that are either induced by or contributed to by the surgery such as pneumothorax, deep venous thrombosis, pulmonary embolism, etc.[16] (Fig. 19-22).

Prolonged conservative care requires careful observation for the occurrence of potential medical complications (Table 19-15) including urinary tract infections (15.1 percent), hypotension (6.8 percent), decubiti (5.5 percent), gastrointestinal bleeding (4.1 percent), and deep venous thrombosis (1.4 percent); adequate numbers of acute beds to allow conservative fracture management in indicated cases; a mature, experienced, and neurologically trained nursing staff; an awareness on the part of the hospital administration that some spinal frac-

Table 19-15. Lumbar versus Sacral: Medical Complications (Northwestern University Acute Spine Injury Center, 1972 to 1986)

Complication[a]	Lumbar		Sacral	
	No.	Percent	No.	Percent
Deep venous thrombosis	1	1.4	2	15.4
Gastrointestinal bleeding	3	4.1	2	15.4
Hypotension	5	6.8	2	15.4
Hyperthermia	3	4.1	3	23.1
Pneumonia	1	1.4	1	7.7
Pressure sore	4	5.5	1	7.7
Urinary tract infection	11	15.1	6	46.2
Other	9	12.3	8	61.5

[a] Listed alphabetically.

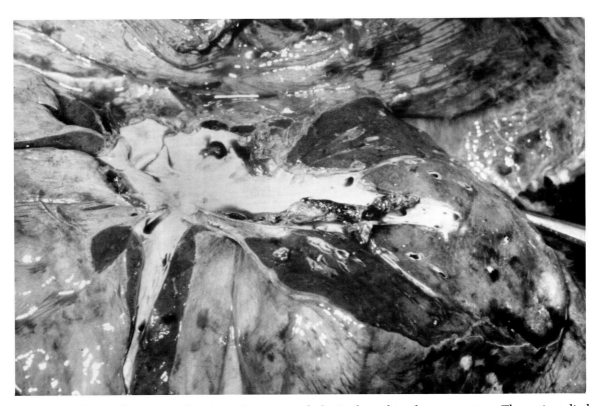

Fig. 19-22. Surgical specimen showing pulmonary embolus in the right pulmonary artery. The patient died of this solitary lesion. The patient also sustained a fracture dislocation L1–L2 in a 40 foot fall from a tree, resulting in complete L1 paraplegia.

tures require only conservative bed care (occasionally up to 4 to 6 weeks). For the patient, there must be an understanding that conservative care does not guarantee that the presence of a spinal deformity (trauma-induced malalignment) will be anatomically reduced, acceptable in its overall alignment, and sufficient for vertical loading when reinstituted. Finally it must be understood that failure of conservative management (failure of the spinal fracture to heal rigidly) may require future spine-stabilizing surgery.

Pillow Fracture Reduction Technique

Radiographs demonstrating anterior displacement of the superior vertebra on the inferior vertebra illustrate vertebral column instability. Although surgical stabilization will ultimately be required, an intervening method of ensuring maintenance of neurologic function (when present) is to prevent either the occurrence of or an increase in spinal column malalignment. When gross instability is obvious, early (or immediate) surgical stabilization is required.

Technique
In the presence of a flexion injury with the patient in the supine position (Fig. 19-23), one pillow is placed transversely across the patient's back, at the level of the gibbus or most prominent lumbar spinous process. This pillow tends to restore or place the thoracolumbar spine in a mild hyperextension position when the patient is supine. When the patient is to be placed in the prone position, two pillows are used; one transversely across the chest at the level of the sternum, and the other transversely across the pelvis at the level of the pubic symphysis. When the patient is prone, these two pillows again maintain the lumbar vertebral column in a position of extension. Frequently, this positioning aid will improve the spine's sagittal alignment. Repeat lateral radiographs with the patient in both the supine and prone position are helpful in evaluating the influence of the pillows and the resulting spinal alignment. These radiographs should be repeated at appropriate intervals to observe for evidence of further spinal instability or malalignment.

A similar technique can be utilized in the presence of an extension injury to the thoracolumbar or lumbar vertebral column. Under these circumstances, the pillow positioning is just the opposite from that used for flexion injuries, and an effort is made to maintain the vertebral column in mild flexion. This is accomplished by placing one or two pillows beneath the abdomen of the prone patient, or use of a single pillow transversely across the superior back and beneath the buttocks, in the supine patient (Fig. 19-24).

It is appropriate to frequently monitor and record the unstable spine-injured patient's neurologic status. This is most reliably obtained by the spinal cord nursing service every 2 hours (at the time of the patient's turning). Should change occur, the attending physician must be immediately notified.

Closed (Manipulative) Reduction Technique

History
The use of closed (manipulative) vertebral column fracture reduction is a technique with considerable controversy. The technique was first utilized by Hippocrates, as early as 400 BC. His technique described the use of an "extension-bench," known by Celsus as *scamnum* in the 1st century AD. Galen, also of the 1st century AD., reported on the effects of trauma to the vertebral column and the spinal cord. He noted that longitudinal incision of the spinal cord produced little apparent neurologic injury, whereas transverse incision across the substance of the cord produced paralysis below the level of incision. These important scientific findings went unnoticed until the 7th century, when Paulus Aegenita first suggested surgery for fractures of the spine. Even then, his advice was ignored.[41,46] Other early authors recommended surgical management of spinal injuries.[47]

Since ancient and medieval times, forceful, brisk manipulative procedures of the spine for spinal deformity (usually secondary to tuberculosis) have been described. The most famous of these writings was by Vidus Vidius in his translation of Orabasuis's *De Laqueiset* (1544). With the victim lying prone on a bench, the spine was pulled from a position of

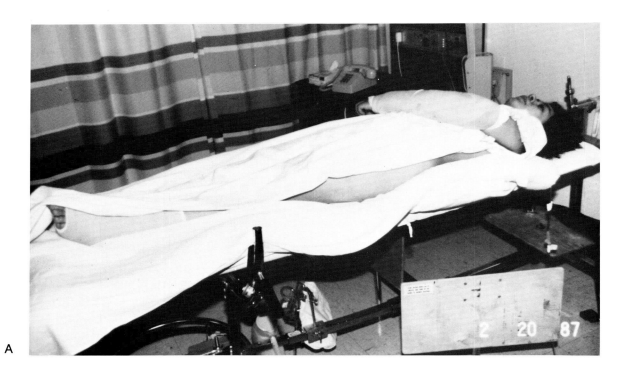

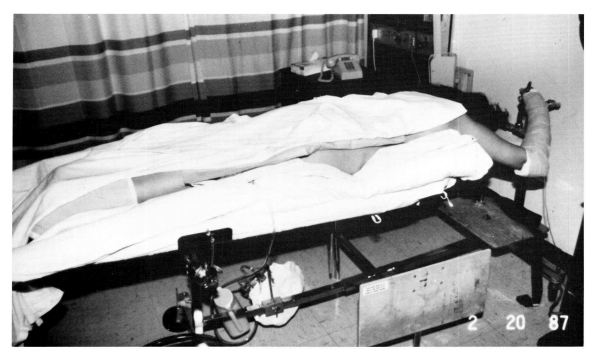

Fig. 19-23. (A) Supine positioning of a patient with a burst fracture of the L4 vertebral body and bilateral fractures of the upper and lower extremities. In the supine position, a pillow is placed transversely at the L1 level to maintain lumbar hyperextension. (B) Prone positioning of patient on Stryker frame. Note maintenance of lumbar spine hyperextension by a transverse pillow beneath the upper chest and pelvis.

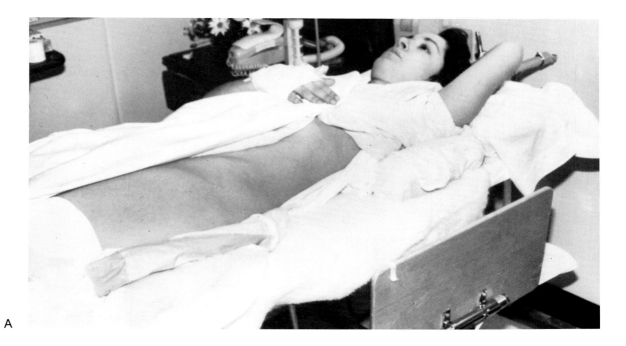

A

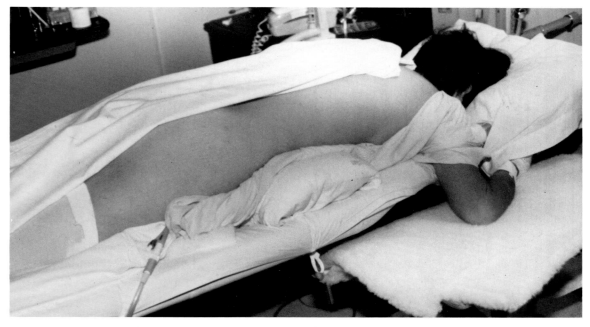

B

Fig. 19-24. (A) Horizontal supine positioning on a Stryker frame of a patient with an extension injury to the lumbar vertebral column. Note transverse pillow placed across upper back and lower pelvis to maintain lumbar kyphosis. (B) Patient maintained in lumbar kyphosis while prone on the Stryker frame by a transverse pillow across the abdomen opposite the vertebral column injury.

kyphosis into extension by means of upward traction in the axilla of the shoulders, and simultaneous traction distally from either the hips or lower extremities. The spinal deformity was approached directly. An attendant applied direct pressure over and across the area of spinal deformity, either standing or sitting on the area of the spinal gibbus or placing direct pressure on the deformity by using a crossbar. Guttmann[44] reported that Jean Francis Calot, in the 1800s, modified the technique by including the use of the hands as the preferred method of manipulation of spinal fracture or dislocation, particularly when associated with paraplegia.[9]

During the 1920s and 1930s, postural reduction of spinal fractures and dislocations (particularly in the area of the dorsolumbar spine) was performed by placing the patient in a position of hyperextension. The patient was placed in a prone position and hyperextended over slings, a frame, or a hammock.[48,49] Another method used was to hang the patient by the ankles in an inverted position, allowing the weight of the body to serve as a means of countertraction. Here again, weights were applied to the inverted patient, tied under the axilla. This method was used by Bohler[50] in the 1930s and Watson-Jones[51] in the 1940s with prone (hyperextension) placement of the patient between two tables. After manipulation, most patients required the application of a plaster jacket, extending from the symphysis pubis to the clavicle, maintaining the vertebral column in hyperextension. Another plaster technique was the use of postural positioning and maintenance in the "plaster bed." This latter technique became a major source of skin pressure sore complications in patients with absent sensation. From these complications came the hyperextension plaster cast, instituted by Bohler[50] in the 1930s for patients with normal or near normal neurologic function. This technique was altered by Guttmann during and after World War II and up until the early 1970s (Frankel et al.[52]) by using pillow positioning for the neurologically injured patient, maintaining the spine in a position of hyperextension until healed.

Considerations

I have used this technique in more than a dozen cases, but only under the most stringent of conditions. When spinal malalignment is significant and neurologic compromise exists, because there exists the possibility that major decompressive (anterior) surgery may be required, multiple service consultation (general surgery, chest surgery, vascular surgery) is requested. For our purposes, the closed reduction procedure is never indicated for fractures of the thoracic spine with preservation of any distal neurologic function. It can be utilized in spinal fractures in which there is a complete neurologic injury distal to the level of thoracic or thoracolumbar injury, or in the incomplete lumbar spine injury below the level of the conus medullaris (L1–L2). The reduction is always conducted with the patient awake.

Technique

After completion of the neurologic and physical assessment, the awake, supine patient, on the Stryker wedge frame, is rotated into the prone position. The patient is always managed while awake.

In the absence of any contraindication, morphine sulfate (2 to 10 mg/70 kg of body weight) or Demerol (meperidine hydrochloride) (50 to 100 mg) is administered for the relief of pain. In the presence of head injury, when there is a history of loss of consciousness, neither drug is administered. Should any complication arise after the administration of either drug, naloxone-(0.4 mg intravenously [IV]) can be given to counteract either drug. Valium (diazepam) (5 to 10 mg IV, given over a 5 to 10 minute period) may be used for muscle relaxation. Because this latter drug can produce respiratory changes that are not reversible by an antagonist drug, care must be exercised in its administration. A known history of associated head injury with loss of consciousness is a contraindication.

A sheet is placed across the anterior chest and out either axilla, so that the tails, when pulled cranially, lie over the posterior shoulders (Fig. 19-25). One attendent maintains traction on these two ends. Inferiorly, traction is applied by two attendents, one at each ankle. Simultaneous with the proximal and distal traction, the surgeon places direct compression over the gibbus and, when indicated, over the appropriate lateral flank (or ribs leading to the level of disability), to attain improved spinal alignment. Follow-up anteroposterior and lateral radiographs are obtained with the patient in the prone position. *Spine fracture manipulation is never conducted for any fracture of the*

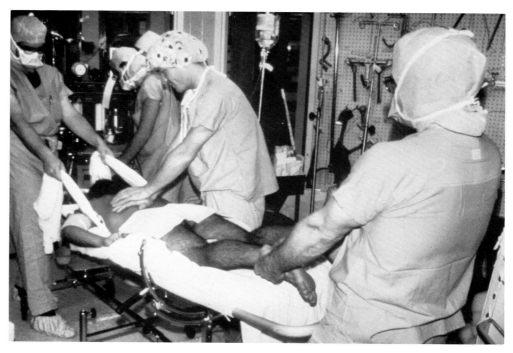

Fig. 19-25. Closed reduction technique used for fracture dislocations involving the thoracolumbar spine with complete neurologic injury. This technique requires traction across the superior chest via the axilla superiorly while bilateral traction is applied to both lower extremities. Pressure over the level of the gibbus is applied manually. This manipulation is performed in the immediate postinjury period, following initial general and neurologic evaluation. The procedure is performed using only an analgesic (meperidine) and muscle relaxant (diazepam). The procedure is never performed in neurologically intact or partially intact patients.

spine (between T1 and the superior surface of L2, i.e., the area containing the spinal cord per se) when there is any evidence of intact neurologic function below the level of injury.

INDICATIONS FOR INTERNAL FIXATION

The indications for surgical stabilization of the spine are varied. As discussed elsewhere, they do not always relate to the type of vertebral column fracture or ligamentous injury present. Occasionally, primary interest is on neurologic function and its preservation, or the concern over managing the patient conservatively, because of the presence of associated injuries. Sometimes, the decision is solely one deemed most appropriate by the manag-

ing physician. The basic guidelines utilized by the Northwestern University spine service are gross spinal malalignment; unreducible fracture-dislocations; evidence of neural tissue compromise in the patient with neurologically incomplete injury (particularly when there is any evidence of neurologic deterioration); instability as defined by the criteria of Denis,[13] Ferguson and Allen,[17] Holdsworth,[14–16] or Kaufer and Hayes:[18]

Comminuted or burst fractures of anterior vertebral elements.

Displacement of bony elements, one upon the other, either in the lateral or anteroposterior plane. Displacement greater than 3.5 mm, or unroofing of intact articular processes by 50 percent,[21] indicates instability in two of the three columns, as described by Denis[13] (Figs. 19-9, 19-11). The presence of a palpable separation between posterior elements of the lumbar spine indicates ligamentous disruption (supraspinous-interspinous ligaments, the facet capsular ligaments, ligamentum flavum, and with a great probability, the posterior longitudinal ligament and the posterior anulus fibrosus).

Instability identified as change in spinal column alignment on serial radiographs.

OPERATIVE STABILIZATION: LUMBAR SPINE

The posterior elements and neural canal of the lumbar spine are large and wide, providing an area or margin of safety for the neural elements contained within the dural sleeve. Nonetheless, the difficult aspects of managing fractures of the lumbar spine include the size (vertical height) of the lumbar vertebra, the available range of motion (flexion) between vertebral elements in the lumbar spine (lying between a "stable" thoracic spine [ribs and sternum] and a stable pelvis), the presence of varying degrees of lumbar and sacral lordosis, and the close proximity of the sacrum (the problems this poses when attempting to manage fractures near the lumbosacral joint).

Frequently, with compression or burst fractures of the vertebral body and loss of the vertical height, there will be a loss of the normal lumbar lordotic curve. Attempts at correcting the deformity by distraction (Harrington distraction rod or AO rod) results in the distraction of vertebral elements at the fracture site. The result is a literal "holding apart" of the fracture. Healing is prolonged owing to distraction at the fracture site and the time required for the vertebral body to be reconstituted.

To gain or maintain vertebral body vertical height reconstitution and maintenance of lumbar lordosis, it is necessary for the internal fixation device to be shaped to the desired curve. Likewise, the extent of the area of the lumbar vertebral column to be instrumented must be of sufficient length for the surgeon to be able to apply the required distractive or corrective force. As long as the fracture involves the midportion of the lumbar curve, this is not a major concern; however, when the fracture involves the upper lumbar spine (L2–

L3) or the lowermost vertebra (L5), fixation of the area of the spine above and below the lumbar segment is required. At the thoracolumbar-lumbar junction, the presence of either kyphosis or lordosis of the spinal segments must be taken into consideration. The presence of either of these deformities also influences the type of internal fixation device chosen. Although the presence of kyphosis or lordosis is not a major consideration when

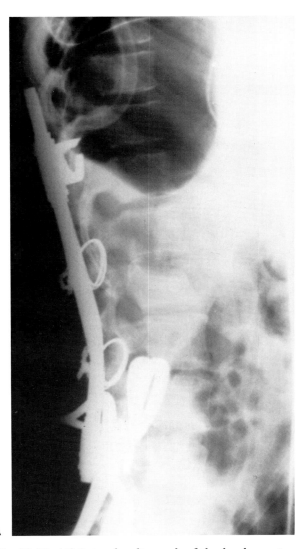

A

Fig. 19-26. **(A)** Lateral radiograph of the lumbar spine showing a fracture of the L2 vertebral body maintained in distracted and reduced position by AO (Jacobs) rods. *(Figure continues.)*

using the Luque rod system (a device which does not permit distraction), the sagittal alignment of the spine is a major consideration when using either the Harrington rod or the Jacob (AO) rod systems. Loss of internal fixation stability in the area of the upper lumbar spine is a frequent complication if the spine undergoes further kyphotic deformation secondary to resorption or collapse of a fractured vertebral body, resulting in excessive biomechanical stresses at the upper hook-bone interface.

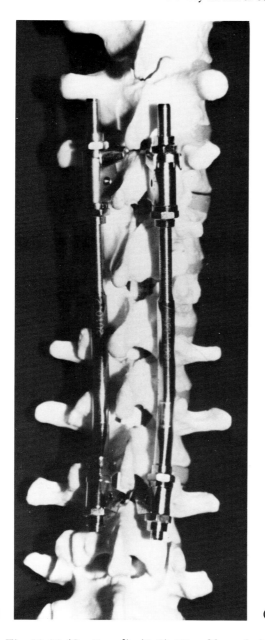
B

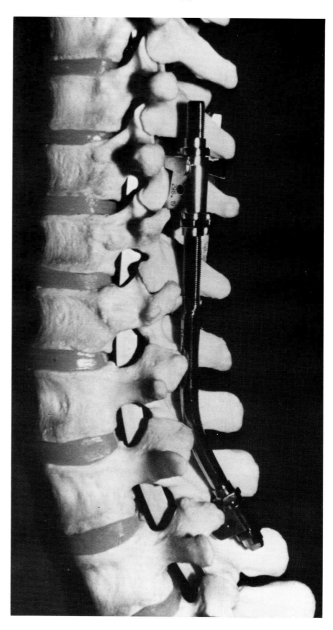
C

Fig. 19-26 *(Continued).* **(B,C)** AP and lateral photographs of AO (Jacobs) rods in place on a skeleton. The rods are thicker, are threaded on the upper end, and have a locking device at the upper end that provides rigid fixation to the lamina.

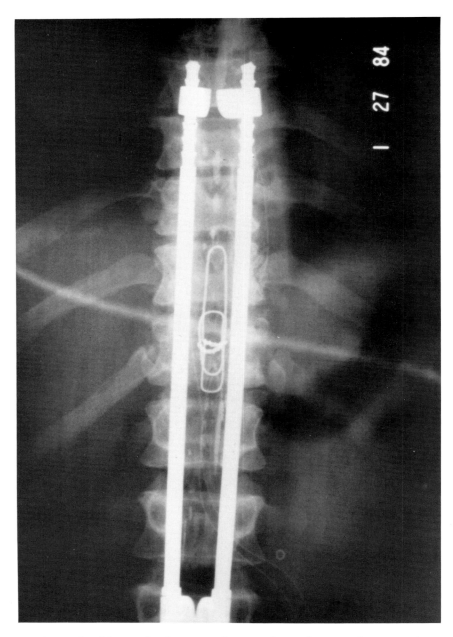

Fig. 19-27. AP radiograph of thoracolumbar spine showing the application of compression across adjacent posterior spinous processes T11–T12–L1 by means of circlage wire through the spinous processes. This wiring technique is most effective for maintaining reduction in posterior facet dislocations at the thoracolumbar junction. It is applied before insertion of other internal fixation apparatus (Harrington distraction rods).

The result is loss of fixation (Fig. 19-38) or fracture of internal fixation (Fig. 19-35).

Harrington distraction rods placed across the lumbosacral joint are capable of producing significant distraction forces across the intervertebral disc space and facet joints (Fig. 19-15C). Because the rods lie posterior to the center of motion for the lumbosacral joint, distraction forces tend to result in distraction of the lumbar vertebral column (with loss of lordotic curve) and vertebral element displacement (Fig. 19-1E). An additional concern in the use of Harrington distraction rods is the displacement of the rod-hook interface when this device is used to cross the lumbosacral joint (Fig. 19-21). This complication is the result of failure to gain stability across the lumbosacral joint (resulting in nonunion) or of flexion of the lumbar spine (with bending), resulting in dislodgment of the rods from the inferior Harrington hooks.

Because of the problem of worsening the distraction deformity across a fracture-dislocation segment when utilizing a Harrington distraction or Jacobs rod system as a method of restoring posterior intersegmental stability, it is helpful to use a

Table 19-16. Lumbar versus Sacral: Surgical Stabilization (Northwestern University Acute Spine Injury Center, 1972 to 1986)

Type of Stabilization	Lumbar		Sacral	
	No.	Percent	No.	Percent
Luque rods	18	24.7	1	7.7
Harrington rod distraction	9	12.3	0	0.0
Weiss springs	9	12.3	0	0.0
Other (Cotrel-Dubousset)	2	2.8	0	0.0
No surgery	35	47.9	12	92.3
Total	73	100.0	13	100.0

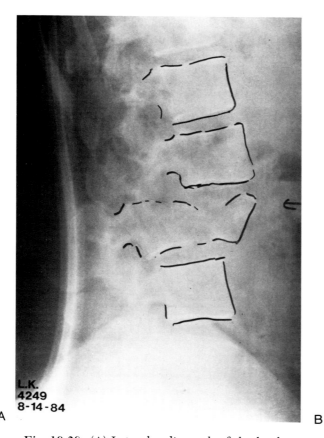

A

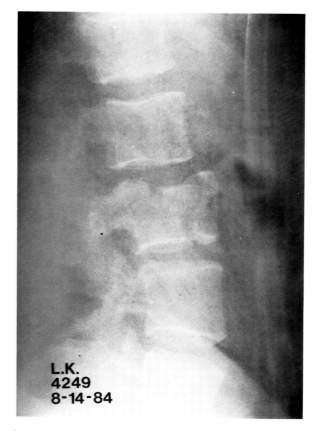

B

Fig. 19-28. (A) Lateral radiograph of the lumbar spine showing fracture dislocation of L4 on L5. Note comminuted fracture of L4 vertebral body. (B) Lateral radiograph showing successful reduction by the closed reduction technique shown in Figure 19-25. *(Figure continues.)*

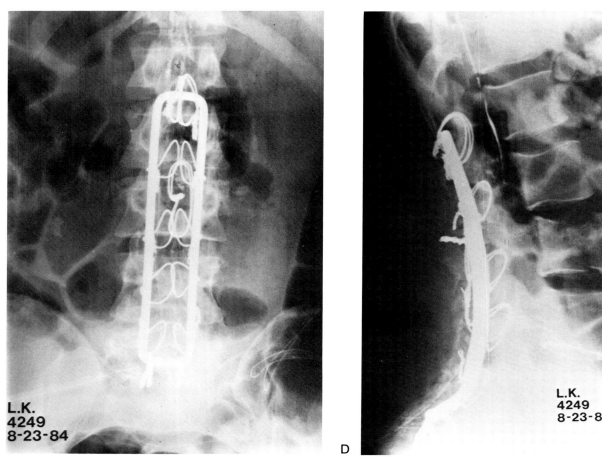

Fig. 19-28 *(Continued)*. **(C,D)** Postoperative AP and lateral radiographs after Luque instrumentation. Note maintenance of anteroposterior and lateral reduction.

circlage wire between (or around) adjacent distracted spinous processes or laminar structures (Fig. 19-27). The wire in this instance replaces the disrupted posterior ligamentous and facet structures.

Luque rod instrumentation is an excellent method of gaining alignment and stability of anterior wedge compression fractures and axial load vertebral body burst fractures, when the integrity of the posterior vertebral wall has been preserved and no evidence of neural canal encroachment exists. The Luque rod stabilization technique is also useful in the management of tumors where there is a loss of anterior bony elements (Fig. 19-28). Their use in this latter example implies that stability remains in the posterior structures.

For those pathological conditions where insufficient posterior laminar structures exist either above or below the level of vertebral column fracture, preventing the use of Harrington, Jacobs, or Luque rods over a reasonable number of segments, a relatively new internal fixation technique now in the early stages of evaluation is being used. It is the transpedicular screw fixation of either the Cotrel-Dubousset instrumentation (Fig. 19-46) or the Synthes AO internal fixator (Fig. 19-29B). Other techniques being used and popularized, particularly in Europe, are plate and pedicular screw fixation of spine fractures (Roy-Camille[2] [Fig. 19-30] or Steffee[10]). The other procedure receiving some notoriety is that described by Magerl.[7,8] The author has not personally seen this latter technique in use.

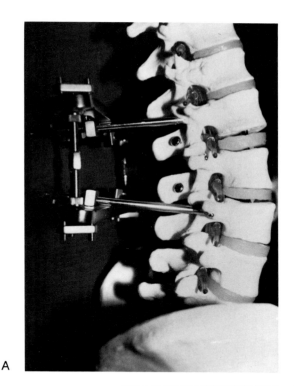
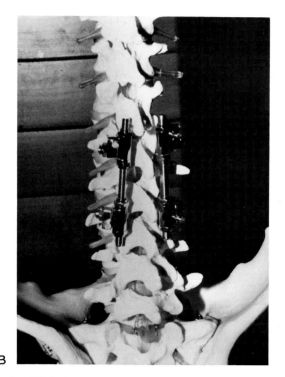

A

B

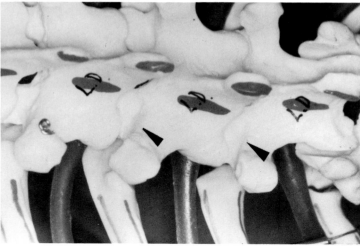

C

Fig. 19-29. (A) Lateral photograph of Magerl device (St. Gallen, Switzerland). Note 6.5 mm Schanz screws entering the posterior vertebral body via the pedicle. The external apparatus of the fixation device is applied externally. This device allows for anteroposterior and lateral reduction of vertebral processes and for the addition of either distraction or compression across the vertebral column. The advantage of this fixation device is the direct application of correcting forces to the fractured area of the vertebral column. A secondary advantage is complete removal of the device upon healing. (B) Internal (AO) fixator applied to the vertebral column via the pedicle. Like the external fixator in Fig. A, this device allows for vertebral column correction over three segments, rather than multiple segments as with other internal fixation devices. (C) Anterior photograph showing thoracic vertebrae T9–T10. Arrows point to the position along the ridge extending across the base of the superior articular facet that overlies the position for placing drill holes through the thoracic lamina into the thoracic pedicle. Note the hole is at the approximate midportion of the superior articular facet. *(Figure continues.)*

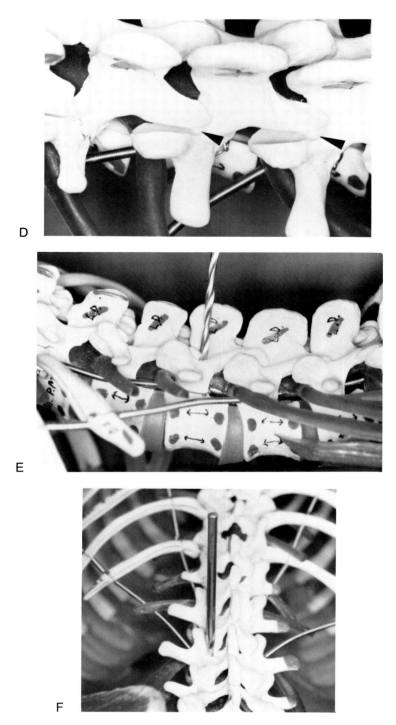

Fig. 19-29 *(Continued)*. (**D**) Posterior view of lumbar vertebral elements L2–L3. Note vertical alignment of facet joint. Drill hole placement (tip of arrow) lies in the midplane of the transverse process and in the midline of facet joint, and slightly proximal to the tip of the inferior articular process of vertebral element above. (**E**) Lateral view of drill hole placement shown in Fig. D. In the lumbar spine, the drill is usually held perpendicular to the tabletop, but the angle will vary with the amount of lordosis or fracture distortion present. Radiographic correlation is required. (**F**) Vertebral column with drill bits placed in lumbar and thoracic drill holes. Note perpendicular position of lumbar drill hole, and 10–15 degree medial angulation of thoracic drill hole.

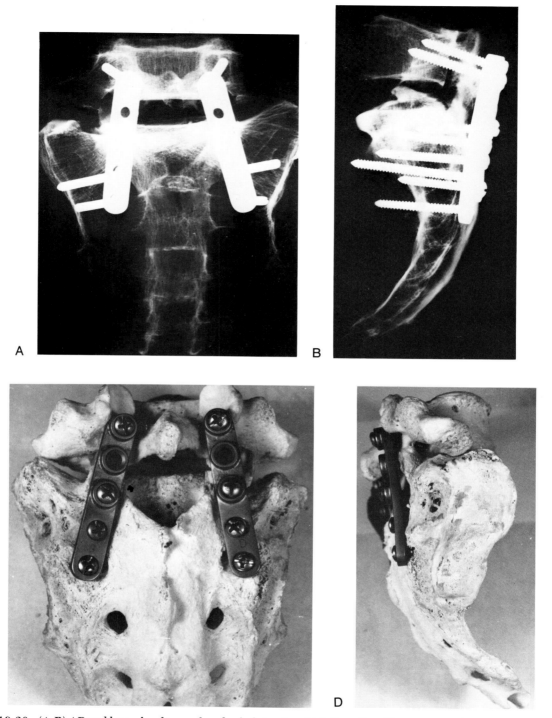

Fig. 19-30. **(A,B)** AP and lateral radiographs of a skeleton in which Roy-Camille posterior plates and screws have been inserted for skeletal fixation at the L5–S1 interface. Note 45° outward angle of the screws in the sacral ala. This screw fixation position is used at the S1 level. An internal angling of the screw by 20 degrees is used at the S2 level. **(C,D)** AP and lateral photographs of the Roy-Camille plate shown in Figs. A and B. *(Figure continues.)*

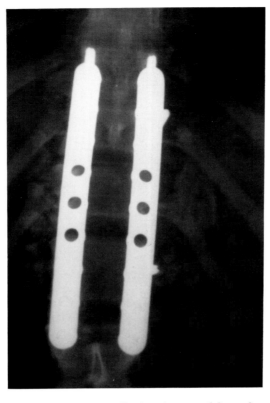
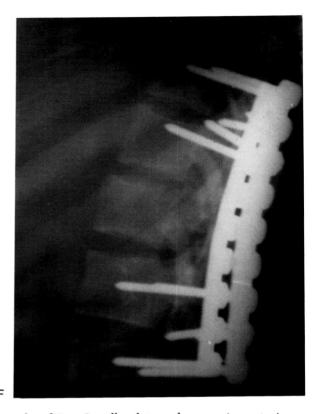

E   F

Fig. 19-30 *(Continued)*. **(E,F)** AP and lateral radiographs of Roy-Camille plate and screws in posterior elements T10–L2. The radiographs show placement of transpedicular screws at four levels and interfragment screws at two levels.

When using L3 as a fractured vertebral process, the considerations which come to mind include the extent of the vertebral body fracture, the involvement of the neural canal and the extent of fractures involving the posterior elements. Assuming for the moment that the posterior elements remain intact, the internal fixation procedures which come to mind (as of 1986–87) include the following:

1. *Harrington Distraction Rods.* Harrington rods are excellent for regaining lost vertebral body height and realigning the vertebral column. The principal flaw in their use is that they induce flattening or loss of lumbar lordosis when used in the lumbar spine and the loss of kyphosis when used in the thoracolumbar junction. To avoid this complication, the Harrington rod must be bent, but bending the rod increases the likelihood for fatigue failure (at the ratchet-shank interface) (Fig. 19-35). If the Harrington-

Moe square-ended rods are not used when the rods are bent, the rods will tend to rotate after insertion, producing loss of fixation and loss of alignment.

2. The *Jacobs "Locking Hook" System (AO-Synthes)* (Fig. 19-26). This device was exhibited at the 1986 AO Spine Course in Davos, Switzerland. It has been used by the author. In the engineering laboratory, it has been described as resulting in the greatest strength-holding capacity except for the external fixator[1] and the Luque sublaminar wire[21] systems. How it compares with the pedicular screw systems is not yet known. Because of the rod's construction and cross-sectional diameter, it is capable of withstanding greater bending loads; therefore, the rod can be bent with less likelihood of fatigue failure. The Jacobs rod system has a "lamina capturing" construction of the proximal locking hook that gives greater holding power at the

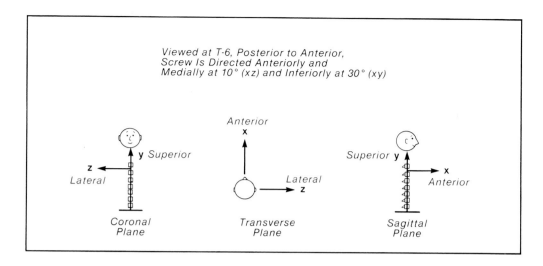

Viewed at T-6, Posterior to Anterior,
Screw Is Directed Anteriorly and
Medially at 10° (xz) and Inferiorly at 30° (xy)

Coronal Plane

y Superior
z
Lateral

Transverse Plane

Anterior
x
Lateral
z

Sagittal Plane

Superior y
x
Anterior

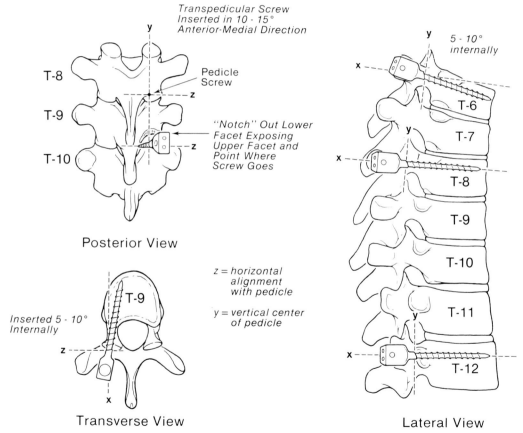

Transpedicular Screw
Inserted in 10 - 15°
Anterior-Medial Direction

T-8

T-9

T-10

Pedicle
Screw

"Notch" Out Lower
Facet Exposing
Upper Facet and
Point Where
Screw Goes

Posterior View

Inserted 5 - 10°
Internally

T-9

z = horizontal
alignment
with pedicle

y = vertical center
of pedicle

A   Transverse View

5 - 10°
internally

T-6

T-7

T-8

T-9

T-10

T-11

T-12

Lateral View

Fig. 19-31. Diagrams showing correct insertion of transpedicular screws in the thoracic and lumbar spine. **(A)** Correct placement of screws in the thoracic spine. Note on the posterior view that the screw insertion point is in the Y or vertical plane at the midpoint of the exposed inferior facet. To permit accurate insertion into the thoracic pedicle, the inferior tip of the inferior facet is removed, and the drill hole is made directly into the base of the superior facet (Z axis). The transverse view shows that the screw or pin is angled 5 to 10 degrees toward the midline as it enters the pedicle of the thoracic vertebra (in the broader lumbar vertebrae, the screws are placed more perpendicularly). As shown in the lateral view, the screw or pin should be parallel to the superior surface of the thoracic vertebra (allowing for thoracic kyphosis as necessary). The screw must not be too long, or it will project from the rounded front of the vertebral body. *(Figure continues.)*

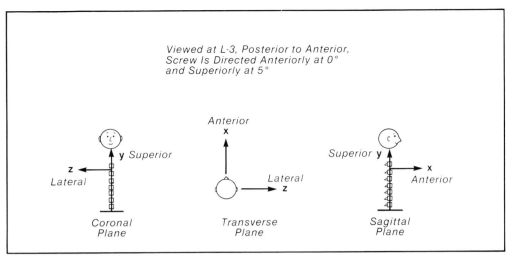

Viewed at L-3, Posterior to Anterior,
Screw Is Directed Anteriorly at 0°
and Superiorly at 5°

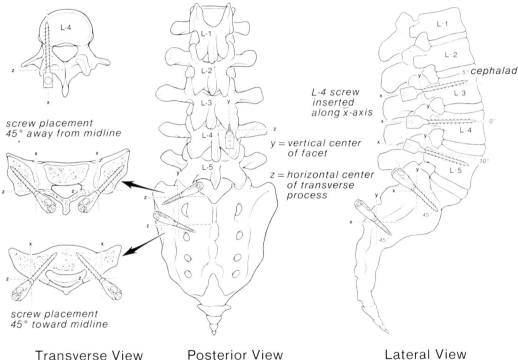

B   Transverse View   Posterior View   Lateral View

Fig. 19-31 *(Continued).* **(B)** Appropriate positioning of screws or pins in the lumbosacral spine. As shown in the posterior view, for lumbar vertebrae the screw is inserted at the point where the midline of the visible inferior facet (**Y** axis) crosses the midline of the lumbar transverse process (**Z** axis). As shown in the transverse view of a lumbar vertebra, the device should lie perpendicular to the **Y** and **Z** axes and directly along the **X** axis. In the S1 segment of the sacrum, the device is inserted just superior to the first sacral foramen, and is angled 45 to 50 degrees inferiorly and 45 degrees externally so that it projects into the sacral ala. In the S2 segment of the sacrum, because of the larger size of the vertebral body at this level, the device is angled 45 to 50 degrees inferiorly and 45 degrees internally, to project into the vertebral body. As shown in the lateral view, lumbar screws should be parallel to the superior border of the vertebra, allowing as necessary for lumbar lordosis. It is important to make sure that the screw is not too long or it will emerge from the spine anteriorly.

superior lamina than does the Harrington distraction hook (see Fig. 18-39). Despite this advantage, loss of fixation can and does occur. The author had loss of fixation using this internal fixation device in two cases in which the rod was bent to reconstitute lumbar lordosis but, because of comminution of the vertebral body, lumbar vertebral column kyphosis occurred during axial loading.

3. The new transpedicular screw fixation systems include the *Cotrel-Dubousset* (Figure 19-46) and the *AO-ASIF Internal Fixator* (Fig. 19-29B; see Fig. 18-40). Both these systems are capable of applying significant distraction forces across as few as three vertebral segments while also allowing maintenance of the lumbar lordosis. The Cotrel-Dubousset screw (6 mm by 40 mm) and the Shanz screw (6.5 mm) used with the AO internal fixator procedure obtain their fixation by direct application to the intact vertebral process, above and below the fracture site transpedicularly (Figs. 19-29, 19-31). Both these techniques can be used in the neurologically injured and intact patient. While some surgeons advocate using them without external support, the author advocates the wearing of an external orthosis postoperatively for 3 months.

4. *Translaminar facet screw*[7] (4.5 mm cortical). This technique has not been used by the author, but it is an adjunctive means of establishing fixation across facet joints to enhance facet joint fixation (Fig. 19-32) in the lumbar spine. Screws are inserted through an untapped drill hole placed opposite the base of the spinous process on the side opposite the facet joint to be stabilized and directed towards the midline of the next lower transverse process on the opposite side (Fig. 19-32). This procedure can be used either alone or in conjunction with other fixation procedures.[7]

5. The *AO-ASIF External Fixator*[7,8,21] (Fig. 19-25A) (Magerl Fixation System). This is an external spine mobilizing device requiring the use of internally placed transpedicular-vertebral body Shanz 6.5 mm screws. This device is not available in the United States and is only recommended for use in the neurologically intact patient. The author has no experience with this device.

Management of wedge compression fractures of the vertebral body where only the anterior aspect of the vertebral process is involved can be stabilized by either a posterior distractive or a posterior compressive device. The author finds the use of a compression device limited to those situations where facet joint dislocation is the primary pathology which exists (Fig. 19-34). Examples of compression devices in use are the Wisconsin Compression System and the Harrington Compression System. In those situations where spine fracture has not resulted in distortion of spinal alignment, stabilization can be gained by the use of any of the procedures listed above.

MANAGEMENT OF FACET DISLOCATIONS

Distraction is relatively uncommon as a mechanism of injury in the lumbar spine. It is usually associated with a flexion component. When seen, these injuries result from rapid deceleration, as in a motor vehicle accident, where the occupant was restrained only by a lap (or pelvic) seat belt. When there is little evidence of a translational (horizontal) type injury, a distraction-type injury is likely to involve facet joint dislocations without facet fracture. Where there is a rotational component (as noted elsewhere in this chapter), because of the restraints placed on the facet joints by their "constraint" design, fracture of the pedicle-facet complex is common (Figs. 19-15, 19-18, 19-19).

While it is rare for lumbar facet joint fractures, subluxations, or dislocations to occur without concomitant injury to the anterior bony complex (vertebral body), the kind of injury involving the vertebral body is an additional issue and must be taken into account. The initial problem becomes the reduction of the facet joint dislocation and decompression of the neural canal. The basic management consideration is whether, after facet reduction, the reduction will be maintained best by a distraction device or a compression device.

Radiologically, in the presence of intact but subluxed or dislocated facets, diastasis of the interspinous space will be present adjacent the level of injury (Figure 19-15). With facet subluxation or

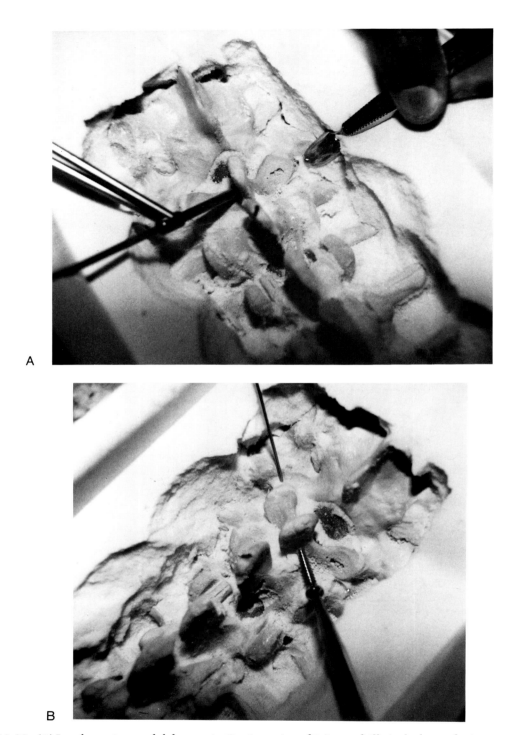

Fig. 19-32. (A) Lumbar spine model demonstrating insertion of 3.2-mm drill via the base of spinous process, through and in line with the associated lamina in the direction of the midportion of the transverse process of the next inferior vertebral element. Note tip of drill opposite instrument. (B) Insertion of cortical screw through the base of the spinous process via the posterior lamina in the direction of the facet joint and the midportion of the transverse process of the next lower element. This view is of the L5–S1 level.

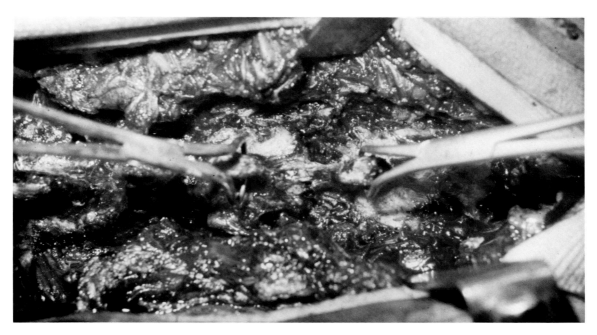

Fig. 19-33. Intraoperative photograph showing the method of regaining facet reduction after facet dislocation. The use of a towel clip and intact spinous processes adjacent to the dislocation site allows vertebral elements to be realigned. To be successful, reduction must be performed within 1 week of trauma. Maintenance of reduction can be achieved by the technique shown in Figure 19-27.

dislocation, the inferior facet of the superior vertebra will be partially or completely displaced on the superior facet of the vertebra below (Figs. 19-16, 19-19). To achieve reduction, the following technique is utilized.

A "towel clip" is placed into the base of each of the two adjacent spinous processes where the subluxation or dislocation has taken place (Fig. 19-33). The spinous processes, with their laminae, are distracted, so as to disengage the overlapping "locked" facets. With traction applied in opposite directions to the spinous processes at the site of injury, the facets are distracted until they are no longer engaged. Downward pressure is applied to the inferior towel clip while upward pressure is applied to the superior towel clip (and lamina). This should allow the inferior facets of the superior vertebral element to be lifted externally over the superior facets of the next inferior vertebral element. The traction on the two adjacent towel clips is then released.

While this "manipulation" appears simple and uncomplicated, it must be remembered that when there is an associated dislocation of the anterior

vertebral segment (body), simultaneous reduction of both segments is only possible when the pedicular attachment between the two is intact. If it is not intact, the posterior element will be easily reduced, but no change in the anterior segment will occur. When the pedicles remain intact, reduction will not occur until both the middle and anterior columns are pulled far enough posteriorly to allow the facets to overlap. To successfully accomplish the reduction, an anterior (ventral) pressure must be applied on the inferior elements, while, simultaneously, a posterior (dorsal) traction force is applied to the posterior elements of the superior element. Because the patient is prone and slightly flexed on the operating table, there is a tendency for the facets to remain in distraction or to redisplace. To assist in maintaining the facet approximation, the two adjacent spinous processes are encircled with a double strand of 18-gauge stainless-steel wire, and the wire is tightened (Fig. 19-27). This will ensure temporary stability until the appropriately selected posterior instrumentation is inserted.

The alternate method of gaining a reduction of

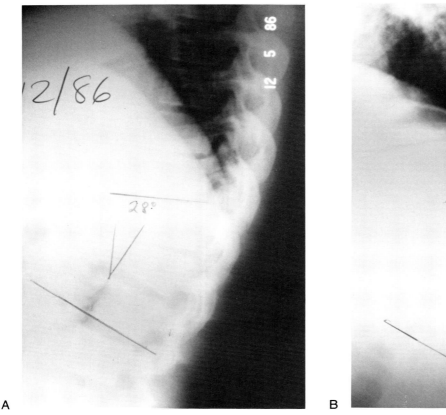
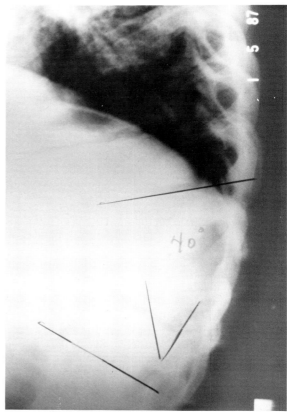

A B

Fig. 19-34. (A,B) Lateral radiographs of the lumbar spine showing loss of correction by 12 degrees during the first month after trauma. Note compression fracture of the L1 vertebral body. *(Figure continues.)*

the dislocated facets is to insert the ends of a lamina spreader (small or medium-size instrument, depending on the level at which one is working) between the two adjacent dislocated lamina-facet complexes. With a distraction force, the facets can be first disengaged, followed by a manipulation similar to that described as above.

With reduction gained, the spinous processes can either be wired "under compression," or the facets can be held in place by the insertion of translaminar screws placed across the respective facets, as noted above[7,8] (Fig. 19-32). This is followed, when indicated, by the insertion of additional stabilizing internal fixation above and below (one or two levels; one level if facet screws are utilized) the level of the facet dislocation.

In the absence of a burst, comminuted, or posterior vertebral body wall fracture, a compression device can be applied posteriorly in the absence of neurologic injury, disc protrusion, or bone fragments in the canal in order to maintain facet joint reduction (Figs. 19-28, 19-34). Devices compatible in this situation include wiring of the two involved adjacent spinous processes alone, and if required, the addition of Harrington compression rods, the Luque rod system, the Wisconsin compression device, or Knodt rods.[53]

If vertebral element dislocation has been present for more than 2 weeks (and particularly if associated with significant fracture of the anterior elements), there is little likelihood that a reduction will be successful unless gross instability persists. The reason is that fractured vertebral elements and soft tissue hematoma undergo rapid fibrosis and become "fixed" (in position) within a matter of 2 to 3 weeks. The presence of displaced vertebral ele-

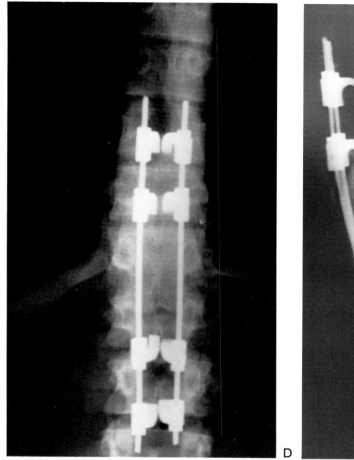
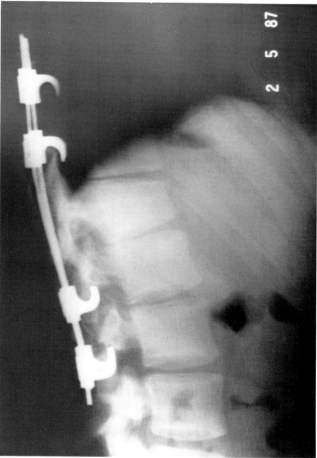

C   D

Fig. 19-34 *(Continued)*. (C,D) AP and lateral radiographs after insertion of compression Harrington apparatus. (Photographs courtesy of Dr. Brian Hayes, Madigan Army Medical Center.)

ments, as noted earlier, is one of two primary indications for early surgical intervention. The other is deterioration of neurologic function in a previously intact patient or in one with an incomplete neurologic injury when additional supporting studies reveal (or suggest) encroachment on neurologic tissue as the probable cause, thus requiring immediate relief.

It is important, when surgically reducing dislocated facets, if at all possible, not to remove portions of adjacent facet surfaces to accomplish reduction. I have found that removing a portion of one of the dislocated facets results in further instability, an increased tendency to dislocate, and difficulty in maintaining facet reduction.

SURGICAL MANAGEMENT OF THE LUMBAR SPINE

Commensurate with residual neurologic function, the ultimate aim of any post-trauma spinal injury management scheme is to maintain spinal mobility while attaining fracture stability. Of the 319 traditional (L1 to L5) lumbar spine fractures occurring in this series of 919 thoracic and lumbar spine fractures, 20 percent resulted in complete neurologic injury, whereas 80 percent resulted in incomplete to normal neurologic injuries. In the group of "redefined" lumbar injuries (L3 to L5), 97 percent were incomplete or normal. The reason

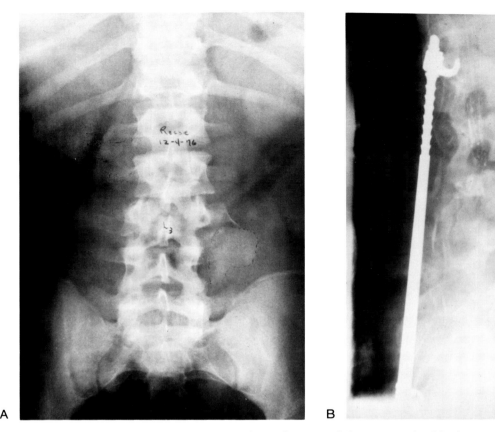

A   B

Fig. 19-35. (A) AP radiograph showing burst fracture of the L3 vertebral body. Patient had a complete L5–S1 neurologic injury. (B) Lateral radiograph of lumbar spine after internal fixation with Harrington distraction apparatus. Note the alignment of the lumbar vertebral column: although the normal lordotic curve is lost, the height of the L3 vertebral body is improved. *(Figure continues.)*

for the 17 percent higher incidence of neurologic injury in the L1 to L5 group versus the L3 to L5 group is the proximity of the injury to the spinal cord (conus medullaris in the former group). In the latter group, peripheral nerve-type neurologic injuries more frequently occurred. Despite the anatomic and neurologic difference that exists between these two areas, the incidence and need for spinal fusion between the two groups were 64.3 and 52.1 percent, respectively. Similarities in the management techniques for these two areas exist for three reasons. First, with additional axial loading to the thoracolumbar junction, where there normally appears a thoracolumbar kyphosis, trauma may induce a progressive vertebral body collapse or posterior structure diastasis secondary

to ligamentous instability. The result is an increase in angular (flexion) deformity at the junction (Fig. 19-34). Second, in the presence of a compression fracture of a lumbar vertebra, progressive axial loading may result in a progressive flexion deformity of the vertebral body, with loss of the lumbar lordosis curve and the onset of a midlumbar kyphosis (Fig. 19-35). Third, with the development of lumbar kyphosis (loss of lordosis or flattening of the lumbar spine), there results a loss of the normal lumbosacral spine "angle" (40 to 50 degrees)[54] and a pronounced alteration in the patient's stance and gait (Fig. 19-21).

Therefore, internal stabilization of fractures of the lumbar spine becomes necessary when there is an unacceptable amount of lumbar kyphotic angu-

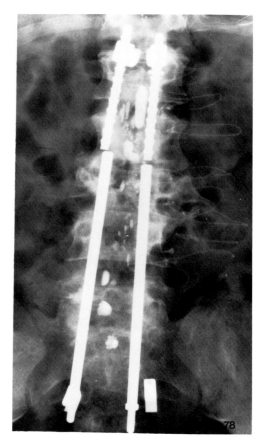
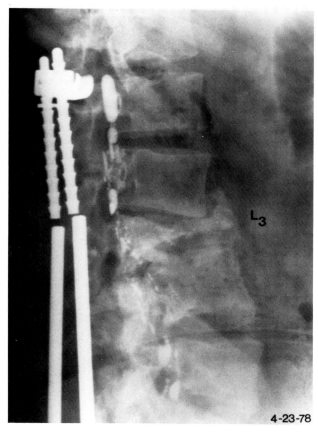

Fig. 19-35 *(Continued).* **(C,D)** AP and lateral radiographs 14 months after operation shows a fracture of the Harrington rods at the shank-ratchet junction adjacent to the L3 vertebral body fracture. *(Figure continues.)*

lar deformity (greater than 30 to 35 degrees of vertebral body compression or angular tilt), resulting in progressive lumbar vertebral column flexion deformity and alterations in the lumbosacropelvic stance angle. The latter effect on gait is a need for the patient to flex at the knees and lean backwards (at the hips) into extension, so as to ambulate in an upright position.

LUMBAR SURGICAL DATA

Review of the methods of internal fixation utilized over the past 14 years for fixation of the lumbar spine describes historically "where we have been and where we are going." Vast changes in the understanding of lumbosacral spine biomechanics and the application of new instrumentation based on these understandings are now under way. While it can be said that the Harrington procedure (1973)[55] was not the first to arrive at a method of spine internal fixation, it was the first to provide stable fixation and correction of vertebral column angular deformities, whether congenital, developmental, or traumatically induced. Weiss in 1975[56] demonstrated the effects of "dynamic" compression on the spine. Luque et al (1982)[4] provided the first introduction to rigid "segmental instrumentation," using first the L rods and later the first rectangular rods. Because of inherent mechanical weaknesses in the Harrington system, Jacobs in 1984[23] developed a new rod-hook system. Long before 1985, Roy-Camille and colleagues[2] demon-

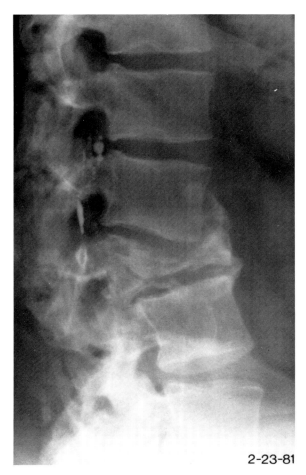

E   2-23-81

Fig. 19-35 *(Continued).* **(E)** Lateral radiograph 3 years after the fracture and 2 years after removal of the internal fixation device. The position of the healed fracture has not changed since removal of the internal fixation device.

strated the beneficial effect of stabilization of the thoracic spine, using plates and transpedicle screws. He now uses these devices in the cervical and lumbar spine. In the United States (1986 to 1987), a similar procedure has been developed by Steffee et al.[10] In Canada, Kostuik and co-workers[9] (1985), and Zielke and colleagues in Germany (1986),[5,6] discussed the use of procedures in which Harrington distraction rods, plates, and transpedicular screws are combined to provide rigid spine fixation in both degenerative and traumatic conditions. Magerl (1985 to 1986)[1,7,8,21] of Switzerland

and colleagues (Germany and the United States) have demonstrated successful use of external and internal fixator methods of managing fractures of the vertebral column. Similar devices await approval for use in the United States.

NORTHWESTERN UNIVERSITY DATA

Of 73 L3 to L5 fractures and dislocations managed between 1972 and 1986, 38 underwent surgical stabilization (Table 19-16). Despite the fact

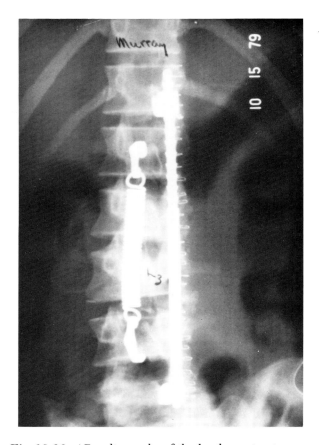

Fig. 19-36. AP radiographs of the lumbar spine in a patient with an "unbalanced" compression fracture of the L3 vertebral body, and a small compression fracture of the anterior superior lip of L2. Radiograph shows Harrington distraction apparatus on the side of the lateral compression vertebral body fracture and Weiss compression spring fixation on side of facet dislocation. This combination is no longer used.

that Luque segmental L or rectangular rod fracture stabilization was introduced into the armamentarium for spinal fracture management 20 years after the introduction of Harrington rods, the procedure was the most frequently utilized stabilization procedure. It was used in 18 patients (24.7 percent) (Fig. 19-28). Before the Harrington instrumentation procedure became a popular fracture fixation method, the Weiss compression springs system (1972 to 1981) was used. This fracture management technique was used in nine patients (12.3 percent). Weiss springs provided dynamic compression across the posterior elements. The criterion for its use was maintenance of continuity of the posterior vertebral body wall (Fig. 19-18). The Harrington distraction rod system, despite prob-

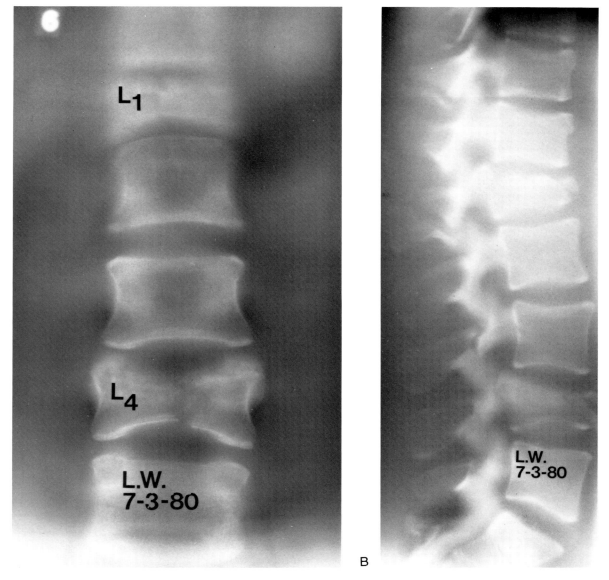

A   B

Fig. 19-37. (A,B) AP and lateral radiographs of the lumbar spine showing fractures of L1 and L4. This fracture pattern coincides with fracture pattern C in Figure 19-20. *(Figure continues.)*

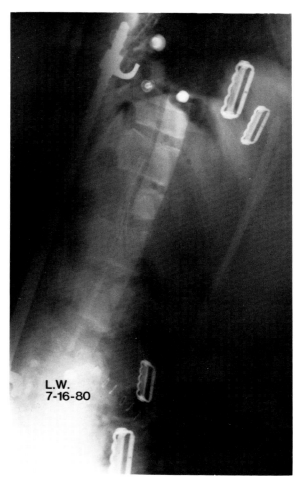

C

Fig. 19-37 *(Continued)*. (C) Lateral radiograph after Harrington distraction rod instrumentation from T10 to L5. Note anterior decompression of L1 with an inlay rib graft across T12–L2.

lems related to the loss or "flattening" of the normal lumbar lordotic curve after insertion, was the procedure of choice in the compression (burst) type of fracture. The device was utilized in nine patients (12.3 percent) (Fig. 19-37).

SURGICAL APPROACH AND NEUROLOGIC IMPROVEMENT

Of the patients undergoing lumbar spine surgical stabilization, 34 (46.6 percent) had posterior stabilization, 1 (1.4 percent) had anterior decompres-

sion and stabilization, and 2 (6.3 percent) had combined (staged) anterior and posterior procedures (Fig. 19-21).

Of the 38 surgically stabilized patients, 1 (2.6 percent) demonstrated loss of one Frankel grade in neurologic function after surgery, 7 patients (18.4 percent) revealed one Frankel grade of neurologic improvement, while 30 (78.9 percent) remained the same neurologically. It is again important to note anatomically that below the level of L1, the neurologic structure present within the lumbar spinal canal is the cauda equina. This structure represents peripheral nerves in as much as they have already exited the spinal cord. It is for this reason that most injuries below L1 are incomplete. In this group of patients, 44 (60.3 percent) were classified as having incomplete injuries, 27 (37.0 percent) were normal and 2 (2.7 percent) revealed a complete neurologic injury on admission (Table 19-5).

OPERATIVE STABILIZATION: LUMBOSACRAL JOINT

Within the 2-year period of 1985 to 1987, the number of advocates of the use of internal fixation devices across the lumbosacral joint increased tremendously. Most of the operative procedures across the lumbosacral joint are procedures recommended for the management of either congenital (spondylolisthesis) or developmental (degenerative) abnormalities. Although trauma at the lumbosacral joint is less often an indication for surgical stabilization, burst or axial load fractures involving either L4 or L5 or facet fractures with subluxation at the L5–S1 level occasionally require surgical stabilization.

As noted above, spinal fusion procedures at the lumbosacral level in the past were primarily recommended for the management of chronic low back pain, recurrent disc disease, back pain due to "instability,"[57] or pathologic processes resulting from tumor. Barr in 1951,[58] Watson Jones in 1952,[59] and Bosworth in 1957[60] each expressed misgivings concerning the value of lumbosacral spinal fusion for the elimination of low back pain and were of the opinion that the failure rate of fusion after surgery was too high. The concern over success and failure of fusion across the lumbosacral joint continues.[53,61] With trauma, instability of the lumbosacral spine is a problem and internal fixation is often precarious. Though screw fixation has been reported as being successful in the nontraumatic back,[62] it alone is not likely to be indicated with spinal trauma.[57] Even Harrington rod-sacral bar stabilization techniques, in conjunction with posterlateral lumbosacral spine fusions, fail.[32]

Of the internal fixation devices and techniques available during the period the above series of patients were managed (1972 to 1986), the internal fixation device most frequently utilized across the lumbosacral joint was the Harrington distraction rod. This technique was used in 6 of 14 (42.9 percent) lumbar or lumbosacral fractures that required stabilization (Table 19-17). As noted in the literature, many varied approaches to the insertion of the fixation device to the posterior pelvis, the sacrum, the lamina of the lumbar spine, etc., have been used. At present, no one procedure has proven most efficacious.[61] Because fracture pathology varies greatly, the same uniform success with the same device, in each instance, is not possible. An excellent example of this occurs with the use of Harrington distraction rods and their fixation to the sacrum. When the lower hooks are secured to the sacrum alone (with the lower hooks in the second sacral foramen), with sublaminar wires, in combination with a sacral bar, or with sacral alae hooks, fixation problems arise. No one procedure is totally reliable.

Because of the unreliability of Harrington hook stability in the sacrum (Figs. 19-5, 19-21F,G, 19-38A) and the loss of the lumbosacral inclination angle when distraction is applied (to less than the normal 40 to 50 degrees), distraction rod-hook

Table 19-17. Lumbar Fractures: Surgical Instrumentation across the Lumbosacral Junction (Northwestern University Acute Spine Injury Center, 1972 to 1986)

Instrumentation across Lumbosacral Junction	No.	Percent
Harrington distraction rods	6	42.9
Compression springs	4	28.6
Luque rods	4	28.6
Total	14	100.0

combinations across the joint have been essentially discontinued. Actually, hook fixation into the second sacral foramen was not the problem, or when necessary, the making of a foramen (in the area of the first or second sacral segment). The problem that arose was that when the patient (after healing of the fracture, and removal of the orthosis, etc.) returned to **flexion** activities at the waist (3 to 6 months postinjury), the patient in essence "became longer" across the lumbosacral area than the Harrington rod-hook combination. The result was loss of fixation of the inferior rod-hook owing to the pulling out of the inferior rod from the (sacral) hook (Fig. 19-38). The upper end of the rod never displaced from the superior hooks or the lamina mechanically. Fracturing of the upper lamina-hook junction did occur, with pulling away, but usually this occurred at the inferior hook. The problem of rod displacement from the lower hook (at the sacrum) is not unique, but seemed to occur with greater frequency below than above the lumbosacral joint. The single remaining indication for use of some sort of distraction device across the lumbosacral joint is in the presence of a burst or comminuted fracture at the level of the fifth lumbar vertebra. Here, distraction is indicated for either fracture reduction of neural canal decompression.

As noted earlier, in the series of 14 spinal fractures that underwent fixation across the lumbosacral junction (between 1972 and 1986), 6 used Harrington rods, 4 used Weiss springs, and 4 used Luque rods. With the lack of stability identified with Weiss compression springs, and with the loss of fixation occurring with the Harrington rod-hook combination, these devices were used less often. Between 1981 and 1986, the three devices above were used with the following frequency: compression springs used, 0; Harrington rod-hook combinations used, 1; and Luque rod systems used, 4. It is readily apparent that a change in philosophy and surgical technique resulted with an evaluation of the surgical results and complications. Although the Luque device has become a more reliable and successful method of attaining stability across the lumbosacral joint (in combination with an external orthosis), its major deficiency is that it cannot be used when dealing with a burst fracture of L4 or L5. The Luque rod fixation technique (to the sacrum) is described below (see Fixation of Luque Rods to the Sacrum).

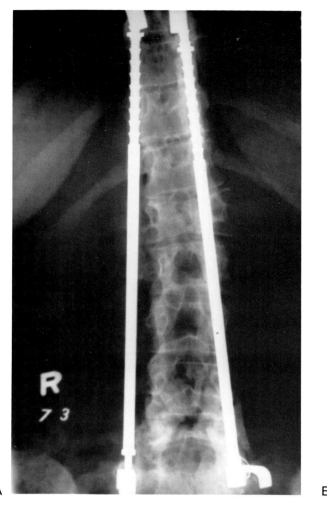

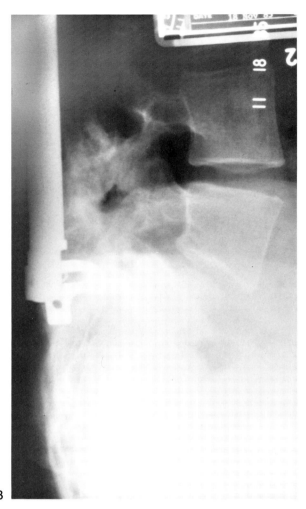

Fig. 19-38. (A) Anterior view of vertebral column after loss of fixation both proximally and distally for a compression fracture of the L1 vertebral body between Harrington rods and Harrington hooks. A most unusual combination. **(B)** Lateral radiograph showing the displacement of the Harrington rods from the sacral ala hooks. *(Figure continues.)*

INTERNAL FIXATION: STABILIZATION PROCEDURES OF THE LUMBOSACRAL JOINT

Complication with Distraction Across the Lumbosacral Junction

A major deficiency with the use of any distraction rod system across the lumbosacral joint is the potential loss of the normal lumbosacral angle (40 to 50 degrees) when distraction forces are applied.

The result is flattening of the lumbosacral angle and reduction of the normally present lordosis. It is important to appreciate that loss of the lumbosacral angle results in disturbances in both patient stance and gait. Nonetheless, distraction rod systems are occasionally indicated in such instances as retrolisthesis of L5 on S1, the presence of burst fractures involving the fifth lumbar vertebra or the first sacral segment, and for stabilization and re-fusion of the L5-S1 interval in those cases in which a previous fusion attempt ended in failure. In each of the

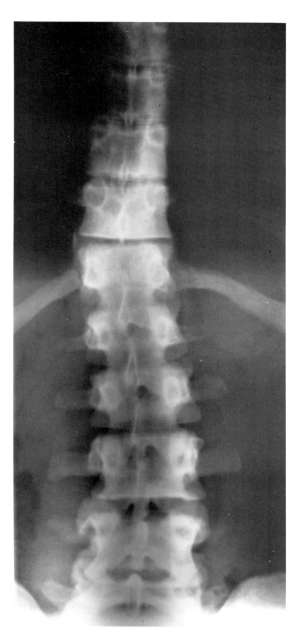

C

Fig. 19-38 *(Continued)*. (C) Postoperative AP view of thoracolumbar spine after removal of internal fixation. (Photographs courtesy of Dr. Brian Hayes, Madigan Army Medical Center.)

above instances, stability of the anterior and posterior longitudinal ligaments must be ensured, otherwise distraction across this junction is likely to contribute to the disability.

Fixation of Harrington hooks to the dorsum of the sacrum is not difficult (Fig. 19-39); however, maintaining fixation is (Fig. 19-38). With forward trunk bending (lumbar spine flexion), the Harrington distraction rod pulls out of the lower hook either at the hook-rod interface or at the hook-sacrum interface (Fig. 19-38A). It may also displace superiorly at the rod-hook interface or hook-lamina attachment.

Fixation of Sublaminar Wires to the Sacrum

With the increased use of Luque instrumentation across the lumbosacral joint for fracture stabilization, rigid fixation of the device to the sacrum is imperative. There exists normally a small first and a slightly larger second sacral foramen (Fig. 19-40). When these are not present or are small in size, a ¼-inch drill (6.8 mm) or a ⅜-inch drill (7.9 mm) can be utilized for either enlargement or placement of two holes (inferior to each other) over the dorsum of the first and the second sacral segments, bilaterally. Placement of the drill holes one-fourth to three-eights of an inch apart provides sufficient distance to pass a curved sublaminar wire and adequate bone stock such that upon tightening, the island of bone will not break. It must be remembered that the internal fixation device being applied across the lumbosacral joint must be bent into an appropriate hyperextended position to maintain or provide for the reconstitution of the normal 50-degree lumbosacral angle. Also, the internal fixation device (rectangular Luque rod system) should be stabilized to the sacrum at two levels to provide maximum fixation and stability. The same fixation principle is true at the level of the lumbar spine.

Placement and Fixation of Sacral Plate and Screws

Screw fixation of devices to the sacrum is becoming an increasingly popular technique. Viewing cross-sections of the sacrum, the thickest portion of

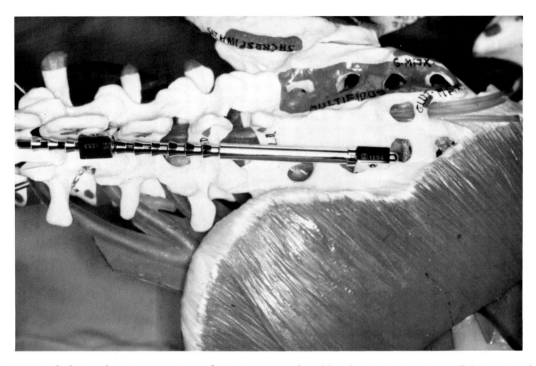

Fig. 19-39. Skeleton showing insertion of Harrington rod and hooks. Note insertion of distraction hook (1254) inferiorly into the second sacral foramen, and of standard (1253) distraction hook proximally into the sublaminar space. This method of hook fixation to the sacrum is an alternative to the transverse sacral bar-Harrington hook fixation. A major complication with this method of stabilization is displacement of the Harrington rod from the inferior Harrington hook upon spine flexion.

the sacrum at the level of the first sacral segment is in the area of the sacral ala. At this level, when inserting a screw from a position parallel with the first sacral foramen, the screw should be inserted with its tip pointed out (into the ala) at a 45-degree angle (Figs. 19-30, 19-31). At the level of the second and third sacral segments, insertion of a screw requires placement into the thicker and more central "body" portion of the sacrum. The screw must be placed from a lateral position parallel to (or slightly lateral to) the sacral foramen and pointed toward the anterior midline (into the body of the respective sacral vertebra). This is an approximate 20-degree angle (Fig. 19-31). Lateral placement of the screw, with internal direction, prevents the screw from entering the sacral canal.

Fixation of Harrington Hooks to the Sacral Alae

The technique by which the Harrington rod system is applied to the superior surface of the sacrum is by means of the sacral alae hook. Visual examination of this hook reveals that the hook is long in its anteroposterior length. For this reason this hook should not be used at any level other than the superior surface of the sacrum. I am aware of the occurrence of paraplegia resulting from the insertion of a sacral alae Harrington hook at the level L5 level. The neurologic complication that occurred was produced indirectly the incorrect use of this hook at this level. When placed into the spinal canal above the lumbosacral junction, the hook extends

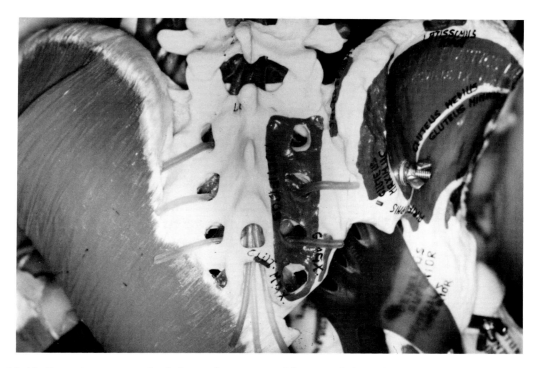

Fig. 19-40. Posterior sacrum of a skeleton showing sacral foramina bilaterally. Exiting each of the foramina are small posterior sensory branches. Small veins accompany these nerve roots.

too far anteriorly, placing pressure on the dura and the cauda equina within the neural canal. This hook should not be used at any level other than the superior surface of the sacrum (Fig. 19-41). Again, this problem is not unique for the sacral alae hook. It has also been reported with the use of a standard (1253) hook.[63]

The reason the sacral alae hook has been used by some surgeons above the level of the lumbosacral junction is that the standard 1253 hook is short in its anteroposterior length. As found in the description of the Harrington distraction rod procedure above, because of the shortness of the hook, and in the presence of a prominent lumbar lordosis, the insertion of the inferior end of the Harrington rod into the hook is simplified by burring a groove across the dorsum (outer table) of the lamina above the level the inferior hook-lamina interface. Making this groove allows the inferior end of the rod to be pushed more anteriorly (into the groove), allowing the rod-hook complex to be more easily united. This technical note applies to the laminae between L2 and L5. As stated, the sacral alae hook is not used above L5 and, in my experience, has not been used on the superior surface of the sacrum. Rather, rod attachment to the pelvis (sacrum) is obtained by the placement of a standard 1253 Harrington hook directly to the sacrum. There is no specific contraindication for the use of a sacral alae hook on the superior surface of the sacrum, rather, a preference exists. My concern is that distraction directly into and across this joint contributes to instability problems encountered at the lumbosacral junction that are not induced by trauma. Regardless, when used, and when in conjunction with a fusion, motion across the junction must not be allowed for 3 months.

Fixation of Harrington Hooks to the Sacrum

A Harrington distraction 1253 hook can be inserted into an already present S1 or S2 sacral foramen, or if these are not present, into a foramen

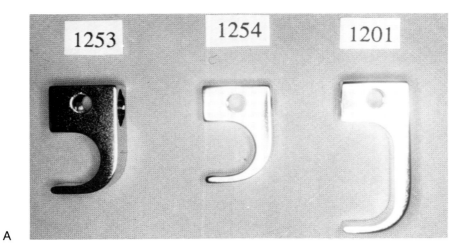

A

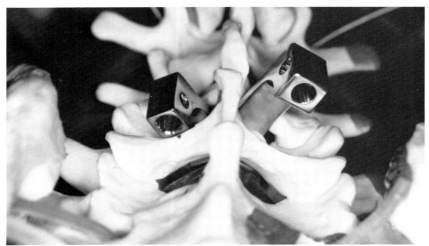

B

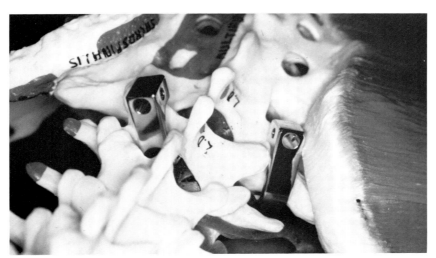

C

Fig. 19-41. (A) Photograph showing the difference in size of the Harrington rod superior distraction hook (1253), inferior hook (1254), and sacral ala hook (1201). Of particular importance is the length of the hook. (B) Inferior-to-superior views of the lumbar spine of a skeleton with the sacral ala hook (1201, right) and standard distraction hook (1254, left) inserted over the superior surface of the L5 lamina. The 1201 hook is inappropriate at any level above the sacral ala. Use of this hook in the lumbar spine is likely to result in increased neurologic injury secondary to nerve root compression by the hook. (C) Lumbar spine of a skeleton showing proper placement of the sacral ala hook (right) and proper placement of the 1254 distraction hook beneath the lamina at L5 (left).

Fig. 19-42. (A,B) Sacrum of a skeleton showing insertion of Luque wire between the first and second sacral foramina. (C) An alternative method of internal fixation stabilization inferiorly to the sacrum using Luque wires. Additional holes for Luque wire placement can be made in the external table of the sacrum (see Figure 19-43).

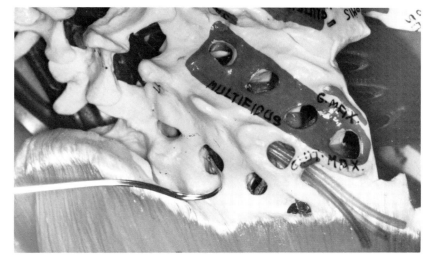

A

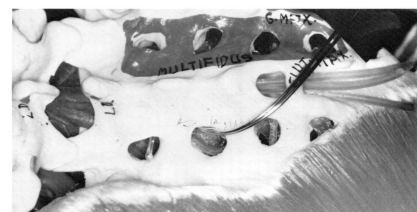

B

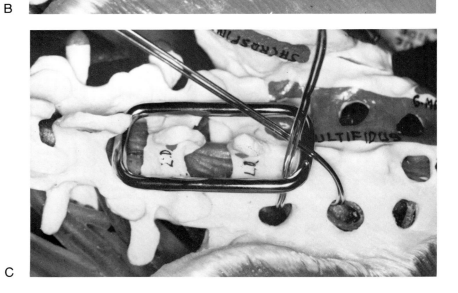

C

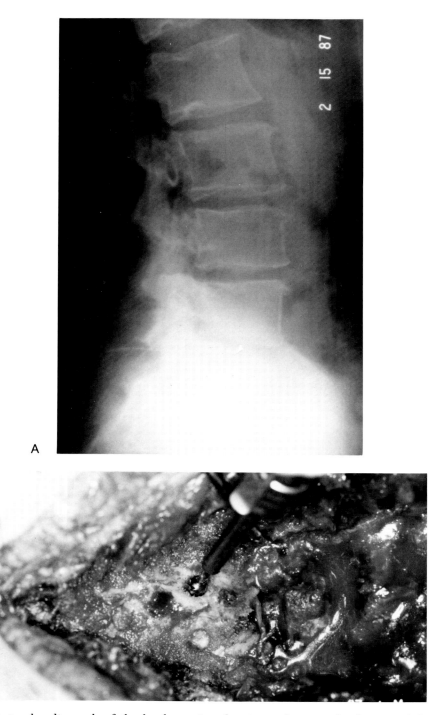

Fig. 19-43. (A) Lateral radiograph of the lumbar spine showing reduction of a fracture dislocation of L5–S1. (B) Surgical view of posterior sacrum. A high-speed burr is being used to make additional holes in the posterior sacrum for insertion of Luque wires. *(Figure continues.)*

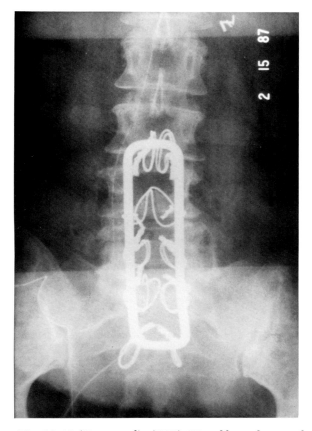
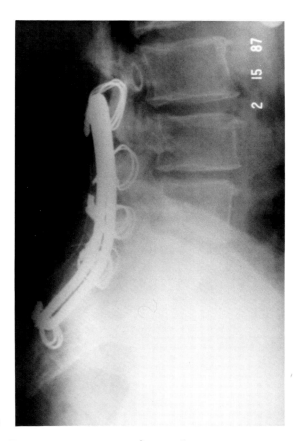

C   D

Fig. 19-43 *(Continued)*. **(C,D)** AP and lateral views showing Luque instrumentation fixation from L3 to S2. Posterolateral spine fusion accompanies the internal fixation stabilization of the lumbosacral spine.

surgically made by drilling ¼-inch holes perpendicularly through the outer table of the sacrum, at or near the position of the anatomic first or second sacral foramen. This is done bilaterally. The Harrington hooks are inserted into the holes, and the remainder of the insertion of the Harrington distraction rod system is performed in the usual manner.

Fixation of Luque Rods to the Sacrum

The technique that I utilize to fix the Luque system to the sacrum is different from that utilized by Allen[64] (Figs. 19-42, 19-43). They shape the lower ends of the Luque rods in such a fashion that the rods can be driven into the space between the inner

and outer tables of the posterior superior iliac crest, along the iliopectineal line. Jacobs et al.,[65] in a comparison test of fixation devices against the posterior iliac crest, was of the opinion that the Allen method of rod fixation was as strong a method of fixation as Harrington hooks into a transinferior iliac spine sacral bar, "backed up with four hole plates and screws into the posterior iliac crests." This latter discussion is academic, for I have yet to find any fixation devices used in such a manner. On the other hand, I have noted that Luque rod fixation to a transverse sacral bar (Fig. 19-44) is very stable. However when the rod is inserted directly into the superoposterior iliac crest, it may undergo fatigue failure at the level of the lumbosacral joint. Failure of the device most likely results from motion "cycling" (Fig. 19-45). Such failure has also

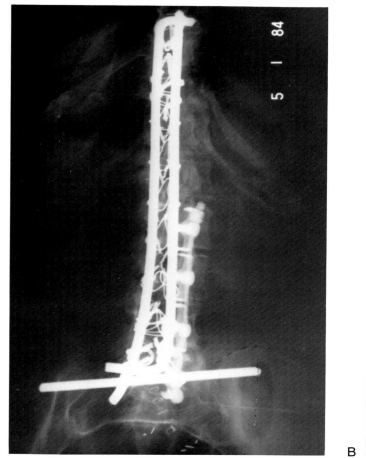
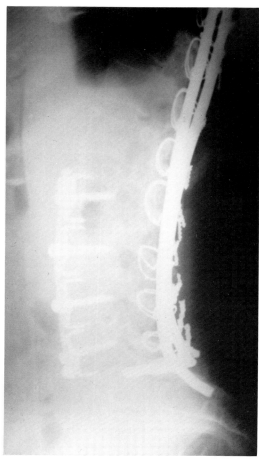

A

B

Fig. 19-44. (A,B) AP and lateral radiographs of the lumbosacral spine after Dwyer anterior instrumentation and Luque instrumentation fixation to a horizontal sacral bar posteriorly. Rapid fusion was achieved by this method of stabilization.

been identified at the other levels.[66] I report such a case at L3.

Sublaminar Wire Fixation: Sacrum

The technique most frequently used is the placement of two ¼-inch holes perpendicularly through the outer table of the sacrum, at or near the position of the anatomic first and second sacral foramina. This procedure is repeated bilaterally. Through these two holes are passed double-strand 18-gauge wires, which later will be tightened around a

Luque rod of appropriate length. This fixation, in addition to that of the lumbar spine (above and below the fracture), provides good rod fixation and stability. Postoperatively, efforts are made to reduce all motion acros the lumbar and lumbosacral joints so that fusion occurs. The patient is protected for 3 months in either a spica plaster of Paris cast or a plastic thoracolumbosacral (TLSO) orthosis mated to a plastic thigh component on one side. Attached to this is an external lock-joint at the hip (Fig. 19-53C). This orthotic device has been found to provide sufficient restriction of motion across the lumbosacral joint to allow fusion to occur in each instance used (five times).

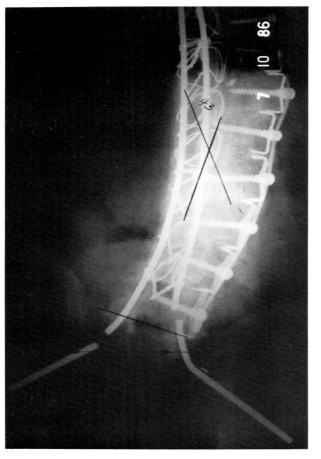 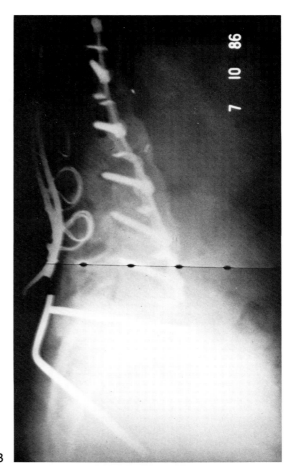

A   B

Fig. 19-45. (A,B) AP and lateral radiographs of a thoracolumbar sacral fusion for scoliosis secondary to neurologic disability. Note fracture of the Luque rods inserted into the iliac wings using the Galveston (Allen) technique. *(Figure continues.)*

Cotrel-Dubousset Posterior Rod-Transpedicular Screw Procedure

The Cotrel-Dubousset internal stabilization technique incorporates the fixation of a posterior spine-stabilizing device (rods and, with other procedures, plates) to the middle and anterior vertebral column by means of screws passed through the posterior lamina into the anterior column via the middle column pedicle[67] (Figs. 19-46, 19-31).

The Cotrel-Dubousset procedure is similar to the Steffee or Roy-Camille plate-screw, the Kostiuk hook-Harrington rod, the Magerl External Fixator, or the Dick Internal Fixator procedure in that fixation of the posterior fixation device to the vertebral column is gained via either screw or Schanz pin placement through the pedicle into the vertebral body (Fig. 19-31).

In the thoracic region, pin or screw hole placement is made 1 to 1.2 mm below the lower border of the inferior facet of the level above, in line with the midlateral point of the facet. In the lumbar region, the hole for the placement of the screw or pin is made in line with the outer (vertical) border of the facet, and at the midpoint of the base of the exposed transverse process at that level (Figs. 19-46, 19-31). Axial alignment of the drill, for

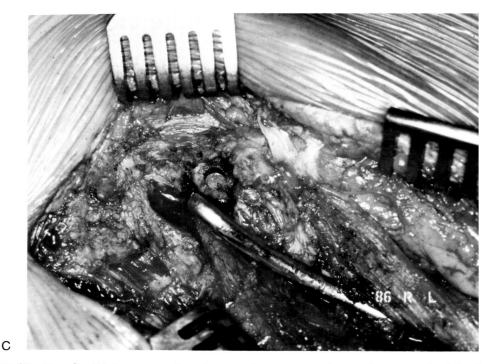

C

Fig. 19-45 *(Continued)*. **(C)** Intraoperative photograph at surgery during the removal of the fractured Luque rod. Note the fracture just above the sacrum. Fracture of internal fixation at this level indicates nonunion of a lumbosacral fusion, and is evidence of "motion cycling."

placement of the pedicle screw into the thoracic or thoracolumbar vertebral column, is an internal angle of approximately 10 to 15 degrees. In the lumbar area, axial alignment of the screw or pin is perpendicular to the horizontal axis. The angle of cephalad or caudad directioning of the drill depends on the degree of thoracic or lumbar kyphosis or lordosis.

In the sacrum, screw fixation at the level of the first sacral segment requires that the placement be in an outward direction of approximately 40 to 50 degrees (Fig. 19-31). This latter angle relates to the extent of lumbosacral lordosis. At the second sacral segment level, screw fixation is best with an internally directed angle of approximately 20 degrees and a caudal direction of approximately 20 degrees. The dorsal entry point of the first sacral screw is just caudal and lateral to the first sacral facet or between the first and second sacral foramina.

Once the Cotrel-Dubousset screws are in place, the posterior rod is appropriately shaped and inserted. When this rod is fixed in place, either distraction or compression can be applied to the vertebral column as required.

Anterior Approach with Bone Graft

The anterior approach to the lumbosacral joint is not easy. It is performed with the surgical assistance of either a general or vascular surgeon. This surgical difficulties encountered with this approach to the L5–S1 interval are the following:

Because the anatomic inclination angle at the lumbosacral promontory is 45 to 50 degrees, good visualization of the intervertebral disc space between L5 and the superior surface of the S1 vertebra is next to impossible (Fig. 19-47). Louis describes positioning the patient on the operating

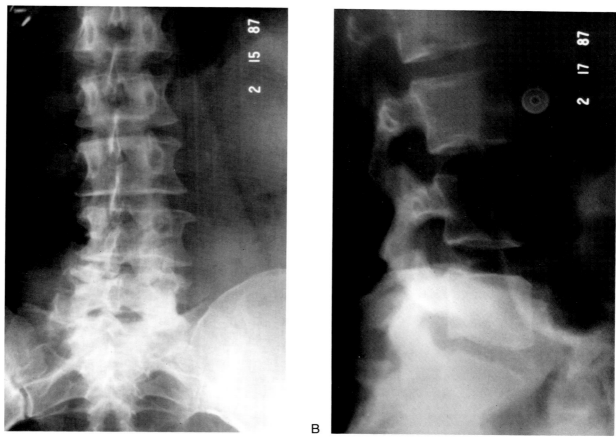

Fig. 19-46. (A,B) AP and lateral radiographs of the lumbosacral spine after trauma to the lumbosacral joint. *(Figure continues.)*

table in a position of hyperlordosis, while the patient is also maintained in cervical head halter traction of 15 to 25 kg (38 to 64 lbs).[3] This position facilitates anterior visualization and excision of the intervertebral disc at the L5–S1 interval in the presence of severe L5 spondylolistheses. This same approach is also utilized for anterior fusion of the L5–S1 interval when previous attempts at posterior fusion at the lumbosacral joint have failed.

In the adult man, segments of the autonomic nervous system (sympathetic and parasympathetic) that innervate the bladder, bowel, and sexual organs, lie in proximity to and within the fatty tissue space between the bifurcation of the common iliac arteries as they exit the aorta. Injury to either of the two plexes may result in impotence. Their

functions are as follows.[68] The parasympathetic nerves (pelvic splanchnic nervi erigentes: S1, S2, S3, S4) provide motor function to bladder emptying, blood vessel dilation, and erection of the penis when stimulated, plus sensory function to the bladder. The sympathetic nerves (through the superior hypogastric presacral plexus), which are responsible for ejaculation of fluid from the seminal vesicles into the urethra, innervate the muscles of the epididymis, ductus deferens, and prostate and also provide some sensory function to the bladder trigon. To prevent injury to either structure during exposure of the anterior L5–S1 area, it is recommended that all dissection be conducted to the right side of the vena cava-aorta complex, with these structures being carefully mobilized (re-

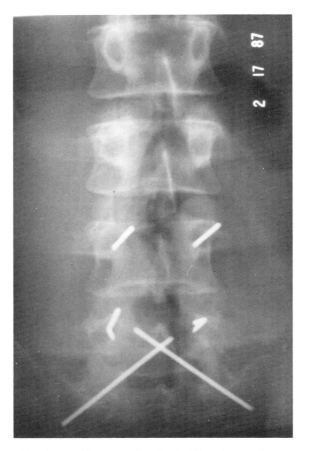
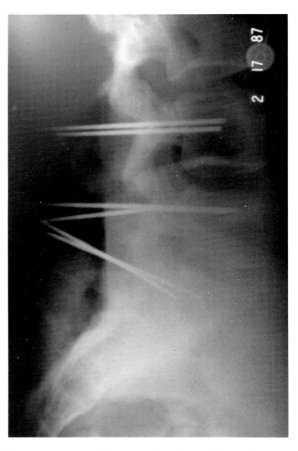

C   D

Fig. 19-46 *(Continued).* **(C,D)** AP and lateral radiographs showing x-ray guide wires placed into the pedicles of L4 and L5 and the sacral ala of S1. *(Figure continues.)*

tracted) toward the left side after careful ligation of each of the lower lumbar segmental veins.

Another hazard encountered during the anterior lumbosacral approach is that which occurs with retraction of the great vessels to the left during the performance of the bone and disc portions of the procedure. Even with careful retraction of the vena cava to the left, temporary (partial to complete) occlusion of the soft-walled, low-pressured vein can occur. Careful monitoring of the cardiac output is suggested (reduction in the arterial blood pressure as a result of reduced cardiac filling and output). Another complication that may result with vena cava occlusion (as identified in one of my patients undergoing a multilevel anterior lumbosacral approach) is the occurrence of pulmonary embolism. The etiology of this complication was thought to be the result of prolonged (partial) occlusion of the vena cava. To prevent this, a conscious effort must be made to remove all vascular retraction for short periods, as often as possible.

After exposure of the lumbosacral promontory, the vena cava and the aorta (or the right common iliac artery) are modestly retracted toward the left, and the intervertebral disc is dissected free by sharp dissection (incising away from the vital structures). A high-speed burr, large pituitary rongeur, and large angled curettes are utilized to clean out the intervertebral disc space. This too is difficult.

If a corporectomy of the L5 vertebra is to be performed, the same technique is used as described under Anterior Approach to the Thoracolumbar Spine. Grooves are placed in the vertebral body above and below S1. Using either split fibular

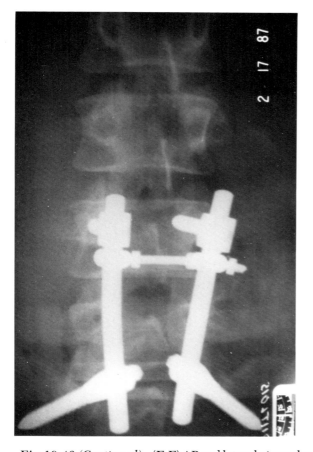
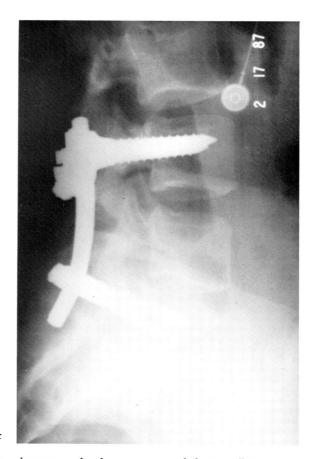

E

F

Fig. 19-46 *(Continued)*. (E,F) AP and lateral views showing the transpedicular–trans-sacral ala Cotrell-Dubousset rod pedicle screw fixation stabilization from L1 to the sacrum.

or rib grafts (as described under Anterior Approach to the Thoracolumbar Spine), the graft is inlaid into the prepared bed. Another technique is the insertion of a bone dowel into a hole placed through the vertebral body (L4, L5, S1) (Fig. 19-48).

If a multiple-level fusion is to be performed, the intervening intervertebral discs are excised. After the placement of appropriate longitudinal grooves into each of the adjacent vertebral bodies, tricortical iliac crest bone block grafts are inserted into each interspace and impacted in place. When the procedure is done at multiple levels (i.e., involving more than three vertebral bodies), bleeding may be brisk from the anterior lumbar intraosseous vertebral vessels. Should rapid administration of blood be required, a technique found useful is the administration of blood via a large bore Intracath catheter

placed directly into the inferior vena cava, with a purse-string suture placed about the catheter during the administration of the blood.

After the performance of an anterior fusion, the method of immobilization routinely utilized is the maintenance of the patient at strict bed rest for 1 to 2 weeks postoperatively, followed by the application of a spica cast or orthosis (as described under Orthotic Management, below) for 3 months.

FRACTURES OF THE SACRUM

Fractures of the sacrum are described as being relatively rare. The literature does not record a relative incidence; however, between 1972 and

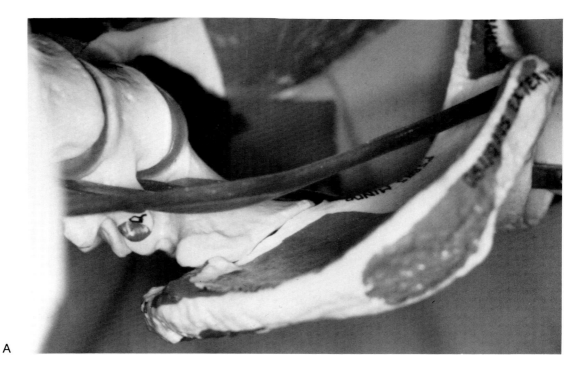

A

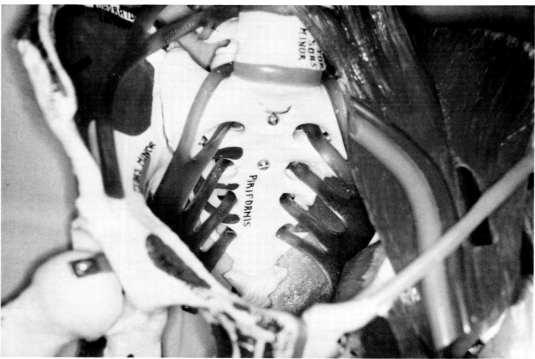

B

Fig. 19-47. **(A)** The sacral promontory as viewed from right superior wing of the ilium. Note that an anterior approach to the disc space at L5 – S1 is difficult when the anatomy is normal, and is very difficult in when there is traumatic or developmental displacement of L5 on S1. **(B)** Anterior photograph of the sacrum showing the relationship of L5 to S1 and the presence of anterior sacral rami, psoas muscles, and iliac arteries that lie in the anterior gutter. An anterior approach to the L5 – S1 interval is facilitated by lateral retraction of the vena cava and aorta rather than surgery between the bifurcation.

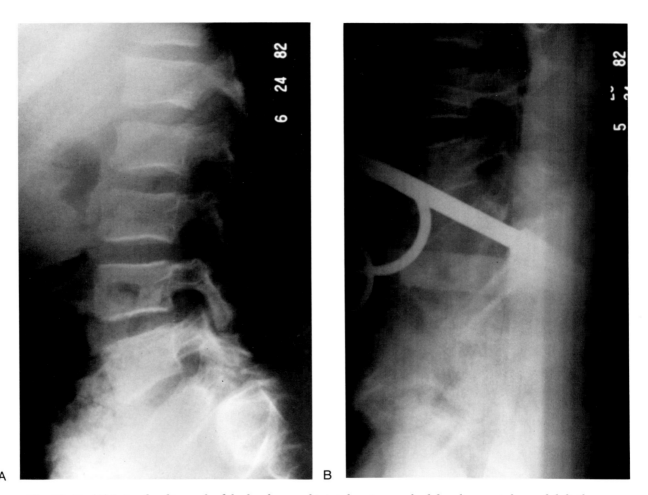

Fig. 19-48. (A) Lateral radiograph of the lumbosacral joint showing marked developmental spondylolisthe-sis (grade IV) of L5 with S1. (B) Lateral radiograph of the lumbar/sacral spine demonstrating placement of the drill bit into the L4 vertebral body through the anteroinferior aspect of vertebral body L4–L5, and into the body of S1. *(Figure continues.)*

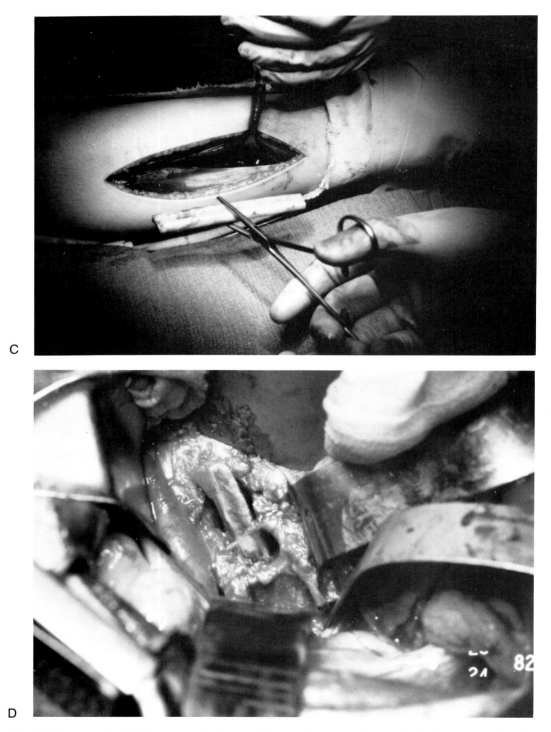

C

D

Fig. 19-48 *(Continued)*. **(C)** Fibular graft obtained from midportion of right fibula. **(D)** Longitudinally split fibula inserted into vertebral bodies L4–L5 and S1. *(Figure continues.)*

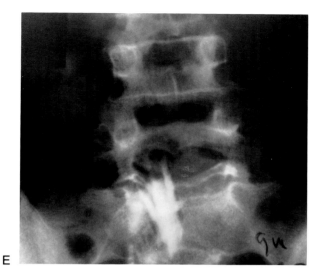

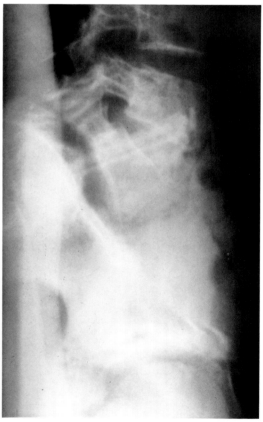

Fig. 19-48 *(Continued).* **(E,F)** AP and lateral radiographs showing anterior fibular graft and fusion of L4 to the sacrum.

1986 in my series of 932 fractures involving the thoracic, thoracolumbar junction, lumbar, and sacral vertebral column, only 13 primary sacral fractures were identified. Other reports on sacral fractures in the medical literature denote the low incidence of sacral fractures.[69,70] Denis and colleagues,[71] in a retrospective analysis of pelvic fractures, noted the presence of 236 associated fractures of the sacrum. Frequently, these fractures go unrecognized in the presence of multiple trauma.

Isolated fractures of the sacrum are less frequent than those associated with lumbar spine fractures, fractures of the transverse processes, fractures of the pelvis[70,71] (personal communication, Denis), or fractures of the lumbosacral joint[69,72] (Fig. 19-49). Roy-Camille et al. reported 13 sacral fractures resulting from falls (frequently suicide related).[2] Denis also has reported a high frequency of sacral fractures related to fractures of the pelvis (personal communication) whereas his series of fractures is more like that of the literature when associating fracture of the sacrum only with fractures of the sacrum alone or in conjunction with fracture of the lumbar spine: 10 of 236 (4 percent) (personal communication).

As already noted, fractures of the sacrum are most frequently associated with major fractures of the pelvis. The mechanism of injury producing isolated fractures of the sacrum is direct trauma. The more common causes for such injuries include: falls,[2] direct injury secondary to a direct blow to the area, motor vehicle-related injuries, etc. Although possible, open fractures of the sacrum (not including gunshot wounds) are rare. In my 13 sacral cases, one fracture was open and required immediate debridement (Fig. 19-2).

RELATIONSHIP OF SACRAL FRACTURES TO NEUROLOGIC INJURIES

Because of the singular presence of elements of the cauda equina in the area of the sacral neural canal, fractures involving the sacrum can, if severe enough, result in cauda equina (peripheral nerve root) injury to S2 through S5 segments. Because of

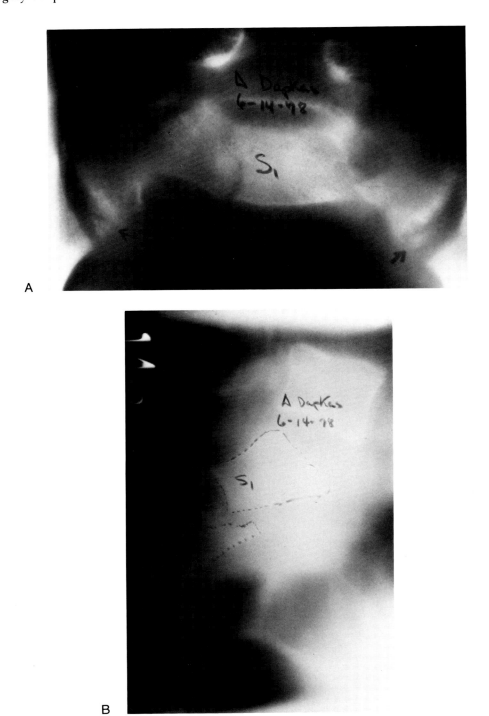

Fig. 19-49. (A,B) Anterior and lateral view of the sacrum showing a comminuted fracture of the sacral body at the level of S2 with moderate anterior displacement of the lower segment.

the bilateral presence of nerve roots, fracture with nerve injury, although not always immediately apparent, is often only unilateral. Prognostically, this fact becomes important from the standpoint of future bowel, bladder, and sexual function. Although this is of concern in the female, from a motor standpoint, it is of major importance in the male. When unilateral nerve discontinuity of a sacral nerve root has occurred (either neurapraxia or axonotmesis), pelvic end organ function is lost on one side only. Because the opposite side remains intact, return of partial function is possible.

Injury to the sacral plexus (S2 to S5) (which are, by virtue of their location, peripheral nerves) results in flaccid motor paralysis and loss of sensory function throughout the perianal "saddle" region. Bulbocavernosus reflex activity is lost, as is voluntary bowel and bladder function.

Types of Nerve Injury

Direct injury to peripheral nerves (in this instance, the sacral nerve root) may produce any one of the following types of injury:

Neurapraxia: temporary loss of motor or sensory nerve function.
Axonotmesis: anatomic discontinuity of the axon cylinder, with maintenance of continuity of the nerve (Schwann cell) sheath. This type of nerve root injury (axon discontinuity) has the potential for axon regeneration, with return of lost motor or sensory function.
Neurotmesis: the complete loss of continuity (or transection) of both the axon cylinder and the nerve (Schwann cell) sheath. Without nerve root repair, loss of neurologic function is permanent.

In the area of the cauda equina (and specifically the sacral area), I am unaware of successful nerve root repairs.

Denis, in a retrospective review of 776 fractures of the pelvis, identified 236 pelvic fractures that also involved the sacrum[71] (personal communication) (Fig. 19-49). Analysis of the fractures resulted in the following sacral fracture classification: a, the fracture type; b, the anticipated neurologic consequence of the fracture; and c, the location of the sacral fracture by "zones":

Zone 1: Fractures through the region of the ala. This segment of the sacrum is thick, articulates with the posterior iliac portion of the pelvic wing, and on occasion is associated with injuries to the L5 nerve root.
Zone 2: Fractures in this area of the sacrum are associated with fractures through the sacral foramen. Although frequently associated with neurologic (nerve root-sciatica) injury, S2-S3 bladder dysfunction is infrequent.
Zone 3: Fractures through the midcentral portion of the sacral canal often result (as anticipated) in injury to the sacral neurologic segments (S2–S3). These nerve roots provide sensory and motor function to the bowel, bladder, vulva, and groin. With perianal paresthesia or anesthesia there will also be loss of bowel and bladder sphincter function. As noted above, the extent of return of neurologic function depends on the type of nerve injury occurring (neurapraxia, axonotomesis, or neurotmesis).

MANAGEMENT OF SACRAL FRACTURES

The overall management scheme for fractures of the sacrum includes only two options: conservative care or surgical intervention. The decision rests on the location of the fracture, whether there is associated neurologic involvement, and the type and extent of the fracture.

Conservative Management

As a rule, most fractures of the sacrum can be managed conservatively. In my series of 13, 10 (77 percent) were managed conservatively. This means that the majority, regardless of the apparent severity, require only observation and careful postfracture management (Fig. 19-50). Fractures qualifying for observation only include transverse fractures with little or no angular or translatory displacement, stellate (nondisplaced comminuted) fractures, fractures of the sacrum with evidence of modest displacement and unilateral isolated nerve

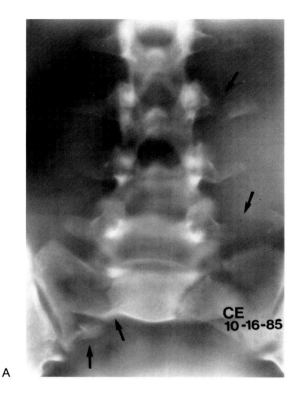

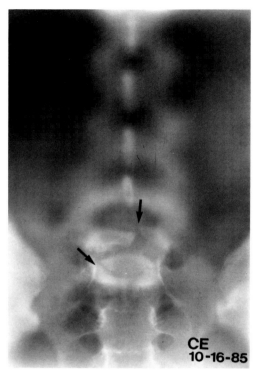

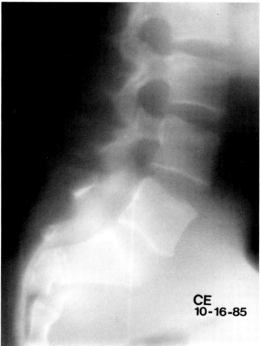

Fig. 19-50. **(A)** Anterior radiograph of lumbosacral spine demonstrating multiple level transverse process fractures and a comminuted fracture involving the sacrum. **(B)** Anterior view of the sacrum showing spina bifida occulta and the loss of symmetrical sacral foramen detail. This later finding is indicative of presence of a sacral fracture. **(C)** Lateral radiograph of the lumbosacral spine showing anterior displacement of the comminuted sacral fracture. *(Figure continues.)*

Fig. 19-50 *(Continued).* **(D)** Intraoperative photograph of posterior sacrum showing retraction of sacral nerve roots away from the fracture fragment, which has extruded posteriorly and is producing nerve root compression. **(E)** View of operative field reveals traumatic avulsion (neurotmesis) of the first sacral nerve root. The nerve stump lies on top of a surgical pledget. The patient's preoperative neurologic examination revealed absence of S2 neurologic function on the left.

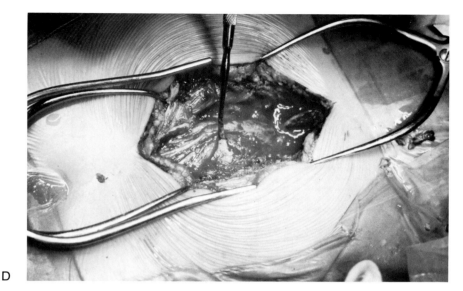

D

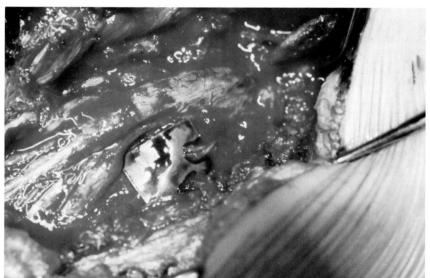

E

root injury with no neurologic injury, and fractures of the sacrum involving the lumbar spine (with normal neurologic function).[63]

Surgical Management

The indication for surgical intervention is clearly based on the existence of incomplete neurologic injury and the presence of a visible and continuing cause for the neurologic deficit. Such cases require open sacral nerve "unroofing" or decompression[73] (Fig. 19-50): fracture-dislocations of the lumbosacral joint with comminution of the sacrum[69]; when alignment is a concern and internal fixation is required[69]; when the fracture of the sacrum is transverse and accompanied by acute anterior displacement of one segment (kyphosis).[70]

In my series of sacral fractures, surgical decompression was required in 3 of 13 cases. One fracture was open (Fig. 19-4), and two required decom-

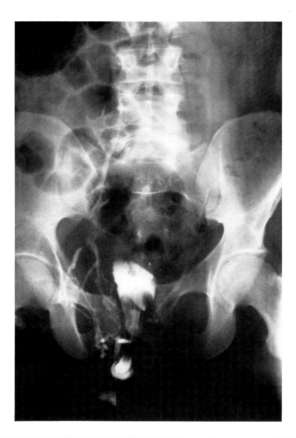

A

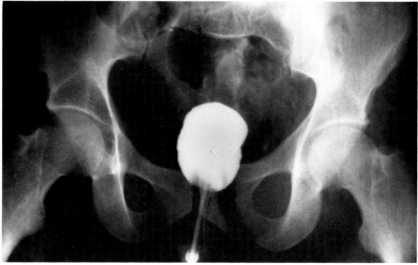

B

Fig. 19-51. **(A)** Transurethral injection of contrast material demonstrating extravasation and retrograde flow through local venous channels, indicating urethral tear. **(B)** AP view of the lower pelvis demonstrating extensive fractures of the left inferior and superior pubic rami and appropriate placement of a transurethral catheter into the bladder. Cystogram revealed no evidence of bladder trauma. Standard sacral radiographs failed to reveal the severe sacral fracture. Note the loss of sacral foramen detail in the sacrum. *(Figure continues.)*

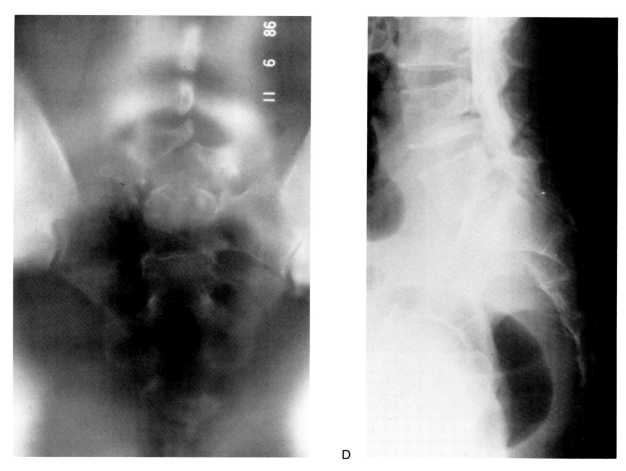

C   D

Fig. 19-51 *(Continued).* **(C,D)** AP and lateral radiographs of the sacrum demonstrating severe comminuted fracture of the sacral body with anterior displacement of the inferior segment. Note the absence of sacral foramen detail in the right sacrum. Note a spina bifida occulta of L5 similar to that seen in Figure 19-50. *(Figure continues.)*

pression (Fig. 19-49). Results from operative decompression remain debatable.[73] When sacral nerve root injury follows fractures of the sacrum, and radiologic examination reveals fracture fragment angulation (malposition), decompression is probably warranted. The nerve injury may be the result of either complete loss of nerve continuity (Fig. 19-49E), or nerve stretch (Fig. 19-49B). Denis is of the opinion that early open decompression is of benefit and likely contributes to the restoring of nerve root function[71] (personal communication). Surgery may contribute, but other factors are of equal importance. First, the nerve root must be in continuity. Second, the neuroanatomic distribution of the sacral plexus to the pelvic organs is bilateral (the bladder, bowel, vulva, rectum). Thus, partial recovery of end organ function is good from the beginning. Therfore, the chance of neurologic recovery after sacral cauda equina injury with neurapraxia is greater than with peripheral nerve involvement in a single lower extremity (Fig. 19-51).

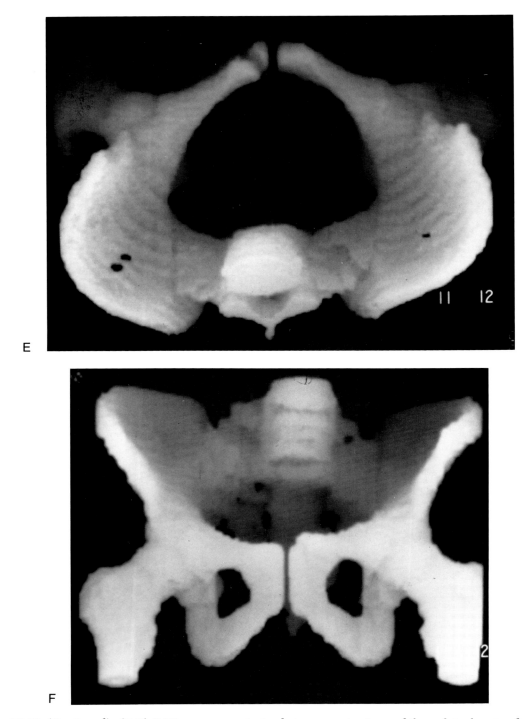

E

F

Fig. 19-51 *(Continued).* **(E,F)** CAT scan computerized stereoscopic views of the pelvis showing fracture through the anterior left pubic symphysis and comminuted fracture through the right sacrum at the sacroiliac joint. *(Figure continues.)*

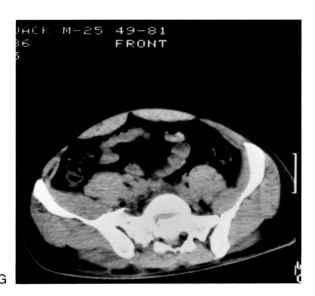

Fig. 19-51 *(Continued).* **(G)** CAT scan of the sacrum showing severe comminution of the sacrum. The patient was managed conservatively.

SACRAL SERIES: SURGICAL DATA

As noted, sacral fractures occur infrequently, though their actual incidence is likely higher than stated because their presence is either insignificant or overlooked when the sacrum is only one of multiple sites traumatized. In the three cases discussed here, anteroposterior radiographs of the pelvis (Fig. 19-52) provided initial visualization of the fracture. Lateral radiographs of the pelvis (sacrum) accurately reflect the extent of both anterior angulation and sacral fracture comminution. Newer radiographic techniques, using multiple CAT computer-generated "three-dimensional" bone imaging, have become a useful method of reconstructing a hip joint[74] or of evaluating the extent of a fracture of the pelvis. This technique makes it possible to identify the extent of a fracture and the direction of its displacement, but, as yet, has not been required in the surgical decision-making process (Fig. 19-52).

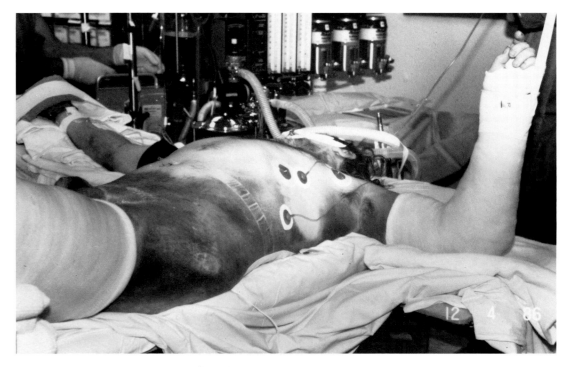

Fig. 19-52. (A) Operating room view of a multiple trauma patient with fractures involving the lumbosacral spine and left upper and lower extremities. Note the extent of subcutaneous ecchymosis secondary to fractures of the pelvis. *(Figure continues.)*

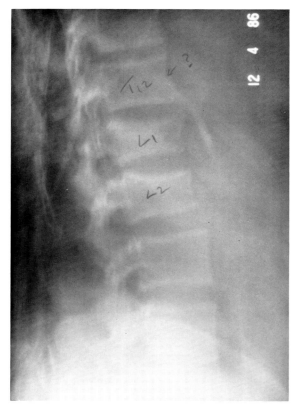

B

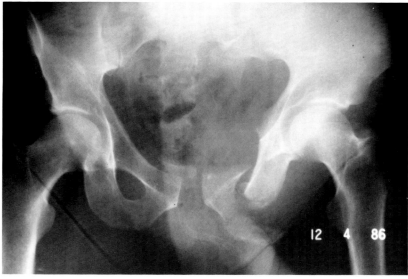

C

Fig. 19-52 *(Continued)*. **(B)** Lateral radiograph of the lumbar spine showing compression fracture of the L1 and L2 vertebral bodies and questionable fracture of the T12 vertebral body. **(C)** Anterior radiograph of the pelvis showing a comminuted fracture involving the superior and inferior pubic rami. Note the lack of detail in the area of the left sacroiliac joint, although fracture was suspected. *(Figure continues.)*

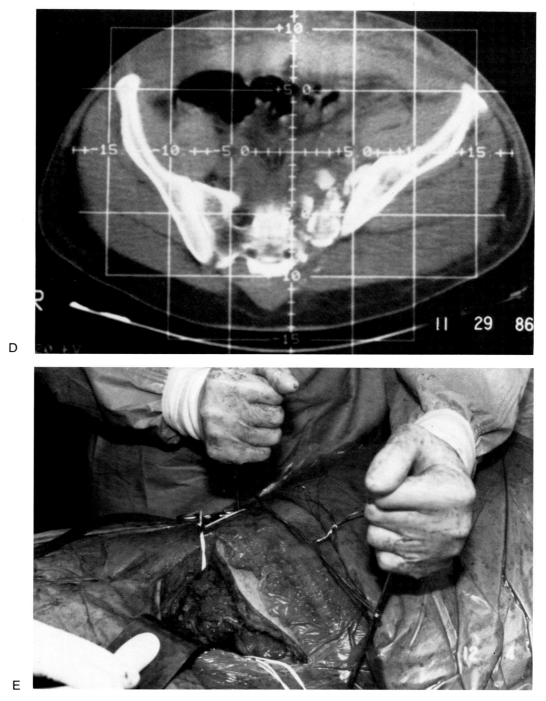

Fig. 19-52 *(Continued).* **(D)** CAT scan of lumbosacral joint graphically reveals the comminuted fracture of the left sacrum and wide diastasis of the pelvic wings. It is important to appreciate the frequent coexistence of fractures of the sacrum with severe fractures involving the pelvic girdle (compare Fig. C). **(E)** Large Steinmann pins are inserted into each anterior superior iliac crest and pulled towards the mid-line. Their position was fixed with #18 gauge wire. Approximation of these pins allowed for maintenance of reduction of the superior pubic rami fractures during internal fixation. The femoral nerve and vessels are tagged with a white cigarette drain. *(Figure continues.)*

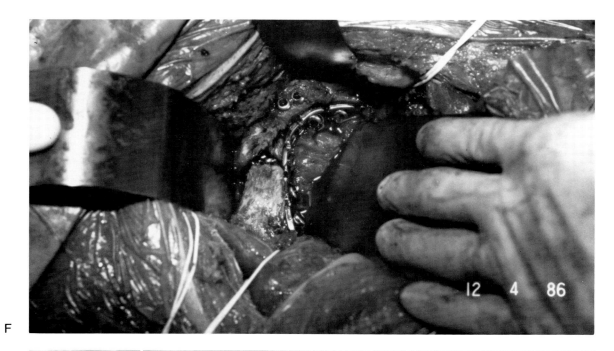

F

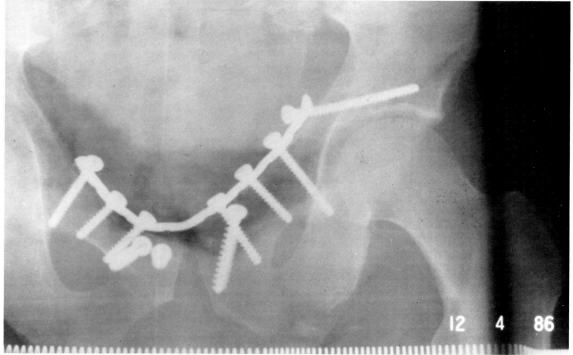

G

Fig. 19-52 *(Continued).* **(F)** Operative view of internal fixation after insertion of malleable plate and screws as well as inter-fragment screws. **(G)** Post-operative radiograph showing internal fixation of the superior pubic rami fractures.

Of the 13 sacral spine fractures and dislocations managed at Northwestern University between 1972 and 1986, the principal etiology was direct trauma or flying objects. One patient had normal neurologic levels on admission and was managed conservatively. Three patients required surgery. One had an open fracture with neurologic injury, and two had overt neurologic injury resulting from fracture comminution and anterior displacement of the lower sacral segment. The three patients revealing neurologic injury demonstrated varying degrees of unilateral and bilateral sacral plexus involvement, primarily at the level of injury (S2, S3). Lost function included voluntary contraction of the perianal muscles, voluntary bladder control, and perianal sensation. The extent of nerve root injury varied, yet uniformly involved S2 and S3.

As noted, most fractures are a combination of transverse and comminuted fractures (Figs. 19-47, 19-48, 19-49, 19-52). As with Denis's (personal communication) and Byrne's[70] findings,[71] the fracture most frequently occurs at the transition between the thickened S1 and slightly thinner S2 segment, and the narrower and thinner (and hollow) midportion of the sacral body. Byrne's review of the literature also noted that fractures of the sacrum were more often associated with angulation at the fracture site than with displacement.[70] Although this was also noted in my series, the number of cases is small.

As noted, 3 of the 13 fractures and dislocations of the sacrum underwent debridement or decompression: The abraded, punctate, open fracture of the sacrum in the first patient required surgical debridement. When the skin was incised sacral nerve roots were found entrapped and acutely "tented" over posteriorly displaced sacral fragments. Neurologic examination revealed bilateral loss of S1–S2 bowel, bladder, and perianal muscle function. Management consisted of nerve root decompression, removal of isolated bone fragments, and primary wound closure. Postoperatively, the patient had neurologic findings as noted on admission. Over the next 8 months, incomplete unilateral return of S2 function occurred.

The second patient required surgical decompression because of an unusually marked comminution and anterior displacement of the lower sacral segment occluding the canal that was associated with loss of unilateral S1–S2–S3 nerve root function (Fig. 19-49). The resulting neurologic injury produced unilateral loss of bowel, bladder, and rectal tone and unilateral hemianesthesia in one labia, along with unilateral weakness in one gastrocnemius muscle. An open unroofing[70] decompression procedure was elected because of the presence of an incomplete neurologic injury and the suspicion that the sacral nerve roots were tented over bone fragments displaced posteriorly, compressing the nerve roots were found contused and entrapped, and one (unilateral, S2) root was transected (Fig. 19-50E).

The third patient requiring decompression was an elderly female victim of multiple sclerosis with osteoporosis, who fell off of a commode, sustaining an acutely angulated fracture of the sacrum. Because of the underlying neurologic disease, the peripheral neurologic examination was mixed. The neurologic examination revealed weakness in the triceps surae (S1–S2) muscle groups, absent bowel and bladder function, and hypoesthesia over the S1–S2 dermatomes, bilaterally. After decompression, nerve root function failed to return.

Postoperative sacral fracture management included protection of the area of the sacral fracture (non-weight bearing with sitting) for 4 to 6 weeks, depending on the type of fracture and neurologic injury present along with ambulation when possible, with the patient going from the supine position to the upright position by using a tilt table. At 6 weeks, patients were allowed to begin gradual weight bearing while sitting. Occasionally, sit supports were applied to the sitting surface so that the two ischial rami carried the sitting weight, not the sacrum. No increase in neurologic deficit occurred.

ORTHOTIC MANAGEMENT

Achieving fusion in the post-traumatic spine is the objective of the management scheme. It requires surgical stabilization, time, and postoperative orthotic protection. Both the surgical group, with conventional internal fixation techniques (omitting plates and transpedicular screw-rod combinations), and the nonoperative, conservatively

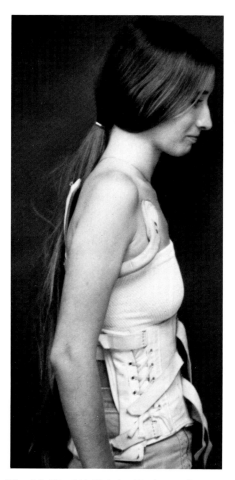
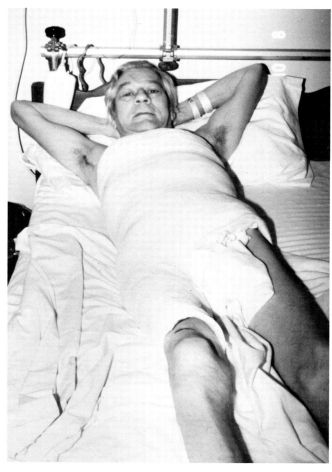

Fig. 19-53. (A) Knight-Taylor orthosis with abdominal corset and pectoral horns. This orthosis maintains the patient in extension. **(B)** A patient with a lumbosacral joint fracture, immobilized in a body cast with a one-legged pantaloon spica. *(Figure continues.)*

managed group received some form of external immobilization for 3 months, until the spine was deemed fused, healed, or stable.

As noted earler, motion in the lumbar spine is great. Whereas the thoracic vertebral column is immobilized by the rib cage and motion between its segments is restricted, the lumbar spine is relatively hypermobile, primarily in flexion, down to and including the lumbosacral joint. Internal fixation achieves an initial stability. An orthosis provides added assurance that fracture healing, without deformity, will occur.

The type of orthosis most frequently applied is the TLSO orthosis of the Knight-Taylor variety

(Fig. 19-53A). Superiorly and anteriorly, "pectoral horns" are added to the spinal uprights. This provides additional support in maintaining the patient in an upright, extended, or semi-hyperextended posture, while also reducing lateral bending. The orthosis crosses over the lumbosacral joint to the level of the coccyx inferiorly and extends proximally to the level of the pectoral muscles anteriorly and the superior border of the scapula posteriorly.

A more conventional method of preventing motion across the lumbosacral joint is with a spica body cast. This cast extends from the sternal notch anteriorly and superiorly to the supracondylar area of one thigh and to the level of the hip joint on the

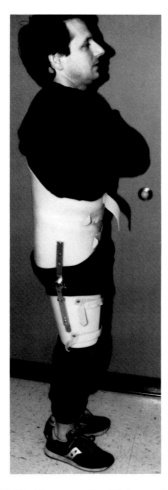
C

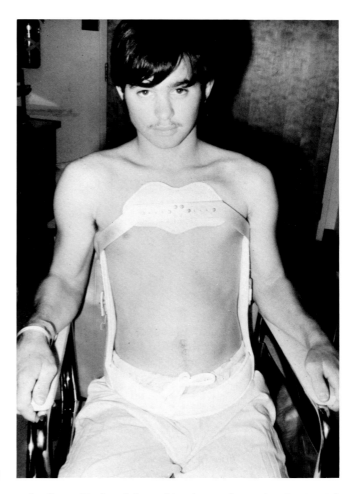
D

Fig. 19-53 *(Continued).* **(C)** Lateral photograph of a molded and shaped lumbar and sacral orthosis with a variable lock external hip joint attached to a unilateral thigh lacer. This orthosis is used when fusion of the lumbar/sacral joint is required. **(D)** Fractures of the lumbar spine at L1–L4 can be managed in a Jewett hyperextension orthosis.

opposite side. This orthosis may be constructed of fiberglass, plaster of paris, or a plastic laminated jacket with thigh socket, fitted together with an external hinge-drop lock at the hip. This lock joint is inserted to block all motion at the hip with sitting or ambulating, while allowing flexion of the hip when supine in bed. As with other forms of orthotic immobilization, it is recommended that the devices be worn up to 3 months postinjury (Fig. 19-50).

Other types of thoracolumbar orthoses can be prescribed for patients with fractures involving the thoracolumbar junction and the lumbar spine. They include the abdominal corset, the body cast

(plaster or fiberglass), the plastic laminated body jacket, and a "three-point" hyperextension orthosis of the Jewett (Fig. 19-53) or the CASH anterior cruciate design.

REFERENCES

1. Wiltse LL (ed): Symposium: internal fixation of the lumbar spine. Clin Orthop 203: February 1986
2. Roy-Camille R, Saillant G, Gagna G, Mazel C: Trans-

verse fractures of the upper sacrum: suicidal jumper's fracture. Spine 10: 838, 1985

3. Louis R: Fusion of the lumbar and sacral spine by internal fixation with screw plates. Clin Orthop 203: 18, 1986

4. Luque ER, Cassis N and Ramirez-Wiella G: Segmental spine instrumentation in the treatment of fractures of the thoracolumbar spine. Spine 7:312, 1982

5. Zielke K, Strempel AV: Posterior lateral distraction spondylodesis using the twofold sacral bar. Clin Orthop 203: 131, 1986

6. Zielke K: VDS system. 45th AO-ASIF Spine Course, Davos, Switzerland, December 17, 1986

7. Magerl FP: Stabilization of the lower thoracic and lumbar spine with external skeletal fixation. Clin Orthop 189:125, 1984

8. Magerl FP: External skeletal fixation. In Weber BG, Magerl FP (eds): The External Fixator. Springer-Verlag, New York, 1985

9. Kostuik JP, Errico TJ, Gleason TF: Techniques of internal fixation for degenerative conditions of the lumbar spine. Clin Orthop 203:219, 1986

10. Steffee AD, Sitkowski PAC, Topham LS: Total vertebral body and pedicle arthroplasty. Clin Orthop 203:203, 1986

11. Chusid JG: Correlative Neuroanatomy and Functional Neurology. 17th Ed. p. 80. Appleton & Lange, 1979

12. Calenoff L, Chessare J, Rogers LF et al.: Multiple levels, spine injuries: importance of early recognition. AJR 130:665, 1979

13. Denis F: The three column spine and its significance in the classification of acute thoracolumbar spine injuries. Spine 8:817, 1983

14. Holdsworth FW, Hardy AG: Early treatment of paraplegics from fracture of the thoracolumbar spine. J Bone Joint Surg 35B:540, 1953

15. Holdsworth FW: Symposium on Spinal Injury. p. 161. Edinburgh Royal College of Surgeons, Edinburgh, 1963

16. Holdsworth FW: Review article — fracture-dislocation and fracture-dislocations of the spine. J Bone Joint Surg 52A:534, 1970

17. Ferguson RL, Allen BL: A mechanistic classification of thoracolumbar spine fractures. Clin Orthop 189:77, 1984

18. Kaufer H, Hayes JT: Lumbar fracture-dislocation. A study of twenty-one cases. J Bone Joint Surg 48A:712, 1966

19. McAfee PC, Yuan HA, Frederickson BE, Lubicky JP: The value of computed tomography in thoracolumbar fractures. J Bone Joint Surg 65A:461, 1983

20. Chance GQ: Note on the type of flexion fracture of the spine. Br J Radiol 21:452, 1948

21. Magerl F, Harms J: Presentation: Classification of Injury and Prognosis — Thoracolumbar Injuries. 45th AO-ASIF Spine Course, Davos, Switzerland, December 16, 1986

22. Frankel HL: Ascending cord lesions in the early stages following spinal injury. Paraplegia 7:111, 1969

23. Jacobs RR: Bilateral fracture of the pedicles through the fourth and fifth lumbar vertebrae with anterior displacement of the vertebral bodies. J Bone Joint Surg 59A: 409, 1977

24. Edmonson AS, Crenshaw AH (eds): The Spine. p. 1939. Campbells Operative Orthopaedics. 6th Ed. Vol. 2. CV Mosby, St. Louis, 1980

25. Meyer PR: Complication of fractures of the dorso-lumbar spine. Complications in Orthopaedic Surgery. 2nd Ed. Vol. 2. JB Lippincott, Philadelphia, 1985

26. White AA, Panjabi MM: Functional spinal unit and mathematical models. Clinical Biomechanics of the Spine. JB Lippincott Philadelphia, 1978

27. Gumley G, Taylor TKF, Ryan MD: Distraction fractures of the lumbar spine. J Bone Joint Surg 64B: 520, 1982

28. Haddad GH, Zickel RE: Intestinal perforations and fractures of lumbar vertebra caused by lap-type seat belts. NY State J Med 67:930, 1967

29. Smith WS, Kaufer H: Patterns and mechanisms of lumbar injuries associated with lap seat belt fractures. J Bone Joint Surg 51A:239, 1969

30. Howland WJ, Curry JL, Buffington CB: Fulcrum fractures of the lumbar spine. JAMA 193:240, 1965

31. Greenbaum E, Harris L, Halloran WX: Flexion fractures of the lumbar spine due to lap-type seat belts. Calif Med 113:361, 1970

32. Olson TH, Selvik G, Willner S: Mobility in the lumbosacral spine after fusion studied with the aid of roentgen stereophotogrammetry. Clin Orthop 129:181, 1977

33. Gelman MI, Umber JS: Fractures of the thoracolumbar spine in ankylosing spondylitis. AJR 130:485, 1978

34. Bergmann EW: Fractures of the ankylosed spine. J Bone Joint Surg 31A:669, 1949

35. Kiwerski J, Wieclawek H, Garwacka L: Fractures of the cervical spine in ankylosing spondylitis. Orthop 8:243, 1985

36. Calenoff L (ed): Radiology in Spinal Cord Injury. CV Mosby, St. Louis, 1981

37. Marie P: Sur la spondylose rhizomelique. Rev Med 18:285, 1898

38. Strümpell A: Bemerkung uber die Chronische Ankylosirende Entzundung der Wirbelsaule und der Huftgelenke. Dsch Z Nervenheilled, p. 338, 1897

39. Brugman JL, Stauffer ES: Spinal fractures in ankylosing spondylitis. Unpublished, 1986
40. Weinstein P, Karpman R, Gall E, Pitt M: Spinal cord injury, spinal fracture and spinal stenosis in Ankylosing spondylitis. J Neurosurg 57:609, 1982
41. Bohler J, Gaudernak T: Anterior plate stabilization for fracture-dislocations of the lower cervical spine. J Trauma 20:203, 1980
42. Johnson CE, Happel LT, Norris R et al.: Delayed paraplegia complicating sublaminar segmental spinal instrumentation. J Bone Joint Surg 68A:556, 1986
43. Nicastro JF, Hartjen CA, Traina J, Lancaster JM: Intraspinal pathways taken by sublaminar wires during removal. An experimental study. J Bone Joint Surg 68A:1206, 1986
44. Guttmann L: Spinal deformities in traumatic paraplegia and tetraplegia following surgical procedures. Paraplegia 7:38, 1969
45. Lewis J, McKibbin B: The treatment of unstable fractures—dislocations of the thoracic-lumbar spine accompanied by paraplegia. J Bone Joint Surg 56B:603, 1974
46. Davis AG: Fractures of the spine. J Bone Joint Surg 11:133, 1929
47. Dick TBS: Traumatic paraplegia pre-Guttmann. Paraplegia 7:173, 1969
48. Hathaway HR: Unusual fractures of the cervical spine with Marie-Strümpell disease. Ohio Med J 46:236, 1950
49. Rogers WA: Cord injury during reduction of thoracic and lumbar vertebral body fracture and dislocation. J Bone Joint Surg 20:689, 1938
50. Bohler L: The Treatment of Fractures. Wright and Son, Bristol, 1935
51. Watson-Jones R: Fracture and Other Bone and Joint Injuries. 1st Ed. p. 641. ES Livingstone, Edinburgh, 1940
52. Frankel HL, Hancock DO, Hystop G et al.: The value of postural reduction in the initial management of closed injuries of the spine with paraplegia and tetraplegia. Part 1. Paraplegia 7:179, 1969
53. Selby D: Internal fixation with Knodt's rods. Clin Orthop. 203:179, 1986
54. Ogilvie JW, Schendel M: Comparison of lumbosacral fixation devices. Clin Orthop 203:179, 1986
55. Harrington PR, Dickson JH: An eleven year clinical investigation of Harrington instrumentation. Clin Orthop 112:113, 1973
56. Weiss M: Dynamic spine alloplasty (spring loading correction device) after fracture and spinal cord injury. Clin Orthop 112:150, 1975
57. Graham CE: Lumbosacral fusion using internal fixation with a spinous process for the graft. Clin Orthop 140:72, 1979
58. Barr JS: Low back and sciatic pain. J Bone Joint Surg 33A:633, 1951
59. Watson Jones R: Reaction of bone to metal. p. 205. In-fractures and Joint Injuries. 4th Ed. Vol. 1. ES Livingston, Edinburg, and Williams & Wilkins, Baltimore, 1952
60. Bosworth DM: Surgery of the spine. AAOS Instructional Course Lectures 14:39, 1957
61. White AH, Zucherman JF, Hsu K: Lumbosacral fusion with Harrington rods and intersegmental wiring. Clin Orthop 203:185, 1986
62. Andrew TA, Brooks S, Piggott H: Long-term follow-up evaluation of screw-and-graft fusion of the lumbar spine. Clin Orthop 203:113, 1986
63. Kornberg M, Herndon WAA, Rechtine GR: Lumbar nerve root compression at the site of hook insertion. Spine 10:853, 1985
64. Allen BL, Ferguson RL: The Galveston technique for L rod instrumentation of the scoliotic spine. Spine 7:276, 1982
65. Jacobs RR, Schlapfer F et al.: A locking hook spinal rod system for stabilization of fracture-dislocations and correction of deformities of the dorsolumbar spine. Clin Orthop 189:168, 1984
66. Cook SD, Harding BS, Whitecloud TS et al.: A clinical and metallurgical analysis of 28 retrieved harrington rods. Contemp Orthop 12:27, 1986
67. 45th AO-ASIF Spine Course, Davos, Switzerland, December 17, 1986
68. Anderson JE: Grant's Atlas of Anatomy. 7th Ed. Williams & Wilkins, Baltimore, 1978
69. Fardon DF: Displaced transverse fracture of the sacrum with nerve root injury: report of a case with successful operative management. J Trauma 19:119, 1979
70. Byrnes DP, Russo GL et al.: Sacrum fractures and neurological damage. J Neurosurg 47:459, 1977
71. Denis F, Davis S, and Comfort T: Sacral fractures, an important problem, though frequently undiagnosed and untreated: retrospective analysis of 236 consecutive cases. Presentation: Federation of Spine Associations, AAOS, January 22, 1987
72. Zoltan JD, Gilula LA, Murphy WA: Unilateral facet dislocation between the fifth lumbar and the first sacral vertebra. J Bone Joint Surg 61A:767, 1979
73. Dowling T, Epstein JA, Epstein NE: S1-S2 sacral fractures involving neural elements of the cauda equina. Spine 10:851, 1985
74. Woolson ST: Three-dimensional bone imaging and preoperative planning of reconstructive hip surgery. Contemp Orthop 12:13, 1986

Bibliography

SPINE TRAUMA SYSTEMS MANAGEMENT

Accidental death and disability: The neglected disease of modern society. Division of Medical Sciences, National Academy of Science, National Research Council, Washington, DC September, 1966

Advanced Trauma Life Support Course, Instructors Manual. Committee on Trauma, American College of Surgeons, 1984

Baxt WG:Aeromedical emergency care.p. 131. In Boyd DR, Edlich RF (eds): Systems Approach to Emergency Medical Care. Appleton-Century-Crofts, Norwalk, CT, 1983

Beal J: Critical Care for Surgical Patients. Macmillan, New York, 1982

Black P: Injuries of the vertebral column and spinal cord: mechanisms and management in the acute phase. In Ballinger WF, et al: The Management of Trauma. 2nd Ed. WB Saunders, Philadelphia, 1973

Bedrook GW: The Care and Management of Spinal Cord Injuries. Springer-Verlag, New York, 1981

Boyd DR, Dunea MM, Flashner BA: The Illinois plan for a statewide system of trauma centers. J Trauma 13:24, 1973

Boyd DR, Edlich RF, Micik SH: The history of EMS in the United States. In Boyd DR,Edlich, RF (eds): Systems Approach to Emergency Medical Care. Appleton-Century-Crofts, Norwalk, CT 1983

Categorization of Hospital Emergency Capabilities: American Medical Association, Chicago, 1971

Covall DA, Clipper IS, Howm TI, Rusk HA: Early management of patients with spinal cord injury. JAMA 151:89, 1953

Boyd DR, Edlich, RF: Systems Approach to Emergency Medical Care. Appleton-Century-Crofts, New York, 1983

Elsberg CA: The Edwin Smith surgical papyrus, and the diagnosis and the treatment of injuries to the skull and spine 5,000 years ago. Amer Med Hist, 3:271,1931

Emergency medical service system act of 1973. Public Law: 93, 1973. Amended 1976, Public Law: 94, 1976

Gehrig R, Michaelis, LS: Statistics of acute paraplegia and tetraplegia on a national scale: Switzerland 1960 – 77. Paraplegia 6:93, 1968

Gschaelder R, Dollfus P, Mole JP, et al: Reflections on the intensive care of acute cervical spinal cord injuries in a general traumatology centre. Paraplegia 17:58, 1979

Guidelines for Facility Categorization and Standards of Care: Spinal Cord Injury. American Spinal Injury Association/Foundation, Chicago, 1981

Heaton LD: Army medical service activities in Vietnam. Mili Med 131:646, 1966

Illinois Categorization Law. Senate Bill 568, Public Act 76 – 1858, 1972

Kraus JF, Franti CE, Riggins RS, et al: Incidence of traumatic spinal cord lesions J Chronic Dis 28:471, 1975

Meyer PR, Carle TV, Hamilton BB: Annual Progress Report. X. Midwest Regional Spinal Cord Injury Care System. Grant 13P – 55864. Department of Education, Washington, DC, 1982

Meyer PR, Raffensperger JG: Special centers for the care of the injured. J Trauma 13:308, 1973

Meyer PR: Trauma Symposium Workshop For Physicians. PHS Contract 232–78–0170. Division of Emergency Medical Services, Department of Health, Education, and Welfare, Washington, DC, 1978

Meyer PR, Rosen JS, Hamilton BB, Hall W: Fracture dislocation of the cervical spine: transportation, assessment and immediate management. In Instructional Course Lectures, American Academy of Orthopaedic Surgeons. p.171 Vol. XXV. CV Mosby, St. Louis, 1976

Meyer PR: Systems approach to the care of the spinal cord injured. p. 404. In Boyd DR, Edlich RF (eds): Systems Approach to Emergency Medical Care. Appleton-Century-Crofts, Norwalk, CT, 1983

Meyer PR: The spinal cord injured patient. p. 311. In Beal JM (ed): Critical Care for Surgical Patients. Macmillan, New York, 1982

Meyer PR: Spinal cord injury. Sect. VI, part (c). Manual of the Trauma Systems Development Workshops. HRA Contract 232–78–0170, Washington, D.C. 1979

Meyer PR, Gireesan GT: Management of acute spinal cord injured patients by the Midwest Regional Spinal Cord Injury Care System. Topics in Acute Care and Trauma Rehabilitation. 1 (3):1, 1987 Aspen Systems Inc.

National Safety Council: Accident facts. National Safety Council, Chicago, 1978

National Safety Council: Body area of motor vehicle occupant injured in motor vehicle accident. National Safety Council, Chicago, 1966

National Safety Council: Part of body injured in work accidents. National Safety Council, Chicago, 1982

Neel S: Helicopter evacuation in Korea. US Armed Forces Med J 6:691, 1955

Neel S: Medical Support of the US Army in Vietnam, 1965–1970. US Government Printing Office, Washington, DC, 1973

Neel, S: Army aeromedical evacuation procedures in Vietnam: implications for rural America. JAMA 204:309, 1968

Rehabilitation Act of 1973. Public Law: 93–112, 93rd Congress, House of Representatives 8070, September 1973

Roy-Camille R, Saillant G, Berteaux D, Marie-Anne S: Early management of spinal injuries. p. 57. In McKibbin, B: Recent Advances in Orthopaedics Vol. 3. Churchill Livingstone, Edinburgh, 1979

Stover S, Fine R: Spinal Cord Injury: The Facts and Figures. National Science Data Center, University of Alabama at Birmingham, Birmingham, Alabama, 1986

Tator CH, Rowed DW: Current concepts in the immediate management of acute spinal cord injuries. Can Med Assoc J 121:1453, 1979

Tong JI, O'Reilly, MJJ, Davison A, Johnston NG: Traffic crash fatalities: injury patterns and other factors. Med J Aust 2:5, 1972

Trunkey DD, Lim RC: Analysis of 425 consecutive trauma fatalities: an autopsy study. J Am Coll Emerg Phys 3:368, 1974

Wannamaker GT: Spinal cord injuries: a review of the early treatment of 300 consecutive cases during the Korean conflict. J Neurosurg 11:517, 1954

West JG, Trunkey DD, Lim RC: Systems of care. Arch Surg 114:455, 1979

Young JS: Initial hospitalization and rehabilitation costs of spinal cord injury. Ortho Clin North Am 9(2):263, 1978

EMBRYOLOGY OF THE SPINE AND NERVOUS SYSTEM

Arey LB: Developmental Anatomy. 6th Ed. WB Saunders, Philadelphia, 1965

Bardeen CR: The development of the thoracic vertebrae in man. Am J Anat 4:163, 1905

LaRocca H: Embryology of the musculoskeletal system. In Lovell WW, Winter RB (eds): Pediatric Orthopaedics. JB Lippincott, Philadelphia, 1978

Last RJ: Innervation of the limbs. J Bone Joint Surg [Am] 31B(3):450, 1949

Ogden JA: The Development and growth of the musculoskeletal system. p. 41. In Albright JA, Brand RA (eds): Scientific Basis of Orthopaedics. Appleton-Century-Crofts, New York, 1979

Parke WW: Development of the spine. p. 1. In Rothman RH, Simeone FA (eds): The Spine. WB Saunders, Philadelphia, 1975

Streeter G, Henser C, Cornor G: Development horizons in human embryos. Contrib Embryol 230 (Reprint II):166, 1951

Winter RB, Lonstein JE, Leonard AS, Smith AE: Spine embryology. p. 1. In Winter RB (ed): Congenital Deformities of the Spine. Thieme-Stratton, New York, 1983

Wyburn GM: Observations on the development of the human vertebral column. J Anat 78:94, 1944

NEUROLOGY AND SPINAL CORD INJURY

Bell HS: Paralysis of both arms from injury of the upper portion of the pyramidal decussation: cruciate paralysis. J Neurosurg 33:376, 1970

Bennett MH, McCallum JE: Experimental decompression of spinal cord. Surg Neurol 8:63, 1977

Breig A: Biomechanics of Central Nervous System. Almqvist and Wiksell Publishers, Stockholm, 1960

Kakulus BA, Bedbrook GM: Pathology of injuries of the vertebral column. p. 27. Vinken PJ, Bruym GW (ed): Handbook of Clinical Neurology. Vol 25. North Holland Publishing Company, Amsterdam, 1976

Chusid JG: Correlative Neuroanatomy and Functional Neurology. 17th Ed. Appleton & Lange, East Norwalk, CT, 1979

Dastur DK, Wadia NH, Desai AD, Singh G: Medullospinal compression due to atlanto-axial dislocation and sudden haematomyelia during decompression. Brain 88:897, 1965

Comarr AE, Kaufman AA: A survey of the neurological results of 858 spinal cord injuries. A comparison of patients with and without laminectomy. J Neurosurg 13:95, 1956

Drew R, McClelland RR, Fisher RF: The dominance of vertebral column fractures associated with neurologic deficits among survivors of light-plane accidents. J Trauma 17:574, 1977

Michaelis LS: International inquiry on neurological terminology and prognosis in paraplegia and tetraplegia. Paraplegia 7:1, 1969

Morgan TH, Wharton G, Ansten G: The results of laminectomy in patients with incomplete spinal cord injuries. Paraplegia 9:14, 1971

Owman C, Sjoberg NO: The importance of short adrenergic neurons in the seminal emission mechanism of rat, guinea-pig and man. J Reprod Fert 28:379, 1972

Pedersen E, Harving H, Klemar B, Toring J: Human anal reflexes. J Neurol Neurosurg Psychiatry 41:813, 1978

Rasmussen AT: The Principal Nervous Pathways. 4th Ed. Macmillian, New York, 1952

Riggins RS: The risk of neurological damage with fractures of the vertebrae. J Trauma 17(2):126, 1977

Rigler LG: Kummell's disease with report of a roentgenologically proved case. AJR 15:749, 1931

Schneider RC, Crosby EC, Russo RH, Gosch HH: Traumatic spinal cord syndromes and their management. Clin Neurosurg 20:424, 1973

Schroder HD: Anatomical and pathoanatomical studies on the spinal efferent systems innervating pelvic structures. J Auton Nerv Syst 14:23, 1985

Sherrington C: The Integrative Action of the Nervous System. Yale University Press, New Haven, CT, 1947

Silver JR, Gibbon NOK: Prognosis in tetraplegia. Br Med J 4:79, 1968

RADIOLOGIC EVALUATION OF SPINE INJURIES

Alker GJ, Young SO, Leslie EV: Postmortem radiology of head and neck injuries in fatal traffic accidents. Radiology 114:611, 1975

Calenoff L, Chessare J, Rogers LF, et al: Multiple levels, spine injuries: importance of early recognition. AJR 130:665, 1979

Calenoff L: Radiologic assessment of the urinary system. p. 327. In Calenoff L (ed): Radiology of Spinal Cord Injury. CV Mosby, St. Louis, 1981

Cooper PR, Ho V: Role of emergency skull x-ray films in the evaluation of the head-injured patient: a retrospective study. Neurosurgery 13:136, 1983

Cummins, RO: Clinicians reasons for overuse of skull radiographs. AJNR 1:339, 1980

Deeb ZL, Martin TA, Kerber CW: Traction device for use with polytome table. AJR 131:732, 1978

Dershner MS, Goodman GA, Perlmutter GS: Computed tomography in the diagnosis of an atlas fracture. AJR 128:688, 1977

Eyes B, Evans AF: Post-traumatic skull radiography: time for a reappraisal. Lancet ii: 85, 1978

French BN, Cobb CA, Dublin AB: Cranial computed tomography in the diagnosis of symptomatic indirect trauma to the carotid artery. Surg Neurol 15:256, 1981

Gehweiler JA, Osborne RL, Becker RF: Radiology of Vertebral Trauma. Monographs in Clinical Radiology. Vol. 16. WB Saunders, Philadelphia, 1980

Harris Jr, JH: The Radiology of Acute Cervical Spine Trauma. Williams & Wilkins, Baltimore, 1978

Hartman JT, Palumbo F, Hill BJ: Cineradiography of the braced normal cervical spine: a comparative study of five commonly used cervical orthoses. Clin Orthop 109:97, 1975

Harwood-Nash DC, Hendrick EB, Hudson AR: The significance of skull fractures in children. A study of 1,187 patients. Radiology 101:151, 1971

Hinck VC, Hopkins CE, Savara BS: Sagittal diameter of the cervical spinal canal in children. Radiology 79:97, 1962

Kattan KR: Backward "displacement" of the spinolaminal line at C2: normal variation AJR 129:289, 1977

Koo AH, LaRoque, RL: Evaluation of head trauma by computed tomography. Radiology 123:345, 1977

Laasonen EM, Riska EB: Preoperative radiological assessment of fractures of the thoracolumbar spine causing traumatic paraplegia. Skeletal Radiol 1:231, 1977

Lusted LB, Keats, TE: Atlas of Roentgenographic Measurement. 2nd Ed. Year Book Medical Publishers, Chicago, 1967

Lusted LB, Keats TE: Atlas of Roentgenographic Measurement. 4th Ed. Year Book Medical Publishers, Chicago, 1978

McAfee PC, Yuan HA, Frederickson BE, Lubicky JP: The value of computed tomography in thoracolumbar fractures. J Bone Joint Surg 65A:461, 1983

Olson TH, Selvik G, Willner S: Mobility in the lumbosacral spine after fusion studied with the aid of roentgen stereophotogrammetry. Clin Orthop 129:181, 1977

Pay NT, George AE, Benjamin MV, Bergeron RT, et al: Positive and negative contrast myelography in spinal trauma. Radiology 123:103, 1977

Penning L: Diagnostic clues by x-ray injuries of the lower cervical spine. Acta Neurol Chir (Wien) 22:234, 1970

Penning L: Prevertebral hematoma in cervical spine injury: incidence and etiologic significance. AJR 136:553, 1981

Resnick D, Niwayama G: Radiographic and pathologic features of spinal involvement in diffuse idiopathic skeletal hyperostosis (DISH). Radiology 119:559, 1976

Shapiro R, Youngberg AS, Rothman SL: The differential diagnosis of traumatic lesions of the occipito-atlanto-axial segment. Radiol Clin North Am 11:505, 1973

Zatzkin HR, Kveton FW: Evaluation of the cervical spine in whiplash injuries. Radiology 75:577, 1960

EFFECTS OF SPINAL INJURY ON ANESTHESIA & RESPIRATORY FUNCTION

Cheshire DJE: Respiratory management in acute traumatic tetraplegia. Paraplegia 1:252, 1964

Clark DL, Rosner BS: Neurophysiologic effects of general anesthetics. I. The electroencephalogram and sensory evoked responses in man. Anesthesiology 38:564, 1973

Derenne H, Macklem PT, Roussos CH: The respiratory muscles: mechanics control and pathophysiology, Part III. Am Rev Resp Dis 118:581, 1978

Frost EAM: The physiopathology of respirations in neurosurgical patients. J Neurosurg 50:699, 1979

Fuglmeyer AR: Effects of respiratory muscle paralysis in tetraplegic and paraplegic patients. Scand J Rehab Med 3:141, 1971

Fuglmeyer AR: Ventilatory function in tetraplegic patients. Scand J Rehab Med 3:151, 1971

Glenn WWL, Holcomb WG, McLaughlin, et al: Total ventilatory support in a quadriplegic patient with radiofrequency electrophrenic respiration. N Eng J Med 286:513, 1972

Glenn WWL, Hogan JF, Loke JSO, et al: Ventilatory support by pacing of the conditioned diaphragm in quadriplegia. N Eng J Med 310:1150, 1984

Gross D, Ladd HW, Riley EJ, et al: The effect of training on strength and endurance of the diaphragm in quadriplegia. Am J Med 68:27, 1980

Ledsome JR, Sharp JM: Pulmonary function in acute cervical cord injury. Am Rev Resp Dis 124:41, 1981

Leigh DE, Bradley M: Ventilatory muscle strength and endurance training. J Appl Physiol 41:508, 1976

Macklem PT: Respiratory muscles: the vital pump. Chest 78:753, 1980

McMichan JC, Piepgras DG, Gracey DR, et al: Electrophrenic respiration. Mayo Clin Proc 54:662, 1979

McMichan JC, Michel L, Westbrook PR: Pulmonary dysfunction following traumatic quadriplegia. JAMA 243:528, 1980

Nunn JF: Applied Respiratory Physiology. 2nd Ed. Butterworth, London, 1977

Ohry A, Molho M, Rozin R: Alterations of pulmonary function in spinal cord injured patients. Paraplegia 13:101, 1975

Ovassapian A, Land P, Schaefer M, et al: Anesthetic management for surgical corrections of severe flexion deformity of the cervical spine. Anesthesiology 58:370, 1983

Quimby CW Jr, Williams RN, Greifenstein FE: Anesthesia problems of the acute quadriplegic patient. Anesth Analg 52:333, 1973

Schonwald G, Fish KJ, Perkash I: Cardiovascular complications during anesthesia in spinal cord injured patients. Anesthesiology 55:550, 1981

Shapiro BA: Clinical Applications of Respiratory Care. 3rd Ed. Year Book Medical Publishers, Chicago, 1985

Shapiro BA, Harrison RA, Walton JR: Clinical Application of Blood Gases. 3rd Ed. Chicago, Year Book Medical Publishers, 1982

Shapiro BA, Cane RD, Harrison RA: Positive end-expiratory pressure therapy in adults with special reference to acute lung injury: a review of the literature and suggested clinical correlations. Crit Care Med 12:127, 1984

Wicks AB, Menter RR: Long-term outlook in quadriplegic patients with initial ventilatory dependency. Chest 90:406, 1986

SURGICAL APPROACHES TO THE CERVICAL AND THORACOLUMBAR SPINE

Ducker TB, Bellegarrique R, Saleman M: Timing of operative care in cervical spinal cord injury. Spine 9:525, 1984

McAfee PC, Bohlman HH, Riley LH, et al: The anterior retropharyngeal approach to the upper part of the cervical spine. J Bone Joint Surg 69A(9):137, 1987

Robinson RA, Southwick WO: Surgical Approaches to the Cervical Spine. p. 299. In American Academy of Orthopaedic Surgeons: Instructional Course Lectures. CV Mosby, St. Louis, 1960

Robinson RA, Smith GW: Anterior lateral cervical disc removal and interbody fusion for cervical disc syndrome (abstract). Bull Johns Hopkins Hospital 96:223, 1955

Robinson RA: Anterior and posterior cervical spine fusion. Clin Orthop 35:34, 1964

Southwick WO, Robinson RA: Surgical approaches to the vertebral bodies in the cervical and lumbar regions. J Bone Joint Surg 39A:631, 1957

Spencer DL: Simultaneous anterior and posterior surgical approach to the thoracic and lumbar spine. Spine 4(1):29, 1979

Vierbiest H: Anterolateral operations for fractures and dislocations in the middle and lower parts of the cervical spine. Report of a series of forty-seven cases. J Bone Joint Surg 51A:1489, 1969

Vierbiest H: Anterior operative approach in cases of spinal cord compression by old irreducible displacement of fresh fractures of the cervical spine. Contributions to operative repair of deformed vertebral bodies. J Neurosurg 19:389, 1962

Vierbiest H: Anterolateral operations for fractures and dislocations of the cervical spine due to injury or previous surgical intervention. Clin Neurosurg 20:334, 1973

Wagner FC, Chehrazi B: Surgical results in the treatment of cervical spinal cord injury. Spine 9:523, 1984

SPINE BIOPSY AND SURGICAL STABILIZATION TECHNIQUES

Allen BL, Ferguson RL: The galveston technique for L. rod instrumentation of the scoliotic spine. Spine 7:276, 1982

Andrew TA, Brooks S, Piggott H: Long-term follow-up evaluation of screw-and-graft fusion of the lumbar spine. Clin Orthop 203:113, 1986

Bailey RW, Badgley, CE: Stabilization of the cervical spine by anterior fusion. J Bone and Joint Surg 42A:565, 1960

Bernhang AM, Rosen H, Leivy D: Internal methyl methacrylate splint provides rapid mobilization in treatment of grossly unstable fracture of cervical spine. Orthop Rev VII:25, 1978

Bloom MH, Raney FL: Anterior intervertebral fusion of the cervical spine, a technical note. J Bone Joint Surg 63A:842, 1981

Bohler J, Gaudernak T: Anterior plate stabilization for fracture-dislocations of the lower cervical spine. J Trauma 20:203, 1980

Brooks AL, Jenkins EB: Atlanto-axial arthrodesis by the wedge compression method. J Bone Joint Surg 60A:279, 1978

Burke DC, Berryman D: The place of closed manipulation in the management of flexion-rotation dislocations of the cervical spine. J Bone Joint Surg 53B:165, 1971

Cloward RB: Treatment of acute fractures and fracture-dislocations by vertebral body fusion. Report of eleven cases. J Neurosurg 18:201, 1961

Cloward R: Surgical treatment of dislocations and compression fractures of the cervical spine by the anterior approach. p. 26. Proceedings of the 17th Veterans Administration Spinal Cord Injury Conference, New York, 1969

Craig FS: Vertebral-body biopsy. J Bone Joint Surg 38A:93, 1956

DeWald R, Faut MM: Anterior and posterior spine fusion for paralytic scoliosis. Spine 4:(5)401, 1979

Dewald RL, Faut MM: Reconstructive spinal surgery as palliation for metastatic malignancies of the spine. Spine 10(1):21, 1985

Dickson JH, Harrington PR, Erwin WD: Results of reduction and stabilization of the severely fractured thoracic and lumbar spine. J Bone Joint Surg 60:799, 1978

Dunn HK, Danials AU, McBride GG: Comparative assessment of spine stability achieved with a new anterior spine fixation device. Orthop Trans 4(2):268, 1980

Dwyer AF, Schafer MF: Anterior approach to scoliosis. J Bone Joint Surg 56B:218, 1974

Edwards CC: The spinal rod sleeve: its rationale and use in thoracic and lumbar injuries. Orthop. Trans., J. Bone Joint Surgery 6(1):11, 1982

Edwards CC: Results using oblique wiring for rotational instability of the cervical spine. Orthop Trans 9(1):142, 1985

Fielding JW: Normal and selected abnormal motion of the cervical spine from the second cervical vertebra to the seventh cervical vertebra based on cineroentgenography. J Bone Joint Surg 46A:1779, 1964

Freeman, G: Correction of severe deformity of the cervical spine in ankylosing spondylitis with the halo device. J Bone Joint Surgery 43A:547, 1961

Harrington PR, Dickson JH: An eleven-year clinical investigation of harrington instrumentation. Clin Orthop 112:113, 1973

Internal fixator for the spine. Bulletin of Synthesis No. 70, Zimmer USA Co, Warsaw IN, 1985

Jacobs RR, Schlaepfer F, Mathys R, et al: A locking hook spinal rod system for stabilization of fracture-dislocations and correction of deformities of dorsolumbar spine. Clin Orthop 189:168, 1984

Louis Rene: Fusion of the lumbar and sacral spine by internal fixation with screw plates. Clin Orthop 203:18, 1986

Luque ER, Cassis N, Ramirez-Wiella G: Segmental spine instrumentation in the treatment of fractures of the thoracolumbar spine. Spine 7(3):313, 1982

Meyer PR: Weiss spring spinal internal fixation. Surgical Technique, p. 22. B–2256, 5M–975, Zimmer USA, Warsaw, IN

Murphy MJ, Odgen JA, Southwick WO: Spinal stabilization in acute spine injuries. Surg Clin North Am 60:1035, 1980

Nachemson A, Elfstrom G: Intravital wireless telemetry of axial forces in harrington distraction rods in patients with idiopathic scoliosis. J Bone Joint Surg 53A:445, 1971

Ogilvie JW, Schendel M: Comparison of lumbosacral fixation devices. Clin Orthop 203:179, 1986

Pinzer MD, Meyer PR, Lautenschlager EP, et al: Measure of internal fixation device support in experimental fixation produced fractures of the dorsolumbar spine. Orthopedics 4(6):28, 1979

Ranawat CS, O'Leary, P, Pellicci, P, et al: Cervical spine fusion in rheumatoid arthritis. J Bone Joint Surg 61A:1003, 1979

Selby D: Internal fixation with knodt's rods. Clin Orthop 203:179, 1986

Spence WT: Internal plastic splint and fusion for stabilization of the spine. Clin Orthop 92:325, 1973

Stagnara P, Fleury D, Pauchet R, et al: Scolioses majeures de l'adulte superieures a 100° − 183 castraites chirurgicalement. Rev Chir Orthop 61:101, 1975

Stagnara P: Scoliosis in Adults: Surgical Treatment of Severe Forms. Excerpta Med Found (International Congress Series) #192, 1969

Steffee AD, Sitkowski PAC, Topham LS: Total vertebral body and pedicle arthroplasty. Clin Orthop 203:203, 1986

Weiss M: Dynamic spine alloplasty (spring loading correction device) after fracture and spinal cord injury. Clin Orthop 112:150, 1975

White AA III, Panjabi MM: The role of stabilization in the treatment of cervical spine injuries. Spine 9:512, 1984

White AH, Zucherman JF, Hsu K: Lumbosacral fusion with Harrington rods and intersegmental wiring. Clin Orthop 203:185, 1986

Wiltse LL: Symposium: Internal Fixation of the Lumbar Spine. Clin Orthop 203:3, 1986

Zielke K, Strempel AV: Posterior lateral distraction spondylodesis using the twofold sacral bar. Clin Orthop 203:131, 1986

CERVICAL SPINE FRACTURES

Abel MS: Occult Traumatic Lesions of the Cervical Vertebra. Warren H. Green, St. Louis, 1970

Ackerson TT, Patzakis MJ, Moore TM, et al: Fractures of the odontoid: a ten-year retrospective study. Contemp Orthop 4(1):54, 1982

Alker GJ, Oh YS, Leslie EV: High cervical spine and cranio-cervical function injuries in fatal traffic accidents: a radiological study. Orthop Clin North Am 9:1003, 1978

Allen BL, Ferguson RL, Lehmann TR, O'Brien RP: A mechanistic classification of closed, indirect fractures and dislocations of the lower cervical spine. Spine 17(1):1, 1982

Anderson LD, d'Alonzo RT: Fractures of the odontoid process of the axis. J Bone Joint Surg 56A(8):1663, 1974

Apuzzo MLJ, Heiden JS, Weiss MH, et al: Acute fractures of the odontoid process. J Neurosurg 48:85, 1978

Babcock JL: Cervical spine injuries: diagnosis and classification. Arch Surg 3:646, 1976

Beatson TR: Fractures and dislocations of the cervical spine. J Bone Joint Surg 45B:21, 1963

Bedbrook GM: Stability of spinal fractures and fracture-dislocations. Paraplegia 9:23, 1971

Bedbrook GM: Spine injuries with tetraplegia and paraplegia. J Bone Joint Surg 61B:267, 1979

Bell W, Meyer P: Non-halo/non-surgical management of C1-C2 fractures. Orthop Trans 7(3):480, 1983

Bohler J: Anterior stabilization for acute fractures and non-union of the dens J Bone Joint Surg 61A(1):18, 1982

Bohler J, Gaudernak T: Anterior plate stabilization for fracture-dislocations of the lower cervical spine. J Trauma 20:203, 1980

Boehler L: The Treatment of Fractures. Bristol, Wright and Son, 1935

Bohlman HH: Acute fractures and dislocations of the cervical spine. J Bone Joint Surg 61A:(8),1119, 1979

Braakman R, Vinken PJ: Unilateral facet interlocking in the lower cervical spine. J Bone Joint Surg 49B:249, 1967

Buckholz RW: Unstable hangman's fractures. Clin Orthop 154:119, 1981

Burke DC: Hyperextension injuries of the spine. J Bone Joint Surg 53B:3, 1971

Burke DC, Tiong TS: Stability of the cervical spine after conservative treatment. Paraplegia 13:191, 1975

Castellano V, Bocconi FL: Injuries of the cervical spine with spinal cord involvement (myelic fractures): statistical considerations. Bull Hosp Jt Dis Orthop Inst 31:188, 1970

Cheshire DJE: The stability of the cervical spine following the conservative treatment of fractures and fracture-dislocations. Paraplegia 7:193, 1969

Clark CR, White AA III: Fractures of the dens. JBJS 67A:1340, 1985

Cloward R: Surgical Treatment of dislocations and compression fractures of the cervical spine by the anterior approach. p. 26. In: Proc 17th Veterans Administration Spinal Cord Injury Conference. Veterans Administration, Washington, D.C., 1969

Cornish BL: Traumatic spondylolisthesis of the axis. J Bone Joint Surg 50B:31, 1968

Coutts MD: Atlanto-epistropheal subluxations. Arch Surg 29:297, 1934

Day GL, Jacoby CG, Dolan KD: Basilar invagination resulting from untreated Jefferson's fracture. AJR 133:529, 1979

DeLorme TL: Axis pedicle fractures. J Bone Joint Surg 49A:1472, 1967

Dolan KD: Cervical spine injuries below the axis. Radiol Clin North Am 15:247, 1977

Effendi B, Roy D, Cornish B, et al: Fractures of the ring of the axis. J Bone Joint Surg 63B:319, 1981

Eismort FJ, Bohlman HH: Posterior atlanto-occipital dislocation with fractures of the atlas and odontoid process. Report of a case with survival. JBJS 60A:397, 1978

Elliott JM, Rogers LF, Wissinger JP, Lee JF: The hangman's fracture. Radiology 104:303, 1972

Fardon DF: Odontoid fracture complicating ankylosing hyperostosis of the spine. Spine 3(2):108, 1978

Forsyth HF: Extension injuries of the cervical spine. J Bone Joint Surg 46A:1792, 1964

Francis WR, Fielding JW, Hawkins et al: Traumatic spondylolisthesis of the axis. J Bone Joint Surg 63B:313, 1981

Funk FJ, Wells RE: Injuries of the cervical spine in football. Clin Orthop 109:50, 1975

Garber JN: Abnormalities of the atlas and axis vertebra —congenital and traumatic. J Bone Joint Surg 46A(8):1782, 1964

Garber JN: Fracture and fracture-dislocation of the cer-

vical spine. p. 18. In American Academy of Orthopaedic Surgeons: Instructional Course Lectures. CV Mosby, St. Louis, 1961

Gerlock AJ, Kischner SG, Heller RM, Kay JJ: The Cervical Spine In Trauma. WB Saunders, Philadelphia, 1978

Grogono BJS: Injuries of the atlas and axis. J Bone Joint Surg 36B:397, 1954

Harviainen S, Lahti P, Davidson L: On cervical spine injuries. Acta Chir Scan 138:349, 1972

Hathaway HR: Unusual fractures of the cervical spine with Marie-Strumpell disease. Ohio State Med J 46:236, 1950

Haughton S: On hanging, considered from a mechanical and physiological point of view. London, Edinburgh and Dublin. Philosophical Magazine and Journal of Science, 4th Series:22, 1866

Hensinger RN, Fielding JW, Hawkins RJ: Congenital anomalies of the odontoid process. Orthop Clin North Am 9(4):901, 1978

Hohl M: Normal motions in the upper portion of the cervical spine. J Bone Joint Surg 46A:1777, 1964

Hohl M, Baker HR: The atlanto-axial joint. J Bone Joint Surg 46A:1739, 1964

Hollin SA, Gross SW, Levin P: Fractures of the cervical spine in rheumatoid spondylitis. Am Surg 31:532, 1965

Jacobs B: Cervical fracture and dislocation (C3-7). Clin Orthop 109:18, 1975

Jacobson G, Adler DC: An evaluation of lateral atlanto-axial displacement in injuries of the cervical spine. Radiology 61:355, 1953

Jacobson G, Adler DC: Examination of the atlanto-axial joint following injury. AJR 76:1081, 1956

Jefferson G: Fracture of the atlas vertebra. Br J Surg 7:407, 1920

Jefferson G: Remarks on fractures of first cervical vertebra. Br Med J 2:153, 1927

Jefferson G: Discussion on spinal injuries. Proc Royal Soc Med 21:625, 1927

Kelly DL, Alexander E, Davis CH, Smith JM: Acrylic

fixation of atlanto-axial dislocation. Technical notes. J Neurosurg 36:366, 1972

Kessler LA: Delayed, traumatic dislocation of the cervical spine. JAMA 224:124, 1973

Kewalramani L, Krauss J: Cervical spine injuries resulting from collision sports. Paraplegia 19:303, 1981

Kewalramani MB, Taylor RG, Albrand OW: Cervical spine injury in patients with ankylosing spondylitis. J Trauma 15(10):931, 1975

Key A: Cervical spine dislocation with unilateral facet interlocking. Paraplegia 13:208, 1975

King DM: Fractures and dislocations of the cervical part of the spine. Aust NZ J Surg 37:57, 1967

Kiwerski J, Wieclawek H, Garwacka, L: Fractures of the cervical spine in ankylosing spondylitis. Int Orthop 8:243, 1985

Lipson SJ: Fractures of the atlas associated with fractures of the odontoid process and transverse ligament ruptures. J Bone Joint Surg 59A:940, 1977

Louis AA, Gupta P, Perkash I: Localization of sensory levels in traumatic quadriplegia by segmental somatosensory evoked potentials. Electroencephalogr Clin Neurophysiol 62:313, 1985

Lyness SS, Simcone, FA: Vascular complications of upper cervical spine injuries. Ortho Clin North Am 9:1029, 1978

Macnab I: Acceleration injuries of the cervical spine. J Bone Joint Surg 56A:1797, 1964

Marar BC: Hyperextension injuries of the cervical spine. J Bone Joint Surg 56A:1655, 1974

Marar BD: The pattern of neurological damage as an aid to the diagnosis of the mechanism in cervical-spine injuries. J Bone Joint Surg 56A:1648, 1974

McCoy SH, Johnson KA: Sagittal fracture of the cervical spine. J Trauma 16:310, 1976

McRae DL: The significance of abnormalities of the cervical spine. AJR 84:3, 1960

Miller MD, Gehweiler JA, Martinez S, et al: Significant new observations on cervical spine trauma. AJR 130:659, 1978

Morizono Y, Sakou T, Kawaidi H: Upper cervical in-

volvement in rheumatoid arthritis. Spine 12:(8) 721, 1987

Norrell H, Wilson CB: Early anterior fusion for injuries of the cervical portion of the spine. JAMA 214:525, 1970

O'Brien JJ, Butterfield WL, Gossling HR: Jefferson fracture with disruption of the transverse ligament. Clin Orthop 126:135, 1977

Olsson O: Fractures of the upper thoracic and cervical vertebral bodies. Acta Chir Scand 102:87, 1951

Osgood RB, Lund CC: Fractures of the odontoid process. N Engl J Med 198:61, 1928

Osgood C, Martin LG, Ackerman E: Fracture-dislocation of the cervical spine with ankylosing spondylitis. J Neurosurg 39:764, 1973

Ovassapian A, Land P, Schaefer M, et al: Anesthetic management for surgical corrections of severe flexion deformity of the cervical spine. Anesthesiology 58:370, 1983

Penning L: Prevertebral hematoma in cervical spine injury: incidence and etiologic significance AJR 136:553, 1981

Penning L: Diagnostic clues by x-ray injuries of the lower cervical spine. Acta Neurol Chir (Wien) 22:234, 1970

Pepin JW, Hawkins RJ: Traumatic spondylolisthesis of the axis: hangman's fracture. Clin Orthop 157:133, 1981

Perret G, Green J: Anterior interbody fusion in the treatment of cervical fracture dislocations. Arch Surg 96:530, 1968

Raynor RB: Severe fractures of the cervical spine treated by early anterior interbody fusion and ambulation. J Neurosurg 28:311, 1968

Richman S, Friedman RL: Vertical fracture of cervical vertebral bodies. Radiology 62:536, 1954

Rogers WA: Fractures and dislocations of the cervical spine. An end result study. J Bone and Joint Surg 39A:341, 1957

Rogers WA: Treatment of fracture-dislocation of the cervical spine. J Bone Joint Surg 24:245, 1942

Roy-Camille R, de la Caffiniere JY, Saillant G: Traumatismes du Rochis Cervical Superieur C1-C2. Masson, Paris, 1973

Roy-Camille R, Saillant G, Sagnet P: Lesions traumatiques durachis cervical sans complication neurologique. Encycl Med Chir A-10:15825, Paris, 1975

Ryan MD, Taylor TKF: Odontoid fractures, a rational approach to treatment. J Bone Joint Surg 64B(4):416, 1982

Schatzker J, Rorabeck CH, Waddell JP: Non-union of the odontoid process: an experimental investigation. Clin Orthop 108:127, 1975

Schatzker J: Fractures of the dens (odontoid process): an analysis of thirty-seven cases. J Bone Joint Surg 53B:392, 1971

Schlicke LH, Callahan RA: A rational approach to burst fractures of the atlas. Clin Orthop 154:18, 1981

Schneider RC, Cherry G, Pantek H: The syndrome of acute central cervical spinal cord injury. J Neurosurg 11:546, 1954

Schneider RC, Livingston KE, Cave AJE, Hamilton G: Hangman's fracture of the cervical spine. J Neurosurg 22:141, 1965

Segal LS, Grimm JO, Stauffer ES: Non-union of fractures of the atlas. J Bone Joint Surg 69A(9):1423, 1987

Selecki BR: Cervical spine and cord injuries: mechanisms and surgical implications. Med J Aust 1:838, 1970

Seljeskog EL, Chou SN: Spectrum of hangman's fracture. J Neurosurg 45:308, 1976

Sherk HH, Pasquariello PS, Watters WC: Multiple dislocations of the cervical spine in a patient with rheumatoid arthritis and Down's Syndrome: Clin Orthop 162:37, 1982

Shrago GG: Cervical spine injuries: association with head trauma. Radiology 118:670, 1973

Shrosbree RD: Neurological sequelae of reduction of fracture dislocations of the cervical spine. Paraplegia 17:212, 1979

Sillivan AW: Subluxation of the atlantoaxial joint: sequel to inflammatory process of the neck. J Pediat 35:451, 1949

Simmons EH: Fracture of the cervical spine in ankylosing spondylitis: analysis of its influence on severe deformity presenting for spinal osteotomy. J Bone Joint Surg 59B:509, 1977

Skold G: Sagittal fractures of the cervical spine. Injury 9:294, 1978

Smith HP, Challa VR, Alexander E: Odontoid compression of the brain in a patient with rheumatoid arthritis: case report. J Neurosurg 53:841, 1980

Southwick WO, Keggi K: The normal cervical spine. Instructional course lecture, American Academy of Orthopaedic Surgeons. J Bone Joint Surg 46A:1767, 1964

Southwick WO: Management of fractures of the dens (odontoid process). J Bone Joint Surg 62A:482, 1980

Spierings ELH, Braakman R: The management of os odontoideum. J Bone Joint Surg 64B:4, 422, 1982

Stauffer ES, Kelly E: Fracture dislocation of the cervical spine. J Bone Joint Surg 59A:45, 1977

Stauffer ES, Kaufer H: Fractures and dislocations of the spine. In Rockwood CA Jr, Green DP (eds): Fractures. Vol. 2. JB Lippincott, Philadelphia, 1975

Surin V: Fractures of the cervical spine in patients with ankylosing spondylitis. Acta Orthop Scan 51:79, 1980

Taylor AR, Blackwood W: Paraplegia in hyperextension cervical injuries with normal radiographic appearances. J Bone Joint Surg 30B:245, 1948

Vermooten VA: Study of the fracture of the epistopheus due to hanging with a note on the possible causes of death. Anat Rec 20:305, 1921

Webb JK, Broughton RBK, McSweeney T, Park WM: Hidden flexion injury of the cervical spine. J Bone Joint Surg 58B:322, 1976

White RJ: Advances in the treatment of cervical cord injuries. Clin Neurosurg 26:556, 1979

Whitley JE, Forsyth HF: The classification of cervical spine injury. AJR 83:633, 1960

Wittek A: Em fall von distension sluxation in atlantoepistropheal. Gelenke, Meurcheuer Med Wochenschr 55:1836, 1908

Woodruff FP, Dewiong FB: Fracture of the cervical spine in patients with ankylosing spondylitis. Radiology 80:17, 1963

Zielinski CJ, Gunther SF, Deeb Z: Cranial-nerve palsies complicating Jefferson fracture. A case report. J Bone Joint Surg 64A(9):1382, 1982

THORACOLUMBAR AND SACRAL SPINE FRACTURES

Andrew TA, Brooks S, Piggott H: Long-term follow-up evaluation of screw-and-graft fusion of the lumbar spine. Clin Orthop 203:113–19, 1986

Bedbrook GM: Treatment of thoracolumbar dislocation and fractures with paraplegia. Clin Orthop 112:27, 1975

Bernini PM, Floman Y, Marvel JP, Rothman, RH: Multiple thoracic spine fractures complicating ankylosing hyperostosis of the spine. J Trauma 21(9):811, 1981

Bonin JG: Sacral fractures and injuries to the cauda equina. J Bone Joint Surg 27A:113, 1945

Bradford DS: Treatment of severe spondylolithesis. A combined approach for reduction and stabilization. Spine, 4(5):423, 1979

Brown HP, Bonnett CC: Spinal deformity subsequent to cord injury. J Bone Joint Surg 55A(2):441, 1973

Bussat P, Rossier AB, Djindjian R, et al: Spinal cord angiography in dorsolumbar vertebral fractures with neurological involvement. Radiology 109:617, 1973

Byrnes DP, Russo GL, Ducker TB, Cowley RA: Sacrum fractures and neurological damage. J Neurosurg 47:459, 1977

Casey BM, Eaton SB, DuBois JJ et al: Thoracolumbar neural arch fractures. JAMA 224:1263, 1973

Chance GQ: Note on the type of flexion fracture of the spine. Br J Radiol 21:452, 1948

Das De S, McCreath SW: Lumbosacral fracture-dislocations. J Bone Joint Surg 63B:58, 1981

Denis F: The three column spine and its significance in the classification of acute thoracolumbar spine injuries. Spine 8(8):817, 1983

Denis F, Davis S, Comfort T: Sacral fractures, an important problem, though frequently undiagnosed and untreated: retrospective analysis of 203 consecutive cases. Presented to the Federation of Spine Assoc., American Academy of Orthopaedic Surgeons, January 1987

Dick TBS: Traumatic paraplegia pre-Guttman. Paraplegia 7:173, 1969

Dowling T, Epstein JA, Epstein NE: S1-S2 sacral fractures involving neural elements of the cauda equina. Spine 10(9):851, 1985

Fardon DF: Displaced transverse fracture of the sacrum with nerve root injury: report of a case with successful operative management. J Trauma 19(2):119, 1979

Ferguson RL, Allen BL: A mechanistic classification of thoracolumbar spine fractures. Clin Orthop 189:77, 1984

Frankel HL, Hancock DO, Hystop G, et al: The value of postural reduction in the initial management of closed injuries of the spine with paraplegia and tetraplegia. Part 1. Paraplegia 7:179, 1969

Fullenlove TM, Wilson JG: Traumatic defects of the pars inter-articularis of the lumbar vertebrae. AJR 122:634, 1974

Gelman MI, Umber JS: Fractures of the thoracolumbar spine in ankylosing spondylitis. AJR 130:485, 1978

Good AE: Nontraumatic fracture of the thoracic spine in ankylosing spondylitis. Arthritis Rheum 10:467, 1967

Graham, CE: Lumbosacral fusion using internal fixation with a spinous process for the graft. Clin Orthop 140:72, 1979

Griffith HB, Gleave JRW, Taylor RG: Changing patterns of fracture in the dorsal and lumbar spine. Brit Med J [Clin Res] 1:891, 1966

Grundy B, Nash CL Jr, Brown RH: Arterial pressure manipulation alters spinal cord function during correction of scoliosis. Anesthesiology 54(3):249, 1981

Gumley G, Taylor TKF, Ryan MD: Distraction fractures of the lumbar spine, J Bone Joint Surg 64B5:520, 1982

Gunterberg B, Petersen I: Sexual function after major resections of the sacrum with bilateral or unilateral sacrifice of sacral nerves. Fertil Steril 27:1146, 1976

Hansen ST, Taylor TKF, Honet JC, Lewis FR: Fracture-dislocations of the ankylosed thoracic spine in rheumatoid spondylitis. J Trauma 7(6):827, 1967

Hardy AG: The treatment of paraplegia due to fracture-dislocations of the dorsolumbar spine. Paraplegia 3:112, 1965

Holdsworth FA, Hardy AG: Early treatment of paraplegics from fracture of the thoracolumbar spine. J Bone Joint Surg 35B:540, 1953

Holdsworth FW: Review article: Fracture-dislocations of the spine. J Bone Joint Surg 52A:1534, 1970

Holdsworth FW: Symposium on Spinal Injury. p. 161. Edinburgh Royal College of Surgeons. 1963

Holdsworth FW: Fractures, dislocations and fracture-dislocations of the spine. J Bone Joint Surg 52A:1534, 1970

Howland WJ, Curry JL, Buffington CB: Fulcrum fractures of the lumbar spine. JAMA 193:240, 1965

Howorth MB: Fracture of the spine. Am J Surg 92:573, 1956

Jacobs RR, Casey MP: Surgical management of thoracic-lumbar spinal injuries: general principles and controversial considerations. Clin Orthop 189:22, 1984

Jacobs RR, Asher MA, Snider RK: Thoracolumbar spine fractures, a comparative study of recumbent and operative treatment in 100 patients. Spine 5:463, 1980

Jacobs, RR: Bilateral fracture of the pedicles through the fourth and fifth lumbar vertebra with anterior displacement of the vertebral bodies. J Bone Joint Surg 59A(3):409, 1977

Jonas, JG: Fracture-dislocation of the dorsal spine. South Med J 69:1502, 1976

Kaufer H, Hayes JT: Lumbar fracture-dislocation. A study of twenty-one cases. J Bone Joint Surg 48A:712, 1966

Keene JS, Drummond DS: Wisconsin Compression System. Surgical Technique, Zimmer USA Co, Warsaw, IN, October, 1981

Kostuik JP, Errico TJ, Gleason TF: Techniques of internal fixation for degenerative conditions of the lumbar spine. Clin Orthop 203:219, 1986

Larson SJ, Holst RA, Hemmy DC, Sances A Jr: Lateral extracavity approach to traumatic lesions of the thoracic and lumbar spine. J Neurosurg 45:628, 1976

Lewis J, McKibbin B: The treatment of unstable fractures-dislocations of the thoracic-lumbar spine accompanied by paraplegia. J Bone Joint Surg 56B:603, 1974

MacEwen GD, Bunnell WP, Sriram K: Acute neurological complications in the treatment of scoliosis: a report of the Scoliosis Research Society. J Bone Joint Surg 57A:404, 1975

Magerl FP: Stabilization of the lower thoracic and lumbar spine with external skeletal fixation. Clin Orthop 189:125, 1984

Magerl F, Harms J: Presentation: Classification of Injury and Prognosis — Thoracolumbar Injuries. 45 AO-ASIF Sping Course, Davos Switzerland, December 16, 1986

Magerl FP: External skeletal fixation. In Weber BG, Magerl FP (eds):The External Fixation. Springer-Verlag, New York, 1985

Martel W: Spinal pseudoarthrosis. Arthritis and Rheum 21:485, 1978

Markolf KL: Deformation of the thoracolumbar intervertebral joint in response to external loads: a biomechanical study using autopsy material. J Bone Joint Surg 54A:511, 1972

McEvoy RD, Bradford DS: The management of burst fractures of the thoracic and lumbar spine. Experience in 53 patients. Spine 10(7):631, 1985

McGuire EJ, Wagner FC: The effects of sacral denervation on bladder and urethral function. Surg Gynecol Obstet 144:343, 1977

Melamed A: Fracture of the pars interarticularis of lumbar vertebra. AJR 94:584, 1965

Meyer PR: Complications of treatment of fractures of the dorsolumbar spine. p. 643 In Epps C (ed):Complications in Orthopaedic Surgery. 1st Ed. Vol.2. JB Lippincott, Philadelphia, 1978

Morris JM, Lucas DB, Bresler B: Role of the trunk in the stability of the spine. J Bone Joint Surg 43A327, 1961

Nash CL, Schatzinger LH, Brown RH, Brodkey J: The unstable stable thoracic compression fracture: Its problems and the use of spinal cord monitoring in the evaluation of treatment. Spine 2:261, 1977

Nicoll EA: Fractures of the dorso-lumbar spine. J Bone Joint Surg 31B:376, 1949

Norton PL, Brown T: The immobilizing effect of back braces: their effect on the posture and motion of the lumbosacral spine. J Bone Joint Surg 39A:111, 1957

Olsson O: Fractures of the upper thoracic and cervical vertebral bodies. Acta Chir Scand 102:87, 1951

Rapp GG, Kernek CB: Spontaneous fracture of the lumbar spine with correction of deformity in ankylosing spondylitis. J Bone Joint Surg 56A:1277, 1974

Rennie W, Mitchell N: Flexion distraction fractures of

the thoraco-lumbar spine. J Bone Joint Surg 55A:386, 1973

Roberts JB, Curtis PH: Stability of the thoracic and lumbar spine in traumatic paraplegia following fracture or fracture-dislocation. J Bone Joint Surg 52A:1115, 1970

Rogers LF, Thayer C, Weinberg PE, Kim KS: Acute injuries of the upper thoracic spine associated with paraplegia. AJR 134:67, 1980

Roy-Camille R, Saillant G, Gagna G, Mazel C: Transverse fractures of the upper sacrum: suicidal jumper's fracture. Spine 10(9):838, 1985

Smith, WS, Kaufer H: Patterns and mechanisms of lumbar injuries associated with lap seat belt fractures J Bone Joint Surg 51A:239, 1969

Smith-Petersen MN, Larson CB, Aufranc, OE: Osteotomy of the spine for correction of flexion deformity in rheumatoid arthritis. J Bone Joint Surg 27:1, 1945

Soreff J, Axdorph G, Bylund P, et al: Treatment of patients with unstable fractures of the thoracic and lumbar spine. A follow-up study of surgical and conservative treatment. Acta Orthop Scand 53:369, 1982

Stauffer ES, Neil JL: Biomechanical analysis of structural stability of internal fixation in fractures of the thoracolumbar spine. Clin Orthop 122:159, 1975

Triscot A, Hallot R: Traumatic paraplegia and associated fractures. Paraplegia 5:211, 1968

White AA, Panjabi MM: Functional spinal unit and mathematical models. p. 35. In: Clinical Biomechanics of the Spine. JB Lippincott, Philadelphia, 1978.

Willen J: Unstable thoracolumbar fractures — an experimental and clinical study. Department of Orthopaedic Surgery and Diagnostic Radiology. University of Goteborg, Sweden, 1984

Wiltse LL, Widell EH, Jackson DW: Fatigue fracture: the basic lesion in isthmic spondylolisthesis. J Bone Joint Surg 57A;17, 1975

SUBLUXATIONS AND DISLOCATIONS OF THE SPINE

Evans DK: Anterior cervical subluxation. J Bone and Joint Surg 58B:318, 1976

Evarts CM: Traumatic occipito-atlantal dislocation. Report of a case with survival. J. Bone Joint Surg 52A:1653, 1970

Farthing JW: Atlantocranial dislocation with survival. A case report. NC Med J 9:34, 1948

Fielding JW, Hawkins RJ: Atlanto-axial rotatory fixation. J Bone Joint Surg, 59A:37, 1977

Fielding JW, Cochran G, Lawsing III JF, Hohl M: Tears of the transverse ligament of the atlas. J Bone Joint Surg, 56A:1683, 1974

Fox, JL, Jerez A: An unusual atlanto-axial dislocation: case report. J Neurosurg 47:115, 1977

Gabrielsen TO, Maxwell JA: Traumatic atlanto-occipital dislocation. With case report of a patient who survived. AJR 97:624, 1966

Gallie WE: Fractures and dislocations of the cervical spine. Am J Surg 46:495, 1939

Hanson TYA, Kraft JP, Adcock DW: Subluxation of the cervical vertebra due to pharyngitis. South Med J 66:427, 1973

Haralson, III RH, Boyd B: Posterior dislocation of the atlas on the axis without fracture. J Bone Joint Surg 51A:561, 1969

Key A: Cervical spine dislocation with unilateral facet interlocking. Paraplegia 13:208, 1975

Kline DG: Atlantoaxial dislocation simulating a head injury: hypoplasia of the odontoid. J Neurosurg 24:1013, 1966

Sherk HH, Pasquariello PS, Watters WC: Multiple dislocations of the cervical spine in a patient with rheumatoid arthritis and Down's syndrome. Clin Orthop 162:37, 1982

Sherk HH, Dawoud S: Congenital os odontoideum with Klippel-Feil anomaly and fatal atlanto-axial instability. Spine 6:42, 1981

von Torklus D, Gehle W: The Upper Cervical Spine: Regional Anatomy, Pathology and Traumatology: A Systematic Radiological Atlas and Textbook. Grune & Stratton, New York; Georg Thieme Verlag, Stuttgart, 1972

Werne S: Studies in spontaneous atlas dislocation. Acta Orthop Scand, Suppl 23, 1957

Wiesel SW, Rothman RH: Atlanto-occipital hypermobility. Orthop Trans 3:283, 1979

Whitesides Jr TE, Kelly RP: Lateral approach to the upper cervical spine for anterior fusion. South Med J 59:879, 1966

Wollin DG: The os odontoideum. Separate odontoid process. J Bone Joint Surg 45A:1459, 1963

Wood-Jones F: The ideal lesion produced by judicial hanging. Lancet 1:53, 1913

Wortzman G, Dewar FP: Rotary fixation of the atlantoaxial joint: rotational atlantoaxial subluxation. Radiology 90:479, 1968

Zolton JD, Gilula LA, Murphy WA: Unilateral facet dislocation between the fifth lumbar and the first sacral vertebra. J Bone Joint Surg 61A(5):767, 1979

ANKYLOSING SPONDYLITIS AFFECTING THE SPINE

Bernini PM, Floman Y, Marvel JP, Rothman RH: Multiple thoracic spine fractures complicating ankylosing hyperostosis of the spine. J Trauma 21(9):811, 1981

Boachie-Adjei O, Bullough P: Incidence of ankylosing hyperostosis of the spine (forestier's disease) at autopsy. Spine 12(8):739, 1987

Brugman JL, Stauffer ES: Spinal fractures in ankylosing spondylitis. unpublished, 1986

Fardon DR: Odontoid fracture complicating ankylosing hyperostosis of the spine. Spine 3(2):108, 1978

Forestier J, Lagier R: Ankylosing hyperostosis of the spine. Clin Orthop 74:65, 1971

Forestier J, Rotes-Querol J: Senile ankylosing hyperostosis of the spine. Ann Rheum Dis 9:321, 1950

Freeman G: Correction of severe deformity of the cervical spine in ankylosing spondylitis with the halo device. J Bone Joint Surg 43A: 547, 1961

Gelman MI, Umber JS: Fractures of the thoracolumbar spine in ankylosing spondylitis. AJR 130:485, 1978

Good AE: Nontraumatic fracture of the thoracic spine in ankylosing spondylitis. Arthritis Rheu 10:467, 1967

Grisolia A, Bell RL, Peltier LF: Fractures and dislocations of the spine complicating ankylosing spondylitis. J Bone Joint Surg 49A:339, 1967

Hansen ST, Taylor TKF, Honet JC, Lewis FR: Fracture-dislocations of the ankylosed thoracic spine in rheumatoid spondylitis. J Trauma 7(6):827, 1967

Hathaway HR: Unusual fractures of the cervical spine with Marie-Strumpell disease. Ohio State Med J 46:236, 1950

Hollingsworth PN, Owen ET, Dawkins RL: Correlation of HLA B27 with radiographic abnormalities of the sacroiliac joints and with other stigmata of ankylosing spondylitis. Clin Rheum Dis 9(2):307, 1983

Hunter T, Dubo H: Spinal fractures complicating ankylosing spondylitis. Arthritis Rheum 26:751, 1983

Kewalramani MB, Taylor RG, Albrand OW: Cervical spine injury in patients with ankylosing spondylitis. J Trauma 15(10):931, 1975

Kiwerski J, Wieclawek H, Garwacka L: Fractures of the cervical spine in ankylosing spondylitis. Orthop 8:243, 1985

Osgood C, Mathews T: Multiple spinal fractures in ankolysing spondylolitis. J Trauma 15:163, 1974

Osgood C, Martin LG, Ackerman E: Fracture-dislocation of the cervical spine with ankylosing spondylitis. J Neurosurg 39:764, 1973

Rapp GG, Kernek CB: Spontaneous fracture of the lumbar spine with correction of deformity in ankylosing spondylitis. J Bone Joint Surg 56A:1277, 1974

Resnick D, Niwayama G: Radiographic and pathologic features of spinal involvement in diffuse idiopathic skeletal hyperostosis (DISH). Radiology 119:559, 1976

Simmons EH: Fracture of the cervical spine in ankylosing spondylitis: analysis of its influence on severe deformity presenting for spinal osteotomy. J Bone Joint Surg 59B:509, 1977

Strumpell A:Bemerkung uber die chronische ankylosirende entzundung der wirbelsaule und der huftgelenke. Deutsche Zeitschrift Nervenh 338, 1897

Surin V: Fractures of the cervical spine in patients with ankylosing spondylitis. Acta Orthop Scan 51:79, 1980

Utsinger PD: Diffuse idiopathic skeletal hyperostosis. Clin Rheum Dis 11:325, 1985

Weinstein P, Karpman R, Gall E, Pitt M: Spinal cord injury, spinal fracture and spinal stenosis in ankylosing spondylitis. J Neurosurg 57:609, 1982

Wilkinson M, Bywaters EGL: Clinical features and course of ankylosing spondylitis. Ann Rheum Dis 17:209, 1958

Woodruff FP, Dewiong FB: Fracture of the cervical spine in patients with ankylosing spondylitis. Radiology 8:17, 1963

Yau ACM, Chan RMW: Stress fracture of the fused lumbodorsal spine in ankylosing spondylitis. J Bone Joint Surg 56B:681, 1974

DEVELOPMENTAL AND CONGENITAL SPINAL DEFORMITIES

Dijck P: Os dontoideum in children: neurological manifestations and surgical management. J Neurol 2:93, 1978

Diokno A, Kass E, Lapides J: New approach to myelodysplasia J Urol 116:771, 1976

Fielding JW, Griffin PP: Os odontoideum: an acquired lesion. J Bone Joint Surg 56A:187, 1974

Fielding JW, Hinsinger RN, Hawkins RJ: Os odontoideum. J Bone Joint Surgery 62A(3):376, 1980

Freiberger RJ, Wilson Jr PD, Nicholas JA: Acquired absence of the odontoid process. J Bone Joint Surg 47A:1231, 1965

Garber JN: Abnormalities of the atlas and axis vertebra —congenital and traumatic. J Bone Joint Surg 46A(8):1782, 1964

Gunther SF; Congenital anomaly of the cervical spine: fusion of the occiput, atlas, odontoid process. J Bone and Joint Surg 62A(8):1377, 1980

Kilfoyle RM, Foley JJ, Norton, PL: Spine and pelvic deformities in childhood and adolescent paraplegia. J Bone Joint Surg 47A:659, 1965

Mathews LS, Vetter WL, Tolo VT: Cervical anomaly simulating hangman's fracture in a child. J Bone Joint Surg 64A(2):299, 1982

Minderhoud JM, Braakman R, Penning L: Os odontoideum: clinical, radiological and therapeutic aspects J Neuro Sci 8:521, 1969

Rivard CH, Narbaitz R, Uithoff HK: Congenital vertebral malformations. Orthop 8:135, 1979

Winter RB, Congential kyphoscoliosis with paralysis following hemivertebra excision. Clin Orthop 119:116, 1976

Whitesides Jr TE, Kelly RP: Lateral approach to the upper cervical spine for anterior fusion. South Med J 59:879, 1966

SPINAL INJURY IN THE PEDIATRIC PATIENT

Anderson JM, Schutt AH: Spinal injury in children: a review of 156 cases seen from 1950 through 1978. Mayo Clin Proc 55:499, 1980

Aufdermauri M: Spinal injuries in juveniles. J Bone Joint Surg 56B:513, 1974

Bailey DK: The normal cervical spine in infants and children. Radiology 59:712, 1952

Bedbrook GM: Correction of scoliosis due to paraplegia sustained in pediatric age group. Paraplegia 15:90, 1977

Burke DC: Spinal cord injury in children. Paraplegia 9:1, 1971

Campbell J, Bonnett C: Spinal cord injury in children. Clin Orthop 112:114, 1975

Cattell HS, Clark Jr GL: Cervical kyphosis and instability following multiple laminectomies in children. J Bone Joint Surg 49A:713, 1967

Cattell HS, Filtzer DL: Pseudosubluxations and other normal variations in the cervical spine in children. J Bone Joint Surg 74A:1295, 1965

Cheshire DJE: The pediatric syndrome of traumatic myelopathy without demonstrable vertebral injury. Paraplegia 15:74, 1977

Davis AT: Principal investigator:proposed research project pilot of multidisciplinary team assessment as a tool in etiologic analysis of childhood pedestrian injury. Northwestern University Medical School, Children's Memorial Hospital, Chicago, 1986

Donovan MM: Atlas-axial lesions in children. Orthop Trans 13(1):11, 1981

Glasauer FE, Cares HL: Traumatic paraplegia in infancy. JAMA 219:38, 1972

Glasauer FE, Cares HL: Biomechanical features of traumatic paraplegia in infancy. J Trauma 13:166, 1973

Hachen HJ: Spinal cord injury in children and adolescents: diagnostic pitfalls and therapeutic considerations in the acute stage. Paraplegia 15:55, 1977

Hegenbarth R, Ebel KD: Roentgen findings in fractures of the vertebral column in childhood: examination of 35 patients and its results. Pediatr Radiol 5:34, 1976

Henrys P, Lyne ED, Lifton C, Salciccioli G: Clincal review of cervical spine injuries in children. Clin Orthop 129:172, 1977

Hensinger RN, Fielding JW, Hawkins RJ: Congenital anomalies of the odontoid process. Orthop Clin N Am 9(4):901, 1978

Holmes JC, Hall JE: Fusion for instability of the cervical spine in children and adolescents. Orthop Clin N Am 9:923, 1978

Horal J, Nachemson A, Scjeller S: Clinical and radiological long term follow-up vertebral fractures in children. Acta Orthop Scan 43:491, 1972

Hubbard DD: Injuries of the spine in children and adolescents. Clin Orthop 100:56, 1974

Jones ET, Hensinger RN: Cervical spine injuries in children. Contemp Orthop 5(4):17, 1982

Kewalramani LS, Tori JA: Spinal cord trauma in children: neurologic patterns, radiologic features, and pathomechanics of injury. Spine 5(1):11, 1980

Leeson MC, Makley JT, Carter JR: Metastatic skeletal disease in the pediatric population. J Pediatr Orthop 5(3):261, 1985

Mayfield JK, Erkkila JC, Winter RB: Spinal deformity subsequent to acquired childhood spinal cord injury. Orthop Trans 3(3):281, 1979

McPhee IB: Spinal fractures and dislocations in children and adolescents. Spine 6(6):533, 1981

Melzak J: Paraplegia among children. Lancet 2:45, 1969

Murphy MJ, Ogden JA, Bucholz RW: Cervical spine injury in the child. Contemp Orthop 3(7):615, 1981

Seimon LP: Fractures of the odontoid process in young children. J Bone Joint Surg 59A:943, 1977

Sherk HH, Schut L, Lang JM: Fractures and dislocations of the cervical spine in children. Orthop Clin N Am 7(3):593, 1976

Sherk HH:, Nicholson JT, Chung SK: Fractures of the odontoid process in young children. J Bone Joint Surg 60A:921, 1978

Sherk HH, Pasquariello PS, Watters WC: Multiple dislocations of the cervical spine in a patient with rheumatoid arthritis and Down's syndrome. Clin Orthop 162:37, 1982

Sullivan CR, Bruwer AJ, Harris LE: Hypermobility of the cervical spine in children, a pitfall in the diagnosis of cervical dislocation. Am J Surg 95:636, 1958

Tachdjian MO, Matson DD: Orthopaedic aspects of intraspinal tumors in infants and children. J Bone Joint Surg 47A:223, 1965

PATHOLOGY, TUMOR AND INFECTION

Barr JS: Low back and sciatic pain. J Bone Joint Surg 33A:633, 1951

Bedbrook GM: Some pertinent observations on the pathology of traumatic spinal paralysis. Paraplegia 1:215, 1963

Bohlman HH, Sachs BL, Carter JR, et al: Primary neoplasms of the cervical spine. Diagnosis and treatment of twenty-three patients. J Bone Joint Surg 68A(4):483, 1986

Cloward RB: Metastatic disc infection and osteomyelitis of the cervical spine. Spine 3(3):194, 1978

Davidson JK, Mucci B: Chordoma. Skeletal Radiol 14:76, 1985

Davis D, Bohlman HH, Walker AE, et al: The pathological findings in fatal craniospinal injuries. J Neurosurg 34:603, 1971

Dewald RL, Faut MM: Reconstructive spinal surgery as palliation for metastatic malignancies of the spine. Spine 10(1):21, 1985

Eismont FJ, Bohlman HH, Prasanna LS, Goldberg et al: Pyogenic and fungal vertebral osteomyelitis with paralysis. J Bone Joint Surg 65A:19, 1983

Fielding, W, Pyle RN, Fietti VG: Anterior cervical body resection and bone-grafting for benign and malignant tumors. J Bone Joint Surg 61A(2):251, 1979

Leeson, MC, Makley JT, Carter JR: Metastatic skeletal disease in the pediatric population. J Pediatr Orthop 5(3):261, 1985

Marie P: Sur la Spondylose Rhizomelique. Rev de Med 18:285, 1898

Mindell ER: Current concepts review—chordoma. J Bone Joint Surg 63A:501, 1981

Roca RP, Yoshikawa TT: Primary skeletal infections in heroin users: a clinical characterization, diagnosis and therapy. Clin Orthop 144:238, 1979

Rana NA: Atlanto-axial subluxation in rheumatoid arthritis. J Bone Joint Surg 55B:458, 1973

Rana NA, Taylor AR: Upward migration of the odontoid peg in rheumatoid arthritis. Proc R Soc Med 64:717, 1971

Ranawat CS, O'Leary P, Pellicci P, et al: Cervical spine fusion in rheumatoid arthritis. J Bone Joint Surg 61A:1003, 1979

Schaberg J, Gainor BJ: A profile of metastatic carcinoma of the spine. Spine 10(1):19, 1985

Sentar HJ, Vennes JL: Loss of autoregulation and post-traumatic ischemia following experimental spinal cord trauma. J Neurosurg 50:198, 1979

Smith HP, Challa VR, Alexander E: Odontoid compression of the brain in a patient with rheumatoid arthritis: case report. J Neurosurg 53:841, 1980

Stone DB, Bonfiglio M: Pyogenic vertebral osteomyelitis. A diagnostic pitfall for the internist. Arch Int Med 112:491, 1963

Sundaresan N, Galicich JH, Lane JM, et al: Treatment of neoplastic epidural cord compression by vertebral body resection and stabilization. J Neurosurg 63(5):676, 1985

Tachdjian, MO, Matson DD: Orthopaedic aspects of intraspinal tumors in infants and children. J Bone Joint Surg 47A:223, 1965

Swischuk LE: Anterior displacement of C2 in children: physiologic or pathologic? Radiology 122:759, 1977

Swischuk LE, Hayden CK, Sarwar M: The dens-arch synchondrosis versus the hangman's fracture. Pediatr Radiol 8:100, 1979

Vermooten VA: Study of the fracture of the epistopheus due to hanging with a note on the possible causes of death. Anat Rec 20:305, 1921

Wiesseman GJ, Wood VE, Kroll LL: Pseudomonas vertebral osteomyelitis in heroin addicts. J Bone Joint Surg 55A:1416, 1973

Wood-Jones F: The examination of the bodies of 100 men executed in Nubia in roman times. Br Med J [Clin Res] 1:736, 1908

WOUND BALLISTICS AND GUNSHOT INJURIES OF THE SPINE

Adams DB: Wound ballistics: a review. Milit Med 147:831, 1982

Berman AT: Low velocity gunshot wounds in police officers. Clin Orthop 192:113, 1985

DeMuth WE: Bullet velocity and design as determinants of wounding capability: an experimental study. J Trauma 6:222, 1966

Haynes WG: Acute war wounds of the spinal cord. Am J Surg 72:424, 1948

Heiden JS, Weiss MH, Rosenberg AW, et al: Penetrating gunshot wounds of the cervical spine in civilians. J Neurosurg 42:575, 1975

Hopkinson DAW: Firearm injuries. Br J Surg 54:344, 1967

Horsley V: The destructive nature of small projectiles. Nature 50:104, 1894

McCravey A: War wounds of the spinal cord. A plea for exploration of spinal cord and cauda equina injuries JAMA 129:152, 1945

Puckett WO: Studies on wounds of the abdomen and thorax produced by high velocity missiles. Milit Surg 98:427, 1946

Rich NM: Missile injuries. Am J Surg 139:414, 1980

Shover RN, Fortson CH, Theodotou CB: Delayed neurological sequelae of a retained foreign body (lead bullet) in the intervertebral disc space. J Bone Joint Sur 42A:595, 1960

Stauffer ES, Wood RW, Kelly EG: Gunshot wounds of the spine:the effects of laminectomy. J Bone Joint Surg 61A:389, 1979

Swan K, Swan RC: Gunshot wounds: pathophysiology and management. PSG, Littleton, MA, 1980

Yashon D, Jane JA, White RJ: Prognosis and management of spinal cord and cauda equina bullet injuries in sixty-five civilians. J Neurosurg 32:163, 1970

Woodruff CE: The cause of the explosive effect of modern small caliber bullets. NY Med J 67:593, 1898

SPINAL CORD VASCULAR ANATOMY AND COMPLICATIONS

Abrams HL: The vertebral and azygos venous system, and some variations in systemic venous return. Radiology 69:5, 1957

Adamkiewicz A: Die blutgefasse des menschlichen ruckenmarkes, IL teil. Die Gefasse der Ruckenmarkoberflache. SB Heidelberg, Akad Wiss 85:101, 1882

Adornato DC, Gildenberg PL, Ferraria CM, et al: Pathophysiology of intravenous air embolism in dogs. Anesthesiology 49:120, 1978

Albin MS, White RJ, Acosta-Rua G, Yashor D: Study of functional recovery produced by delayed localized cooling after spinal cord injury in primates. J Neurosurg 29:113, 1968

Albin MS, Carroll RG, Maroon JC: Clinical consideration concerning detection of venous air embolism. Neurosurgery 3:380, 1978

Basta JW, Niedjalik K, Pallares V: Autonomic hyperreflexia: intraoperative control with pentolinium tartarate. J Anesth 49:1087, 1977

Batson OV: The function of the vertebral vein and their role in the spread of metastases. Ann Surgery 112:138, 1940

Batson OV: The vertebral vein system as a mechanism for the spread of metastasis. Am J Roentgen Radium Ther 6(48):715, 1942

Batzdorf U, Bentson JR, Machleder HI: Blunt trauma to the cervical carotid artery. Neurosurgery 5:195, 1979

Bernini FP, Elefante R, Smaltino F, Tedeschi G: Angiographic study on the vertebral artery in cases of deformities of the occipital joint. AJR 107:526, 1969

Bunegin L, Albin MS, Helsel PE: Positioning the right atrial catheter: a model for re-appraisal. Anesthesiology 55:343, 1981

Bussat P, Rossier AB, Djindjian R, et al: Spinal cord angiography in dorsolumbar vertebral fractures with neurological involvement. Radiology 109:617, 1973

Carpenter S: Injury of neck as cause of vertebral artery thrombosis. J Neurosurg 18:849, 1961

Christenson PR, Oritt TW, Fisher HD, et al: Intravenous angiography using digital video subtraction: intravenous cervicocerebrovascular angiography. AJNR 1:379, 1980

Cordobes F, Lobato R, Rivas JJ: Observations of 82 patients with extradural hematoma. J Neurosurg 54:179, 1981

Dichiro G, Fried LC, Doppman JL: Experimental spinal cord angiography. Br J Radiol 43:19, 1970

Djindjian R, Houdart R, Hurth M: Angiography of the Spinal Cord. p. 52. University Park Press, Baltimore, 1970

Dommisse CF: The blood supply of the spinal cord. J Bone Joint Surg 56B:225, 1974

Dommisse GF: The Arteries and Veins of the Human Spinal Cord from Birth. Churchill Livingstone, Edinburgh, 1975

Dragon R, Saranchak H, Lakin P et al: Blunt injuries to the carotid and vertebral arteries. Am J Surg 141:497, 1981

Feeney JF, Watterson RL: The development of the vascular pattern within the walls of the central nervous system of the chick embryo. J Morphol 78:231, 1946

French BN, Cobb CA, Dublin AB: Cranial computed tomography in the diagnosis of symptomatic indirect trauma to the carotid artery. Surg Neurol 15:256, 1981

Harris WH, Salzman EW, Desanctis RW: The prevention of thromboembolic disease by prophylactic anticoagulants. J Bone Joint Surg 49A:81, 1967

Hart RG, Easton JD: Dissection of cervical and cerebral arteries. Neurol Clin N Am 1:155, 1983

Herlihy WF: Revision of venous system: the role of the vertebral veins. Med J Aust 22:661, 1947

Higazi, I: Post-traumatic carotid thrombosis. J Neurosurg 20:354, 1963

Jamieson KG, Yelland JDN: Extradural hematoma. Report of 167 cases. J Neurosurg 129:13, 1968

Kassell NF, Boarini DJ, Adams Jr HP: Intracranial and cervical vascular injuries. p. 275 In Cooper PR (ed): Head Injuries. Williams & Wilkins, Baltimore, 1982

Kobrine AI, Evans DE, Rizzoli H: Correlation of spinal cord blood flow and function in experimental compression. Surg Neurol 10:54, 1978

Kruger BR, O'Kazaki H: Vertebral-basilar distribution infarction following chiropractic cervical manipulation. Mayo Clin Proc 55:322, 1980

Lazorthes G, Gouaze A, Zadeh JO, et al: Arterial vascularization of the spinal cord. J Neurosurg 35:253, 1971

Lyness SS, Simeone FA: Vascular complications of upper cervical spine injuries. Ortho Clin N Am 9:1029, 1978

Marshall LF, Bruce DA, Bruno L, Langfitt TW: Vertebrobasilar spasm: a significant cause of neurological deficit in head injury. J Neurosurg 48:560, 1978

McLaurin RL, Ford LE: Extradural hematoma. Statistical survey of 47 cases. J Neurosurg 21:364, 1964

Murray DS: Post-traumatic thrombosis of the internal carotid and vertebral arteries after nonpenetrating injuries of the neck. Br J Surg 44:556, 1957

Phonprasert C, Suwanwela C, Hongsaprabhas D, et al: Extradural hematoma: Analysis of 138 cases. J Trauma 20:679, 1980

Richards T, Hoff J: Factors affecting survival from acute subdural hematoma. Surgery 75:253, 1974

Schermann BM, Tucker WS: Bilateral traumatic thrombosis of the internal carotid arteries in the neck: a case report with review of the literature. Neurosurgery 10:751, 1982

Schneider RC, Schemm, GW: Vertebral artery insufficiency in acute and chronic spinal trauma. J Neurosurg 18:348, 1961

Sherman DG, Hart RG, Easton JD: Abrupt change in head position and cerebral infarction. Stroke 12:2, 1981

Shull JR, Rose DL: Pulmonary embolism in patients with spinal cord injury. Arch Phys Med Rehab 47:444, 1966

Stephen RB, Stillwell DL: Arteries and Veins of the Human Brain. Charles C Thomas, Springfield, Illinois, 1969

Suh TH, Alexander L: Vascular system of the human spinal cord. Arch Neurol Psych 41:659, 1939

Turnbull IM: Blood supply of the spinal cord: normal and pathological considerations. Clin Neurosurg 20:56, 1973

Watson N: Venous thrombosis and pulmonary embolism in spinal cord injury. Paraplegia 6:113, 1968

Woolam DHM, Millen JW: Discussion on the vascular disease of the spinal cord. Proc Royal Soc Med 51:540, 1958

CORTICAL AND SPINAL EVOKED POTENTIAL MONITORING

Baust W, Ilsen HW, Jorg W, Wambach G: A neurophysiological method for the localization of transverse lesions of the spinal cord. Acta Neurochir (Wien) 26:352, 1972

Bohlman, HH, Behniuk E, Field G, Raskulinecz G: Spinal cord monitoring of experimental incomplete cervical spinal cord injury. Spine 6:428, 1981

Brown RH, Nash Jr CL: Current status of spinal cord monitoring. Spine 4:466, 1979

Chehrazi B, Parkinson J, Bucholz R: Evoked somatosensory potentials to common peroneal nerve stimulation in man. J Neurosurg 55:733, 1981

Chiappa, KH, Ropper AH: Evoked potentials in clinical medicine: Part 1. N Eng J Med 306:1140, 1982

Chiappa KH: Evoked Potentials in Clinical Medicine. Raven Press, New York, 1983

Clark, DL, Rosner BS: Neurophysiologic effects of general anesthetics: I. The electroencephalogram and sensory evoked responses in man. Anesthesiology 38:564, 1973

Cohen AR, Young W, Ransohoff J: Intraspinal localization of the somatosensory evoked potential. Neurosurgery 9:157, 1981

Croft TJ, Brodkey JS, Nulsen FE: Reversible spinal cord trauma: a model for electrical monitoring of spinal cord function. J Neurosurg 36:402, 1972

D'Angelo CM, Van Gilder JC, Taub A: Evoked cortical potentials in experimental spinal cord trauma. J Neurosurg 38:332, 1973

Dawson GD: A summation technique for detecting small signals in a large irregular background. J Physiol 115:2P, 1951

Dawson GD: A summation technique for the detection of small evoked potentials. Electroencephalogr Clin Neurophysiol 6:65, 1954

Dorfman LJ, Perkash I, Bosley TM, Cummins KL: Use of cerebral evoked potentials to evaluate spinal somatosensory function in patients with traumatic and surgical myelopathies. J Neurosurg 52:654, 1980

Eisen A, Elleker G: Sensory nerve stimulation and evoked cerebral potentials. Neurology 30:1097, 1980

Eisen A, Hoirch M, Moll A: Evaluation of radiculopathies by segmental stimulation and somatosensory evoked potentials. Can J Neurol Sci 10:178, 1983

Engler GL, Spielholz NI, Bernhard WN, et al: Somatosensory evoked potentials during harrington instrumentation for scoliosis. J Bone Joint Surg 60A:528, 1978

Ertekin C, Mutlu R, Sarica Y, Uckardesier L: Electrophysiological evaluation of the afferent spinal roots and nerves in patients with conus medullaris and cauda equina lesions. J Neurol Sci 48:419, 1980

Giblin DR: Somatosensory evoked potentials in healthy subjects and in patients with lesions of the nervous system. Ann NY Acad Sci 112:93, 1964

Girard B, Minaire P, Casteran J, et al: Anal and urethral sphincter electromyography in spinal cord injured patients. Paraplegia 16:244, 1979

Green J, Gildemeister R, Hazelwood C: Dermatomally stimulated somatosensory cerebral evoked potentials in the clinical diagnosis of lumbar disc disease. Clin Electroencephalogr 14:152, 1983

Greenberg RP, Mayer DJ, Becker DP, Miller JD: Evaluation of brain function in severe human head trauma with multimodality evoked potentials. Part 1: evoked brain-injury potentials and analysis. J Neurosurg 47:150, 1977

Greenberg RP, Mayer DJ, Becker DP, Miller JD: Evaluation of brain function in severe human head trauma with multimodality evoked potentials. Part 2: localization of brain dysfunction and correlation with post traumatic neurological conditions. J Neurosurg 47:163, 1977

Greenberg RP, Miller JD, Becker DP: Clinical findings associated with brainstem dysfunction: an electrophysiological study in severe human head trauma. p.229. In Popp, AJ, Bourke RS, Nelson AR, Kimelberg HK (eds): Neural Trauma. Raven Press, New York, 1979

Grossman RG, Lindquist C, Feinstein R, Eisenberg HM: Monitoring of the excitability of the cerebral cortex in brain injury with the direct cortical response. p. 237. In Popp, AJ, Bourke RS, Nelson AR, Kimelberg HK (eds): Neural Trauma. Raven Press, New York, 1979

Grundy BL: Monitoring of sensory evoked potentials during neurosurgical operations: methods and applications. Neurosurgery 11:556, 1982

Grundy BL, Heros RC, Tung AS, Doyle E: Intraoperative hypoxia detected by evoked potential monitoring. Anesth Analg 60:437, 1981

Grundy BD, Procopio PT, Janetta PJ, Line, et al: Evoked potential changes produced by positioning for retromastoid craniectomy. Neurosurgery 10:766, 1982

Grundy BL: Intraoperative monitoring of sensory-evoked potentials. Anesthesiology 58:72, 1983

Hahn, JF, Lesser R, Klem G, Leuders H: Simple technique for monitoring intraoperative spinal cord function. Neurosurgery 9:692, 1981

Halliday AM, Wakefield GS: Cerebral evoked potentials in patients with dissociated sensory loss. J Neurol Neurosurg Psychiatry 26:211, 1963

Halliday AM: Changes in the form of cerebral evoked responses in man associated with various lesions of the nervous system. Ann NY Acad Sci 112:93, 1964

Hargadine JR, Branston NM, Symon L: Central conduction time in primate brain ischemia—a study in baboons. Stroke 11:637, 1980

Hattori S, Seiki K, Kawai S: Diagnosis of the level and severity of cord lesion in cervical spondylotic myelopathy: spinal evoked potentials. Spine 4:478, 1979

Hume AL, Cant BR: Central somatosensory conduction after head injury. Ann Neurol 10:411, 1981

Hutch JA, Elliott H: Electromyographic study of electrical activity in the paraurethral muscles prior to and during voiding. J Urol 99:759, 1968

Jorg J: Die Electrosensible Diagnostik in der Neurologie. Springer-Verlag, Berlin, 1977

Jorg J, Dullberg W, Koeppen S: Diagnostic value of segmental somatosensory evoked potentials in cases with chronic progressive para- or tetraspastic syndromes. p. 347. In Courjon J , Manguiere F, Revol M (eds): Clinical Applications of Evoked Potentials in Neurology. Raven Press, New York, 1982

Katz S, Blackburn JG, Perot PL, Lam CF: The effects of slow spinal injury on somatosensory evoked potentials from forelimb stimulaion. Electroencephalogr Clin Neurophysiol 44:236, 1978

Koht A, Sloan T, Ronai A, Toleikis JR: Intraoperative deterioration of evoked potentials during spinal surgery. p. 161. In Schramm Jr, Jones SJ (eds): Spinal Cord Monitoring, Springer-Verlag, Berlin, 1985

Kojima Y, Yamamoto T, Ogino H, et al: Evoked spinal potentials as a monitor of spinal cord viability. Spine 4:471, 1979

Krane R, Siroky M: Studies on sacral-evoked potentials. J Urol 124:872, 1980

Leuders H, Gurd A, Hahn J, et al: A new technique for intraoperative monitoring of spinal cord function: multichannel recording of spinal cord and subcortical evoked potentials. Spine 7:110, 1982

Levy, WJ, York DH, McCaffrey M, Tanzer F: Motor evoked potentials from transcranial stimulation of the motor cortex in humans. Neurosurgery 15:287, 1984

Levy WJ, McCaffrey M, York DH, Tanzer F: Motor evoked potentials from transcranial stimulation of the motor cortex in cats. Neurosurgery 15:214, 1984

Levy, WJ, York DH: Evoked potentials from the motor tracts in humans. Neurosurgery 12:422, 1983

Low, MD, Purves S, Purves BL: A critical assessment of the use of evoked potentials in diagnosis of peripheral nerve, spinal cord and cerebral disease. p. 169. In Marley TP. (ed): Current Controversies in Neurosurgery. WB Saunders, Philadelphia, 1976

Macon JB, Poletti CE: Conducted somatosensory evoked potentials during spinal surgery. Part 1: control conduction velocity measurements. J Neurosurg 57:349, 1982

Macon JB, Poletti CE, Sweet WH, et al: Conducted somatosensory evoked potentials during spinal surgery.

Part 2: clinical applications. J Neurosurg. 57:354, 1982

McCallum JE, Bennett MH: Electrophysiologic monitoring of spinal cord function during intraspinal surgery. Surgical Forum 26:469, 1975

Merton PA, Morton HB, Hill DK, Maisen DC: Scope of a technique for electrical stimulation of human brain, spinal cord and muscle. Lancet 2:597, 1982

Merton PA, Morton HB: Stimulation of the cerebral cortex in the intact human subject. Nature 285:287, 1980

Merton PA, Morton HB: Electrical stimulation of human motor and visual cortex through the scalp. J Physiol (Lond) 355:9, 1980

Nash, CL, Lorig RA, Schatzinger LR, Brown RH: Spinal cord monitoring during operative treatment of the spine. Clin Orthop 126;100, 1977

Nash CL, Schatzinger, LH, Brown RH, Brodkey J: The unstable thoracic compression fracture: its problems and the use of spinal cord monitoring in the evaluation of treament. Spine 2:261, 1977

Nordling J, Anderson JT, Walter S, et al: Evoked response of the bulbocavernosus reflex. Eur Urol 5:36, 1979

Nordwall A, Axelgaard J, Harado Y, et al: Spinal cord monitoring using evoked potentials recorded from feline vertebral bone. Spine 4:486, 1979

Pedersen E: Electromyography of the sphincter muscles. In Cobb WA, Van Duijn H: Contempoary Clinical Neurophysiology. Elsevier, Amsterdam, 405, 1978

Perot PL: The clinical use of somatosensory evoked potentials in spinal cord injury. Clin Neurosurg 20:367, 1973

Perot PL: Somatosensory evoked potentials in the evaluation of patients with spinal cord injury. p. 160. In Marley, TP (ed): Current Controversies in Neurosurgery. WB Saunders, Philadelphia, 1976

Perot PL, Vera CL: Scalp-recorded somatosensory evoked potentials to stimulation of nerves in the lower extremities and evaluation of patients with spinal cord trauma. Ann NY Acad Sci 388:359, 1982

Raudzens PA: Intraoperative monitoring of evoked potentials. Ann NY Acad Sci 388:308, 1982

Reger SI, Henry DT, Whitehall R, et al: Spinal evoked potentials from the cervical spine, Spine 4:495, 1979

Robertson FC, Kisheri, PRS, Miller JD: The value of serial CT in the management of severe head injury. Surg Neurol 12:161, 1979

Rowed DW, McLean JAG, Taot CH: Somatosensory evoked potentials in acute spinal cord injury: prognostic value. Surg Neurol 9:203, 1978

Rowed DW: Value of somatosensory evoked potentials for prognosis in partial cord injuries. p. 167. In Tator CD (ed): Early Management of Acute Spinal Cord Injury. Raven Press, New York, 1982

Royal College of Radiologists: A study of the utilization of skull radiography in 9 accident-and-emergency units in the UK. Lancet ii:1234 1980.

Russin LD, Guinto Jr, FC: Multidirectional tomography in cervical spine injury. J Neurosurg 45:9, 1976

Scarff T, Toleikis JR, Bunch W, Parrish S: Dermatomal somatosensory evoked potentials in children with myelomeningocele. Z Kinderchir, 28:384, 1980

Scarff TB, Dallmann DE, Toleikis JR, Bunch WH: Dermatomal somatosensory evoked potentials in the diagnosis of lumbar root entrapment. Surgical Forum 32:489, 1981

Scher AT: Double fractures of the spine — an indication for routine radiographic examination of the entire spine after injury. S Afr Med J 53:411, 1978

Schramm J, Oettle GJ, Pichert T: Clinical application of segmental somatosensory evoked potentials (SEP) — experience in patients with nonspace-occupying lesions. p. 455. In Barber C (ed): Evoked Potentials.MTP Press, Leichester, 1980

Sedgewick EM, El-Negamy E, Frankel H: Spinal cord potentials in traumatic paraplegia and quadriplegia. J Neurol Neurosurg Psychiatry 43:823, 1980

Sheldon JJ, Sersland T, Leborgne J: Computed tomography of the lower lumbar vertebral column. Radiology 124:113, 1977

Shimoji K, Higashi H, Kano T: Epidural recording of spinal electrogram in man. Electroencephalogr Clin Neurophysiol 30:236, 1971

Shimoji K, Kano T, Morioka T, Ikezono E: Evoked spinal electrogram in a quadriplegic patient. Electroencephalogr Clin Neurophysiol 35:659, 1973

Simha RP, Ducker TB, Perot PL: Arterial oxygenation. Findings and its significance in central nervous system trauma patients. JAMA 224:1258, 1973

Singer JM, Russell GV, Coe JE: Changes in evoked potentials after experimental cervical spinal cord injury in the monkey. Exp Neurol 29:449, 1970

Sloan TB, Koht A: Depression of cortical somatosensory evoked potentials by nitrous oxide. Br J Anaesth 57:849, 1985

Sloan TB, Ronai AK, Koht A: Reversible loss of somatosensory evoked potentials during cervical spine fusion. Anesth Analg 65:96, 1986

Spielholz NI, Benjamin MV, Engler G, Ransohoff J: Somatosensory evoked potentials and clinical outcome in spinal cord injury. p. 217. In Popp AJ, Bourke RS, Nelson LR, Kimelberg HK (eds): Neural Trauma. Raven Press, New York, 1979

Stochard JJ, Sharbrough FW: Unique contributions of short-latency auditory and somatosensory evoked potentials to neurologic diagnosis. Prog Clin Neurophysiol 7:231, 1980

Tadmor R, Davis KR, Roberson GH, New PFJ, Taveras JM: Computed tomographic evaluation of traumatic spinal injuries. Radiology 127:825, 1978

Tamaki T: Clinical benefits of SEP. Seikagaku, 29:681, 1977

Toleikis JR, Scarff TB, Dallmann DE: Dermatomal somatosensory evoked potentials in the diagnosis of lumbosacral root entrapment. Nicolet Potentials: 16, Fall, 1982

Toleikis JR, Sloan T, Schrader S, Koht A: Scalp distribution of dermatome evoked potentials. p. 59. In Schramm Jr, Jones SJ(eds): Spinal Cord Monitoring. Springer-Verlag, Berlin, 1985

Waldman J, Kaufer H, Heuringer RH, Callaghan ML: Wake-up technique during Harrington rod procedure. A case report. Anesth Anal 56:733, 1977

Woolson ST: Three-dimensional bone imaging and preoperative planning in reconstructive hip surgery. Contemp Orthop 12(5):13, 1986

Young W, Tomasula J, DeCrescito V, et al: Vestibulospinal monitoring in experimental spinal trauma. J Neurosurg 52:64, 1980

Young W: Correlation of somatosensory evoked potentials and neurological findings in spinal cord injury. p. 153. In Tator CH (ed): Early Management of Acute Spinal Cord Injury. Raven Press, New York, 1982

UROLOGIC CONSEQUENCES OF SPINAL INJURY

Abel B, Gibbon N, Jameson R, Krishnan K: The neuropathic urethra. Lancet ii:1229, 1974

Abrams PH: Perfusion urethral profilometry. Urol Clin North Am 6:103, 1979

Anderson RU: Non sterile intermittent catheterization with antibiotic prophylaxis in the acute spinal cord injured male patient. J Urol 124:392, 1980

Bors E, Comarr AE: Neurological Urology. University Park Press, Baltimore, 1971

Boyce W, Elkins I: Reconstructive renal surgery following anatrophic nephrolothotomy: follow-up of 100 consecutive cases. J Urol 111:307, 1974

Bradley WE, Rockswold G, Timm G, Scott FB: Neurology of micturition. J Urol 115:481, 1976

Brindley GS: Electroejaculation: its technique, neurological implications and uses J Neurol Neurosurg Psychiatry 44:9, 1981

Broecker B, Klein F, Hackler R: Cancer of the bladder in spinal cord paients. J Urol 125:196, 1981

Clarke S, Thomas DG: Characteristics of the urethral pressure profile in flaccid male paraplegics. Brit J Urol 53:157, 1981

Comarr AE: Sexual function among patients with spinal cord injury. Urol Int 25:134, 1970

David A, Ohry A, Rozin R: Spinal cord injuries: male infertility aspects. Paraplegia 2:1511, 1977

DeGroat WC, Booth A: Physiology of male sexual function. Ann Intern Med 92(2):329, 1980

DeGroat WC, Booth AM: Physiology of the urinary bladder and urethra. Ann Int Med 92(2): 312, 1980

Donovan W, Stolov W, Clowers D, Clowers M: Bacteriuria during intermittent catheterization following spinal cord injury. Arch Phys Med Rehabil 59:351, 1978

Donovan WH, Clowers DE, Kiviat M, Macri D: Anal sphincter stretch: a technique to overcome detrusor-sphincter spasticity dyssynergia. Arch Phys Med Rehabil 58:320, 1977

Ertekin C, Reel F: Bulbocavernosus reflex in normal men and in patients with neurogenic bladder and/or impotence. J Neruol Sci 28:1, 1976

Fisher C, Sonda L, Dickno A: Use of cryoprecipitate coagulum in extracting renal calculi. Urology 15:6, 1980

Foster WM, Bergofsky EH, Bohning DE, et al: Effect of adrenergic agents and their mode of action on mucociliary clearance in man. J Appl Physiol 41:146, 1976

Francois N, Maury M, Jovannet D, Et al: Electroejaculation of a complete paraplegic followed by pregnancy. Paraplegia 16:248, 1978

Gibbon N, Parsons K, Woolfenden K: The neuropathic urethra. Lancet 2:129, 1974

Gibbon N: Management of the bladder in acute and chronic disorders of the nervous system. Acta Neurol Scand Suppl 20(42):133, 1966

Gjone R, Ween E: Results of bladder training 1966-74. Paraplegia 15:47, 1977

Gosling J, Dixon J, Critchley H, and Thompson S: A comparative study of the human external sphincter and periurethral levator and muscles. Brit J Urol 53:35, 1981

Guttmann L, Frankel H: The value of intermittent catheterization in the early management of traumatic paraplegia and tetraplegia. Paraplegia 4:63, 1966

Hachen HJ, Krucker V: Clinical and laboratory assessment of the efficacy of baclofen or urethral sphincter spasticity in patients with traumatic paraplegia. Eur Urol 3:237, 1977

Hachen HJ, Ott R: Late results of bilateral endoscopic sphincterotomy in patients with upper motor neuron lesions. Paraplegia 13:268, 1976

Hachen HJ: Clinical and urodynamic assessment of alpha-adrenolytic therapy in patients with neurogenic bladder function. Paraplegia 18:299, 1980

Hackler R, Klein F, Hackler R: Cancer of the bladder in spinal cord patients. J Urol 125:196, 1981

Hutch JA, Elliott H: Electromyographic study of electrical activity in the paraurethral muscles prior to and during voiding. J Urol 99:759, 1968

Hutch JA: Anatomy and Physiology of the Bladder, Trigone and Urethra. Appleton-Century-Crofts, New York, 1972

Kaufman JM, Fam B, Jacobs S, et al: Bladder cancer and squamous metaplasia in spinal cord patients. J Urol 125:196, 1981

Kiviat M: Transurethral sphincterotomy: relationship of site of incision to postoperative potency and delayed hemorrhage. J Urol 114:339, 1975

Krane RJ, Olsson CA: Phenoxybenzamine in neurogenic bladder dysfunction. J Urol 110:653, 1973

Krane R, Siroky M: Studies on sacral-evoked potentials. J Urol 124:872, 1980

Lapides J, Diokno AC, Gould F, Lowe, B: Further observations on self-catheterization. J. Urol 116:169, 1979

Lieskovsky G, Skinner DC: Use of intestinal segments in the urinary tract. p. 2620. In Walsh PC et al (eds): Campbell's Urology, WB Saunders, Philadelphia, 1986

Madersbacher H, Scott FB: The twelve o'clock sphincterotomy: technique, indications, results. Paraplegia 13:261, 1976

Naftchi NE, Viao A, Sell GH, Lowman EW:Pituitary-testicular axis dysfunction in spinal cord injury. Arch Phys Med Rehabil 61:402, 1980

Nanninga J, Meyer PR: Urethral sphincter activity following acute spinal cord injury. J Urol 123:528, 1980

Nanninga J, Rosen J, O'Conor Jr VJ: Experience with transurethral external sphincterotomy in patients with spinal cord injury. J Urol 112:72, 1974

Nanninga JB, Wu Y, and Hamilton B: Long-term intermittent catheterization in the spinal cord injury patient. J Urol 128:760, 1982

Newman H, Northrup J: Mechanism of human penile erection: an overview. Urology 17:399, 1981

Nordling J, Meyhoff H, Hald T: Neuromuscular dysfunction of the lower urinary tract with special reference to the influence of the sympathetic nervous system. Scand J Urol Nephrol 15:7, 1981

O'Flynn, JD: An assessment of surgical treatment of vesical outlet obstruction in spinal cord injury: a review of 471 cases. Brit J Urol 48:657, 1976

O'Flynn JD: Neurogenic bladder in spinal cord injury. Urol Clin North Am 1:155, 1974

Ott R, Rossier AB: Intermittent catheterization in bladder rehabilitation in traumatic acute spinal cord lesions. Urol Int 27:51, 1972

Price M, Kottke F, Olson M: Renal function in patients with spinal cord injury: the eight year of a ten year continuing study. Arch Phys Med Rehabil 56:76, 1975

Rosen JS, Nanninga J, O'Conor Jr VJ: Silent hydronephrosis: a hazard revisited. Paraplegia 14:124, 1976

Ross, JC, Gibbon N, Sunder G: Division of the external urethral sphincter in the neuropathic bladder: a twenty year review. Brit J Urol 48:649, 1976

Rossier A, Ott R: Bladder and urethral recordings in acute and chronic spinal cord injury patients. Urol Int 31:49, 1976

Schellhammer P, Hackler RH, Bunts RC: External sphincterotomy: rationale for the procedure and experience with 150 patients. Paraplegia 12:5, 1974

Schoenfeld, L, Carrion H, Politano V: Erectile impotence. Urology 4:681, 1974

Sher AT: Changes in the upper urinary tract as demonstrated on intravenous pyelography and micturating cystourethrography in patients with spinal cord injury. Paraplegia 13:157, 1975

Stover, S, Lloyd LK, Nepomuceno C, Gale L: Intermittent catheterization: follow-up studies. Paraplegia 15:38, 1977

Sunder GS, Parsons KF, Gibbon N: Outflow obstruction in neuropathic bladder dysfunction: the neuropathic urethra. Brit J Urol 50:190, 1978

Tanago, EA: Membrane and microtransducer catheters: their effectiveness for profilometry of the lower urinary tract. Urol Clin North Am 6:110, 1979

Thomas D: Clinical urodynamics in neurogenic bladder dysfunction. Urol Clin North Am 6:237, 1979

Thomas DG, Smallwood R, Graham D: Urodynamic observations following spinal trauma. Brit J Urol 47:161, 1975

Vivian J, Bors E: Experience with intermittent catheterization in the southwest regional system for treament of spinal injury. Paraplegia 12:158, 1974

Warren J, Muncie H, Bergquist E, Hoopes J: Sequelae and management of urinary infection in the patient requiring chronic catheterization. J Urol 125:1, 1981

Warren J, Muncie H, Bergquist E, Hoopes J: Sequelae and management of urinary infection in the patient requiring chronic catheterization. J Urol 125:1, 1981

Weiss HD: Physiology of penile erection. Ann Inter Med 76:793, 1972

Wu Y, Hamilton B, Boyink M, Nanninga J: Reusable catheter for longterm sterile intermittent catheterization. Arch Phys Med Rehabil 62:39, 1981

SPINE INJURIES WITH SEATBELTS

Dehner JR: Seatbelt injuries of the spine and abdomen. AJR 111:833, 1971

Epstein BS, Epstein JA, Jones MD: Lap-sash three-point seat belt fractures of the cervical spine. Spine 3:189, 1978

Fletcher B, Brogdon BG: Seat-belt fractures of the spine and sternum. JAMA 200:167, 1967

Greenbaum E, Harris L, Halloran WX: Flexion fractures of the lumbar spine due to lap-type seat belts. Calif Med 113:361, 1970

Haddad, GH, Zickel RE: Intestinal perforations and fractures of lumbar vertebra caused by lap-type seat belts. NY State J MEd 67:930, 1967

Rogers LF: The roentgenographic appearance of transverse or chance fractures of the spine: the seat belt fracture. AJR 111:844, 1971

Smith WS, Kaufer H: Patterns and mechanisms of lumbar injuries associated with lap seat belt fractures. J Bone Joint Surg 51A:239, 1969

NON-SPINAL COMPLICATIONS RESULTING FROM SPINE AND HEAD TRAUMA

Bellamy R, Pitts FW, Stauffer ES: Respiratory complications in traumatic quadriplegia: analysis of 20 years' experience. J Neurosurg 39:596, 1973

Bergofsky EH: Respiratory failure in disorders of the thoracic cage. Am Rev Respir Dis 119:643, 1979

Bergofsky EH: Mechanism for respiratory insufficiency after cervical cord injury. A source of alveolar hypoventilation. Ann Inter Med 61:435, 1964

Bohlman HH: Complications of treatment of fractures and dislocations of the cervical spine. p. 681. In Epps C (Ed): Complications in Orthopaedic Surgery. 2nd Ed. Vol 2. JB Lippincott, 1985

Bulger RF, Rejowski JE, Beatty RA: Vocal cord paralysis associated with anterior cervical fusion: Considerations for prevention and treatment. J Neurosurg 26:657, 1985

Carpenter S: Injury of neck as cause of vertebral artery thrombosis. J Neurosurg 18:849, 1961

Cerullo LJ, Raimondi AJ: Neurological emergencies. In Beal JM (ed): Critical Care for Surgical Patients. p. 297 Macmillan, New York, 1982

Cooperman LH, Strobel GE, Kennel EM: Massive hyperkalemia after administration of succinylocholine. Anesthesiology 32:161, 1970

Crompton MR: Visual lesions in closed head injuries. Brain 93:785, 1970

Delavelle J, Lalanne B, Megret M: "Man-In-The-Barrel." Neurology 29:501, 1987

Elisevich KV, Ford RM, Anderson DP, et al: Visual abnormalities with multiple trauma. Surg Neurol 22:565, 1984

Epps CH: Complications in Orthopaedic Surgery. JB Lippincott, Philadelphia, 1978

Epstein HC: Traumatic dislocations of the hip. Clin Orthop 92:116, 1973

Erickson RP: Autonomic hyperreflexia: pathophysiology and medical management. Arch Phys Rehabil 61:431, 1980

Frankel HL: Ascending cord lesions in the early stages following spinal injury. Paraplegia 7:111, 1969

Gregory CF: Early complications of dislocation and fracture dislocation of the hip joint. In American Academy of Orthopaedic Surgeons: Instructional Course Lectures. Vol. 22. CV Mosby, St. Louis, 1973

Guttmann L: Spinal deformities in traumatic paraplegia and tetraplegia following surgical procedures. Paraplegia 7:38, 1969

Harris P: Associated injuries in traumatic paraplegia and tetraplegia. Paraplegia 5:215, 1968

Harris WH, Salzman, EW, Desanctis RW: The prevention of thromboembolic disease by prophylactic anticoagulats. J Bone Joint Surg 49A:81, 1967

Henry RC, Taylor PH: Cerebrospinal fluid otorrhea and otorhinorrhea following closed head injury. J Laryongol Otolaryngol 192:743, 1978

Higazi I: Post-traumatic carotid thrombosis. J Neurosurg 20:3543, 1963

Hinchley JE, Areno A, Benoit AR, et al: The stress ulcer syndrome p. 325. In Welch C(ed): Advances in Surgery. Vol. 4. Year Book Medical Publishers, Chicago, 1970

Jamieson KG, Yelland JDN: Extradural hematoma. Report of 167 cases. J Neurosurg 129:13, 1968

Jefferson A: Ocular complications of head injuries. Trans Ophthal Soc UK 81:595, 1961

Jennett B, Murray A, MacMillan R, et al: Head injuries in Scottish hospitals. Lancet ii:696, 1977

Jennett B, Snock J, Bond MR, Brooks N: Disability after severe head injury. Observations of the use of the Glasgow Outcome Scale. J Neurol Neurosurg Psychiatry 44:285, 1981

Johnson CE, Happel LT, Norris R, et al: Delayed paraplegia complicating sublaminar segmental spinal instrumentation. J Bone Joint Surg 68A(4):556, 1986

Kahanovitz N, Mehringer M, Johanson P: Intracranial entrapment of the atlas—complicating an untreated fracture of the posterior arch of the atlas. J Bone Joint Surg 63A:831,1981

Kewalramani LS, Taylor RG: Multiple non-contiguous injuries to the spine. Acta Orthop Scan 47:52, 1976

Kobrine AI, Timmins E, Rajjoub RK, Rizzoni, HV, Davis, et al: Demonstration of massive traumatic brain swelling with 20 minutes after injury. J Neurosurg 46:256, 1977

Kornberg M, Herndon WAA, Rechtine GR: Lumbar nerve root compression at the site of hook insertion. Spine 10(9):853, 1985

Kruger BR, O'Kazaki H: Vertebral-basilar distribution infarction following chiropractic cervical manipulation. Mayo Clin Proc 55:322, 1980

Kurnick NB: Autonomic hyperreflexia and its control in patients with spinal cord lesions. Ann Inter Med 44:678, 1956

Lindenberg R: Significance of the tentorium in head injuries from blunt forces. Clin Neurosurg 12:129, 1966

Malcolm, BW, Bradford DS, Winter RB, Chou SN: Post-traumatic kyphosis. J Bone Joint Surg 63A;891, 1981

Marshall LF, Bruce DA, Bruno L, Langfitt TW: Vertebrobasilar spasm: a significant cause of neurological deficit in head injury. J Neurosurg 48:560, 1978

McAfee, PC, Bohlman HH, Ducker T, Eismont FJ: Failure of fixation of the spine with methylmethacrylate. A retrospective analysis of twenty-four cases. J Bone Joint Surg, 68A(8):1145, 1986

McLaurin RL, Ford LE: Extradural hematoma. Statistical survey of 47 cases. J Neurosurg 21:364, 1964

Meeks, LW, Renshaw, TS: Vertebral osteophytosis and dysphagia. J Bone Joint Surg 55A(1):197, 1973

Merkel KD, Brown ML, Dewanjee MK, Fitzgerald RH: Comparison of indium-labeled-leukocyte imaging with sequential technetium-gallium scanning in the diagnosis of low grade musculoskeletal sepsis. A prospective study. J Bone Joint Surg 76A:465, 1985

Meyer, PR: The Decubitus Ulcer is Still With Us. (film). Stryker Corporation. Frank J Corbett, Inc, Chicago, November, 1979

Murray DS: Post-traumatic thrombosis of the internal carotid and vertebral arteries after nonpenetrating injuries of the neck. Br J Surg 44:556, 1957

Nicastro JF, Hartjen, CA, Traina J, Lancaster JM: Intraspinal pathways taken by sublaminar wires during removal. An experimental study. J Bone Joint Surg 68A(8):1206, 1986

Richards T, Hoff J: Factors affecting survival from acute subdural hematoma. Surgery 75:253, 1974

Rogers WA: Cord injury during reduction of thoracic and lumbar vertebral body fracture and dislocation. J Bone Joint Surg 20:689, 1938

Rose J, Valtonen S, Jennett B: Avoidable factors contributing to death after head injury. Br Med J 2:615, 1977

Schneider RC: Transposition of compressed spinal cord in kyphoscoliosis patient with neurological deficits. With special reference to vascular supply of the cord. J Bone Joint Surg 42A:1027, 1960

Schneider RC, Gosch HH, Norrell H, et al: Vascular insufficiency and differential distortion of brain and cord caused by cervicomedullary football injuries. J Neurosurg 33:363, 1970

Schneider RC, Crosby EC: Vascular insufficiency of brain stem and spinal cord in spinal trauma. Neurology 9:643, 1969

Schneider RC, Kahn EA: Chronic neurological sequelae of acute trauma to the spine and spinal cord. Part II. The syndrome of chronic anterior spinal cord injury or compression. Herniated intervertebral discs. J Bone Joint Surg 41A:449, 1959

Schneider RC, Schemm, GW: Vertebral artery insufficiency in acute and chronic spinal trauma. J Neurosurg 18:348, 1961

Schneider RC, Johnson FC: Bilateral traumatic abducens palsy. A mechanism of injury suggested by the study of associated fractures. J Neurosurg 34:33, 1971

Seibel R, LaDuca J, Hassett J, Babikian G et al: Blunt trauma, femur traction and the pulmonary failure-septic state. Ann Surg 202(3):283, 1985

Shover RN, Fortson CH, Theodotou CB: Delayed neurological sequelae of a retained foreign body (lead bullet) in the intervertebral disc space. J Bone Joint Surg 42A;595, 1960

Shrago GG: Cervical spine injuries: association with head trauma. Radiology 118:670, 1973

Silver JR, Morris WR, Ottinowski JS: Associated injuries in patients with spinal injury. Injury 12:219, 1976

Stone WA, Beach TP, Hamelberg W: Succinylcholine: danger in spinal cord injured patient. Anesthesiology 32:168, 1970

Stringer WL, Kelly Jr DJ: Traumatic dissection of the extra cranial internal carotid artery. Neurosurgery 6:123, 1980

Sumner D: On testing the sense of smell. Lancet ii:895, 1962

Summers CG, Wirthschafter JD: Bilateral trigeminal and abducens neuropathies following low velocity, crushing head injury. J Neurosurg 50:508, 1979

Thomas ET: Circulatory collapse following succinylcholine: report of a case. Anesth Analg 48:333, 1969

Tobey RE: Paraplegia, succinylocholine and cardiac arrest. Anesthesiology 32:359, 1970

Turner JWA: Indirect injuries of the optic nerve. Brain 66:140, 1943

Woodhurst WB, Robertson WD, Thompson GB: Carotid injury due to intraoral trauma: case report and review of the literature. Neurosurgery 6:599, 1980

Wright RL: Traumatic hematomas of the posterior cranial fossa. J Neurosurg 25:402, 1966

HEAD INJURY AND RESEARCH

Bolender N, Cromwell LD, Wendling L: Fracture of the occipital condyle. AJR 131:729, 1978

Brown FD, Mullan S, Duda EE: Delayed traumatic intracerebral hematomas. J Neurosurg 48:1019, 1978

Caton R: The electric currents of the brain. Br Med J 2:278, 1875

Caton R: Interim report on investigation of the electric currents of the brain. Br Med J (Supp) 1:62, 1877

Cerullo LJ, Raimondi AJ: Neurological emergencies. p. 297. In Beal JM (ed): Critical Care for Surgical Patients. Macmillan, New York, 1982

Cooper PR, Ho V: Role of emergency skull x-ray films in the evaluation of the head-injured patient: A retrospective study.

Cordobes F, Lobato R, Rivas JJ: Observations of 82 patients with extradural hematoma. J Neurosurg 54:179, 1981

Einhorn A, Mizrahi, EM: Basilar skull fractures in children the incidence of CNS infection and the use of antibiotics. Am J Dis Child 132:1121, 1978

Eismont FJ, Bohlman, HH: Posterior atlanto-occipital dislocation with fractures of the atlas and odontoid process. Report of a case with survival. J Bone Joint Surg 60A:397, 1978

Gabrielsen TO, Maxwell JA: Traumatic atlanto-occipital dislocation. With case report of a patient who survived. AJR 97:624, 1966

Galbraith S, Murray WR, Patel AR, Knill-Jones R: The relationship between alcohol and head injury and its effect on the conscious level. Br J Surg 63:128, 1976

Gennarelli TA: Cervical concussion and diffuse brain injuries. p 83. In Cooper, PR (ed): Head Injuries. Williams & Wilkins, Baltimore, 1982

Gianotta SL, Weiss MH, Apuzzo MLJ, Martin E: High dose glococorticoids in the management of severe head injury. Neurosurgery 15:497, 1984

Harding-Smith J, MacIntosh, PK, Sherbon KJ: Fracture of the occipital condyle. J Bone Joint Surg 63A(7):1170, 1981

Ingelzi RJ, Vander Ark GD: Analysis of the treatment of basilar skull fractures with and without antibiotics. J Neurosurg 43:721, 1975

Jacoby CG: Fracture of the occipital condyle. AJR 132:500, 1979

Marshall LF, Smith RW, Shapiro HM: Outcome with aggressive treatment in severe head injuries. II. Acute and chronic barbiturate administration in the management of head injury. J Neurosurg 50:26, 1979

Miller JD, Sakalas R, Ward JD, et al: Methyleprednisolone treatment in the patient with brain tumors. Neurosurgery 1:114, 1977

Miller JD, Sweet RC, Narayan R, Becker DP: Early insults to the injured brain. JAMA 240:439, 1978

Newlon, PG, Greenberg RP, Hyatt MS, et al: The dynamics of neuronal dysfunction and recovery following severe head injury assessed with serial multimodality evoked potentials. J Neurosurg 57:168, 1982

Phonprasert C, Suwanwela C, Hongsaprabhas D, et al: Extradural hematoma: analysis of 138 cases. J Trauma 20:679, 1980

Plum F, Posner JB: The Diagnosis of Stupor and Coma. 3rd Ed. EA Davis, Philadelphia, 1980

Porter RW: Some problems in the management of the spinal cord injury patient with associated head or facial trauma. Proc Veterans Administration Spinal Cord Injury Conf 19:29, 1973

Robinson BP:, Seeger JF, Zak, SM: Rheumatoid arthritis and position vertebrobasilar insufficiency. J Neurol 65:111, 1986

Rockoff MA, Marshall LF, Shapiro HM: High dose barbiturate therapy in humans: A clinical review of 60 patients. Ann Neurol 3:83, 1979

Rosenbluth, PR, Arias B, Quartetti EV, Carney AL: Current management of subdural hematoma. Analysis of 100 consecutive cases JAMA 179:759, 1962

Rovit RL, Murali R: Injuries of the cranial nerves. p. 99. In Cooper, PR (ed): Head Injury. Williams & Wilkins, Baltimore, 1982

Russell WR, Smith A: Post-traumatic amnesia in closed head injury. Arch Neurol 5:16, 1961

Rutherford WH: Diagnosis of alcohol ingestion in mild head injuries. Lancet i:1021, 1977

Sage JI, Van Uitert RL: "Man-In-The-Barrel" syndrome. Neurology 26:1102, 1986

Smith HP, Challa VR, Alexander E: Odontoid compression of the brain in a patient with rheumatoid arthritis: Case report. J Neurosurg 53:841, 1980

Sherman DG, Hart RG, Easton JD: Abrupt change in head position and cerebral infarction. Stroke 12:2, 1981

Teasdale G, Jennett B: Assessment of coma and impaired consciousness. A practical scale. Lancet ii:81, 1974

Teasdale G, Jennett B: Assessment and prognosis of coma after head injury. Acta Neurochir (Wien) 34:45, 1976

Weiss MH: Head trauma and spinal cord injuries: diagnostic and therapeutic criteria. Crit Care Med 2:311, 1974

Wertheim SB, Bohlman HH: Occipitocervical fusion, indications, technique and long-term results of thirteen patients. J Bone Joint Surg 69A(6):833, 1987

RELATED RESEARCH IN SPINAL CORD INJURY

Albin MS, White RJ, Acosta-Rua G, Yashor D: Study of functional recovery produced by delayed localized cooling after spinal cord injury in primates. J Neurosurg 29:113, 1968

Allen AR: Surgery of experimental lesions of spinal cord equivalent to crush injury of fracture dislocation of spinal column. JAMA 57:878, 1911

Bowman, WC, Nott MW: Actions of sympathomimetic amines and their antagonists on skeletal muscle. Pharm. Rev 21:27, 1969

Brachken, MB, Collins WF, Freeman DF, et al: Efficacy of methylprednisolone in acute spinal cord injury JAMA (1)251:45, 1984

Cook SD, Harding BS, Whitecloud TS, et al: A clinical

and metallurigical analysis of 28 retrieved harrington rods. Contemp Orthop 12(5):27, 1986

De la Torre JC, Johnson CM, Goode DJ, et al: Pharmacologic treatment and evaluation of permanent experimental spinal cord trauma. Neurology 25:508, 1975

Dichiro G, Fried LC, Doppman JL: Experimental spinal cord angiography. Br J Radiol 43:19, 1970

Ducker TB, Hamit HF: Experimental treatment of acute spinal cord injury. J Neurosurg 30:693, 1969

Ducker TB, Saleman M, Perot Jr PL, Ballentine D: Experimental spinal cord trauma. I: Correlation of blood flow, tissue oxygen and neurologic status in the dog. Surg Neurol 10:60, 1978

Ducker TB, Saleman M, Lucas J, et al: Experimental spinal cord trauma. II. Blood flow, tissue oxygen, evoked potentials in both paretic and plegic monkeys. Surg Neurol 10:64, 1978

Ducker TB, Saleman M, Daniell HB: Experimental spinal cord trauma. III. Therapetuic effects of immobilization and pharmacologic agents. Surg Neurol 10:71, 1978

Faden AI, Jacobs TP, Holaday JW: Thyrotropin-releasing hormone improves neurologic recovery after spinal trauma in cats. N Engl J Med 305:1063, 1981

Flamm, ES, Young W, Demopoulos HB, et al: Experimental spinal cord injury: treatment with naloxone. Neurosurg 10:227, 1982

Gosch HH, Gooking E, Schneider RC: An experimental study of cervical spine and cord injuries. J Trauma 12:570, 1972

Gudeman, SK, Miller JD, Becker D: Failure of high-dose steroid therapy to influence intracranial pressure in patients with severe head injury. J Neurosurg 51:301, 1979

Hall ED, Braughler JM: Glucocorticoids mechanisms in the acute spinal cord injury. A review and therapeutic rationale. Surg Neurol 18:320, 1982

Kobrine AL, Evans DE, Rizzoli HV: Experimental acute balloon compression of the spinal cord. J Neurosurg 51:841, 1979

Lucas DB, Bresler B: Stability of the Ligamentous Spine. Technical Report 40. P. 312. Biomechanics Laboratory, University of California, San Francisco, 1961. The Laboratory 312-317, 1982

Markolf, KL: Deformation of the thoracolumbar inter-

vertebral joint in response to external loads: a biomechanical study using autopsy material. J Bone and Joint Surg 54A:511, 1972

Martin SH, Bloedel JR: Evaluation of experimental spinal cord injury using cortical evoked potentials. J Neurosurg 39:75, 1973

Osterholm J, Matthews GJ: Altered norepinephrine metabolism following experimental spinal cord injury. Part I: relationship to hemorrhagic necrosis and postwounding neurological deficits. J Neurosurg 36:384, 1972

Osterholm J, Matthews GJ: Altered norepinephrine metabolism following experimental spinal cord injury. Part II: protection against traumatic spinal cord hemorrhagic necrosis by norepinephrine synthesis blockade with alpha methyl tyrosine. J Neurosurg 36:395, 1972

Osterholm JL: The pathophysiological response to spinal cord injury: the current status of related research. J Neurosurg 40:3, 1974

Pardy RL, Leigh DE: Ventilaory muscle training. Respir Care 29:278, 1984

Roaf R: A study of the mechanics of spinal injuries. J Bone Joint Surg 42B:810, 1960

Saowski HS, Geyer JR, Harman PO, Cane RD: Use of myoelectric and volume-linked feedback for breathing training in a patient with spinal cord injuries. Respir Care 26:130, 1981

Stauffer ES, Neil JL: Biomechanical analysis of structural stability of internal fixation in fractures of the thoracolumbar spine. Clin Orthop 122:159, 1975

White AA, Hirsch C: The significance of the vertebral posterior elements in the mechancis of the thoracic spine. Clin Orthop 81:2, 1971

White AA, Panjabi MM: Clinical Biomechanics of the Spine. JB Lippincott, Philadelphia, 1978

White R: Current status of spinal cord cooling. Clin Neurosurg 20:400, 1973

TEXTBOOKS: ANATOMY AND SPINE

Anderson JE: Grant's Atlas of Anatomy. 7th Ed. Williams & Wilkins, Baltimore, 1978

Bosworth DM: Surgery of the spine. American Academy

of Orthopaedic Surgeons. Instructional Course Lectures 14:39, 1957

Calenoff L (ed.): Radiology in Spinal Cord Injury. CV Mosby, St. Louis, 1981

Carpenter MB: Core Text of Neuroanatomy. 2nd ed. Williams & Wilkins, Baltimore, 1978

Edmonson AS, Crenshaw, AH: The Spine. P. 1939. Campbell's Operative Orthopaedics. 6th Ed. Vol. 2. CV Mosby St. Louis, 1980

Gerlock AJ, Kischner SG, Heller RM, Kay JJ: The Cervical Spine in Trauma. WB Saunders, Philadelphia, 1978

Guttmann L: Spinal cord injuries: comprehensive management and research. Blackwell Scientific Publications, Oxford and FA Davis, Philadelphia, 1973

Hanafee W, Crandall P: Trauma of the spine and its contents. Radiology Clinics N A 4:365, 1966

Louis R: Surgery of the Spine. Surgical Anatomy and Operative Approaches. Springer-Verlag, Berlin, Heidelberg, New York, 1983

Martin J: Positioning in Anesthesia and Surgery. WB Saunders, 1978

Norell HA: Fractures and dislocations of the spine. In Rothman, RH, Simeone FA (eds): The Spine. Vol. 2 Philadelphia, WB Saunders, 1975

Numoto M, Flanagan M, Wallman L, Donaghy R: Proceedings of the 18th Veterans Administration Spinal Injury Conference. Veterans Administration, Washington, D.C., 1971, p. 227

Popp AJ, Bourke RS, Nelson AR, Kimelberg HK: Neural Trauma, Raven Press, New York, 1979

Ruge D, Wiltse L: Spinal Disorders: Diagnosis and Treatment. Lea & Febiger, Philadelphia, 1977

Schaeffer JP: Morris' Human Anatomy: A Complete Systematic Treatise. 11th Ed. The Blakiston Company, New York, 1953

Thorek P: Anatomy in Surgery. JB Lippincott, Philadelphia, 1955

Watson-Jones R: Reaction of bone to metal. p. 205. In Fractures and Joint Injuries, 4th Ed. Vol 1. Williams & Wilkins, Baltimore, 1952

Watson-Jones, R: Fracture and Other Bone and Joint Injuries. p. 641. 1st Ed. ES Livingstone, Edinburgh, 1940

Index

Page numbers followed by *f* represent figures; those followed by *t* represent tables

A

AAOS. *See* American Academy of Orthopaedic Surgeons (AAOS)
Abducens nerve, injury to, 149
Abducens palsy, 149
Accidents
  motor vehicle
    extrication of victim of, 11f, 12
    spinal injury caused by, 531, 531t
    patient transport after, 19–20
  water, preventing spinal injuries in victim of, 12–13, 13f, 14f
Adamkiewicz, artery of, 89, 553
  angiographic visualization of, 258
  with complete neurologic injury, 576f
  injury of
    neurologic function and, 94
    with thoracic spine fracture, 56
  level of entry of, 100, 104–105
Airway
  assessment of, 7
  maintenance of, 7, 157, 161–165
Algorithm, treatment, for spinal cord-multiple trauma management, 40–44
Alkaline phosphatase, in skeletal development, 62
American Academy of Orthopaedic Surgeons (AAOS), Committee on Orthotics and Prosthetics of, technical analysis form for nomenclature, 279
Amipaque. *See* Metrizamide
Anal stretch technique, 272
Anal wink, in assessment of neurologic injury, 10, 10t
Anemia, preoperative, thoracolumbar spine surgery and, 659
Anencephaly, developmental origin of, 69
Anesthesia
  evoked potentials and, 172
  patient position and, 159–160
  for spinal cord injury, 157–172
  technique modifications of, in spinal cord surgery, 171–172

Angiography
  for brain injury evaluation, 152
  in spinal trauma evaluation, 256–260
  for suspected vascular injury, 143, 145
Ankylosing spondylitis, spinal fractures in, 250
Anoxia, in head-injured patients, 147
Antibiotics
  thoracic spine surgery and, 606
  thoracolumbar spine surgery and, 709
Anulus fibrosus
  development of, 72, 77
  removal of, 671
AO-ASIF External Fixator, 770f–772f, 774, 777
AO-ASIF Internal Fixator, 777
AO internal fixator system, in thoracolumbar spine surgery, 696, 699f–700f, 701
AO Synthes-Jacobs rods, 777
  in burst fracture management, 652
  lumbar spine fixation with, 766f–767f, 774
  in thoracic spine surgery, 616–617
  in thoracolumbar spine stabilization, 676
  in thoracolumbar spine surgery, 692–696, 694f–695f, 697f–698f
Aorta, rupture of, radiographic evidence of, 188–189
Aplasia, of odontoid process, 445
Arachnoiditis, associated with iophendylate use, 251
Areflexia, detrusor, 267, 270
Arrhythmia, after spinal cord injury, 166
Arteries
  of Adamkiewicz. *See* Adamkiewicz, artery of
  of anterior cervical spinal cord, 98f
  anterior spinal, 97, 99, 100, 101, 104
    tributaries of, 553
  aortic segmental, 101
  carotid. *See* Carotid artery
  catheterization of, 258

  intercostal. *See* Arteries, segmental
  lateral sacral, 101
  medullary feeder, 101
  posterior inferior cerebellar, 99
  posterior spinal, 99–100, 100f, 101, 104
  segmental, 97
  spinal cord, injury to, 85
  superior intercostal, 100, 104
  of thoracolumbar and sacral spinal cord, 88f
  vertebral, injury to, 143, 144f
    treatment of, 153
Arthritis
  of cervical spine, spine immobility and, 517
  rheumatoid. *See* Rheumatoid arthritis
Articular pillar, fractures of, 223–224
Aspirin, and coagulation failure during surgery, 706, 707–708
Assessment
  neurologic. *See* Neurologic assessment
  patient. *see* Patient assessment
Atlantoaxial joint
  dislocations involving, 381–382
  injuries of, 380–381
Atlas
  anatomy of, 210
  fractures of, 212–213, 213f, 377, 378f, 379
    complications of, 434–435
  radiographic examination of, 204, 207
  transverse ligament injuries involving, 435, 436f, 437, 437f
Atropine, for blocking side effects of vagal nerve stimulation, 166
Autonomic nervous system. *See* Nervous system, autonomic
Avulsion fractures, of vertebral body, 648
Axial load injuries
  effects of, 735
  of thoracic spine, 583
Axis
  anatomy of, 210–211
  fractures of, 213, 215, 216f, 218

Axis (continued)
neural arch of. See Neural arch
odontoid process of. See Dens;
Odontoid process
radiographic examination of, 204,
207
Axonotmesis, defined, 807

B

Back pain, lumbosacral spinal fusion
and, 786–787
Baclofen, in treatment of bladder
dysfunction, 272
Bacteriuria, during catheterization, 270
Balanced forearm orthoses (BFO),
316, 319f
Batson's plexus, 102–105
Bell-Magendie law, 116
Betz cells, 107, 108f
BFO. See Balanced forearm orthoses
(BFO)
Biomechanical forces
and extent of spinal injury, 353,
355, 355t
in lumbar spine injuries, by injury
level, 719t
in lumbar vs. sacral injuries, 718t,
718–719
in spinal injuries, 734–736
in thoracic spine fractures, 574–
575, 575t
in thoracic spine injuries, 531t,
532–534, 534t, 566–567
in thoracolumbar spine fractures,
627, 630t, 631t
neurologic injury and, 630t
in thoracolumbar spine injuries, 722t
Bladder
assessment of, 267–268
cancer of, long-term catheterization
and, 273
distended, autonomic hyper-reflexia
caused by, 166–167
dysfunction of, 267–269
drugs for, 272
management of, 270–273
nervous system control of, 266f
normal function of, 265–267
Bladder training, risks of, 270–271
Bleeding. See also Hemorrhage
rate of, according to type of injury, 8
in spinal surgery, 167–169
in thoracic spine surgery, management of, 606
in thoracolumbar spine surgery,
706–707
Blood flow, spinal cord. See Spinal
cord blood flow (SCBF)
Blood gases, monitoring of, 34
Blood supply, of thoracic spine, 575
Blood transfusion
complications of, 168–169
during spinal surgery, 167–169

Blood vessels, spinal cord. See Vascular
injury; Vascular supply
Body jacket. See Thoracolumbosacral
orthosis (TLSO)
Bohler approach to anterior cervical
stabilization, 469, 470f–474f,
475
Bone
cancellous, bleeding from, 707
injuries of, 290–295
membrane-derived, formation of,
62–63
ossification of, 61, 63
Bone grafts
anterior, dislodgement of, 709
anterior interbody inlay, 406f, 407f
anterior tricortical iliac, 508, 508f
cortical, 409f
direct, 512, 513f–514f
donor procedures for, 505, 508–
509, 510f–511f, 512
effects of, 411, 411f, 412f–413f
iliac crest, in thoracolumbar spine
surgery, 703, 704f–705f,
705–706
of lumbosacral spine, 798–801,
802f–805f
methyl methacrylate and, 503–504
posterior iliac, 440f, 508–509
in thoracic spinal fusion, 607–608
in thoracolumbar spine surgery,
bleeding at site of, 707–708
in thoracolumbar vertebral body,
672f, 673, 673f, 674f
tibial, 509, 510f–511f, 512
tricortical interbody, 589f
Bowel conduit, urinary diversion into,
complications of, 273
Bradycardia
in autonomic hyper-reflexia, 166
with cervical spine injury, 39–40
preganglionic nerve fiber injury and,
114, 116
after spinal cord injury, 165, 166
Brain, topography of, 116f
Brain injury
angiography in evaluation of, 152
primary, 139
secondary, 141
Brainstem auditory evoked response,
122
Breathing
ataxic, 149
difficulties with. See Respiratory
distress
work of, 177–178, 178f
signs of increasing, 182
Breathing exercises, 181
Brooks fusion technique, 500–501,
501f
Callahan modification of, 501
Brown-Séquard syndrome, 203, 353,
363
Bulbocavernosus reflex
in assessment of lumbosacral spinal
injury, 726

in assessment of neurologic injury,
657–658
as indicator of extent of neurologic
injury, 9–10, 10t
interpreting significance of, 93
Burst fractures, 220, 221f
axial load injuries and, 735
as indication for internal fixation, 765
of lumbar spine, 239–241, 240f,
241f–243f, 680f, 743,
756f–759f
of lumbosacral spine, 720f–721f
of thoracic spine, 578, 580
of vertebral body, 616f, 649, 652
distraction-fixation techniques for,
615

C

Cadaver contracture, 306, 307f
Calculi, urinary tract, 273–274
Camp polyethylene collar, 285, 287f
Cancer
bladder, long-term catheterization
and, 273
fractures caused by metastasis of,
248–249, 251f
prostate, metastasis of, to spinal
column, 102
Cardiovascular system, spinal cord
injury and, 165–166
Carotid artery injury to
symptoms of, 143
treatment of, 153
CASH. See Cruciform anterior spinal
hyperextension (CASH) orthosis
Casts, plaster, 285, 288f
Catheter, indwelling, 273
Catheterization
long-term, bladder cancer and, 273
risks of, 272
of spinal cord-injured patient, 38
during spinal shock, 270
Cauda equina, neuroanatomy of, 655
Cell Saver, 167, 167f, 168
in thoracic spine surgery, 606
Cell(s), Betz, 107, 108f
Central cord syndrome, 429, 517, 519f
in thoracolumbar spine surgery, 708
Cerebral edema, computed tomography evaluation of, 151
Cerebral injuries, types of, 137
Cerebral swelling, 140
Cervical hemivertebra, 351, 352f–
353f
Cervical kyphosis, 411
Cervical orthoses, 15f–17f, 41f, 283,
284f, 285, 286f–287f, 288,
288f–289f, 290, 290f
Cervical spine
bony injuries of, 290–295
congenital abnormalities of, 344f,
344–345, 483–484, 485f
conservative management of,
341–395

dislocations of
  delayed traumatic, 230
  facet joint, 45f, 46f, 47f–48f,
      400f–401f, 401, 404f
    anatomic consequences of, 402f
  without fracture, 386, 387f
facet joint of. *See* Facet joints, cervical
fracture-dislocation of, 91f
fractures of, 353, 355
  assessment for, 341–343
  C1 ring, 432, 433f–434f, 434. *See
      also* Atlas, fractures of;
      Jefferson fracture
  compression, 451, 452, 452f,
      453f–454f, 454
  C3 to C7, management of, 386–390
  emergency room reduction of,
      44–49
  extension, 389, 389f
  facet joint, 400f–401f, 401
    unilateral, 453f–454f, 454
  hangman's. *See* Hangman's fracture
  hyperextension, 216, 218, 218f
  medical complications with, 390t,
      390–391
  multiple-level, 387, 388f, 419
  occipital condyle, 375–376
  treatment of, by type, 369t
    by type and extent, 435t
    by type and surgery site, 443t
infection involving, 345f, 345–346,
    374f, 375
injuries of. *See* Cervical spine injuries
instability of, 91, 93, 491
  measurement of, 371, 371f, 372f,
      373–375
lateral tomogram of, 191f
lower, dislocations and fracture-dis-
    locations of, 225–231
manipulation of, 401–403
normal, 205f–206f
  lateral view of, 210f
normal motion of, 370–371
occipitoatlantoaxial area of. *See*
    Occipitoatlantoaxial junction
orthotic management of, 283–295
osteoarthritis of, 344
pathologic processes involving,
    483–484
radiographic examination of, 190,
    204, 205f–206f, 207
radiographs of, difficulty obtaining,
    187, 190f
realignment of, after trauma,
    45–46, 49
reduction of, in emergency room,
    44–46, 49
rheumatoid arthritis of, 373, 373f
splinting of, inappropriate, 18f
spondylosis of, 344, 346, 405, 405f
support of
  during initial assessment, 41f
  during patient transport, 15f, 16f
surgical stabilization of, 391–392,
    397–523. *See also* Cervical
    spine surgery

tear-drop fracture of, with complete
    quadriplegia, 200
theories of structure of, 368
tumor of, 346, 347f–350f
Cervical spine injuries, 26f, 28f–32f
airway management and, 7
altered consciousness from, 147–148
at atlantoaxial joint, 380–381
causes of, 343–350
classification of, 17, 368–370, 397
complications associated with,
    157–158
ear pain with, 389–390
emergency intubation with, 161f
emergency room management of,
    355–359
evoked potentials in evaluation of,
    366–367
extension
  in elderly, 429
  stable and unstable, 419, 424f–
      428f, 429
extrication of patient with, 12,
    13f–16f
flexion, 387–388
  stable, 414, 415f–417f
  unstable, 414, 418f
flexion distraction, 90f
with gross instability, 49f
with head trauma, 138f
hyperextension, 356f, 357f
initial management of, 398–401
isotope scanning in evaluation of,
    367–368
levels of, in quadriplegic patient, 325t
lower, 220–231
magnetic resonance imaging in
    evaluation of, 365–366
management of, factors influencing,
    451
monitoring and limiting neurologic
    injury in first 24 hours,
    361–362
multiple-level, 419
myelography in evaluation of, 412
neurologic assessment with, 357, 359
neurologic trauma and, 351–355
  at occipitoatlantal junction, 376, 376f
polytomography in evaluation of,
    364–365
pulmonary dysfunction associated
    with, 34, 36f
radiographic evaluation of, 364, 365f
respiratory assessment with, 357
rotary fixation, 437–438, 438f–441f
stable, 412, 414
unstable, 412
upper, neurologic syndromes
    accompanying, 429–430
ventilation and, 165
vital signs changes associated with,
    39–40
Cervical spine surgery. *See also*
    specific techniques; Spinal
    fusion
anterior procedures, 462–483

anterior stabilization in, indications
    for, 464, 469
bone graft, effects of, 411, 411f–413f
CO_2 laser for supine dissection in,
    497–498
in elderly patient, 405
immobilization after, 512, 514
with internal fixation techniques,
    397, 398f, 399f, 405,
    406f–409f
neurologic complications of, 514,
    517, 517t
nonunion rate after, 514
occiput-cervical fusion, 484–485,
    488f–489f, 489–492
posterior procedures, 483–505
preoperative considerations in, 404–
    405, 411
sublaminar wire stabilization, 491f,
    491–492, 493f, 494f,
    495–498, 495f–499f
three-level fusion, with anterior
    cervical AO plate-screws,
    475, 479
Cervical traction, application of, 358f,
    359, 360f, 361, 398, 401
  preceding injury diagnosis, 17
Cervicothoracic junction
  radiographs of, difficulty obtaining,
      188
  swimmer's view of, 190, 204, 207f
Cervicothoracic orthosis (CTO), 285
  indications for use of, 290–291
  for thoracic spine injuries, 297
Cervicothoracolumbosacral orthosis
    (CTLSO), 622
  with thoracic spine fracture, 568,
      569f
Chance fractures, 244, 247f
  distraction-flexion, of lumbar spine,
      745f
  of lumbar spine, 743, 743f,
      749f–750f, 750
  of thoracic spine, 611f
Chest
  incision site for, 662, 663f, 664
  injuries of
    minilaparotomy in evaluation of,
        34, 34f–35f
  monitoring of, 545
Cheyne-Stokes respiration, after head
    injury, 149
Chondrification centers, development
    of, 76–77, 78f
Chondroitin sulfate, in skeletal
    development, 62
Chondrosis, neurocentral, 77, 78f
Chordoma, developmental origin of, 82
Circulation, maintenance of, 7–8
Clavicle, ossification of, 63
Clay shoveler's fracture, 222–223,
    225f
Coagulation
  in thoracic spine surgery, 606
  in thoracolumbar spine surgery, 669
Cocaine, during intubation, 161

Coma, Glasgow Scale for assessing, 8, 8t, 148, 148t
Coma vigil, 430
Compression fractures
anterior wedge, 220, 220f
of thoracic spine, 575, 578
of cervical spine, 451, 452, 452f–454f, 454
with retropulsion of C5 vertebral body, 513f–514f
three-level sublaminar wiring to correct, 492f
effects of, 735
flexion injuries and, 735
of lumbar spine, 35f, 697f
of thoracic spine, 532, 532f, 540f, 568, 578, 579f, 679f
Murig-Williams plates in management of, 594f–595f
of thoracolumbar spine, 237, 237f, 239, 645f–646f
unbalanced, of lumbar spine, 784f
of upper dorsal spine, 233, 235
of vertebral body, distraction-fixation techniques for, 615
Compression rods, in thoracic spine surgery, 617–619, 618f, 619f
Computed tomography (CT)
advantages, disadvantages, and indications for, 192
for brain injury evaluation, 151, 151f, 152f
in cervical spine injury evaluation, 364–365
in lumbar spine injury assessment, 729
Concussion, 139
Congenital deformities, spinal, developmental causes of, 80–82
Consciousness
altered
with elevated intracranial pressure, 141
with head injury, 152–153
with intracranial mass, 143
level of
assessment of, 8–9, 148, 148t
with head injury, 147–148
Contracture, cadaver, 306, 307f
Contusion, 140
Conus medullaris, 57f
anastomotic loop of, 95f, 97, 101
arterial vascular supply to, 95f
defined, 655
Corporectomy
cervical, and three-level spinal fusion, 479, 480f–481f, 482–483
of L5 vertebra, 800
of thoracic vertebra, 677–678
of vertebral body, inappropriate use of, 403
Corset, thoracolumbar, 296f, 297
Cortical evoked potentials, in cervical spine injury evaluation,

366–367
Corticobulbar fasciculus motor tract, 108, 108f
Corticospinal fasciculus motor tract, 108, 108f, 109
Corticospinal motor system. See Pyramidal system
Corticosteroids, for head injury treatment, 154
Costochondritis, 558
Cotrel-Dubousset internal stabilization technique, 777, 797–798, 799f–801f
Coughing, with spinal cord injury, 180
Coughing exercises, 181
Craig-Scott knee-ankle-foot orthosis, 335
Cranial nerves, assessment of, 148–149
Cranial vault, development of, 63, 63f
Cranioatlantoaxial articulation, stability of, 370
Craniovertebral angle, injury of, 370
Craniovertebral junction
atlantoaxial dislocation and subluxation involving, 219, 219f
atlantooccipital dislocation involving, 218, 218f
radiographic evaluation of, 210–212
Cranium, stabilization of, 283
Cruciform anterior spinal hyperextension (CASH) orthosis, 296f, 297
Cruciform ligament, rupture of, 343f
Crutchfield tongs, 44f
CTO. See Cervicothoracic orthosis (CTO)
Cushing reflex, 141
Cystometrogram for bladder evaluation, 267–268
Cystourethrograms, of normal and abnormal bladder and urethra, 269f

D

Decadron. See Dexamethasone
Deep venous thrombosis
with cervical spine fracture, 390, 390t
postoperative, prevention of, 520–521
prevention of, 391
with thoracolumbar spinal instability, 633
Dejerine effect, 145f, 149, 430
Demerol. See Meperidine hydrochloride
Denis, Francis, 631–633
Denis theory of spine instability, 601
Dens. See also Odontoid process
anatomy of, 211
apophyseal separations of, 216
fractures of, 215–216, 217f
DEP. See Dermatomal evoked potentials (DEP)

Dermatomal evoked potentials (DEP), 122
in spinal cord injury, 127f, 127–128, 129
Dermatome, development of, 72
Detrusor areflexia, 267, 270
Dexamethasone (Decadron)
for preventing spinal cord edema, 362
for vascular injury management, 87
Diaphragm
innervation of, 165
inadequate, 157
rupture of, with thoracic spine injury, 547f–548f
sensory areas of, 112
Diastasis, spinal, with distraction-type internal fixation, 604
Diazepam (Valium), in initial management of cervical spine injury, 398
Disc, cervical
extrusion of, 589f
herniated, 517, 518f
Disc spaces, intervertebral, radiographic evaluation of, 208
DISH. See Disseminated interstitial spine hyperostosis
Dislocations
of atlantoaxial junction, 381–382
of cervical facet joints, 45f–48f, 402f, 404f, 454–455, 456f–460f, 460–461, 461f–462f, 493f
of cervical spine, 230, 386, 387f
classification criteria for, 634–635
of craniovertebral junction, 211–212
of dorsal spine, 233f–234f, 235, 236f
of lower cervical spine, 225–231
of lumbar spine, 634f
of lumbosacral joint, 56
radiographic interpretation of, 207–210
of thoracic facet joints, 533
Disseminated interstitial spine hyperostosis (DISH), 424f, 427f, 639f–641f
Distraction-extension injuries, effects of, 735
Diuretics, osmotic, for treatment of increased intracranial pressure, 153–154
Dorsal spine
fractures of, 232
radiographic evidence of, 188–189
and multiple-level injuries, 198
radiologic examination of, 232–233
upper
compression fractures of, 233, 235
fracture dislocations of, 233f, 233f–234f, 235, 236f
fractures of, 231–235
Drug abuse, screening patient for, 38
Drugs
for autonomic hyper-reflexia, 166–167

hemorrhage resulting from preoperative use of, 706
for preventing deep venous thrombosis, 391
in treatment of bladder dysfunction, 272
Dunn internal fixator, 710f–711f
loss of, 709
Dura mater
formation of, 63
tears of, 256

E

Ectoderm, development of, 64, 65f, 76
Edema
cerebral, computed tomography evaluation of, 151
spinal cord, prevention of, 362
Ejaculation, in spinal cord-injured patient, 274–275
Elderly patient
cervical spine extension injury in, 429
cervical spine surgery in, 405
Electroejaculation, 274
Embolus, pulmonary, 760f
Embryo, 65f, 66f–69f
development of
major stages of, 65t
stages of, 64–77
Emergency room
assessment of spinal cord and related injuries in, 23–60
cervical spine injury management in, 355–359
protocol for, 31–38
Endochondral ossification, 61, 63
Engen orthosis system, 308, 310f
Entoderm, development of, 64, 66f, 76
Epinephrine, for reducing blood loss during surgery, 167
ERV. See Expiratory reserve volume (ERV)
Esophagus, trauma of, 114
Ethanol, altered consciousness from, 147
Evoked potentials
as adjunct to clinical examination, 132
in cervical spine injury evaluation, 366–367
compared with other diagnostic tools, 129
future applications of, 132–133
in head injury evaluation, 128–129
inhalation agents and, 172
in monitoring experimental animal surgery, 130–131
in monitoring spinal surgery, 129–132
multimodality, in head trauma evaluation, 129
in multiple trauma evaluation, 128–129
over lumbar spine, 123
over scalp, 123–124

principles of, 121–124
in spinal cord function evaluation, 121–136
from stimulation of posterior tibial nerve, 123f
system for measurement of, 122, 122f
typical, waveforms of, 123f
Expiratory reserve volume (ERV), 173, 176, 176f
with spinal cord injury, 179
Extension-dislocations
classification criteria for, 638–639, 641
management of, 641–642
neurologic injuries with, 641
Extension fractures, 542–543
Extension injury, of thoracic spine, 583
Eyes, injury to, 148

F

Facet joints
cervical
dislocation of, 493f, 520, 520f
anatomic consequences of, 402f
bilateral, 460–461, 461f–462f
unilateral, 454–455, 456f–459f, 460
fracture of, 400f–401f, 401
radiographic evaluation of, 208
unilateral dislocation of, pathologic consequences of, 456f, 459f
dislocation of
flexion-distraction forces and, 734
management of, 777, 779–780
fractures of, 223–224, 243
unilateral, 581–583, 584f–586f
of lumbosacral spine, bilateral dislocation of, 753f–754f
midlumbar spine, dislocation of, 748f
thoracic
dislocation of, 533
rotational injury and, 629f
Facet locking
bilateral, of lower cervical spine, 225–226, 226f
unilateral, 226–227, 227f
of upper dorsal spine, 235
Femur, comminuted transverse fracture of, 591f
Fetus, development of, 64–80
major stages of, 65t
FEV₁. See Forced expiratory volume
Flexion-dislocations
classification criteria for, 635
with neurologic injury, 635
treatment of, 635, 638
Flexion-distraction injuries, effects of, 735
Flexion injuries
of cervical spine, 90f, 387–388, 414, 415f–417f, 418
sternal occipital mandibular immobilizer (SOMI) in treatment of, 421f–423f

effects of, 735
of lumbar spine, 719
neurologic, 341
of thoracic spine, 538–539, 567, 576f
of thoracolumbar spine, 719
Follicle-stiumulating hormone (FSH), in spinal cord-injured patient, 274
Fontanels, closure of, 63
Foot orthoses, 338f
Forced expiratory spirogram, 174, 175f
Forced expiratory volume (FEV₁), 175
with spinal cord injury, 179
Forced vital capacity (FVC), 175, 175f
with spinal cord injury, 179
Four-poster orthosis, 285, 288, 291f
Fracture-dislocations
of cervical spine, 225–231
hyperextension, 231
classification criteria for, 642–643
management of, 643, 647–648
neurologic injuries with, 643
of thoracic spine, 637f–638f
of thoracolumbar spine, Harrington rod-sublaminar wire in management of, 642f
Fractures
in ankylosing spondylitis, 250
of anterior arch, 212–213
avulsion, of vertebral body, 648
burst. See Burst fractures
of cervical spine. See Cervical spine, fractures of
Chance. See Chance fractures
compression. See Compression fractures
of craniovertebral junction, 211–212
hangman's. See Hangman's fracture
Jefferson, 212–213, 214f–215f, 373, 377, 378f, 379
Kaufer and Hayes classification of, 745–747
multiple-level, 419
multiple-level noncontiguous, 198, 202f
of neural arch, 212–213
radiographic interpretation of, 207–210
of sacral spine, 801, 805, 806f
skull, types of, 139
spinal, mechanism of, 198–199, 203
tear-drop, 218f, 220, 222f
of cervical spine, 200
of thoracic spine. See Thoracic spine, fractures of
of thoracolumbar spine. See Thoracolumbar spine, fractures of
unilateral laminar, 429
wedge compression. See Wedge compression fractures
Frankel scale of neurologic function, 712, 712t, 713t, 714t
FRC. See Functional residual capacity (FRC)

FSH. *See* Follicle-stimulating hormone (FSH)
Functional residual capacity (FRC), 174, 174f, 176, 176f
  with spinal cord injury, 179, 180
Fusion, spinal. *See* Spinal fusion
FVC. *See* Forced vital capacity

G

Galen, spinal trauma reports of, 761
Gallie fusion technique, 498, 500
Gallium-67, in cervical spine injury evaluation, 367
Ganglion, spinal, development of, 76
Garber fusion technique, Meyer modification of, 496–497, 499f
Garber-Meyer fusion technique, 440f, 494f, 499f
Gardner-Wells tong traction, 41f, 42f, 43f, 45–46, 47f–48f, 291, 292, 293f, 358f, 361f, 479
  for cervical spine realignment, 425f
  in initial management of cervical spine injury, 398
  with rotary fixation injury, 438, 438f–439f
  with unilateral facet joint dislocation, 455, 460
Gas myelography, 251, 254
Gastric ulceration, prophylactic management of, 391
Genu valgum, orthotic management of, 331
Genu varum, orthotic management of, 331
Germ layers, development of, 64, 64f
Gestation, stages of, 64–77
Glasgow Coma Scale, 8, 8t, 148, 148t
  with quadriplegic patients, 148t
Guilford two-poster orthosis, 285, 288, 291f
Gunshot wounds
  angiographic examination after, 258, 258f–259f
  paraplegia caused by, 248f, 249f
  spinal injury caused by, 531, 531t, 532
  of thoracic spine, 567
    neurologic injuries and, 555f, 557
  of thoracolumbar spine, 652, 653f, 743f–744f

H

Halo vest orthosis
  with Jefferson fracture, 434
  low-profile, 292, 293f
  during occiput-cervical spine fusion, 491
  postoperative indications for, 512
Hand
  orthoses for, 309f–310f
  resting position of, 306, 306f

Hangman's fracture, 28f, 213, 215, 216f, 447–451, 448f, 449f, 450f
  of cervical spine, 36f, 162f–164f
    transient quadriparesis with, 200
  classification of, 448–449
  Effendi classification of, 383, 383f, 384
  mechanism of, 447
Harrington compression rods, 621, 777
  in thoracic spine surgery, 617
Harrington distraction-compression rods, in thoracic fracture management, 598f–599f
Harrington distraction rods, 621, 777
  in burst fracture management, 652
  for fracture-dislocations, 644f
  insertion of, 790f
  loss of, 709, 711–712
  for lumbar burst fracture stabilization, 784, 785f–786f
  lumbar spine fixation with, 768f, 774
  procedure for, 615–616, 616f
  in scoliosis management, problems with, 593, 596
  in thoracolumbar spine surgery, 678, 680f–683f, 683, 684f–687f, 688, 694f
  for unilateral compression fracture treatment, 582, 586f, 588f
Harrington hooks
  sacral alae fixation of, 790–791, 791f
  sacral fixation of, 791, 795
  in sacral spine, unreliability of, 787
Harrington rods, in thoracolumbar spine stabilization, 676–677, 677f
Head injuries
  assessment of patient with, 146–152
  closed, 137
  definitions of, 137
  evoked potentials in evaluation of, 128–129
  hysteria with, 150
  incidence of, 145–146
  neurologic assessment and management of, 137–156
  primary, definitions pertaining to, 139–141
  radiologic evaluation of, 150–152
  respiratory assessment after, 149–150
  somatosensory evoked potentials in evaluation of, 126
  with spinal cord injury, 25f
  with spinal injury, 145–146
  treatment of, 152–154
  vascular injury mimicking, 143, 145
  vital sign changes associated with, 40
Heart, loss of sympathetic nervous system function and, 114, 119
Hematology evaluation, in differential diagnosis, 38
Hematoma, 249
  at bone graft site, 707–708

computed tomography evaluation of, 151f, 151–152, 152f
  epidural, with skull fracture, 139
  extradural, 140–141
    myelographic finding of, 254
  with head injury, 150
  indications of, 203
  mediastinal, and fracture or fracture-dislocation of dorsal spine, 233, 233f
  paraspinal, 577f
  retropharyngeal, as indication of hyperextension injury, 210
  after spinal cord injury, 544
  subdural, traumatic acute, 140
  treatment of, 153
Hematomyelia, 235, 256
  myelographic view of, 256f–257f
Hemimelia, developmental causes of, 80
Hemivertebra
  cervical, 351, 352f–353f
  developmental origin of, 81
Hemodilution, for reducing blood loss, 167–168
Hemopneumothorax
  with cervical spine injury, 34, 36f
  thoracolumbar spine surgery and, 659
Hemorrhage. *See also* Bleeding
  control of, 8
  in thoracolumbar spine surgery, 706
Hemothorax, 4f
  with cervical spine injury, 36f
  with spinal cord injury, 547f
  with thoracic spine fracture, 53f, 545
  with thoracic spine injury, 551f, 579f
Hip, basilar neck-intertrochanteric fracture of, 591f
Hip-knee-ankle-foot orthoses (HKAFOs), 329, 331f
  for hip stability, 335–336
  for paraplegic patient, 334
Hippocrates, extension-bench technique of, 761
HKAFO. *See* Hip-knee-ankle-foot orthoses
Holdsworth, Frank, 627, 631–632
Horner's syndrome, 149
Hyaluronic acid, in skeletal development, 62
Hydronephrosis, bladder training and, 270–271
Hyper-reflexia, autonomic, spinal surgery and, 166–167
Hyperemia, after spinal cord injury, 124
Hypertension
  in autonomic hyper-reflexia, 166
  after spinal cord injury, 166
Hyperventilation
  central neurogenic (CNH), 149
  for reducing intracranial pressure, 153
Hypoplasia, of odontoid process, 445

Hypotension
  deliberate, for reducing blood loss, 167
  preganglionic nerve fiber injury and, 114, 116
  with spinal cord injury, 39, 165
Hypothermia
  with cervical spine injury, 39–40
  preganglionic nerve fiber injury and, 114, 116
  for preventing spinal cord edema, 362
  after spinal cord injury, 165
Hypovolemia, vital sign changes with, 40
Hypoxemia, with spinal cord injury, 179–180
Hysteria, with head injury, 150

I

IC. See Inspiratory capacity (IC)
ICP. See Intracranial pressure (ICP)
Illinois Categorization Law of 1972, 3
Illinois State Emergency Medical Service (Trauma) Program, 23
Incontinence, 267
Indium-111, in cervical spine injury evaluation, 367
Infection
  of cervical spine, 345f, 345–346, 374f, 375
  pulmonary, thoracolumbar spine surgery and, 659
  in thoracolumbar spine surgery, 708–709
Inspiratory capacity (IC), 174, 174f
Inspiratory reserve volume (IRV), 173, 174, 174f
Internal fixation techniques. See also specific devices
  blood loss by type of, 708t
  in cervical spine surgery, 397, 398f, 399f, 405, 406f, 407f
  distraction-type
    diastasis with, 604
    in lumbosacral spine, 788–789
    in thoracic spine surgery, 615–617
    in thoracolumbar spine surgery, 678, 679f–683f, 683, 684f–687f, 688
  indications for, 765–766
  for lumbosacral spine, 788–801
  neurologic injury with, 603–604
  in thoracic spine surgery, 603–604
Intracranial pressure (ICP)
  increased
    brain injury caused by, 141
    treatment of, 153–154
  monitoring of, 154
Intracranial pressure-compliance curve, 141f
Intubation
  nasotracheal
    awake blind, 163f, 164, 164f

awake fiberoptic, 161, 161f, 163f, 164, 164f
  rigid oral, 165
Iophendylate (Pantopaque), adverse effects of, 251
IRV. See Inspiratory reserve volume (IRV)
Ischemia
  brain stem, altered consciousness with, 147
  cerebral, 143
  spinal cord, 544, 544f
  vascular. See Vascular ischemia
Isotope scanning, in cervical spine injury evaluation, 367–368

J

Jackets, plaster, 294f
Jefferson fracture, 212–213, 214f–215f, 373, 377, 378f, 379, 432, 433f–434f, 434
Jewett hyperextension orthosis, with lumbosacral spine fracture, 819f
Jewett orthosis, 295, 295f

K

KAFO. See Knee-ankle-foot orthoses
Kefzol, in thoracolumbar spine surgery, 709
Kidney stones, 273–274
Kirschner wires, for determining anterior longitudinal ligament integrity, 582f–583f
Klippel-Feil syndrome, 351, 352f–353f, 483
Kümmell phenomenon, 241
Knee, excessive flexion of, orthotic management of, 331
Knee-ankle-foot orthoses (KAFO), 329, 331f
  for genu valgum, 334f
  for paraplegic patient, 335
Knight lumbosacral orthosis, 301, 301f
Knight-Taylor orthosis, 297, 297f, 298, 298f–299f
  with lumbosacral joint fracture, 818f–819f
  with thoracic spine fracture, 568, 569f
  after thoracic spine surgery, 609, 609f
Kyphosis
  of cervical spine, 411
  of lumbar spine, 782
    secondary to vertebral collapse, 632f
  of thoracic spine, 567
  with thoracolumbar spine fracture, 683
  with unilateral vertebral body fracture, 582

L

Laminae, fractures of, 223f, 224
Laminar fracture, unilateral, 429
Laminectomy, posterior, inappropriate use of, 403
Laparotomy, exploratory, 34f–35f
Larynx, trauma of, 114
Laser, CO_2, in cervical spine surgery, 497–498
Lateral flexion injuries, effects of, 735
Lehneis orthosis system, 308, 309f
Lesions, posterior fossa, 150
Ligament
  anterior longitudinal
    electrocautery dissection of, 669, 671f
    with thoracolumbar and lumbar spinal injuries, 580–581, 582f–583f
  cruciform, rupture of, 343f
  injury of, after spinal fusion, 519–520
  transverse, atlas injuries involving, 435, 436f, 437, 437f
Limbs. See Lower limb; Upper limb
Lipomeningocele, 81f
Litholapaxy, 274
Lithotripsy
  electrohydraulic, 274
  extracorporeal shock wave, 273
Locked-in syndrome, 430
Low-temperature-plastic orthosis system, 308, 310f
Lower limb
  alignment of, 326–328
  biomechanics of, 328–333
  orthotic management of, 325–326
  Technical Analysis Form for, 326–328, 327f–330f
Lumbar spine
  burst compression fracture of, 756f–759f
  Chance fracture of, 742, 742f
  compression fracture of, 202f, 237, 238f, 239
    unbalanced, 784f
  defined, 525, 717
  disc space infection in, 102
  dislocation of, 634f
  emergency room reduction of, 56
  evoked potentials over, 123
  extension fracture-dislocation of, 737f–738f
  extension injuries of, 752–753
  flexion-distraction injury of, 747f–748f, 748, 748f, 750
  fracture-dislocation of, 769f
  fracture-dislocation reduction in, 794f–795f
  fractures of, 237–246
    burst, 680f
    Chance, 746f
    classification of, 744–754
    compared with sacral fractures, 744t

Lumbar spine (continued)
  fulcrum, 244
  initial evaluation of, 724, 726–727
  management of
    conservative, 756–765
    by fracture type, 749t
    multiple trauma with, 723t,
      723–724
    transfer of patient with, 727
    transverse, 244–246, 247f
  fusion in development of, 77, 79
  injuries of
    biomechanical, etiologic, and
      fracture patterns of, 741–744
    biomechanical forces involved in,
      718–719
    bone scanning of, with technetium
      99m, 733
    complications associated with, 158
    distraction-type, 777, 779
    extension, 740f–742f
    magnetic resonance imaging in
      assessment of, 731
    medical complications with, 760t
    paraplegia resulting from, 337
    radiographic evaluation of,
      727–730
    somatosensory evoked potentials
      in assessment of, 732
    statistics on, 718t, 718–719, 719t
  loss of correction in, 780f–781f
  with lower-extremity injuries, 724
  orthotic management of, after
    surgery, 817–819
  radiographic examination of,
    190–191, 237
  stability of, 744–754
  stabilization of
    compared with sacral spine
      stabilization, 769t
    surgical, 766–777
      neurologic function and, 786
  surgical management of, 780–786
  transpedicular screw insertion in,
    774f–775f
  tumor of, 732f–733f
Lumbosacral orthosis (LSO), 301f, 303f
  indications for, 300
Lumbosacral spine
  bone graft of, 798–801, 802f–805f
  dislocation of, 56
  distraction rod systems and,
    complications with, 788–789
  flexion-distraction dislocation of,
    751f–752f, 752
  fractures of, 813f–816f
    axial load burst, 720f–721f
    multiple-level, 808f–809f
    neurologic injuries with, 719,
      722t, 722–723, 723t
  internal fixation procedures for,
    788–801
  orthotic management of, 300–302
  stabilization of, surgical, 786–787
Lung capacity, total (TLC), 174, 174f

defined, 173
  with spinal cord injury, 179
Lung compliance, 177, 177f
Lungs
  bleeding from, in thoracolumbar
    spine surgery, 707
  elastic forces of, 176–177
  relationship of, to thorax, 176, 176f
Luque rods
  applications of, in thoracic spine
    surgery, 610, 612f, 612–615,
    613f, 614f
  in burst fracture management, 652
  with cervical extension fracture-dis-
    location, 738f
  indications and hazards with, 604
  loss of, 709, 711–712
  sacral fixation of, 795–796, 796f,
    797f
  scoliosis management with, spinal
    fractures and, 596
  in thoracolumbar spine surgery,
    676, 688–689, 691f,
    691–692
Luque wire, sacral insertion of, 793f
Luteinizing hormone (LH), in spinal
  cord-injured patient, 274

M

Magerl, Fritz, 397
Magerl device, 397, 398f, 777
  lumbar spine fixation with, 770f–
    772f
Magnetic resonance imaging (MRI)
  in cervical spine injury evaluation,
    365–366
  in lumbar spine injury assessment,
    730
Man-in-the-barrel syndrome, 430
Mandible, ossification of, 63
Manipulation, cervical spine, 401–403
Marie-Strümpell rheumatoid spondy-
  litis, 411, 631
  with cervical hyperextension
    fracture-dislocation, 736f
  cervical reduction with, 410f
  with pattern A spinal injury, 755
  postoperative immobilization of pa-
    tients with, 512, 515f
Mechanical forces. See Biomechanical
  forces
Meninges, tears of, 256
Meningocele, 81f, 82
Menstrual cycle, in spinal cord-injured
  patient, 275
Meperidine hydrochloride (Demerol),
  in initial management of
    cervical spine injury, 398
Mesoderm, development of, 65f,
  66–67, 76
Metastatic disease, fractures caused
  by, 248–249, 251f
Methyl methacrylate, bone graft
  technique and, 503–504

Metrizamide (Amipaque), adverse effects of, 251
Meyer cervical orthosis, 41f, 283, 284f
Meyer fusion technique, 462f
Micturition, nervous system control of,
  265–266
Midazolam hydrochloride (Versed), in
  initial management of cervical
  spine injury, 398
Midwest Regional Spinal Cord Injury
  Care System (MRSCICS), 1,
  27, 197, 198
  catchment area for, 2f, 3
  history of, 23
Minilaparotomy, with signs of lower
  chest trauma, 34, 34f–35f
Morphine, in management of cervical
  spine injury, 398, 401
MRSCICS. see Midwest Regional
  Spinal Cord Injury Care System (MRSCICS)
Murig-Williams plates, 593, 594f, 595f
Muscle relaxants
  in initial management of cervical
    spine injury, 398
  spinal cord injury and, 166
Muscles
  extraocular, assessment of, 149
  intercavitary paraspinous, 558, 562
  of thorax and thoracic spine,
    557–562
  of ventilation, 175–176
  ventilatory
    fatigue of, 178–179, 182
    increasing strength of, 181
Myelography
  in cervical spine injury evaluation,
    412
  gas, 251, 254
  indications for, 254, 732–735
  in lumbar spine injury evaluation,
    729–730
  in neurologic injury evaluation, 363
  in spinal injury evaluation, 250–256
Myelomeningocele, 81f, 82
  developmental origin of, 69
Myotome, development of, 72

N

Neck, anterior, injury to, 28f–30f
Neo-Synephrine. See Phenylephrine
  hydrochloride
Nerve fibers
  conduction speeds of, 117–118
  preganglionic, injury of, 116
  types of, 117
Nerve palsy
  with cervical injuries, 148
  cranial, as complication of atlas
    fracture, 434
Nerve roots
  avulsions of, myelographic finding
    of, 254, 254f–255f, 256

disease of, dermatomal evoked potentials in evaluation of, 127–128
distribution of, 9f
embryonic development of, 69–70
injuries of, 540
spinal, 117
Nerves
abducens, injury to, 149
cranial, assessment of, 148–149
laryngeal, 462–463, 463f
oculomotor, injury to, 148
olfactory, assessment of, 148
optic, injury to, 148
parasympathetic, lumbosacral spine surgery and, 799–800
phrenic. *See* Phrenic nerve
pudendal, in bladder function, 266
spinal, 37f
sympathetic, lumbosacral spine surgery and, 799–800
vagus, relationship of, to carotid artery, 462–463, 463f
Nervous system
anatomy of, 107–119
autonomic, 107
embryonic development of, 69–70
in bladder function, 265–266, 266f
central, and communication with peripheral nervous system, 92f
embryonic and fetal developmental events of, sequence of, 62t
embryonic development of, 69–70, 70f–71f
parasympathetic autonomic, 118
prenatal development of, 61–62
sympathetic
loss of function of, 114, 116
overactivity of, 158
spinal cord injury and, 165
Neural arch
failed fusion of, 82
fractures of, 212, 447–451. *See also* Hangman's fracture
sacral, fusion of, 79
Neural crest, development of, 76
Neural tube
development of, 67
differentiation of, 69–70
failed closure of, 82
Neurapraxia, defined, 807
Neuroanatomy, 107–119
of respiratory system, 112–114, 113f
Neuroectoderm, differentiation of, 71f
Neurologic assessment, 8–9, 357, 359
in emergency room, 9–10
form for, 730f
with head injury, 147
perianal, 9–10, 10t
Neurologic function
level of, 8t, 9
lumbar spine surgical stabilization and, 786
myelography in evaluation of, 412
potential for loss of, from cervical

spine surgery, 404
with thoracic spine fracture, 568–569
after thoracolumbar vs. lower spine surgery, 712t
Neurologic injuries
with cervical spine fracture, 390, 390t
cervical spine injury and, 44–45, 351–355
complete vs. incomplete, defined, 158–159
with extension-dislocations, 641
extent of, and level of spine fracture, 27t
from flexion-dislocations, 635
with fracture-dislocations, 643
with internal fixation devices, 603–604
with lumbar spine fractures, 722–723
with lumbar vs. sacral fractures, 722t
with lumbosacral fractures, 719, 722t, 722–723, 723t
monitoring and limiting of, in first 24 hours, 361–362
myelography in evaluation of, 363
with rotation injuries, 540
with sacral fractures, 805, 807
secondary to vascular changes, 89–94
with spine trauma, 51t
symptoms of, 89
of thoracic spine, 579f
without fracture, 575, 577f
with thoracic spine injuries, 554–557, 555f, 567, 573
of thoracolumbar spine, 654–658
in thoracolumbar spine surgery, 708
types of, 807
Neurologic shock, preventing, 362–363
Neurotmesis, defined, 807
Nitroglycerine, for autonomic hyper-reflexia, 166
Nitrous oxide, somatosensory evoked potentials and, 172
Northwestern University, 1, 23, 31
Northwestern University Medical School, approach to evoked potential evaluation of spinal cord injury, 128
Northwestern University Spine Injury Center, 137
Notochord
development of, 64, 65f, 66, 66f
mucoid degeneration of, 77
Nucleus pulposus, development of, 72, 77

O

Occipital condyle, fractures of, 375–376

Occipitoatlantal joint
injuries of, 376, 376f
instability of, 489
Occipitoatlantoaxial junction, injury to, 429–432, 432f
Occiput-cervical spine
fusion of, 484–485, 488f–489f, 489–492
ligamentous anatomy of, 436f
Oculomotor nerves, injury to, 148
Odontoid process. *See also* Dens
amputation of, 485, 489
deformities involving, 445, 446f
displacement of, neurologic deficit from, 517
erosion of, 344
failure of union of, 80f
fractures of, 439f–442f, 440, 442–443, 444f, 470f–474f, 736f
classification of, 442
conservative management of, 385–386
flexion-extension, Roy-Camille fusion technique for, 498f, 501–503
nonunion of, 469
Olfactory nerves, assessment of, 148
Ondine's curse, 430, 484
Optic nerve, injury to, 148
Orthoses
cervical, 15f, 16f–17f, 41f, 283, 284f, 285, 286f–287f, 288, 288f, 289f, 290, 290f
force systems of, 306–307
Jewett, 295, 295f
lower limb, 325–327, 329, 331, 331f, 332f, 333, 333f
lumbosacral, 300–302
materials for, 308
for paraplegic patient, 333–338
purposes of, 307
for quadriplegic patient, 312, 315–325
thoracic, 295–300
Orthotics. *See also* specific orthoses
for cervical spine, 283–295
after lumbar spine surgery, 817–819
spinal, 279–304
for thoracic spine, 569–570
after thoracic spine surgery, 609, 609f, 621–622
upper limb, 306–312
Orthotist, role of, 283
Os odontoideum, 80f, 81, 345, 346, 351f, 371, 445, 446f
etiology of, 385
management of, 384–385
Ossification
endochondral, 61, 63
intramembranous, 61
sequence of, 77
Ossification centers
development of, 77, 78f
primary, expansion of, 63
in spinal atlas, axis, and sacrum, 79

Osteoarthritis. *See* Arthritis
Oxygen-delivering capacity, defined,
    167–168
Oxygenation, maintenance of, 7–8

P

Pain
    back, lumbosacral spinal fusion and,
        786–787
    route of stimuli for, 109–111, 110f
Palsy, abducens, 149
Pantopaque. *See* Iophendylate
Paraplegia
    fractures of thoracic spine associated
        with, 236f
    from gunshot wounds, 248f, 249f
    with knee hyperextension, orthotic
        management of, 330
    lesion levels in, 338t
    orthotic management of, 333–338
    thoracic fracture-dislocation with,
        252f–253f
    with thoracic spine injuries, 567
    as vascular surgery complication, 89,
        90
Parasympathetic nerves, lumbosacral
        spine surgery and, 799–800
Parasympathetic nervous system,
        bladder function and,
        265–266
Pars interarticularis, fractures of, 243
Patient, transfer of
    with cervical spine injury, 342
    with lumbar spine injury, 727
    protocol for, 19–20, 20f
Patient assessment, 7–9
    ABCs of, 7
    in emergency room, 23–60
Paulus Aegenita, spinal surgery recom-
        mendations of, 761
PEEP. *See* Positive end-expiratory
        pressure
Perianal assessment, in evaluation of
        neurologic function, 9–10, 10t
Perianal reflex
    in assessment of lumbosacral spinal
        injury, 726
    in assessment of neurologic function,
        10, 10t, 657
Pericardiocentesis, 32f
Periosteum, osteogenic function of, 63
Peripheral nervous system, and
        communication with central
        nervous system, 92f
Peripheral perfusion, maintenance of,
        7–8
Peripheral vascular system, vasodilata-
        tion of, hypotension caused
        by, 39
Phenylephrine hydrochloride
        (Neo-Synephrine), during
        intubation, 161
Philadelphia collar, 285, 286f, 516f

extended, 285, 288f
    after operative intervention, 291
Phrenic nerve, 112, 113f
    respiration and, 165
Pillar views, 224
Pillow fracture reduction technique,
        761
Plaster casts, 285, 288f
Plaster jackets, 294f
Pneumonia
    with cervical spine fracture, 390,
        390t
    with spinal cord injury, 180, 181t
Pneumothorax
    with spinal cord injury, 547f
    tension, initial management of, 7
    with thoracic spine fracture, 545
    with thoracic spine injury, 551f
Poikilothermia, 158
Polytomography, in cervical spine
        injury evaluation, 364–365
Posterior elements
    fractures of, 240, 243–244, 246f,
        528f, 529f
    of lumbar spine, displacement of, as
        indication for internal
        fixation, 765–766
    thoracic confused with lumbar, 596,
        599
    thoracolumbar, fractures of, 652
Postive end-expiratory pressure
        (PEEP), 182
Potassium, levels of
    muscle relaxants and, 166
    succinylcholine administration and,
        171
Priapism, in assessment of neurologic
        injury, 9–10, 10t, 657
Proprioception, pathways of, 111f,
        111–112
Prostate, carcinoma of, metastasis of,
        to spinal column, 102
Pudendal nerve, in bladder function,
        266
Pulmonary compliance, 177, 177f
Pulmonary embolus, 760f
Pulmonary function
    acute spinal cord injury and,
        173–183
    components of, 173
Pulmonary system, monitoring of, with
        cervical spine injury, 34, 36f
Pulse rate, after spinal cord injury,
        165–166
Pupillary response, factors affecting, 149
Pyramidal system, 107–109, 108f,
        116–117
    as pathway for light touch, pain, and
        temperature, 110–111

Q

Quadriparesis, transient, with
        hangman's fracture of cervical
        spine, 200

Quadriplegia
    bilateral facet lock with, 226f
    with hyperextension strain, 232f
    lesion levels in, 325t
    with occipitoatlantoaxial junction
        injury, 432f
    orthotic management of, 312,
        315–325
    with tear-drop fracture of cervical
        spine, 200
Queen Anne plaster cast, 285, 288f

R

Radiographs
    cross-table lateral, deficiencies of,
        186–187
    flexion-extension, 729
    interpretation of, 203–210
Radiography
    in acute neurologic and vertebral
        injury assessment, 185–263
    in cervical spine injury evaluation,
        364, 365f
    in lumbar spine injury evaluation,
        727–730
    portable equipment for, 187
    role of, 185
Rancho orthosis system, 308, 309f
Reciprocating gait orthosis (RGO), 334
Reduction techniques
    closed (manipulative), 761,
        764–765, 765f
    pillow fracture, 761, 762f, 763f
    spinal, in emergency room, 44–56
Reflex, bulbocavernosus. *See* Bulboca-
        vernosus reflex
Rehabilitation Institute of Chicago, 1,
        23
Rehabilitation Institute of Chicago
        (RIC) orthosis, 320, 324f
Renal failure, in spinal cord-injured
        patients, 274
Residual volume (RV), 173, 174, 174f,
        176f
    with spinal cord injury, 179
Respiration
    assessment of, after head injury,
        149–150
    thoracic spine fracture and, 545
Respiratory distress, diagnosing cause
        of, 7
Respiratory system
    evaluation of, 357
    innervation of, 112–114, 113f
Rheumatoid arthritis
    of cervical spine, 373, 373f
    postoperative immobilization of
        patients with, 512
Ribs
    11th
        excision of, 664f, 665, 666f
        resection of, 665, 665f, 668f
    ossification of, 79

Ring of atlas fracture, 377, 378f, 379, 382, 383f, 384
Robinson-Southwick anterior fusion technique, 408f
Rotational injuries, effects of, 735
Roy-Camille device, 774
  lumbar spine fixation with, 773f–774f
  in thoracolumbar spine internal fixation, 648f
Roy-Camille fusion technique, 498f, 500f, 500–503
RV. *See* Residual volume (RV)

S

Sacral cord, injury of, 267, 268, 270f
  sexual function and, 274
Sacral plexus, injury of, 807
Sacral spine
  defined, 525
  fixation of Harrington hooks to, 791, 795
  fractures of, 801, 805, 806f
    classification of, 807
    compared with lumbar fractures, 744t
    management of, 807, 809, 811
    neurologic injuries and, 805, 807
    statistics on, 813, 817
  Harrington hook stability in, 787
  injuries of
    medical complications with, 760t
    paraplegia resulting from, 337
  Luque rod fixation to, 795–796, 796f–797f
  stabilization of, compared with lumbar spine stabilization, 769t
  sublaminar wire fixation of, 789, 791f
Sacrum
  fractures of, 725f–726f
  ossification of, 79
Scalp, evoked potentials over, 123–124
SCBF. *See* Spinal cord blood flow (SCBF)
Sclerotome, development of, 72
Scoliosis
  as complication of spinal trauma, 558, 562
  congenital, developmental origin of, 81
  Harrington distraction rods in management of, problems with, 593, 596
  iatrogenic, from compression of unilateral vertebral body fracture, 582
  lumbar, 560f
  paralytic
    after thoracic fracture dislocation, 564f
    of thoracolumbar spine, 610f, 690f
Seatbelt syndrome, 245–246

Sensory afferent pathways, 109, 110f
Sensory evoked potentials. *See* Evoked potentials; specific types
Sexual function, in spinal cord-injured patient, 274–275
Shear force, effects of, 735
Sherrington's all-or-none law, 117
Shock
  neurologic, preventing, 362–363
  spinal, 158
    of thoracolumbar spine, 656–658
Shock wave lithotripsy, extracorporeal, 273
Skin, breakdown of
  during patient transfer, 31, 342
  thoracolumbar spine surgery and, 659
Skull, measurement of base of, 372f, 373
Skull fracture
  depressed, 140f
    treatment of, 153
  linear, 139f, 142f
    treatment of, 153
  radiologic evaluation of, 150–151
  types of, 139
Sleep apnea syndrome, 430
Sodium nitroprusside, for autonomic hyper-reflexia, 166
Soft collar cervical orthosis, limitations of, 283, 285
Soft tissue
  injuries to, 283, 285, 286f–287f, 288, 290
  retropharyngeal, in cervical spine evaluation, 209–210
Somatosensory evoked potentials (SSEP), 122
  in cervical spine injury evaluation, 366–367
  clinical examination compared to, 126
  in experimental spinal cord injury, 124–125
  inhalation agents and, 172
  for intraoperative monitoring, 159, 159f
  limitations of, 126, 128
  loss of, during thoracic spine surgery, 607
  in lumbar spine injury assessment, 732
  in monitoring experimental animal surgery, 130
  during occiput-cervical spine fusion, 490
  in spinal cord injury evaluation, 125–126, 128–129
  surgical monitoring with, 87, 169f, 170f, 171, 171f
SOMI. *See* Sternal occipital mandibular immobilizer (SOMI)
Somites
  embryonic development of, 71–72, 73f
  formation of, 73f, 73–74

Sperm count, after spinal cord injury, 274
Sphincter, external striated (periurethral)
  in bladder function, 266
  evaluation of, 268, 268f
Sphincterotomy
  indications for, 272–273
  technique for, 273
Spina bifida occulta, 82
Spinal block, myelographic finding of, 254
Spinal cord. *See also* Spinal cord injuries
  blood flow in, factors affecting disturbance of, 85–86
  cervical
    arterial vascular supply to, 97–99, 98f
    arteries of, 98f
  compression of, lateral view of, 466f
  conus medullaris portion of, 57f
  critical vascular zone of, 93f, 94
  edema of, preventing, 362
  embryonic development of, 69–70
  functional loss of, diagnosis of, 89
  ischemia of, 544, 544f
  neurologic functional loss in, factors affecting, 85–86
  posterior, arterial vascular supply to, 94f
  posterior cervicothoracic, arterial vascular supply to, 101f
  posterior vascular supply to, 99–100, 100f
  prenatal development of, 61–62
  ratio of, to spinal canal, 352–353, 354f
  sacral, vascular supply of, 88f, 100–101, 101f
  sensory evoked potentials in evaluation of, 121–136
  swelling of, 577f
    myelographic finding of, 256
  thoracic
    diameter of, 554
    measurement of, in sagittal plane, 538t
    susceptibility of, 573
    vascular injuries to, 546, 548, 553–554
  thoracolumbar, vascular supply of, 88f, 100–101, 101f
  tumors of, 89
  vascular anatomy of, 85–106
  vascular insult of, indications of, 89
  vascular ischemic changes in, neuropathologic processes secondary to, 90–91
  vascular supply of, 95–96, 96f, 97
    clinical support of, 553–554
  venous drainage of, 102–103, 105
Spinal cord blood flow (SCBF)
  factors affecting disturbance of, 85–86
  injury and, 124, 125

Spinal cord injuries
  acute, 1–21
  age of, evaluation of, 158
  anesthesia for, 157–172
  anesthesia technique modifications
      in, 171–172
  ascending neurologic loss after,
      544f, 544–545
  bladder dysfunction and, 267–269
  from bullet or knife wounds, 246,
      248, 248f, 249f
  cardiovascular considerations in,
      165–166
  complete vs. incomplete, 158–159
  defined, 24
  dermatomal evoked potentials in
      evaluation of, 127–128
  emergency room assessment of, 23–
      60
  evoked potentials in evaluation of,
      Northwestern University
      approach to, 128
  experimental, somatosensory evoked
      potentials in, 124–125
  extrication of patient with, 11–19
  factors affecting extent of, 107
  with fracture dislocations of spine,
      203
  incidence and distribution of,
      192–193, 197
  level of
      evaluation of, 157–158
      and extent of neurologic injury,
          27t
  mortality statistics for, 1–3
  with multiple trauma, 547f–548f
  muscle relaxants and, 166
  neurologic injury secondary to, 51t
  primary causes of, 12
  pulmonary complications with, 180
  pulmonary effects of, 173–183
  pulmonary trauma associated with,
      25f
  without radiographic evidence of
      vertebral injury, 193
  sexual function and, 274–275
  somatosensory evoked potentials in
      evaluation of, 125–126
  with spinal fracture, 192
  sport-related, 157
  stable vs. unstable, 158
  trauma center facilities and, 3, 7
  trauma sites associated with, 27
  treatment algorithm for management
      of, 40–44
  ventilation in, 165
  ventilatory muscle fatigue and,
      178–179
  vital sign changes associated with,
      38–43
Spinal cord injury syndrome
  anterior, 200, 203
  central, 200
Spinal cord trauma team, 31
Spinal fractures. *See* Fractures

Spinal fusion
  anterior techniques, 476–483
  anteroposterior techniques,
      504–505, 506f–507f
  Brooks technique, 500–501, 501f
  cervical, 476f–479f, 589f
      corporectomy and, 479, 480f–
          481f, 482–483
  failed, 82
  Gallie technique, 498, 500
  Garber-Meyer technique, 440f, 499f
  lumbar, 77, 79
  of lumbosacral joint, 786–787
  Meyer technique, 462f
  nonunion rate after, 514
  posterior techniques, 483–505
      for thoracic spine, 607–608, 608f
  Robinson-Southwick technique, 408f
  Roy-Camille technique, 498f, 500f
  of sacral spine, 79, 801
  sports participation after, 519–520
  with thoracolumbar fracture
      dislocation, 560f–561f
  three-level, with anterior cervical
      AO plate-screws, 475, 479
Spinal ganglia, development of, 76
Spinal injuries
  angiography in evaluation of,
      256–260
  biomechanical force causing, and
      extent of injury, 353, 355,
      355t
  from bullet or knife wounds, 246,
      248, 248f, 249f
  emergency surgery for, indications
      and protocol for, 57, 59
  etiology of, 343t, 531, 531t
  with head injury, 145–146
  initial radiographs of, 186–190,
      187f–188f, 189f, 190f
  mechanism of, 198–199, 203
  multiple-level, 197–198, 530
      distribution of, by level of injury,
          199f
      incidence of, 342–343
      patterns of, 198, 198f, 754f,
          754–756
  myelography in evaluation of,
      250–256
  radiologic assessment after, 342
  stability of, 204
Spinal nerves, 37f
Spinal shock, 158
  of thoracolumbar spine, 656–658
Spinal stenosis, dermatomal evoked
      potentials in evaluation of,
      127–128
Spine
  atlas-axis (C1-C2) anlage develop-
      ment in, 74, 76
  axis ossification centers of, 79, 79f
  bony injuries of, 290–295
  cervical. *see* Cervical spine
  column theory of, 593t, 631t,
      631–632

congenital deformities of, develop-
      mental causes of, 80–82
  development of, 72–76, 75f
  dorsal. *See* Dorsal spine
  fracture dislocations of, incidence of
      spinal cord injuries associated
      with, 203
  fractures of, incidence of, by level of
      injury, 197t
  injuries of, classification of,
      634–635, 638–643,
      647–648
  instability of, Denis theory of, 601
  lumbar. *See* Lumbar spine
  malalignment of, conservative vs.
      surgical management of, 601
  nerve roots of, 117
  orthotic management of, 279–304
  pathologic fractures of, from
      metastatic disease, 248–249,
      251f
  posterior elements of. *See* Posterior
      elements
  reduction of, in emergency room,
      44–56
  sacral. *See* Sacral spine
  soft tissue injuries of, 283, 285,
      286f–287f, 288, 290
  stability of
      column theory and, 593t, 631t,
          631–632
      interim techniques for maintain-
          ing, 761, 764–765
      scheme for determining, 746, 746t
  thoracic. *see* Thoracic spine
  thoracolumbar. *See* Thoracolumbar
      spine
  three-column model of, 725f
Spinous processes
  fractures of, 243, 414, 415f–417f
  isolated fractures of, 222–223, 225f
  radiographic evaluation of, 208–209
  separation of, 227f–230f
  thoracic, 566
      malalignment of, 535f
      posterior wiring of, 619–620,
          621f
Spondylitis
  ankylosing, of cervical spine, 483
  cervical, 518f
  Marie-Strümpell rheumatoid. *See*
      Marie-Strümpell rheumatoid
      spondylitis
  rheumatoid, 476f–479f
Spondylolisthesis
  cause of, 79
  with hyperflexion strain, 228–229
Spondylosis, cervical, 344, 346, 405,
      405f, 483, 736f
  extensive, 517, 518f, 519
SSEP. *See* Somatosensory evoked
      potentials (SSEP)
Steffee plate transpedicular screw
      system, 777
Stenosis, spinal. *See* Spinal stenosis

Sternal occipital mandibular immobi-
    lizer (SOMI), 285, 289f–
    290f, 516f
  after cervical spine surgery, 512
  for cervical spine stabilization, 403,
    404f
  with flexion injury of cervical spine,
    421f, 422f, 423f
  after operative intervention, 291
  for stable cervical posterior flexion
    injuries, 414, 415f–417f
  with tracheostomy, 292f
  with unilateral laminar fracture,
    429
Steroids
  spinal cord edema and, 362
  for vascular injury management, 87
Stiffness, torsional, thoracic spine
    fractures and, 526, 527f, 528
Strain
  hyperextension, 230–231, 232f
  hyperflexion, 208f–209f, 228–230,
    231f
Stryker wedge frame, 342, 358f, 359
  in initial management of cervical
    spine injury, 398
  lumbar spine fracture management
    with, 56
  thoracic spine fracture management
    with, 51
Subluxation, radiographic interpreta-
    tion of, 208
Substance abuse, screening patient for,
    38
Succinylcholine
  contraindications for, 158
  effects of, 166
  potassium levels and, 171
Surgery. See also Spinal fusion
  autonomic hyper-reflexia and,
    166–167
  blood loss and transfusion during,
    167–169
  cervical spine. See Cervical spine
    surgery
  emergency, indications for, 57, 59,
    403–405, 411
  experimental animal, evoked
    potentials in monitoring,
    130–131
  fracture vs. scoliosis, 593, 596
  monitoring of, 168f, 169, 169f, 170f,
    171, 171f
    evoked potentials in, 129–130,
    129–132
  patient evaluation preceding,
    157–159
  patient position during, 159–160
  and spinal cord vascular embarrass-
    ment, 85–87
  vascular, complications of, 89–95
  vascular injury during, management
    of, 87
Swiss AO-ASIF plate and pedicle
    screw system, 774

Sympathetic nerves, lumbosacral spine
    surgery and, 799–800
Sympathetic nervous system
  bladder function and, 266–267
  sexual function and, 274

T

Tactile discrimination, pathways of,
    111f, 111–112
TAF. See Technical Analysis Form
    (TAF)
Tear-drop fracture, 220, 222f
  hyperextension, 222, 230
Technetium 99 (^{99}Tc) scanning, in
    cervical spine injury evalua-
    tion, 367
Technetium 99m, bone scanning with,
    in lumbar spine injuries, 732
Technical Analysis Form (TAF), 279,
    280f–282f
  lower limb, 326–328, 327f–330f
  for upper limb, 308, 311f–314f, 312
Temperature, route of stimuli for,
    109–111, 110f
Tension pneumothorax, initial
    management of, 7
Testosterone, in spinal cord-injured
    patient, 274–275
Thomas collar, 285, 286f
Thoracic spine
  biomechanical features of, 295
  blood supply of, 575
  comminuted fracture of, 202f
  compression fracture of
    CT scan of, 195f–196f
    radiograph of, 193f–194f
  decompression of, 662f
  defined, 525
  flexion injury of, 576f
  fracture-dislocations of, 4f–6f,
    200f–201f, 235, 562f–564f,
    637f–638f
  fractures of, 52f, 53f–56f, 525–571
    anterior wedge compression, 575,
      578
    associated with paraplegia, 236f
    axial load-compression, 534, 537f,
      537–538, 590f
    biomechanical forces contributing
      to, 531t, 532, 533–534,
      534t, 534–543, 566–567,
      574–575, 575t
    burst, 578, 580
    Chance, 611f
    compression, 679f
    conservative management of,
      566–570
    conservative vs. surgical manage-
      ment of, 622, 622t
    emergency room reduction of,
      50–56
    extension and bending, 541–543,
      542f, 543f
    injuries accompanying, 545

    multiple-level, 568, 583, 587f–
      592f
    neurologic function and, 568–569
    orthotic management of, 569–570
    patterns of, 528, 530, 531–534
    posterior fixation devices for,
      620–621
    reduction of, 606–607
    rotation (torsion), 539–541, 541f
    by type and by treatment, 578t
    by type and extent, 581t
    vascular injury associated with, 56
  injury of
    complications associated with, 158
    delayed, 185–186, 187f
    flexion, 538–539
    neurologic, without fracture, 575,
      577f
    neurologic injuries associated
      with, 554–557, 555f, 567
    paraplegia resulting from,
      334–337
  instability of, 574–575
  measurement of diameter of, 573
  muscular anatomy of, 557–562
  orthotic management of, 295–300
  osteology of, 562–566
  radiographic examination of, 190
  rigidity of, 573
  transpedicular screw insertion in,
    774f–775f
  vascular anatomy of, 89
Thoracic spine surgery, 573–624
  anatomic considerations in, 596,
    597f, 599–600
  anterior approach, 600–601,
    602f–603f
  AO Synthes-Jacobs locking hook-spi-
    nal rod system in, 616–617
  distraction-fixation techniques in,
    615–617
  fracture reduction in, 606–607
  Harrington compression rods in, 617
  Harrington distraction rod proce-
    dure in, 615–616, 616f
  incision for, 605–606
  instrumentation for, 610–621
  with internal fixation devices, com-
    plications of, 603–604
  myelogram during, 607
  orthotic management after, 609,
    609f, 621–622
  outcomes of
    by instrumentation, 622–623,
      623t
    by surgical approach, 623t,
      623–624
  patient positioning in, 605, 605f
  posterior approach, 604
  posterior element preparation in, 606
  somatosensory evoked response loss
    in, 607
Wisconsin compression rod system
    in, 617–618
wound closure in, 608–609

Thoracic vertebra, anatomy of, 565f
Thoracolumbar corset, 296f, 297
Thoracolumbar spine
  anatomic landmarks of, 600f
  anteroposterior surgical approach to, 625–715, 663f
  defined, 525
  exposure of, 668f, 669f
  fracture-dislocations of, 241–243, 244f, 245f, 559f–561f
    apophyseal joint abnormalities associated with, 236f
  fractures of, 237–246, 627–633
    biomechanical forces associated with, 627, 630t, 631t
    blood loss in, by approach type, 678t
    classification of, 627, 630–631, 631t
    compression, 237f, 645f–646f
    injuries associated with, 625–626, 626t
    management of, by type, 647t
    medical complications of, 635t
    multiple-level, 652, 654
    neurologic injury and, 630t
    patient positioning and, 635, 636f
  injuries of
    etiology of, 627, 627t
    extrication of patient with, 19
    instability of, 632f, 633, 633f, 634f
      after internal fixation removal, 789f
    musculoskeletal structures of, 558f
    neuroanatomy of, 655
    neurologic assessment of, 655–656, 656t
    neurologic injury of, 654–658
    posterior stabilization of, 662, 662f
    radiograph of, 187–188
    radiographic examination of, 237
    relationship of lumbar plexus and conus medullaris to, 628f
    spinal shock of, 656–658
    stabilization of, 675t, 675–676
Thoracolumbar spine surgery, 658–714
  anterior corporectomy, 677–678
  anterior (transthoracic-transabdominal) approach, 659
  complications of, 706–712
  iliac crest bone graft in, 703, 704f–705f, 705–706
  incision site selection in, 659, 662, 664
  infection in, 708–709
  instrumentation in, 678–706
  neurologic function after, 712t
  neurologic injury in, 708
  posterior approach, 675
  results of, 713, 713t, 714t
  Wisconsin compression rods in, 688
Thoracolumbosacral orthosis (TLSO)
  indications for, 292, 293f
  Knight-Taylor, 297, 297f, 298, 298f–299f

for quadriplegic patient, 315, 315f
  for thoracic spine injuries, 297
Thoracostomy tube, insertion of, in patient with cervical spine injury, 39f
Thoracotomy, transpleural, in lumbar spine surgery, 59
Thorax
  muscular anatomy of, 557–558, 562
  relationship of, to lungs, 176, 176f
Thrombosis, venous. See Deep venous thrombosis
Tidal volume (V_T), 173, 174, 174f, 176f
Tietze's syndrome, 558
TLC. See Lung capacity, total
TLSO. See Thoracolumbosacral orthosis (TLSO)
Tomography
  advantages, disadvantages, and indications for, 191–192
  computed. See Computed tomography (CT)
Torsion injuries, effects of, 735
Torsional stiffness, thoracic spine fractures and, 526, 527f, 528
Touch, light, route of stimuli for, 109–111, 110f
Tourniquets, indications for use of, 8
Trachea, trauma of, 114
Tracheostomy, in-place, in cervical spine surgery, 463–464
Traction
  cervical. See Cervical traction
  Gardner-Wells. See Gardner-Wells tong traction
Transfusion, blood. See Blood transfusion
Translaminar-facet screws, 777
Transportation, patient, after accident, 19–20
Trauma
  abdominal, 33f
  chest, minilaparotomy in evaluation of, 34, 34f–35f
  head. See Head injuries
  multiple
    with cervical spine injuries, 451
    evaluation of, 25f–26f
    evoked potentials in evaluation of, 128–129
    incidence of, 3, 7
    with lumbar spine fractures, 723t, 723–724
    mortality statistics for, 1–3
    as recovery factor in spinal cord injury, 137
    with spinal cord injury, 547f–548f
    in spine-injured patients, 4f–6f, 342
    with thoracic spine fracture, 545
    treatment algorithm for management of, 40–44
  spine. See Spine injuries
  vital sign changes associated with, 27t

Trauma centers
  for acute spinal cord injuries, 1
  classification of, 3, 7
  components of, 23, 24f
  controversy over, 23
  coordinator of, 27, 30
  survival rate following injury and, 3
Trauma coordinator, 27, 30
Trauma team, 31
Treatment algorithm, for spinal cord-multiple trauma management, 40–44
Trimethaphan, for autonomic hyperreflexia, 166
Trochlear nerves, injury to, 149
Tumors
  of cervical spine, 346, 347f–350f
  fractures caused by metastasis of, 248–249, 251f
  of lumbosacral vertebral body, 633, 633f
  of spine, 89

U

Ulceration, gastric, prophylactic management of, 391
Upper limb
  evaluation of injuries to, 308, 311f–314f, 312
  orthotic management of, 306–312
  Technical Analysis Form for, 308, 311f–314f, 312
Urethra, pressure in, measurement of, 268
Urinary bladder. See Bladder
Urinary diversion, into bowel conduit, complications of, 273
Urinary tract
  calculi of, 273–274
  infection of, with cervical spine fracture, 390, 390t

V

Valium. See Diazepam
Vascular injury
  head injury mimicked by, 143, 145
  with thoracic spine injuries, 546, 548, 553–554
Vascular ischemia, of spinal cord, neuropathologic processes secondary to, 90–91
Vascular supply
  arterial, of thoracic and lumbar vertebra, 95–96, 96f
  of spinal cord, 85–106
    clinical support of, 553–554
Vascular surgery, complications of, 89–95
VC. See Vital capacity (VC)
Veins
  extradural vertebral, metastatic emboli and, 103

medullary, 103
of spinal cord, 102–103
Venous reflux, 103
Venous thrombosis, deep. *See* Deep
    venous thrombosis
Ventilation
    alveolar, impaired, 158
    methods of, at accident scene, 7
    muscles of, 175–176
        increasing strength of, 181
    pulmonary, detection of problems
        with, 34
    in spinal cord injury, 165
Ventilation/perfusion (V/Q) ratios,
    with spinal cord injury, 180
Ventilatory failure
    acute, with spinal cord injury, 180,
        181t
    with cervical neurologic injury, 182
VEP. *See* Visual evoked potentials (VEP)
Versed. *See* Midazolam hydrochloride
Vertebra(e)
    anterior segmental vessels of,
        interruption of, 86, 87f
    cleft, developmental origin of, 81
    rotational displacement of, radio-
        graphic evaluation of, 209,
        227f–228f
    rotational injuries and, 735
    thoracic, anatomy of, 565, 565f
Vertebral arches, ossification of, 79
Vertebral body
    arterial vascular supply to, 97
    burst fractures of, 649, 652
        distraction-fixation techniques for,
            615
    cervical
        corporectomy and three-level
            fusion of, 479, 480f–481f,
            482–483
        retropulsion of, 513f–514f
        unstable flexion-axial load-induced
            bilaminar injury of, 419,
            420f–423f

comminuted compression fracture
    of, 86f
compression fractures of, distrac-
    tion-fixation techniques for,
    615
congenital fusion of, 73
corporectomy of, inappropriate use
    of, 403
formation of, 75f, 79
fractures of, 220f, 220–222, 221f,
    222f
    unilateral, 581–583, 584f–586f
injury of, with flexion-axial load,
    452, 453f–454f, 454
lumbrosacral, tumors of, 633, 633f
maintaining height of, 766
ossification of, 77
post-traumatic collapse in, 241
sagittal split of, 222, 223f
thoracic, corporectomy of, 677–678
thoracolumbar
    bone graft of, 672f, 673, 673f, 674f
    excision of, 669, 671f, 672f
    fractures of, 648–652
    normal architecture of, 632f
    unilateral fractures of, distraction-
        fixation techniques for, 615
vascular supply of, development of,
    76
wedge compression fractures of,
    648–649, 649f–651f
Vertebral column. *See* Spine
Vertebral process, formation of, 75f
Vertebrobasilar insufficiency, signs of,
    143
Vesicosphincter dyssynergy, 267, 272f
Vessels
    of Adamkiewicz. *See* Adamkiewicz,
        artery of
    segmental, 100
Vidus Vidius, spinal manipulations
    techniques of, 761, 764
Visual evoked potentials (VEP), 122,
    123f, 133

Vital capacity (VC), 174, 174f
    measurement of, 182
    as reflection of ventilatory reserve,
        178
Vital signs
    changes in, in trauma patients, 27t
    interpretation of, with multitrauma,
        38–43
    neurologically altered, 114
Vocal cords, trauma of, 114
V_T. *See* Tidal volume (V_T)

W

Wake-up test, for surgical monitoring,
    169
Wedge compression fractures, of
    vertebral body, 648–649,
    649f–651f
    axial load injuries and, 735
    stabilization of, 777
Weiss compression springs, 593, 595f
    in thoracic spine surgery, 618, 620f
    in thoracolumbar spine stabilization,
        676
    in thoracolumbar spine surgery,
        689f, 701, 702f–703f, 703
Wheelchairs, 315, 316, 317f, 319, 320
Whiplash, management of, 283, 285
White rami communicantes. *See*
    Preganglionic fibers
WHO. *See* Wrist-hand orthoses (WHOs)
Wisconsin compression rods, 777
    in thoracic spine surgery, 617–618
    in thoracolumbar spine surgery, 688
Work of breathing, 177–178, 178f
    increasing, signs of, 182
Wound closure, in thoracic spine
    surgery, 608–609
Wrist-hand orthoses (WHOs), for
    quadriplegic patient, 315,
    316f, 319, 320, 321f, 322f,
    323f

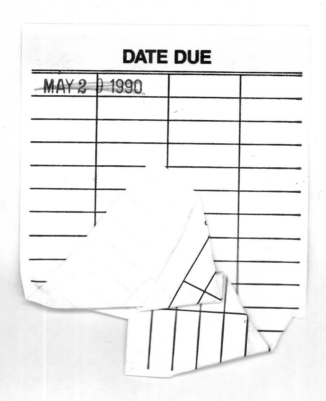